The GALE ENCYCLOPEDIA of ALTERNATIVE MEDICINE

SECOND EDITION

The GALE
ENCYCLOPEDIA *of*
ALTERNATIVE
MEDICINE

SECOND EDITION

VOLUME

2

D-K

JACQUELINE L. LONGE, PROJECT EDITOR

THOMSON

GALE

Detroit • New York • San Francisco • San Diego • New Haven, Conn. • Waterville, Maine • London • Munich

THOMSON
★
GALE

The Gale Encyclopedia of Alternative Medicine, Second Edition

Project Editor
Jacqueline L. Longe

Editorial
Deirdre S. Blanchfield, Laurie Fundukian, Erin Watts

Editorial Support Services
Andrea Lopeman

Rights Acquisition Management
Margaret Abendroth, Ann Taylor

Imaging
Randy Bassett, Lezlie Light, Dan W. Newell, Robyn V. Young

Product Design
Michelle DiMercurio, Tracey Rowens

Composition and Electronic Prepress
Evi Seoud, Mary Beth Trimper

Manufacturing
Wendy Blurton, Dorothy Maki

Indexing
Synapse Corp. of Colorado

LIBRARY OF CONGRESS CATALOGING-IN-PUBLICATION DATA

The Gale encyclopedia of alternative medicine / Jacqueline L. Longe, project editor.-- 2nd ed.
    p. ; cm.
    Includes bibliographical references and index.
    ISBN 0-7876-7424-9 (set hardcover : alk. paper) -- ISBN 0-7876-7425-7 (v. 1 : alk. paper) -- ISBN 0-7876-7426-5 (v. 2 : alk. paper) -- ISBN 0-7876-7427-3 (v. 3 : alk. paper) -- ISBN 0-7876-7428-1 (v. 4 : alk. paper)
    1. Alternative medicine--Encyclopedias.
    [DNLM: 1. Complementary Therapies--Encyclopedias--English. 2. Internal Medicine--
Encyclopedias--English. WB 13 G1507 2005] I. Title: Encyclopedia of alternative medicine. II. Longe, Jacqueline L.
    R733.G34 2005
    615.5'03--dc22
                                       2004022502

This title is also available as an e-book
ISBN 7876-9396-0 (set)
Contact your Gale sales representative for ordering information

ISBN 0-7876-7424-9(set)
0-7876-7425-7 (Vol. 1)
0-7876-7426-5 (Vol. 2)
0-7876-7427-3 (Vol. 3)
0-7876-7428-1 (Vol. 4)

Printed in the United States of America
10 9 8 7 6 5 4 3 2

CONTENTS

LIST OF ENTRIES

Marijuana
Marsh mallow
Martial arts
Massage therapy
McDougall diet
Measles
Meditation
Mediterranean diet
Medium-chain triglycerides
Melatonin
Memory loss
Meniere's disease
Meningitis
Menopause
Menstruation
Mercurius vivus
Mercury poisoning
Mesoglycan
Metabolic therapies
Methionine
Mexican yam
Migraine headache
Milk thistle
Mind/Body medicine
Mistletoe
Mononucleosis
Morning sickness
Motherwort
Motion sickness
Movement therapy
Moxibustion
MSM
Mugwort
Mullein
Multiple chemical sensitivity
Multiple sclerosis
Mumps
Muscle spasms and cramps
Music therapy
Myopia
Myotherapy
Myrrh

N

Narcolepsy
Native American medicine

Natrum muriaticum
Natural hormone replacement
    therapy
Natural hygiene diet
Naturopathic medicine
Nausea
Neck pain
Neem
Nettle
Neuralgia
Neural therapy
Neurolinguistic programming
Niacin
Night blindness
Noni
Nosebleeds
Notoginseng root
Nutmeg
Nutrition
Nux vomica

O

Oak
Obesity
Obsessive-compulsive disorder
Omega-3 fatty acids
Omega-6 fatty acids
Ophiopogon
Oregano essential oil
Ornish diet
Ortho-bionomy
Orthomolecular medicine
Osha
Osteoarthritis
Osteopathy
Osteoporosis
Ovarian cancer
Ovarian cysts
Oxygen/Ozone therapy

P

Pain
Paleolithic diet

Panchakarma
Pancreatitis
Panic disorder
Pantothenic acid
Parasitic infections
Parkinson's disease
Parsley
Passionflower
Past life therapy
Pau d'arco
Pelvic inflammatory disease
Pennyroyal
Peppermint
Peripheral neuropathy
Periwinkle
Pet therapy
Phlebitis
Phobias
Phosphorus
Pilates
Pinched nerve
Pine bark extract
Pinellia
Pityriasis rosea
Placebo effect
Plantain
Pleurisy
Pneumonia
Polarity therapy
Postpartum depression
Post-traumatic stress disorder
Potassium
Pranic healing
Prayer and spirituality
Pregnancy
Pregnancy massage
Premenstrual syndrome
Prickly heat
Prickly pear cactus
Pritikin diet
Probiotics
Prolotherapy
Prostate cancer
Prostate enlargement
Psoriasis
Psychoneuroimmunology
Psychophysiology
Psychosomatic medicine
Psychotherapy

PLEASE READ – IMPORTANT INFORMATION

The Gale Encyclopedia of Alternative Medicine is a medical reference product designed to inform and educate readers about a wide variety of complementary therapies and herbal remedies and treatments for prevalent conditions and diseases. Thomson Gale believes the product to be comprehensive, but not necessarily definitive. It is intended to supplement, not replace, consultation with a physician or other healthcare practitioner. While Thomson Gale has made substantial efforts to provide information that is accurate, comprehensive, and up-to-date, Thomson Gale makes no representations or warranties of any kind, including without limitation, warranties of merchantability or fitness for a particular purpose, nor does it guarantee the accuracy, comprehensiveness, or timeliness of the information contained in this product. Readers should be aware that the universe of complementary medical knowledge is constantly growing and changing, and that differences of medical opinion exist among authorities. They are also advised to seek professional diagnosis and treatment for any medical condition, and to discuss information obtained from this book with their healthcare provider.

ABOUT THE ENCYCLOPEDIA

The Gale Encyclopedia of Alternative Medicine (GEAM) is a one-stop source for alternative medical information that covers complementary therapies, herbs and remedies, and common medical diseases and conditions. It avoids medical jargon, making it easier for the layperson to use. The Gale Encyclopedia of Alternative Medicine presents authoritative, balanced information and is more comprehensive than single-volume family medical guides.

Scope

Over 800 full-length articles are included in The Gale Encyclopedia of Alternative Medicine. Many prominent figures are highlighted as sidebar biographies that accompany the therapy entries. Articles follow a standardized format that provides information at a glance. Rubrics include:

Therapies

- Origins
- Benefits
- Description
- Preparations
- Precautions
- Side effects
- Research & general acceptance
- Resources
- Key terms

Herbs/remedies

- General use
- Preparations
- Precautions
- Side effects
- Interactions
- Resources
- Key terms

Diseases/conditions

- Definition
- Description
- Causes & symptoms
- Diagnosis
- Treatment
- Allopathic treatment
- Expected results
- Prevention
- Resources
- Key terms

Inclusion criteria

A preliminary list of therapies, herbs, remedies, diseases, and conditions was compiled from a wide variety of sources, including professional medical guides and textbooks, as well as consumer guides and encyclopedias. The advisory board, made up of three medical and alternative healthcare experts, evaluated the topics and made suggestions for inclusion. Final selection of topics to include was made by the medical advisors in conjunction with Thomson Gale editors.

About the Contributors

The essays were compiled by experienced medical writers, including alternative healthcare practitioners and educators, pharmacists, nurses, and other complementary healthcare professionals. GEAM medical advisors reviewed over 95% of the completed essays to insure that they are appropriate, up-to-date, and medically accurate.

How to Use this Book

The Gale Encyclopedia of Alternative Medicine has been designed with ready reference in mind:

- Straight **alphabetical arrangement** allows users to locate information quickly.

- Bold faced terms function as *print hyperlinks* that point the reader to related entries in the encyclopedia.

- A list of **key terms** is provided where appropriate to define unfamiliar words or concepts used within the context of the essay. Additional terms may be found in the **glossary**.

- **Cross-references** placed throughout the encyclopedia direct readers to where information on subjects without their own entries can be found. Synonyms are also cross-referenced.

- A **Resources section** directs users to sources of further complementary medical information.

- An appendix of alternative medical organizations is arranged by type of therapy and includes valuable **contact information**.

- A comprehensive **general index** allows users to easily target detailed aspects of any topic, including Latin names.

Graphics

The Gale Encyclopedia of Alternative Medicine is enhanced with over 450 images, including photos, tables, and customized line drawings. Each volume contains a color insert of 64 important herbs, remedies, and supplements.

ADVISORY BOARD

An advisory board made up of prominent individuals from complementary medical communities provided invaluable assistance in the formulation of this encyclopedia. They defined the scope of coverage and reviewed individual entries for accuracy and accessibility. We would therefore like to express our appreciation to them:

CONTRIBUTORS

Margaret Alic, PhD
Medical Writer
Eastsound, WA

Greg Annussek
Medical Writer
American Society of Journalists and Authors
New York, NY

Barbara Boughton
Health and Medical Writer
El Cerrito, CA

Ruth Ann Prag Carter
Freelance Writer
Farmington Hills, MI

Linda Chrisman
Massage Therapist and Educator
Medical Writer
Oakland, CA

Gloria Cooksey, CNE
Medical Writer
Sacramento, CA

Amy Cooper, MA, MSI
Medical Writer
Vermillion, SD

Sharon Crawford
Writer, Editor, Researcher
American Medical Writers Association
Periodical Writers Association of Canada and the Editors'
    Association of Canada
Toronto, ONT Canada

Sandra Bain Cushman
Massage Therapist
Alexander Technique Practitioner and Educator
Charlottesville, VA

Tish Davidson, MA
Medical Writer
Fremont, CA

Lori DeMilto, MJ
Medical Writer
Sicklerville, NJ

Doug Dupler, MA
Medical Writer
Boulder, CO

Paula Ford-Martin, PhD
Medical Writer
Warwick, RI

Rebecca J. Frey, PhD
Medical Writer
New Haven, CT

Lisa Frick
Medical Writer
Columbia, MO

Kathleen Goss
Medical Writer
Darwin, CA

Elliot Greene, MA
former president, American Massage Therapy Association
Massage Therapist
Silver Spring, MD

Peter Gregutt
Medical Writer
Asheville, NC

Clare Hanrahan
Medical Writer
Asheville, NC

David Helwig
Medical Writer
London, ONT Canada

Beth A. Kapes
Medical Writer, Editor
Bay Village, OH

Katherine Kim
Medical Writer
Oakland, CA

Erika Lenz
Medical Writer
Lafayette, CO

Lorraine Lica, PhD
Medical Writer
San Diego, CA

Whitney Lowe, LMT
Orthopedic Massage Education & Research Institute
Massage Therapy Educator
Bend, OR

Mary McNulty
Freelance Writer
St.Charles, IL

Katherine E. Nelson, ND
Naturopathic physician
Naples, FL

Teresa Odle
Medical Writer
Ute Park, NM

Jodi Ohlsen Read
Medical Writer
Carver, MN

Carole Osborne-Sheets
Massage Therapist and Educator
Medical Writer
Poway, CA

Lee Ann Paradise
Freelance Writer
Lubbock, TX

Patience Paradox
Medical Writer
Bainbridge Island, WA

Belinda Rowland, PhD
Medical Writer
Voorheesville, NY

Joan M. Schonbeck, RN
Medical Writer
Marlborough, MA

Gabriele Schubert, MS
Medical Writer
San Diego, CA

Kim Sharp, M Ln
Medical Writer
Houston, TX

Kathy Shepard Stolley, PhD
Medical Writer
Virginia Beach, VA

Judith Sims, MS
Science Writer
Logan, UT

Patricia Skinner
Medical Writer
Amman, Jordan

Genevieve Slomski, PhD
Medical Writer
New Britain, CT

Jane E. Spear
Medical Writer
Canton, OH

Liz Swain
Medical Writer
San Diego, CA

Judith Turner, DVM
Medical Writer
Sandy, UT

Samuel Uretsky, PharmD
Medical Writer
Wantagh, NY

Ken R. Wells
Science Writer
Laguna Hills, CA

Angela Woodward
Science Writer
Madison, WI

Kathleen Wright, RN
Medical Writer
Delmar, DE

Jennifer L. Wurges
Medical Writer
Rochester Hills, MI

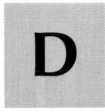

Damiana

Description

Damiana, of the Turneraceae plant family, is an aromatic shrub with small yellow flowers that grows on dry, sunny, rocky hillsides in south Texas, Southern California, Mexico, and Central America. The two species used in herbal healing, both of which are referred to as damiana, are *Turnera aphrodisiaca* and *Turnera diffusa*. Damiana usually grows to a height of about 24 in (60 cm). Its pale green leaves, which turn yellow-brown when dried, are 0.5–1 in (15–25 mm) long and quite narrow. They have serrated (jagged) edges. The leaves and sometimes the stems of the plant have medicinal uses. Other names for damiana include old woman's broom, Mexican damiana, pastorata, hierba del venado, oreganello, and the bourrique.

General use

Damiana affects primarily the urinary and reproductive systems. It has been used as an aphrodisiac and to boost sexual potency in men by the native peoples of Mexico, including the Mayan Indians, for thousands of years. It is said to act as a sexual stimulant and produce a feeling of general well being. Damiana is sometimes used in men to treat spermatorrhea, premature ejaculation, sexual sluggishness, and prostate complaints. It is often used in combination with other herbs to treat **impotence**.

In the past 100 years, damiana has shifted from being primarily a male sexual remedy to also being prescribed for women. In women it is used to treat painful **menstruation**, **menopause** disorders, and headaches caused by menstruation.

Today both men and women may use damiana to relieve **anxiety**, nervousness, and mild **depression**, especially if these symptoms have a sexual component. The herb is also used as a general tonic to improve wellness. As a general tonic it is said to act as a stimulant, improve circula-

tion, and regulate hormonal activity. Some herbal practitioners also use it as a diuretic. Damiana tonic should be used moderately, and not be taken on a long-term basis.

Damiana has also been used traditionally to improve digestion and to treat **constipation**, as in larger doses it has a mild laxative effect. Other uses include treatment of **asthma**, **cough** and flu, and nephritis. During the 1960s, damiana was touted as a recreational drug. Some users claimed that damiana produced a mild "high" or hallucinogenic effect similar to **marijuana** that lasts an hour to an hour and a half.

In addition to its medicinal uses, damiana is used in Mexico to flavor liqueurs, tea, and other beverages and foods. It tastes slightly bitter, and the leaves have a strong resinous aroma when crushed. Damiana is approved for food use by the United States Food and Drug Administration (FDA).

Despite its long history and frequent use in many different cultures, scientists have been unable to isolate any active ingredients that would account for damiana's aphrodisiac, stimulant, or hallucinogenic properties. The herb contains a volatile oil that may mildly irritate the genitourinary system. This volatile oil may be at the root of damiana's reputation as an aphrodisiac.

The German Federal Health Agency's Commission E, which was established in 1978 to independently review and evaluate scientific literature and case studies pertaining to herb and plant medications, found no proof that damiana acts either as a sexual stimulant or as a hallucinogen. On the other hand, they also found no proof that damiana was likely to cause harm. A 1999 study on rats conducted in Italy found that extracts of *Turnera diffusa* had no effect on sexually potent rats, but did increase the performance of sexually sluggish or impotent rats. There have been no clinical trials involving humans.

Preparations

The leaves and occasionally the stems of damiana are used medicinally. They are normally harvested while the plant is in flower and then are dried. Dried leaves turn a yellow-brown color and may be powdered, used in capsules, or steeped in water or alcohol. Damiana is always used internally, never topically.

Traditionally damiana has been prepared as a tea or infusion. Although folk recipes vary, generally about 1 cup (250 ml) of boiling water is added to 1/2 cup (1 g) of dried leaves, and allowed to steep about 15 minutes. One cup of this infusion is drunk two to three times daily. This infusion is slightly bitter and has an astringent quality.

Damiana is also available as a tincture of which 1–3 ml is taken two or three times a day. If taken in capsule or tablet form, 3–8 g twice a day may be taken. Damiana is also available in concentrated drops. Damiana is often used in conjunction with other herbs having similar properties, and is often found as an ingredient in herbal mixtures or formulas.

Precautions

Scientific evidence indicates that damiana is one of the safest substances commonly taken for sexual enhancement. It has a long history of traditional medicinal and food use with no harmful consequences reported. It is believed to be unlikely to cause harm or have negative side effects when taken in the designated doses. However, no rigorous scientific studies have examined the effects of long-term use of this herb.

Side effects

Large doses of damiana may cause loose stools because of the herb's laxative properties. Otherwise, no unwanted side effects have been reported.

Interactions

Damiana is often used in combination with other herbs without any negative effects. It is not known to interact with any other herbs or pharmaceuticals, although few, if any, scientific studies have been done on its interactions.

Resources

BOOKS

Peirce, Andrea. *The American Pharmaceutical Association Practical Guide to Natural Medicines.* New York: William Morrow and Company, 1999.

PDR for Herbal Medicines. Montvale, NJ: Medical Economics Company, 1998.

OTHER

"Damiana." www.rain-tree.com/damiana.htm.

"Turnera diffusa aphrodisiaca." Plants for a Future. http://www.pfaf.org.

Tish Davidson

Dance therapy

Definition

Dance therapy is a type of **psychotherapy** that uses movement to further the social, cognitive, emotional, and physical development of the individual. Dance therapists work with people who have many kinds of emotional problems, intellectual deficits, and life-threatening illnesses. They are employed in psychiatric hospitals, day care centers, mental health centers, prisons, special schools, and private practice. They work with people of all ages in both group and individual therapy. Some also engage in research.

Dance therapists try to help people develop communication skills, a positive self-image, and emotional stability.

Origins

Dance therapy began as a profession in the 1940s with the work of Marian Chace. A modern dancer, she began teaching dance after ending her career with the Denishawn Dance Company in 1930. In her classes, she noticed that some of her students were more interested in the emotions they expressed while dancing (loneliness, shyness, fear, etc.) than the mechanics of the moves. She began encouraging them by emphasizing more freedom of movement rather than technique.

In time, doctors in the community started sending her patients. They included antisocial children, people with movement problems, and those with psychiatric illnesses. Eventually, Chace became part of the staff of the Red Cross at St. Elizabeth's Hospital. She was the first dance therapist employed in a formal position by the federal government. Chace worked with the emotionally troubled patients at St. Elizabeth's and tried to get them to reach out to others through dance. Some of them were schizophrenics and others were former servicemen suffering from **post-traumatic stress disorder**. Success for these patients meant being able to participate with their class in moving to rhythmic music. "This rhythmic action in unison with others results in a feeling of well-being, **relaxation**, and good fellowship," Chace said once.

Chace eventually studied at the Washington School of Psychiatry and began making treatment decisions about her patients along with other members of the St. Elizabeth's medical team. Her work attracted many followers and the first dance therapy interns began learning and teaching dance therapy at St. Elizabeth's in the 1950s.

Other dancers also began using dance therapy in the 1940s to help people feel more comfortable with themselves and their bodies. These dancers included Trudi Schoop and Mary Whitehouse. Whitehouse later became a Jungian analyst and an influential member of the dance therapy community. She developed a process called "movement in-depth," an extension of her understanding of dance, movement, and depth psychology. She helped found the contemporary movement practice called "authentic movement." In this type of movement, founded on the principles of Jungian analysis, patients dance out their feelings about an internal image, often one that can help them understand their past or their current life struggles. One of Whitehead's students, Janet Alder furthered Whitehead's work in authentic movement by establishing the Mary Starks Whitehouse Institute in 1981.

In 1966, dance therapy became formally organized and recognized when the American Dance Therapy Association (ADTA) was formed.

Benefits

Dance therapy can be helpful to a wide range of patients—from psychiatric patients to those with **cancer** to lonely elderly people. Dance therapy is often an easy way for a person to express emotions, even when his or her experience is so traumatic he or she can't talk about it. It is frequently used with rape victims and survivors of sexual abuse and incest. It can also help people with physical deficits improve their self-esteem and learn balance and coordination.

Dance therapists also work with people who have chronic illnesses and life-threatening diseases to help them deal with **pain**, fear of death, and changes in their

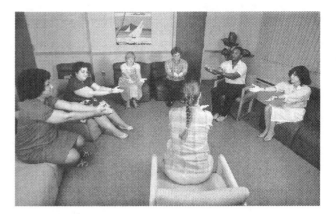

Dance therapy in a mental health unit. *(Photo Researchers, Inc. Reproduced by permission.)*

body image. Many people with such illnesses find dance therapy classes to be a way to relax, get away from their pain and emotional difficulties for a while, and express feelings about taboo subjects (such as impending death).

Dance therapy is suitable even for people who are not accomplished dancers, and may even be good for those who are clumsy on the dance floor. The emphasis in dance therapy is on free movement, not restrictive steps, and expressing one's true emotions. Children who cannot master difficult dances or can't sit still for traditional psychotherapy often benefit from free-flowing dance therapy. Even older people who cannot move well or are confined to wheelchairs can participate in dance therapy. All they need to do is move in some way to the rhythm of the music.

Dance therapy can be useful in a one-on-one situation, where the therapist works with only one patient to provide a safe place to express emotions. Group classes can help provide emotional support, enhanced communication skills, and appropriate physical boundaries (a skill that is vital for sexual abuse victims).

Description

There are currently more than 1,200 dance therapists in 46 states in the United Sates and in 29 foreign countries. Like other mental health professionals, they use a wide range of techniques to help their patients. Some of the major "schools of thought" in dance therapy include the Freudian approach, Jungian technique, and object relations orientation. Many therapists, however, do not ascribe to just one school, but use techniques from various types of dance therapy.

The authentic movement technique is derived from the Jungian method of analysis in which people work with recurring images in their thoughts or dreams to derive meaning in their life. Instead of asking the patient to dance out certain emotions, the therapist instructs the patient to move when he or she feels "the inner impulse." The moves are directed by the patient and the therapist is a noncritical witness to the movement. The moves are supposed to emerge from a deep level within the patient.

In Freudian technique, dance therapists work with patients to uncover feelings hidden deep in the subconscious by expressing those feelings through dance.

In object relations technique, the therapist often helps the patient examine problems in his or her life by considering the primary initial relationship with the parents. Emotions are expressed in a concrete, physical way. For instance, a patient would work out his fears of abandonment by repeatedly coming close to and dancing at a distance from the therapist.

Dance therapists sometimes use other types of therapy along with dance, such as art or drama. Therapists also discuss what happens during a dancing session by spending time in "talk therapy." Dance therapists use visualizations during sessions, too. For example, the therapist might instruct patients to imagine they are on a beautiful, peaceful beach as they dance.

In one frequently used technique, the therapist mirrors the movements of the patient as he or she expresses important emotions. This is especially powerful in private one-on-one therapy. It is thought that this device provides a sense of safety and validates the patient's emotions.

The underlying premise of dance therapy is that when people dance, they are expressing highly significant emotions. A fist thrust out in anger into the air or a head bent in shame has deep significance to a dance therapist. Through dance therapy, the theory goes, patients are able to more easily express painful, frightening emotions, and can progress from there. After experiencing dance therapy, they can talk about their feelings more freely and tear down the barriers they have erected between themselves and other people. The hope is that eventually they can go on to live more psychologically healthy lives.

Preparations

People who want to use dance therapy should find a qualified therapist. The ADTA provides lists of qualified therapists. The person should begin dance therapy with an open mind and a willingness to participate so he or she can get the most benefit.

Precautions

A qualified dance therapist should have completed a graduate program in dance therapy approved by the ADTA and should be registered with the ADTA. He or she should not just be a dancer, but should also have extensive training in psychology.

Side effects

No known side effects.

Research & general acceptance

Dance therapy was once dismissed as simply an ineffective, "feel good" treatment, but it is now more respected. Many research studies have proven that dance therapy can be an effective tool to help people overcome psychological problems.

In a 1993 study, older people with cognitive deficits showed that dance therapy could significantly increase their functional abilities. Patients improved their balance, rhythmic discrimination, mood, and social interaction.

In 1999, a pilot study of 21 university students showed that those who took a series of four to five group dance therapy sessions in a period of two weeks significantly reduced their test **anxiety** as measured by a well-known exam called the Test Anxiety Inventory. Afterwards, the subjects reported that their dance movement experience was positive and provided them with psychological insight. The researchers concluded that dance therapy could be a viable method of treatment for students who suffer from overwhelming test anxiety, and should be researched further.

In another 1999 study presented at the ADTA national conference in November 1999, dance therapist Donna Newman-Bluestein reported success in using techniques of dance therapy with cardiac patients. In a **stress** reduction class, health professionals used dance therapy methods to teach body awareness, relaxation, self-expression, creativity, and empathy. According to Newman-Bluestein, the dance therapy techniques helped the patients deal with such stressful emotions as anger, increased their self-awareness, made them more relaxed, and helped them adjust emotionally to having **heart disease**.

Training & certification

Dance therapists should have dance experience and a liberal arts background with coursework in psychology for their undergraduate degree. Professional dance therapy training takes place on the graduate level. A qualified dance therapist has received a graduate degree from a school approved by the ADTA, or has a master's degree in dance or psychology and has taken additional dance therapy credits.

Authentic movement—A type of movement that is influenced heavily by Jungian analysis, and works by analyzing the internal images of the patient. Patients are also urged to dance only when they feel the "impulse" to move.

Freudian analysis—A type of psychological treatment where the therapist seeks to help the patient resolve conflicts and traumas buried in the subconscious.

Jungian analysis—A method of psychological treatment where the patient strives to understand the internal, often mythic images in his or her thoughts and dreams.

Psychotherapy—A medical treatment that seeks to resolve psychological traumas and conflicts, often by discussing them and emotionally reliving difficult events in the past.

Test anxiety—A name for the stress and anxiousness that commonly occur in students before they take exams.

After graduation, dance therapists can become registered with the ADTA, meaning that they are qualified to practice. After two years they may receive an additional recognition when they become an Academy of Dance Therapist Registered. They can then teach dance therapy and can supervise interns.

Dance therapists can also obtain psychological credentials by taking a test and becoming registered by the National Board for Certified Counselors, Inc.

Resources

BOOKS

Halprin, Anna. *Dance as a Healing Art: Returning to Health Through Movement and Imagery.* Mendocino, CA: LifeRhythm, 2000.

Levy, Fran J., ed. *Dance and Other Expressive Art Therapies: When Words Are Not Enough.* New York: Routledge, 1995.

Pallaro, Patrizia, ed. *Authentic Movement: Essays by Mary Starks Whitehouse, Jane Adler and Joan Chodorow.* London: Jessica Kingsley Publishers, 1999.

PERIODICALS

Brody, Jane. "Dancing Shoes Replace the Therapist's Couch." *New York Times* (10 October 1995): C13.

"Dance/Movement Therapy Opens Communication Pathways." *Brown University Long-Term Quality Advisor* (July 15, 1996).

Erwin-Grabner, et al. "Effectiveness of Dance/Movement Therapy on Reducing Test Anxiety." *American Journal of Dance Therapy* 21, no. 1 (Spring/Summer 1999).

ORGANIZATIONS

American Dance Therapy Association. (410) 997-4040. info@adta.org. http://www.adta.org.

OTHER

Newman-Bluestein, Donna. "You Gotta Have Heart: Integrating Dance Therapy into Cardiac Rehabilitation Stress Management." Presented at the ADTA National Conference. (November 1999).

Barbara Boughton

Dandelion

Description

Dandelion (*Taraxacum officinale*) is a common meadow herb of the Asteraceae or sunflower family. There are about 100 species of dandelion, and all are beneficial. This sun-loving beauty is a native of Greece, naturalized in temperate regions throughout the world, and familiar to nearly everyone. The perennial dandelion grows freely wherever it can find a bit of earth and a place in the sun. Dandelion's nutritive and medicinal qualities have been known for centuries.

Dandelion's common name is derived from the French *dent de lion*, a reference to the irregular and jagged margins of the lance-shaped leaves. There are numerous folk names for this widely-used herb. They include pissabed, Irish daisy, blow ball, lion's tooth, bitterwort, wild endive, priest's crown, doonheadclock, yellow gowan, puffball, clock flower, swine snort, fortune-teller, and cankerwort. The generic name is thought to be derived from the Greek words *taraxos*, meaning disorder, and *akos*, meaning remedy. Another possible derivation is from the Persian *tark hashgun*, meaning wild endive, one of dandelion's common names. The specific designation *officinale* indicates that this herb was officially listed as a medicinal. Dandelion held a place in the United States *National Formulary* from 1888 until 1965, and the dried root of dandelion is listed in the *United States Pharmacopoeia* (USP).

Dandelion may be distinguished from other similar-looking herbs by the hollow, leafless flower stems that contain a bitter milky-white liquid also found in the root and leaves. The dark green dandelion leaves, with their irregular, deeply jagged margins, have a distinctive hairless mid-rib. The leaves are arranged in a rosette pattern, and may grow to 1.5 ft (45.7 cm)in length. They have a

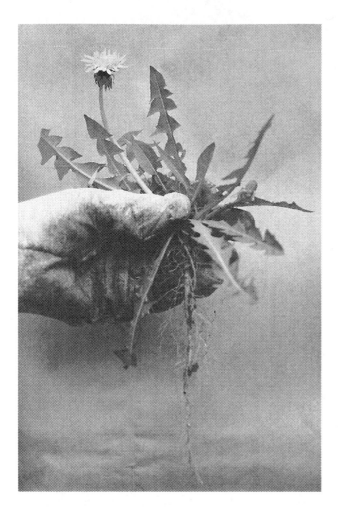

A dandelion plant with flower. *(Photograph by Robert J. Huffman/Field Mark Publications. Reproduced by permission.)*

lovely magenta tint that extends up along the inner rib of the stalkless leaf. When the plant is used as a dye, it yields this purple hue. Dandelion blossoms are singular and round, with compact golden-yellow petals. They bloom from early spring until well into autumn atop hollow stalks that may reach from 4–8 in (10.2ndash;20.3 cm) tall. The golden blossoms yield a pale yellow dye for wool. After flowering, dandelion develops a round cluster of achenes, or seed cases. As many as 200 of these narrow seed cases, each with a single seed, form the characteristic puffball. Each achene is topped with a white, feathery tuft to carry it on the breeze. Dandelion's tap root may grow fat, and reach as deep as 1.5 ft (45.7 cm) in loose soil. The root has numerous hairy rootlets. Dandelion is a hardy herb and will regrow from root parts left in the ground during harvest.

General use

Dandelion has a long history of folk use. Early colonists brought the herb to North America. The native people soon recognized the value of the herb and sought it out for its medical and nutritious benefits. The entire plant is important as a general tonic, particularly as a liver tonic. It may be taken as an infusion of the leaf, a juice extraction, a root decoction, or a tincture. Fresh leaves may be added to salads or cooked as a potherb. The juice extracted from the stem and leaf is the most potent part of the plant for medicinal purposes. It has been used to eradicate **warts** and soothe calluses, bee stings, or sores. Infusions of dandelion blossoms have been used as a beautifying facial, refreshing the skin.

Dandelion is a nutritive herb rich in **potassium**, calicum, and **lecithin**, with **iron**, **magnesium**, **niacin**, **phosphorus**, proteins, silicon, **boron**, and **zinc**. Dandelion provides several B vitamins along with vitamins C and E as well as vitamin P. Chemical constituents in the leaf include bitter glycosides, **carotenoids**, terpenoids, choline, potassium salts, iron, and other minerals. The root also has bitter glycosides, tannins, triterpenes, sterols, volatile oil, choline, asparagin, and inulin.

Many herbalists regard the dandelion as an effective treatment for liver disease, useful even in such extreme cases as **cirrhosis**. It cleanses the bloodstream and increases bile production, and is a good remedy for gall bladder problems as well. The herb is also a boon to such other internal organs as the pancreas, kidneys, stomach, and spleen. The dried leaf, taken as a tea, is used as a mild laxative to relieve **constipation**. Dandelion leaf is also a good natural source of potassium, and will replenish any potassium that may be lost due to the herb's diuretic action on the kidneys. This characteristic makes dandelion a safe diuretic in cases of water retention due to heart problems.The herb is useful in cases of **anemia** and **hepatitis**, and may lower elevated blood pressure. Dandelion may also provide relief for rheumatism and arthritis. Dandelion therapy, consisting of therapeutic doses of dandelion preparations taken over time, may help reduce stiffness and increase mobility in situations of chronic degenerative joint disease. The root, dried and minced, can used as a coffee substitute, sometimes combined with roasted acorns and rye.

Preparations

All parts of the dandelion have culinary and medicinal value. It is best to harvest fresh young dandelion leaves in the spring. The small, young leaves are less bitter, and may be eaten uncooked in salads. Larger leaves can be lightly steamed to reduce bitterness. Leaves gathered in the fall are naturally less bitter. Dandelion blossoms, traditionally used in wine making, may be gathered throughout the flowering season. The deep, fleshy taproot should be gathered in the fall. It takes careful digging and loosening to extract the root intact, although any root parts left in the soil will eventually produce another plant. The root should be washed. Thicker roots should be sliced down their length to facilitate drying. The pieces should be spread out on a paper-lined tray in a light, airy room out of direct sunlight and stored in tightly sealed dark glass containers. Dried dandelion root may be somewhat less potent than the fresh root.

Leaf infusion: Place 2 oz of fresh dandelion leaf, less if dried, in a warmed glass container. Bring 2.5 cups of fresh nonchlorinated water to the boiling point and add it to the herbs. Cover the mixture and steep for 15–20 minutes, then strain. Drink the infusion warm or cold throughout the day, up to three cups per day. The prepared tea can be kept for about two days in the refrigerator.

Tincture: Combine 4 oz of finely-cut fresh dandelion root and leaf (or 2 oz of dry powdered herb) with 1 pt of brandy, gin, or vodka in a glass container. The alcohol should be enough to cover the plant parts and have a 50/50 ratio of alcohol to water. Cover and store the mixture away from light for about two weeks, shaking several times each day. Strain and store in a tightly capped dark glass bottle. A standard dose is 10–15 drops of the tincture in water, up to three times a day.

Precautions

Dandelion acts as a cholagogue, which means that it increases the flow of bile. It should not be used by persons with closure of the biliary ducts and other biliary ailments.

Side effects

Dandelion is a safe and nutritious herb widely used throughout the world. No health hazards have been reported when dandelion is used in designated therapeutic doses. According to the *PDR For Herbal Medicine*, however, some "superacid gastric complaints" could be triggered by using the herb. Dandelion stems contain a liquid latex substance that may be irritating to the skin of senstitive persons.

Interactions

No interactions have been reported between dandelion and standard medications.

Resources

BOOKS

Duke, James A., Ph.D. *The Green Pharmacy*. Emmaus, PA: Rodale Press, 1997.

Foster, Steven, and James A. Duke. *Peterson Field Guides, Eastern/Central Medicinal Plants*. Boston-New York: Houghton Mifflin Company, 1990.

KEY TERMS
. . . .

Achene—Any small, dry, hard seed case or fruit that does not split open at maturity to discharge the seed. Dandelion seeds are held inside achenes.

Cholagogue—A substance that stimulates the flow of bile.

Infusion—The most potent form of extraction of an herb into water. Infusions are steeped for a longer period of time than teas.

Tincture—The extraction of a herb into an alcohol solution for either internal or external use.

Hoffmann, David. *The New Holistic Herbal*. 2nd ed. Boston: Element, 1986.

Hutchens, Alma R. *A Handbook of Native American Herbs*. Boston: Shambhala Publications, Inc., 1992.

PDR for Herbal Medicines. Montvale, NJ: Medical Economics Company, 1998.

Tyler, Varro E., Ph.D. *Herbs of Choice*. New York: The Haworth Press, Inc., 1994.

Weiss, Gaea, and Shandor Weiss. *Growing & Using the Healing Herbs*. New York: Wings Books, 1992.

OTHER

Hoffmann, David L. "Dandelion." In *Herbal Materia Medica*. Health World Online. http://www.healthy.net.

Clare Hanrahan

Dandruff

Definition

Dandruff is the common name for a mild form of seborrheic **dermatitis** of unknown cause. It is a natural and harmless scalp condition in which the shedding of dead skin cells occurs at an unusually fast rate. Because of the oily skin often associated with this condition, these cells clump together and flake off as dandruff.

Description

Dandruff is very common. Up to one-third of the U.S. population is affected by this condition. While it is not considered a disease, dandruff is a cosmetic concern for many people.

The following problems tend to exacerbate dandruff:

• cold weather

• dry indoor heating

• **stress** (physical or emotional)

• food allergies

• nutritional deficiencies (B-complex vitamins or **omega-3 fatty acids**)

• use of hair spray and gels

• use of hair-coloring chemicals

• use of electric hair curlers or blow dryers

Causes & symptoms

Dandruff is caused by an overgrowth of skin cells that make up the scalp. It is not known what accelerates this cell growth. However, scientists have suggested that dandruff may be a hypersensitive reaction to the proliferation of *Pityrosporum ovale*, a yeast that occurs naturally on the scalp. Another theory that held for some time linked dandruff to a fungus. A 2002 report said that scientists had identified new fungi of the Malassezia that seem to exist in overabundance on the scalps of those affected with the disease.

Diagnosis

Dandruff is easy to diagnose. The condition is characterized by the appearance of white flakes on the hair or on the shoulders and collar. People with oily hair tend to have dandruff more often. Dandruff usually does not require medical treatment. However, if, in addition to dandruff, a person also has greasy scaling on the face, eyebrows and eyelashes and thick, red patches on the body, he or she may have the more severe form of seborrheic dermatitis. This condition may require medical advice and treatment.

Treatment

Alternative treatments for dandruff include nutritional therapy, herbal therapy and **relaxation** therapy.

Nutritional therapy

The following nutritional changes may be helpful:

• Identification and avoidance of potential allergenic foods.

• Limited intake of milk and other dairy products, seafoods and fatty treats. These foods tend to exacerbate dandruff.

• Reduction or elimination of animal proteins and eating mostly whole grains, fresh vegetables, beans and fruit.

• Avoiding citrus until dandruff clears.

• Diet supplemented with B-complex vitamins which may alleviate dandruff condition.

• Avoiding excess salt, sugar, and alcohol.

• Taking 1 tablespoon of **flaxseed** oil per day. Flaxseed oil is rich in omega-3 fatty acids, which may be effective in treating a variety of skin conditions including dandruff.

From a traditional medical approach, dandruff may be the body's way of eliminating excess protein accumulated but not assimilated in the system. It may also be a symptom of liver and kidney imbalances. A more stabilizing diet is needed, reducing highly acidic foods such as tomatoes and certain spices.

Herbal therapy

Massaging **tea tree oil** (*Melaleuca alternifolia*) into the scalp may help prevent or relieve dandruff. This oil can relieve scaling and **itching**. Ayurvedic treatment also includes various oil therapies, called *suehana* for the head. Increased **exercise** can increase circulation and help eliminate fats and oils.

Relaxation therapies

Relaxation techniques such as **meditation** or **yoga** may help relieve stress, which exacerbates dandruff.

Allopathic treatment

There is no cure for this natural harmless skin condition. Because a greasy scalp is associated with dandruff condition, more frequent hair washing using regular shampoo is usually all that is needed. In more severe cases, medicated shampoo may be necessary.

The two most commonly used anti-dandruff shampoos are **selenium** sulfide and **zinc** pyrithione. Both of these are cytostatic agents. Cytostatic drugs slow down the growth and formation of top skin layer on the scalp. To get the best result, one should leave the shampoo on for as long as possible. It is recommended that a person lather the anti-dandruff shampoo at the beginning of the shower, leave it on until the end of the shower, then rinse, lather, and rinse again. As a result of treatment with any of these drugs, dandruff will become less noticeable. Because it can be irritating, shampoo containing selenium sulfide should not be used if the skin is cut or abraded.

Products containing salicylic acid and **sulfur** are reserved for more severe cases. Salicylic acid loosens the dead skin cells so that they can be sloughed off more easily. Sometimes, antibacterial shampoos are used to reduce bacteria on the scalp.

Recently, antifungal products, such as ketoconazole (Nizoral) shampoos, are available over-the-counter (1% preparation) and by prescription (2% preparation). These shampoos are often prescribed by dermatologists to reduce the growth of *P. ovale*. These preparations may be helpful if dandruff is not relieved by other shampoo treatments.

The most severe and recalcitrant dandruff conditions may require tar shampoos. These shampoos reduce the growth of top skin cells on the scalp. It is recommended that the shampoo be left on the hair for at least 10 minutes for best results. Coal tar shampoos can be messy and can stain blond or white hair. Coal tar also can be carcinogenic (causing **cancer**). However, the FDA approves this product because when used as shampoo, because it contacts the scalp for only a short period of time. Still, it is a good idea to use alternative treatments for this relatively harmless condition.

Because anti-dandruff shampoos may lose effectiveness after a while, it may be helpful to rotate between a medicated shampoo and a regular shampoo or try a different type of anti-dandruff shampoo.

Expected results

While one can not cure dandruff, it can be easily managed. A mild dandruff condition often responds to more frequent hair washes with regular shampoo. More severe conditions may require anti-dandruff preparations.

Prevention

Preventive measures include regular hair washing, reducing stress, eating healthy foods and increasing humidity inside the house. In addition, excessive use of hair curlers, hair sprays and gels, and frequent hair coloring should be avoided. These tend to irritate the scalp and may worsen dandruff.

Resources

BOOKS
"Dandruff." In *The Medical Advisor: The Complete Guide to Alternative & Conventional Treatments*, home edition. Alexandria, VA: Time-Life, Inc., 1997.
Murray, Michael T. and Joseph E. Pizzorno. "Seborrheic Dermatitis." In *Encyclopedia of Natural Medicine*. 2nd ed. Roseville, CA: Prima Publishing, 1998.

PERIODICALS
Johnson, Betty Anne and Julia R. Nunley. "Treatment of Seborrheic Dermatitis." *American Family Physician* 61 (2000): 2703-2710.
"P&G Scientists Pinpoint Cause of Dandruff" *Health &Medicine Week* (August 12, 2002). 11.

Cytostatic—Suppressing the growth and multiplication of cells.
Flake—A small, thin skin mass.
Scale—Any thin, flaky, plate-like piece of dry skin.
Seborrheic dermatitis—An inflammatory condition of the skin of the scalp, with yellowish greasy scaling of the skin and itching. Other areas of the body may also be affected. Mild seborrheic condition is called dandruff.

Snyder, Karyn. "Is OTC Dandruff Shampoo As Effective As Rx?" *Drug Topics Archive* (September 16, 1996). http://www.pdr.net.

ORGANIZATIONS
American Academy of Dermatology. P.O. Box 4014, Schaumburg, IL 60168. (888) 462-DERM. Fax: (847) 330-8907. http://www.aad.org.

OTHER
"Seborrheic Dermatitis." *The Merck Manual of Diagnosis and Therapy*. http://www.merck.com/pubs/manual/section101 chapter111/111d.htm.
Sorgen, Carol. "Go Hug a Tree: Tea Tree Oil Treats Skin Conditions." *CBSHealthWatch*. http://cbs.medscape.com.

Mai Tran
Teresa G. Odle

Deadly nightshade *see* **Belladonna**

Deglycyrrhizinated licorice
Description

Deglycyrrhizinated **licorice**, or DGL, is a specific type of preparation derived from the licorice root. It is used differently than herbal licorice because it is much higher in agents that soothe or heal mucous membranes, and lower in other constituents found in licorice root and full extracts of licorice root. DGL may also be spelled, deglycyrrhizinated liquorice. The herb, licorice, from which DGL is derived, is known by the names *Glycyrrhiza*, sweet root, and *Yasti-madhu* with the glycyrrhizin removed.

Licorice is a perennial herb, which is native to the Middle East, and widely cultivated in Europe, the Middle East, and Asia. The root has a long history of use as a medicament and flavoring agent. Its name, *Glycyrrhiza* (sweet root) has been attributed to the first century Greek physician, Dioscorides.

Glycyrrhizin is the cause of pseudoaldosteronism, a condition mimicking the effects of excessive levels of the adrenal hormone aldosterone. The deglycyrrhizinated product was developed to concentrate the demulcent and healing aspects of licorice, while avoiding excess exposure to glycerrhizin and its adverse effects when taken in high doses.

General use

Deglycyrrhizinated licorice is used to soothe and protect the lining of the stomach and duodenum (upper small intestine)— the common sites of gastric ulcers. Ulcers in the stomach are known as peptic ulcers, while those in the small intestine are duodenal ulcers. DGL has been studied for the treatment of peptic and duodenal ulcers, and appears to be both safe and effective for long-term maintenance therapy for certain patients who have these ulcers. Some marketers claim that DGL has anti-inflammatory, antimicrobial, and antioxidant activities. However these claims are unsubstantiated.

One study, using a mouthwash containing deglycyrrhizinated licorice, showed dramatic improvement in the healing and **pain** of mouth ulcers.

Preparations

DGL is available as:

• capsules, 250 milligrams (mg)

• chewable tablets (with or without sugar), 140 and 380 mg

• lozenges, 400 mg

• wafers, 380 mg

• liquid, various concentrations

Precautions

Deglycyrrhizinated licorice appears to be very safe. However, severe allergic reactions are possible. There has been one report of a case of nilk alkali syndrome in a patient who was drinking unusually large amounts of milk. This has led to a caution against taking **calcium** supplements and deglycyrrhizinated licorice at the same time. However, it is usually safe at normal dose levels.

Although there have been few studies conducted to determine whether interactions between deglycyrrhizinated licorice and conventional drugs exist, research has failed to identify problems.

KEY TERMS

Aldosterone—A hormone produced by the adrenal gland, instrumental in the regulation of sodium and potassium resorption by the kidney.

Demulcent—An oily or sticky substance used to soothe irritation in mucous membranes.

Expectorant—A medication that promotes the secretion or expulsion of phlegm, mucus, or other matter from the respiratory tract.

Gastritis—Inflammation of the stomach, particularly of its mucous membrane.

Lozenge—A medicated candy intended to be dissolved slowly in the mouth to soothe irritated tissues of the throat.

Milk Alkali Syndrome—A disorder of the kidneys caused by long-term treatment of ulcers with antacids, particularly alkaline compounds such as sodium bicarbonate, and large amounts of calcium.

Side effects

Gastritis, **nausea**, and **diarrhea** are reported side effects.

Interactions

All clinically significant adverse interactions with licorice have been due to the effects of the glycyrrizic acid. They would not be anticipated with this component removed. DGL reportedly reduces the gastric ulceration caused by aspirin and other nonsteroidal anti-inflammatory drugs.

Resources

BOOKS

Blumenthal, M., ed. *The Complete German Commission E Monographs.* Austin, TX: The American Botanical Council, 1998.

Blumenthal, M., A. Goldberg, and J. Brinckmann, eds. *Herbal Medicine: Expanded Commission E Monographs.* Austin, TX: The American Botanical Council, 2000.

PERIODICALS

Gibbs, C. J., and H. A. Lee. "Milk-Alkali Syndrome Due to Caved-S." *J R Soc Med* (August 1992): 498–9.

Petry, J. J., and S. K. Hadley. "Medicinal Herbs: Answers and Advice, Part 2." *Hospital Practice* (August 15, 2001): 55–9.

Rees, W. D., J. Rhodes, J. E. Wright, L. F. Stamford, and A. Bennett. "Effect of Deglycyrrhizinated Liquorice on Gastric Mucosal Damage by Aspirin." *Scandinavian Journal of Gastroenterol* (1979:605–7.

Samuel Uretsky, Pharm.D.

Dehydroepiandrosterone *see* **DHEA**

Dementia

Definition

Dementia is a loss of mental ability severe enough to interfere with normal activities of daily living, lasting more than six months, not present since birth, and not associated with a loss or alteration of consciousness.

Description

Dementia is a group of symptoms caused by gradual death of brain cells. The loss of cognitive abilities that occurs with dementia leads to impairments in memory, reasoning, planning, and personality. While the overwhelming number of people with dementia are elderly, it is not an inevitable part of **aging**. Instead, dementia is caused by specific brain diseases. **Alzheimer's disease** is the most common cause, followed by vascular or multi-infarct dementia.

The prevalence of dementia has been difficult to determine, partly because of differences in definition among different studies, and partly because there is some normal decline in functional ability with age. Dementia affects 5–8% of all people between ages 65 and 74, and up to 20% of those between 75 and 84. Estimates for dementia in those 85 and over range from 30–47%. Between two and four million Americans have Alzheimer's disease; that number is expected to grow to as many as 14 million by the middle of the twenty-first century as the population as a whole ages.

The cost of dementia can be considerable. While most people with dementia are retired and do not suffer income losses from their disease, the cost of care is often enormous. Financial burdens include lost wages for family caregivers, medical supplies and drugs, and home modifications to ensure safety. Nursing home care may cost several thousand dollars a month or more. The psychological cost is not as easily quantifiable but can be even more profound. The person with dementia loses control of many of the essential features of his life and personality, and loved ones lose a family member even as they continue to cope with the burdens of increasing dependence and unpredictability.

Causes & symptoms

Causes

Dementia is usually caused by degeneration of brain cells in the cerebral cortex, the part of the brain responsible for thoughts, memories, actions, and personality. Death of brain cells in this region leads to the cognitive impairment that characterizes dementia.

The most common cause of dementia is Alzheimer's disease (AD), accounting for half to three quarters of all cases. The brain of a person with AD becomes clogged with two abnormal structures, called neurofibrillary tangles and senile plaques. Neurofibrillary tangles are twisted masses of protein fibers inside nerve cells, or neurons. Senile plaques are composed of parts of neurons surrounding a group of proteins called beta-amyloid deposits. Why these structures develop is unknown. Current research indicates possible roles for inflammation, blood flow restriction, and accumulation of aluminum in the brain and toxic molecular fragments known as free radicals or oxidants.

Several genes have been associated with higher incidences of AD, although the exact role of these genes is still unknown. In 2001, investigators discovered a rare mutation in the amyloid precursor protein (APP) that is linked to early-onset Alzheimer's. The discovery points scientists to new ideas for targeting and treating the disease.

Vascular dementia is estimated to cause from 5–30% of all dementias. It occurs from a decrease in blood flow to the brain, most commonly due to a series of small strokes (multi-infarct dementia). Other cerebrovascular causes include: vasculitis from **syphilis**, **Lyme disease**, or **systemic lupus erythematosus**; subdural hematoma; and subarachnoid hemorrhage. Because of the usually sudden nature of its cause, the symptoms of vascular dementia tend to begin more abruptly than those of Alzheimer's dementia. Symptoms may progress stepwise with the occurrence of new strokes. Unlike AD, the incidence of vascular dementia is lower after age 75.

Other conditions which may cause dementia include:

- AIDS
- Parkinson's disease
- Lewy body disease
- Pick's disease
- Huntington's disease
- Creutzfeldt-Jakob disease
- brain tumor
- hydrocephalus

- head trauma

- multiple sclerosis

- prolonged abuse of alcohol or other drugs

- vitamin deficiency: thiamin, **niacin**, or B$_{12}$

- hypothyroidism

- hypercalcemia

Symptoms

Dementia is marked by a gradual impoverishment of thought and other mental activities. Losses eventually affect virtually every aspect of mental functioning. The slow progression of dementia is in contrast with delirium, which involves some of the same symptoms, but has a very rapid onset and fluctuating course with alteration in the level of consciousness. However, delirium may occur with dementia, especially since the person with dementia is more susceptible to the delirium-inducing effects of may types of drugs.

Symptoms include:

- Memory losses. Short-term **memory loss** is usually the first symptom noticed. It may begin with misplacing valuables such as a wallet or car keys, then progress to forgetting appointments, where the car was left, and the route home, for instance. More profound losses may eventually follow, such as forgetting the names and faces of family members.

- Impaired abstraction and planning. The person with dementia may lose the ability to perform familiar tasks, to plan activities, and to draw simple conclusions from facts.

- Language and comprehension disturbances. The person may be unable to understand instructions, or follow the logic of moderately complex sentences. Later, he or she may not understand his or her own sentences, and have difficulty forming thoughts into words.

- Poor judgment. The person may not recognize the consequences of his or her actions or be able to evaluate the appropriateness of behavior. Behavior may become crude or offensive, overly-friendly, or aggressive. Personal hygiene may be ignored.

- Impaired orientation ability. The person may not be able to identify the time of day, even from obvious visual clues; or may not recognize his or her location, even if familiar. This disability may stem partly from losses of memory and partly from impaired abstraction.

- Decreased attention and increased restlessness. This may cause the person with dementia to begin an activity and quickly lose interest, and to wander frequently. Wandering may cause significant safety problems, when combined with disorientation and memory losses. The person may begin to cook something on the stove, then become distracted and wander away while it is cooking.

- Personality changes and psychosis. The person may lose interest in once-pleasurable activities, and become more passive, depressed, or anxious. Delusions, suspicion, paranoia, and hallucinations may occur later in the disease. Sleep disturbances may occur, including **insomnia** and sleep interruptions.

Diagnosis

Since dementia usually progresses slowly, diagnosing it in its early stages can be difficult. Several office visits over several months or more may be needed. Diagnosis begins with a thorough physical exam and complete medical history, usually including comments from family members or caregivers. A family history of either Alzheimer's disease or cerebrovascular disease may provide clues to the cause of symptoms. Simple tests of mental function, including word recall, object naming, and number-symbol matching, are used to track changes in the person's cognitive ability. Recent studies suggest that positron emissions tomography (PET) scans of the brain might be able to identify those at risk for Alzheimer's. As these tests become more widely available, they may offer hope for earlier detection of dementia.

Depression is common in the elderly and can be mistaken for dementia; therefore, ruling out depression is an important part of the diagnosis. Distinguishing dementia from the mild normal cognitive decline of advanced age is also critical. The medical history includes a complete listing of drugs being taken, since a number of drugs can cause dementia-like symptoms.

Determining the cause of dementia may require a variety of medical tests, chosen to match the most likely etiology. Cerebrovascular disease, hydrocephalus, and tumors may be diagnosed with x rays, CT or MRI scans, and vascular imaging studies. Blood tests may reveal nutritional or metabolic deficiencies or hormone imbalances.

Treatment

Nutritional supplements

Some nutritional supplements may be helpful, especially if dementia is caused by deficiency of these essential nutrients:

- Acetyl-L-carnitine: improves brain function and increases attention span, enhances ability to concentrate and increases energy in patients with Alzheimer's disease.

- **Antioxidants** (**vitamin E**, **vitamin C**, beta-carotene, or **selenium**): may slow down disease progression by preventing the damaging effects of free radicals.

- B-complex vitamins and **vitamin B$_{12}$**: may significantly improve mental function in patients who have low levels of these essential nutrients.

- **Coenzyme Q$_{10}$:** helps deliver more oxygen to the brain

- DHEA: may increase brain function in old people.

- **Magnesium**: may be helpful if the dementia is caused by magnesium deficiency and/or accumulation of aluminum in the brain

- Phosphotidylserine: Deficiency of this nutrient may decrease mental function and cause depression.

- Zinc: may boost short-term memory and increase attention span

Herbal treatment

Herbal remedies that may be helpful in treating dementia include Chinese or **Korean ginseng, Siberian ginseng, gotu kola**, and *Ginkgo biloba*. Of these, **ginkgo biloba** is the most well known and widely accepted by Western medicine. Ginkgo extract, derived from the leaves of the *Ginkgo biloba* tree, interferes with a circulatory protein called platelet-activating factor. It also increases circulation and oxygenation to the brain. Ginkgo extract has been used for many years in China and is widely prescribed in Europe for treatment of circulatory problems. A 1997 study of patients with dementia appeared to show that gingko extract could improve their symptoms. Some scientists believe that, taken early enough in the process, *Ginkgo biloba* can delay the onset of Alzheimer's, but this claim has not yet been sufficiently backed by enough supportive studies.

Homeopathy

A homeopathic physician may prescribe patient-specific homeopathic remedies to alleviate symptoms of dementia.

Acupressure

This form of therapy uses hands to apply pressure on specific **acupressure** points to improve blood circulation and calm the nervous system.

Aromatherapy

Aromatherapists use **essential oils** as inhalants or in baths to improve mental performances and to calm the nerves.

Chelation therapy

This is a controversial treatment that may provide symptomatic improvement in some patients. However, its effectiveness has not been supported by clinical stud-

ies. In addition, this form of therapy may cause kidney damage. Therefore, it should only be given under watchful eyes of a qualified physician.

Allopathic treatment

There are no therapies that can reverse the progression of Alzheimer's disease. Therefore, treatment of dementia begins with treatment of the underlying disease when possible. Aspirin, estrogen, vitamin E, selegiline, propentofylline and milameline are currently being evaluated for their ability to slow the rate of progression.

Care for a person with dementia can be difficult and complex. The patient must learn to cope with functional and cognitive limitations, while family members or other caregivers assume increasing responsibility for the person's physical needs.

Symptoms of dementia may be treated with a combination of **psychotherapy**, environmental modifications and medication. Behavioral approaches may be used to reduce the frequency or severity of problem behaviors, such as aggression or socially inappropriate conduct.

Modifying the environment can increase safety and comfort while decreasing agitation. Home modifications for safety include removal or lock-up of hazards such as sharp knives, dangerous chemicals, and tools. Child-proof latches or Dutch doors may be used to limit access as well. Lowering the hot **water** temperature to 120°F (48.9°C) or less reduces the risk of scalding. Bed rails and bathroom safety rails can be important safety measures, as well. Confusion may be reduced with simpler decorative schemes and presence of familiar objects. Covering or disguising doors (with a mural, for example) may reduce the tendency to wander. Positioning the bed in view of the bathroom can decrease incontinence.

Two drugs, tacrine (Cognex) and donepezil (Aricept), are commonly prescribed for Alzheimer's disease. These drugs inhibit the breakdown of acetylcholine in the brain, prolonging its ability to conduct chemical messages between brain cells. They provide temporary improvement in cognitive functions for about 40% of patients with mild-to-moderate AD. Hydergine is sometimes prescribed as well, though it is of questionable benefit for most patients. Other drugs that are frequently used in dementia patients include antianxiety (for agitation and **anxiety**) and antipsychotics (for paranoia, delusions or hallucinations) and antidepressants (for depressive symptoms). Evaluation of any medical side effects from the medications should be ongoing.

Long-term institutional care may be needed for the person with dementia, as profound cognitive losses often precede death by a number of years. Early planning for the financial burden of nursing home care is critical. Useful information about financial planning for long-term care is available through the Alzheimer's Association.

Expected results

The prognosis for dementia depends on the underlying disease. On average, people with Alzheimer's disease live eight years past their diagnosis, with a range from one to twenty years. Vascular dementia is usually progressive, with death from **stroke**, infection, or **heart disease**.

Prevention

There is no known way to prevent Alzheimer's disease, although several of the drugs under investigation may reduce its risk or slow its progression. Nutritional supplements, including antioxidants, may also help protect against Alzheimer's disease. New studies also show that use of nonsteroidal anti-inflammatory agents (over-the-counter **pain** relievers like ibuprofen and naproxen) may lower risk of Alzheimer's. The risk of developing multi-infarct dementia may be reduced by reducing the risk of stroke. Sources of aluminum, which can be found in aluminum cookware, canned sodas, and certain antacids and deodorants, should be avoided.

Resources

BOOKS

Halpern, Georges. *Ginkgo: A Practical Guide.* Garden City Park, NY: Avery Publishing Group, 1998.

Jacques, Alan. *Understanding Dementia.* New York: Churchill Livingstone, 1992.

Mace, Nancy L. and Peter V. Rabins. *The 36-Hour Day.* Baltimore: Johns Hopkins University Press, 1995.

Murray, Michael and Joseph Pizzorno. "Alzheimer's Disease." In *Encyclopedia of Natural Medicine.* 2nd ed. Rocklin, CA: Prima Publishing, 1998.

Zand, Janet, Allan N. Spreen, and James B. LaValle. "Alzheimer's Disease." In *Smart Medicine for Healthier Living: A Practical A-to-Z Reference to Natural and Conventional Treatments for Adults.* Garden City Park, NY: Avery Publishing Group, 2000.

PERIODICALS

Gottlieb, Scott R. "NSAIDs Can Lower Risk of Alzheimer's." *British Medical Journal* 323 no.7324(December 1, 2001):1269.

Mitka M. "PET and Memory Impairment." *JAMA, Journal of the American Medical Association* 286 no. 16(October 24, 2001):1961.

Stephenson Joan. "Alzheimer Treatment Target?" *JAMA, Journal of the American Medical Association* 286 no. 14(October 10, 2001):1704.

ORGANIZATION

Alzheimer's Association. 919 North Michigan Ave., Suite 1000, Chicago, IL 60611. (800) 272-3900 (TDD: (312) 335-8882). http://www.alz.org/.

Mai Tran
Teresa G. Odle

Depression

Definition

Depression, also known as depressive disorders or unipolar depression, is a mental illness characterized by a profound and persistent feeling of sadness or despair and/or a loss of interest in things that once were pleasurable. Disturbance in sleep, appetite, and mental processes are a common accompaniment.

Description

Everyone experiences feelings of unhappiness and sadness occasionally. However, when these depressed feelings start to dominate everyday life without a recent loss or trauma and cause physical and mental deterioration, they become what is known as depression. Each year in the United States, depression affects an estimated 17 million people at an approximate annual direct and indirect cost of $53 billion. One in four women is likely to experience an episode of severe depression in her lifetime, with a 10–20% lifetime prevalence, compared to 5–10% for men. The average age a first depressive episode occurs is in the mid-20s, although the disorder strikes all age groups indiscriminately, from children to the elderly.

There are two main categories of depression: major depressive disorder and dysthymic disorder. Major depressive disorder is a moderate to severe episode of depression lasting two or more weeks. Individuals experiencing this major depressive episode may have trouble sleeping, lose interest in activities in which they once took pleasure, experience a change in weight, have difficulty concentrating, feel worthless and hopeless, or have a preoccupation with death or suicide. In children, major depression may appear as irritability.

While major depressive episodes may be acute (intense but short-lived), dysthymic disorder is an ongoing, chronic depression that lasts two or more years (one or more years in children) and has an average duration of 16 years. The mild to moderate depression of dysthymic disorder may rise and fall in intensity, and those afflicted with the disorder may experience some periods of normal, non-depressed mood of up to two months in length. Its onset is gradual, and dysthymic patients may not be able to pinpoint exactly when they started feeling depressed. Individuals with dysthymic disorder may experience a change in sleeping and eating patterns, low self-esteem, fatigue, trouble concentrating, and feelings of hopelessness.

Depression also can occur in **bipolar disorder**, an affective mental illness that causes radical emotional changes and mood swings, from manic highs to depressive lows. The majority of bipolar individuals experience alternating episodes of mania and depression.

Causes & symptoms

The causes behind depression are complex and not yet fully understood. While an imbalance of certain neurotransmitters, the chemicals in the brain that transmit messages between nerve cells, is believed to be key to depression, external factors such as upbringing (more so in dysthymia than major depression) may be as important. For example, it is speculated that, if an individual is abused and neglected throughout childhood and adolescence, a pattern of low self-esteem and negative thinking may emerge, and from that, a lifelong pattern of depression may follow. A 2003 study reported that two-thirds of patients with major depression say they also suffer from chronic **pain**.

SYMPTOMS OF ADULT DEPRESSION
Longterm sadness
Feelings of worthlessness or guilt
Lack of interest in sex
Loss of concentration
Loss of interest in activities
Fatigue
Weight loss or gain
Insomnia or oversleeping
Anxiety
Suicidal thoughts
Slowed speech and physical movement

Heredity seems to play a role in who develops depression. Individuals with major depression in their immediate family are up to three times more likely to have the disorder themselves. It would seem that biological and genetic factors may make certain individuals predisposed or prone to depressive disorders, but environmental circumstances may often trigger the disorder.

External stressors and significant life changes, such as chronic medical problems, death of a loved one, divorce or estrangement, miscarriage, or loss of a job also can result in a form of depression known as adjustment disorder. Although periods of adjustment disorder usually resolve themselves, occasionally they may evolve into a major depressive disorder.

Major depressive episode

Individuals experiencing a major depressive episode have a depressed mood and/or a diminished interest or pleasure in activities. Children experiencing a major depressive episode may appear or feel irritable, rather than depressed. In addition, five or more of the following symptoms will occur on an almost daily basis for a period of at least two weeks:

• Significant change in weight

• insomnia or hypersomnia (excessive sleep)

• psychomotor agitation or retardation

• fatigue or loss of energy

• feelings of worthlessness or inappropriate guilt

• diminished ability to think or to concentrate, or indecisiveness

• recurrent thoughts of death, or suicidal and/or suicide attempts

SYMPTOMS OF CHILDHOOD/ADOLESCENT DEPRESSION

Drop in school performance
Weight loss or gain
Stomachaches
Insomnia
Social withdrawal
Drug or alcohol abuse
Isolation
Apathy
Fatigue
Lack of concentration

Dysthymic disorder

Dysthymia commonly occurs in tandem with other psychiatric and physical conditions. Up to 70% of dysthymic patients have both dysthymic disorder and major depressive disorder, known as double depression. Substance abuse, panic disorders, personality disorders, social **phobias**, and other psychiatric conditions also are found in many dysthymic patients. Dysthymia is prevalent in patients with certain medical conditions, including **multiple sclerosis**, **AIDS**, **hypothyroidism**, **chronic fatigue syndrome**, **Parkinson's disease**, diabetes, and postcardiac transplantation. The connection between dysthymic disorder and these medical conditions is unclear, but it may be related to the way the medical condition and/or its pharmacological treatment affects neurotransmitters. Dysthymic disorder can lengthen or complicate the recovery of patients also suffering from medical conditions.

Along with an underlying feeling of depression, people with dysthymic disorder experience two or more of the following symptoms on an almost daily basis for a period for two or more years (most suffer for five years), or one year or more for children:

- under or overeating
- insomnia or hypersomnia
- low energy or fatigue
- low self-esteem
- poor concentration or trouble making decisions
- altered libido
- altered appetite
- altered motivation
- feelings of hopelessness

Diagnosis

The guidelines for diagnosis of major depressive disorder and dysthymic disorder are found in the *Diagnostic and Statistical Manual of Mental Disorders, Fourth Edition (DSM IV)*. In addition to an interview, several clinical inventories or scales may be used to assess a patient's mental status and determine the presence of depressive symptoms. Among these tests are: the Hamilton Depression Scale (HAM-D), Child Depression Inventory (CDI), Geriatric Depression Scale (GDS), Beck Depression Inventory (BDI), and the Zung Self-Rating Scale for Depression. These tests may be administered in an outpatient or hospital setting by a general practitioner, social worker, psychiatrist, or psychologist.

Treatment

A variety of alternative medicines have proven to be helpful in treating depression. A recent report from Great Britain emphasized that more physicians should encourage alternative treatments such as behavioral and self-help programs, supervised **exercise** programs, and watchful waiting before subscribing antidepressant medications for mild depression. Chocolate, coffee, sugar, and alcohol can negatively affect mood and should be avoided. **Essential fatty acids** may reduce depression and boost mood. Expressing thoughts and feelings in a journal is therapeutic. **Aromatherapy**, particularly citrus fragrance, has had a positive effect on depression. **Psychotherapy** or counseling is an integral component of treatment because it can find and treat the cause of the depression.

Psychosocial therapy

Psychotherapy explores a person's life to bring forth possible contributing causes of depression. During treatment, the therapist helps the patient to become aware of his or her thinking patterns and how they originated. There are several different subtypes of psychotherapy, but all have the common goal of helping the patient develop healthy problem solving and coping skills.

Cognitive-behavioral therapy assumes that the patient's faulty thinking is causing the current depression and focuses on changing thought patterns and perceptions. The therapist helps the patient identify negative or distorted thought patterns and the emotions and behavior that accompany them, and then retrains the patient to recognize the thinking and react differently to it.

Chinese medicine and herbals

The principle of treatment of depression involves regulating qi, reducing phlegm, calming the mind, and promoting mental resuscitation. The Chinese medicine

Bai Jin Wan (White Metal Pill) is used to treat depression (5 g twice daily). A practitioner may prescribe a variety of treatments—including lifestyle changes—depending on the type and severity of the depression.

There is some evidence that **acupuncture** is a helpful treatment for depression. One double-blind study found that patients who received acupuncture specific for depression were significantly less depressed than control patients who had either nonspecific acupuncture or no treatment.

St. John's wort (*Hypericum perforatum*) is the most widely used antidepressant in Germany. Many studies on the effectiveness of St. John's wort have been performed. One review of the studies determined that St. John's wort is superior to placebo and comparable to conventional antidepressants. In early 2000, well designed studies comparing the effectiveness of St. John's wort versus conventional antidepressants in treating depression were underway in the United States. Despite uncertainty concerning its effectiveness, a 2003 report said acceptance of the treatment continues to increase. A poll shoed that about 41% of 15,000 science professionals in 62 countries said they would use St. Johnís wort for mild to moderate depression. Although St. John's wort appears to be a safe alternative to conventional antidepressants, care should be taken, as the herb can interfere with the actions of some pharmaceuticals. The usual dose is 300 mg three times daily.

Orthomolecular therapy

Orthomolecular therapy refers to therapy that strives to achieve the optimal chemical environment for the brain. The theory behind this approach is that mental disease is caused by low concentrations of specific chemicals. Linus Pauling believed that mental disease was caused by low concentrations of the B vitamins, **biotin**, **vitamin C**, or **folic acid**. Supplementation with vitamins B_1, B_2, and B_6 improved the symptoms of depression in geriatric patients taking tricyclic antidepressants. The **amino acids** tryptophan, tyrosine, and phenylalanine have been shown to have positive effects on depression, although large, controlled studies need to be carried out to confirm these findings.

S-ADENOSYL-METHIONINE. In several small studies, S-adenosyl-methionine (SAM, SAMe) was shown to be more effective than placebo and equally effective as tricyclic antidepressants in treating depression. The usual dosage is 200 mg to 400 mg twice daily. In 2003, a U.S. Department of Health and Human Services team reviewed 100 clinical trials on SAMe and concluded that it worked as well as many prescription medications with-

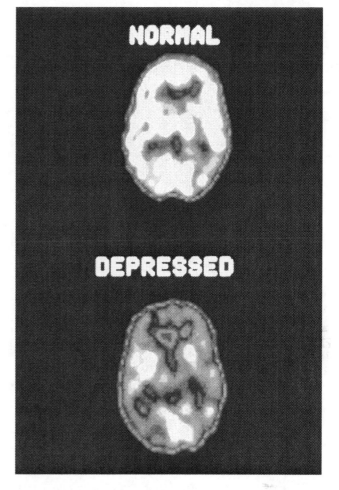

Positron emission tomography (PET) scans comparing a normal brain with that of someone with a depressed mental disorder. *(Photo Researchers, Inc. Reproduced by permission.)*

out the side effects of stomach upset and decreased sexual desire.

5-HYDROXYTRYPTOPHAN. 5-hydroxytryptophan (5-HT, **5-HTP**) is a precursor to serotonin. Most of the commercially available 5-HT is extracted from the plant *Griffonia simplicifolia*. In several small studies, treatment with 5-HT significantly improved depression in more than half of the patients. One review of these studies suggests that 5-HT has antidepressant properties, however, large studies must be performed to confirm this finding. The usual dose is 50 mg three times daily. Side effects include **nausea** and gastrointestinal disturbances.

Homeopathic remedies

Homeopathic remedies can be helpful treatments for depression. A homeopathic practitioner should be consulted for dosages, but common remedies are:

• *Arum metallicum* for severe depression

• Ignatia for adjustment disorder

• *Natrum muriaticum* for depression of long duration.

Light therapy

Light therapy is helpful in controlling the depression of **seasonal affective disorder** (SAD). Treatment consists of exposure to light of a high intensity and/or specific spectra for an hour per day from a light box placed on the floor or on a table. The light intensity is usually 10,000 lux which is similar to the light of a sunny day. The opposite may be used, as well, which is the use of a dawn simulator for those patients who have an overdose of light exposure and require more sleep with less light. Most persons will see an effect within three to four weeks. Side effects include headaches, eyestrain, irritability, and insomnia. A week or more in a sunny climate may improve SAD.

Allopathic treatment

Depression usually is treated with antidepressants and/or psychosocial therapy. When used together correctly, therapy and antidepressants are a powerful treatment plan for the depressed patient.

Drugs

Selective serotonin reuptake inhibitors (SSRIs), such as fluoxetine (Prozac) and sertraline (Zoloft), reduce depression by increasing levels of serotonin, a neurotransmitter. Some clinicians prefer SSRIs for treatment of dysthymic disorder. Anxiety, **diarrhea**, drowsiness, **headache**, sweating, nausea, poor sexual functioning, and insomnia all are possible side effects of SSRIs. A recent study shows this generation of drugs increases patients' risk of gastrointestinal bleeding.

Tricyclic antidepressants (TCAs) are less expensive than SSRIs, but have more severe side effects including persistent **dry mouth**, sedation, **dizziness**, and cardiac arrhythmias. Because of these side effects, caution is taken when prescribing TCAs to elderly patients. TCAs include amitriptyline (Elavil), imipramine (Tofranil), and nortriptyline (Aventyl, Pamelor). A 10-day supply of TCAs can be lethal if ingested all at once, so these drugs may not be a preferred treatment option for patients at risk for suicide.

Monoamine oxidase inhibitors (MAO inhibitors), such as tranylcypromine (Parnate) and phenelzine (Nardil), block the action of monoamine oxidase (MAO), an enzyme in the central nervous system. Patients taking MAOIs must avoid foods high in tyramine (found in aged cheeses and meats) to avoid potentially serious hypertensive side effects.

Heterocyclics include bupropion (Wellbutrin) and trazodone (Desyrel). Bupropion is prescribed to patients with a seizure disorder. Side effects include agitation, anxiety, confusion, tremor, dry mouth, fast or irregular heartbeat, headache, low blood pressure, and insomnia. Because trazodone has a sedative effect, it is useful in treating depressed patients with insomnia. Other possible side effects of trazodone include dry mouth, gastrointestinal distress, dizziness, and headache. In 2003, Wellbutrin's manufacturer released a once-daily version of the drug that offered low risk of sexual side effects or weight gain.

Electroconvulsive therapy

ECT, or electroconvulsive therapy, usually is employed after all therapy and pharmaceutical treatment options have been explored and exhausted. However, it is sometimes used early in treatment when severe depression is present and the patient refuses oral medication, or when the patient is becoming dehydrated, extremely suicidal, or psychotic.

The treatment consists of a series of electrical pulses that move into the brain through electrodes on the patient's head. ECT is given under general anesthesia and patients are administered a muscle relaxant to prevent convulsions. Although the exact mechanisms behind the success of ECT therapy are not known, it is believed that the electrical current modifies the electrochemical processes of the brain, consequently relieving depression. Headaches, muscle soreness, nausea, and confusion are possible side effects immediately following an ECT procedure. **Memory loss**, typically transient, has also been reported in ECT patients. ECT causes severe memory problems for months or years in one out of every 200 patients treated.

Late in 2001, a study reported on a pacemaker-like device used to treat **epilepsy** adapted for patients with depression. An implanted electronic device sends intermittent signals to the vagus nerve, which in turn carries the signals to the brain, connecting in areas known to regulate mood. Although still experimental at this time, early results in treating depression have been encouraging.

Expected results

Untreated or improperly treated depression is the number one cause of suicide in the United States. Proper treatment relieves symptoms in 80–90% of depressed patients. After each major depressive episode, the risk of recurrence climbs significantly—50% after one episode, 70% after two episodes, and 90% after three episodes. For this reason, patients need to be aware of the symptoms of recurring depression and may require long-term maintenance treatment.

Overall, recent recommendations from mental health clinicians suggest that the recovery process for patients with depression works best when mental health professionals focus on the whole person behind the disorder. In addition to prescribing medications, they also should address a patient's self-esteem, feeling of control, and determination. They emphasize that patients with depression need a sense of optimism and should be encouraged to seek the support of family members and friends.

Prevention

Patient education in the form of therapy or self-help groups is crucial for training patients with depressive disorders to recognize early symptoms of depression and to take an active part in their treatment program. Extended maintenance treatment with antidepressants may be required in some patients to prevent relapse. Early intervention with children with depression is effective in halting development of more severe problems.

Resources

BOOKS

American Psychiatric Association. *Diagnostic and Statistical Manual of Mental Disorders.* 4th ed. Washington, DC: American Psychiatric Press, Inc., 1994.

Peightel, James A., Thomas L. Hardie, and David A. Baron. "Complementary/Alternative Therapies in the Treatment of Psychiatric Illnesses." In *Complementary/Alternative Medicine: An Evidence Based Approach.* John W. Spencer and Joseph J. Jacobs, eds. St. Louis: Mosby, 1999.

Thompson, Tracy. *The Beast: A Reckoning with Depression.* New York: G. P. Putnam, 1995.

Ying, Zhou Zhong and Jin Hui De. "Psychiatry and Neurology." In *Clinical Manual of Chinese Herbal Medicine and Acupuncture.* New York: Churchill Livingston, 1997.

PERIODICALS

"A Natural Mood-booster that Really Works: a Group of Noted Researchers Found that the Supplement SAMe Works as Well as Antidepressant Drugs." *Natural Health* (July 2003): 22.

"Antidepression 'Pacemaker' Demonstrates Long-Term Benefits." *Medical Devices and Surgical Technology Week.* (December 30, 2001): 34.

Deltito, Joseph, and Doris Beyer. "The Scientific, Quasi-scientific and Popular Literature on the Use of St. John's Wort in the Treatment of Depression." *Journal of Affective Disorders* 51 (1998): 345-351.

"FDA Approves Once-daily Supplement." *Biotech Week* (September 24, 2003): 6.

Head, Kathi. "Conquer Depression Without Drugs." *Let's Live* 68 (2000): 72+.

KEY TERMS

Hypersomnia—Excessive sleeping (can be from 9–20 hours, or more); a symptom of dysthymic and major depressive disorder.

Neurotransmitter—A chemical in the brain that transmits messages between neurons, or nerve cells. Changes in the levels of certain neurotransmitters, such as serotonin, norepinephrine, and dopamine, are thought to be related to depressive disorders.

Psychomotor agitation—Disturbed physical and mental processes (e.g., fidgeting, wringing of hands, racing thoughts); a symptom of major depressive disorder.

Psychomotor retardation—Slowed physical and mental processes (e.g., slowed thinking, movement, and talking); a symptom of major depressive disorder.

Seasonal affective disorder (SAD)—Depression caused by decreased daylight during the winter months.

Jancin, Bruce. "Chronic Pain Affects 67% of Patients With Depression: 'Stunning' Finding in Primary Care Study." *Internal Medicine News* (September 15, 2003): 4.

Miller, Mark D. "Recognizing and Treating Depression in the Elderly." *Medscape Mental Health* 2, no.3 (1997). http://www.medscape.com.

Miller, Sue. "A Natural Mood Booster." *Newsweek* (May 5, 1997): 74-5.

"New Depression and Anxiety Treatment Goals Defined." *Health and Medicine Week.* (December 31, 2001): 24.

Salmans, Sandra. "More on Treatments." *Depression: Questions You Have..Answers You Need* (1997): 145+.

Sansone, Randy A. and Lori A. Sansone. "Dysthymic Disorder: The Chronic Depression." *American Family Physician* 53, no. 8 (June 1996): 2588-96.

"St. John's Wort Healing Reputation Upheld?" *Nutraceuticals International.* (September 2003).

"Try Alternatives Before Using Antidepressants." *GP.* (September 29, 2003): 12.

ORGANIZATIONS

American Psychiatric Association (APA). Office of Public Affairs, 1400 K Street NW, Washington, DC 20005. (202) 682-6119. http://www.psych.org/.

American Psychological Association (APA). Office of Public Affairs, 750 First St. NE, Washington, DC 20002-4242. (202) 336-5700. http://www.apa.org/.

National Alliance for the Mentally Ill (NAMI). 200 North Glebe Road, Suite 1015, Arlington, VA 22203-3754. (800) 950-6264. http://www.nami.org.

National Depressive and Manic-Depressive Association (NDMDA). 730 N. Franklin St., Suite 501, Chicago, IL 60610. (800) 826-3632. http://www.ndmda.org.

National Institute of Mental Health (NIMH). 5600 Fishers Lane, Rm. 7C-02, Bethesda, MD 20857. (301) 443-4513. http://www.nimh.nih.gov/.

Belinda Rowland
Teresa G. Odle

Dermatitis

Definition

Dermatitis is a general term used to describe inflammation of the skin.

Description

Most types of dermatitis are characterized by a pink or red rash that itches.

Contact dermatitis is an allergic reaction to something that irritates the skin and is manifested by one or more lines of red, swollen, blistered skin that may itch or weep. It usually appears within 48 hours after coming into contact with a substance to which the skin is sensitive. The condition is more common in adults than in children.

Contact dermatitis can occur on any part of the body, but it usually affects the hands, feet, and groin. Contact dermatitis usually does not spread from one person to another, nor does it spread beyond the area exposed to the irritant unless affected skin comes into contact with another part of the body. However, in the case of some irritants, such as poison ivy, contact dermatitis can be passed to another person or to another part of the body.

Stasis dermatitis is characterized by scaly, greasy looking skin on the lower legs and around the ankles. Stasis dermatitis is most apt to affect the inner side of the calf.

Nummular dermatitis, which is also called nummular eczematous dermatitis or nummular **eczema**, generally affects the hands, arms, legs, and buttocks of men and women older than 55 years of age. This stubborn, inflamed rash forms circular, sometimes itchy, patches and is characterized by flares and periods of inactivity.

Atopic dermatitis is characterized by **itching**, scaling, swelling, and sometimes blistering. In early childhood it is called infantile eczema and is characterized by redness, oozing, and crusting. It is usually found on the face, inside the elbows, and behind the knees.

Seborrheic dermatitis may be dry or moist and is characterized by greasy scales and yellowish crusts on the scalp, eyelids, face, external surfaces of the ears, underarms, breasts, and groin. In infants it is called **cradle cap**.

Causes & symptoms

Allergic reactions are genetically determined, and different substances cause contact dermatitis to develop in different people. A reaction to resin produced by poison ivy, poison **oak**, or poison sumac is the most common source of symptoms. It is, in fact, the most common allergy in this country, affecting one of every two people in the United States.

Flowers, herbs, and vegetables can also affect the skin of some people. **Burns** and **sunburn** increase the risk of dermatitis developing, and chemical irritants that can cause the condition include:

- chlorine
- cleansers
- detergents and soaps
- fabric softeners
- glues used on artificial nails
- perfumes
- topical medications

Contact dermatitis can develop when the first contact occurs or after years of use or exposure.

Stasis dermatitis, a consequence of poor circulation, occurs when leg veins can no longer return blood to the heart as efficiently as they once did. When that happens, fluid collects in the lower legs and causes them to swell. Stasis dermatitis can also result in a rash that can break down into sores known as stasis ulcers.

The cause of nummular dermatitis is not known, but it usually occurs in cold weather and is most common in people who have dry skin. Hot weather and **stress** can aggravate this condition, as can the following:

- **allergies**
- fabric softeners
- soaps and detergents
- wool clothing
- bathing more than once a day

Atopic dermatitis can be caused by allergies, **asthma**, or stress, and there seems to be a genetic predisposition for atopic conditions. It is sometimes caused by an allergy to nickel in jewelry.

Seborrheic dermatitis (for which there may also be a genetic predisposition)is usually caused by overproduction of the oil glands. In adults it can be associated with

diabetes mellitus or gold allergy. In infants and adults it may be caused by a **biotin** or vitamin B deficiency.

Diagnosis

The diagnosis of dermatitis is made on the basis of how the rash looks and its location. The doctor may scrape off a small piece of affected skin for microscopic examination or direct the patient to discontinue use of any potential irritant that has recently come into contact with the affected area. Two weeks after the rash disappears, the patient may resume use of the substances, one at a time, until the condition recurs. Eliminating the substance most recently added should eliminate the irritation.

If the origin of the irritation has still not been identified, a dermatologist may perform one or more patch tests. This involves dabbing a small amount of a suspected irritant onto skin on the patient's back. If no irritation develops within a few days, another patch test is performed. The process continues until the patient experiences an allergic reaction at the spot where the irritant was applied.

Treatment

Herbal treatments for dermatitis

Some herbal therapies can be useful for skin conditions. Among the herbs most often recommended are:

• burdock root (*Arctium lappa*)
• calendula (*Calendula officinalis*) ointment
• chamomile (*Matricaria recutita*) ointment
• cleavers (*Galium* ssp.)
• evening primrose oil (*Oenothera biennis*)
• nettles (*Urtica dioica*)

Treatments for contact dermatitis

Contact dermatitis can be treated botanically and homeopathically. Specific homeopathic remedies are designed for individuals. Grindelia (*Grindelia* spp.) and **sassafras** (*Sassafras albidum*) can help when applied topically. Determining the source of the problem and eliminating it is essential. Oatmeal baths are very helpful in relieving the itch. Bentonite clay packs or any mud pack draws the fluid and helps dry up the lesions. Cortisone creams are not recommended by practitioners of natural medicine as they suppress the reaction rather than clear it.

Treatments for atopic dermatitis

NUTRITIONAL THERAPY. Because most cases of atopic dermatitis are caused by food allergy, the following dietary changes are often recommended:

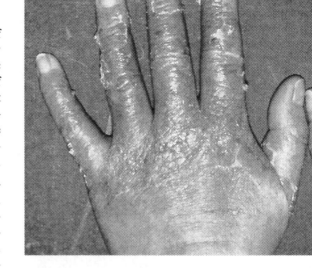

Dermatitis on hands and fingers. *(Custom Medical Stock Photo. Reproduced by permission.)*

• Identification and avoidance of allergenic foods. Foods that often cause allergy in infants include milk, eggs, peanuts, tomatoes, seafoods, wheat, and soybean.

• Supplementing daily diet with **vitamin A** (5,000 U), **vitamin E** (400 IU) and **zinc** (45-60 mg) or alternatively, taking multivitamin-and-mineral supplement one tablet once daily.

• Taking fish oils supplements. Adults should take 540 mg of EPA and 360 mg of DHA per day.

Additionally, flavonoids such as quercetin, grapeseed extract and **green tea** extract, and **ginkgo biloba** may be helpful for some people.

HERBAL THERAPY. The following herbal preparations may be helpful:

• *Glycyrrhiza glabra* (licorice)
• *Arctium lappa* (burdock, gobo)
• *Taraxacum officinale* (dandelion)

Treatments for seborrheic dermatitis

Treatments for this common skin disorder include topical applications and nutritional therapy.

NUTRITIONAL THERAPY. Diet is one of the major causes of seborrheic dermatitis especially in infants. Therefore, the following dietary changes and nutritional supplements are often necessary:

- Identification and avoidance of foods that may cause allergies. Common allergenic foods in infants are wheat, corn, citrus, peanuts, eggs and seafoods.

- Eating biotin-rich foods (soy foods, sesame, barley) or taking biotin supplements. Seborrheic dermatitis may be caused by biotin deficiency. Infants often respond well to biotin treatment alone (without vitamin B-complex supplementation).

- Taking daily multivitamin and mineral supplement which provides high amounts of vitamin B-complex, especially vitamin B_6, and zinc. Seborrheic adults often require both vitamin B-complex and biotin supplements.

- One tablespoon per day (for adults). **Flaxseed** oil is a good source of **omega-3 fatty acids** that help moisturize the skin and decrease inflammation.

TOPICAL TREATMENT. Selenium-based shampoos are often used to treat greasy scales and crusts on the scalp. Some adults with seborrheic scales on the scalp, nose, brow around the mouth respond well to topical treatment with **pyridoxine** (50 mg/g) ointment.

Stasis dermatitis

Stasis dermatitis should be treated by a trained practitioner. This condition responds well to topical herbal therapies, however, the cause must also be addressed.

Allopathic treatment

Treating contact dermatitis begins with eliminating or avoiding the source of irritation. Prescription or over-the-counter corticosteroid creams can lessen inflammation and relieve irritation. Creams, lotions, or ointments not specifically formulated for dermatitis can intensify the irritation. Oral antihistamines are sometimes recommended to alleviate itching, and antibiotics are prescribed if the rash becomes infected. Medications taken by mouth to relieve symptoms of dermatitis can make skin red and scaly and cause **hair loss**.

Patients who have a history of dermatitis should remove their rings before washing their hands. They should use bath oils or glycerine-based soaps and bathe in lukewarm saltwater.

Patting rather than rubbing the skin after bathing and thoroughly massaging lubricating lotion or nonprescription cortisone creams into still-damp skin can soothe red, weepy nummular dermatitis. Highly concentrated cortisone preparations should not be applied to the face, armpits, groin, or rectal area.

Coal-tar salves can help relieve symptoms of nummular dermatitis that have not responded to other treatments, but these ointments have an unpleasant odor and stain clothing.

Patients who have stasis dermatitis should elevate their legs as often as possible and sleep with a pillow between the lower legs.

Tar or zinc paste may also be used to treat stasis dermatitis. Because these compounds must remain in contact with the rash for as long as two weeks, the paste and bandages must be applied by a nurse or a doctor.

Coal-tar shampoos may be used for seborrheic dermatitis that occurs on the scalp. Sun exposure after the use of these shampoos should be avoided because the risk of sunburn of the scalp is increased.

Expected results

Dermatitis is often chronic, but symptoms can generally be controlled.

Prevention

Contact dermatitis can be prevented by avoiding the source of irritation. If the irritant cannot be avoided completely, the patient should wear gloves and other protective clothing whenever exposure is likely to occur.

Immediately washing the exposed area with soap and water can stem allergic reactions to poison ivy, poison oak, or poison sumac, but because soaps can dry the skin, patients susceptible to dermatitis should use them only on the face, feet, genitals and underarms.

Clothing should be loose fitting and 100% cotton. New clothing should be washed in dye-free, unscented detergent before being worn.

Injury to the lower leg can cause stasis dermatitis to ulcerate (form open sores). If stasis ulcers develop, a doctor should be notified immediately.

Yoga and other **relaxation** techniques may help prevent atopic dermatitis caused by stress.

Avoidance of sweating may aid in preventing seborrheic dermatitis.

A patient who has dermatitis should also notify a doctor if any of the following occurs:

- Fever develops

- Skin oozes or other signs of infection appear

- Symptoms do not begin to subside after seven days treatment

- Contact with someone who has a wart, **cold sore**, or other viral skin infection

KEY TERMS

· ·

Allergic reaction—An inappropriate or exaggerated genetically determined reaction to a chemical that occurs only on the second or subsequent exposures to the offending agent, after the first contact has sensitized the body.

Corticosteroid—A group of synthetic hormones that are used to prevent or reduce inflammation. Toxic effects may result from rapid withdrawal after prolonged use or from continued use of large doses.

Patch test—A skin test that is done to identify allergens. A suspected substance is applied to the skin. After 24–48 hours, if the area is red and swollen, the test is positive for that substance.

Rash—A spotted, pink or red skin eruption that may be accompanied by itching and is caused by disease, contact with an allergen, food ingestion, or drug reaction.

Ulcer—An open sore on the skin, resulting from tissue destruction, that is usually accompanied by redness, pain, or infection.

Resources

BOOKS

Editors of Time-Life Books. *The Medical Advisor: The Complete Guide to Conventional and Alternative Treatments.* Alexandria, VA: Time-Life, Inc., 1996.

Gottlieb, B., ed. *New Choices in Natural Healing.* Emmaus, PA: Rodale Press, Inc.,1995.

Murray, Michael T. and Joseph E. Pizzorno. "Seborrheic Dermatitis." In *Encyclopedia of Natural Medicine.* Rev. 2nd ed. Rocklin, CA: Prima Publishing, 1998.

Murray, Michael T. and Joseph E. Pizzorno. "Eczema (Atopic Dermatitis)." *Encyclopedia of Natural Medicine.* Rev. 2nd ed. Rocklin, CA: Prima Publishing, 1998.

OTHER

Allergic Contact Dermatitis. http://www.skinsite.com/info_allergic.htm. (10 April 1998).

Dermatitis, Contact. http://www.thriveonline.com.health/Library/illsymp/illness162.html. (10 April 1998).

Nummular Dermatitis. http://www.skinsite.com/info_nummular_dermatitis.htm. (7 April 1998).

Poison ivy, oak, sumac. http://www.thriveonline.com/health/Library/illsymp/illness413.html. (10 April 1998).

Stasis Dermatitis. http://www.skinsite.com/info_stasis_dermatitis.htm. (7 April 1998).

Mai Tran

Detoxification

Definition

Detoxification is one of the more widely used treatments and concepts in alternative medicine. It is based on the principle that illnesses can be caused by the accumulation of toxic substances (toxins) in the body. Eliminating existing toxins and avoiding new toxins are essential parts of the healing process. Detoxification utilizes a variety of tests and techniques.

Origins

Detoxification methods of healing have been used for thousands of years. **Fasting**, a method used often in detoxification treatments, is one of the oldest therapeutic practices in medicine. Hippocrates, the ancient Greek known as the father of Western medicine, recommended fasting as a means for improving health. **Ayurvedic medicine**, a traditional healing system that has developed over thousands of years, utilizes detoxification methods to treat many chronic conditions and to prevent illness.

Detoxification treatment has become one of the cornerstones of alternative medicine. Conventional medicine notes that environmental factors can play a significant role in many illnesses. Environmental medicine is a field that studies exactly how those environmental factors influence disease. Conditions such as **asthma, cancer, chronic fatigue syndrome, multiple chemical sensitivity**, and many others are strongly influenced by exposure to toxic or allergenic substances in the environment. The United States Centers for Disease Control estimate that over 80% of all illnesses have environmental and lifestyle causes.

Detoxification has also become a prominent treatment as people have become more aware of environmental pollution. It is estimated that one in every four Americans suffers from some level of **heavy metal poisoning**. Heavy metals, such as lead, mercury, cadmium, and arsenic, are by-products of industry. Synthetic agriculture chemicals, many of which are known to cause health problems, are also found in food, air, and water. American agriculture uses nearly 10 pounds of pesticides per person on the food supply each year. These toxins have become almost unavoidable. Pesticides that are used only on crops in the southern United States have been found in the tissue of animals in the far north of Canada. DDT, a cancer-causing insecticide that has been banned for decades, is still regularly found in the fatty tissue of animals, birds, and fish, even in extremely remote regions such as the North Pole.

The problem of toxins in the environment is compounded because humans are at the top of the food chain

COMMON HERBS USED FOR DETOXIFICATION

Antibiotics	Anticatarrhals (Help Eliminate Mucus)	Blood Cleansers
Clove	Boneset	Burdock root
Echinacea	Echinacea	Dandelion root
Eucalyptus	Garlic	Echinacea
Garlic	Goldenseal root	Oregon grape root
Myrrh	Hyssop	Red clover blossoms
Prickly ash bark	Sage	Yellow dock root
Propolis	Yarrow	
Wormwood		

Diaphoretics/Skin Cleaners	Diuretics	Laxatives
Boneset	Cleavers	Buckthorn
Burdock root	Corn silk	Cascara sagrada
Cayenne pepper	Horsetail	Dandelion root
Elder flowers	Juniper berries	Licorice root
Ginger root	Parsley leaf	Rhubarb root
Goldenseal root	Uva ursi	Senna leaf
Peppermint	Yarrow dock	Yellow dock
Oregon grape root		
Yellow dock		

Common herbs used for detoxification. *(Stanley Publishing. Reproduced by permission.)*

and are more likely to be exposed to an accumulation of toxic substances in the food supply. For instance, pesticides and herbicides are sprayed on grains that are then fed to farm animals. Toxic substances are stored in the fatty tissue of those animals. In addition, those animals are often injected with synthetic hormones, antibiotics, and other chemicals. When people eat meat products, they are exposed to the full range of chemicals and additives used along the entire agricultural chain. Detoxification specialists call this build up of toxins *bioaccumulation*. They assert that the bioaccumulation of toxic substances over time is responsible for many physical and mental disorders, especially ones that are increasing rapidly (like asthma, cancer, and mental illness). As a result, detoxification therapies are increasing in importance and popularity.

Benefits

Detoxification is helpful for those patients suffering from many chronic diseases and conditions, including **allergies**, **anxiety**, arthritis, asthma, chronic **infections**, **depression**, diabetes, headaches, **heart disease**, high **cholesterol**, low blood sugar levels, digestive disorders, mental illness, and **obesity**. It is helpful for those with conditions that are influenced by environmental factors, such as cancer, as well as for those who have been exposed to high levels of toxic materials due to accident or occupation. Detoxification therapy is useful for those suffering from allergies or immune system problems that conventional medicine is unable to diagnose or treat, including chronic **fatigue** syndrome, environmental illness/multiple chemical sensitivity, and **fibromyalgia**. Symptoms for those suffering these conditions may include unexplained fatigue, increased allergies, hypersensitivity to common materials, intolerance to certain foods and **indigestion**, aches and pains, low grade **fever**, headaches, **insomnia**, depression, sore throats, sudden weight loss or gain, lowered resistance to infection, general malaise, and disability. Detoxification can be used as a beneficial preventative measure and as a tool to increase overall health, vitality, and resistance to disease.

Description

Toxins in the body include heavy metals and various chemicals such as pesticides, pollutants, and food additives. Drugs and alcohol have toxic effects in the body. Toxins are produced as normal by-products in the intestines by the bacteria that break down food. The digestion of protein also creates toxic by-products in the body.

The body has natural methods of detoxification. Individual cells get detoxified in the lymph and circulatory systems. The liver is the principle organ of detoxification, assisted by the kidneys and intestines. Toxins can be excreted from the body by the kidneys, bowels, skin, and lungs. Detoxification treatments become necessary when the body's natural detoxification systems become overwhelmed. This can be caused by long-term effects of improper diet, **stress**, overeating, sedentary lifestyles, illness, and poor health habits in general. When a build up of toxic substances in the body creates illness, it's called toxemia. Some people's digestive tracts become unable to digest food properly, due to years of overeating and **diets** that are high in fat and processed foods and low in fiber (the average American diet). When this happens, food cannot pass through the digestive tract efficiently. Instead of being digested properly or eliminated from the bowel, food can literally rot inside the digestive tract and produce toxic by-products. This state is known as toxic colon syndrome or intestinal toxemia.

Detoxification therapies try to activate and assist the body's own detoxification processes. They also try to eliminate additional exposure to toxins and to strengthen the body and immune system so that toxic imbalances won't occur in the future.

Testing for toxic substances

Detoxification specialists use a variety of tests to determine the causes contributing to toxic conditions. These causes include infections, allergies, addictions, toxic chemicals, and digestive and organ dysfunction. Blood, urine, stool, and hair analyses, as well as allergy tests, are used to measure a variety of bodily functions that may indicate problems. Detoxification therapists usually have access to laboratories that specialize in sophisticated diagnostic tests for toxic conditions.

People who have toxemia are often susceptible to infection because their immune systems are weakened. Infections can be caused by parasites, bacteria, viruses, and a common yeast. Therapists will screen patients for underlying infections that may be contributing to illness.

Liver function is studied closely with blood and urine tests because the liver is the principle organ in the body responsible for removing toxic compounds. When the liver detoxifies a substance from the body, it does so in two phases. Tests are performed that indicate where problems may be occurring in these phases, which may point to specific types of toxins. Blood and urine tests can also be completed that screen for toxic chemicals such as PCBs (environmental poisons), formaldehyde (a common preservative), pesticides, and heavy metals. Another useful blood test is a test for **zinc** deficiency, which may reveal heavy metal poisoning. Hair analysis is used to test for heavy metal levels in the body. Blood and urine tests check immune system activity, and hormone levels can also indicate specific toxic compounds. A 24-hour urine analysis, where samples are taken around the clock, allows therapists to determine the efficiency of the digestive tract and kidneys. Together with stool analysis, these tests may indicate toxic bowel syndrome and digestive system disorders. Certain blood and urine tests may point to nutritional deficiencies and proper recovery diets can be designed for patients as well.

Detoxification therapists may also perform extensive allergy and hypersensitivity tests. Intradermal (between layers of the skin) and sublingual (under the tongue) allergy tests are used to determine a patient's sensitivity to a variety of common substances, including formaldehyde, auto exhaust, perfume, tobacco, chlorine, jet fuel, and other chemicals.

Food allergies require additional tests because these allergies often cause reactions that are delayed for several days after the food is eaten. The RAST (radioallergosorbent test) is a blood test that determines the level of antibodies (immunoglobulins) in the blood after specific foods are eaten. The cytotoxic test is a blood test that determines if certain substances affect blood cells, including foods and chemicals. The ELISA-ACT (enzyme-linked immunoserological assay activated cell test) is considered to be one of the most accurate tests for allergies and hypersensitivity to foods, chemicals, and other agents. Other tests for food allergies are the elimination and rotation diets, in which foods are systematically evaluated to determine the ones that are causing problems.

Detoxification therapists usually interview and counsel patients closely to determine and correct lifestyle, occupational, psychological, and emotional factors that may also be contributing to illness.

Detoxification therapies

Detoxification therapists use a variety of healing techniques after a diagnosis is made. The first step is to eliminate a patient's exposure to all toxic or allergenic substances. These include heavy metals, chemicals, radiation (from x rays, power lines, cell phones, computer screens, and microwaves), smog, polluted water, foods, drugs, **caffeine**, alcohol, perfume, excess noise, and stress. If mercury poisoning has been determined, the patient will be advised to have mercury fillings from the teeth removed, preferably by a holistic dentist.

Specific treatments are used to stimulate and assist the body's detoxification process. Dietary change is immediately enacted, eliminating allergic and unhealthy foods, and emphasizing foods that assist detoxification and support healing. Detoxification diets are generally low in fat, high in fiber, and vegetarian with a raw food emphasis. Processed foods, alcohol, and caffeine are avoided. Nutritional supplements such as vitamins, minerals, **antioxidants**, **amino acids**, and **essential fatty acids** are often prescribed. **Spirulina** is a sea algae that is frequently given to assist in eliminating heavy metals. Lipotropic agents are certain vitamins and nutrients that promote the flow of bile and fat from the liver.

Many herbal supplements are used in detoxification therapies as well. **Milk thistle** extract, called silymarin, is one of the more potent herbs for detoxifying the liver. Naturopathy, Ayurvedic medicine, and **traditional Chinese medicine** (TCM) recommend numerous herbal formulas for detoxification and immune strengthening. If infections or parasites have been found, these are treated with herbal formulas and antibiotics in difficult cases.

For toxic bowel syndrome and digestive tract disorders, herbal laxatives and high fiber foods such as **psyllium** seeds may be given to cleanse the digestive tract and promote elimination. Colonics are used to cleanse the lower intestines. **Digestive enzymes** are prescribed to improve digestion, and **acidophilus** and other friendly bacteria are reintroduced into the system with nutritional supplements.

Fasting is another major therapy in detoxification. Fasting is one of the quickest ways to promote the elimination of stored toxins in the body and to prompt the healing process. People with severe toxic conditions are supervised closely during fasting because the number of toxins in the body temporarily increases as they are being released.

Chelation therapy is used by detoxification specialists to rid the body of heavy metals. Chelates are particular substances that bind to heavy metals and speed their elimination. In 2002, a new five-year clinical trial was funded to explore the use of chelation therapy in patients with heart disease. Homeopathic remedies have also been shown to be effective for removing heavy metals.

Sweating therapies can also detoxify the body because the skin is a major organ of elimination. Sweating helps release those toxins that are stored in the subcutaneous (under the skin) fat cells. Saunas, therapeutic baths, and **exercise** are some of these treatments. Body therapies may also be prescribed, including **massage therapy**, **acupressure**, **shiatsu**, manual lymph drainage, and **polarity therapy**. These body therapies seek to improve circulatory and structural problems, reduce stress, and promote healing responses in the body. Mind/body therapies such as **psychotherapy**, counseling, and stress management techniques may be used to heal the psychological components of illness and to help patients overcome their negative patterns contributing to illness.

Practitioners and treatment costs

The costs of detoxification therapies can vary widely, depending on the number of tests and treatments required. Detoxification treatments can be lengthy and involved since illnesses associated with toxic conditions usually develop over many years and may not clear up quickly. Detoxification treatments may be lengthy because they often strive for the holistic healing of the body, mind, and emotions.

Practitioners may be conventionally trained medical doctors with specialties in environmental medicine or interests in alternative treatment. The majority of detoxification therapists are alternative practitioners, such as naturopaths, homeopaths, ayurvedic doctors, or traditional Chinese doctors. Insurance coverage varies, depending on the practitioner and the treatment involved. Consumers should review their individual insurance policies regarding treatment coverage.

Preparations

Patients can assist diagnosis and treatment by keeping detailed diaries of their activities, symptoms, and contact with environmental factors that may be affecting their health. Reducing exposure to environmental toxins and making immediate dietary and lifestyle changes may speed the detoxification process.

Side effects

During the detoxification process, patients may experience side effects of fatigue, malaise, aches and pains, emotional duress, **acne**, headaches, allergies, and symptoms of colds and flu. Detoxification specialists claim that these negative side effects are part of the healing process. These reactions are sometimes called *healing crises*, which are caused by temporarily increased levels of toxins in the body due to elimination and cleansing.

Research & general acceptance

Although environmental medicine is gaining more respect within conventional medicine, detoxification

KEY TERMS

Allergen—A foreign substance, such as mites in house dust or animal dander that, when inhaled, causes the airways to narrow and produces symptoms of asthma.

Antibody—A protein, also called immunoglobulin, produced by immune system cells to remove antigens (the foreign substances that trigger the immune response).

Fibromyalgia—A condition of debilitating pain, among other symptoms, in the muscles and the myofascia (the thin connective tissue that surrounds muscles, bones, and organs).

Hypersensitivity—The state where even a tiny amount of allergen can cause severe allergic reactions.

Multiple chemical sensitivity—A condition characterized by severe and crippling allergic reactions to commonly used substances, particularly chemicals. Also called environmental illness.

treatment is scarcely mentioned by the medical establishment. The research that exists on detoxification is largely testimonial, consisting of individual personal accounts of healing without statistics or controlled scientific experiments. In the alternative medical community, detoxification is an essential and widely accepted treatment for many illnesses and chronic conditions.

Resources

BOOKS

Goldberg, Burton. *Chronic Fatigue, Fibromyalgia and Environmental Illness*. Tiburon, CA: Future Medicine, 1998.

Lappe, Marc. *Chemical Deception: The Toxic Threat to Health and the Environment*. San Francisco: Sierra Club, 1991.

Lawson, Lynn. *Staying Well in a Toxic World*. Chicago: Noble, 1993.

Randolph, Theron G., M.D. *Environmental Medicine: Beginnings and Bibliographies of Clinical Ecology*. Fort Collins, CO: Clinical Ecology Publications, 1987.

PERIODICALS

Alternative Therapies Magazine. P.O. Box 17969, Durham, NC 27715. (919) 668-8825. www.alternative-therapies.com.

Journal of Occupational and Environmental Medicine. 1114 N. Arlington Heights Rd., Arlington Heights, IL 60004. (847) 818-1800.

"Physician Group Backs New NIH Chelation Therapy Study for Heart Disease." *Heart Disease Weekly* (September 29, 2002): 13.

ORGANIZATIONS

American Holistic Medical Association. 4101 Lake Boone Trail, Suite 201, Raleigh, NC 27607.

Cancer Prevention Coalition. 2121 West Taylor St., Chicago, IL 60612. (312) 996-2297. http:\\www.preventcancer.com.

Center for Occupational and Environmental Medicine.7510 Northforest Dr., North Charleston, SC 29420. (843) 572-1600. http:\\www.coem.com.

Northeast Center for Environmental Medicine. P.O. Box 2716, Syracuse, NY 13220. (800) 846-ONUS.

Northwest Center for Environmental Medicine. 177 NE 102nd St., Portland, OR 97220. (503) 561-0966.

OTHER

A Citizens Toxic Waste Manual. Greenpeace USA, 1436 U St. NW, Washington, DC 20009. (202) 462-1177.

Douglas Dupler
Teresa G. Odle

Devil's claw

Description

Devil's claw (*Harpagophytum procumbens*) is an African plant whose fruit looks like a giant claw. The plant grows in an arid climate and is found in Namibia, Madagascar, the Kalahari Desert, and other areas on the African continent. The tuberous roots are used in traditional medicine. The root is collected when the rainy season ends. The root is chopped and dried in the sun for three days. Devil's claw is also known as grapple plant and wood spider.

General use

Devil's claw has been used for numerous conditions in several areas of the world. In South Africa, the root and tuber have been used for centuries as an all-purpose folk remedy. Devil's claw has been used to reduce **fever** and **pain**, to treat **allergies** and **headache**, and to stimulate digestion. Traditional healers also used devil's claw to treat inflammatory conditions such as arthritis, rheumatism, and lower back pain. Devil's claw has also been used as a remedy for liver and kidney disorders.

Devil's claw root was also used in folk medicine as a pain reliever and for complications with pregnancies. In addition, an ointment made from devil's claw was used for skin injuries and disorders.

European colonists brought the African plant back to their continent where it was used to treat arthritis. In the United States, use of devil's claw dates back to the time of slavery. The slaves brought herbs and herbal knowledge with them to the new continent.

Devil's claw has been used as an herbal remedy in Europe for a long time. Current uses for devil's claw are much the same as they were centuries ago. In Europe, the herb is still a remedy for arthritis and other types of joint pain, such as **rheumatoid arthritis**, **osteoarthritis**, and **gout** (a painful joint inflammation disease).

Devil's claw is also used for soft tissue conditions with inflammation, like **tendinitis** and **bursitis**. The bitter herb is also used as a remedy for loss of appetite and mildly upset stomach.

The herb is currently used for other conditions such as problems with **pregnancy**, **menstruation**, and **menopause**. Devil's claw is also regarded as a remedy for headaches, **heartburn**, liver and gallbladder problems, allergies, skin disorders, and nicotine poisoning.

European research during the late 1990s indicated that devil's claw relieved arthritis and joint pain conditions. The herb also helped with soft muscle pain such as tendinitis. However, there is no evidence that proves devil's claw is an effective remedy for other conditions such as difficulties during pregnancy and skin disorders.

Preparations

Several forms of devil's claw are used. In Europe, doctors treat some conditions like arthritis with an injection of devil's claw extract. The herb is taken internally as a tea or in capsule form. When taken for pain relief, devil's claw must be taken regularly for up to one month before results are seen. An ointment form of devil's claw can be applied to the skin to treat **wounds** or scars.

Herbal tea and tincture

Devil's claw tea is prepared by pouring 1.25 cups (300 ml) boiling water over 1 tsp (4.5 g) of the herb. The mixture, which is also called an infusion, is steeped for eight hours and then strained. The daily dosage is 3 cups of warm tea.

For most conditions, the average daily dosage is 1 tsp (4.5 g) of devil's claw herb. However, the amount is reduced to 1/3 tsp (1.5 g) when devil's claw is taken for appetite loss.

In a tincture, the herb is preserved with alcohol. The tincture steeps for two weeks and is shaken daily. It is then strained and bottled. When devil's claw tincture is used as a remedy, the dosage is 1 tsp (4.5 g) taken three times per day for a specified period.

Tea and tincture should be consumed 30 minutes before eating. This allows for better absorption of the herb.

Devil's claw capsules

The anti-inflammatory properties of devil's claw are attributed to two constituents, harpagoside and beta sitoserol. If a person takes devil's claw capsules or tablets as a remedy, attention should be paid to the harpagoside content. The daily amount of harpagoside in capsules should total 50 mg.

Combinations

For arthritis treatment, devil's claw can be combined with anti-inflammatory or cleansing herbs. In addition, devil's claw can be combined with bogbean or meadowsweet. An herbalist, naturopathic doctor, or traditional healer can provide more information on herb combinations appropriate for a specific condition.

Precautions

Devil's claw is safe to use when proper dosage recommendations are followed, according to sources including the *PDR (Physician's Desk Reference) for Herbal Medicines*, the 1998 book based on the 1997 findings of Germany's Commission E.

Although devil's claw has not undergone the FDA research required for approval as a remedy, other studies in Europe confirm that devil's claw is safe for most people. However, people with ulcers should be cautious because the herb stimulates the production of stomach acid.

Furthermore, it is not known if devil's claw is safe for people with major liver or kidney conditions. In addition, devil's claw could cause an allergic reaction.

There is some debate in the alternative medicine community about whether pregnant women can use devil's claw as a remedy. Some researchers say that the herb is safe to use; others say that not enough research has been done to prove that the herb is safe for pregnant women. There appears to be no scientific proof that using devil's claw could result in miscarriages.

Side effects

Devil's claw could cause an allergic reaction or mild gastrointestinal difficulties.

Interactions

No interactions between other medications and devil's claw have been reported according to the *PDR for Herbal Medicines*. However, the herb may possibly block the effect of medication taken to correct abnormal heart rhythms.

Resources

BOOKS

Duke, James A. *The Green Pharmacy.* Emmaus, PA: Rodale Press, Inc., 1997.

Gottlieb, Bill. *New Choices in Natural Healing.* Emmaus, PA: Rodale Press, Inc., 1995.

Keville, Kathi. *Herbs for Health and Healing.* Emmaus, PA: Rodale Press, Inc., 1996.

PDR for Herbal Medicines. Montvale, NJ: Medical Economics Company, 1998.

Ritchason, Jack. *The Little Herb Encyclopedia.* Pleasant Grove, UT: Woodland Health Books, 1995.

Squier, Thomas Broken Bear, with Lauren David Peden. *Herbal Folk Medicine.* New York: Henry Holt and Company, 1997.

Tyler, Varro, and Steven Foster. *Tyler's Honest Herbal.* Binghamton, NY: The Haworth Herbal Press, 1999.

ORGANIZATIONS

American Botanical Council. PO Box 201660, Austin TX, 78720. (512) 331-8868. www.herbalgram.org/.

Arthritis Foundation. 1330 W. Peachtree St., Atlanta, GA 30309. http://www.arthritis.org.

Herb Research Foundation. 1007 Pearl St., Suite 200, Boulder, CO 80302. (303) 449-2265. http://www.herbs.org.

Liz Swain

DGL *see* **Deglycyrrhizanated licorice**

DHEA

Description

DHEA is the acronym for dehydroepiandrosterone, a hormone produced naturally from **cholesterol** in the adrenal glands of males and females. It is a precursor to the male sex hormone testosterone. It is also sold as an over-the-counter dietary supplement.

The human body produces very little DHEA until about the age of seven, when production soars. It peaks in the mid-20s and starts to decline in the early 30s. By the mid-70s, DHEA production has dropped by about 80-90%. At all ages, DHEA levels are slightly higher in men than women. The optimum DHEA level in a healthy adult is 750-1,250 milligrams per deciliter of blood (mg/dL) for men and 550-980 mg/dL for women.

DHEA was first identified in 1934 and was sold over the counter mainly as a weight loss aid until the late 1980s. Then the federal Food and Drug Administration (FDA) classified DHEA as a drug, making it available by prescription only. The FDA reversed itself in 1994, re-classifying DHEA as a dietary supplement obtainable without a prescription.

A 1994 study by researchers at the University of California, San Diego looked at 30 middle-age men and women who took 50 mg of DHEA a day for three months. The test subjects generally reported an improved sense of well-being, increased energy, enhanced sex drive, and an improved ability to deal with **stress**. The results were widely reported by the mass media, with several referring to DHEA as the "fountain of youth hormone."

Despite hundreds of studies of DHEA over the past three decades, researchers are still unclear on how the hormone works or exactly what it does in the body. Although it is know DHEA decreases with age, it is not known whether this constitutes a deficiency or is because the body needs less DHEA as it ages.

The main reason so little is known about DHEA is because the hormone is not patentable, so drug companies are unwilling to spend money doing further research on it. Much of the research today in funded through universities and the National Institute on Aging that maintains a skeptical philosophy about DHEA supplementation.

General use

Originally marketed as a weight loss supplement, DHEA is now promoted as being beneficial for treating a wide variety of medical conditions, including **cancer**, **heart disease**, Alzheimer's, and **AIDS**. It is also purported to have anti-aging qualities. Studies in rodents and test tubes have shown daily doses of DHEA can prevent or benefit such conditions as cancer, heart disease, **osteoporosis**, diabetes, lupus, **obesity**, and viral **infections**. Far fewer long-term studies have been done in humans and the results are often conflicting. In general, DHEA supplementation seems to be more beneficial to men than women.

Proponents of DHEA also say the hormone has anti-aging properties that can slow the aging process and lead to longer life. In his book, *The DHEA Breakthrough: Look Younger, Live Longer, Feel Better,* biochemist Stephen Cherniske, states that DHEA supplementation along with proper diet, vitamins, and **exercise**, can prolong life. "After all, the human body is designed to last about 120 years, and with proper care they can all be vibrantly healthy years. What DHEA provides is the missing link in your longevity program. It gives you a better-than-fighting chance against the diseases that cause more than 75 percent of premature deaths."

Preparations

Most DHEA is derived from Mexican wild yams through a chemical process. Eating the yams will not produce the hormone. DHEA is generally taken once daily. Dosage recommendations vary. Allopathic physicians who support DHEA supplementation usually recommend 5-10 milligrams (mg) once a day. Some homeopathic health practitioners recommend 10-50 mg a day. Dr. Ray Sahelian, a physician and author of several books on dietary supplements, also recommends "hormone holidays." With this approach, persons would take DHEA every other day, five days in a row and two days off, or go off it one or two weeks a month. DHEA commonly is sold in tablets of 5mg, 10mg, 25mg, and 50mg. It also comes in available as a cream, ointment, lozenge, and herbal tea. A bottle of 90 25-mg capsules costs $12-24.

Precautions

Several studies have shown DHEA may increase the risks of **prostate cancer** in men and endometrial cancer in women. Medical experts suggest before taking DHEA supplements, individuals should have a blood test to determine existing DHEA and other hormone (testosterone or estrogen) levels. Also, men taking the supplement should have regular PSA tests and women should have periodic mammograms since DHEA may promote the growth of **breast cancer**.

There are several warnings associated with DHEA use. It should not be taken by men who have a history of prostate problems or by women with a history of breast, ovarian, or **uterine cancer**. It is not recommended for anyone under age 40, or by women who are pregnant, nursing, or who can still bear children. Women who are taking an estrogen replacement, who have a history of heart disease, and anyone with other significant health problems should consult their doctor before taking DHEA.

Side effects

Some side effects have been reported and are usually associated with doses of 5 mg a day or more. These include **acne**, body and facial hair growth in women, enlarged breasts in men, scalp **hair loss**, **anxiety**, **insomnia**, headaches, mood changes, and **fatigue**. It can cause menstrual irregularities in women under age 50, and may decrease HDL (good cholesterol) in women. A few cases of irregular heart rhythm have been reported in people taking 25-50 mg a day of DHEA.

Interactions

DHEA functions similarly to pregnenolone, so the two should not be taken together in full doses.

KEY TERMS

Adrenal glands—A pair of endocrine organs near the kidneys that produce steroids such as sex hormones, hormones associated with metabolic functions, and epinephrine.

Cholesterol—A fatty substance manufactured in the liver and carried throughout the body in the bloodstream.

Endometrial—Pertaining to the endometrium, a mucous membrane lining the uterus.

Estrogen—A hormone that stimulates development of female secondary sex characteristics.

Lupus—A group of diseases characterized by skin lesions.

Osteoporosis—A condition or disease characterized by high density and fragility of the bones.

Pregnenolone—A steroid ketone formed by the oxidation of other steroids, such as cholesterol, and is a precursor to the hormone progesterone.

PSA test—A blood test to determine prostate specific antigen levels in men, which can help determine the risk for prostate cancer.

Testosterone—A male hormone produced in the testes or made synthetically that is responsible for male secondary sex characteristics.

Resources

BOOKS

Cherniske, Stephen A. *The DHEA Breakthrough: Look Younger, Live Longer, Feel Better.* New York: Ballantine Books, 1998.

Greenberg, Beverly. *DHEA Discovery: Wonder Hormone of the '90s.* Los Angeles: Majesty Press, 1997.

Ley, Beth M. *DHEA: Unlocking the Secrets to the Fountain of Youth.* Newport Beach, CA: BL Publications, 1997.

Moore, Neecie. *Bountiful Health, Boundless Energy, Brilliant Youth: The Facts About DHEA.* Seattle: Validation Press. 2000.

Sahelian, Ray. *All About DHEA: Frequently Asked Questions.* New York: Avery Publishing Group, 1999.

Watson, Ronald Ross, ed. *Health Promotion and Aging: Dehydroepiandrosterone (DHEA).* Newark, NJ: Harwood Academic Publishing, 1999.

PERIODICALS

Firshein, Richard. "On the DHEA Watch." *Psychology Today* (November/December 1998): 24.

Marandino, Cristin. "Is Time Running Out for Longevity Supplements?" *Vegetarian Times* (October 1997): 20-21.

Miller, Richard A. "Lifelong Treatment With Oral DHEA Does Not Preserve Immune Function, Prevent Disease, or Im-

---

prove Survival in Genetically Heterogeneous Mice." *The Journal of the American Medical Association* (October 6, 1999): 1,212.

Russell, Dr. Robert. "Should You Start Taking Over-the-Counter Hormones? A Closer Look at DHEA and Melatonin." *Tufts University Health & Nutrition Newsletter* (July 1997): 4-5.

Sadovsky, Richard. "Dehydroepiandrosterone Replacement in Older Patients." *American Family Physician* (October 1, 1999): 1,538.

Sahalian, Ray. "DHEA & Other Hormones .. An Update." *Better Nutrition* (March 1999): 66.

Sahalian, Ray. "DHEA: The Promise of Hormones." *Better Nutrition* (May 1998): 58-61.

Silberman, Alex. "Forever Young?" *Vegetarian Times* (February 2000): 66.

OTHER

"Should I Take DHEA?" drkoop.com. http://www.drkoop.com/news/sports/news/stories/dhea.html. (2000).

Ken R. Wells

Diabetes mellitus

Definition

Diabetes mellitus is a condition in which the pancreas no longer produces enough insulin or when cells stop responding to the insulin that is produced, so that glucose in the blood cannot be absorbed into the cells of the body. Symptoms include frequent urination, tiredness, excessive thirst, and hunger.

Description

Diabetes mellitus is a chronic disease that causes serious health complications including renal (kidney) failure, **heart disease**, **stroke**, and blindness. Approximately 14 million Americans (about 5% of the population) have diabetes. Unfortunately, as many as one-half of them are unaware that they have it.

Background

Every cell in the human body needs energy in order to function. The body's primary energy source is glucose, a simple sugar resulting from the digestion of foods containing carbohydrates (sugars and starches). Glucose from the digested food circulates in the blood as a ready energy source for cells. Insulin is a hormone or chemical produced by cells in the pancreas, an organ located behind the stomach. Insulin binds to receptor sites on the outside of cells and acts like a key to open a door-

SYMPTOMS OF DIABETES MELLITUS
Excessive thirst
Increased appetite
Increased urination
Weight loss
Fatigue
Nausea
Blurred vision
Frequent vaginal infections in women
Impotence in men
Frequent yeast infections

way into the cell through which glucose can enter. Some of the glucose can be converted to concentrated energy sources like glycogen or fatty acids and saved for later use. When there is not enough insulin produced or when the doorway no longer recognizes the insulin key, glucose stays in the blood instead of entering the cells.

The body will attempt to dilute the high level of glucose in the blood, a condition called hyperglycemia, by drawing water out of the cells and into the bloodstream. The excess sugar is excreted in the urine. It is not unusual for people with undiagnosed diabetes to be constantly thirsty, to drink large quantities of water, and to urinate frequently as their bodies try to get rid of the extra glucose. This creates high levels of glucose in the urine.

At the same time that the body is trying to get rid of glucose from the blood, the cells are starving for glucose and sending signals to the body to eat more food, thus making patients extremely hungry. To provide energy for the starving cells, the body also tries to convert fats and proteins to glucose. The breakdown of fats and proteins for energy causes acid compounds called ketones to form in the blood. Ketones also will be excreted in the urine. As ketones build up in the blood, a condition called ketoacidosis can occur. If left untreated, ketoacidosis can lead to coma and death.

Types of diabetes mellitus

Type I diabetes, sometimes called juvenile diabetes, begins most commonly in childhood or adolescence. In this form of diabetes, the body produces little or no insulin. It is characterized by a sudden onset and occurs more frequently in populations descended from northern European countries (Finland, Scotland, Scandinavia)

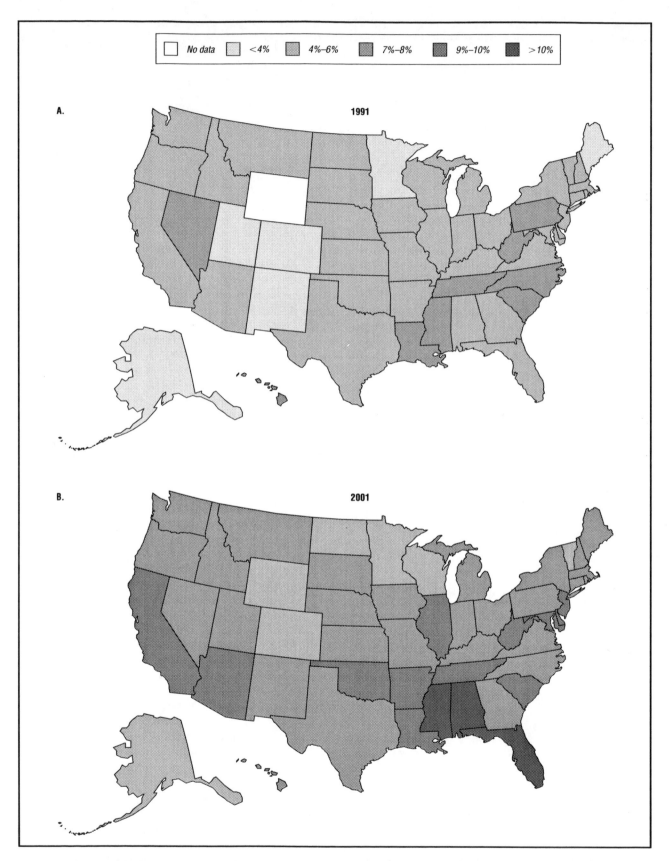

| | No data | <4% | 4%–6% | 7%–8% | 9%–10% | >10% |

A.
1991

B.
2001

Maps of 1991 and 2001 diagnosed diabetes cases in the United States shows the rapid spread of the disease in one decade. (*Map by GGS Information Services, Inc. The Gale Group.*)

than in those from southern European countries, the Middle East, or Asia. In the United States, approximately 3 people in 1,000 develop Type I diabetes. This form also is called insulin-dependent diabetes because people who develop this type need to have injections of insulin 1–2 times per day.

Brittle diabetics are a subgroup of Type I where patients have frequent and rapid swings of blood sugar levels between hyperglycemia (a condition where there is too much glucose or sugar in the blood) and **hypoglycemia** (a condition where there are abnormally low levels of glucose or sugar in the blood). These patients may require several injections of different types of insulin or an insulin pump during the day to keep their blood sugar within a fairly normal range.

The more common form of diabetes, Type II, occurs in approximately 3–5% of Americans under 50 years of age, and increases to 10–15% in those over 50. More than 90% of the diabetics in the United States are Type II diabetics. In 2003, a report noted that nearly one-third of the U.S. population over age 20 has this form of diabetes but remains undiagnosed. Sometimes called age-onset or adult-onset diabetes, this form of diabetes occurs most often in people who are overweight and do not **exercise**. It also is more common in people of Native American, Hispanic, and African-American descent. People who have migrated to Western cultures from East India, Japan, and Australian Aboriginal cultures are also more likely to develop Type II diabetes than those who remain in their original countries.

Type II is considered a milder form of diabetes because of its slow onset (sometimes developing over the course of several years) and because it can usually be controlled with diet and oral medication. The consequences of uncontrolled and untreated Type II diabetes, however, are just as serious as those for Type I. This form also is called noninsulin-dependent diabetes, a term that is somewhat misleading. Many people with Type II diabetes can control the condition with diet and oral medications, however, insulin injections sometimes are necessary.

Another form of diabetes, called gestational diabetes, can develop during **pregnancy** and generally resolves after the baby is delivered. This diabetic condition develops during the second or third trimester of pregnancy in about 2% of pregnancies. The condition usually is treated by diet, however, insulin injections may be required. Women who have diabetes during pregnancy are at higher risk for developing Type II diabetes within 5–10 years.

Diabetes also can develop as a result of pancreatic disease, **alcoholism**, malnutrition, or other severe illnesses that stress the body.

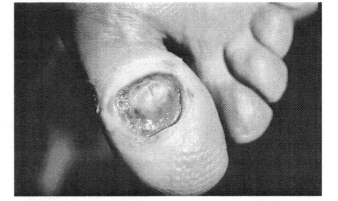

Persons with diabetes often suffer from foot ulcers, as shown above. *(Custom Medical Stock Photo. Reproduced by permission.)*

Causes & symptoms

The causes of diabetes mellitus are unclear, however, there seem to be both hereditary (genetic factors passed on in families) and environmental factors involved. Research has shown that some people who develop diabetes have common genetic markers. In Type I diabetes, an autoimmune response is believed to be triggered by a virus or another microorganism that destroys the cells that produce insulin. In Type II diabetes, age, **obesity**, and family history of diabetes play a role.

In Type II diabetes, the pancreas may produce enough insulin, however, cells have become resistant to the insulin produced and it may not work as effectively. Symptoms of Type II diabetes can begin so gradually that a person may not know that he or she has it. Early signs are tiredness, extreme thirst, and frequent urination. Other symptoms may include sudden weight loss, slow wound healing, urinary tract infections, **gum disease,** or blurred vision. It is not unusual for Type II diabetes to be detected while a patient is seeing a doctor about a health concern that was caused by the yet undiagnosed diabetes.

Individuals who are at high risk of developing Type II diabetes mellitus include people who:

- are obese (more than 20% above their ideal body weight)

- have a relative with diabetes mellitus

- belong to a high-risk ethnic population (African-American, Native American, Hispanic, or Native Hawaiian)

- have been diagnosed with gestational diabetes or have delivered a baby weighing more than 9 lb (4 kg)

- have high blood pressure (140/90 mmHg or above)

- have a high density lipoprotein **cholesterol** level less than or equal to 35 mg/dL and/or a triglyceride level greater than or equal to 250 mg/dL

- have had impaired glucose tolerance or impaired **fasting** glucose on previous testing

Several common medications can impair the body's use of insulin, causing a condition known as secondary diabetes. These medications include treatments for high blood pressure (furosemide, clonidine, and thiazide diuretics), drugs with hormonal activity (oral contraceptives, thyroid hormone, progestins, and glucocorticorids), and the anti-inflammation drug indomethacin. Several drugs that are used to treat mood disorders (such as **anxiety** and **depression**) also can impair glucose absorption. These drugs include haloperidol, lithium carbonate, phenothiazines, tricyclic antidepressants, and adrenergic agonists. Other medications that can cause diabetes symptoms include isoniazid, nicotinic acid, cimetidine, and heparin.

Symptoms of diabetes can develop suddenly (over days or weeks) in previously healthy children or adolescents, or can develop gradually (over several years) in overweight adults over the age of 40. The classic symptoms include feeling tired and sick, frequent urination, excessive thirst, excessive hunger, and weight loss.

Ketoacidosis, a condition due to starvation or uncontrolled diabetes, is common in Type I diabetes. Ketones are acid compounds that form in the blood when the body breaks down fats and proteins. Symptoms include abdominal **pain**, **vomiting**, rapid breathing, extreme tiredness, and drowsiness. Patients with ketoacidosis will also have a sweet breath odor. Left untreated, this condition can lead to coma and death.

With Type II diabetes, the condition may not become evident until the patient presents for medical treatment for some other condition. A patient may have heart disease, chronic infections of the gums and urinary tract, blurred vision, numbness in the feet and legs, or slow-healing **wounds**. Women may experience genital **itching**.

Diagnosis

Diabetes is suspected based on symptoms. Urine tests and blood tests can be used to confirm a diagnosis of diabetes based on the amount of glucose in the urine and blood. Urine tests also can detect ketones and protein in the urine which may help diagnose diabetes and assess how well the kidneys are functioning. These tests also can be used to monitor the disease once the patient is under treatment.

Urine tests

Clinistix and Diastix are paper strips or dipsticks that change color when dipped in urine. The test strip is compared to a chart that shows the amount of glucose in the urine based on the change in color. The level of glucose in the urine lags behind the level of glucose in the blood. Testing the urine with a test stick, paper strip, or tablet is not as accurate as blood testing, however it can give a fast and simple reading.

Ketones in the urine can be detected using similar types of dipstick tests (Acetest or Ketostix). Ketoacidosis can be a life-threatening situation in Type I diabetics, so having a quick and simple test to detect ketones can assist in establishing a diagnosis sooner.

Another dipstick test can determine the presence of protein or albumin in the urine. Protein in the urine can indicate problems with kidney function and can be used to track the development of renal failure. A more sensitive test for urine protein uses radioactively tagged chemicals to detect microalbuminuria, small amounts of protein in the urine, which may not show up on dipstick tests.

Blood tests

Fasting glucose test. Blood is drawn from a vein in the patient's arm after the patient has not eaten for at least eight hours, usually in the morning before breakfast. The red blood cells are separated from the sample and the amount of glucose is measured in the remaining plasma. A plasma level of 7.8 mmol/L (200 mg/L) or greater can indicate diabetes. The fasting glucose test is usually repeated on another day to confirm the results.

Postprandial glucose test. Blood is taken right after the patient has eaten a meal.

Oral glucose tolerance test. Blood samples are taken from a vein before and after a patient drinks a sweet syrup of glucose and other sugars. In a non-diabetic, the level of glucose in the blood goes up immediately after the drink and then decreases gradually as insulin is used by the body to metabolize, or absorb, the sugar. In a diabetic, the glucose in the blood goes up and stays high after drinking the sweetened liquid. A plasma glucose level of 11.1 mmol/L (200 mg/dL) or higher at two hours after drinking the syrup and at one other point during the two-hour test period confirms the diagnosis of diabetes.

A diagnosis of diabetes is confirmed if a plasma glucose level of at least 11.1 mmol/L, a fasting plasma glucose level of at least 7 mmol/L; or a two-hour plasma glucose level of at least 11.1 mmol/L during an oral glucose tolerance test.

In 2002, scientists announced that a new simple blood test to screen for diabetes had been developed. Prior to that time, community-wide screening procedures had not proven cost-effective. The new screening test proved cost-effective if conducted in physician offices on patients with three known risk factors of obesity, self-reported high blood pressure, and family history of diabetes.

Home blood glucose monitoring kits are available so diabetics can monitor their own levels. A small needle or lancet is used to prick the finger and a drop of blood is collected and analyzed by a monitoring device. Some patients may test their blood glucose levels several times during a day and use this information to adjust their diet or doses of insulin.

Treatment

There is currently no cure for diabetes. Diet, exercise, and careful monitoring of blood glucose levels are the keys to manage diabetes so that patients can live a relatively normal life. Diabetes can be life-threatening if not properly managed, so patients should not attempt to treat this condition without medical supervision. Treatment of diabetes focuses on two goals: keeping blood glucose within normal range and preventing the development of long-term complications. Alternative treatments cannot replace the need for insulin but they may enhance insulin's effectiveness and may lower blood glucose levels. In addition, alternative medicines may help to treat complications of the disease and improve quality of life.

Diet

Diet and moderate exercise are the first treatments implemented in diabetes. For many Type II diabetics, weight loss may be an important goal to help them to control their diabetes. A well-balanced, nutritious diet provides approximately 50–60% of calories from carbohydrates, approximately 10–20% of calories from protein, and less than 30% of calories from fat. The number of calories required depends on the patient's age, weight, and activity level. The calorie intake also needs to be distributed over the course of the entire day so surges of glucose entering the blood system are kept to a minimum. In 2002, a Korean study demonstrated that eating a combination of whole grains and legume powder was beneficial in lowering blood glucose levels in men with diabetes.

Keeping track of the number of calories provided by different foods can be complicated, so patients are usually advised to consult a nutritionist or dietitian. An individualized, easy-to-manage diet plan can be set up for each patient. Both the American Diabetes Association and the American Dietetic Association recommend **diets** based on the use of food exchange lists. Each food exchange contains a known amount of calories in the form of protein, fat, or carbohydrate. A patient's diet plan will consist of a certain number of exchanges from each food category (meat or protein, fruits, breads and starches, vegetables, and fats) to be eaten at meal times and as snacks. Patients have flexibility in choosing the foods they eat as long as they don't exceed the number of exchanges prescribed. The food exchange system, along with a plan of moderate exercise, can help diabetics lose excess weight and improve their overall health. Certain foods will be emphasized over others to promote a healthy heart as well.

Supplements

CHROMIUM PICOLINATE. Several studies have had conflicting results on the effectiveness of **chromium** picolinate supplementation for control of blood glucose levels. In one study, approximately 70% of the diabetics receiving 200 micrograms of chromium picolinate daily reduced their need for insulin and medications. While some studies have shown that supplementation caused significant weight loss, and decreases in blood glucose and serum triglycerides, others have shown no benefit. Chromium supplementation may cause hypoglycemia and other side effects.

MAGNESIUM. Magnesium deficiency may interfere with insulin secretion and uptake and worsen the patient's control of blood sugar. Also, magnesium deficiency puts diabetics at risk for certain complications, especially **retinopathy** and cardiovascular disease.

VANADIUM. Vanadium has been shown to bring blood glucose to normal levels in diabetic animals. Also, people who took vanadium were able to decrease their need for insulin.

Chinese medicine

Non-insulin dependent diabetics who practiced daily **qigong** for one year had decreases in fasting blood glucose and blood insulin levels. **Acupuncture** may relieve pain in patients with diabetic neuropathy. Acupuncture also may help to bring blood glucose to normal levels in diabetics who do not require insulin.

Best when used in consultation with a Chinese medicine physician, some Chinese patent medicines that alleviate symptoms of or complications from diabetes include:

• *Xiao Ke Wan* (Emaciation and Thirst Pill) for diabetics with increased levels of sugar in blood and urine.

• *Yu Quan Wan* (Jade Spring Pill) for diabetics with a deficiency of Yin.

• *Liu Wei Di Huang Wan* (Six Ingredient Pill with Rehmannia) for stabilized diabetics with a deficiency of Kidney Yin.

• *Jin Gui Shen Wan* (Kidney Qi Pill) for stabilized diabetics with a deficiency of Kidney Yang.

Herbals

Herbal medicine can have a positive effect on blood glucose and quality of life in diabetics. The results of clinical study of various herbals are:

- Wormwood (*Artemisia herba-alba*) decreased blood glucose.

- Gurmar (*Gymnema sylvestre*) decreased blood glucose levels and the need for insulin.

- *Coccinia indica* improved glucose tolerance.

- Fenugreek seed powder (*Trigonella foenum graecum*) decreased blood glucose and improved glucose tolerance.

- Bitter melon (*Momordica charantia*) decreased blood glucose and improved glucose tolerance.

- Cayenne pepper (*Capsicum frutescens*) can help relieve pain in the peripheral nerves (a type of diabetic neuropathy).

Other herbals that may treat or prevent diabetes and its complications include:

- **Bilberry** (*Vaccinium myrtillus*) may lower blood glucose levels and maintain healthy blood vessels.

- Garlic (**Allium sativum**) may lower blood sugar and cholesterol levels.

- Onions (**Allium cepa**) may help lower blood glucose levels.

- Ginkgo (*Ginkgo biloba*) improves blood circulation.

Yoga

Studies of diabetics have shown that practicing **yoga** leads to decreases in blood glucose, increased glucose tolerance, decreased need for diabetes medications, and improved insulin processes. Yoga also enhances the sense of well-being.

Biofeedback

Many studies have been performed to test the benefit of adding **biofeedback** to the diabetic's treatment plan. **Relaxation** techniques, such as visualization, usually were included. Biofeedback can have significant effects on diabetes including improved glucose tolerance and decreased blood glucose levels. In addition, biofeedback can be used to treat diabetic complications and improve quality of life.

Allopathic treatment

Traditional treatment of diabetes begins with a well balanced diet and moderate exercise. Medications are prescribed only if the patient's blood glucose cannot be controlled by these methods.

Oral medications

Oral medications are available to lower blood glucose in Type II diabetics. Drugs first prescribed for Type II diabetes are in a class of compounds called sulfonylureas and include tolbutamide, tolazamide, acetohexamide, chlorpropamide, glyburide, glimeperide, and glipizide. The way that these drugs work is not well understood, however, they seem to stimulate cells of the pancreas to produce more insulin. New medications that are available to treat diabetes include metformin, acarbose, and troglitizone. These medications are not a substitute for a well planned diet and moderate exercise. Oral medications are not effective for Type I diabetes, in which the patient produces little or no insulin.

Insulin

Patients with Type I diabetes need daily injections of insulin to help their bodies use glucose. Some patients with Type II diabetes may need to use insulin injections if their diabetes cannot be controlled. Injections are given subcutaneously—just under the skin, using a small needle and syringe. Purified human insulin is most commonly used, however, insulin from beef and pork sources also is available. Insulin may be given as an injection of a single dose of one type of insulin once a day. Different types of insulin can be mixed and given in one dose or split into two or more doses during a day. Patients who require multiple injections over the course of a day may be able to use an insulin pump that administers small doses of insulin on demand. In 2002, reports announced that early research shows a synthetic insulin called insulin glargine might show promise for patients at risk for hypoglycemia from insulin therapy. Clinical trials showed that when used in combination with certain other short-acting insulins, it safely regulated blood glucose for longer durations and was well tolerated by patients.

Hypoglycemia, or low blood sugar, can be caused by too much insulin, too little food (or eating too late to coincide with the action of the insulin), alcohol consumption, or increased exercise. A patient with symptoms of hypoglycemia may be hungry, sweaty, shaky, cranky, confused, and tired. Left untreated, the patient can lose consciousness or have a seizure. This condition is sometimes called an insulin reaction and should be treated by giving the patient something sweet to eat or drink like candy, sugar cubes, or juice.

Surgery

Transplantation of a healthy pancreas into a diabetic patient is a successful treatment, however, this transplant usually is done only if a kidney transplant is performed at the same time. It is not clear if the potential benefits of transplantation outweigh the risks of the surgery and subsequent drug therapy.

Expected results

Uncontrolled diabetes is a leading cause of blindness, end-stage renal disease, and limb amputations. It also doubles the risk of heart disease and increases the risk of stroke. Eye problems including **cataracts, glaucoma**, and retinopathy also are more common in diabetics. Kidney disease is a common complication of diabetes and may require kidney dialysis or a kidney transplant. Babies born to diabetic mothers have an increased risk of birth defects and distress at birth.

Diabetic **peripheral neuropathy** is a condition where nerve endings, particularly in the legs and feet, become less sensitive. Diabetic foot ulcers are a problem since the patient does not feel the pain of a blister, callous, or other minor injury. Poor blood circulation in the legs and feet contributes to delayed wound healing. The inability to sense pain along with the complications of delayed wound healing can result in minor injuries, **blisters**, or calluses becoming infected and difficult to treat. Severely infected tissue breaks down and rots, often necessitating amputation of toes, feet, or legs.

Prevention

Research continues on ways to prevent diabetes and to detect those at risk for developing diabetes. While the onset of Type I diabetes is unpredictable, the risk of developing Type II diabetes can be reduced by maintaining ideal weight and exercising regularly. The physical and emotional stress of surgery, illness, and alcoholism can increase the risks of diabetes, so maintaining a healthy lifestyle is critical to preventing the onset of Type II diabetes and preventing further complications of the disease.

In early 2002, researchers announced that patients at high risk for developing diabetes who took an ACE inhibitor called ramipril reduced their risk of developing diabetes substantially. Another report at Duke University showed that sustained intensive exercise could forestall development of diabetes or cardiovascular disease in high-risk patients. The benefits of long-term exercise even continue one month after exercising stops. In 2003, advances in genetics found a key gene that may explain why some people are more susceptible to the disease than others.

Resources

BOOKS

Foster, Daniel W. "Diabetes Mellitus." In *Harrison's Principles of Internal Medicine*. 14th ed. Edited by Anthony S. Fauci, et al. New York: McGraw-Hill, 1998.

Garber, Alan J. "Diabetes Mellitus." In *Internal Medicine*. Edited by Jay H. Stein, et al. St. Louis: Mosby, 1998.

Karam, John H. "Diabetes Mellitus & Hypoglycemia." In *Current Medical Diagnosis & Treatment 1998*. 37th ed. Edited by L.M. Tierney, Jr., S.J. McPhee, and M.A. Papadakis. Stamford, CT: Appleton & Lange, 1998.

McGrady, Angele and James Horner. "Complementary/Alternative Therapies in General Medicine: Diabetes Mellitus." In *Complementary/Alternative Medicine: An Evidence Based Approach*. Edited by John W. Spencer and Joseph J. Jacobs. St. Louis: Mosby, 1999.

Sherwin, Robert S. "Diabetes Mellitus." In *Cecil Textbook of Medicine*. 20th ed. Edited by J. Claude Bennett and Fred Plum. Philadelphia, PA: W.B. Saunders Company, 1996.

Smit, Charles Kent, John P. Sheehan, and Margaret M. Ulchaker. "Diabetes Mellitus." In *Family Medicine, Principles and Practice*. 5th ed. Edited by Robert B. Taylor. New York: Springer-Verlag, 1998.

Ying, Zhou Zhong and Jin Hui De. "Endocrinology." In *Clinical Manual of Chinese Herbal Medicine and Acupuncture*. New York: Churchill Livingston, 1997.

PERIODICALS

"Exercise Can Forestall Diabetes in At-Risk Patients." *Diabetes Week* (March 25, 2002):2.

Fox, Gary N., and Zijad Sabovic. "Chromium Picolinate Supplementation for Diabetes Mellitus." *The Journal of Family Practice* 46 (1998): 83-86.

Hartnett, Terry. "Early Results Show Promise for Synthetic Insulin." *Diabetes Week* (March 18, 2002):4.

Jenkins, David JA, et al. "Type 2 Diabetes and the Vegetarian Diet." *American Journal of Clinical Nutrition* (September 2003):610S.

"Mouse, Stripped of a Key Gene, Resists Diabetes." *Biotech Week* (September 24, 2003):557.

"Nearly One-third of Diabetes Undiganosed, According to New Government Data." *Medical Letter on the CDC & FDA* (September 28, 2003):13.

"Ramipril Cuts Diabetes Risk." *Family Practice News* 32, no. 3 (February 1, 2002):10.

"Simple Blood Test Could Detect New Cases of Diabetes." *Diabetes Week* (January 21, 2002):4.

"Whole Grain and Legume Powder Diet Benefits Diabetics and the Healthy." *Diabetes Week* (January 7, 2002):8.

"Trends in the Prevalence and Incidence of Self- Reported Diabetes Mellitus-United States, 1980-1994." *Morbidity & Mortality Weekly Report* 46 (1997): 1014-1018.

"Updated Guidelines for the Diagnosis of Diabetes in the US." *Drugs & Therapy Perspectives* 10 (1997): 12-13.

ORGANIZATIONS

American Diabetes Association. 1660 Duke Street, Alexandria, VA 22314. (703) 549-1500. Diabetes Information and Action Line: (800) DIABETES. http://www.diabetes.org.

American Dietetic Association. 430 North Michigan Avenue, Chicago, IL 60611. (312) 822-0330. http://www.eatright. org.

KEY TERMS

. . . .

Cataracts—A condition in which the lens of the eye becomes cloudy.

Diabetic peripheral neuropathy—The sensitivity of nerves to pain, temperature, and pressure is dulled particularly in the legs and feet.

Diabetic retinopathy—The tiny blood vessels to the retina, the tissues that sense light at the back of the eye, are damaged, leading to blurred vision, sudden blindness, or black spots, lines, or flashing light in the field of vision.

Glaucoma—A condition in which pressure within the eye causes damage to the optic nerve, which sends visual images to the brain.

Hyperglycemia—A condition of having too much glucose or sugar in the blood.

Hypoglycemia—A condition of having too little glucose or sugar in the blood.

Insulin—A hormone produced by the pancreas that is needed by cells of the body to use glucose (sugar), the body's main source of energy.

Ketoacidosis—A condition due to starvation or uncontrolled Type I diabetes. Ketones are acid compounds that form in the blood when the body breaks down fats and proteins. Symptoms include abdominal pain, vomiting, rapid breathing, extreme tiredness, and drowsiness.

Kidney dialysis—A process by which blood is filtered through a dialysis machine to remove waste products that would normally be removed by the kidneys. The filtered blood is then circulated back into the patient. This process is also called renal dialysis.

Pancreas—The organ that produces insulin.

Juvenile Diabetes Foundation International. 120 Wall Street, New York, NY 10005-4001. (212) 785-9595. (800) JDF-CURE.

National Diabetes Information Clearinghouse. 1 Information Way, Bethesda, MD 20892-3560. (301) 654-3327.

National Institutes of Health. National Institute of Diabetes, Digestive and Kidney Diseases. 9000 Rockville Pike, Bethesda, MD 20892. (301) 496-3583. http://www.niddk.nih.gov.

OTHER

Centers for Disease Control and Prevention Diabetes. http://www.cdc.gov/nccdphp/ddt/ddthome.htm.

"Insulin-Dependent Diabetes." National Institute of Diabetes and Digestive and Kidney Diseases. National Institutes of Health, NIH Publication No. 94-2098.

"Noninsulin-Dependent Diabetes." National Institute of Diabetes and Digestive and Kidney Diseases. National Institutes of Health, NIH Publication No. 92-241.

Belinda Rowland
Teresa G. Odle

Diamond diet

Definition

The Diamond diet, popularly known as the Fit for Life Program, is a way of eating designed to be employed as a health lifestyle. Developed by Harvey and Marilyn Diamond, it is a set of dietary principles intended to serve as a blueprint for habits that can easily become routine, allowing individuals to take control of their health.

Origins

Harvey Diamond was an ill and underweight child with chronic and painful stomach problems. As a young adult, his health problems continued as he became overweight. After experiencing the dieting merry-go-round of losing and regaining his weight, Diamond decided that dieting does not work and that he needed to learn how to best care for his body. In 1970, Diamond found his answer in the concept of natural hygiene, an approach to the care and upkeep of the body that focuses on prevention of disease and healthful living. As described by Diamond, the concept of natural hygiene teaches that the body is self-cleansing, self-healing, and self-maintaining. Healing powers are contained within the body itself. He states "the body is always striving for health and .. achieves this by continuously cleansing itself of deleterious waste material." In combination with an overall healthful lifestyle of adequate rest, **exercise**, sunshine, **stress** management, and interpersonal relationships, understanding how food impacts this cleansing process allows individuals to eliminate the cause of their health problems.

Almost immediately upon Diamond's introduction to this concept, his lifelong stomach pains ceased. Within one month, he had lost 50 pounds (a loss he was able to maintain). Diamond became a proponent of natural hygiene and, in 1981, began a seminar program known as The Diamond Method. In 1983, he earned a doctorate in nutritional science from the American College of Health Science, a non-accredited college in Austin, Texas. It is the basic fundamentals of natural hygiene that Harvey and Marilyn Diamond synthesized into the dietary and lifestyle principles of the Fit for Life Program.

Benefits

Although popularly discussed as a weight loss program, Fit for Life is not a diet. True to the tenets of natural hygiene, the approach to eating laid out in the Fit for Life books is designed to provide for optimal body functioning by internal cleansing of illness-producing toxins. Although weight loss and energy enhancements are positive results, the underlying goal is cleansing. Disease, as understood in this approach, is "nothing more than the body's own effort to cleanse itself of toxins." These toxins are the products of metabolic imbalance, or toxemia, resulting from wastes. Dead cells, food residue, and additives build up in the bodies and cannot be eliminated at the same rate they are produced. Understanding and minimizing this level of toxemia is the key to healthy longevity. The dietary guidelines of the Fit for Life program are designed to generate a minimum of toxic food residue within the body and to enable the body to continuously expel the toxic waste that is produced. An additional intent is that the dietary guidelines incorporate good food and enjoyable meals rather than strict, hard-to-follow regimens. If the program is stopped for any reason, according to Diamond, it can be re-started with almost immediate results.

Description

The Fit for Life program places an emphasis not only on what foods are eaten, but also in what combinations and at what time of day those foods are eaten. Three general principles guide Diamond's hygienic approach to eating.

The Principle of High-Water-Content Food

Water is vital to cleansing the inside of the body of accumulated wastes. Consuming sufficient high-water-content foods, fruits, and vegetables is crucial to accomplish this cleansing. Unlike drinking water, the water found in fruits and vegetables provides for the transport of the nutrients found in those foods. It then flushes waste matter from the body.

The Principle of Proper Food Combining

According to this principle, foods should be eaten in combinations that are most compatible with digestive chemistry. Otherwise, the food will remain in the stomach longer than it should and cause digestive problems. Proteins and starches should not be eaten together because the stomach cannot digest both efficiently at the same time. For optimal digestion, proteins should be combined with vegetables at mealtime or a starch combined with vegetables.

The Principle of the Correct Consumption of Fruit

Fruit should be fresh and ripe when eaten. It should be eaten alone on an empty stomach, not with or after anything else. The reason is that fruit requires no digestion in the stomach and should be able to pass through the stomach quickly to help the body in its **detoxification** efforts. Additionally, because fruit requires so little digestive energy, it should be eaten in the morning to best work with natural body cycles of food utilization and elimination. The body needs to spend its energy on proper cleansing during the morning hours rather than diverting crucial energy to digestive processes. According to Diamond, the most beneficial habit a person can develop is consuming exclusively fresh fruit and fresh fruit juice from awakening until noon.

Research & general acceptance

Proponents, including some **nutrition** and medical professionals, claim benefits include weight loss, improved energy, and overall better health from following the program. M.D.s, including Edward Taub, an Assistant Clinical Professor at the University of California, Irvine, and Kay S. Lawrence, contributed to the first Fit for Life book. Critics contend that the principles of the program disagree with much established nutritional advice such as that provided by the American Dietetic Association (ADA). The regimen does not, for example, advocate weight loss by counting calories, recommend the basic food groups, or call to attention the health benefits of milk. Although the emphasis on fresh fruits and vegetables is generally seen as positive, it is also called extreme by some reviewers. Reviewers in nutritional publications have raised concerns about inadequate protein intake, the possibility of deficiencies in **calcium**, **zinc**, some B vitamins (notably **riboflavin** and **thiamine**), and **iron** deficiency **anemia**. Some nutritionists have also argued that rigorously following the Fit for Life dietary guidelines could lead to inadequate nutrition for the proper development of growing children or fetuses. Critical reviews range from Environmental Nutrition's assessment that the Fit for Life regimen is "probably not dangerous, [but] has the potential to be unhealthy and therefore is not recommended" to the position of J. Lynne Brown, Ph.D., R.D. that if "followed rigorously, it could lead to serious health problems." Diamond rebuffs his critics, ADA guidelines and nutritional advice in particular, calling for a broader understanding of science, a quest for truth and less emphasis on credentials which are, he argues, the way organizations such as the ADA maintain power over dissenting opinions.

Resources

BOOKS

Diamond, Harvey and Marilyn. *Fit for Life*. New York, Warner Books. 1985.

Diamond, Harvey and Marilyn. *Fit for Life II: Living Health*. New York, Warner Books. 1987.

PERIODICALS

Brown, J. Lynne. "Fit for Life." *Journal of Nutrition Education* (1986): 18, 6.

Kenny, James J. "Fit for Life." *Nutrition* (1986): 3, 8.

ORGANIZATIONS

American Dietetic Association. 216 Jackson Blvd., Chicago, Illinois 60606.(312) 899-0040. adaf@eatright.org. http://www.eatright.org.

American Natural Hygiene Society. P.O. Box 30630, Tampa, FL 33630. (813) 855-6607. anhs@anhs.org. http://www.anhs.org/index.html.

OTHER

Healthcare Reality Check. http://www.hcrc.org.

Quackwatch: Your guide to Health Fraud, Quackery, and Intelligent Decisions. http://www.quackwatch.com/index.html.

Kathy Stolley

Diaper rash

Definition

Dermatitis of the buttocks, genitals, lower abdomen, or thigh folds of an infant or toddler is commonly referred to as diaper rash.

Description

The outside layer of skin normally forms a protective barrier that prevents infection. One of the primary causes of dermatitis in the diaper area is prolonged skin contact with wetness. Under these circumstances, natural oils are stripped away, the outer layer of skin is damaged, and there is increased susceptibility to infection by bacteria or yeast.

Diaper rash is a term that covers a broad variety of skin conditions that occur on the same area of the body. Some babies are more prone to diaper rash than others.

Causes & symptoms

Frequently a flat, red rash is caused by simple chafing of the diaper against tender skin, initiating a friction rash. This type of rash is not seen in the skin folds. It may be more pronounced around the edges of the diaper, at the waist and leg bands. The baby generally doesn't appear to experience much discomfort. Sometimes the chemicals or detergents in the diaper are contributing factors and may result in **contact dermatitis**. These **rashes** should clear up easily with proper attention. Ignoring the condition may lead to a secondary infection that is more difficult to resolve.

Friction of skin against itself can cause a rash in the baby's skin folds, called intertrigo. This rash appears as reddened areas that may ooze, and is often uncomfortable when the diaper is wet. Intertrigo can also be found on other areas of the body where there are deep skin folds that tend to trap moisture.

Seborrheic dermatitis is the diaper area equivalent of **cradle cap**. It is scaly and greasy in appearance and may be worse in the folds of the skin.

Yeast, or candidal dermatitis, is the most common infectious cause of diaper rash. The affected areas are raised and quite red with distinct borders, and satellite lesions may occur around the edges. Yeast is part of the normal skin flora, and is often an opportunistic invader when simple diaper rash is untreated. It is particularly common after treatment with antibiotics, which kill the good bacteria that normally keep the yeast population in check. Usual treatments for diaper rash will not clear it up. Repeated or difficult to resolve episodes of **yeast infection** may warrant further medical attention, since this is sometimes associated with diabetes or immune problems.

Another infectious cause of diaper rash is **impetigo**. This bacterial infection is characterized by **blisters** that ooze and crust.

Diagnosis

The presence of skin lesions in the diaper area means that the baby has diaper rash. However, there are several types of rash that may require specific treatment in order to heal. It is useful to be able to distinguish them by appearance as described above.

A baby with a rash that does not clear up within two to three days, or a rash with blisters or bleeding, should be seen by a healthcare professional for further evaluation.

Treatment

Good diaper hygiene will prevent or clear up many simple cases of diaper rash. Diapers should be checked very frequently and changed as soon as they are wet or soiled. Good air circulation is also important for healthy skin. Babies should have some time without wearing a diaper, and a waterproof pad can be used to protect the bed or other surface. Rubber pants, or other occlusive fabrics, should not be used over the diaper area. Some cloth-like disposable diapers promote better air circulation than plastic-type diapers. It may be necessary for mothers to experiment with diaper types to see if the baby's skin reacts better to cloth or disposable ones. If disposable diapers are used, the baby's skin may react differently to various brands. If the baby is wearing cloth diapers, they should be washed in a mild detergent and double rinsed.

The diaper area should be cleaned with something mild, even plain water. Some wipes contain alcohol or chemicals that can be irritating for some babies. Plain water may be the best cleansing substance when there is a rash. Using warm water in a spray bottle (or giving a quick bath) and then lightly patting the skin dry can produce less skin trauma than using wipes. In the event of suspected yeast, a tablespoon of cider vinegar can be added to a cup of warm water and used as a cleansing solution. This is dilute enough that it should not burn, but acidifies the skin pH enough to hamper the yeast growth.

Barrier ointments can be valuable to treat rashes. Those that contain **zinc** oxide are especially effective. These creams and ointments protect already irritated skin from the additional insult of urine and stool, particularly if the baby has **diarrhea**. Cornstarch powder may be used on rashes that are moist, such as impetigo.

Nutrition

What the baby eats can make a difference in stool frequency and acidity. Typically, breast-fed babies will have fewer problems with rashes. When adding a new food to the diet, the baby should be observed closely to see whether rashes are produced around the baby's mouth or anus. If this occurs, the new food should be discontinued.

Babies who are taking antibiotics are more likely to get rashes due to yeast. To help bring the good bacterial counts back to normal, *Lactobacillus bifidus* can be added to the diet. It is available in powder form from most health food stores.

Herbal treatment

Some herbal preparations can be useful for diaper rash. **Calendula** reduces inflammation, tightens tissues, and disinfects. It has been recommended for seborrheic dermatitis as well as for general inflammation of the skin. The ointment should be applied at each diaper change. **Chickweed** ointment can also be soothing for irritated skin and may be applied once or twice daily.

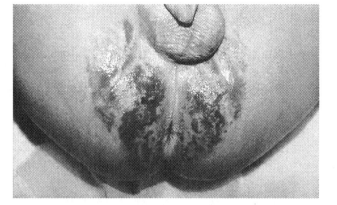

Baby with severe diaper rash. *(Custom Medical Stock Photo. Reproduced by permission.)*

Allopathic treatment

Antibiotics are generally prescribed for rashes caused by bacteria, particularly impetigo. This may be a topical or oral formulation, depending on the size of the area involved and the severity of the infection.

Over-the-counter antifungal creams, such as Lotrimin, are often recommended to treat a rash resulting from yeast. If topical treatment is not effective, an oral antifungal may be prescribed.

Mild steroid creams, such as 0.5-1% hydrocortisone, can be used for seborrheic dermatitis and sometimes intertrigo. Prescription strength creams may be needed for short-term treatment of more stubborn cases.

Expected results

Treated appropriately, diaper rash will resolve fairly quickly if there is no underlying health problem or skin disease.

Prevention

Frequent diaper changes are important to keep the skin dry and healthy. Application of powders and ointments is not necessary when there is no rash. Finding the best combination of cleansing and diapering products for the individual baby will also help to prevent diaper rash.

Resources

BOOKS

Eisenberg, Arlene, Heidi Murkoff, and Sandee Hathaway. *What to Expect the First Year.* New York: Workman Publishing, 1989.

Sears, William, and Martha Sears. *The Baby Book.* Boston: Little, Brown and Company, 1993.

OTHER

Greene, Alan. "Diaper Rash." *Dr. Greene's HouseCalls* http://drgreene.com/960430.asp. (1996).

Judith Turner

Diarrhea

Definition

To most persons, diarrhea means an increased frequency or softer consistency of bowel movements; however, the medical definition is more exact than this. Diarrhea best correlates with an increase in stool weight; stool weights above 300 g per day generally indicates diarrhea. This is mainly due to excess water, which normally makes up 60-85% of fecal matter. In this way, true diarrhea is distinguished from diseases that cause only an increase in the number of bowel movements (hyperdefecation), or incontinence (involuntary loss of bowel contents).

Diarrhea is also classified by physicians into acute, which lasts one to two weeks, and chronic, which continues for longer than 23 weeks. Viral and bacterial **infections** are the most common causes of acute diarrhea.

Description

In many cases, acute infectious diarrhea is a mild, limited annoyance. However, acute infectious diarrhea has a huge impact worldwide, causing over five million deaths per year. While most deaths are among children under five years of age in developing nations, the impact, even in developed countries, is considerable. For example, over 250,000 persons are admitted to hospitals in the United States each year because of diarrhea. Rapid diagnosis and proper treatment can prevent much of the suffering associated with this illness.

Chronic diarrhea also has a considerable effect on health, as well as on social and economic well being. Patients with **celiac disease, inflammatory bowel disease**, and other prolonged diarrheal illnesses develop nutritional deficiencies, which diminish growth and immunity. They affect social interaction and result in the loss of many working hours.

Causes & symptoms

Diarrhea occurs because more fluid passes through the large intestine (colon) than can be absorbed. As a rule, the colon can absorb several times more fluid than is required on a daily basis. However, when this reserve capacity is overwhelmed, diarrhea occurs.

Diarrhea is caused by infections or illnesses that either lead to excess production of fluids or prevent absorption of fluids. Also, certain substances in the colon, such as fats and bile acids, can interfere with water absorption and cause diarrhea. In addition, rapid passage of material through the colon can cause diarrhea.

Symptoms related to diarrheal illness are often those associated with any injury to the gastrointestinal tract, such as **fever, nausea, vomiting**, and abdominal **pain**. All or none of these may be present depending on the cause of diarrhea. The number of bowel movements can vary with up to 20 or more per day. In some patients, blood or pus is present in the stool. Bowel movements may contain undigested food material.

The most common causes of acute diarrhea are infections (the cause of traveler's diarrhea), **food poisoning**, and medications. Medications are a frequent and often overlooked cause, especially antibiotics and antacids. Both prescription and over-the-counter medications can contain additives, such as lactose and sorbitol, that will produce diarrhea in sensitive persons. Less often, various sugar-free foods, which sometimes contain poorly absorbable materials, cause diarrhea. Review of **allergies** or skin changes may also point to a cause.

Chronic diarrhea is frequently due to many of the same things that cause the shorter episodes (infections, medications, etc.); symptoms just last longer. Some infections can become chronic. This occurs mainly with **parasitic infections** (such as *Giardia*), or when patients have altered immunity (such as **AIDS**).

The following are the more usual causes of chronic diarrhea:

- AIDS
- colon **cancer** and other bowel tumors
- endocrine or hormonal abnormalities (thyroid, **diabetes mellitus**, etc.)
- food allergy
- inflammatory bowel disease (**Crohn's disease** and ulcerative colitis)
- lactose intolerance
- malabsorption syndromes (celiac and Whipple's disease)
- other (alcohol, microscopic colitis, radiation, surgery)

Complications

The major effects of diarrhea are dehydration, malnutrition, and weight loss. Signs of dehydration can be hard to notice but include thirst, **dry mouth**, weakness or lightheadedness (particularly if worsening on standing), urine darkening, or a decrease in urination. Severe dehydration leads to changes in the body's chemistry and could become life-threatening. Dehydration from diarrhea can result in kidney failure, neurological symptoms, arthritis, and skin problems.

Diagnosis

Most cases of acute diarrhea never need diagnosis or treatment, as many are mild and produce few problems. But patients with fever over 102°F (38.9°C), signs of dehydration, bloody bowel movements, severe abdominal pain, known immune disease, or recent use of antibiotics need prompt medical evaluation.

When diagnostic studies are needed, the most useful are stool culture and examination for parasites; however these are often negative and a cause cannot be found in a large number of patients. The earlier cultures are performed, the greater the chance of obtaining a positive result. Stool samples of patients who had used antibiotics in the preceding two months need to be examined for the toxins that cause antibiotic-associated colitis. Tests are also available to check stool samples for microscopic amounts of blood and for cells that indicate severe inflammation of the colon. Examination with an endoscope is sometimes helpful in determining severity and extent of inflammation. Tests to check changes in blood chemistry (**potassium**, **magnesium**, etc.) and a complete blood count (CBC) may be performed.

Chronic diarrhea is quite different, and most patients with this condition will receive some degree of testing. Many exams are the same as for an acute episode, as some infections and parasites cause both types of diarrhea. A careful history to evaluate medication use, dietary changes, family history of illnesses, and other symptoms is necessary. Key points in determining the seriousness of symptoms are weight loss of over 10 lb (4.5 kg), blood in the stool, and nocturnal diarrhea (symptoms that awaken the patient from sleep). A combination of stool, blood, and urine tests may be needed in the evaluation of chronic diarrhea; in addition a number of endoscopic and x-ray studies are frequently required.

Treatment

Diet

Treatment is ideally directed toward correcting the cause; however, the first aim is to prevent or treat dehydration and nutritional deficiencies. When possible, food intake should be continued even in patients with acute diarrhea. A physician should be consulted as to what type and how much food is permitted. Low-fat **diets** or more easily digestible fat is useful in some patients. The BRAT diet, which limits food intake to bananas, rice, applesauce, and toast, can help to resolve diarrhea. These foods provide soluble and insoluble fiber without irritation. If the toast is slightly burnt, the charcoal can help sequester toxins and pull them from the body.

The patient should drink plenty of fluids, however, in severe cases hospitalization to provide intravenous fluids may be necessary. A physician should be notified if the patient is dehydrated, and if oral replacement is suggested then commercial (Pedialyte and others) or homemade preparations can be used. The World Health Organization (WHO) has provided this easy recipe for home preparation, which can be taken in frequent small sips:

- table salt: 3/4 teaspoon
- baking powder: 1 teaspoon
- orange juice: 1 cup
- water: 1 quart or liter

Supplements

Nutrient replacement also plays a role in preventing and treating diarrhea. **Zinc** especially appears to have an effect on the immune system, and deficiency of this mineral can lead to chronic diarrhea. Also, zinc replacement improves growth in young patients.

Dietary supplements that are generally beneficial in the treatment of digestive disorders include:

- vitamin C: 50-500 mg daily
- vitamin B_6: 50-150 mg daily
- magnesium aspartate: 400 mg daily
- vitamin E: 400 IU daily
- glutamine: 3,000 mg daily
- garlic, deodorized: 2,000 mg daily
- deghycirrhizinated **licorice**: chew as needed

Probiotics

Probiotics refers to treatment with beneficial microbes either by ingestion or through a suppository. Studies and the clinical use of probiotics have shown their utility in the resolution of diarrhea, especially antibiotic-associated diarrhea. Beneficial microbes include the bacteria *Lactobacillus acidophilus* and *L. bifidus* and the yeast *Saccharomyces boulardii*. To treat diarrhea, the patient can eat one cup of yogurt (containing active *Lactobacillus acidophilus* cultures) daily. Alternatively, one or two **acidophilus** capsules may be taken at each meal or at bedtime.

Acupuncture

Shallow **acupuncture**, when the needles are inserted superficially and rapidly removed, was more therapeutic than drugs in children with acute or chronic diarrhea. In another study, acupuncture eliminated symptoms and normalized stools in children with chronic diarrhea who had not responded to conventional or Chinese medicines.

Herbals and Chinese medicines

Herbal remedies for diarrhea include meadowsweet, **goldenseal**, and **chamomile** taken as an infusion throughout the day.

Chinese patent medicines used for treating diarrhea include:

- *Xiang Sha Liu Jun Wan* (Six-Gentlemen Pill with **Aucklandia** and Amomum)
- *Fu Zi Li Zhong Wan* (Prepared **Aconite** Pill to Regulate the Middle)
- *Si Shen Wan* (Four-Miracle Pill)
- *Wu Mei Wan* (Mume Pill)
- *Jian Pi Wan* (Strengthen the Spleen Pill)
- *Shen Ling Bai Zhu Wan* (Ginseng, Poria, and **Atractylodes** Macrocephala Pill)

Allopathic treatment

Anti-motility agents (loperamide, diphenoxylate) are useful for persons with chronic diarrhea; their use is limited or even contraindicated in patients with acute diarrhea, especially in those with high fever or bloody bowel movements. They should not be taken without the advice of a physician. Other treatments that are available, depending on the cause of diarrhea, include the bulk agent **psyllium** and the binder cholestyramine. Also, new antidiarrheal drugs that decrease excessive secretion of fluid by the intestinal tract are available.

Expected results

Prognosis is related to the cause of the diarrhea; for most individuals in developed countries, a bout of acute, infectious diarrhea is at best uncomfortable. However, in both industrialized and developing areas, serious complications and death can occur.

Prevention

Proper hygiene and food handling techniques will prevent many cases. Traveler's diarrhea can be avoided

---

KEY TERMS

Anti-motility medications—Medications such as loperamide (Imodium), diphenoxylate (Lomotil), or medications containing codeine or narcotics that decrease the ability of the intestine to contract. These can worsen the condition of a patient with dysentery or colitis.

Colitis—Inflammation of the colon.

Endoscope—A thin flexible tube that uses a lens or miniature camera to view various internal organs including the gastrointestinal tract. Both diagnosis and therapeutic procedures can be done with this instrument.

Endoscopy—The performance of an exam using an endoscope.

Lactose intolerance—An inability to properly digest milk and dairy products.

Probiotics—The use of beneficial microbes to treat various diseases, including diarrhea.

---

by use of Pepto-Bismol and/or antibiotics, if necessary. The most important action is to prevent dehydration, as outlined above.

Resources

BOOKS

Fine, Kenneth D. "Diarrhea." In *Sleisenger & Fordtran's Gastrointestinal and Liver Disease.* Edited by Mark Feldman, et al. Philadelphia: W. B. Saunders Company. 1997.

Friedman, Lawrence S., and Kurt J. Isselbacher. "Diarrhea." In *Harrison's Principles of Internal Medicine.* Edited by Anthony S. Fauci, et al. New York: McGraw Hill, 1998.

Thielman, Nathan M. and Richard L. Guerrant. "Food-Borne Illness." In *Conn's Current Therapy, 1996.* Edited by Robert E. Rakel. Philadelphia: W. B. Saunders Company, 1996.

Ying, Zhou Zhong and Jin Hui De. "Gastrointestinal Diseases." In *Clinical Manual of Chinese Herbal Medicine and Acupuncture.* New York: Churchill Livingston, 1997.

PERIODICALS

Donowitz, Mark, Freddy T. Kokke, and Roxan Saidi. "Evaluation of Patients with Chronic Diarrhea." *New England Journal of Medicine* 332 (March 16, 1995): 725-729.

Dupont, Herbert L. and The Practice Parameters Committee of the American College of Gastroenterology. "Guidelines on Acute Infectious Diarrhea in Adults." *American Journal of Gastroenterology* 92 (1977): 1962-1975.

Penny, Mary E. and Claudio F. Lanata. "Zinc in the Management of Diarrhea in Young Children." *New England Journal of Medicine* 333 (September 28, 1995): 873-874.

"Traveler's Diarrhea: Don't Let It Ruin Your Trip." *Mayo Clinic Health Letter* (January 1997).

"When Microbes Are on the Menu." *Harvard Health Letter* (December 1994): 4-5.

ORGANIZATIONS

World Health Organization (WHO). CH-1211 Geneva 27, Switzerland. +41 22 791 2111. Fax: +41 22 791 0746. Telex: 45 415416. postmaster@who.ch. http://www.who.ch.

OTHER

Directory of Digestive Diseases Organizations for Patients. http://www.niddk.nih.gov/DigDisOrgPat/DigDisOrgPat.html (January 17, 2001).

Selected publications and documents on diarrhoeal diseases (including cholera). World Health Organization (WHO). http://www.who.ch/chd/pub/cdd/cddpub.htm (January 17, 2001).

Belinda Rowland

Diathermy

Definition

In diathermy, high-frequency electrical currents are used to heat deep muscular tissues. The heat increases blood flow, speeding up recovery. Doctors also use diathermy in surgical procedures by sealing blood vessels with electrically heated probes.

The term diathermy is derived from the Greek words *therma,* meaning heat, and *dia,* meaning through. Diathermy literally means heating through.

Origins

The therapeutic effects of heat have long been recognized. More than 2,000 years ago, the Romans took advantage of heat therapies by building hot-spring bathhouses. Since then, various methods of using heat have evolved. In the early 1890s, French physiologist Arséne d'Arsonval began studying the medical application of high-frequency currents. The term diathermy was coined by German physician Carl Franz Nagelschmidt, who designed a prototype apparatus in 1906. Around 1925, United States doctor J. W. Schereschewsky began studying the physiological effects of high-frequency electrical currents on animals. It was several years, however, before the fundamentals of the therapy were understood and put into practice.

Benefits

Diathermy can be used to treat arthritis, **bursitis,** and other conditions involving stiff, painful joints. It is also used to treat pelvic **infections** and sinusitis. A benefit of diathermy is that it is a painless procedure that can be administered at a clinic. Also, if the treatment relieves **pain,** then patients can discontinue pain killers and escape their high cost and side effects.

Description

Diathermy involves heating deep muscular tissues. When heat is applied to the painful area, cellular metabolism speeds up and blood flow increases. The increased metabolism and circulation accelerates tissue repair. The heat helps the tissues relax and stretch, thus alleviating stiffness. Heat also reduces nerve fiber sensitivity, increasing the patient's pain threshold.

There are three methods of diathermy. In each, energy is delivered to the deep tissues, where it is converted to heat. The three methods are:

• Shortwave diathermy. The body part to be treated is placed between two capacitor plates. Heat is generated as the high-frequency waves travel through the body tissues between the plates. Shortwave diathermy is most often used to treat areas like the hip, which is covered with a dense tissue mass. It is also used to treat pelvic infections and sinusitis. The treatment reduces inflammation. The Federal Communications Commission regulates the frequency allowed for short-wave diathermy treatment. Most machines function at 27.33 megahertz.

• Ultrasound diathermy. In this method, high-frequency acoustic vibrations are used to generate heat in deep tissue.

• Microwave diathermy. This method uses radar waves to heat tissue. This form is the easiest to use, but the microwaves cannot penetrate deep muscles.

Diathermy is also used in surgical procedures. Many doctors use electrically heated probes to seal blood vessels to prevent excessive bleeding. This is particularly helpful in neurosurgery and eye surgery. Doctors can also use diathermy to kill abnormal growths, such as tumors, **warts,** and infected tissues.

Preparations

To keep patients from sweating, patients are usually asked to remove clothing from the body part being treated. If a patient sweats, the electrical currents may pool in the area, causing **burns.** Also, clothing containing metal must be removed, as must earrings, buttons, barrettes, or zippers that contain metal. Watches and hearing aids should be removed because the therapy may affect their function.

Practitioners of surgical diathermy should steer clear of alcohol-based solutions to prepare and cleanse the skin. These preparations can create a flammable vapor and cause burns and fires.

Precautions

Patients with metal implants should not undergo diathermy treatment because the metal can act as a conductor of heat and result in serious internal burns. Female patients with metallic uterine implants, such as an IUD, should avoid treatment in the pelvic area. Diathermy should not be used in joints that have been replaced with a prosthesis or in those with sensory impairment who may not be able to tell if they are burning. Furthermore, pulsed shortwave diathermy should be avoided during **pregnancy**, as it can lead to abnormal fetal development.

Patients with hemophilia should avoid the treatment because the increased blood flow could cause them to hemorrhage.

Side effects

Some patients may experience superficial burns. Since the therapy involves creating heat, care must be taken to avoid burns, particularly in patients whose injuries have caused decreased sensitivity to heat. Also, diathermy may affect pacemaker function.

Female patients who receive treatment in the lower back or pelvic area may experience an increased menstrual flow.

Research & general acceptance

For years, physiotherapists and physical therapists have used diathermy as a routine part of physical rehabilitation.

Training & certification

It is recommended that those who treat patients with diathermy complete a course in shortwave therapy and should retake courses every five years to stay updated on procedures. Physiotherapists should also stay updated by reading appropriate medical journals.

Resources

BOOKS

Magill's Medical Guide. Englewood Cliffs, NJ: Salem Press Inc., 1998.

The Merck Manual. Whitehouse Station, NJ: Merck Research Laboratories, 1999.

Michlovitz, Susan L. *Thermal Agents in Rehabilitation.* Philadelphia: F.A. Davis Company, 1996.

Thom, Harald. *Introduction to Shortwave and Microwave Therapy.* Springfield, IL: Charles C. Thomas, 1966.

KEY TERMS

. . . .

Bursitis—Pain and swelling in a joint, often the elbow, hip, knee or shoulder. In bursitis, the bursa (a sac-like membrane that acts as a pillow between the bones and tissues) becomes inflamed.

Capacitor plates—An apparatus that can carry electricity and stores an electrical charge.

Hemophilia—A blood-clotting disorder that can lead to serious hemorrhage from minor cuts and injuries.

OTHER

"Diathermy." *Surgical-tutor.org.uk.* http://www.surgical-tutor.org.uk/core/preop1/diathermy.htm. (19 June 2000).

Lisa Frick

Diets

Definition

Humans may alter their usual eating habits for many reasons, including weight loss, disease prevention or treatment, removing toxins from the body, or to achieve a general improvement in physical and mental health. Others adopt special diets for religious reasons. In the case of some vegetarians and vegans, dietary changes are made out of ethical concerns for the rights of animals.

Origins

The practice of altering diet for special reasons has existed since antiquity. For example, Judaism has included numerous dietary restrictions for thousands of years. One ancient Jewish sect, the Essenes, is said to have developed a primitive **detoxification** diet aimed at preparing the bodies, minds, and spirits of its members for the coming of a "messiah" who would deliver them from their Roman captors. Preventative and therapeutic diets became quite popular during the late twentieth century. Books promoting the latest dietary plan continue to make the bestseller lists, although not all of the information given is considered authoritative.

Benefits

People who are moderately to severely overweight can derive substantial health benefits from a weight-loss

UNHEALTHY FOOD ADDITIVES		
Name	**Description**	**Example products**
Aspartame	An artificial sweetener associated with rashes, headaches, dizziness, depression, etc.	Diet sodas, sugar substitutes, etc.
Brominated vegetable oil (BVO)	Used as an emulsifier and clouding agent. Its main ingredient, bromate, is a poison.	Sodas, etc.
Butylated hydroxyanisole (BHA)/ butylated hydroxytoluene (BHT)	Prevents rancidity in foods and is added to food packagings. It slows the transfer of nerve impulses, effects sleep, aggressiveness and weight in test animals.	Cereal and cheese packaging
Citrus red dye #2	Used to color oranges, it is a probable carcinogen. The FDA has recommended it be banned.	Oranges
Monosodium gltamate (MSG)	A flavor enhancer that can cause headaches, heart palpitations, and nausea.	Fast food, processed and packaged food
Nitrites	Used as preservatives, nitrites form cancer-causing compounds in the gastrointestinal tract and have been associated with cancer and birth defects.	Cured meats and wine
Saccharin	An artificial sweetener that may be carcinogenic.	Diet sodas and sugar substitutes
Sulfites	Used as a food preservative, sulfites have been linked to atleast four deaths reported to the FDA in the United States.	Dried fruits, shrimp, and frozen potatoes
Tertiary butyhydroquinone (TBHQ)	It is extremely toxic in low doses and has been linked to childhood behavioral problems.	Candy bars, baking sprays, and fast foods
Yellow dye #6	Increases the number of kidney and adrenal gland tumors in lab rats. It has been banned in Norway and Sweden.	Candy and sodas

diet. A weight reduction of just 10 to 20 pounds can result in reduced **cholesterol** levels and lower blood pressure. Weight-related health problems include **heart disease**, diabetes, high blood pressure, and high levels of blood sugar and cholesterol.

In individuals who are not overweight, dietary changes may also be useful in the prevention or treatment of a range of ailments including acquired immunodeficiency syndrome (**AIDS**), cancer, **osteoporosis, inflammatory bowel disease**, chronic pulmonary disease, renal disease, **Parkinson's disease**, seizure disorders, and food **allergies** and intolerances.

Description

The idea of a healthful diet is to provide all of the calories and nutrients needed by the body for optimal performance, at the same time ensuring that neither nutritional deficiencies nor excesses occur. Diet plans that claim to accomplish those objectives are so numerous they are virtually uncountable. These diets employ a variety of approaches, including the following:

- Fixed-menu: Offers little choice to the dieter. Specifies exactly which foods will be consumed. Easy to follow, but may be considered "boring" to some dieters.

- Formula: Replaces some or all meals with a nutritionally balanced liquid formula or powder.

- Exchange-type: Allows the dieter to choose between selected foods from each food group.

- Flexible: Doesn't concern itself with the overall diet, simply with one aspect such as fat or energy.

Diets may also be classified according to the types of foods they allow. For example, an omnivorous diet consists of both animal and plant foods, whereas a lacto-ovo-vegetarian diet permits no animal flesh, but does include eggs, milk, and dairy products. A vegan diet is a stricter form of **vegetarianism** in which eggs, cheese, and other milk products are prohibited.

A third way of classifying diets is according to their purpose: religious, weight-loss, detoxification, lifestyle-related, or aimed at prevention or treatment of a specific disease.

Precautions

Dieters should be cautious about plans that severely restrict the size of food portions, or that eliminate entire food groups from the diet. It is highly probable that they will become discouraged and drop out of such programs. The best diet is one that can be maintained indefinitely without ill effects, that offers sufficient variety and balance to provide everything needed for good health, and that is considerate of personal food preferences.

Fad diets for quick weight loss are coming under increasing fire, since dieters seldom maintain the weight loss. In 2001, researchers found that three times as many people on moderate fat weight loss diets stuck to their plan compared to those on traditional low-fat diets. Not only do many diets offer only short-term and rapid weight loss, some can be bad for the dieter's health. For instance, the American Heart Association made a statement in late 2001 questioning the value of high-protein, low-carbohydrate diets. The association said that the diets don't work over the long term and that they can pose some health risks to dieters. In 2003, these statements were largely supported. Though clinical trials showed that these types of diets worked in lowering weight without raising cholesterol for the short-term, many of the participants gained a percentage of the weight back after only one year. A physician group also spoke out about high protein diets' dangers for people with decreased kidney function and the risk of bone loss due to decreased **calcium** intake.

Low-fat diets are not recommended for children under the age of two. Young children need extra fat to maintain their active, growing bodies. Fat intake may be gradually reduced between the ages of two and five, after which it should be limited to a maximum of 30% of total calories through adulthood. Saturated fat should be restricted to no more than 10% of total calories.

Weight-loss dieters should be wary of the "yo-yo" effect that occurs when numerous attempts are made to reduce weight using high-risk, quick-fix diets. This continued "cycling" between weight loss and weight gain can slow the basal metabolic rate and can sometimes lead to eating disorders. The dieter may become discouraged and frustrated by this success/failure cycle. The end result of yo-yo dieting is that it becomes more difficult to maintain a healthy weight.

Caution should also be exercised about weight-loss diets that require continued purchases of special prepackaged foods. Not only do these tend to be costly and over-processed, they may also prevent dieters from learning the food-selection and preparation skills essential to maintenance of weight loss. Further, dieters should consider whether they want to carry these special foods to work, restaurants, or homes of friends.

Concern has been expressed about weight-loss diet plans that do not include **exercise**, considered essential to long-term weight management. Some diets and supplements may be inadvisable for patients with special conditions or situations. In fact, use of the weight loss supplement **ephedra** was found to cause serious conditions such as **heart attack** and **stroke**. In 2003, the U.S. Food and Drug Administration (FDA) was considering controlling or banning the supplement. In short, most physician organizations see fad diets as distracting from learning how to achieve weight control over the long term through healthy lifestyle changes such as eating smaller, more balanced meals and exercising regularly.

Certain fad diets purporting to be official diets of groups such as the American Heart Association and the Mayo Clinic are in no way endorsed by those institutions. Patients thinking of starting such a diet should check with the institution to ensure its name has not been misappropriated by an unscrupulous practitioner.

Side effects

A wide range of side effects (some quite serious) can result from special diets, especially those that are nutritionally unbalanced. Further problems can arise if the dieter is taking high doses of dietary supplements. Food is essential to life, and improper **nutrition** can result in serious illness or death.

Research & general acceptance

It is agreed among traditional and complementary practitioners that many patients could substantially benefit from improved eating habits. Specialized diets have proved effective against a wide variety of conditions and diseases. However, dozens of unproved but widely publicized "fad diets" emerge each year, prompting widespread concerns about their usefulness, cost to the consumer, and their safety.

Training & certification

A wide variety of practitioners provide advice on dietary matters. These range from unregulated, uncertified alternative practitioners, to registered dietitians, medical doctors, and specialists. Nutritional advice can also be obtained from home economists and from college or university nutrition departments.

Resources

PERIODICALS

"American College of Preventive Medicine Weighs in Against Fad Diets." *Obesity and Diabetes Week* (March 17, 2003): 7.

"Atkins Diet Vindicated But Long-term Success Questionable." *Obesity, Fitness and Wellness Week* (June 14, 2003): 25.

Cerrato, Paul C. "AHA Questions High-protein Weight-loss Diets" *Contemporary OB/GYN* 46, no. 12 (December 2001): 107-112.

"Healthy Fat Superior to Low-fat diet for Long-term Weight Loss" *Obesity, Fitness and Wellness Week* (November 10, 2001): 2.

"High-protein Diets Risky for Bones and Kidneys." *Health Science* (Spring 2003): 9.

Kirn, Timothy F. "FDA Probes Ephedra, Proposes Warning Label (Risk of Heart Attack, Seizure, Stroke)." *Clinical Psychiatry News* (April 2003):49.

ORGANIZATIONS

American Dietetic Association. 216 West Jackson Blvd., Chicago, IL 60606-6995. (312) 899-0040. http://www.eatright.org.

David Helwig
Teresa G. Odle

Digestive enzymes

Description

Enzymes are catalysts for virtually every biological and chemical reaction in the body, and digestive enzymes are crucial for the breakdown of food into nutrients that the body can absorb. Digestive enzymes, of which a variety are herbs, are used to treat a number of digestive problems and other conditions.

General use

Digestive enzymes are used for relief of a number of digestive conditions, including:

- flatulence
- **heartburn**
- **diarrhea**
- spasms
- inflammation
- **constipation**
- gastroesophageal reflux
- peptic ulcers
- **indigestion**

Minor digestive complaints can be relieved by these mild digestive enzymes, rather than the more pharmacologically active ones.

Digestive enzymes also may be used to treat and to provide relief to other conditions, such as anorexia, **Crohn's disease**, ulcerative colitis, **parasitic infections**, cystic fibrosis, and **pancreatitis**.

Carminative herbs

Carminative herbs are considered to be mild and are rich in volatile oils, which have antibacterial properties. These herbs include **peppermint** (*Mentha spicata*), **ginger** (*Zingiber officinale*), **fennel** (*Foeniculum vulgare*), **anise** (*Pimpinella anisum*), and **lemon balm** (*Melissa officinalis*). Carminative herbs help to stimulate peristalsis, which is the wave-like action that pushes food through the digestive tract. These herbs can also help to relax the smooth muscle of the digestive tract, helping to reduce spasms. The antibacterial properties of the volatile oils aid in reducing **gas** pains that result from bacteria in the intestines acting on pieces of food that have not been digested fully.

Peppermint is one of the oldest medicinal herbs. Peppermint has three major actions in the body: it reduces **nausea** and **vomiting**, it encourages the liver to produce bile, and it clears the stomach of imbalanced bacteria. It is particularly useful for treating spastic colon, **irritable bowel syndrome** and diarrhea. Peppermint is also useful for reducing gas **pain** and indigestion.

Demulcent herbs can help ease heartburn, another bothersome digestive condition. These herbs are rich in mucilage, soothing irritated or inflamed tissue. Examples of demulcent herbs include **marsh mallow** root (*Althaea officinalis*), Irish moss (*Chondrus crispus*), and **slippery elm** (*Ulmus rubra*).

Herbs, known as **bitters**, can relieve constipation and assist the stomach in acid digestion. Bitter herbs stimulate bile production, and bile is the body's natural laxative. Taking bitters in a capsule or pill form will not work because in order for the liver to produce bile, the bitters must be tasted, not just ingested. Some examples of a bitter herb are **dandelion** root (*Taraxacum officinale*), ginger, and **aloe** (*Aloe vera*).

Ginger has been found to be particularly useful in treating nausea. In a 1988 study involving 80 Danish naval cadets who were unaccustomed to sailing heavy seas, ginger capsules were found to be very beneficial in reducing seasickness. Another study in 1990 at Bartholomew Hospital in London found ginger to be effective in reducing post-operative nausea. Ginger has stimulating and antiemetic properties that warm the stomach to reduce intestinal and gas pain.

Aloe can be a powerful laxative when used internally. It takes 10-15 hours to work in the body, so it is best used in the evening before bedtime. Do not use aloe for an extended period of time, or dependency can develop. Overuse of aloe can result in loss of intestinal tone. Overdoses of aloe can result in diarrhea, intestinal distress, and kidney problems, so caution should be taken when using this herb.

Astringent herbs are beneficial in slowing down diarrhea. These herbs contain tannin, a substance that causes protein in body tissues to tighten up. When an astringent herb is taken, the proteins in the digestive tract tighten up to form a protective barrier that reduces fluid and electrolyte loss.

Preparations

A few suggestions apply before using any of the various herbal supplements to aid digestion. It is best not to overeat, and snacking between meals on anything other than fruit should be avoided. Increase the consumption of fruit, vegetables and whole grains, and try to decrease the amount of fatty foods, red meat, dairy products, nuts, and nut butters from the diet. Try to relax while eating, chew food 10–20 times, and avoid distractions while eating, such as reading or watching television. Drink at least eight glasses of water each day.

Many of these herbs make delicious teas, and are commonly available as packaged teas. Those who wish to make their own tea should try steeping one teaspoon of dry herb per cup of boiled water for five to 10 minutes. Be sure to cover the tea so that the volatile oils do not evaporate. An Indian custom that is also helpful for digestion is to keep fennel or anise seed available at the table to pass around following a meal.

Precautions

There have been very few scientific studies to prove either the adverse or the beneficial health effects of the 1,500-plus herbal products that are available throughout the United States. Furthermore, under the Dietary Supplement Health and Education Act of 1994, herbal products are not required to be proven safe before they are marketed. After the product is marketed, the U.S. Food and Drug Administration (FDA) must prove the dietary supplement unsafe before it can be removed from the shelves. Many people associate the term "natural" with "safe," and that is not always the case. Anyone taking herbal products of any kind should be certain to discuss this with their physician. As is the case with some prescription medications, dependency on some herbal supplements is possible. No herbal supplements should be taken for extended periods of time without discussing this with a physician first.

Herbal preparations can vary widely from one brand to another, and within the same brand from one purchase to the next, making inconsistency in the concentration of ingredients a potential risk. Anyone using herbal products should be careful and try to use well-known brands because these products are largely unregulated.

Side effects & interactions

Anyone taking herbal products should always discuss this with their physician. Herbs have the potential to interact with any prescription medication, as well as with other herbs. So, persons wishing to take digestive enzymes should consult a physician.

Resources

PERIODICALS

Starbuck, J. "3 Herbs for Good Digestion: Ginger, Peppermint and Aloe." *Better Nutrition* (1999): 44-49.

Sullivan, K. "Oh, What a Relief It Is." *Vegetarian Times* (1996): 94-99.

ORGANIZATIONS

Alternative Medicine Foundation, Inc. 5411 W. Cedar Lane, Suite 205-A, Bethesda, MD 20814. (301) 581-0116.

American Botanical Council. P.O. Box 144345, Austin, TX 78714-4345. (512) 926-4900. Fax: (512) 926-2345. http://www.herbalgram.org.

National Center for Complementary and Alternative Medicine. P.O. Box 8218, Silver Spring, MD 20907-8218. (888) 644-6226.

Kim Sharp

Digitalis purpurea see **Foxglove**

Diverticulitis

Definition

Diverticulitis refers to the development of inflammation and infection in one or more *diverticula*. Diverticula are outpouchings or bulges which occur when the inner, lining layer of the large intestine (colon) bulges out (herniates) through the outer, muscular layer. The presence of diverticula indicates a condition called diverticulosis.

Description

Diverticula tend to occur most frequently in the last segment of the large intestine, the sigmoid colon. They occur with decreasing frequency as an examination moves toward the beginning of the large intestine. The chance of developing diverticula increases with age, so that by the age of 50, about 20–50% of all people will have some diverticula. By the age of 90, virtually everyone will have developed some diverticula. Most diverticula measure 3–30 mm in diameter. Larger diverticula, termed giant diverticula, are quite infrequent, but may measure as large as 15 cm in diameter.

The great majority of people with diverticulosis will remain symptom-free. Many diverticula are quite accidentally discovered during examinations for other conditions of the intestinal tract.

Causes & symptoms

Diverticula are believed to be caused by overly forceful contractions of the muscular wall of the large intestine. As areas of this wall spasm, they become weaker and weaker, allowing the inner lining to bulge through. The anatomically weakest areas of the intestinal wall occur next to the blood vessels that course through the wall, so diverticula commonly occur in these locations.

Diverticula are most common among the populations of the developed countries of the West (North America, Great Britain, and northern and western Europe). This is thought to be due these countries' **diets**, which tend to be quite low in fiber. A diet low in fiber results in the production of smaller volumes of stool. In order to move this smaller stool along the colon and out of the rectum, the colon must narrow itself significantly, and does so by contracting down forcefully. This causes an increase in pressure, which, over time, weakens the muscular wall of the intestine and allows diverticular pockets to develop.

Diverticulitis is believed to occur when a hardened piece of stool, undigested food, and bacteria (called a fecalith) becomes lodged in a diverticulum. This blockage interferes with the blood supply to the area, and infection sets in.

Diverticulitis is three times more likely to occur in the left side of the large intestine. Since most diverticula are located in the sigmoid colon (the final segment of the large intestine which empties into the rectum), most diverticulitis also takes place in the sigmoid. The elderly have the most serious complications from diverticulitis, although very severe **infections** can also occur in patients under the age of 50. Men are three times more likely than women to be stricken with diverticulitis.

An individual with diverticulitis will experience **pain** (especially in the lower left side of the abdomen) and **fever**. In response to the infection and the irritation of nearby tissues within the abdomen, the abdominal muscles may begin to spasm. About 25% of all patients with diverticulitis will have some rectal bleeding, al-

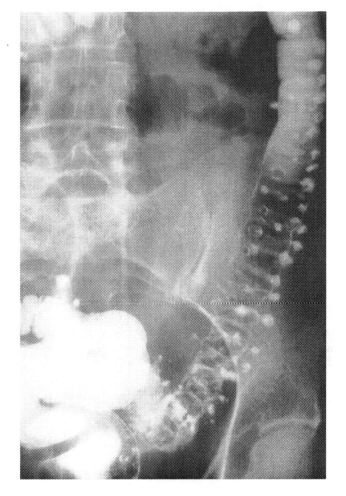

A barium study x ray showing colonic diverticulosis. *(Custom Medical Stock Photo. Reproduced by permission.)*

though this rarely becomes severe. Walled-off pockets of infection, called abscesses, may appear within the wall of the intestine, or even on the exterior surface of the intestine. When a diverticulum weakens sufficiently, and is filled to bulging with infected pus, a perforation in the intestinal wall may develop. When the infected contents of the intestine spill out into the abdomen, a severe infection called peritonitis may occur. Peritonitis is an infection and inflammation of the lining of the abdominal cavity, the peritoneum. Other complications of diverticulitis include the formation of abnormal connections, called fistulas, between two organs which normally do not connect (for example, the intestine and the bladder), and scarring outside of the intestine that squeezes off and obstructs a portion of the intestine.

Diagnosis

When diverticula are suspected because a patient begins to have sudden rectal bleeding, the location of the bleeding can be studied by performing angiography. Angiography involves inserting a tiny tube (catheter) through an artery in the leg, and moving it up into one of the major arteries of the gastrointestinal system. A dye (contrast medium) which will show up on x-ray films, is injected into the catheter, and the area of bleeding is located by looking for an area where the contrast is leaking into the interior (lumen) of the intestine.

A procedure called colonoscopy provides another method for examining the colon and locating the site of bleeding. In colonoscopy, a small, flexible scope (colonoscope) is inserted through the rectum and into the intestine. A fiber-optic camera that projects to a nearby television screen is mounted in the colonoscope, which allows the physician to view the interior of the colon and locate the source of bleeding.

Diagnosis of diverticulitis is not difficult in patients with previously diagnosed diverticulosis. The presence of abdominal pain and fever in such an individual would make the suspicion of diverticulitis quite high. Examination of the abdomen will usually reveal tenderness to touch, with the patient's abdominal muscles contracting strongly to protect the tender area. During a rectal exam, a doctor may be able to feel an abnormal mass. Touching this mass may prove painful to the patient.

When a practitioner is suspicious of diverticulitis as the cause for the patient's symptoms, he or she will most likely avoid the types of tests usually used to diagnose gastrointestinal disorders. These include barium enema and colonoscopy (although colonoscopy may have been used earlier to diagnose the diverticulosis). The concern is that the increased pressure exerted on the intestine during these exams may increase the likelihood of intestinal perforation. After medical treatment for the diverticulitis, these examinations may be performed in order to learn the extent of the patient's disease.

Treatment

Treatment for uncomplicated diverticulitis usually requires hospitalization, but some physicians will agree to try treatment at home for very mildly ill patients. These patients will be put on a liquid diet and receive oral antibiotics. Although **relaxation**, **guided imagery**, and **acupuncture** treatment may be helpful in alleviating pain symptoms, a course of antibiotics is necessary to treat the infection itself.

An infusion of herbs with anti-inflammatory and soothing properties, such as **Mexican yam** (*Dioscorea villosa*), German **chamomile** (*Matricaria recutita*), **marsh mallow** (*Althaea officinalis*), and calamus (*Acorus calamus*, or sweet flag) may be helpful in treating the inflammation of diverticulitis. **Ginger** (*Zingiber*

officinale) can also be helpful in relieving gastrointestinal **gas** that may be symptomatic of the disorder.

Allopathic treatment

"Resting the bowel" is a mainstay of treatment, and involves keeping the patient from eating or sometimes even drinking anything by mouth. Therefore, a patient hospitalized for diverticulitis will need to receive fluids through a needle in the vein (intravenous or IV fluids). Antibiotics will also be administered through the IV. In cases of severe bleeding (hemorrhaging), blood transfusion may be necessary. Medications that encourage clotting may also be required.

While there are almost no situations when uncomplicated diverticulosis requires surgery, giant diverticula always require removal. This is due to the very high chance of infection and perforation of these diverticula. When giant diverticula are diagnosed, the usual treatment involves removing that portion of the intestine.

The various complications of diverticulitis need to be treated aggressively, because the death rate from problems such as perforation and peritonitis is quite high. Abscesses can be drained of their infected contents by inserting a needle through the skin of the abdomen and into the **abscess**. When this is unsuccessful, open abdominal surgery will be required to remove the piece of the intestine containing the abscess. Fistulas require surgical repair, including the removal of the length of intestine containing the origin of the fistula, followed by immediate reconnection of the two free ends of intestine. Peritonitis requires open surgery. The entire abdominal cavity is cleaned by being irrigated (washed) with a warmed sterile saltwater solution, and the damaged piece of intestine is removed. Obstructions require immediate surgery to prevent perforation. Massive, uncontrollable bleeding, while rare, may require removal of part or all of the large intestine.

During any of these types of operations, the surgeon must make an important decision regarding the quantity of intestine that must be removed. When the amount of intestine removed is great, it may be necessary to perform a colostomy. A colostomy involves pulling the end of the remaining intestine through the abdominal wall, to the outside. This bit of intestine is then fashioned so that a bag can be fit over it. The patient's waste (feces) collect in the bag, because the intestine no longer connects with the rectum. This colostomy may be temporary, in which case another operation will be required to reconnect the intestine, after some months of substantial healing has occurred. Other times, the colostomy will need to be permanent, and the patient will have to adjust to living permanently with the colostomy bag. Most people with colostomies are able to go on with a very active life.

Occasionally, a patient will have such severe diverticular disease that a surgeon recommends planning ahead, and schedules removal of a portion of the colon. This is done to avoid the high risk of surgery performed after a complication has set in. Certain developments will identify those patients who are at very high risk of experiencing dangerous complications, such as those with a history of diverticulitis.

Surgery for chronic (recurring) diverticulitis remains controversial. Some surgeons say that surgery prevents recurrence of problems, while others say it does not. In 2002, a report to family physicians said that elective surgery in cases of severe diverticulitis produces good outcomes and low rates of recurrence. However, patients should be cautioned about possible postoperative complications such as bleeding, abscess, and bowel obstruction. The risk of depends on functional bowel symptoms before surgery.

Expected results

The prognosis for people with diverticula is excellent, with only 20% of such patients ever seeking any medical help for their condition.

While diverticulitis can be a difficult and painful disease, it is usually quite treatable. Prognosis is worse for individuals who have other medical problems, particularly those requiring the use of steroid medications, which increase the chances of developing a serious infection. Prognosis is also worse in the elderly.

Prevention

While there is no absolutely certain way to prevent the development of diverticula, it is believed that high-fiber diets may help. Foods that are recommended for their high fiber content include whole grain breads and cereals, and all types of fruits and vegetables. Most experts suggest that individuals take in 20–35 grams of fiber daily. If this is not possible to achieve through diet, an individual may supplement with fiber products that are mixed into juice or water.

Resources

BOOKS
Hoffman, David. *The Complete Illustrated Herbal.* New York: Barnes & Noble Books, 1999.
Isselbacher, Kurt J., and Alan Epstein. "Diverticular, Vascular, and Other Disorders of the Intestine and Peritoneum." In *Harrison's Principles of Internal Medicine.* Edited by Anthony S. Fauci, et al. New York: McGraw-Hill, 1998.

PERIODICALS
Cerda, James J., et al. "Diverticulitis: Current Management Strategies." *Patient Care* 31, no. 12 (July 15, 1997): 170+.

> ## KEY TERMS
> **Angiography**—X ray imaging of the arteries in a particular part of the body. Angiography is often performed in order to localize internal bleeding.
>
> **Bowel obstruction**—A blockage in the intestine that prevents the normal flow of waste down the length of the intestine.
>
> **Colonoscopy**—Examination of an area of the gastrointestinal tract by putting a lighted scope, usually bearing a fiber-optic camera, into the rectum, and passing it through the intestine.
>
> **Colostomy**—A procedure performed when a large quantity of intestine is removed. The end piece of the intestine leading to the rectum is closed.
>
> **Fistula**—An abnormal connection formed between two organs which usually have no connection at all.
>
> **Sigmoid colon**—The final portion of the large intestine which empties into the rectum.

Cunningham, Mark A., et al. "Medical Versus Surgical Management of Diverticulitis in Patients Under Age 40." *American Journal of Surgery* 174, no. 6 (December 1997): 733+.
"Diet for Diverticulosis." *Consumer Reports on Health* 8, no. 11 (November 1996): 132.
"Keeping Diverticulosis Silent." *Berkeley Wellness Letter* 12, no. 4 (January 1996): 6+.
Walling, Anne D. "Surgical Treatment of Severe Diverticular Disease." *American Family Physician* (June 1, 2002): 2366.

ORGANIZATIONS
National Digestive Diseases Information Clearinghouse. 2 Information Way, Bethesda, MD 20892-3570. (301)654-3810. http://www.niddk.nih.gov/health/digest/nddic.htm.

Paula Ford-Martin
Teresa G. Odle

Diverticulosis *see* **Diverticulitis**

Dizziness

Definition

Dizziness is classified into three categories—vertigo, syncope, and nonsyncope nonvertigo. Each category has a characteristic set of symptoms, all related to the sense of balance. In general, syncope is defined by a brief loss of consciousness (fainting) or by dimmed vision and feeling uncoordinated, confused, and lightheaded. Many people experience a sensation like syncope when they stand up too fast. Vertigo is the feeling that either the individual or the surroundings are spinning. This sensation is like being on a spinning amusement park ride. Individuals with nonsyncope nonvertigo dizziness feel as though they cannot keep their balance. This sensation may become worse with movement.

Description

The brain coordinates information from the eyes, the inner ear, and the body's senses to maintain balance. If any of these sources of information is disrupted, the brain may not be able to compensate. For example, people sometimes experience **motion sickness** because the information from their body tells the brain that they are sitting still, but information from the eyes indicates that they are moving. The messages don't correspond and dizziness results.

Vision and the body's senses are the most important systems for maintaining balance, but problems in the inner ear are the most frequent cause of dizziness. The inner ear, also called the vestibular system, contains fluid that helps to fine tune the information the brain receives from the eyes and the body. When fluid volume or pressure in the inner ear changes, information about balance is altered. The discrepancy gives conflicting messages to the brain about balance and induces dizziness.

Certain medical conditions can cause dizziness because they affect the systems that maintain balance. For example, the inner ear is very sensitive to changes in blood flow. Because such medical conditions as high blood pressure or low blood sugar can affect blood flow, these conditions are frequently accompanied by dizziness. Circulation disorders are the most common causes of dizziness. Other causes are head injuries, ear **infections**, **allergies**, and nervous system disorders.

Dizziness often disappears without treatment or with treatment of the underlying problem, but it can be long-term or chronic. According to the National Institutes of Health, 42% of Americans will seek medical help for dizziness at some point in their lives. The costs may exceed a billion dollars and account for five million visits to physicians annually. Episodes of dizziness increase with age. Among people aged 75 or older, dizziness is the most frequent reason for seeing a doctor.

Causes & symptoms

Careful attention to symptoms can help determine the underlying cause of the dizziness. The underlying problems may be benign and easily treated, or they may be dangerous and require intensive therapy. Not all cases of dizziness can be linked to a specific cause. More than one type of dizziness can be experienced at the same time and symptoms may be mixed. Episodes of dizziness may last for a few seconds or for days. The length of an episode is related to the underlying cause.

The symptoms of syncope include dimmed vision, loss of coordination, confusion, lightheadedness, and sweating. These symptoms can lead to a brief loss of consciousness or fainting. They are related to a reduced flow of blood to the brain; they often occur when a person is standing up and can be relieved by sitting or lying down. Vertigo is characterized by a sensation of spinning or turning, accompanied by **nausea**, **vomiting**, ringing in the ears, **headache**, or **fatigue**. An individual may have trouble walking, remaining coordinated, or keeping balance. Nonsyncope nonvertigo dizziness is characterized by a feeling of being off balance that becomes worse if the individual tries moving or performing detail-intense tasks.

A person may experience dizziness for many reasons. Syncope is associated with low blood pressure, heart problems, and disorders in the autonomic nervous system, which controls such involuntary functions as breathing. Syncope may also arise from emotional distress, **pain**, and other reactions to outside stressors. Nonsyncope nonvertigo dizziness may be caused by rapid breathing, low blood sugar, or **migraine headache**, as well as by more serious medical conditions.

Vertigo is often associated with inner ear problems called vestibular disorders. A particularly intense vestibular disorder, **Ménière's disease**, interferes with the volume of fluid in the inner ear. This disease, which affects approximately one in every 1,000 people, causes intermittent vertigo over the course of weeks, months, or years. Ménière's disease is often accompanied by ringing or buzzing in the ear, **hearing loss**, and a feeling that the ear is blocked. Damage to the nerve that leads from the ear to the brain can also cause vertigo. Such damage can result from head injury or a tumor. An acoustic neuroma, for example, is a benign tumor that wraps around the nerve. Vertigo can also be caused by disorders of the central nervous system and the circulation, such as hardening of the arteries (arteriosclerosis), **stroke**, or **multiple sclerosis**.

Some medications cause changes in blood pressure or blood flow. These medications can cause dizziness in some people. Prescription medications carry warnings of such side effects, but common drugs such as **caffeine** or nicotine can also cause dizziness. Certain antibiotics can damage the inner ear and cause hearing loss and dizziness.

Diet may cause dizziness. The role of diet may be direct, as through alcohol intake. It may be also be indirect, as through arteriosclerosis caused by a high-fat diet. Some people experience a slight dip in blood sugar and mild dizziness if they miss a meal, but this condition is rarely dangerous unless the person is diabetic. Food sensitivities or allergies can also be a cause of dizziness. Such chronic conditions as **heart disease** and serious acute problems such as seizures and strokes can cause dizziness. These conditions, however, usually exhibit other characteristic symptoms.

Diagnosis

During the initial medical examination, an individual with dizziness should provide a detailed description of the type of dizziness experienced, when it occurs, and how often each episode lasts. A diary of symptoms may help to track this information. The patient should report any symptoms that accompany the dizziness, such as ringing in the ear or nausea, any recent injury or infection, and any medication taken.

The examiner will check the patient's blood pressure, pulse, respiration, and body temperature as well as the ear, nose, and throat. The sense of balance is assessed by moving the individual's head to various positions or by tilt-table testing. In tilt-table testing, the person lies on a table that can be shifted into different positions and reports any dizziness that occurs.

Further tests may be indicated by the initial examination. Hearing tests help assess ear damage. X rays, computed tomography scan (CT scan), and magnetic resonance imaging (MRI) can pinpoint evidence of nerve damage, tumors, or other structural problems. If a vestibular disorder is suspected, a technique called electronystagmography (ENG) may be used. ENG measures the electrical impulses generated by eye movements. Blood tests can determine diabetes, high **cholesterol**, and other diseases. In some cases, a heart evaluation may be useful. Despite thorough testing, however, an underlying cause cannot always be determined.

Doctors caution that childhood syncope (fainting), although rarely serious, can indicate a serious cardiac. If the fainting is abrupt or happens with exertion, it may indicate a more serious problem.

Treatment

Because dizziness may arise from serious conditions, it is advisable to seek medical treatment. Alternative treatments can often be used alongside conventional medicine without conflict. Potentially beneficial therapies include nutritional therapy, herbal remedies, **homeopathy**, **aromatherapy**, **osteopathy**, **acupuncture**, **acupressure**, and **relaxation** techniques.

Nutritional therapy

To prevent dizziness, nutritionists often advise eating smaller but more frequent meals and avoiding caffeine, nicotine, alcohol, foods high in fat or sugar, or any substances that cause allergic reactions. A low-salt diet may also be helpful to some people. Nutritionists may also recommend certain dietary supplements:

• **Magnesium** citrate, aspartate or maleate: for dizziness caused by magnesium deficiency.

• B-complex vitamins, especially **vitamin B$_{12}$**: for dizziness caused by deficiency of these essential vitamins.

Herbal remedies

The following herbs have been used to treat dizziness symptoms:

• Ginger: for treatment of dizziness caused by nausea.

• Ginkgo biloba: may decrease dizziness by increasing blood flow to the brain.

Homeopathy

Homeopathic therapies can work very effectively for dizziness, and are especially applicable when no organic cause can be identified. They are chosen according to the patient's specific symptom profile:

• Aconite: for feeling light-headed from postural hypotension (getting up too quickly)

• Coccolus: for motion sickness or syncope

• *Conium maculatum:* for feeling dizzy while looking at rapidly-moving images.

• Gelsemium: for feeling light-headed and out of balance, often associated with **influenza** or stage fright.

• Petroleum: for dizziness upon standing up too fast and headache before and after a storm.

Aromatherapy

Aromatherapists recommend a warm bath scented with **essential oils** of **lavender**, geranium, and sandalwood as treatment for dizziness. This therapy can have a calming effect on the nervous system.

Osteopathy

An osteopath or chiropractor may suggest manipulations or adjustments of the head, jaw, neck, and lower back to relieve pressure on the inner ear.

Acupressure

Acupressure may be able to improve circulation and decrease the symptoms of vertigo. The Neck Release, which involves pressing on five pairs of points on the shoulder blades and neck, is helpful for dizziness associated with migraine headaches.

Relaxation techniques

Relaxation techniques, such as **yoga**, **meditation**, and **massage therapy** for relieving tension, are popularly recommended methods for reducing **stress**.

Allopathic treatment

Treatment of dizziness is determined by the underlying cause. If an individual has a cold or influenza, a few days of bed rest is usually adequate to resolve dizziness. Other causes of dizziness, such as mild vestibular system damage, may resolve without medical treatment. If dizziness continues, drug therapy may be required to treat such underlying illnesses as high blood pressure, arteriosclerosis, nervous conditions or diabetes. A physician may also prescribe antibiotics if ear infections are suspected. Selective serotonin reuptake inhibitors (SSRIs) have recently been shown to relieve dizziness in patients who have psychiatric symptoms. When other measures have failed, surgery may be suggested to relieve pressure on the inner ear. If the dizziness is not treatable by drugs, surgery, or other means, physical therapy may be used and the patient may be taught coping mechanisms for the problem.

Expected results

The outcome of treatment depends on the cause of dizziness. Controlling or curing the underlying factors usually relieves the dizziness itself. In some cases, the symptoms disappear without treatment. In a few cases, dizziness can become a permanent disabling condition.

Prevention

Most people learn through experience that certain activities will make them dizzy and they learn to avoid them. For example, if reading in a car produces motion sickness, reading should be postponed until after the trip. Changes in diet can also cut down on episodes of dizziness in susceptible people. For example, persons with Ménière's disease may avoid episodes of vertigo by leaving salt, alcohol, and caffeine out of their **diets**. Reducing blood cholesterol can help diminish arteriosclerosis and indirectly treat dizziness. Daily multiple vitamin and mineral supplements may help prevent dizziness caused by deficiencies of these essential nutrients. Relaxation techniques can help ward off tension and **anxiety** that can cause dizziness.

Some cases of dizziness cannot be prevented. Acoustic neuromas, for example, are not predictable or preventable.

KEY TERMS

Acoustic neuroma—A benign tumor that grows on the nerve leading from the inner ear to the brain. As the tumor grows, it exerts pressure on the inner ear and causes severe vertigo.

Autonomic nervous system—The part of the nervous system that controls such involuntary body functions as breathing and heart beat.

Electronystagmography—A method for measuring the electricity generated by eye movements. Electrodes are placed on the skin around the eye and the individual is subjected to a variety of stimuli so that the quality of eye movements can be assessed.

Ménière's disease—A disease of the labyrinth in the ear, characterized by dizziness, hearing loss, ringing in the ears, and nausea.

Syncope—Dizziness or brief loss of consciousness resulting from an inadequate flow of oxygenated blood to the brain.

Vertigo—Dizziness associated with a sensation of whirling or spinning.

Vestibular system—The area of the inner ear that helps maintain balance.

Alternative approaches designed to rebalance the body's energy flow, such as acupuncture and constitutional homeopathy, may be helpful in cases where the cause of dizziness cannot be pinpointed.

Resources

BOOKS

Cameron, Myra. *Lifetime Encyclopedia of Natural Remedies.* Paramus, NJ: Prentice Hall, 1993.

Yardley, Lucy. *Vertigo and Dizziness.* New York: Routledge, 1994.

Zand, Janet, Allan N. Spreen, and James B. LaValle. *Smart Medicine for Healthier Living: A Practical A-Z Reference to Natural and Conventional Treatments for Adults.* Garden City Park, NY: Avery Publishing Group, 1999.

PERIODICALS

Ohnson, Kate. "Fainting Usually is Benign, but it can be Fatal." *Pediatric News* (July 2002):25.

PERIODICALS

"SSRIs Relieve Dizziness in Psyciatric Patients." *Critical Care Alert* (August 2002):2.

ORGANIZATIONS

Ménière's Network. 2000 Church St., P.O. Box 111, Nashville, TN 37236. (800) 545-4327.

The Vestibular Disorders Association. P.O. Box 4467, Portland, OR 97208-4467. (503) 229-7705. http://www.teleport.com/~veda/.

Mai Tran
Teresa G. Odle

Dolomite

Description

Physical characteristics

Dolomite is a common mineral. It is also known as $CaMg(CO_3)_2$ and is a type of compact limestone consisting of a **calcium magnesium** carbonate. In combination with calcite and aragonite, dolomite makes up approximately 2% of the earth's crust. The mineral was first described by and then named after the French mineralogist and geologist Deodat de Dolomieu (1750–1801).

Dolomite is a fairly soft mineral that occurs as crystals as well as in large sedimentary rock beds several hundred feet thick. The crystals—usually rhombohedral in shape—are transparent to translucent and are colorless, white, reddish-white, brownish-white, gray, or sometimes pink. In powdered form, dolomite dissolves readily with effervescence in warm acids.

Although rock beds containing dolomite are found throughout the world, the most notable quarries are located in the Midwestern United States; Ontario, Canada; Switzerland; Pamplona, Spain; and Mexico.

Formation

Although dolomite does not form on the surface of the earth at the present time, massive layers of dolomite can be found in ancient rocks. Dolomite is one of the few sedimentary rocks that undergoes a significant mineralogical change after it is deposited. Dolomite rocks are originally deposited as calcite/aragonite-rich limestone, but during a process called diagenesis, the calcite and/or aragonite is transformed into dolomite. Magnesium-rich ground water containing a significant amount of salt is thought to be essential to dolomite formation. Thus, warm, tropical marine environments are considered the best sources of dolomite formation.

Chemical components

Dolomite is composed of 52.06% oxygen, 13.03% carbon, 13.18% magnesium, and 21.73% calcium. **Iron** and **manganese** carbonates, barium, and lead are sometimes present as impurities.

General use

Dolomite is commonly used in a variety of products. A few of these are listed below:

- antacids (neutralizes stomach acid)
- base for face creams, baby powders, or toothpaste
- calcium/magnesium nutritional supplements for animals and humans
- ceramic glazes on china and other dinnerware (dolomite is used as source of magnesia and calcia)
- fertilizers (dolomite added as soil nutrient)
- glass (used for high refractive optical glass)
- gypsum impressions from which dental plates are made (magnesium carbonate)
- mortar and cement
- plastics, rubbers, and adhesives

Although calcium carbonate (the kind found in dolomite) has the highest concentration of calcium by weight (40%) and is the most common preparation available, this form of calcium is relatively insoluble and can be difficult to break down in the body. In contrast, calcium citrate, although containing about half as much calcium by weight (21%), is a more soluble form. Since calcium citrate does not require gastric acid for absorption, it is considered a better source of supplemental calcium, particularly for the elderly, whose stomach acid secretions are decreased.

Calcium supplements offer many benefits and recent research even reports that calcium supplements can help prevent formation of **kidney stones** when combined with a fairly low animal protein, low salt diet. Doctors once advised a low-calcium diet to prevent kidney stones.

Preparations

Dolomite is generally ground into coarse or finely-grained powder and made into calcium/magnesium capsules or antacids for human consumption. The powdered form is also used in animal feed, fertilizers, and a variety of other applications.

Precautions

Nutritional supplements

Not all commercially prepared calcium supplements are tested for heavy metal contamination. In 1981 the Federal Drug Administration (FDA) cautioned the public to limit the intake of calcium supplements made from dolomite or bone meal (ground up cow's bones) because of potentially hazardous lead levels. Additional studies show that other calcium supplements, such as carbonates and various chelates, may also contain hazardous amounts of lead.

When purchasing calcium supplements, products marked as purified (especially those made from dolomite, bone meal, or oyster shells) or those containing the USP (*United States Pharmacopoeia*) symbol are considered the safest. The symbol means that the vitamin and mineral manufacturer's product has voluntarily met the USP's criteria for quality, strength, and purity.

New research also encourages consumers to tell their doctors when they take antacids and calcium supplements so that physicians can watch for possible side effects or interactions with medications. Some antacids can cause side effects that eventually put patients at risk for serious problems. If a patient has a complicating problem like renal dysfunction, he or she can suffer from aluminum toxicity from certain antacids.

Ceramic glazes

Another potential health risk associated with dolomite arises from storing food in or eating or drinking from dinnerware or cups made with glazes containing dolomite. Although it is not possible to detect a lead glaze on china with the naked eye, corroded glaze, or a dusty or chalky, gray residue on the glaze after the piece has been washed is a good indication of lead content. Although high lead toxicity is rare, trace amounts may be present. If possible, it is best to purchase dinnerware that is labeled lead-free. Also, stoneware, unless painted with decorations on the surface, are normally coated with a material that contains no lead. Glass dishes, with the exception of leaded glass and glass painted with decorations or decals, are also considered safe.

The problem is intensified if the food or beverage consumed is acidic, since acid increases lead leaching. Although other additives in glazes may contribute to the lead content (such as lead oxide or cadmium) leaching out, dolomite is a potential cause for lead toxicity.

Glazes on bathtubs also may contain harmful amounts of lead, which may leach out into the bathwater, especially if the glaze is worn. Information regarding lead content can be obtained from the manufacturer. Lead testing kits are also available by mail order or at most home and garden centers.

Fertilizers and animal feed

Dolomite and bone meal in fertilizers and animal feed may contaminate the soil, animals, and humans with lead and other toxic metals.

Side effects

Indirect side effects may occur if more than the recommended dosage of any calcium supplement is taken over an extended period of time. If more than 2,000 mg/day of calcium is consumed, gastrointestinal problems can occur.

Some of the short-term symptoms of low-level lead exposure (which is particularly harmful to the young and elderly) include:

- decreased appetite
- stomachache
- sleeplessness
- constipation
- vomiting
- diarrhea
- fatigue
- irritability
- headaches

Some of the long-term effects of low-level lead exposure include:

- learning disabilities
- brain damage
- loss of IQ points
- attention deficit disorder
- hyperactive behavior
- criminal or antisocial behavior
- neurological problems

Interactions

Research on the interactions of dolomite with other drugs, vitamins, minerals, or foods is limited.

Resources

BOOKS

Deer, W. A., R. A. Howie, and J. Zussman. "Dolomite." In *An Introduction to Dolomite*. Essex, England: Longman Group, 1966.

Haas, Elson M. "Calcium." In *Staying Healthy With Nutrition*. Berkeley, CA: Celestial Arts, 1992.

PERIODICALS

"Unrestricted Calcium Intake Protects Against Recurrent Kidney Stones Better than a Restricted Calcium Diet." *Environmental Nutrition* (March 2002): 3.

Wooten, James W. "Know Your Antacids—and Who's Taking Them." *RN* (March 2002): 92.

ORGANIZATIONS

National Lead Information Center. 801 Roeder Road, Suite 600, Silver Spring, MD 20910. (800) 424-LEAD. <http://www.epa.gov/lead/nlic.htm>.

National Osteoporosis Foundation. 1232 22nd Street NW, Washington, DC 20037-1292. (202) 223-2226. <http://www.nof.org>.

Genevieve Slomski
Teresa G. Odle

Dong quai

Description

Dong quai (*Angelica sinensis*), also called Chinese **angelica**, is a member of the Umbelliferae (Apiaceae), or carrot family. This Oriental medicinal herb is sometimes called the empress of herbs, or female ginseng.

Dong quai grows best in such damp places as moist meadows, river banks, and mountain ravines. It may be biennial or perennial. The bitter-sweet root, described by some herbalists as resembling carved ivory, is used medicinally. Dong quai, variously known as dang gui or tang kuei, produces a round, hollow, grooved stem that grows as high as 7 ft. The lower leaves are large and tri-pinnate, each further divided into two or three leaflets. The smaller upper leaves are pinnate, which means that the leaflets are arranged in opposite rows along the leaf stalk. The leaves of dong quai resemble those of carrot, celery, or **parsley** and emerge from dilated sheaths surrounding a bluish-colored stem that is branched at the top. Honey-scented, greenish-white flowers grow in large compound flat-topped clusters and bloom from May to August.

General use

Dong quai is one of the most extensively researched Chinese medicinal herbs. It is well known as a female remedy thought to benefit women throughout the menstrual cycle and during the transition to **menopause**. A recent study indicates that dong quai is a popular herbal remedy among women being treated for **ovarian cancer**. Dong quai has been used in China for thousands of years to treat ailments of the female reproductive system and as a tonic herb to treat **fatigue**, mild **anemia**, high blood pressure and poor circulation in both men and women. Chinese herbalists prepare dong quai in combination with other herbs, including **astragalus** (*Astragalus membranaceus*) as a fatigue tonic, **mugwort** (*Artemesia vulgaris*), bai shao (white peony), chai hu (bupleurum root),and rou gui (**cinnamon bark**) in medicinal formulas for women. Secondary herbs are used to enhance the action of the primary ingredient or to provide additional properties that work synergistically with the primary ingredient. Research in the United States indicates that dong quai has no demonstrable estrogen-like effect on menopausal women when it is used alone. However, other research has shown that dong quai, when used in combination with other herbs, resulted in a reduction of the severity of **hot flashes**, vaginal dryness, **insomnia**, and mood changes. Dong quai should not be regarded as a replacement for natural estrogen. Its unique mechanism of action reportedly promotes the synthesis of natural progesterone, a hormone whose production declines during menopause. Dong quai's ability to relieve menstrual problems has been attributed to its muscle-relaxing properties and its ability to quiet spasms in the internal organs. Dong quai has a tonic effect on all female reproductive organs and increases blood flow to the uterus. It acts to increase vaginal secretions and to nourish vaginal tissue. Dong quai root's analgesic properties help diminish uterine **pain** and have been found to be as much as 1.7 times as effective as aspirin. The herb has also been useful in the treatment of migraine headaches.

One recent Western study, however, has called into question the value of dong quai for treating menopausal symptoms. The authors of the study found that **black cohosh** appears to be a more effective herbal remedy for hot flashes and other symptoms associated with menopause.

Research in China indicates that dong quai stimulates production of the red blood cells that carry oxygen throughout the body. Its sedative properties relieve emotional distress and irritability. It is used to treat mild anemia and as a liver tonic. The herb is beneficial to the endocrine and circulatory systems, promoting healthful blood circulation. Its laxative properties ease **constipation**, particularly in the elderly. This beneficial herb has also been proven effective against certain fungi, such as *Candida albicans*, the primary cause of vaginal **yeast infection**. Dong quai also helps to dissolve **blood clots**.

Dong quai contains high amounts of **vitamin E, iron**, cobalt, and other vitamins and minerals important to women, including **niacin, magnesium, potassium**, and vitamins A, C, and B$_{12}$. The plant contains numerous

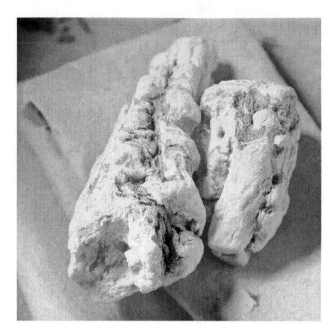

Dong quai root. *(© Steven Mark Needham/Getty Images. Reproduced by permission.)*

phytochemicals, including coumarins, phytosterols, polysaccharides, and flavonoids.

European angelica (*A. archangelica*) stimulates secretion of gastric juices and has been used to treat digestive problems, flatulence, and loss of appetite. The root of European angelica has sometimes been used in cases of prolonged labor or to treat problems with retention of the placenta after **childbirth**.

American angelica (*A. atropurpurea*) has also been used by some herbalists for menstrual complaints, though the Chinese dong quai is most often used in formulas for women.

Preparations

The medicinal part of the angelica plant is the root. Dong quai root can be prepared as an infusion or decoction, tincture, tablet, or capsule. It is also available dried, either whole, diced, or sliced. The herb is nontoxic, but recent findings suggest caution in using it over an extended period of time. The dried root may be chewed in quarter inch segments two to three times daily, up to three to four grams per day.

Infusion or decoction: Research indicates that extracts of dong quai that retain the volatile constituents act to raise blood pressure and relax uterine muscles. An infusion of the root, steeped in hot **water**, retains the volatile constituents and is useful to treat **dysmenorrhea** and to quiet uterine spasm. For amenorrhea, where stimulation of the uterine muscles is sought, a decoction is the indicated.

Simmer the root in water to evaporate the volatile constituents. Most Chinese herbalists use dong quai in combination with other herbs depending on the problems being addressed and these are prepared together.

Alcohol tincture: Combine fresh or dry, chopped root with enough alcohol to cover in a glass container. Alcohol should be of good quality. A 50/50 alcohol/water ratio is optimal. If the alcohol is not 100 proof, add pure water to obtain a 50/50 ratio. Brandy, vodka, and gin are often used. Seal the mixture in an air-tight container and set aside in a dark place for about two weeks. Shake daily. Strain through cheesecloth or muslin and store in dark containers for up to two years. Dosage: 10-40 drops of the fresh root tincture one to three times daily.

Precautions

Pregnant or lactating women are advised not to use dong quai. Menstruating women who are experiencing unusually heavy bleeding should discontinue use of dong quai without advice of a qualified herbal practitioner, because in certain preparations the herb may act to increase the blood flow. Consult a qualified herbalist before use if fibroids are present, or when there is unusual breast tenderness.

Dong quai should not be used as a substitute for hormonal replacement therapy, or HRT. Women who are concerned about the possible side effects of HRT should consider fo-ti or such other herbs as **licorice** and **hops**.

Side effects

Dong quai has been considered quite safe; however, it may cause minor gastric upset in sensitive individuals. Stomach upset can be eliminated if dong quai is combined with other herbs in preparation. The herb may also increase sensitivity to the sun and other ultraviolet exposure in fair-skinned individuals.

More seriously, a study published in 2002 reported that dong quai appears to encourage the growth of **breast cancer** cells independent of its estrogenic activity. The researchers recommend cautious use of dong quai until definitive studies can be performed. Interestingly, two teams of researchers in the United States and China respectively reported in 2003 that dong quai appears to suppress the growth of human **prostate cancer** cells.

Interactions

Some herbalists suggest that fruit consumption be decreased when using dong quai.

As of 2003, dong quai has been reported to interact with some prescription medications, particularly anticoagulant and antiplatelet drugs. Dong quai appears to have an additive effect with these medications, increasing bleeding time. In May 2002 the FDA added dong quai to the list of herbal products not to be used together with **sodium** warfarin (Coumadin).

Dong quai has also been reported to interact with bleomycin (Blenoxane), an anticancer drug used to treat tumors of the cervix, uterus, testicle, and penis, as well as certain types of lymphoma.

Resources

BOOKS

The Alternative Advisor, The Complete Guide to Natural Therapies and Alternative Treatments. Alexandria, VA: Time-Life, Time Warner, Inc., 1997.

Gladstar, Rosemary. *Herbal Healing for Women.* New York: Simon & Schuster, 1993.

The PDR Family Guide To Natural Medicines And Healing Therapies. New York: Three Rivers Press, 1999.

PDR for Herbal Medicines. Montvale, NJ: Medical Economics Company, 1998.

Werbach, Melvyn R., M.D., and Michael T. Murray, N.D. *Botanical Influences on Illness, A Sourcebook of Clinical Research.* 2nd ed. Tarzana, CA: Third Line Press, 2000.

PERIODICALS

Amato, P., S. Christophe, and P. L. Mellon. "Estrogenic Activity of Herbs Commonly Used as Remedies for Menopausal Symptoms." *Menopause* 9 (March-April 2002): 145-150.

Huntley, A. L., and E. Ernst. "A Systematic Review of Herbal Medicinal Products for the Treatment of Menopausal Symptoms." *Menopause* 10 (September-October 2003): 465–476.

Ng, S. S., and W. D. Figg. "Antitumor Activity of Herbal Supplements in Human Prostate Cancer Xenografts Implanted in Immunodeficient Mice." *Anticancer Research* 23 (September-October 2003): 3585–3590.

Oerter Klein, K., M. Janfaza, K. A. Wong, and R. J. Chang. "Estrogen Bioactivity in Fo-Ti and Other Herbs Used for Their Estrogen-Like Effects as Determined by a Recombinant Cell Bioassay." *Journal of Clinical Endocrinology and Metabolism* 88 (September 2003): 4077–4079.

Powell, C. B., S. L. Dibble, J. E. Dall'Era, and I. Cohen. "Use of Herbs in Women Diagnosed with Ovarian Cancer." *International Journal of Gynecologic Cancer* 12 (March-April 2002): 214-217.

Scott, G. N., and G. W. Elmer. "Update on Natural Product-Drug Interactions." *American Journal of Health-System Pharmacists* 59 (February 2002): 339-347.

Shang, P., A. R. Qian, T. H. Yang, et al. "Experimental Study of Anti-Tumor Effects of Polysaccharides from *Angelica sinensis.*" *World Journal of Gastroenterology* 9 (September 2003): 1963–1967.

ORGANIZATIONS

National Center for Complementary and Alternative Medicine (NCCAM) Clearinghouse. P.O. Box 7923, Gaithersburg, MD 20898-7923. (888) 644-6226. <http://nccam.nih.gov>.

KEY TERMS

Decoction—A medication or herbal preparation made by boiling.

Infusion—A medicine or herbal preparation made by steeping plant parts or other substances in water to extract their medicinal principles.

Volatile—Evaporating readily at room temperature. The essential oils of a plant are sometimes called volatile oils for this reason.

U. S. Food and Drug Administration (FDA). 5600 Fishers Lane, Rockville, MD 20857. (888) 463-6332. <http://www.fda.gov>.

OTHER

Herbal Hall: Home for Herbs. http://www.herb.com/herbal.html.

Khalsa, Karta Purkh Singh. "The Chinese Way to Women's Health." *Delicious Magazine* http://www.delicious.online.com. (March 1997).

Life Extension Foundation. "Female Hormone Modulation Therapy." *Nutrition Science News* http://www.lef.org. (March 1998).

Walker, Christy, Amy Bigus, and Deanna Massengil. "Dong Quai." http://www.geocities.com/chadrx/dong.html.

Clare Hanrahan
Rebecca J. Frey, PhD

Dowsing *see* **Radiesthesia**

Drug abuse *see* **Substance abuse and dependence**

Dry mouth

Definition

Dry mouth, known medically as xerostomia, is the abnormal reduction of saliva due to medication, disease, or medical therapy.

Description

Dry mouth due to the lack of saliva can be a serious medical problem. Decreased salivation can make swallowing difficult, decrease taste sensation, and promote tooth decay.

Causes & symptoms

Dry mouth, resulting from thickened or reduced saliva flow, can be caused by a number of factors: medications, both prescription and over-the-counter; systemic diseases, such as **anemia** or diabetes, manifestations of syndromes such as **rheumatoid arthritis**, lupus, chronic hardening and thickening of the skin, or chronic and progressive inflammation of skeletal muscles; **infections** of the salivary glands; blockage of the salivary ducts caused by stones or tumors forming in the ducts through which the saliva passes; dehydration; medical therapies, such as local surgery or radiation; secretion reduction due to the normal **aging** process; and emotional **stress**.

Dry mouth, together with dry eyes, is a core symptom of **Sjögren's syndrome**, named for the Swedish physician who first described it. Sjögren's syndrome is an autoimmune disorder in which the body's white cells attack the glands that produce saliva and tears. It is a common cause of dry mouth in the elderly.

Although psychiatric disorders involving dry mouth are unusual, several cases have been reported of somatoform disorders in which dry mouth is a central symptom. Somatoform disorders are psychiatric disturbances characterized by external physical symptoms or complaints that are related to psychological problems rather than organic illness.

Diagnosis

The diagnosis of dry mouth is not difficult. The patient will state that his or her saliva is very thick or nonexistent. Finding the cause of the dry mouth may be more difficult and require some laboratory testing. Salivary gland biopsy for stones or tumors should be performed if indicated.

Treatment

To treat dry mouth, the use of caffeine-containing beverages, alcoholic beverages, and mouthwashes containing alcohol should be minimized. Drinking water and fruit juices will decrease dry mouth problems. Chewing gum and lemon drops can be used to stimulate saliva flow. **Bitters** also can initiate salivary flow as long as the salivary glands and ducts are functional. Commercial saliva substitutes are available without prescription and can be used as frequently as needed. Use of a humidifier in the bedroom reduces nighttime oral dryness.

Herbal therapy

There are several herbal remedies that may be effective in increasing saliva production and preventing dry mouth. Drinking **ginger**, **chamomile**, or Chinese **green tea** at frequent intervals stimulates salivary flow. A Chinese herbal mix of ophiopogois, pinelliae tuber, zizyphi fructus, glycyrrhiaze, ginseng radix, and oryzae semen

has been evaluated as treatment for dry mouth. Studies have shown this formula is effective in relieving dry mouth in half of those tested, including severe cases, such as **cancer** patients undergoing radiation therapy.

Nutritional therapy

Because dry mouth often causes **gum disease**, patients should take **vitamin C** and beta-carotene supplements as a preventive measure.

Acupuncture

Acupuncture has been tried since the late 1990s as a treatment for dry mouth caused by cancer treatments. Practitioners at a California clinic that offers acupuncture to cancer patients use a total of eight needles, to stimulate three points on each ear and one on each index finger. Of the 50 patients who have been treated with acupuncture in this clinic, 35 reported significant improvement in their salivation, and 13 reported that the improvement lasted for over three months before they required another treatment.

Allopathic treatment

Treatment of dry mouth involves management of the underlying condition. If dry mouth is caused by medication, the medication should be changed. If dry mouth is caused by blockage of the salivary ducts, the cause of the blockage should be investigated. When such systemic diseases as diabetes and anemia are brought under control, dry mouth problems may decrease.

Some new medications have been developed to treat dry mouth associated with cancer therapy and Sjögren's syndrome. Amifostine (Ethyol), a medication that protects the cells of the mouth against radiation and chemotherapy agents, has been approved by the Food and Drug Administration (FDA) as a treatment for dry mouth related to cancer therapy. Pilocarpine hydrochloride (Salagen) is a drug that was approved in 1998 for treating dry mouth associated with Sjögren's syndrome; it works by stimulating the salivary glands to produce more moisture. A study published in 2002 indicates that pilocarpine also relieves dry mouth in cancer patients. Cevimeline (Evoxac) is a newer drug that was approved by the FDA in February 2000 for the treatment of dry mouth associated with Sjögren's syndrome. All three medications appear to give good results and to be well tolerated by patients.

Expected results

The prognosis for patients with xerostomia due to medication problems is good, if the offending agent can

KEY TERMS

. . . .

Salivary duct—Tube through which saliva is carried from the salivary gland to the mouth.

Salivary gland—Gland in which saliva is formed.

Sjögren's syndrome—An autoimmune disorder in which the body's white cells attack the glands that produce saliva and tears. Dry mouth is a core symptom of Sjögren's syndrome.

Xerostomia—The medical term for dry mouth.

be changed. Dry mouth due to systemic problems may be eliminated or improved once the disease causing the dry mouth is under control. Persistent xerostomia can be managed well with saliva substitutes.

Prevention

A patient needs to ask his or her health care provider if any medication to be prescribed will cause dry mouth. Patients with persistent xerostomia need to practice good oral hygiene and visit a dentist on a regular basis; the lack of adequate saliva can cause severe dental decay. The salivary glands are very sensitive to radiation, so any patient scheduled for radiation therapy of the head and neck should discuss minimizing exposure of the salivary glands to radiation with the radiation therapy provider.

Resources

BOOKS

Lee, K. J., ed. *Essential Otolaryngology.* 7th ed. New York: McGraw-Hill, 1998.

Rakel, Robert, ed. *Conn's Current Therapy.* Philadelphia: W.B. Saunders Company, 1997.

PERIODICALS

Johnstone, P. A., R. C. Niemtzow, and R. H. Riffenburgh. "Acupuncture for Xerostomia: Clinical Update." *Cancer* 94 (February 15, 2002): 1151–1156.

Koukourakis, M. I. "Amifostine in Clinical Oncology: Current Use and Future Applications." *Anticancer Drugs* 13 (March 2002): 181–209.

Leek, H., and M. Albertsson. "Pilocarpine Treatment of Xerostomia in Head and Neck Patients." *Micron* 33 (2002): 153–155.

Petrone, D., J. J. Condemi, R. Fife, et al. "A Double-Blind, Randomized, Placebo-Controlled Study of Cevimeline in Sjögren's Syndrome Patients with Xerostomia and Keratoconjunctivitis Sicca." *Arthritis Rheum* 46 (March 2002): 748–754.

Ship, J. A., S. R. Pillemer, and B. J. Baum. "Xerostomia and the Geriatric Patient." *Journal of the American Geriatric Society* 50 (March 2002): 535–543.

Sugano, Sumio, Isamu Takeyama, Sadao Ogino, et al. "Effectiveness of Formula Ophiopogoins in the Treatment of Xerostomia and Pharyngoxerosis." *Acta Otolanryngol (Stockh)* 252 (1996): 124–129.

Votta, T. J., and L. Mandel. "Somatoform Salivary Complaints. Case Reports." *New York State Dental Journal* 68 (January 2002): 22–26.

ORGANIZATIONS

American Dental Association. 211 E. Chicago Ave. Chicago, IL 60611. (312) 440-2500. <http://www.ada.org>.

American Medical Association. 515 N. State Street, Chicago, IL 60612. (312) 464-5000. <http://www.ama-assn.org>.

Mai Tran
Rebecca J. Frey, PhD

Dyslexia

Definition

Dyslexia is a kind of learning disability noted for spatial reversals and shifts and is sometimes described as a neurological disorder. It manifests as difficulties with reading, writing, spelling and sometimes math. Occasionally, balance, movement, and rhythm are affected. Persons with dyslexia frequently display above average to superior intelligence, gifted creativity and genius. Leonardo da Vinci, Albert Einstein, Walt Disney, and the Olympic multi-Gold Medal diving champion, Greg Louganis, are noted examples of persons with dyslexia.

Description

Genetics is believed to be a deciding factor in whether or not a person develops dyslexia. The condition may appear as early as three months. One report suggested that as many as 5–15% of Americans are affected. The National Institute of Health (NIH) reports that up to 8% of American elementary school children may have the unique characteristics described originally in 1920 by Dr. Samuel Torrey Orton. Believing it first a condition of "cross lateralization of the brain," by which he meant that functions normally processed on the right side of the brain are processed on the left side in the person with dyslexia, Dr. Orton later modified his description of the condition as being a "mixed hemispheric dominance," by which he meant that the alteration of functions to the opposite side of the brain occurred sometimes, but not all the time.

Since the advent of Magnetic Resonance Imaging (MRIs), scientists have been able to view dyslexia from

SYMPTOMS OF DYSLEXIA
inability to associate symbols with sounds and vice versa
frequent word guessing
confusion with verbal instructions without visual cues
confused handedness
difficulty sequencing items
slow, soft spoken reading
frequent mispronounciation of words when reading
misperception of words, letters, and numbers moving or disappearing on a written page

another vantage point, ironically, a process imitating what happens inside the mind of a dyslexic individual, according to one educator with dyslexia, Ronald D. Davis. He describes the ordinary ability of the person with dyslexia to visualize an object from multiple points of view, a process which has a moving point of view and which is spatially unanchored. When presented with a word that is easily visualized as a known object, like horse, the dyslexic mind easily imagines the horse from multiple perspectives, and, so rapidly—somewhere between 400 to 2,000 times faster than those without dyslexia— visual cues are processed 'almost intuitively,' demonstrating great mastery of the objectified visual world. However, when it comes to processing sound, language, speaking, handwriting and understanding verbalized communication not associated with an object, like the words the or and, a series of non-image disconnections leads to confusion, disorientation, and an inability to adequately make sense of key pieces of visual information. To the person with dyslexia, a simple seven word sentence may look like a three word sentence with four blank spaces here and there.

Causes & symptoms

Although an exact cause has not been identified, studies have identified differences in the way sound and visual information are processed between persons with and without dyslexia. In the dyslexic individual these differences create what one NIH scientist refers to as a "physiologic signature"—a unique brain pattern— perhaps the result of emphasized activity along dopamine related neuro-pathways. Dopamine is a neurotransmitter, a chemical substance acting in the brain that facilitates certain kinds of messages. According to one author, when dopamine levels are high, the person with dyslexia experiences time as moving very slowly outside themselves, and very fast inside. As if time stands still. This author also notes that when the person with dyslexia experiences

episodes of disorientation, *when words or sounds do not create a visual picture for them* and their mind continues to try and solve the confusion visually, dopamine levels shift and change. This would seem to be consistent with some of the symptoms of dyslexia, such as *inaccurate perceptions of time and a lot of day dreaming.*

Symptoms may include:

- poor ability to associate symbols with sounds and vice versa

- frequent word guessing when reading, and an inability to retain meaning

- confusion when given verbal instructions unaccompanied by visual cues

- confused sense of spatial orientation, especially by reversing letters and numbers, and losing one's place frequently while reading, or skipping lines

- having the perception that words, letters and numbers move around, disappear, or get bigger or smaller

- overlooking punctuation marks or other details of language

- slow, labored reading and speech may be difficult to understand, words often mispronounced and softly spoken

- confused sense of right and left handedness

- math concepts are difficult to learn, excessive daydreaming, and difficulty with time

- difficulty sequencing items

- difficulty with jigsaw puzzles; walking a chalk line straightly or other fine motor skill tasks.

Other more positive characteristics common with dyslexia include:

- primary ability of the brain to alter and create perceptions

- highly aware of their environment, intelligent, and above average curiosity

- intuitive, insightful, and having the extraordinary ability of thinking in pictures

- multi-dimensional perception (from various viewpoints almost simultaneously)

- vivid imagination

- experiencing thought as reality (confusing what they see with what they think they see), thereby being abundantly creative.

Diagnosis

Diagnosis is difficult in part because symptoms can also result from other conditions and because no two individuals display the same symptoms. As a result, dyslexia can be viewed as a developmental condition, a "self-created condition," rather than as a disease. As each individual baby interprets visual data, and adapts to the environment accordingly, developing their own individual and unique brain patterns. It is that developmental pattern that is consistent among people with dyslexia. When the individual's mind cannot make sense of the data, confusion and disorientation result; incorrect data is incorporated, causing the individual to make mistakes that leads to emotional reactions, primarily frustration. A behavior is adopted that constitutes a learning disability because it disables future learning and, ultimately, affects self esteem.

Sometimes the learning disorder of dyslexia is inaccurately paralleled to Attention Deficit Disorder (ADD) or Attention Deficit Hyperactivity Disorder (ADHD). In a 2003 study, distinguishable differences between the two **learning disorders** were readily apparent. Comparing 105 boys between the ages of eight and ten, from three different schools and cross divided into three different groups—35 boys diagnosed with ADHD not taking stimulant medication, 35 boys with dyslexia, and 35 boys without learning disabilities—the study found clear and diagnostically useful differences in speech related patterns between all groups. However, since diagnosis of a learning disability may be made between parents and teacher or other school administrators on the basis of symptoms rather than clinical diagnostic testing, careful diagnosis, as always, is advisable.

Treatment

Ronald D. Davis, writing in *The Gift of Dyslexia* outlines an alternative and complementary treatment consistent with the "moving point of view" model. According to this model, and the reason why letters seem to change shape and float, why lines of print appear to move, and why words appear to be other than they are is that the dyslexic individual sees the world predominantly through his or her "mind's eye," rather than through his or her physiologic eye. In other words, the person with dyslexia more than all others, sees what he or she 'thinks' they see, rather than what their eyeballs see. To further complicate matters, they do this so quickly, they easily become confused when the multiple facets do not produce a solid view. The object of treatment proposed by Ronald Davis, a dyslexic individual himself, is to train the mind's eye to return to a learned, anchored, viewpoint when they realize they are seeing with their mind, and not with their eyeballs. This is accomplished with assessment testing, followed by one-on-one exercises that retrain mental perception pathways. Using the gifts of the dyslexic individual—their imagination and curiosity—these exercises involve creative physical activities, including the use of modeling clay, "koosh" balls, and movement training. Davis founded the Reading Research Council's Dyslexia Correction Center in 1982, and the Davis Dyslexia Association International, which trains educators and therapists, in 1995.

Another alternative treatment option seeks to address unmastered learning skills needed for reading and math. This system, called Audioblox, may be used one-on-one (especially for children) or in groups, and involves a series of mental exercises that address learning, focussing on the "deficits" of dyslexia. Treatment involves the purchase of a kit online that contains a book entitled *The Right to Read,* a supplementary manual, a computer program on CD to supplement Audioblox training, and teaching materials. The book is in two parts; first, an explanation of theory; second, the program itself, with exercises. The supplementary manual contains specialized programs for areas of deficit, including handwriting, spelling, math, pre-school readiness, and high school or adult learning. The teaching materials include 96 colored blocks, representing each of six colors on each of the six sides of the block; a view blocking screen; colored cards with preprinted patterns; letter cards; a reading book with a story written in the 800 most common English words, and word cards; and, a demonstration video. The kit originates in England; pricing in America ranges approximately between $135 and $150.

Special education recommendations include helping a child stay organized and on task by keeping their desk and workplace free of extraneous, distracting materials; making more frequent, shorter assignments to increase confidence; providing positive, "immediate gratification" feedback; and short conferences or work contracts as needed.

Allopathic treatment

Allopathic medical treatment for dyslexia includes use of anti-motion drugs, addressing the symptoms of balance and coordination which results from visual per-

Dyslexia

Acetylcholine—A chemical of nerve transmission involved with movement.

Attention Deficit Disorder (ADD)—A learning disability characterized by an inability to pay attention. It may be different from dyslexia in that dyslexic individuals are highly aware and able to pay attention, but unable to make sense of their perceptions.

Attention Deficit with Hyperactivity Disorder (ADHD)—A learning disability characterized by an inability to sit still or concentrate well. It has been demonstrated to be diagnostically different from dyslexia by speech and vocalization patterns.

Cross lateralization—A term used to describe what was believed to be a difference in the way the mind works in persons with and without dyslexia. It was believed that functions processed in the right half of the brain by a person without dyslexia were processed in the left half by a person with dyslexia.

Dopamine—A chemical of nerve transmission involved with pleasure and pain and some forms of movement.

Dyslexia—A term applied to a kind of learning disability particularly noted for reversals and spatial shifts, making reading, writing, spelling and math very difficult.

Koosh ball—A lightweight, "furry" ball of rubber band material used in Davis technique exercises

for retraining neuropathways in the brain of a person with dyslexia.

Mind's eye—A term referring to an imaginary point from which the mind views what the eyes look at or what the imagination presents. In dyslexia, the mind's eye is unanchored to one location, and sends many signals to the brain about what it sees, which causes disabling confusion.

Mixed hemispheric dominance—A term later used to describe what was believed to be a difference in the way the mind works in persons with and without dyslexia. It was believed that functions processed in the right half of the brain by a person without dyslexia were sometimes processed in the left half by a person with dyslexia.

Monoamine oxidase (MAO) inhibitors—A group of anti-depressant drugs.

Neurotransmitter—A chemical substance which facilitates the passing of messages along nerve pathways. There are several different neurotransmitters used in the human nervous system, each with distinct effects on mood, movement and perception.

Point of view—In a person with dyslexia, this term is used to describe the angle from which their mind's eye views an object. This point of view may be unanchored and moving about, as if several different people were telling what they see all at the same time.

ception alterations; stimulant drugs such as Cylert or Ritalin, to address symptoms of low self esteem, restlessness, and distractibility, and 'nootropics' drugs, a class of drugs believed to improve cognitive function. The stimulant drugs may be more effective for learning disorders related to ADHD or ADD than for dyslexia. The drug Piracetam, a nootropic, although reported as a possible treatment for dyslexia, is also reported to have legal issues because it has not been approved for use in the United States by the Food and Drug Administration (FDA). Reported potential side effects of the stimulants include nervousness and **insomnia**, and are contra-indicated with **epilepsy, allergies**, blood pressure problems, or with use of monoamine oxidase (MAO) inhibitors. Long-term use of stimulants in children are reported to adversely affect growth, may ironically depress the nervous system or lead to loss of consciousness. By reducing natural levels of stimulants in the brain, they may

also cause dependence. The stimulants and nootropics are said to increase the effects of alcohol and amphetamines. Other possible interactions include use of anticonvulsants or anti-epileptics; tricyclic anti-depressants; anti-coagulants, like Coumadin; and "atropine-like drugs" that blocks the neurotransmitter acetylcholine.

Prognosis

If left unaddressed, a person with dyslexia may become "functionally illiterate," able to function limited by their ability to read, spell, have their handwriting understood, or do arithmetic. Recognizing that dyslexia is a developed learning disorder affecting people of extraordinary curiosity, imagination and intelligence—people of genius, often—from a productive or functional point of view, dyslexia may contribute significantly, positively or negatively, to performance levels. From an emotional or psychological point of view, dyslexia affects self esteem, and promotes confusion and frustration, that may contribute to under achievement.

Prevention

No method of preventing dyslexia is currently known. However, existing methods of treatment may prevent or reduce the secondary or indirect losses to individuals, society and culture that might otherwise occur. As the genetic aspects of dyslexia are revealed, genetic chromosomal modifications may prevent the expression of dyslexia in future generations. Wise use of present and future understandings will allow individuals with dyslexic gifts, individuals such as Leonardo daVinci, Albert Einstein, Walt Disney and Greg Louganis, to continue to contribute their genius and talents.

Resources

BOOKS

Clayman, M.D., Charles B., ed. *The American Medical Association Guide to Prescription and Over-The-Counter Drugs.* New York: Random House, 1988.

Davis, Ronald D., with Edlon M. Braun. *The Gift of Dyslexia, Why Some of the Smartest People Can't Read and How They Can Learn.* New York: Berkley Publishing Group, 1997.

Pierangelo, Ph.D., Roger and Robert Jacoby. *Parents' Complete Special Education Guide.* New York: Simon Schuster, 1996.

Thomas, M.D., Clayton L., ed. *Taber's Cyclopedic Medical Dictionary, 16th edition.* Philadelphia: Davis Co., 1989.

OTHER

Audioblox U.K. *Audioblox Program* [Cited May 12, 2004]. <http://www.audiblox2000.com/uk/program.htm>.

Audioblox U.K. *Dyslexia* [Cited May 12, 2004]. <http://www.audiblox2000.com/uk/dyslexia.htm>.

Breznitz, Zvia. "The Speech and Vocalization Patterns of Boys with ADHD Compared with Boys with Dyslexia and Boys Without Learning Disabilities." *Journal of Genetic Psychology.* 164.4. December 2003. [Cited May 10, 2004]. <http://galenet.galegroup.com/servlet/HWRC>.>

"Dyslexia" *The Dyslexia File, Center for Current Research.* [Cited May 12, 2004]. <http://www.lifestages.com/health/dyslexia.html>.

Schoon, Chris. *Piracetam FAQ* Version 0.6. Dated 2/1/03. Last modified, March 14, 2004. [Cited May 10, 2004]. <http://www.erowid.org/smarts/piracetam/piracetam faq.shtml>.

Katy Nelson, N.D.

Dysmenorrhea

Definition

Dysmenorrhea is the occurrence of painful cramps during **menstruation**.

Description

More than half of all girls and women suffer from dysmenorrhea (cramps), a dull or throbbing **pain** that usually centers in the lower mid-abdomen, radiating toward the lower back or thighs. Menstruating women of any age can experience cramps.

While the pain may be only mild for some women, others experience severe discomfort that can significantly interfere with everyday activities for several days each month. In fact, about 43 % of women in the United States suffer pain so severe that it disrupts their daily lives and about 18% miss one or more days or work, school, or other activities each year because of menstrual cramps.

Causes & symptoms

Dysmenorrhea is called "primary" when there is no specific abnormality, and "secondary" when the pain is caused by an underlying gynecological problem. It is believed that primary dysmenorrhea occurs when prostaglandins, hormone-like substances produced by uterine tissue, trigger strong muscle contractions in the uterus during menstruation. However, the level of prostaglandins does not seem to correlate with how strong a woman's cramps are. Some women have high levels of prostaglandins and no cramps, whereas other women with low levels have severe cramps. This is why experts assume that cramps must also be related to other causes, such as **diets**, genetics, **stress**, and different body types, in addition to prostaglandins. The first year or two of a girl's periods are not usually very painful. However, once ovulation begins, the blood levels of the prostaglandins rise, leading to stronger contractions.

Secondary dysmenorrhea may be caused by **endometriosis**, fibroid tumors, or an infection in the pelvis.

The likelihood that a woman will have cramps increases if she:

• has a family history of painful periods

• leads a stressful life

• doesn't get enough **exercise**

• uses **caffeine**

• has **pelvic inflammatory disease** (PID)

Symptoms include a dull, throbbing cramping in the lower abdomen that may radiate to the lower back and thighs. In addition, some women may experience **nausea** and **vomiting**, **diarrhea**, irritability, sweating, or **dizziness**. Cramps usually last for two or three days at the beginning of each menstrual period. Many women often notice their painful periods disappear after they have their first child, probably due to the stretching of the opening of the uterus or because the birth improves the uterine blood supply and muscle activity, although others do not notice a change.

Diagnosis

A doctor should perform a thorough pelvic exam and take a patient history to rule out any underlying condition that could cause cramps.

Treatment

Nutritional therapy

The following dietary changes may help prevent or treat menstrual pain:

• Increased dietary intake of foods such as fiber, **calcium**, soy foods, fruits and vegetables.

• Decreased consumption of foods that exacerbate PMS. They include caffeine, salt and sugar.

• Quitting **smoking**. Smoking has been found to worsen cramps.

• Taking daily multi-vitamin and mineral supplements that contain high doses of **magnesium** and vitamin B_6 (**pyridoxine**), and **flaxseed** or **fish oil** supplements. Recent research suggests that vitamin B supplements, primarily vitamin B_6 in complex, magnesium, calcium, **zinc**, **vitamin E**, and fish oil supplements (**omega-3 fatty acids**) also may help relieve cramps.

Herbal therapy

An herbalist may recommend one of the following herbal remedies for menstrual pain:

• Chasteberry (*Vitex agnus-castus*) for women who also experience breast pain, irregular periods, and ovarian cysts.

• Dong quai (*Angelica sinensis*) for women with typical menstrual pain.

• Licorice (*Glycyrrhiza glabra*) for abdominal bloating and cramping.

• Black cohosh (*Cimifuga racemosa*) for relief of menstrual pain as well as mood swing and depression.

Yoga

Several **yoga** positions are popular as methods to ease menstrual pain. In the "cat stretch" position, the woman rests on her hands and knees, slowly arching the back. The pelvic tilt is another popular yoga position, in which the woman lies with knees bent, and then lifts the pelvis and buttocks.

Exercise

Exercise may be a way to reduce the pain of menstrual cramps through the brain's production of endorphins, the body's own painkillers.

Other remedies

Acupuncture and Chinese herbs are other popular alternative treatments for cramps. There are particular formulas depending on the pattern of imbalance. **Aromatherapy** and massage may ease pain for some women. Transcutaneous Electrical Nerve Stimulation (TENS) has been touted as a safe and practical way to relieve the pain of dysmenorrhea. It works by using electrodes to stimulate nerve fibers. Some women find relief through visualization, concentrating on the pain as a particular color and gaining control of the sensations. Others find that imagining a white light hovering over the painful area can actually lessen the pain for brief periods. Simply changing the position of the body can help ease cramps. The simplest technique is assuming the fetal position with knee pulled up to the chest while hugging a heating pad or pillow to the abdomen. Also, orgasm can make a woman feel more comfortable by releasing tension in the pelvic muscles.

Allopathic treatment

Several drugs can lessen or completely eliminate the pain of primary dysmenorrhea. Most popular are the non-steroidal anti-inflammatory drugs (NSAIDs), which prevent or decrease the formation of prostaglandins. These include aspirin, ibuprofen (Advil), and naproxen (Aleve). For more severe pain, prescription strength ibuprofen (Motrin) is available. These drugs are usually begun at the first sign of the period and taken for a day or two.

If an NSAID is not available, acetaminophen (Tylenol) may also help ease the pain. Heat applied to the painful area may bring relief, and a warm bath twice a day also may help.

Studies of a drug patch containing glyceryl trinitrate to treat dysmenorrhea suggest that it also may help ease pain. This drug has been used in the past to ease preterm contractions in pregnant women.

In 2002, an intrauterine device (IUD) was introduced to help eliminate the pain of menstrual cramps related to endometriosis. The IUD, known as Mirena, is approved for use in the Untied States as a contraceptive.

Expected results

Treatments should lessen or eliminate pain.

Prevention

Avoidance of caffeine, alcohol, and sugar prior to onset of period and NSAIDs taken a day before the period begins should eliminate cramps for some women.

Resources

BOOKS

Carlson, Karen J., Stephanie Eisenstat, and Terra Ziporyn. *The Harvard Guide to Women's Health*. Cambridge: Harvard University Press, 1996.

Murray, Michael T and Joseph E. Pizzorno. "Premenstrual syndrome." In *Encyclopedia of Natural Medicine*. Rev. 2nd ed. Rocklin, CA: Prima Publishing, 1998.

PERIODICALS

Hale, Ellen. "Taming menstrual cramps." *FDA Consumer* 25, no. 5 (June 1991): 26–29.

Harel, Z., et.al. "Supplementation with omega-3 polyunsaturated fatty acids in the management of dysmenorrhea in adolescents." *American Journal of Obstetrics and Gynecology* 174 (April 1996): 13, 335–8.

McDonald, Claire, and Susan McDonald. "A Woman's Guide to Self-care." *Natural Health* (January–February 1998): 121–142.

"Menstrual Pain Severely Affects almost Half of U.S. Women." *AORN Journal* (April 2002): 121–778.

"More Power, Less Pain." *Chemist & Druggist* (April 6, 2002): 36.

"The Mirena IUD May Diminish Endometriosis –related Dysmenorrhea (Results of Two Small Studies)." *OB GYN News* (May 15 2002): 16.

ORGANIZATIONS

American College of Obstetricians and Gynecologists. 409 12th St. SW, Washington, DC 20024. (202) 638-5577.

Federation of Feminist Women's Health Centers. 633 East 11th Ave., Eugene, OR 97401. (503) 344-0966.

National Women's Health Network. 1325 G St. NW, Washington, DC 20005. (202) 347-1140.

Katy Nelson, N.D.

Dyspepsia *see* **Indigestion**

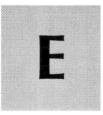

E

Ear acupuncture *see* **Auriculotherapy**

Earache

Definition

An earache is a commonly used term for ear **pain** or discomfort that is a symptom of disease or injury.

Description

An earache itself is not a disease, but it is a symptom of disease or injury in the external or middle ear. It may also be a symptom of problems in the mouth, nose, or throat. Infants or very young children may be unable to say that they are in pain. Increased irritability or pulling at the ears is often a sign of ear pain in infants.

Causes & symptoms

The most common cause of an earache is a buildup of pressure in the eustachian tube. Among other functions, the eustachian tube drains fluids out of the middle ear via the back of the throat. A cold, allergy, or **sore throat** can cause the eustachian tube to swell shut. Infants and young children are especially susceptible to earaches caused by problems with the eustachian tube, since the structure is still underdeveloped in that age group. When the normal drainage of fluid is prevented, it can accumulate in the middle ear, causing pressure, pain, stagnation, and possibly infection.

An earache may be due to a perforated, or broken, eardrum. The eardrum can be broken as a result of a blow to the head, infection in the inner ear, suction applied to the ear, or the insertion of a foreign object into the ear. **Infections** of the middle and outer ears are often associated with earaches. Other causes of an earache may be the obstruction of the ear canal with a foreign object or excessive ear wax, **boils** in the ear canal, a her-

pes zoster infection of the ear, keratosis of the ear, tumors, an infection of the mastoid process, "swimmer's ear," and the aftermath of surgical procedures. Ear pain can also be caused by a rapid descent from high altitudes, during air travel or travel in the mountains. A **sinus infection**, arthritis of the jaw, sore throat, **tonsillitis**, and dysfunction of the temporomandibular joint (TMJ) may be the source of referred pain to the ears.

Diagnosis

A history of the illness should be obtained, including information about the symptoms accompanying the earache. A physical exam should be performed, which may include an examination of the ears, the nasal passages and sinuses, and the throat. An otoscope may be used to see more deeply into the ears, nose, and throat. In addition, the teeth, tongue, tonsils, salivary glands, and TMJ should be examined for problems that might be causing referred pain to the ears. A culture and sensitivity test should be done if there is any discharge from the ears. X rays or a computed tomography (CT) scan may be required to diagnose the problem. Hearing and balancing tests are important to the diagnosis of an earache.

Treatment

Three to five drops of the warmed oil extract of **mullein** flowers (*Verbascum thapsus*), **garlic** (*Allium sativa*), or **St. John's wort** (*Hypericum perforatum*), or a combination of any of the three should be placed into the affected ear. The oil of *Calendula officinalis* may be used in the same manner. If there is a persistent **ear infection**, **goldenseal** (*Hydrastis canadensis*) salve or tincture can be placed directly onto the outer ear or into the ear canal three to four times per day. Glycerin can be introduced into the ear if it is suspected that excessive earwax or **water** in the ear is causing the problem.

Food and environmental **allergies** should be considered as contributors to the development of ear pain and infections, especially if the earache is chronic or recurrent. Allergy testing should be done, and then the allergens should be avoided. Alcohol, dairy products, **smoking, caffeine**, sugary foods, and processed foods should also be avoided to keep from stressing the immune system. One or two cloves of raw garlic daily may help end chronic episodes of earache, since garlic can kill many of the pathogens that cause earaches. If there is trouble tolerating raw garlic, a daily garlic supplement can be taken instead. Daily supplementation of **vitamin C, bioflavonoids, zinc**, and **beta carotene** is recommended to treat some of the underlying conditions causing ear pain and bolster general immune function.

Several homeopathic remedies may also be helpful in treating earaches. Depending upon the symptoms, a 6C or 12C dose of **Pulsatilla**, Mercurius, or *Hepar sulphuris,* or a 30C dose of **Belladonna** can be taken for up to four doses. If there is no symptom relief, a homeopath or other healthcare practitioner should be consulted.

Hydrotherapy treatment for earaches includes the use of hot compresses. To make a compress, a large cloth soaked in hot water should be placed over both ears and the throat for about five minutes. A hot water bottle or smaller compress can also be used. A new hot compress can be used every three to five minutes until the earache is relieved for a maximum of 30 minutes. This treatment is best when the feet are in a hot footbath while the compresses are being applied. Hot water can be added as needed to keep the water comfortably hot. The soak can be repeated two or three times a day as needed.

Massage such as tui na or **reflexology** can be helpful in clearing up ear pain, congestion, and TMJ dysfunction. A knowledgeable practitioner should be consulted.

Allopathic treatment

If an earache is accompanied by any of the following symptoms, a healthcare provider should be consulted as soon as possible:

- severe pain
- discharge from the ear
- a **fever** of 102°F (38.8°C) or higher
- a sudden change in hearing
- a sudden onset of dizziness
- an inability to concentrate
- facial muscle weakness
- earache lasts for more than a few days
- earache is worse during chewing
- sudden or severe ear pain without any other accompanying symptoms

- does not respond to home treatment
- appears to be getting worse
- pain, tenderness, or redness of the over the area of the mastoid process, which often indicates a serious infection

Antibiotics, decongestants, and antihistamines are often prescribed to halt the infection and inflammation that may be the cause of ear pain. The insertion of ear tubes may be recommended for children who have persistent ear infections to reestablish proper functioning of the middle ear. However, the effectiveness of this treatment is still widely debated. Repeated swallowing or gum-chewing can relieve ear pain caused by changes in pressure secondary to changes in altitude. Allowing infants and young children to suck on a bottle during descent can help relieve popping and ear pain. TMJ dysfunction should be evaluated by a dentist. Anti-inflammatory medication, tranquilizers, or muscle relaxants may be prescribed for temporary relief. Other treatments for TMJ problems include braces to correct the bite or a bite plate to wear when sleeping.

Expected results

Earaches can generally be relieved by attending to the underlying problem. Untreated problems may lead to serious ear damage and possible **hearing loss**. Most children with chronic earaches due to infections tend to outgrow the condition.

Prevention

A hair dryer or other method should be used after swimming if there is a tendency for the ears to retain water. Earplugs should be worn while swimming and cotton or wool should be loosely inserted into the outer ear canal during showers or when the hair is being washed. Objects such as cotton swabs should not be inserted into the ear canal. A healthy immune system should be maintained to reduce the opportunity for infections.

Resources

OTHER

Merck & Co., Inc. *The Merck Manual of Diagnosis and Therapy.* (http://www.merck.com/pubs/mmanual/section7/chapter82/82a.htm.

WebMD, Inc. *Earache.* (http://webmd.lycos.com/content/article/3172.10330.

Patience Paradox

Ear infection

Definition

Otitis media is an infection of the middle ear space, which lies behind the eardrum (tympanic membrane). It is characterized by **pain**, **dizziness**, and partial loss of hearing.

Description

A little knowledge of the basic anatomy of the middle ear will be helpful for understanding the development of otitis media. The external ear canal is a tube that leads from the outside opening of the ear to a structure called the tympanic membrane. Behind the tympanic membrane is the space called the middle ear. Within the middle ear are three tiny bones called ossicles. These are the malleus, the incus, and the stapes. Their shapes are often described as a hammer, an anvil, and a stirrup. Sound in the form of vibration causes movement in the eardrum, and then in the chain of ossicles. The ossicles transmit the sound to the cochlea within the inner ear, which sends it to the brain for processing.

The nasopharynx is the passageway behind the nose that takes inhaled air into the breathing tubes leading to the lungs. The eustachian tube is a canal that runs between the middle ear and the nasopharynx. One of the functions of the eustachian tube is to keep the air pressure in the middle ear equal to that outside. This equalization of the air pressure allows the eardrum and ossicles to vibrate appropriately, so that hearing is normal.

By age three, almost 85% of all children will have had otitis media at least once. It is the most common pediatric complaint. Babies and children between the ages of six months and six years are most likely to develop otitis media. Children at higher risk for otitis media include boys, children from poor families, those with **allergies**, Native Americans, Native Alaskans, children born with cleft palate or other defects of the structures of the head and face, and children with Down syndrome. Babies whose first ear infection occurs prior to six months of age are more prone to chronic problems with otitis media. There also appears to be some genetic predisposition towards otitis media, which may be related to the structure and function of the area in and around the middle ear. Exposure to cigarette smoke significantly increases the risk of ear **infections**, as well as other problems affecting the respiratory system. In addition, children who enter daycare at an early age have more upper respiratory infections (URIs or colds), and thus more cases of otitis media. Although the ear infection itself is not contagious, the URIs that predispose children to them certainly are. The most common times of year for otitis media to strike are winter and early spring, which are the same times that URIs are most common.

Otitis media is an important medical problem, because it often results in fluid accumulation within the middle ear. This is known as otitis media with effusion (OME). The effusion can last for weeks to months. Effusion within the middle ear can cause significant hearing impairment. When such hearing impairment occurs in a young child, it may interfere with the development of normal speech and language processing. A chronic effusion also increases the risk for subsequent infections, as the fluid provides a growth medium for bacteria.

In adults, acute otitis media can lead to such complications as paralysis of the facial nerves. Recovery from these complications may take from two weeks to as long as three months.

Causes & symptoms

The first precondition for the development of acute otitis media is exposure to an organism capable of causing the infection. Otitis media can be caused by either viruses or bacteria. Virus infections account for about 15% of cases. The three most common bacterial pathogens are *Streptococcus pneumoniae*, *Haemophilus influenzae*, or *Moraxella catarrhalis*. As of 2003, about 75% of ear infections caused by *S. pneumoniae* are reported to be resistant to penicillin.

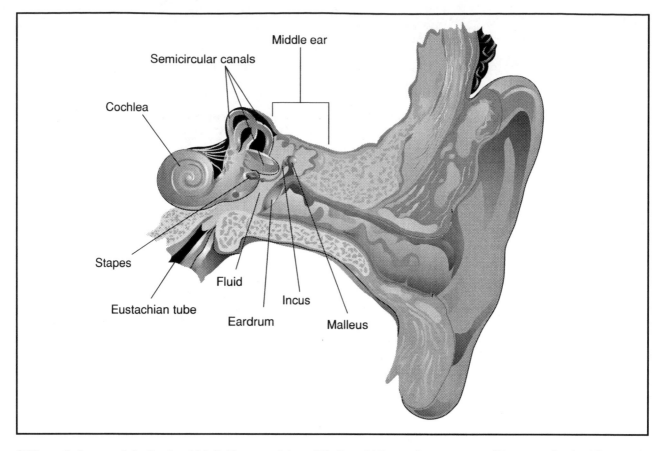

Semicircular canals

Middle ear

Cochlea

Stapes

Fluid

Eustachian tube

Incus

Eardrum

Malleus

Otitis media is an ear infection in which fluid accumulates within the middle ear. A common condition occurring in childhood, it is estimated that 85% of all American children will develop otitis media at least once. *(Illustration by Electronic Illustrators Group. The Gale Group.)*

Otitis media may also be caused by other disease organisms, including *Bordetella pertussis*, the causative agent of **whooping cough**, and *Pneumocystis carinii*, which often causes opportunistic infections in patients with **AIDS**.

There are other factors that make the development of an ear infection more likely. Because the eustachian tube has a more horizontal orientation and is considerably shorter in early childhood, material from the nasopharynx can easily reach the middle ear. Discharges from the nasopharynx include infection-causing organisms. Children also have a lot of lymph tissue, some of which makes up the adenoids, in the area of the eustachian tube. The adenoids may enlarge with repeated respiratory tract infections, ultimately blocking the eustachian tubes. When the eustachian tube is blocked, the middle ear is more likely to fill with fluid. This fluid increases the risk of infection, and the corresponding risks of **hearing loss** and delayed speech development.

Recent advances in gene mapping have led to the discovery of genetic factors that increase a child's susceptibility to otitis media. Researchers are hoping to de-velop molecular diagnostic assays that will help to identify children at risk for severe ear infections.

Most cases of acute otitis media occur during the course of a URI. Symptoms may include cold symptoms, **fever**, ear pain, irritability, and problems with hearing. Babies may have difficulty feeding. When significant fluid is present within the middle ear, pain can increase depending on position. Lying down may cause an increase in painful pressure within the middle ear, so that babies often fuss if not held upright. Older children sometimes complain of a full sensation in the affected ear. If the fluid build-up behind the eardrum is sufficient, the eardrum may develop a hole (perforate), causing bloody fluid or greenish-yellow pus to drip from the ear. Although the pain may be severe before the eardrum perforates, the pain is usually relieved by the reduction of pressure brought on by a perforation.

Diagnosis

Diagnosis is usually made simply by looking at the eardrum through a special lighted instrument called an otoscope. The eardrum will appear red and swollen, and may appear either abnormally drawn inward, or bulging outward. Under normal conditions, the ossicles create a particular pattern on the eardrum, referred to as "landmarks." These landmarks may be obscured in the course of an infection. Normally, the light from the otoscope reflects off the eardrum in a characteristic fashion. This is called the "cone of light." In an infection, this cone of light may be shifted or absent.

A special attachment to the otoscope allows the examiner to blow a puff of air gently into the ear. Normally, this should cause movement of the eardrum. In an infection, or when there if fluid behind the eardrum, this movement may be decreased or absent. Movement of the eardrum can also be assessed by a tympanogram. A tympanogram is a quick, painless test. If there is fluid in the middle ear, the tympanogram reading will be flat. If the middle ear is filled with air, as it is normally, the test will also show whether it is at higher or lower pressure than it should be. This measurement could be an indicator of abnormal function of the eustachian tube.

Hearing tests, or audiograms, are sometimes used to determine whether hearing loss has occurred because of infection or persistent fluid, and whether the loss is severe. A hearing screen for children old enough to describe their own hearing reliably can be performed in schools or at the pediatrician's office. More accurate testing is done in a soundproof booth by an audiologist. This method can also be modified for use with children who can't give a verbal indication that they have heard a sound, but are old enough to turn their heads to see the source of a noise.

Fluid or pus draining from the ear can be collected. This sample can then be processed in a laboratory to allow any organisms present to multiply sufficiently (cultured) to permit the organisms to be viewed under a microscope and identified. Cultures are also used to determine the sensitivity of the organisms to specific antibiotics.

Treatment

Chiropractic

One particular **chiropractic** procedure, known as the endonasal technique, is thought to help the eustachian tube to open and thus improve drainage of the middle ear. The tube is sometimes blocked off due to exudates or inflammatory processes. The endonasal technique can offer significant relief from **earache**.

Craniosacral therapy and osteopathy

Craniosacral therapy uses gentle manipulation of the bones of the skull to relieve pressure and improve eustachian tube function. This treatment may also help the

eustachian tubes to assume a position in which they can drain on their own. The pressure exerted on a baby's head during the birth process sometimes contributes to the tubes being in a position in which it is hard for them to drain. Osteopaths practice a similar gentle manipulation of the bones of a child's head. One osteopathic study of children from kindergarten through third grade in a Missouri school district found a direct correlation between abnormal head shape at birth and susceptibility to otitis media during the early elementary school years. As of 2003 there are pediatric osteopaths who specialize in cranial work.

Herbal therapy

A number of herbal treatments for otitis media have been recommended, including eardrops made with **goldenseal** (*Hydrastis canadensis*), **mullein** (*Verbascum thapsus*), **St. John's wort** (*Hypericum perforatum*), and **echinacea** (*Echinacea* spp.). Tinctures of echinacea, **thyme** (*Thymus vulgaris*), and elderflower (*Sambucus nigra*) are often recommended for oral treatment of otitis media due to chronic congestion. Warm **garlic** oil can be instilled directly into the ear. Steam inhalation infused with **eucalyptus** or **chamomile** may reduce the congestion of the URIs that often accompany otitis media.

Homeopathy

Homeopathic remedies that may be prescribed for middle ear infections include **aconite**, *ferrum phosphoricum*, **belladonna**, chamomilla, **lycopodium**, **pulsatilla**, or **silica**.

Nutrition

Some practitioners believe that food allergies may increase the risk of ear infections, and they suggest eliminating suspected food allergens from the diet. The top food allergens are wheat, dairy products, corn, peanuts, citrus fruits, and eggs. Elimination of sugar and sugar products can allow the immune system to work more effectively. Other nutritionists have noted that children who were breastfed as babies are less susceptible to ear infections.

Acupuncture

Acupuncture can help to reestablish a normal flow of fluids within the head. This form of treatment may also enhance the immune system.

Allopathic treatment

Medications

Antibiotics are the treatment of choice for acute otitis media (AOM). Different antibiotics are used depending on the type of bacteria most likely to be causing the infection. This decision involves knowledge of the types of antibiotics that have worked on other ear infections occurring within a particular community at a particular time. Options include sulfa-based antibiotics, as well as a variety of penicillins, cephalosporins, and others. The patient's sensitivity to certain medications, as well as previously demonstrated resistant strains, also contributes to the choice of antibiotic. As of 2003, an 0.3% topical solution of ofloxacin has been recommended as a more effective medication than other oral or topical antibiotics.

Following a course of antibiotic treatment, approximately 40% of children will continue to have fluid behind the eardrum, resulting in otitis media with effusion (OME). The eardrum is no longer red or infected. The fluid may take weeks to months to resolve. Generally, it is safe to allow this condition to continue with observation for up to 12 weeks. At that time, hearing should be tested. If hearing loss is insignificant or only in one ear, observation can continue for up to a total of 4–6 months, at which time placement of ventilation tubes in the eardrum is often recommended. The tube functions as an accessory eustachian tube until it falls out. If hearing loss is significantly affecting both ears at any time after six weeks from diagnosis of OME, antibiotic treatment or tube placement should be considered.

The overuse of antibiotics is contributing to some strains of bacteria—particularly *S. pneumoniae*—developing resistance and becoming more difficult to treat. Research is being done to try to help determine whether there may be some ear infections that would resolve without antibiotic treatment. One pediatrician has suggested some changes in usage of antibiotics for otitis media. He describes five factors to use to determine whether antibiotic treatment can be limited to five days or perhaps avoided altogether. The factors to consider are the age of the child; time of year; severity of the infection; frequency of infection; and rapidity of response to antibiotics. Generally, otitis media clears more readily when it occurs in an older child, in the summer, and causes relatively mild symptoms in a child who has not experienced frequent infections in the past. Given these factors, it may be possible to avoid antibiotic use. The patient must be monitored to be sure the infection clears without complication. If antibiotic treatment is initiated and the infection clears quickly, a five-day course of medication may be all that's needed.

Whether or not antibiotics are used, such pain relievers as Tylenol or Motrin can be very helpful in reducing the pain and inflammation associated with otitis media.

The use of decongestants and antihistamines does not appear to shorten the course of infection.

Surgery

In a few rare cases, a surgical perforation to drain the middle ear of pus may be performed. This procedure is called a myringotomy. The hole created by the myringotomy generally heals itself in about a week. In 2002 a new minimally invasive procedure was introduced that uses a laser to perform the myringotomy. It can be performed in the doctor's office and heals more rapidly than the standard myringotomy.

Although some doctors have recommended removing the adenoids to prevent recurrent otitis media in young children, recent studies indicate that surgical removal of the adenoids does not appear to offer any advantages over a myringotomy as a preventive measure.

Expected results

With treatment, the prognosis for acute otitis media is very good. Long-lasting accumulations of fluid within the middle ear, however, place the patient at risk both for difficulties with hearing and speech, and for the repeated development of ear infections. Furthermore, without treatment, otitis media occasionally leads to serious complications, including an infection within the nearby mastoid bone, called mastoiditis.

Prevention

Although otitis media seems inevitable in childhood, some measures can be taken to decrease the chance of repeated infections and fluid accumulation. Breastfeeding provides some protection against URIs, which in turn protects against the development of otitis media. If a child is bottle-fed, parents should be advised to feed him or her upright, rather than allowing the baby to lie down with the bottle. General good hygiene practices (especially hand washing) help to decrease the number of upper respiratory infections in a household or daycare center. Hand sanitizers are preferable to antibacterial soaps, which may contribute to bacterial resistance.

The use of pacifiers should be avoided or limited. They may act as fomites, particularly in a daycare setting. In children who are more susceptible to otitis media, pacifier use can increase by as much as 50% the number of ear infections experienced.

Two vaccines can prevent otitis media associated with certain strains of bacteria. One is designed to prevent **meningitis** and other diseases, including otitis media, that result from infection with *Haemophilus influenzae* type B. Another is a vaccine against *Streptococcus pneumoniae*, a very common cause of otitis media. Children who are at high risk or have had severe or chronic infections may be good candidates for these vaccines; in fact, a recent consensus report among pediatricians recommended routine administration of the pneumococcal conjugate vaccine to children younger than two years, as well as those at high risk for AOM. Parents should consult a healthcare provider concerning the advisability of this treatment.

Another vaccine that appears to lower the risk of AOM in children is the intranasal vaccine that was recently introduced for preventing **influenza**. Although the flu vaccine was not developed to prevent AOM directly, one team of researchers found that children who were given the vaccine before the start of flu season were 43% less likely to develop AOM than children who were not vaccinated.

As of early 2003, there is no vaccine effective against *M. catarrhalis*. Researchers are working on developing such a vaccine, as well as a tribacterial vaccine that would be effective against all three pathogens that commonly cause otitis media.

A nutrition-based approach to preventive treatment is undergoing clinical trials as of late 2002. This treatment involves giving children a dietary supplement of lemon-flavored cod liver oil plus a multivitamin formula containing **selenium**. The pilot study found that children receiving the supplement had fewer cases of otitis media, and that those who did develop it recovered with a shorter course of antibiotic treatment than children who were not receiving the supplement.

After a child has completed treatment for otitis media, a return visit to the practitioner should be scheduled. This visit should occur after the course of antibiotic has been completed. It allows the practitioner to evaluate the patient for the persistent presence of fluid within the middle ear. In children who have a problem with recurrent otitis media, a small daily dose of an antibiotic may prevent repeated full attacks of otitis media. In children who have frequent bouts of otitis media or persistent fluid, a procedure to place ventilation tubes within the eardrum may help to equalize pressure between the middle ear and the outside, thus preventing further fluid accumulation.

Resources

BOOKS

Duran, Marlene, et al. "Infections of the Upper Respiratory Tract." In *Harrison's Principles of Internal Medicine,* 14th ed., edited by Anthony S. Fauci, et al. New York: McGraw-Hill, 1998.

"Otitis Media and its Complications." In *Nelson's Textbook of Pediatrics,* edited by Richard Behrman. Philadelphia: W.B. Saunders Co., 1996.

Pelletier, Kenneth R., MD. *The Best Alternative Medicine,* Part I: Chiropractic and Osteopathy. New York: Simon & Schuster, 2002.

KEY TERMS

Adenoid—A collection of lymph tissue located in the nasopharynx.

Effusion—A collection of fluid that has leaked out into some body cavity or tissue.

Eustachian tube—A small tube that runs between the middle ear space and the nasopharynx.

Fomite—An inanimate object that can transmit infectious organisms.

Myringotomy—A surgical procedure performed to drain an infected middle ear. A newer type of myringotomy uses a laser instead of a scalpel.

Nasopharynx—The part of the airway leading into the nose.

Ossicles—Tiny bones located within the middle ear that convey the vibrations of sound through to the inner ear.

Perforation—A hole that develops in a body tissue. In otitis media, the eardrum sometimes perforates because of the pressure of fluid behind it.

Topical—Referring to a medication applied to the skin or outward surface of the body. Ear drops are one type of topical medication.

Ray, C. George. "Eye, Ear, and Sinus Infections." In *Sherris Medical Microbiology: An Introduction to Infectious Diseases,* edited by Kenneth J. Ryan. Norwalk, CT: Appleton and Lange, 1994.

PERIODICALS

Abes, G., N. Espallardo, M. Tong, et al. "A Systematic Review of the Effectiveness of Ofloxacin Otic Solution for the Treatment of Suppurative Otitis Media." *ORL* 65 (March-April 2003): 106–116.

Bucknam, J. A., and P. C. Weber. "Laser Assisted Myringotomy for Otitis Media with Effusion in Children." *ORL-Head and Neck Nursing* 20 (Summer 2002): 11-13.

Cripps, A. W., and J. Kyd. "Bacterial Otitis Media: Current Vaccine Development Strategies." *Immunology and Cell Biology* 81 (February 2003): 46–51.

Decherd, M. E., R. W. Deskin, J. L. Rowen, and M. B. Brindley. "*Bordetella pertussis* Causing Otitis Media: A Case Report." *Laryngoscope* 113 (February 2003): 226–227.

Goodwin, J. H., and J. C. Post. "The Genetics of Otitis Media." *Current Allergy and Asthma Reports* 2 (July 2002): 304-308.

Hoberman, A., C. D. Marchant, S. L. Kaplan, and S. Feldman. "Treatment of Acute Otitis Media Consensus Recommendations." *Clinical Pediatrics* 41 (July-August 2002): 373-390.

Linday, L. A., J. N. Dolitsky, R. D. Shindledecker, and C. E. Pippinger. "Lemon-Flavored Cod Liver Oil and a Multivitamin-Mineral Supplement for the Secondary Prevention of Otitis Media in Young Children: Pilot Research." *Annals of Otology, Rhinology, and Laryngology* 111 (July 2002): 642-652.

Marchisio, P., R. Cavagna, B. Maspes, et al. "Efficacy of Intranasal Virosomal Influenza Vaccine in the Prevention of Recurrent Acute Otitis Media in Children." *Clinical Infectious Diseases* 35 (July 15, 2002): 168-174.

Mattila, P. S., V. P. Joki-Erkkila, T. Kilpi, et al. "Prevention of Otitis Media by Adenoidectomy in Children Younger Than 2 Years." *Archives of Otolaryngology—Head and Neck Surgery* 129 (February 2003): 163–168.

Menger, D. J., and R. G. van den Berg. "*Pneumocystis carinii* Infection of the Middle Ear and External Auditory Canal. Report of a Case and Review of the Literature." *ORL* 65 (January-February 2003): 49–51.

Redaelli de Zinis, L. O., P. Gamba, and C. Balzanelli. "Acute Otitis Media and Facial Nerve Paralysis in Adults." *Otology and Neurotology* 24 (January 2003): 113–117.

Weiner, R., and P. J. Collison. "Middle Ear Pathogens in Otitis-Prone Children." *South Dakota Journal of Medicine* 56 (March 2003): 103–107.

ORGANIZATIONS

American Academy of Otolaryngology, Head and Neck Surgery, Inc. One Prince Street, Alexandria, VA 22314-3357. (703) 836-4444.

American Academy of Pediatrics (AAP). 141 Northwest Point Boulevard, Elk Grove Village, IL 60007. (847) 434-4000. <www.aap.org>.

American Osteopathic Association (AOA). 142 East Ontario Street, Chicago, IL 60611. (800) 621- 1773. <www.aoa-net.org>.

Judith Turner
Rebecca J. Frey, PhD

Eastern red cedar *see* **Juniper**

Eating disorders *see* **Anorexia nervosa; Binge eating disorder; Bulimia nervosa**

Echinacea

Description

Echinacea, commonly known as the purple coneflower, is a perennial herb of the Composite family, commonly known as the daisy family. Most often referred to as the purple coneflower, this hardy plant is also known as Sampson root, Missouri snakeroot, and rudbeckia. The prominent, bristly seed head inspired the generic name of the plant, taken from the Greek word, *echinos* meaning hedgehog.

Echinacea is a North American prairie native, abundant in the mid west and cultivated widely in ornamental and medicinal gardens. The purple-pink rays of the blossom droop downward from a brassy hued center cone composed of many small, tubular florets. The conspicuous flowers bloom singly on stout, prickly stems from mid-summer to autumn. Flower heads may grow to 4 in (10.16 cm) across. The dark green leaves are opposite, entire, lanceolate, toothed, and hairy with three prominent veins. The narrow upper leaves are attached to the stem with stalks. The lower leaves are longer, emerging from the stem without a leaf stalk, and growing to 8 in (20.32 cm) in length. The plant develops deep, slender, black roots. Echinacea propagates easily from seed or by root cuttings. However, due to its increasing popularity as an herbal supplement, echinacea is numbered among the 19 medicinal plants considered at risk by the Vermont nonprofit organization United Plant Savers.

General use

Three species of echinacea are useful medicinally: *Echinacea augustifolia, Echinacea purpurea,* and *Echinacea pallida.* The entire plant has numerous medicinal properties that act synergistically to good effect. Echinacea is most often used to boost the immune system and fight infection. Research has shown that echinacea increases production of interferon in the body. It is antiseptic and antimicrobial, with properties that act to increase the number of white blood cells available to destroy bacteria and slow the spread of infection. As a depurative, the herbal extract cleanses and purifies the bloodstream, and has been used effectively to treat **boils**. Echinacea is vulnerary, promoting wound healing through the action of a chemical substance in the root known as caffeic acid glycoside. As an alterative and an immuno-modulator, echinacea acts gradually to promote beneficial change in the entire system. It has also been used to treat urinary infection and *Candida albicans* **infections**. Echinacea is a febrifuge, useful in reducing fevers. It is also useful in the treatment of **hemorrhoids**. A tincture, or a strong decoction of echinacea serves as an effective mouthwash for the treatment of pyorrhea and gingivitis.

Native American plains Indians relied on echinacea as an all-purpose antiseptic. The Sioux tribe valued the root as a remedy for snake bite, the Cheyenne tribe chewed the root to quench thirst, and another tribe washed their hands in a decoction of echinacea to increase their tolerance of heat. European settlers learned of the North American herb's many uses, and soon numerous echinacea-based remedies were commercially available from pharmaceutical companies in the United States. Echinacea was a popular remedy in the United

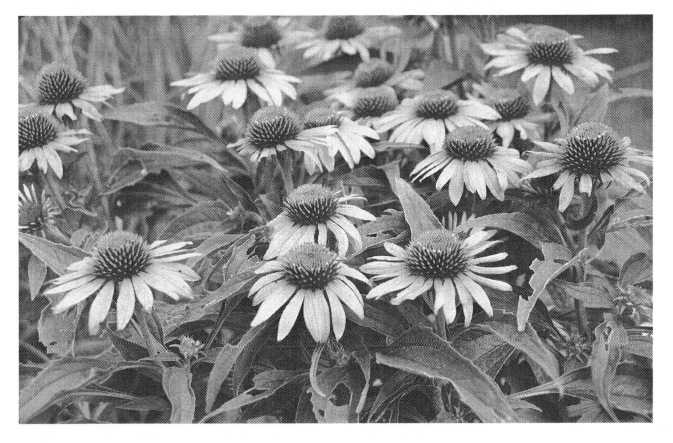

Echinacea flowers, also called purple coneflowers. *(Photo Researchers, Inc. Reproduced by permission.)*

States through the 1930s. It was among many medicinal herbs listed in the *U.S. Pharmacopoeia*, the official U.S. government listing of pharmaceutical raw materials and recipes. The herb fell out of popular use in the United States with the availability of antibiotics. In West Germany, more than 200 preparations are made from the species *E. purpurea*. Commercially prepared salves, tinctures, teas, and extracts are marketed using standardized extracts. Echinacea is regaining its status in the United States as a household medicine-chest staple in many homes. It is one of the best-selling herbal supplements in U.S. health food stores.

Clinical studies have found that the entire plant possesses medicinal properties with varying levels of effectiveness. Echinacea is of particular benefit in the treatment of upper respiratory tract infections. Some research has shown that echinacea activates the macrophages that destroy **cancer** cells and pathogens. When taken after cancer treatments, an extract of the root has been found to increase the body's production of white blood cells. Echinacea has been shown to be most effective when taken at the first sign of illness, rather than when used as a daily preventative. Other research has demonstrated the significant effect of *E. purpurea* root on reducing the du-

ration and severity of colds and flu. Some herbal references list only the root as the medicinal part, others include the aerial parts of the plant, particularly the leaf. Most research has been done on the species *E. pallida* and *E. purpurea*. All three species of echinacea are rich in vitamins and minerals. Echinacea is an herbal source of **niacin**, **chromium**, **iron**, **manganese**, **selenium**, silicon, and **zinc**.

While echinacea has proven effective for treating or preventing upper respiratory tract infections, scientific research proving its effectiveness for other uses still lacks, according to a report released in early 2002. The report says that data for other uses of the herb are inconclusive or don't exist.

Preparations

The quality of any herbal supplement depends greatly on the conditions of weather and soil where the herb was grown, the timing and care in harvesting, and the manner of preparation and storage.

Decoction is the best method to extract the mineral salts and other healing components from the coarser herb materials, such as the root, bark, and stems. It is prepared by adding 1 oz (0.028 kg) of the dried plant materials, or 2 oz (560 g) of fresh plant parts, to one pint of pure, unchlorinated, boiled water in a non-metallic pot. The mixture is simmered for about one half hour, then strained and covered. A decoction may be refrigerated for up to two days and retain its healing qualities.

An infusion is the method used to derive benefits from the leaves, flowers, and stems in the form of an herbal tea. Twice as much fresh, chopped herb as dried herb should be used. It is steeped in one pint of boiled, unchlorinated water for 10-15 minutes. Next, it is strained and covered. The infusion is drunk warm and sweetened with honey if desired. A standard dose is three cups per day. An infusion will keep for up to two days in the refrigerator and retain its healing qualities.

A tincture is the usual method to prepare a concentrated form of the herbal remedy. Tinctures, properly prepared and stored, will retain medicinal potency for two years or more. Combine 4 oz (112 g) of finely cut fresh or powdered dry herb with one pint of brandy, gin, or vodka, in a glass container. The alcohol should be enough to cover the plant parts and have a 50/50 ratio of alcohol to water. The mixture should be placed away from light for about two weeks and shaken several times each day. It should be strained and stored in a tightly capped, dark glass bottle. A standard dose is one 4 ml of the tincture three times a day.

Precautions

Echinacea is considered safe in recommended doses. Pregnant or lactating women, however, are advised not to take echinacea in injection form. Because the plant has proven immuno-modulating properties, individuals with systemic lupus erythmatosus, **rheumatoid arthritis, tuberculosis, leukemia, multiple sclerosis,** or **AIDS** should consult their physician before using echinacea. Echinacea should not be given to children under two years of age and it should only be given to children over two in consultation with a physician. Research indicates that echinacea is most effective when taken at first onset of symptoms of cold or flu, and when usage is continued no longer than eight weeks. There is some indication that the herb loses its effectiveness when used over a long period of time. It is necessary to interrupt use for a minimum of several weeks in order to give the body's immune system the opportunity to rest and adjust.

Side effects

No side effects are reported with oral administration of echinacea, either in tincture, capsule, or as a tea, when taken according to recommended doses. **Chills, fever,** and

KEY TERMS

Alterative—A medicinal substance that acts gradually to nourish and improve the system.

Antimicrobial—A plant substance that acts to inhibit the growth of harmful microorganisms, or acts to destroy them.

Febrifuge—A plant substance that acts to prevent or reduce fever.

Glycoside—An herbal carbohydrate that exerts powerful effect on hormone-producing tissues. The glycoside breaks down into a sugar and a non-sugar component.

Lanceolate—Narrow, leaf shape that is longer than it is wide, and pointed at the end.

Macrophage—Specialized cells present throughout the lymphoid tissues of the body that circulate in the bloodstream. Macrophages have a surface marker that stimulates other cells to react to an antigen.

allergic reactions have been reported in some research studies using an injection of the plant extract. Different brands of echinacea vary considerably in effectiveness.

Interactions

Those taking drugs to suppress the immune system should check with their doctors before taking Echinacea. When used in combination with other herbs, dosage should be lowered.

Resources

BOOKS

Foster, Steven and James A. Duke. *A Field Guide to Medicinal Plants.* New York: The Peterson Field Guide Series, Houghton Mifflin Company, 1990.

Hoffmann, David. *The New Holistic Herbal.* Massachusetts: Element Books Inc., 1986.

Kowalchik, Claire and William H. Hylton, editors. *Rodale's Illustrated Encyclopedia of Herbs.* Pennsylvania: Rodale Press Inc., 1987.

McIntyre, Anne. *The Medicinal Garden.* Henry Holt and Company Inc., 1997.

Official Proceedings. *Medicines from the Earth, Protocols for Botanical Healing.* Massachusetts: Gaia Herbal Research Institute, 1996.

Ondra, Nancy, editor. "200 Herbal Remedies." Excerpted from *The Complete Book of Natural & Medicinal Cures.* Pennsylvania: Rodale Press Inc., 1994.

Weed, Susun S. *Wise Woman Ways, Menopausal Years.* New York: Ash Tree Publishing, 1992.

PERIODICALS

Deneen, Sally and Tracey C. Rembert. "Stalking Medicinal Plants, An International Trade Imperils Wild Herbs." *E Magazine* (July/August 1999).

Schardt, David and Barbara Sorkin. "Echinacea." *Nutrition Action Newsletter* 29, no. 2 (March 2002):1–6.

Wallace, Phil. "Popular Herbal Supplements Get Mixed Reviews in Journal." *Food Chemical News* (January 7, 2002):30.

OTHER

Herb World News Online, Research Reviews. http://www.herbs.org. Herb Research Foundation, 1999.

Clare Hanrahan
Teresa G. Odle

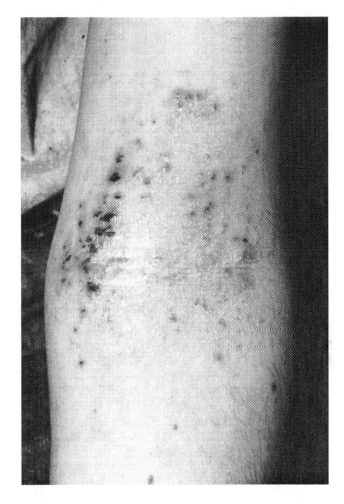

A close-up view of atopic dermatitis in the crook of the elbow of a 12-year-old patient. This condition commonly occurs in childhood. *(Custom Medical Stock Photo. Reproduced by permission.)*

Eczema

Definition

Eczema, also called atopic dermatitis (AD), is a noncontagious inflammation of the skin that is characteristically very dry and itchy. The condition is frequently related to some form of allergy, which may include foods or inhalants.

Description

Atopic dermatitis is sometimes described as "the itch that rashes"—the scratching of the irritated areas may very well initiate the rash in some patients. The skin of those affected by AD is abnormally dry because of excessive loss of moisture. Chronic or severe cases of it can cause the affected areas to form thick plaques (patches of slightly raised skin), develop serous (watery) exudates, or become infected.

The areas of the body that are affected by AD tend to vary with age. Children under five years old most commonly have AD, but it can occur at any age. It can be mild and intermittent, or severe and chronic. Infants frequently experience it on the face and other areas of the head. They frequently rub their heads with their hands or on the crib bedding. The stomach and limbs may also become involved. Older children commonly have the worst spots on flexor surfaces, namely the inner wrists and elbows, backs of knees, and tops of ankles. The hands and feet are other common sites. The knees, elbows, hands, and feet may continue to be a problem into adulthood.

Causes & symptoms

Genetic predisposition plays a large role in who will get AD or other **allergies**. The condition is not contagious. A child who has one parent with some form of allergic, or atopic, disease has somewhere between a 25–60% chance of also experiencing allergies, whether AD or some other form. There is approximately a 50–80% chance that a child of two parents with allergies will also develop some form of atopy. The genetic predisposition of the individual, combined with such factors such as early exposure to strong antigens, will determine whether and to what extent that person will develop allergies. Aside from a predisposition to eczema, increased use of soapy detergents and baby wipes is probably responsible for higher incidence of childhood eczema as well.

The hallmark sign of AD is a red, itchy rash. The age of the patient determines what regions are most likely affected, as described above, but exceptions do occur.

Diagnosis

No laboratory test can reliably diagnose AD, although some patients will be reactive to tests designed to diagnose allergy. These would include skin tests by intradermal injection, scratch, or patch tests. There is also a blood test available that measures levels of antibodies to suspected allergens. Diagnosis is generally made by the appearance and location of the rash. A personal or family history of allergy of any type, including food allergy, **asthma**, or **hay fever** also supports the diagnosis of AD.

Other types of dermatitis that may be described as eczematous include **contact dermatitis**, nummular dermatitis, and stasis dermatitis. The stasis type is related to poor circulation, which may also be a factor in nummular dermatitis. These forms generally occur in older adults, whereas AD is primarily a disease of children. Contact dermatitis can occur at any age. It results from skin contact with either an irritant or an allergen. The area affected is limited to the area in contact with the offending substance.

Treatment

The basis of treatment for AD is keeping the skin moist and clean, as well as avoiding irritants and known allergens as much as possible. Further measures become necessary if the case is particularly severe, or if the skin becomes infected.

Conventional wisdom has been that minimal bathing of the patient with AD is ideal. The rationale was that bathing would break down the natural oil barrier of the skin and cause further drying. It actually appears now that frequent long, tepid soaks are beneficial to hydrate the very dry skin that this condition produces. Adding a muslin bag filled with milled oats or the commercially available preparation Aveeno bath to the water can be soothing. The bath water should cover as much of the skin as possible. Wet towels may be draped around the shoulders, upper trunk, and arms if they are above the water level. The face should be dabbed frequently during bathing to keep it moist. The use of soap should be minimized, and limited to very mild agents such as Cetaphil. The bath must be followed within two or three minutes by a gentle patting dry, and a thick application of a water barrier ointment, such as Aquaphor, Unibase, or Vaseline. Lotions are not generally recommended as they almost universally contain alcohol, which is drying and may burn when applied. Soaking in plain water can be painful during severe episodes of AD. Adding one-half cup of table salt to one-half tub of water creates a normal saline solution, similar to what is naturally present in the tissues, and may relieve the burning. Commercial Domeboro powder may also be helpful.

One alternative to bathing is to use soaking wraps. For this method, cotton towels or other cloths are soaked in tepid water, with table salt or Domeboro powder added for comfort if desired. The patient's bed is covered with something waterproof, and the bare skin is covered as thoroughly as possible with the wet wrappings. The body should then be covered by a waterproof covering to slow evaporation. Vinyl sheeting and plastic wrap are two alternatives. The wraps should be left in place for as long as possible, but at least for 30 minutes, before the water barrier and any topical medications are applied.

Environmental improvement affords some relief for many patients. Pet dander and cigarette smoke are potential aggravating factors. Keeping these out of the home is probably for the best, but at minimum, they should not be allowed in the room of the allergic person. Clothing and bedding should be 100% soft cotton, and laundered in detergent with no perfumes. These items should also be washed before the initial use in order to rid them of potentially irritating residues. Clothes should fit loosely to prevent irritation from rubbing. Washing bedding in hot water will help to kill dust mites. Running laundry through a double rinse cycle will help to remove any vestiges of detergent. Avoiding the use of fabric softener or dryer sheets helps, as these are frequently scented and may be irritating. Drying clothes or bedding outdoors should be avoided, because pollen and other potential allergens are likely to cling to them. Mattresses and pillowcase can be covered by special casings that are impervious to the microscopic dust mites that infest them. Under normal circumstances, these mites cause no problem, but they can be a major irritant for the individual with asthma or AD.

Temperature extremes can make AD worse, so heating and cooling should be employed as appropriate, along with adding humidity if needed. Patients tend to have abnormal regulation of body temperature, and sometimes feel warmer or colder than other people in similar circumstances. Sweating will frequently aggravate AD. Room temperature should be adjusted for comfort. Central air conditioning is the best option for cooling the home. Evaporative cooling brings a large amount of potential irritants into the house, as do open windows. Air conditioning rather than open windows should also be used to cool the car. Electrostatic filters and vent covers are available to remove irritants from the air in the house. These should be frequently changed or cleaned as recommended by the manufacturer.

In the patient's room, dust-collecting items such as curtains, carpeting, and stuffed animals are best minimized. Vacuuming and dusting should be done regularly when the affected person is not in the room. A HEPA filter unit, and a vacuum with a built-in HEPA filter remove a high percent of dust and pollen from the environment.

Some simple mechanical measures will reduce the amount of skin damage done by scratching. It is important to keep fingernails short. Using a nail file will produce a smoother nail edge than scissors or clippers. It is particularly difficult to keep children from scratching irritated and itchy skin, but using pajamas and clothing with maximum skin coverage will help to protect the bare skin from fingernails. Mittens or socks may be used to cover the hands at night to reduce the effects of scratching. Infant gowns with hand coverings are useful for the very young patient.

In addition to the skin care and environmental measures to relieve eczema, there are some complementary therapies that may prove helpful.

Acupuncture

Any type of therapy that relieves **stress** can also help to manage AD. Acupuncturists also claim to be able to treat blood and energy deficiencies, and to counteract the effects of detrimental elements, including heat, dampness, and wind.

Autogenic training

Autogenic training is similar to methods of **meditation** and self-hypnosis. Instructors help the patient to achieve and maintain a relaxed state of positive concentration. This is eventually done independently. Even ten minutes of practice per day can produce beneficial results for mind and body. Research has shown AD to be one of the conditions that is improved by this technique.

Aromatherapy/massage

Massage is another therapy that can be effective in reducing stress. The oils that are used in the treatment can also make a difference in AD. Some patients get relief from the topical use of **evening primrose oil** (EPO) diluted in carrier oil. Aromatherapists may use small amounts of **essential oils** from **lavender**, bergamot, and geranium. These are promoted to decrease both **itching** and inflammation. Improper dilutions, however, can worsen the condition.

Herbal therapy

Some herbal therapies can be useful for skin conditions. Among the herbs most often recommended are:

• Calendula (*Calendula officinalis*) ointment, for anti-inflammatory and antiseptic properties.

• Chickweed (*Stellaria media*) ointment, to soothe itching.

• Evening primrose oil (*Oenograceae*) topically to relieve itching, and internally to supplement fatty acids.

• German **chamomile** (*Chamomilla recutita*) ointment, for anti-inflammatory properties.

• Nettle (*Urtica dioica*) ointment, to relieve itching.

• Peppermint (*Menta piperita*) lotion, for antibacterial and antiseptic properties.

• Chinese herbal medicine. In **traditional Chinese medicine**, there are formulas used to treat eczema that nourish the blood, moisten the skin, stop itching, and encourage healing. Some formulas are used topically and others taken internally.

There is individual variation in the effectiveness of the topical treatments. Some experimentation may help to find the combination that most benefits an individual. When the condition is chronic, severe, or infected, guidance from a health care professional should be sought before attempting self-treatment.

Hypnotherapy

Hypnotherapy has the potential to improve AD through using the power of suggestion to reduce itching. Since mechanical damage to the skin done by scratching may irritate, or actually cause, the rash, any measure that reduces scratching can prove helpful.

Nutritional supplements

There are several nutrients that can prove helpful for treating AD. Oral doses of EPO, which contains gamma-linolenic acid, have been shown to significantly reduce itching. The amount used in studies was approximately six grams of EPO per day. **Fish oil** has also been shown to improve AD, at an approximate dose of 1.8 g per day. **Vitamin C** can affect both skin healing and boost the immune system. Doses of 50–75 mg per kilogram of body weight have been proven to relieve symptoms of AD. Additional **copper** may be required in supplemental form when high doses of vitamin C are taken. **Vitamin E** is reportedly useful, but there are no documented studies of its benefits.

Reflexology

The areas of the foot that receive attention from a reflexologist when a patient has AD include the ones relating to the affected areas of the body, as well as those for the solar plexus, adrenal glands, pituitary gland, liver, kidneys, gastrointestinal tract, and reproductive glands.

Allopathic treatment

Allopathic treatment involves use of oral antihistamines to decrease itching, topical water barriers as mentioned above, mild topical corticosteroids when indicated, and topical antibiotics if needed. The water barrier should be applied generously; the corticosteroids and antibiotics used sparingly, and only on areas where indicated. The person applying the topical medications can wear gloves to minimize exposure to the steroids and antibiotics. Oral antibiotics may also be used when widespread infection is present. On rare occasions, oral corticosteroids are prescribed to reduce severe itching and inflammation, but this course is best avoided due to its potential side effects. In 2001, the U.S. Food and Drug Administration (FDA) approved a new nonsteroid prescription cream for patients age two and older called Elidel.

Expected results

There is no cure for AD, although most patients will experience improvement with age. Perhaps half of children will have no further trouble past the age of five years. However, as many as 75% of those who have AD in childhood will go on to have other allergic manifestations such as asthma, food allergies, and hay **fever**. Diligent daily care of the skin and avoidance of known triggers will control most cases of AD to a large extent.

Prevention

One of the best things a mother can do to help keep her child from getting AD is to breastfeed. It is best for the baby to have breast milk exclusively for at least six months, particularly when there is a family history of AD or other types of allergy. There also appears to be an advantage to the breastfeeding mother avoiding foods known to be commonly allergenic, particularly if there is a family history. This would include wheat, eggs, products made from cow's milk, peanuts, and fish. If breastfeeding is not possible, a hypoallergenic formula should be used if there is family history of allergy. Consult a health care provider for help with determining the best type.

The patient already diagnosed with AD can minimize flare-ups by avoiding known triggers and following the skin care program outlined above. It is important to continue to follow guidelines for a daily emollient routine (moistening skin twice daily) even when skin is under control to prevent flare-ups. Eczematous skin is also more susceptible to **infections**. Patients should try to stay away from people with chicken pox, cold sores, and other contagious skin infections.

Resources

BOOKS

Chevallier, Andrew. *The Encyclopedia of Medicinal Plants.* New York: DK Publishing, Inc., 1996.

Editors of Time-Life Books. *The Medical Advisor: The Complete Guide to Conventional and Alternative Treatments.* Alexandria, VA: Time-Life, Inc., 1996.

Gottlieb, Bill, editor. *New Choices in Natural Healing.* Emmaus, PA: Rodale Press, Inc., 1995.

Shealy, C. Norman. *The Complete Illustrated Encyclopedia of Alternative Healing Therapies.* Boston: Element Books, Inc., 1999.

PERIODICALS

PERIODICALS

"Detergents Linked to Rise in Infant Eczema." *Australian Nursing Journal* (July 2002): 29.

"Eczema Guidelines to Make up for Inadequate Training." *Practice Nurse* (September 27, 2002): 9.

PERIODICALS

"Guidelines for the Effective Use of Emollients." *Chemist & Druggist* (September 14, 2002): 22.

PERIODICALS

"Prescription Cream Treats Atopic Eczema." *Critical Care Nurse* (August 2002): 76.

OTHER

Food Allergy Network. *Food Allergy and Atopic Dermatitis* Fairfax, VA: Food Allergy Network, 1992.

Hollandsworth, Kim et. al. *Atopic Dermatitis.* Pediatric Clinical Research Unit, 1994.

Judith Turner
Teresa G. Odle

Edema

Definition

Edema is a condition of abnormally large fluid volume in the circulatory system or in tissues between the body's cells (interstitial spaces).

Description

Normally the body maintains a balance of fluid in tissues by ensuring that the same amount of water entering the body also leaves it. The circulatory system transports fluid within the body via its network of blood vessels. The fluid, which contains oxygen and nutrients needed by the cells, moves from the walls of the blood vessels into the body's tissues. After its nutrients are used up, fluid moves back into the blood vessels and returns to the heart. The lymphatic system (a network of channels in the body that carry lymph, a colorless fluid containing white blood cells to fight infection) also absorbs and transports this fluid. In edema, either too much fluid moves from the blood vessels into the tissues, or not enough fluid moves from the tissues back into the blood vessels. This fluid imbalance can cause mild to severe swelling in one or more parts of the body.

Causes & symptoms

Many ordinary factors can upset the balance of fluid in the body to cause edema, including:

- Immobility. The leg muscles normally contract and compress blood vessels to promote blood flow with walking or running. When these muscles are not used, blood can collect in the veins, making it difficult for fluid to move from tissues back into the vessels.

- Heat. Warm temperatures cause the blood vessels to expand, making it easier for fluid to cross into surrounding tissues. High humidity also aggravates this situation.

- Medications. Certain drugs, such as steroids, hormone replacements, nonsteroidal anti-inflammatory drugs (NSAIDs), and some blood pressure medications may affect how fast fluid leaves blood vessels.

- Intake of salty foods. The body needs a constant concentration of salt in its tissues. When excess salt is taken in, the body dilutes it by retaining fluid.

- Menstruation and **pregnancy**. The changing levels of hormones affect the rate at which fluid enters and leaves the tissues.

Some medical conditions may also cause edema, including:

- Heart failure. When the heart is unable to maintain adequate blood flow throughout the circulatory system, the excess fluid pressure within the blood vessels can cause shifts into the interstitial spaces. Left-sided heart failure can cause pulmonary edema, as fluid shifts into the lungs. The patient may develop rapid, shallow respirations, shortness of breath, and a **cough**. Right-sided heart failure can cause pitting edema, a swelling in the tissue under the skin of the lower legs and feet. Pressing this tissue with a finger tip leads to a noticeable momentary indentation.

- Kidney disease. The decrease in **sodium** and water excretion can result in fluid retention and overload.

- Thyroid or liver disease. These conditions can change the concentration of protein in the blood, affecting fluid movement in and out of the tissues. In advanced liver disease, the liver is enlarged and fluid may build up in the abdomen.

- Malnutrition. Protein levels are decreased in the blood, and in an effort to maintain a balance of concentrations, fluid shifts out of the vessels and causes edema in tissue spaces.

Some conditions that may cause swelling in just one leg include:

- Blood clots. Clots can cause pooling of fluid and may be accompanied by discoloration and **pain**. In some instances, clots may cause no pain.

- Weakened veins. **Varicose veins**, or veins whose walls or valves are weak, can allow blood to pool in the legs. This is a common condition.

- Infection and inflammation. Infection in leg tissues can cause inflammation and increasing blood flow to the area. Inflammatory diseases, such as **gout** or arthritis, can also result in swelling.

- Lymphedema. Blocked lymph channels may be caused by infection, scar tissue, or hereditary conditions. Lymph that can't drain properly results in edema. Lymphedema may also occur after **cancer** treatments, when the lymph system is impaired by surgery, radiation, or chemotherapy.

- Tumor. Abnormal masses can compress leg vessels and lymph channels, affecting the rate of fluid movement.

Symptoms vary depending on the cause of edema. In general, weight gain, puffy eyelids, and swelling of the legs may occur as a result of excess fluid volume. Pulse rate and blood pressure may be elevated. Hand and neck veins may be observed as fuller.

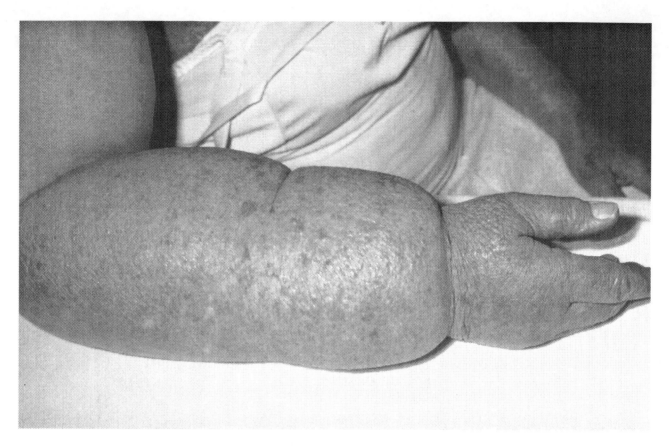

Gross lymphoedema in the arm of an elderly woman following radiotherapy treatment for breast cancer. *(Photograph by Dr. P. Marazzi. Photo Researchers.)*

Diagnosis

Edema is a sign of an underlying problem, rather than a disease unto itself. A diagnostic explanation should be sought. Patient history and presenting symptoms, along with laboratory blood studies, if indicated, assist the health professional in determining the cause of the edema.

Treatment

Simple steps to lessen fluid build-up may include:

• reducing sodium intake

• maintaining proper weight

• exercise

• elevation of the legs

• use of support stockings

• massage

• travel breaks

Nutritional therapy

A naturopath or a nutritionist may recommend the following dietary changes:

• Reduction of salt intake, including salty foods such as olives, soy sauce, or pickles. Cutting back the amount of sodium eaten may help reduce edema.

• Limited use of alcohol, **caffeine**, sugar, and dairy products.

• Increased consumption of whole grain foods, cucumbers, apples, potatoes, grapes, onions, cabbage, and oranges.

• Daily vitamin and mineral supplements.

Herbal therapy

Diuretic herbs can also help relieve edema. One of the best herbs for this purpose is **dandelion** (*Taraxacum mongolicum*), since, in addition to its diuretic action, it is a rich source of **potassium**. (Diuretics flush potassium from the body, and it must be replaced to avoid potassium deficiency.)

Hydrotherapy

Hydrotherapy using daily contrast applications of hot and cold (either compresses or immersion) may also be helpful.

KEY TERMS

Digitalis—A naturally occurring compound used in the preparation of the medication digoxin, prescribed to increase the heart rate and strengthen the force of the heart's contractions.

Diuretics—Medications used in the treatment of fluid overload, to promote excretion of sodium and water.

Interstitial spaces—Areas of the body occurring outside the vessels or organs, between the cells.

Pitting edema—A swelling in the tissue under the skin, resulting from fluid accumulation, that is measured by the depth of indentation made by finger pressure over a boney prominence.

Other alternative treatments

Other alternative therapies may also reduce edema. They include **traditional Chinese medicine**, Ayurveda, juice therapy, and bodywork. Traditional Chinese medicine and **acupuncture** have an elaborate diagnostic system to determine the pattern causing the edema. Thus treatment, if done correctly, results not only in the removal of fluid, but also with the correction of the problem.

Allopathic treatment

The three "Ds"—diuretics, digitalis, and diet—are frequently prescribed for medical conditions that result in excess fluid volume. Diuretics are medications that promote urination of sodium and water. Digoxin is a digitalis preparation that is sometimes needed to decrease heart rate and increase the strength of the heart's contractions. One dietary recommendation includes less sodium in order to decrease fluid retention. Consideration of adequate protein intake is also made.

For patients with lymphedema, a combination of therapies may prove effective. Combined decongestive therapy includes the use of manual lymph drainage (MLD), compression bandaging, garments and pumps, and physical therapy.

Resources

BOOKS
The Burton Goldberg Group. "Edema." in *Alternative Medicine: The Definitive Guide*. Tiburon, CA: Future Medicine Publishing, Inc., 1999.

Monahan, Frances D., and Marianne Neighbors. *Medical-Surgical Nursing: Foundation for Clinical Practice*, 2nd ed. Philadelphia: W. B. Saunders, 1998.

ORGANIZATIONS
Lymphedema and Wound Care Clinic of Austin. 5750 Balcones Dr., Ste. 110, Austin, TX 78731. (512) 453-1930. <www.lymphedema.com.>

Mai Tran

Elder

Description

Gaining popularity in modern times as a cold and flu medicine, elder flower has been an important folk remedy for centuries. The Roman naturalist Pliny wrote about the therapeutic value of this flowering tree in the first century A.D. Native Americans used elder as a treatment for respiratory **infections** and **constipation** as well as an herbal pad for healing **wounds**. Black elder (*Sambucus nigra*) is the most popular variety of the plant, though there are other species known to have similar chemical ingredients. Elder grows in Europe, Asia, North Africa, and the United States. Most medicinal elder is obtained from the former Soviet Union, Eastern Europe, and the United Kingdom. The Latin word *sambucus* is thought to be derived from the Greek *sambuca*, which refers to a stringed musical instrument popular among the Ancient Romans. In fact, some modern day Italians still make a primitive pipe called a *sampogna* from the branches of the tree, which also produces fragrant, cream-colored flowers and deep-violet berries. The flowers and berries are used most often in the drug of commerce, though the leaves, bark, and roots are also considered to have therapeutic effects. The berries traditionally have been used to make elderberry wine as well as pies and jellies, although no value has yet been found in these products.

The German Commission E, considered an authoritative source of information on alternative remedies, determined that elder has the ability to increase bronchial secretions as well as perspiration. These properties can be useful in helping to alleviate symptoms of the **common cold** or the flu. Even more interesting is the possibility that elder, like another herbal remedy called **echinacea**, may have the power to shorten the duration of colds by up to a few days. While it is not known exactly how elder produces its therapeutic effects, study has focused on several naturally occurring chemicals in the plant. Elder's flavonoids and phenolic acids are thought to be responsible for its ability to increase perspiration. The triterpenes in elder may also be potential "active ingredients," though more study is required to confirm this. The remaining chemical constituents of medicinal elder usually include **potassium** and other minerals; sterols;

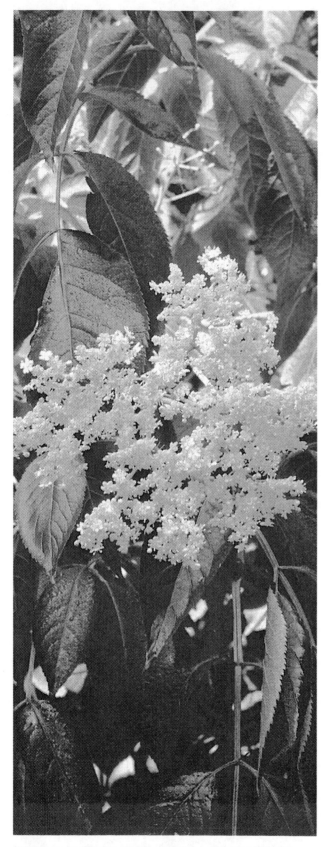

Elderflowers. (© PlantaPhile, Germany. Reproduced by permission.)

volatile oils containing linoleic, linolenic, and palmitic acid; mucilage; pectin; protein; sugar; and tannins.

A number of other properties have been ascribed to elder as well, including anti-inflammatory, diuretic, antiviral, and antispasmodic activities. A 1997 study published in the *Journal of Ethnopharmacology*, which studied black elder in the test tube, indicates that the herb has some activity as an anti-inflammatory. While this may help to partially explain elder's success in treating colds, it also suggests that the herb may have potential as a treatment for inflammatory diseases such as rheumatism. Elder has also been described in the history of folk medicine as a laxative and a sedative.

General use

While not approved by the FDA, black elder flower is primarily used in the United States and Europe for colds and the flu. When taken internally, elder flower is approved by the Commission E for colds. In Germany, elder flower tea is licensed by the government to treat the common cold and other upper respiratory problems. By increasing bronchial secretions as well as perspiration, elder is believed to help ease symptoms such as **cough** and **fever** and may even shorten a cold's duration. In the United States and Canada, elder is often combined with **peppermint** leaf and **yarrow** flower in preparations intended to alleviate cold-related fever.

In a study published in the *Journal of Alternative and Complementary Medicine* in 1995, use of a standardized elderberry extract shortened the duration of the flu by about three days. The placebo-controlled, double-blind study involved the residents of an Israeli kibbutz. "A significant improvement of the symptoms, including fever, was seen in 93.3% of the cases in the SAM-treated group [elder-treated group] within 2 days," the researchers reported, "whereas in the control group 91.7% of the patients showed an improvement within 6 days." About 90% of the people treated with elder were considered flu-free in two to three days, while the majority of patients in the placebo group only got well after about 6 days. The authors of the study recommended elder as a possible treatment for **influenza** A and B based on the herbal remedy's effectiveness, lack of side effects, and low cost. By way of comparison, over-the-counter synthetic drugs may offer some measure of symptomatic relief for a cold but have not been proven to actually speed recovery. Elder is also being investigated as a treatment for other viral infections such as human immunodeficiency virus (HIV) and herpes.

Throughout its long history, elder has been used to treat a variety of other diseases and medical problems. These include liver disease, kidney disorders, rheumatism, **insomnia**, toothaches, **measles**, **asthma**, **cancer**, chafing, epilepsy, **gout**, headaches, **neuralgia, psoriasis, syphilis**, and **laryngitis**. It has also been used topically as an herbal pad to reduce external swelling and heal wounds. Some women have used elder to increase the amount of milk produced during breastfeeding. However, as of early 2000, sufficient scientific evidence to support these additional uses is lacking. While elder has been used as a folk remedy for treating diabetes, studies in rodents suggest that it has no effects on blood sugar regulation.

Preparations

Dosage of elder generally ranges from 10-15 g per day, divided into three equal doses. The drug, which is recommended for internal use only, is usually taken as a tea or liquid extract. Elder tea can be prepared by steeping 3-4 g (2 teaspoonfuls) of dried elder flower in 150 ml of hot (not boiling) water. The mixture should be strained after about 5 minutes. The tea works best when it is consumed at a temperature as hot as can be safely tolerated. Dosage is several cups of tea a day (do not exceed the daily maximum of 15 g of elder), taken in the afternoons and evenings. When using a standardized liquid extract of elder, follow the package directions for proper use.

Precautions

Taken in recommended dosages, elder is not known to be harmful. It should be used with caution in children, women who are pregnant or breastfeeding, and people with kidney or liver disorders because its effects in these groups have not been sufficiently studied.

Be careful not to confuse black elder with a more toxic species of the plant called dwarf elder (*Sambucus ebulus*). Dwarf elder is generally not recommended for medical purposes and may cause **vomiting** and **diarrhea** in large dosages.

Side effects

Side effects are considered rare. Mild abdominal distress or allergic reactions may occur.

Interactions

Elder is not known to interact adversely with other medications or herbal remedies. Preparations that combine elder with yarrow flower and peppermint leaf have been used without apparent harm.

Resources

BOOKS

Fetrow, Charles W. and Avila, Juan R. *Professional's Handbook of Complementary and Alternative Medicine*. Pennsylvania: Springhouse, 1998.

> ## KEY TERMS
>
> **Antispasmodic**—An agent with the ability to prevent or relieve convulsions or muscle spasms.
>
> **Diuretic**—An agent that increases the production of urine.
>
> **Echinacea**—A popular herbal remedy used to treat colds, the flu, and urinary tract infections.
>
> **Edema**—Abnormal swelling of tissue due to fluid buildup. Edema, which typically occurs in the legs, liver, and lungs, is often a complication of heart or kidney problems.

Gruenwald, Joerg. *PDR for Herbal Medicines*. New Jersey: Medical Economics, 1998.

Sifton, David W. *PDR Family Guide to Natural Medicines and Healing Therapies*. New Jersey: Medical Economics, 1999.

PERIODICALS

Yesilada E., Ustun O., Sezik E., et al. "Inhibitory effects of Turkish folk remedies on inflammatory cytokines: interleukin-1alpha, interleukin-1beta and tumor necrosis factor alpha." *J Ethnopharmacol* (1997) 58(1):59-73.

Zakay-Rones Z., Varsano N., Zlotnik M., et al. "Inhibition of several strains of influenza virus in vitro and reduction of symptoms by an elderberry extract *(Sambucus nigra L.)* during an outbreak of influenza B Panama." *J Altern Complement Med* (1995) 1(4):361-9.

ORGANIZATIONS

American Botanical Council. PO Box 144345, Austin, TX 78714-4345.

Herb Research Foundation. 1007 Pearl Street, Suite 200, Boulder, CO 80302.

OTHER

Herb Research Foundation. http://www.herbs.org (January 17, 2001).

OnHealth. http://www.onhealth.com (January 17, 2001).

Discovery Health. http://www.discoveryhealth.com (January 17, 2001).

Greg Annussek

Electroacupuncture

Definition

Electroacupuncture is an **acupuncture** technique that applies small electrical currents to needles that have been inserted at specific points on the body.

Origins

Acupuncture originated thousands of years ago in China as a healing technique. Electroacupuncture was developed in 1958 in China, when acupuncturists there began experimenting with it as surgical anesthesia, or **pain** control. After several years of testing during surgery, acupuncturists began applying electroacupuncture in clinical practice for many conditions.

Benefits

Electroacupuncture can be used to treat the same variety of health conditions that regular acupuncture treats, and for conditions that do not respond to conventional acupuncture. It is effectively used as surgical anesthesia, as a means of reducing chronic pain and muscle spasms, and as a treatment for neurological (nerve) disorders.

Description

Acupuncturists begin treatment by diagnosing a patient. Diagnosis is performed with interviews, close examinations (such as of the tongue and **pulse diagnosis**), and other methods. Acupuncture strives to balance and improve the flow of *chi*, or life energy, which travels throughout the body in channels called *meridians*. According to **traditional Chinese medicine** (TCM), illness is caused when chi does not move properly in the body. Acupuncturists are trained to determine where chi is stagnated, weak, or out of balance, which indicates where and how acupuncture points on the body should be stimulated. Electroacupuncture is often recommended for cases of accumulation of chi, such as in chronic pain, and in cases where the chi is difficult to prompt or stimulate.

Patients usually lie down for acupuncture treatment. Thin, sterilized needles are used, and the surface of the skin where they will be inserted is sterilized, as well. One advantage of electroacupuncture is that the margin of error for needle placement is greater than for regular acupuncture, because the electrical current stimulates a larger area around the needle. Electroacupuncture works with two needles at a time in order for electrical current to pass through the body from one needle to another. Small devices are used to create and regulate a pulsing electric charge, which is sent to the needles by attaching small clips to their ends. The electric charge is very small, and can be adjusted by the acupuncturist or patient. Both the voltage (intensity) and the frequency of the electric charge can be adjusted for healing effects. Voltage levels should be raised slowly. Several pairs of needles may be stimulated at one time, for up to 30 or more minutes of electrical stimulation along the meridians. Another similar, though conventional, medical tech-

nique is called *transcutaneous electrical nerve stimulation* (TENS), which uses electrodes that are taped to the surface of the skin instead of attached to inserted needles, which may be advantageous for patients for whom needles pose risks or problems. This technique stimulates along nerve and muscle groups.

Precautions

Electroacupuncture should not be used on people who have seizures, **epilepsy**, histories of **heart disease** or strokes, or those with heart pacemakers. Electroacupuncture should not be performed on the head, throat, or directly over the heart, and should be per-

---

REINHOLD VOLL 1909–1989

German physician Reinhold Voll initially studied architecture in school and had no intention to become a physician. He decided to study medicine when various treatments to restore the health of his father failed. He spent much of his early career specializing in tropical diseases, sports medicine, and public health, and set up a practice in Plochingen in southern Germany. He was introduced to methods of Chinese acupuncture by a doctor who worked in the tropics and was a firm believer in the practice. By the 1950s, Voll was engaging in the ancient Chinese practice. He had an idea that modern technology might enhance acupuncture in the treatment of various chronic diseases such as allergies, chronic fatigue, migraines, and chronic liver, kidney or pancreatic diseases. His research led him to electroacupuncture (EAV), using electric currents to enhance manipulation of the traditional acupuncture points. In addition to that, he realized that there were even more points, or meridians, that corresponded directly with particular organs. Voll then developed a system to measure the degree of inflammation these organs suffered.

Voll focused on certain criteria by which to treat these points. He determined that conditions were either inflammable, chronic, or subchronic. By the use of nosodes, remedies composed of bacteria or viruses, and based on the causes of those diseases and using other homeopathic agents, he was able to test for drugs before the patient ingested them. It was Voll who also discovered the relationship between teeth and the inner organs, an important key to understanding health and disease.

The Institute for ElectroAcupuncture & ElectroDiagnostics is based on Voll's original methods is located in Munich, Germany. The website for additional information can be located at: http://www.eavnet.com.

Jane Spear

KEY TERMS

Anesthesia—Method of controlling pain during surgery.

Epilepsy—Condition characterized by sudden seizures and other symptoms.

Pacemaker—Device that is surgically implanted in those suffering from heart disease or disorders, which regulates the beating of the heart.

formed with care on spastic muscles. Another recommended precaution is that electrical current should not be sent across the midline of the body, which is the line running from the nose to the navel.

Side effects

During electroacupuncture, patients report sensations of tingling, warmth, and mild aches. Bruising and bleeding may occur, as the needles may hit small blood vessels.

Resources

BOOKS

Kakptchuk, Ted. *The Web That Has No Weaver: Understanding Chinese Medicine.* New York: Congdon and Weed, 1983.

Requena, Yves, M.D. *Terrains and Pathology in Acupuncture.* Massachusetts: Paradigm, 1986.

OTHER

American Association of Oriental Medicine. http://www.aaom.org.

North American Society of Acupuncture and Alternative Medicine. http://www.nasa-altmed.com.

Douglas Dupler

Eleutherococcus senticosus see **Ginseng, Siberian**

Elimination diet

Definition

An elimination diet functions as a test, determining whether patients may have a sensitivity to certain foods. Initially, patients stop eating foods suspected of causing illness. Then, after a suitable period of time (often 10–14 days), they review the patients' symptoms. If significant improvement has occurred, it is assumed that an allergy or intolerance to certain foods may be involved. These suspect foods are then reintroduced into the diet, one by one.

When symptoms return (usually within three days), the problematic food is identified and removed from the diet.

Benefits

Elimination **diets** are potentially useful in identifying hard-to-detect food intolerances that proponents believe are responsible for a wide range of ailments. These include **constipation**, headaches, migraine, **infections** of the ear or sinuses, frequent colds, post nasal drip, chronic nasal congestion, sore throats, chronic **cough**, **eczema**, **hives**, **acne**, **asthma**, **pain** or stiffness in the muscles or joints, heart palpitations, **indigestion**, ulcers of the mouth, stomach, or duodenum, **Crohn's disease**, **diarrhea**, yeast infections, urticaria, **edema**, **depression**, **anxiety**, hyperactivity, weight change, and generalized **fatigue**.

Description

The following lists of appropriate and inappropriate foods for an elimination diet represent general guidelines. Elimination diets vary according to practitioner and the specific symptoms or allergy.

Foods that may be prohibited in an elimination diet include those containing:

- Additives: monosodium glutamate, artificial preservatives, sweeteners, flavors, or colors.
- Alcohol: beer, ale, stout, porter, malt liquors, wine, coolers, vodka, gin, rum, whiskey, brandy, liqueurs, and cordials.
- Citrus fruits: oranges, calamondins, tangerines, clementines, tangelos, satsumas, owaris, lemons, limes, kumquats, limequats, and grapefruit.
- Commonly eaten foods: anything consumed more than three times weekly, as well as foods that are craved, or that cause a feeling of weakness.
- Corn: as well as corn syrup or sweetener, corn oil, vegetable oil, popcorn, corn chips, corn tortillas.
- Dairy products: milk, milk solids, cheese, butter, sour cream, yogurt, cottage cheese, whey, and ice cream.
- Eggs: both yolks and whites.
- Gluten: any pasta, breads, cakes, flour, or gravies containing wheat.
- Honey.
- Maple syrup.
- Sugar: candy, soft drinks, fruit juices with added sugar or sweetener, cakes, cookies, sucrose, fructose, dextrose, or maltose.

Foods that may be allowed include:

- Cereals: puffed rice or millet, oatmeal, or oat bran.

- Daily multivitamin: this is especially important during extended dieting to replace missing nutrients.

- Fats and oils: soy, soy milk, soy cheese, sunflower oil, safflower oil, **flaxseed** oil, olive oil, and sesame oil.

- Fruits and vegetables: typically, anything except corn and citrus fruits. Some practitioners suggest fruit be consumed in moderation, and preferably whole as opposed to juices.

- Grain and flour products: rice cakes or crackers, rye or spelt bread (both must be 100% with no added wheat), kasha, rice, amaranth, quinoa, millet, oriental noodles, other exotic grains.

- Legumes: soybeans, string beans, black beans, navy beans, kidney beans, peas, chickpeas, lentils, tofu. Canned beans should be avoided unless they are free of preservatives and sugar.

- Seeds and nuts: must not contain sugar or salt. Nut butters are allowed if they meet this requirement and are organic.

- Water: two quarts daily. Preferably bottled, as tap water contains potential allergens including fluoride and chlorine.

- Other: honey, white vinegar, salt, pepper, **garlic**, onions, **ginger**, herbal teas, coffee substitutes, spices or condiments (mustard, ketchup) that are free from sugar, preservatives, and citrus. These products can commonly be found at health food stores.

An important complement to any elimination diet is a food diary, in which all dietary consumption is recorded, along with any subsequent symptoms. Patterns should be evident after about one month of record keeping.

Precautions

As with all therapies, anyone considering an elimination diet should weigh the potential benefits against the risks. The decision, according to some, is comparable to deciding to take a prescribed medication, and should be done only under the supervision of a competent medical practitioner.

Elimination diets should never be used by individuals with severe food **allergies**, as reintroducing a suspect food may provoke an asthma attack, anaphylactic shock, or other dangerous reaction. Generally, an elimination diet will only be used when symptoms are believed to be related to just one or two suspect foods.

Patients need to know that following a strict elimination diet is not an easy matter. It is extremely important to read packaged-food labels carefully, because many processed foods contain monosodium glutamate, sugar, and other substances that may be prohibited. It is almost impossible for elimination-diet patients to eat in restaurants, at school, or at the homes of friends. The resulting isolation must be considered as part of the decision to undertake an elimination diet. Patients should also consider whether they have sufficient time for the extra planning, shopping, and food preparation involved.

Elimination-diet patients should be vigilant to replace any nutrients missing from their restricted diet. For example, **calcium** supplements may be advisable for someone eliminating dairy products from the diet. Needless to say, any prescribed medications should be continued during any diet.

Putting a very young child on an elimination diet may endanger the child's **nutrition** and normal growth. A breastfeeding mother may harm both her own health and that of her infant if she undertakes an elimination diet during lactation.

Side effects

The most significant side effects of an elimination diet are nutritional disorders resulting from a prolonged, highly restrictive diet, and the risk of a serious reaction as suspect foods are re-introduced to the diet. Some proponents also caution that patients consuming a very limited variety of foods risk becoming allergic to those very foods. For these reasons, both professional supervision and substitution of missing nutrients both essential.

Research & general acceptance

Elimination diets are widely used by medical doctors, but considerable differences of opinion exist over the range of illnesses that may be caused by food allergies or intolerances. Many physicians and researchers question the role of allergies in migraine, **rheumatoid arthritis**, **osteoarthritis**, and other conditions. Some doctors suggest that elimination diets should be used only after other diagnostic methods have been tried, including history-taking, skin tests, blind food challenges, and radioallergosorbent testing.

Training & certification

Because of the risks involved, elimination diets should be undertaken only under competent medical supervision. Some patients may wish to consult an allergy specialist.

Resources

BOOKS

Brostoff, Jonathan, and Linda Gamlin. *Food Allergies and Food Intolerance: The Complete Guide to Their Identifi-*

cation and Treatment. Rochester, Vt.: Inner Traditions Intl. Ltd., 2000.

David Helwig

Emphysema

Definition

Emphysema is a progressive, incurable chronic lung condition. The air sacs (alveoli) are destroyed and oxygen uptake is restricted due to the loss of elasticity of lung tissue.

Description

As of 1998 there were an estimated two million people suffering from emphysema in America. Between three and five percent were attributed to genetic factors, the remainder being a result of environmental pollution, with **smoking** ranking far and away as the main cause.

Normally functioning lungs are elastic, and efficiently expand and recoil as air passes freely through their passageways (bronchus) to the alveoli, where oxygen is moved into the blood and carbon dioxide is filtered out. When a person inhales cigarette smoke or airborne pollutants, his or her immune system responds by releasing substances that are meant to defend the lungs against the smoke. These substances can also attack the cells of the lungs, but the body normally inhibits such action with the release of other substances.

When individuals are exposed to pollution over a long period of time the lung tissue is damaged in such a way that it loses its elasticity. When damage has occurred to the alveoli, sufferers have difficulty making a complete exhalation, which causes residual volume—air trapped inside the lungs. With the passage of time, this causes the chest to permanently expand and become barrel shaped.

As the disease progresses, increasingly more effort is needed to breathe. Emphysema frequently occurs with one or more other respiratory diseases, such as **bronchitis** and **asthma**. It is one of the diseases that are collectively referred to as chronic obstructive pulmonary disease (COPD). As a cause of death, it ranks fourth after **heart disease**, **cancer** and **stroke**.

Causes & symptoms

People who smoke or live in polluted atmospheres are possible candidates for emphysema. People with a genetic defect (alpha 1-antitrypsin deficiency) are also at risk. The early stages of emphysema may go undiagnosed, but the main symptoms are breathlessness, blueness of the lips and fingernails, and exhaustion. Sufferers of chronic bronchitis and asthma are also at risk. People who develop emphysema as a result of their work often develop asthma prior to symptoms of their condition.

Emphysema is traditionally a disease suffered by miners, particularly coal miners, as the fine dust that results from mining attacks the alveoli over a period of time. Most miners suffer from emphysema to some degree after a lifetime "down in the pit." In fact, emphysema is sometimes referred to as miner's lung or black lung.

The situation has somewhat improved in recent years due to awareness of the causes of emphysema and improved work conditions for many workers. Others who may be at risk for emphysema include sand blasters, metal grinders, anyone whose job exposes him or her to **silica** (silicosis), asbestos (asbestososis), or **iron** filings (siderosis). In addition, dust from wood, cotton, talc, cereal grains coffee, pesticides, drug or enzyme powders, or fiberglass may cause emphysema. People who use their lungs in their work are also susceptible (such as trumpet players and glass blowers). Any worker who is exposed to abnormal levels of dust, fumes, smoke, gases, vapors, or mists over a long period of time may be at risk for emphysema.

Sufferers typically complain that they "can't get enough air" as stale air builds up inside the lungs and the patient becomes starved of oxygen. Coughing, **wheezing,** and chronic mucous production are other common symptoms.

Diagnosis

A diagnosis of emphysema will not be made on the basis of the above symptoms alone. A detailed medical history will be taken along with x rays and pathology examinations. Peak flow tests will also be conducted.

Treatment

Damage to the lungs as a result of emphysema cannot be reversed, so preventative measures to limit its progres-

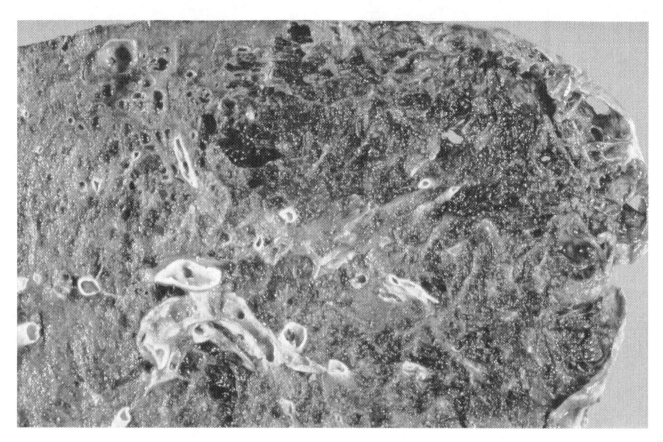

Cross section of a smoker's lung affected by emphysema. *(Photograph by Dr. E. Walker. Science Photo Library/Photo Researchers, Inc. Reproduced by permission.)*

sion are essential. The following measures and treatments are regarded as beneficial for emphysema sufferers.

Herbalism

Herbs can be beneficial in relieving the symptoms of emphysema, helping the body to ward off infection, and easing the asthmatic symptoms that often accompany emphysema.

Some of them are:

- Lobelia: This is a mild sedative, also having strong expectorant properties. It is widely used for chest complaints, including emphysema and bronchitis, and can help to cut an asthma attack short.

- **Thyme**: A tea made with thyme is recommended for overcoming shortness of breath. It is also a powerful antiseptic.

- Mullein: This is another traditional remedy for chest complaints. Boil two tablespoons of the dried leaves with a glass of milk and drink.

- **Echinacea**: Echinacea is a powerful immune system stimulant and will strengthen the body in general, warding off colds and **infections**.

- Lungwort: A member of the borage family, this herb is very healing for the lungs. It should be taken as an infusion.

- Black cohosh: This herb is an expectorant and astringent. It relieves coughing.

- Sage: This is one of the most useful of all herbs and is said to be good for whatever it is taken for. It is antiviral and bactericidal.

- **Garlic**: A very powerful anti-viral, garlic can be of real help to those trying to avoid infections and lung congestion.

Chinese herbal medicine

Qing Qi Hua Tan Wan (**Pinellia** expectorant pills) are the Chinese herbalists' treatment for chronic lung complaints, particularly bronchitis and asthma.

Juices for emphysema

Herbalist Kitty Campion recommends the following juices for the treatment of emphysema: equal parts of carrot juice, parsnip juice, watercress juice and potato juice, or equal parts of orange juice and lemon juice, diluted half and half with a strong decoction of rosehip tea.

Aromatherapy

Aromatherapy involves massaging the patient with potent plant **essential oils**, which have been proven to enter the circulation through the skin. The constituents of the oils can have a powerful effect on a variety of illnesses, but since their beneficial qualities are also transported through the air, they are considered to be doubly beneficial to those who suffer from respiratory ailments.

Aromatherapy oils for respiratory disease:

• *Canada balsam* may alleviate respiratory symptoms and is an expectorant. It is also a bactericide and recommended for those suffering from chronic chest ailments.

• *Tolu balsam* is an excellent treatment for chest infections.

• *Frankincense* is good for infection and catarrhal discharge.

• *Niaouli* is a very strong antiseptic and beneficial for pulmonary trouble.

• *Rose damascena* is recommended for bronchial complaints, and also uplifts the spirits.

• *Tea tree oil* was recently discovered to be one of the most potent anti-viral, anti-bacterial and anti-fungal agents known to medicine. Therefore highly beneficial as a preventative measure against chest infection.

Acupuncture

This ancient Chinese system of holistic treatment works on the principal that illness is the result of blockage in the flow of life force. The practitioner aims to stimulate relevant meridians in the body, and so release trapped life force, returning bodily functions to normal. The treatment is virtually painless.

Treatment can be expected to improve blood circulation and the capacity of the body to restore itself. Research has indicated that **acupuncture** can produce changes in the electrical fields of body cells, promoting a return to the body's normal state. Consequently, few negative side effects are associated with acupuncture treatment.

Breathing techniques

Very few people actually breathe correctly, and if lung function is not up to par, the difference between breathing fully and taking shallow ineffective, breaths can make a remarkable difference in the way a person feels and the way his or her body functions. Oxygen shortage in the body promotes disease, and ensuring that oxygen levels are kept up can avert disaster, even with the existence of lung-impairment. Improved breathing techniques can rid the body of free radicals, neutralize environmental toxins, and destroy many harmful microbes that cannot exist in an oxygen-rich environment. Without sufficient oxygen, the body cannot fully utilize nutrients from food, and bodily functions generally become less efficient. Every effort must be made to promote proper breathing,in order to offset the effects of reduced lung function.

In cases of emphysema, it is particularly important to ensure that the out-breath expels all of the previous in-breath. When exhalation is incomplete, wastes produced by breathing are not expelled from the body in the normal way, and residual volume, which is a common occurrence with progressive emphysema, may cause chest enlargement.

Homeopathy

Homeopathy is the treatment of illness according to a system of "like cures like" that stimulates the body to heal itself. While it could definitely contribute to the successful treatment of emphysema, Homeopathy requires a qualified practitioner, as the patient's condition must be accurately assessed in order that the correct remedy be prescribed. Even for the same disorder, no two patients will receive the same treatment.

Lifestyle

For lung dysfunction of any kind, it is vital to take steps to ensure that a person's lifestyle is not contributing to the problem. Pollution must be avoided at all costs, and steps should be taken to ensure that the living environment is free of chemical irritants. This may involve avoiding fragrances, as they can overburden damaged lungs. Some unscented products use a masking fragrance which only increases toxicity. Common household products, such as fabric softeners, bleach, scented detergents, and furniture polish, can harm the body and the environment.

It must be noted that pesticides, fungicides, herbicides, and fertilizers are all neurotoxins, (poisonous to the nervous system). Natural alternatives are obtainable for most household cleaning products. Personal care products can also cause damage, so only natural sources should be used. Chlorinated pools should be avoided.

Every effort should be made to obtain food that is organically grown, in order to avoid pesticides and chemicals. Processed foods should be avoided because they often contain chemicals, dyes, and preservatives, and because the food is stripped of most of its nutritional value. Notably, artificial sweeteners, particularly aspartame, break down into deadly poisons in the body.

Clothing should be all natural fibers, as permanent press and wrinkle-resistant clothes have often been treated with formaldehyde which does not wash out. For the same reasons, synthetic fiber bed coverings should also be avoided. All plastic products should be avoided as far as possible as they all have toxic elements. Windows should be open as often as possible to increase oxygen in the atmosphere. Some houseplants should be acquired, as they give off oxygen.

It is also very important to undertake some form of gentle, regular **exercise** as this can do much to improve symptoms. Suitable forms of exercise may be swimming, walking and gentle rebounding. If an emphysema patient is very weak, he or she could sit on a mini-trampoline while a helper does the strenuous bit; very real benefits will still be obtained in this way. Strenuous activities are not suitable for anyone with lung impairment.

Naturopathy

According to the principles of naturopathy, the body has the power to heal itself. Treatment should focus on providing the system with optimum **nutrition** so it can carry out all repairs necessary. This involves ensuring that all food that is eaten is of the highest quality.

Naturopaths advocate dietary supplements to assist with this process, and certain dietary supplements can be very valuable in arresting the progress of Emphysema. Trials have been conducted involving treating emphysema patients with **vitamin A**, which is known to play an important role in healthy body tissue. **Vitamin E** can also be helpful, and **vitamin C** should always be taken, as it is a catalyst for other nutrients. For best results, it is advised to consult a practitioner.

Allopathic treatment

Prior to any other treatment, it is essential that emphysema sufferers who smoke take steps to give up the habit. Otherwise, damage to the lungs will continue to go unchecked and other measures will be very limited in their success. Apart from lifestyle changes, physicians generally recommend avoidance of infection, and antibiotics may be prescribed as a preventative measure.

A physician may also prescribe bronchodilator medicines, which are usually prescribed for asthma patients, if there is any obstruction of the airways. For the same reason, anti-inflammatories may also be prescribed.

Chest physiotherapy, breathing exercises, and a program of physical exercise (collectively referred to as pulmonary rehabilitation) are considered beneficial to all emphysema patients, regardless of the degree of impairment. Supplementary oxygen may be required at some stage.

In extreme cases, lung volume reduction surgery may be recommended. If successful, this can eliminate

KEY TERMS

Acupuncture—An ancient Chinese system of treatment, which involves the painless insertion of very fine needles under the skin at certain key points on the body.

Catalyst—An agent that helps other substances to do their work.

Free radicals—The result of oxidization in the body, these molecules are chemically unbalanced and cause a chain reaction of damage to other molecules in the body. One of the prime causes of aging symptoms and deterioration in body funtions.

Naturopathy—A medical paradigm of diagnosis and healing based on "removing the obstacles to cure" and using as modalities: diet, therapeutic nutrition, botanical medicine, homeopathy, physical medicine and counseling.

Residual volume—The amount of air trapped inside the lungs as a result of incompletely exhaling.

the need for supplemental oxygen and improves breathing function. In this procedure, the damaged parts of the lung are removed in order to allow healthy lung tissue to expand. Careful evaluation of patients is carried out prior to this procedure. A final resort is lung transplant surgery. Because of the relatively large risk involved, this is carried out in only a small minority of patients.

Expected results

It is generally accepted that emphysema is incurable. Physicians and alternative medicine practitioners assert that they can relieve sufferers greatly from symptoms and halt the progress of the disease with appropriate management and preventative measures.

Prevention

Any person who feels that his/her work conditions are likely to be a possible cause of emphysema should take steps to protect him/herself. A respirator should be worn, at least until work conditions can be improved. Several steps may be taken to improve conditions, primary of which should be to improve ventilation.

Early diagnosis is vital to the successful management of emphysema. If preventative and therapeutic measures are taken at the early onset of symptoms, damage can be restricted and the outlook can be positive. At all times, care should be taken to eliminate sources of pollution or chemical irritants from the environment, both in the home and elsewhere. The first step in overcoming emphysema for any patient should be to remove the cause, whether working conditions, polluted atmosphere or smoking.

Resources

BOOKS

Ryman, Daniele. *Aromatherapy* London: Piatkus Books, 1999.
Treacher, Sylvia. *Practical Homeopathy* UK: Parragon Books, 2000.

ORGANIZATIONS

The National Emphysema Foundation <http://emphysemafoundation.org/>

OTHER

"Progress in Emphysema Research. <" http://www.lrri.org/gobmasso.html> (January 17, 2001).

Patricia Skinner

Encopresis *see* **Constipation**

Endometriosis

Definition

Endometriosis is a condition in which bits of tissue similar to the lining of the uterus (endometrium) grow in other parts of the body (and within the uterus). Like the uterine lining, this tissue builds up and sheds in response to monthly hormonal cycles. The blood discarded from these implants falls onto surrounding organs, causing swelling and inflammation. This repeated irritation leads to the development of scar tissue and adhesions.

Description

Endometriosis is estimated to affect 7% of women of childbearing age in the United States. It most commonly strikes between the ages of 25 and 40. Endometriosis can also appear in the teen years, but never before the start of **menstruation**. It is seldom seen in postmenopausal women.

Endometriosis was once called the "career woman's disease" because it was thought to be a product of delayed childbearing. The statistics defy such a narrow generalization; however, **pregnancy** may slow the progress of the condition. Women whose periods last longer than a week with an interval of less than 27 days between them seem to be more prone to the condition.

Endometrial implants are most often found on the pelvic organs, including the ovaries, uterus, fallopian

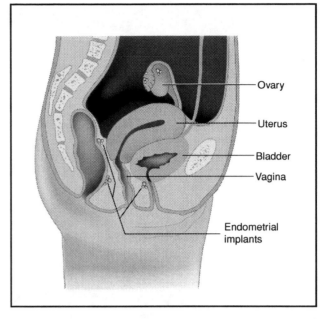

Endometrial tissue is normally flushed out of the uterus as part of the menstrual cycle. However, some tissue may become implanted in other organs of the pelvic cavity, causing endometriosis. *(Illustration by Electronic Illustrators Group. The Gale Group.)*

tubes, and in the cavity behind the uterus. Occasionally, this tissue grows in such distant parts of the body as the lungs, arms, and kidneys. **Ovarian cysts** may form around endometrial tissue (endometriomas) and may range from pea to grapefruit size. Endometriosis is a progressive condition that usually advances slowly over the course of many years. Doctors rank cases from minimal to severe based on factors such as the number and size of the endometrial implants, their appearance and location, and the extent of the scar tissue and adhesions in the vicinity of the growths.

Causes & symptoms

Although the exact cause of endometriosis is unknown, a number of theories have been put forward. Some of the more popular ones are:

• Implantation theory. This theory states that a reversal in the direction of menstrual flow sends discarded endometrial cells into the body cavity where they attach to internal organs and seed endometrial implants. There is considerable evidence to support this explanation. Reversed menstrual flow occurs in 70-90% of women and is thought to be more common in women with endometriosis.

• Vascular-lymphatic theory. This theory suggests that the lymph system or blood vessels (vascular system) are the vehicles for distribution of endometrial cells out of the uterus.

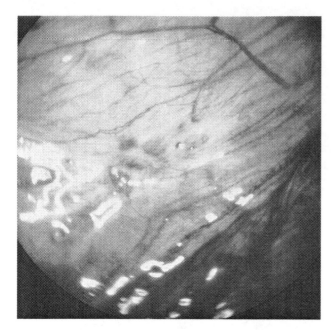

An endoscopic view of endometriosis on pelvic wall. *(Custom Medical Stock Photo. Reproduced by permission.)*

• Coelomic metaplasia theory. According to this hypothesis, remnants of tissue left over from prenatal development of the woman's reproductive tract transform into endometrial cells throughout the body.

• Induction theory. This explanation postulates that an unidentified substance found in the body forces cells from the lining of the body cavity to change into endometrial cells.

In addition to these theories, the following factors are thought to influence the development of endometriosis:

• Heredity. A woman's chance of developing endometriosis is seven times greater if her mother or sisters have the disease.

• Immune system function. Women with endometriosis may have lower functioning immune systems that have trouble eliminating stray endometrial cells. This would explain why a high percentage of women experience reversed menstrual flow while relatively few develop endometriosis.

• Dioxin exposure. Some research suggests a link between the exposure to dioxin (TCCD), a toxic chemical found in weed killers, and the development of endometriosis.

While many women with endometriosis suffer debilitating symptoms, others have the disease without knowing it. Strangely, there does not seem to be any re-lation between the severity of the symptoms and the extent of the disease. The most common symptoms are:

• Menstrual **pain**. Pain in the lower abdomen that begins a day or two before the menstrual period starts and continues until the end is typical of endometriosis. Some women also report lower back aches, and pain during urination and bowel movement, especially during their periods.

• Painful sexual intercourse. Pressure on the vagina and cervix causes severe pain for some women.

• Abnormal bleeding. Heavy menstrual periods, irregular bleeding, and spotting are common features of endometriosis.

• **Infertility**. There is a strong association between endometriosis and infertility, although the reasons for this have not been fully explained. It is thought that the build-up of scar tissue and adhesions blocks the fallopian tubes and prevents the ovaries from releasing eggs. Endometriosis may also affect fertility by causing hormonal irregularities and a higher rate of early miscarriage.

Diagnosis

The first step is to perform a pelvic exam to try to feel if implants are present. Very often there is no strong evidence of endometriosis from a physical exam. The only way to make a definitive diagnosis is through minor surgery called a laparoscopy. A laparoscope, a slender scope with a light on the end, is inserted into the woman's abdomen through a small incision near her belly button. This allows the doctor to examine the internal organs. Often, a sample of tissue is taken for later examination in the laboratory. Endometriosis is sometimes discovered when a woman has abdominal surgery for another reason such as tubal ligation or hysterectomy.

Various imaging techniques such as ultrasound, computed tomography scan (CT scan), or magnetic resonance imaging (MRI) can offer additional information but aren't useful in making the initial diagnosis. A blood test may also be ordered because women with endometriosis have higher levels of the blood protein CA125. Testing for this substance before and after treatment can predict a recurrence of the disease, but is not reliable as a diagnostic tool.

Treatment

Although severe endometriosis should not be self-treated, many women find they can help relieve symptoms through alternative therapies. In a survey conducted by the Endometriosis Association, 40-60% of the women who used alternative medicines reported relief of pain and other symptoms.

Diet

A **high-fiber diet**, particularly from grains and beans, may decrease cramping and inflammation. The oils in seeds, nuts, and certain fish (cod, salmon, mackerel, and sardines) may help to relieve cramping. Carrots, beets, lemons, cauliflower, brussels sprouts, cabbage, onions, **garlic**, citrus fruits, vegetables, **chicory**, radicchio, and yogurt may help to reduce symptoms. Some women have found relief when they turned to a **macrobiotic diet** (one that is very restrictive and intended to prolong life). Occasionally, an allergy **elimination diet** may be recommended.

Sugar and animal fats can increase inflammation and aggravate pain. Milk and meat may contain hormones so they should be avoided. Vegetarian or vegan **diets** may be recommended for those with endometriosis.

Supplements

The following can be used to treat endometriosis:

- vitamin B complex to help the liver break down excess estrogen
- vitamin C to reduce heavy menstrual bleeding
- calcium
- bioflavonoids to help reduce heavy menstrual bleeding
- magnesium to relieve pain and flush out toxins
- vitamin E to heal inflamed tissues
- iron for **anemia** resulting from heavy bleeding
- lipotropic factors (Choline, **methionine**, and inositol enhance liver function.)
- fish oil capsules, flax oil, or any essential fatty acid to reduce cramping

Several herbal remedies for endometriosis exist. The first four in this list are the most commonly used remedies:

- Genistein (soy/isoflavone) helps the body excrete excess estrogen and possibly blocks estrogen's effect.
- Cramp bark (*Viburnum opulus*) helps ease cramping.
- Dong quai (*Angelica sinensis*) balances hormone levels and reduces inflammation.
- Black cohosh (*Cimicifuga racemosa*) helps the body excrete excess estrogen and improves the health of pelvic organs.
- Red clover (*Trifolium pratense*) balances hormone levels.
- Milk thistle (*Silybum marianum*) helps the liver.
- Life (*Senecio aureus*) root may improve the health of pelvic organs.

- Feverfew (*Chrysanthemum parthenium*) eases pain and cramping.
- Dandelion eases pain and cramping and supports the liver.
- Yarrow (*Archillea millefolium*) eases cramping and restores hormonal balance.
- Evening primrose oil (*Oenothera biennis*) relieved endometriosis symptoms in 90% of patients in a study.
- Shepherd's purse (*Capsella bursa-pastoris*) reduces heavy menstrual bleeding and tones the uterus.
- Meadowsweet (*Filipendula ulmaria*) reduces pain.

Other treatments

Other remedies for endometriosis include **acupuncture** or **acupressure** to relieve pain, visualization, **guided imagery**, naturopathy, **homeopathy** (Lilium tigrum, **sepia**, and **belladonna**), **hydrotherapy**, **exercise**, and **meditation**.

Allopathic treatment

How endometriosis is treated depends on the woman's symptoms, her age, the extent of the disease, and her personal preferences. The condition cannot be fully eradicated without surgery. Treatment focuses on managing pain, preserving fertility, and delaying the progress of the condition.

Medication

Over-the-counter pain relievers such as aspirin, acetaminophen (Tylenol), ibuprofen (Motrin, Advil), and naproxen (Aleve, Naprosyn) are useful for mild cramping and menstrual pain. If pain is severe, a doctor may prescribe narcotic medications, although these can be addicting and are rarely used.

Hormonal therapies effectively tame endometriosis but also act as contraceptives. They include oral contraceptives, synthetic male hormones (danazol, gestrinone), progestins, and gonadotropin-releasing hormone antagonists.

Surgery

Endometrial implants and ovarian cysts can be removed with laser surgery performed through a laparoscope. For women with minimal endometriosis, this technique is usually successful in reducing pain and slowing disease progress. It may also help infertile women increase their chances of becoming pregnant.

Removing the uterus, ovaries, and fallopian tubes (a hysterectomy) is the only permanent method of eliminating endometriosis. This is an extreme measure that deprives a woman of her ability to bear children and forces her body into **menopause**.

Expected results

Most women who have endometriosis have minimal symptoms and do well. Overall, endometriosis symptoms come back in an average of 40% of women over the five years following treatment. A 2002 review found that teenagers and young women under the age of 22 years have almost twice the chance of symptom recurrence after surgical removal of endometriosis compared with older women. Some researchers now believe that younger women may have a different form of endometriosis than that found in older women.

With hormonal therapy, pain returned after five years in 37% of patients with minimal symptoms and 74% of those with severe cases. The highest success rate from conservative treatment followed complete removal of implants using laser surgery. Of these women, 80% were still pain-free five years later. Hysterectomy may be necessary should other treatments fail.

Prevention

There is no proven way to prevent endometriosis. One study, however, indicated that girls who begin participating in aerobic exercise at a young age are less likely to develop the condition.

Resources

BOOKS

Ballweg, Mary Lou. *The Endometriosis Sourcebook.* Chicago: Congdon & Weed, 1995.

D'Hooghe, Thomas M. and Joseph A. Hill. "Endometriosis" in *Novak's Gynecology,* edited by Jonathan S. Berek, et al., 12th ed. Baltimore, MD: Williams & Wilkins, 1996.

Malesky, Gail. "Endometriosis." *Nature's Medicines: from Asthma to Weight Gain, from Colds to High Cholesterol— the Most Powerful All-Natural Cures.* Emmaus, PA: Rodale Press, 1999.

Trickey, Ruth. *Women, Hormones & The Menstrual Cycle: Herbal & Medical Solutions From Adolescence to Menopause.* St. Leonards, Australia: Allen & Unwin, 1998.

PERIODICALS

Aesoph, Lauri M. "Nature's Rx for Endometriosis." *Let's Live* 67 (June 1999): 70+.

Drexler, Madeline. "What Can You Do About Endometriosis?" *Self* 17 (January 1995):122+.

Johnson, Kate. "Endometriosis Symptoms often Recur in Teens (Postsurgery Complaints)." *Pediatric News* (September 2002):43.

KEY TERMS

Adhesions—Web-like scar tissue that may develop as a result of endometriosis and bind organs to one another.

Endometrial implants—Growths of endometrial tissue that attach to organs, primarily in the pelvic cavity.

Endometrium—The tissue lining the uterus that grows and sheds each month during a woman's menstrual cycle.

Estrogen—A female hormone that promotes the growth of endometrial tissue.

Laparoscopy—Procedure used to diagnose and treat endometriosis. It is performed by inserting a slender, wand-like instrument through a small incision in the woman's abdomen.

Menopause—The end of a woman's menstrual periods when the body stops making estrogen.

Retrograde menstruation—Menstrual flow that travels into the body cavity rather than out through the vagina.

ORGANIZATIONS

Endometriosis Association International Headquarters. 8585 North 76th Place, Milwaukee, WI 53223. (800) 992-3636. http://EndometriosisAssn.org.

Belinda Rowland
Teresa G. Odle

Endometrial cancer *see* **Uterine cancer**

Energy medicine

Definition

Energy medicine is based upon the belief that changes in the "life force" of the body, including the electric, magnetic, and electromagnetic fields, affect human health and can promote healing.

Origins

The notion of a life force or energy is shared by people around the world. Since ancient times, traditional cultures have believed that a special energy vitalizes all life. This energy is known as chi, prana, pneuma, orgone, mana, ether, odyle, élan vital, bio-cosmic energy, and many other names.

Early Ayurvedic references to a life force, or prana, go back to the eighth century B.C. In the West, as early as the sixth century B.C., Pythagoras conceived of a life energy, or pneuma, visible in a luminous body. A century later, Hippocrates, the father of modern medicine, recognized the body's natural capacity for healing, or *Vis medicatrix naturae*. He instructed physicians to find the blocking influences both within a patient and between them and the cosmos, in order to restore the healing life force. Nature, not the doctor, is the source of healing.

In the sixteenth century, the Swiss alchemist and physician Paracelsus reported "a healing energy that radiates within and around man like a luminous sphere." He believed this energy could cause and cure disease and could work from a distance. He also thought that magnets, planets, and stars could influence this energy. There are echoes of these beliefs in some theories and practices of contemporary energy medicine. However, the ideas of Francis Bacon and the French philosopher and mathematician René Descartes have had a much greater impact on Western medicine as a whole.

Bacon applied logical mathematical concepts to analyze humans and the world. He believed that the laws of science should be used to "master rather than become harmonious with nature." Descartes proposed that the body, which was measurable, and the mind, which was immeasurable, were firmly separate. The body could influence the mind but the mind could not influence the body. These notions promoted the search for physical causes of human illness. They also led to a denial of the mind's ability to affect physical health. As a result, mainstream science came to devalue or reject any phenomenon that cannot be measured or objectively proved.

From the seventeenth century onward, Western medicine has focused primarily upon the physical aspects of disease. Scientists who studied forces within the body that were difficult to measure were often ignored or ridiculed. The Austrian psychiatrist Wilhelm Reich, who had been a student and colleague of Sigmund Freud, was jailed and his books publicly burned because of his theories about "orgone" energy. His views, however, have influenced the development of many body-mind approaches, particularly bioenergetics.

The 1990s brought a new emerging scientific paradigm in relation to medicine and health care. According to biophysicist Beverly Rubik, this emerging paradigm "... celebrates the creative, subtle, empowering, wise, and enduring features of life that were never acknowledged during the age of machines and mechanistic thought. Living systems are self-organizing systems that

CAROLINE MYSS 1953–

Caroline Myss graduated with a B.A. in Journalism in 1974 from St. Mary of the Woods College in Terre Haute, Indiana. Working as a journalist in her native Chicago, Myss interviewed Dr. Elisabeth Kubler-Ross, M.D., who was devoted to the study of death and the dying. She credits Kubler-Ross with inspiring her to go on to Loyola-Mundelein University, a Jesuit school in Chicago, to get an M.A. in Theology in 1979. Myss then started a small New Age publishing company, consulted with holistic doctors, and gave individuals intuitive readings. It was her pairing with Dr. C. Norman Shealy, founder of the American Holistic Medical Association, in 1984, that began to thrust her into the limelight in energy medicine. With television appearances on such high-profile shows as *Oprah*, Myss is the best-known intuitive on the circuit of holistic practitioners. Her belief stems from a principle that the mind and body work together to contribute to a person's well-being. While the traditional medical community is skeptical of the scientific basis for her claims, her international popularity continues to rise.

Her first book, *Anatomy of the Spirit*, was published in 1996, followed in the fall of 1997 with *Why People Don't Heal and How They Can*. Those, along with an audiotape series called *Energy Anatomy*, are bestsellers. By 2000, Myss discontinued private readings and devoted herself to workshops and seminars worldwide.

Myss can be contacted at her office, at 7144 N Harlem Avenue, Chicago, IL 60631, or through her website: <http://www.myss.com>.

Jane Spear

expend energy in order to maintain their coherence and integrity...Healing is ultimately self-healing, a natural response to internal dynamic shifts or external challenges." This new paradigm also conveys that "...very small or subtle stimuli applied to the body-mind can have profound effects and set a person on the road to recovery."

Benefits

In a 1990 review of more than 131 controlled scientific studies of healers from around the world, Dr. Daniel Benor found evidence of healing for a wide range of human conditions. These include changes in immune system functioning as well as improvement of skin-wound healing, blood pressure, nearsightedness, **leukemia**, **anxiety**, **asthma**, **bronchitis**, **epilepsy**, tension **headache**, neck and back **pain**, post-operative pain, self-esteem, **heart disease**, and relationships.

Patients have also reported spontaneous healing of a variety of conditions including **cancer** and paralysis. Spiritual awakenings or new attitudes and a fresh sense of meaning in life can also result from energy healing.

Description

Energy medicine is a broad term that includes touch therapies, movement therapies, spiritual healing, **meditation**, magnetic field therapy, **homeopathy**, **acupuncture**, **light therapy**, and other innovative methods of healing. What these various approaches have in common is an energetic understanding of health and healing. These therapies may affect the patient's internal energy, external energy (aura, or other energy fields surrounding the body) or both. Many of these therapies fall into several different categories at once and their benefits may not be exclusively due to changes in life force. Energetic touch therapies include, but are not limited to, **reiki**, **therapeutic touch** (although the physical body is not touched), watsu, **polarity therapy**, Ayurvedic massage, zero balancing, **reflexology**, Jin Shin Jyutsu, **lomilomi**, **breema** bodywork, **Thai massage**, **shiatsu**, amma, Chi Nei Tsang, Jin Shin Do, Shen, and **Chinese massage**, and **acupressure**. Energetic movement therapies include **qigong**, **t'ai chi** chuan, aikido, karate, and **yoga** (there are many different forms of yoga). Spiritual healing includes distance healing, laying on of hands, meditation, ceremony, ritual, and other shamanic practices.

Some of the methods of energy medicine involve gentle physical touch, while others work with the energy around the body with the practitioner holding his or her hands several inches away. Some methods can be applied from a distance, others require attendance at a ceremony and may include family and friends. The movement modalities may require learning and practicing a particular movement or breath sequence. Other therapies may involve wearing magnets, being exposed to various kinds of light rays, or receiving energy stimulation with needles and heat.

The duration and cost of an energy medicine session vary greatly depending upon the method and the healer. Some methods are expensive while others are free or offered for a modest donation. These modalities are not covered by insurance unless administered by a licensed health care professional.

Preparations

The amount and type of preparation vary. While some forms of energy medicine require no specific preparations, others do. These preparations may range from wearing loose clothing for yoga and other movement therapies, to an hour-long diagnostic interview with a practitioner of **traditional Chinese medicine** prior to receiving certain types of Chinese massage. In general, people with heart problems, recent surgery, or back problems should consult a physician before attempting any of the movement therapies.

Precautions

Other treatments besides, or instead of, energy medicine may be needed for a particular disease or condition. In addition, persons who have experienced physical violence or abuse may have strong emotional reactions to therapies that involve physical contact; they should consult a knowledgeable counselor before undertaking these forms of treatment.

Side effects

The side effects can vary depending upon the modality. It is not unusual for people to experience some soreness or stiffness after a session of bodywork or movement therapies, particularly if they have not been accustomed to regular physical **exercise**. Some people experience headaches after light therapy. Lastly, some people find that energy therapies bring up painful emotions and memories.

Research & general acceptance

Over the course of the past three decades, energy medicine has moved from being a marginal area of research to gaining a large measure of mainstream acceptance. The Human Potential movement of the 1960s and the counterculture of the early 1970s helped to stimulate popular interest in Eastern practices and belief systems, while the feminist movement of the same period led many women to explore mind/body connections and question the masculine assumptions and values of Western science and medicine. In recent years, the medical establishment has shown a new openness to research in the area of energy medicine, as was shown by the funding of the Office of Alternative Medicine at the National Institutes of Health. At present, there are a number of clinical trials that have been designed to measure the effectiveness of alternatives to conventional treatment.

Despite over 300 studies during the past 40 years showing the efficacy of energy healing, however, these findings are still ignored or rejected by many scientists. Benor details many reasons for this rejection, including the fact that healers have not been able to produce results with reliability and consistency in a laboratory setting. Benor writes, "The time has come to accept that healing is the way it is. It appears to be influenced by multiple

KEY TERMS

Aura—A light or radiance that is claimed to emanate from the body and to be visible to certain persons with psychic or spiritual powers.

Bioenergetics—The study of energy transformation in living systems.

Paradigm—A pattern or model.

factors—so many, in fact, that it is virtually impossible to establish a repeatable experiment in which all would occur in the same combination more than once...We will have to be content with our human limitations and settle for approximate results, measured in probabilities over large numbers of trials. No apologies are needed. These are the limitations of healing."

Training & certification

There is no course of training leading to certification or licensure for energy medicine as such. Various schools of touch and **movement therapy**, as well as energy healing, offer their own forms of certification. The requirements vary according to each modality and each school. Spiritual healers may be certified through a school of energy healing, recognized within a particular religious tradition for their healing aptitude, or initiated into healing by another means. Many healers develop their healing gifts on their own. The evidence suggests that any caring person can develop a certain amount of healing ability through meditation, prayer, study with other experienced healers, and practice.

Resources

BOOKS

Becker, Robert O., et al. *The Body Electric: Electromagnetism and the Foundation of Life.* New York: William Morrow and Company, 1987.

Benford, Sue, et al. "Exploring the Concept of Energy in Touch-Based Healing" in *Clinician's Complete Reference to Complementary and Alternative Medicine,* ed. Donald Novey. St. Louis, MO: Mosby, 2000.

Collinge, William, PhD. *Subtle Energy: Awakening to the Unseen Forces in Our Lives.* New York: Warner Books, Inc., 1998.

Dossey, Larry, M.D. *Reinventing Medicine: Beyond Mind-Body to a New Era of Healing.* New York: HarperCollins Publishers, 1999.

Gerber, Richard. *Vibrational Medicine for the 21st Century: The Complete Guide to Energy Healing and Spiritual Transformation.* Eagle Books, 2000.

Rubik, Beverly. *Life at the Edge of Science.* Oakland, CA: The Institute of Frontier Science, 1996.

ORGANIZATIONS

Barbara Brennan School of Healing. P.O. Box 2005. East Hampton, NY 11937. (516) 329-0951. Fax: (516) 324-9745. e-mail: bbshoffice@barbarabrennan.com.

Healing Light Center Church. 261 E. Alegria Ave. #12. Sierra Madre, CA 91024. (626) 306-2170. Fax: (626) 355-0996.

Institute for Frontier Science. 6114 LaSalle Ave. Oakland, CA 94611. (510) 531-5767. E-mail: brubik@compuserve.com. <http://www.healthy.net/frontierscience/>

International Society for the Study of Subtle Energies and Energy Medicine (ISSSEEM). 356 Goldco Circle. Golden, CO 80401. (303) 278-2228. <http://www.vitalenergy.com/ISSSEEM>.

Linda Chrisman

English plantain *see* **Plantain**

Enuresis *see* **Bedwetting**

Environmental therapy

Definition

Environmental therapy, also known as environmental medicine and formerly called clinical ecology, is the diagnosis and treatment of conditions caused by environmental factors.

Origins

The founder of environmental medicine was Theron G. Randolph, M.D., who was a trained specialist in internal medicine, immunology, and **allergies**. Several decades ago, Randolph became concerned with chronically ill patients who had symptoms of allergies and immune system disorders, but didn't respond to conventional medical care. Randolph believed that patients were getting sick from environmental substances and pollutants that allergy specialists could not determine or did not recognize as causing illness. Conventional allergy specialists in Randolph's time believed that allergies could only be detected by measuring the response of immunoglobulin E (IgE). IgE is a particular antibody produced by the immune system when an antigen (foreign substance) triggers a reaction. Randolph believed that testing for allergies using only this technique limited the determination of immune system problems. Using other tests and techniques, he found that many substances that didn't necessarily cause increased amounts of IgE could create allergic symptoms and complications in the body. Research has since shown that food allergies cause increases in immunoglobulin G (IgG) and not in IgE. Scientists now recognize that the immune system is too complex to be measured by only one test.

Randolph also found that allergic and toxic substances often produce subtle reactions in the body that may accumulate into major illnesses and problems. Many of these substances were not previously thought of as allergenic or toxic, including numerous common foods and chemicals (particularly petrochemicals and by-products of industry). Randolph determined that environmental agents could cause mental and behavioral disturbances as well as physical symptoms. Randolph and other doctors developed and used new diagnostic techniques, including intradermal (between skin layers) and sublingual (under the tongue) allergy tests, to determine exactly which environmental factors were influencing illnesses. Environmental doctors were able to heal many patients, simply by removing certain foods and chemicals from their environments.

Randolph went on to dedicate his work to studying the interaction between patients and their environments. He and his colleagues called this new field of medicine clinical ecology, which was later changed to environmental medicine. The field's basic ideas are that doctors must consider both the patient and the patient's environment in treatment, and that there are cause and effect relationships between environmental factors and illness. Environmental factors include food, air, water, living arrangements, and workplace environments. For illnesses that are caused by exposure to negative environmental factors, healing can be induced not by drugs, but by testing for and removing the environmental causes of illness and by strengthening the patient's resistance.

Environmental therapists have isolated many substances that cause illness and adverse reactions in people, including chemicals, car exhaust, tobacco smoke, pesticides, drugs, food additives, and common allergens like dust, mold, animal dander, and pollen. Many people may also have allergic and negative reactions to common foods such as dairy products, corn syrup, sugar, wheat, certain fruits and vegetables, nuts, and meat. Exposure to toxic and allergenic substances may exert a cumulative effect on the body, weakening and taxing the immune system over time so that the body becomes hypersensitive (more susceptible) to substances that were once tolerated.

In 2002, a Harvard University study demonstrated that global warming was adding to the presence of airborne allergens like ragweed pollen. Atmospheric carbon dioxide concentration is up 29 percent since industrial times began and is expected to double again in the next 50 to 100 years. The heavy carbon dioxide concentration helps plants grow faster and larger, producing more allergens.

Environmental medicine has become increasingly popular in the last few decades as the public has become more aware of environmental pollution. Every year, more than 700,000 different chemicals are released into the environment, and the figure has been growing by 10% or more per year. Toxic or allergenic chemicals can be found in everything from common household materials like carpet and furniture to basic items like food and water. Environmental therapists believe that new medical problems have arisen due to the immune system's inability to handle all of the new pollutants and synthetic chemicals to which it is exposed. Environmental illness is the cumulative effect of lengthy or constant exposure to these toxins. Those with environmental illness become hypersensitive to even minute quantities of common materials. Environmental hypersensitivity can cause severe disability in many people.

Environmental medicine recognizes that some new and baffling illnesses have appeared that conventional medicine either does not recognize or is unable to treat, sometimes called "twentieth century diseases." These conditions include environmental illness/multiple chemical sensitivity (EI/MCS), **chronic fatigue syndrome**, **fibromyalgia**, **Gulf War syndrome**, and **sick building syndrome**. Furthermore, diseases for which environmental causes are believed to be major factors are also increasing (like **cancer** and **asthma**), making environmental medicine increasingly important.

Benefits

Environmental medicine is helpful for those patients suffering from chronic allergies, asthma, chronic **fatigue** syndrome, EI/MCS, fibromyalgia, Gulf War syndrome, and sick building syndrome. It is helpful for those with conditions that are influenced by environmental factors, such as cancer, as well as for those who have been exposed to high levels of toxic materials due to accident or occupation. Environmental medicine is also used for people suffering allergic or immune system problems that conventional medicine is unable to diagnose or treat. Symptoms for those suffering environmental illness include unexplained fatigue, increased allergies, hypersensitivity to common materials, intolerance to certain foods and **indigestion**, aches and pains, low-grade **fever**, headaches, **insomnia**, **depression**, sore throats, sudden weight loss or gain, lowered resistance to infection, general malaise, and disability.

Description

Environmental therapy treats patients by first identifying the environmental causes of illness. The next step is removing environmental causes and reducing exposures to all potential toxins. Cleansing and detoxifying the body of toxic substances and supporting overall (holistic) healing and recovery are the other components of the treatment process.

The cost of treatment by a practitioner of environmental medicine can vary depending on the education of the practitioner. Costs are generally comparable to visits to trained medical specialists. Practitioners may be conventionally trained medical doctors, researchers with graduate degrees in environmental medicine, or alternative medicine practitioners such as homeopaths, **Ayurvedic medicine** practitioners, **traditional Chinese medicine** practitioners, and naturopaths. Treatment costs vary, depending on the type and number of tests required to identify problems and the subsequent healing therapies required. Many insurance policies cover costs of environmental therapy, particularly when the practitioner is a certified medical doctor. Consumers should be aware of their insurance company's policies on coverage.

Diagnosing environmental illness

Environmental therapists use extensive testing to determine the environmental factors that may be causing illness. These factors include infection, allergy, addictions, and toxic chemicals. **Infections** that often plague those with environmental illness can be caused by parasites, bacteria, viruses, and yeast. Blood, urine, stool, and hair analyses are used to measure a variety of bodily functions that may indicate problems. Environmental therapists have access to laboratories that specialize in sophisticated blood, urine, and other diagnostic tests.

In testing for environmental illness, liver function is studied closely because the liver is the principle organ in the body responsible for removing toxic compounds. Another useful blood test is a test for **zinc** deficiency, which may indicate **heavy metal poisoning**. Heavy metal poisoning can be caused by lead, mercury, arsenic, cadmium, and aluminum, all of which are present in the environment. Hair analysis is also used to test for heavy metal toxicity. Blood and urine tests can also be completed that screen for toxic chemicals such as PCBs (environmental poisons), formaldehyde (a common preservative), pesticides, and heavy metals. Immune system tests, which show levels of particular antibodies, can also indicate specific environmental factors. Hormone levels also may indicate environmental illness. Certain blood and urine tests may suggest nutritional deficiencies and proper recovery **diets** can be designed for patients.

Environmental therapists also perform extensive allergy and hypersensitivity tests. Intradermal and sublingual allergy tests are used to determine a patient's sensitivity to a variety of common substances, including formaldehyde, auto exhaust, perfume, tobacco, chlorine, jet fuel, and other chemicals.

Food allergies require additional tests because these allergies often have reactions that are delayed for several days after eating the food. The RAST (radioallergosorbent test) is a blood test that determines the level of immunoglobulins in the blood after specific foods are eaten. The cytotoxic test is a blood test that determines whether certain substances affect blood cells, including foods and chemicals. The ELISA-ACT (enzyme-linked immunoserological assay activated cell test) is considered one of the most accurate tests for allergies and hypersensitivity to foods, chemicals, and other agents. Other tests for food allergies are the elimination and rotation diets, where foods are systematically evaluated to isolate those that are causing problems.

Therapies used in environmental medicine

After environmental causes of illness are identified, the next step is to reduce or eliminate the patient's exposure to them to reduce the burden on the immune system. Patients are advised to immediately remove toxic and allergic agents from the home and workplace, to make lifestyle and dietary changes to reduce exposure, and to improve general physical and mental health.

Detoxification methods are used by alternative practitioners in treating environmental illnesses. These methods try to rid the body of accumulated toxic substances and to restore efficient functioning. Detoxification methods include dietary therapies, **fasting, exercise**, sweating, laxatives, enemas, and other techniques that stimulate and support the body's natural detoxification mechanisms. Nutritional and herbal supplements are used in the detoxification and strengthening process. These supplements include **antioxidants** and vitamins, numerous herbs that detoxify the body and stimulate the immune system, and enzymes to improve digestion. Natural and holistic treatments are used to rebuild and strengthen the patient's overall health and resistance. Traditional healing systems such as traditional Chinese medicine, naturopathy, ayurveda, and **homeopathy** may be used as therapeutic programs for environmental illness.

Preparations

Patients can assist diagnosis and treatment by keeping detailed diaries of their activities, symptoms, and contact with environmental factors that may be affecting their health.

Side effects

If detoxification treatments are used, patients may experience side effects of fatigue, malaise, aches and pains, emotional duress, **acne**, headaches, allergies, and symptoms of colds and flu. Detoxification specialists claim that these negative side effects are part of the healing process. These reactions are sometimes called *healing crises*, which are caused by temporarily increased levels of toxins in the body due to elimination and cleansing.

Research & general acceptance

Environmental medicine is gaining more respect in the medical community and is now a field in conventional medicine. Many leading medical schools and universities offer programs or specialties in environmental medicine. Research in environmental medicine is being widely funded and conducted by mainstream organizations such as the National Institutes of Health, the Environmental Protection Agency, as well as alternative medical schools. The National Academy of Science recognizes that many illnesses are caused or influenced by environmental factors, including cancer and **multiple chemical sensitivity**. The U.S. Centers for Disease Control have estimated that up to 82% of diseases may be due to environmental and lifestyle factors.

Training & certification

The American College of Occupational and Environmental Medicine is the world's largest organization for environmental medicine. Its members include certified and practicing doctors. The American Academy of Environmental Medicine certifies environmental medicine practitioners. The National Institute of Environmental Health Sciences is affiliated with the National Institutes of Health. It conducts research in environmental medicine and supports several academic programs of study in environmental medicine, including those at Harvard, Oregon State University, Vanderbilt, University of California, and MIT.

Resources

BOOKS

Goldberg, Burton. *Chronic Fatigue, Fibromyalgia and Environmental Illness.* Tiburon, CA: Future Medicine, 1998.

Lawson, Lynn. *Staying Well in a Toxic World.* Chicago: Noble, 1993.

Randolph, Theron G., M.D. *Environmental Medicine: Beginnings and Bibliographies of Clinical Ecology.* Fort Collins, CO: Clinical Ecology Publications, 1987.

Steinman, David, and Samuel Epstein. *The Safe Shopper's Bible.* New York: IDG, 1993.

PERIODICALS

"Global Warming May Significantly Increase Airborne Allergies." *Immunotherapy Weekly* (April 10, 2002):4.

> ## KEY TERMS
>
> **Allergen**—A foreign substance, such as mites in house dust or animal dander that, when inhaled, causes the airways to narrow and produces symptoms of asthma.
>
> **Antibody**—A protein, also called immunoglobulin, produced by immune system cells to remove antigens.
>
> **Fibromyalgia**—A condition of debilitating pain, among other symptoms, in the muscles and the myofascia (the thin connective tissue that surrounds muscles, bones, and organs).
>
> **Hypersensitivity**—The state where even a tiny amount of allergen can cause severe allergic reactions.
>
> **Multiple chemical sensitivity**—A condition characterized by severe and crippling allergic reactions to commonly used substances, particularly chemicals. Also called environmental illness.

Health Connections Quarterly 7510 Northforest Dr., North Charleston, SC 29420. (843) 572-1600. http:\\www.coem.com.

Journal of Occupational and Environmental Medicine 1114 N. Arlington Heights Rd., Arlington Heights, IL 60004. (847) 818-1800.

ORGANIZATIONS

American Academy of Environmental Medicine. 23121 Verdugo Dr., Suite 204, Laguna Hills, CA 92653. (714) 583-7666.

Center for Occupational and Environmental Medicine. 7510 Northforest Dr., North Charleston, SC 29420. (843) 572-1600. http:\\www.coem.com.

Northwest Center for Environmental Medicine.177 NE 102nd St., Portland, OR 97220. (503) 561-0966.

Douglas Dupler
Teresa G. Odle

Enzyme therapy

Definition

Enyzme therapy is a plan of dietary supplements of plant and animal enzymes used to facilitate the digestive process and improve the body's ability to maintain balanced metabolism.

Origins

Enzymes are protein molecules used by the body to perform all of its chemical actions and reactions. The body manufactures several thousands of enzymes. Among them are the **digestive enzymes** produced by the stomach, pancreas, small intestine, and the salivary glands of the mouth. Their energy-producing properties are responsible for not only the digestion of nutrients, but their absorption, transportation, metabolization, and elimination as well.

Enzyme therapy is based on the work of Dr. Edward Howell in the 1920s and 1930s. Howell proposed that enzymes from foods work in the stomach to pre-digest food. He advocated the consumption of large amounts of plant enzymes, theorizing that if the body had to use less of its own enzymes for digestion, it could store them for maintaining metabolic harmony. Four categories of plant enzymes are helpful in pre-digestion: protease, amylase, lipase, and cellulase. Cellulase is particularly helpful because the body is unable to produce it.

Animal enzymes, such as pepsin extracted from the stomach of pigs, work more effectively in the duodenum. They are typically used for the treatment of nondigestive ailments.

The seven categories of food enzymes and their activities

• amylase: breaks down starches

• cellulase: breaks down fibers

• lactase: breaks down dairy products

• lipase: breaks down fats

• maltase: breaks down grains

• protease: breaks down proteins

• sucrase: breaks down sugars

Enzyme theory generated further interest as the human diet became more dependent on processed and cooked foods. Enzymes are extremely sensitive to heat, and temperatures above 118°F (48°C) destroy them. Modern processes of pasteurization, canning, and microwaving are particularly harmful to the enzymes in food.

Benefits

In traditional medicine, enzyme supplements are often prescribed for patients suffering from disorders that affect the digestive process, such as cystic fibrosis, Gaucher's disease, diabetes, and **celiac disease**. A program of enzyme supplementation is rarely recommended for healthy patients. However, proponents of enzyme therapy believe that such a program is beneficial for everyone. They point to enzymes' ability to purify the blood, strengthen the immune system, enhance mental capacity, cleanse the colon, and maintain proper pH balance in urine. They feel that by improving the digestive process, the body is better able to combat infection and disease.

Some evidence exists that pancreatic enzymes derived from animal sources are helpful in **cancer** treatment. The enzymes may be able to dissolve the coating on cancer cells and may make it easier for the immune system to attack the cancer.

A partial list of the wide variety of complaints and illnesses that can be treated by enzyme therapy includes:

• AIDS

• anemia

• alcohol consumption

• anxiety

• acute inflammation

• back pain

• cancer

• colds

• chronic **fatigue** syndrome

• colitis

• constipation

• **diarrhea**

• food **allergies**

• gastritis

• gastric duodenal ulcer

• gout

• headaches

• hepatitis

• hypoglycemia

• infections

• mucous congestion

• multiple sclerosis

• nervous disorders

• nutritional disorders

• obesity

• premenstrual syndrome (PMS)

• stress

In 2002, a biopharmaceutical company received consideration from the U.S. Food and Drug Administration (FDA) to apply for approval of a new enzyme replacement therapy that would provide long-term treatment for patients with Fabry's disease, a condition characterized by defective digestion. Fabry's disease patients don't digest fat properly and as a result, develop kidney and heart problems in adulthood. The therapy under development is called Replagal (agalsidase alfa).

Description

Enzyme supplements are extracted from plants like pineapple and papaya and from the organs of cows and pigs. The supplements are typically given in tablet or capsule form. Pancreatic enzymes may also be given by injection. The dosage varies with the condition being treated. For nondigestive ailments, the supplements are taken in the hour before meals so that they can be quickly absorbed into the blood. For digestive ailments, the supplements are taken immediately before meals accompanied by a large glass of fluids. Pancreatic enzymes may be accompanied by doses of **vitamin A**.

Preparations

No special preparations are necessary before beginning enzyme therapy. However, it is always advisable to talk to a doctor or pharmacist before purchasing enzymes and beginning therapy.

Precautions

People with allergies to beef, pork, pineapples, and papaya may suffer allergic reactions to enzyme supplements. Tablets are often coated to prevent them from breaking down in the stomach, and usually shouldn't be chewed or crushed. People who have difficulty swallowing pills can request enzyme supplements in capsule form. The capsules can then be opened and the contents sprinkled onto soft foods like applesauce.

Side effects

Side effects associated with enzyme therapy include **heartburn**, **nausea** and **vomiting**, diarrhea, bloating, **gas**, and **acne**. According to the principles of therapy, these are temporary cleansing symptoms. Drinking eight to ten glasses of water daily and getting regular **exercise** can reduce the discomfort of these side effects. Individuals may also experience an increase in bowel movements, perhaps one or two per day. This is also considered a positive effect.

Plant enzymes are safe for pregnant women, although they should always check with a doctor before using enzymes. Pregnant women should avoid animal enzymes. In rare cases, extremely high doses of enzymes can result in a build up of uric acid in the blood or urine and can cause a break down of proteins.

KEY TERMS

Celiac disease—A chronic disease characterized by defective digestion and use of fats.

Cystic fibrosis—A genetic disease that causes multiple digestive, excretion, and respiratory complications. Among the effects, the pancreas fails to provide secretions needed for the digestion of food.

Duodenum—The first part of the small intestine.

Gaucher's disease—A rare genetic disease caused by a deficiency of enzymes needed for the processing of fatty acids.

Metabolism—The system of chemical processes necessary for living cells to remain healthy.

Research & general acceptance

In the United States, the FDA has classified enzymes as a food. Therefore, they can be purchased without a prescription. However, insurance coverage is usually dependent upon the therapy resulting from a doctor's orders.

Training & certification

There is no specific training or certification required for practicing enzyme therapy.

Resources

BOOKS

Cassileth, Barrie R. *The Alternative Medicine Handbook.* New York: W.W. Norton, 1998.

PERIODICALS

"FDA to Review TKT's Application for Replagal to Treat Fabry Disease." *Proteomics Weekly* (August 26, 2002): 9.

Lee, Lita. "Life-threatening Health Issues: The Enzyme/Hormonal Connection." *Share Guide* (September-October 2002): 32-42.

OTHER

Enzyme Therapy for Your Health. http://members.tripod.com/~colloid/enzyme.htm.

Questions and Answers about Food Enzymes and Nutrition. http://www.enzymes.com/.

Therapies: Enzyme Therapy. http://library.thinkquest.org/24206/enzyme-therapy.html.

Mary McNulty
Teresa G. Odle

EPA *see* **Fish oil**

Ephedra

Description

Ephedra, also known as Ma Huang, is an herb utilized by Chinese medicine for more than 2,500 years due to its ability to remedy symptoms of **asthma** and upper respiratory **infections**. A member of the Ephedracae family of herbs (*Ephedra sinica*), ephedra is native to northern China and Inner Mongolia where it thrives in desert areas as a jointed, barkless plant with branches that bear few leaves and tiny yellow-green flowers that bloom in summer. While varieties of ephedra grow throughout the world, the United States version flourishes in the dry southwest.

Ephedra became popular to Mormon settlers in the early 1800s as a stimulant consumed in the form of tea in place of the coffee and black tea from which they abstained, giving the plant one of its many names, Mormon Tea. Other folk names that have resulted over time include Desert Tea, Desert Herb, and Squaw Tea. The herbal drink was named Whorehouse Tea after it was served in brothels during the 1800s due to unproven beliefs that it cured **gonorrhea** and **syphilis**.

The medicinal herb Ma Huang is made of the dried, young branchlets of ephedra. Harvested in the autumn, ephedra is reproduced from seed or by root division and the stems are dried in the sun throughout the year for production. The herb should be stored away from light. Ephedra gains its strength primarily from the alkaloid ephedrine, pseudephedrine, and norpseudephedrine. These active ingredients produce central nervous system stimulation. Other key components of ephedra include:

- tannin, an acidic substance found in the bark
- saponin, originating in the roots
- flavone, the chemical from which natural colors of many plants originate
- volatile oil

General use

A bitter-tasting herb that has been relied upon by the Chinese throughout centuries to heal ailments from fevers and **chills**, to nasal and chest congestion, ephedra also maintains its prominence as a strong stimulant. Contrary to its reputation, Zen monks used the herb to promote calm concentration during **meditation**. However, larger amounts can make a person jittery. Today, ephedra is used in the United States as an herbal medicine to treat asthma and **hay fever**, and the begin-

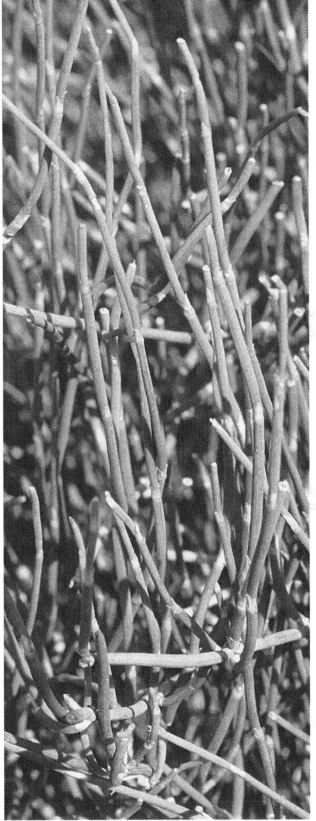

Ephedra. (*© PlantaPhile, Germany. Reproduced by permission.*)

nings of colds and flu. The herb is also used to raise blood pressure, cool fevers, and ease the **pain** of rheumatism.

While ephedrine was used in various decongestant and bronchodilator products in the United States beginning in the late 1920s through the 1940s, its potential for causing dangerous side effects led to the creation of a chemical substitute. Scientists created the equally effective, but safer, pseudephedrine that remains the active ingredient in many over-the-counter (OTC) products such as Sudafed. Primatene Mist, an OTC that contains ephedrine, is used regularly to treat asthma.

The body responds to ephedra as one of its key ingredients, ephedrine, opens bronchial passages, activating the heart and raising blood pressure while increasing metabolism. Due to its stimulating effect on the nervous system, many weight loss and energy products contain ephedra. Ephedrine increases basal metabolic rate (BMR), causing the body to burn calories faster. Dieters use ephedra-based products because they suppress the appetite and stimulate metabolism. While these diet products prove to be effective, their results are rarely permanent, and long-term use can be quite harmful. Chinese sources only recommended its use for acute situations.

As an "energy" product, ephedra increases alertness and perception. The use of ephedra in this way dates back to bodyguards of Genghis Khan, who, legend has it, fearful of being beheaded if they fell asleep on duty, consumed tea containing ephedra to stay alert. **Caffeine** products, such as coffee, tea, chocolate, and cola drinks, enhance the effect of energy products containing ephedra. Additional medicinal uses of ephedra include the promotion of **menstruation**, the decreased desire for cigarettes, and the promotion of uterine contractions. Ma Huang is also known for its ability to increase sexual sensation.

Some controversy surrounds the extended use of ephedra. It is recommended that products containing ephedra be taken only for short periods of time. Tachyphylaxis, or becoming immune to a drug's effectiveness due to overuse, and dependence on the drug may develop when taken consistently over time. Both ephedrine and Ma Huang are considered doping substances. In April 1996, the United States Food and Drug Administration (FDA) issued a warning on dietary supplements containing ephedra that were labeling themselves as safe substitutes for "street drugs," such as the illegal drug ecstasy. The FDA stated that these products could have "potentially dangerous effects on the nervous system and heart."

Ephedra is classified as a dietary supplement, and unlike pharmaceutical companies that must follow strict rules regarding safety, efficacy, and quality set by the FDA, manufacturers of supplements are not held to these guidelines. In 1994, the regulation of herbal medicine-type products in the United States changed with the passage of the Dietary Supplement Health and Education Act (DSHEA). At this time, herbal products were reclassified, along with vitamins and minerals, as dietary supplements. When classified in this grouping that falls somewhere between food and over-the-counter drugs, herbal supplement manufacturers were then able to begin making "structure-function" claims for a product on its label if there is scientific evidence supporting these claims. When appropriate, supplement manufacturers are allowed to use three types of claims: nutrient-content claims, disease claims, and **nutrition** support claims. These claims are made to guide the buyers of supplements, but supplement manufacturers may use the claims without FDA authorization, and are not required by law to conduct scientific studies on their products. In March 1999, the placement of a "Supplement Facts" panel became a requirement on the labels of most dietary supplements. In January 2002, The United States Pharmacopeial Convention announced it would launch a dietary supplement verification program. Though voluntary, the program would allow supplement manufacturers to provide documentation that they had a quality standard system in place, the organization would audit that system, then verify the quality of the supplement as long as the manufacturer continued to meet the criteria.

While questions surround the correct use of ephedra in the United States, the German government's Federal Institute for Drugs and Medical Devices (Commission E) certifies that ephedra herba, ephedra, and Ma Huang is an approved remedy for diseases of the respiratory tract with mild bronchospasms. Approval from Commission E, however, is not equivalent to the FDA's higher standards of drug approval. Some states in the United States have limited the use of ephedra, or banned the drug completely.

Preparations

Ephedra is available over the counter as a fluid extract, in tablet form, or as a dried bulk herb at Chinese pharmacies, Asian markets, and health food stores where it is permitted throughout the United States. When purchasing the herb, be certain to avoid those that look dry or have a greenish-brown cross section.

Chinese herbalists prepare ephedra for use by combining one part honey, four parts dried herb in combination with other herbs, and a small amount of water in a wok. The herbs are simmered over low heat until the water has evaporated and the herb begins to turn brown. Other forms of preparation include frying ephedra in vinegar or wine to improve its tonic effect on blood circulation, and toasting it to an ash so that it may increase its ability to stop bleeding.

To treat **fever** and chills, Chinese herbalists recommend combining ephedra with cinnamon twig and other herbs. Coughing and **wheezing** are remedied with a mixture of ephedra and **apricot seed**, while **licorice** is added to the herb for **stomachaches**. An upper respiratory infection, or congestion, is treated with a combination of ephedra and **ginger**. The powder form, mixed with rehmannia, is also used by the Chinese to treat kidney energy (yin) deficiency. It is recommended to consult a Chinese medicine practitioner, or physician for detailed information on mixtures of ephedra and doses of the herb.

As the United States has adopted the herb for its healing properties, the variety of ephedra preparations has increased. The average single dose of ephedrine for adults is 15–30 mg, with a maximum allowed daily dose of 300 mg per day. When consumed as a tea, 1 teaspoon (5 ml) of ephedra is boiled with 1 cup (250 ml) water for 15–20 minutes, with up to 2 cups (500 ml) of the tea allowed per day. This tea (also known as a decoction) is prescribed by herbalists for asthma. The tincture preparation is used in treatments to ease the aches and joint pains caused by rheumatism. The amount of tincture recommended is 1/4 teaspoon (1.25 ml)–1 teaspoon (5 ml) in combination with other herbs, up to three times a day.

As a dietary supplement, there is no FDA control over the manufacturing of ephedra, including what is in the pill, additional ingredients added to the pill, how it is produced, or what part of the plant it is made from. For example, when the whole ephedra plant is used for treatment, the side effects are minimal. When key ingredients, such as ephedrine, are isolated from the herb, the strength of the drug increases, therefore increasing the side effects. The potencies and purity within supplements vary greatly by brand and by bottle, resulting in the difficulty of exact dosage recommendations. It is recommended that directions on the product's label are followed exactly for proper use.

Precautions

While ephedra may be taken safely in the correct doses, the supplement has shown to be harmful to children, adolescents, older or chronically ill people, and pregnant women or women who are breastfeeding. Those with **heart disease**, high blood pressure, **prostate enlargement**, pheochromocytoma, diabetes, **glaucoma**, thyrotoxicosis, overactive thyroid gland (**hyperthyroidism**), nervousness, anorexia, **insomnia**, suicidal ten-

dencies, stomach ulcers, or bulimia should not take ephedra. It is also recommended that the herb be avoided by those with **diarrhea** or abdominal bloating.

It should be noted that ephedra is an ingredient in many weight-loss aids. While it is effective for a dieter's purpose as it accelerates his/her metabolism, the excess stimulation can cause dangerous consequences. The strength of the herb is extremely powerful as a stimulant, with its active ingredient epinephrine mimicking the effects of adrenaline. The molecular structure of epinephrine is close to methampetamine, also known as speed, and the use of ephedra can result in a positive test for amphetamines in the urine. Regular use of ephedra has shown to lead to dependence on the herb.

Many cases of Ma Huang toxicity have been reported to the FDA and possibly serious cardiovascular effects have been associated with its use. Health Canada issued a recall for products containing more than recommended levels of ephedra in early 2002 because of serious, possibly fatal, side effects. The dose limits set by Canadian authorities were more than 8 mg of ephedrine or a label that recommended more than 8 mg per dose or 32 mg per day. It also included products recommended use exceeding seven days.

A 2002 study concluded that use of Ma Huang could be associated with serious complications including increased risk of **stroke**, **heart attack** or even sudden death and that the effects were not limited to massive doses.

Side effects

Side effects of ephedra include insomnia, **dry mouth**, nervousness, irritability, **headache**, and **dizziness**. The following side effects are considered serious: increased blood pressure, increased heart rate, and heart palpitations. If these develop, the use of ephedra should be stopped and a physician should be consulted immediately.

In 2000, the FDA reported that the herb ephedra when used as a weight-loss product could result in serious side effects, including heart attack, stroke, and high blood pressure. These potentially life-threatening outcomes, especially to those people with heart problems, are a result of those products that combine ephedra with other stimulants, such as caffeine. At this time it is estimated that four million people safely use products that contain the combined ingredients of ephedra and caffeine.

Ephedra may be life threatening if taken in very high dosages (over 100 g, lethal dosage when taken orally corresponding to approximately 1–2 g L-ephedrine). Signs of poisoning by the herb include severe outbreaks of sweating, enlarged pupils, spasms and elevated body temperature, with heart failure and asphyxiation causing death. To treat the symptoms of poisoning caused by ephedra, seek medical attention immediately.

Interactions

While ephedra may be taken safely on its own, several adverse effects may result from taking the herb along with other drugs.

Drugs that may cause adverse effects if combined with ephedra include:

- methyl xanthines, such as caffeine
- beta blockers
- Dexamthasone
- Reserpine
- Amitriptyline
- urinary alklinizers, such as **sodium** bicarbonate
- unrinary acidifiers, for example, ammonium chloride
- monoamine oxidase inhibitors, such as heart glycosides
- secale alkaloid derivatives, such as oxytocin
- Yohimbine
- Gaunethidine, which leads to the enhancement of the sympathomimetic effect, or stimulation of the nervous system

Those who are taking any of the aforementioned drugs should avoid ephedra. The isolated drug ephedrine (the active ingredient of ephedra) has also been shown to cause side effects if combined with other drugs, including: antidepressants that increase the overall effect of ephedrine; methyldopa, due to possible increased blood pressure; and ergot preparations that may lead to serious blood pressure problems. Other substances that may cause alarming circumstances if combined with any form of ephedra include cocaine, **marijuana**, and caffeinated drinks. While it is known that Ma Huang taken with certain drugs and other substances may causes adverse effects, overall drug interactions with the supplement ephedra have not been thoroughly studied. It is recommended that a physician be notified before beginning the use ephedra in any form, or of any herbal supplement.

Resources

BOOKS

Chevallier, Andrew. "Ephedra sinica." In *The Encyclopedia of Medicinal Plants.* New York: DK Publishing Inc., 1996.

The Editors of Time-Life Books. "Conventional and Natural Medicines." In *The Medical Advisor: The Complete Guide to Alternative & Conventional Treatments.* Richmond, VA: Time-Life Inc., 1996.

KEY TERMS

Central nervous system—Consisting of the brain and spinal cord, with their nerves and end organs that control voluntary acts. Includes sensory and motor nerve fibers controlling skeletal muscles.

Dietary supplement—According to the United States Food and Drug Administration (FDA), any product intended for ingestion as a supplement to the diet.

Ergot preparations—A classification of drugs made from a fungus, used primarily for the treatment of migraines.

Metabolism—The result of all physical and chemical changes that take place within an organism, for example, the human body.

Pheochromocytoma—A tumor of the sympatho-adrenal system that produces hypertension resulting in excessive headaches, sweating, and palpitation, apprehension, flushing of the face, nausea, and vomiting.

Thyrotoxicosis—Toxic condition due to hyperactivity of the thyroid gland.

Fleming, Thomas. "Ephedra sinica." In *PDR for Herbal Medicines.* Montvale, NJ: Medical Economics Company Inc., 1998.

Griffith, H. Winter. "Ephedrine." In *Complete Guide to Prescription & Nonprescription Drugs.* New York: Berkley Publishing Group, 1998.

PERIODICALS

Binkley, Alex. "Health Canada Issues Ephedra Recall." *Food Chemical News* 43, no.49 (January 21, 2002):19.

Kurtzwell, Paula. "An FDA Guide to Dietary Supplements." *FDA Consumer* no. 99 (September/October 1998): 2323.

Levy, Sandra. "Watch for New Seal of Approval on Dietary Supplements." *Drug Topics* 146, no.29 (January 7, 2002):29.

Samenuk, David. "Adverse Cardiovascular Events Temporarily Associated with Ma Huang, an Herbal Source of Ephedrine." *JAMA, Journal of the American Medical Association* 287, no. 12:1506.

Taylor, David. "Herbal Medicine at a Crossroads." *Environmental Health Perspectives* 104, no.9 (September, 1996).

ORGANIZATIONS

American Botanical Council. PO Box 201660, Austin, TX 78720–1660.

Food and Drug Administration, Office of Consumer Affairs. HFE-88, Rockville, MD 20857.

Herb Research Foundation. 1007 Pearl Street, Suite 200, Boulder, CO 80302.

OTHER

Drug Digest. http://www.drugdigest.org (January 17, 2001).
The Ephedra Site. http://ephedra.demon.nl/index.html
WebMD. http://WebMD.com

Beth Kapes
Teresa G. Odle

Epididymitis

Definition

Epididymitis is the inflammation or infection of the epididymis, the long coiled tube that attaches to the upper part of each testicle. The epididymis functions as a storage, transport, and maturation place for sperm before ejaculation.

Description

In adults, epididymitis is the most common cause of **pain** in the scrotum, and in adolescents, the second most common cause. The acute form is usually associated with the most severe pain and swelling. If symptoms last for more than six weeks after treatment begins, the condition is considered chronic.

Epididymitis is most common between the ages of 18 and 40, but children can get it, too. Boys who experience painful urination, have a history of urinary tract **infections**, abnormal bladder function, or abnormalities of the genitals and urinary structures are more inclined to get epididymitis. It is seldom found in adolescents who aren't sexually active.

The infection is especially common among members of the military who **exercise** for extended periods without emptying their bladders.

Factors that increase the risk of developing epididymitis include:

- infection of the bladder, kidney, prostate, or urinary tract

- other recent illness

- narrowing of the urethra (the tube that drains urine from the bladder)

- use of a urethral catheter

The infection doesn't start in the epididymis. It is an ascending infection that most often starts in the urethra or urinary tract before spreading to the epididymis.

Causes & symptoms

Among men under age 35 who are sexually active, *Chlamydia trachomatis* or *Neisseria gonorrhoeae* are the most common causes of epididymitis.

Nonsexually transmitted epididymitis is associated with urinary tract infections and is more common in men who have undergone surgery for urinary tract problems or who have anatomical abnormalities.

Although epididymitis is often caused by and associated with some of the same organisms that cause some sexually transmitted diseases, there are other causes as well. The condition can also be attributed to pus-generating bacteria associated with infections in other parts of the body. This cause, however, is rare.

Epididymitis can also be caused by injury or infection of the scrotum or by irritation from urine that has accumulated in the vas deferens (the duct through which sperm travels after leaving the epididymis).

Epididymitis is characterized by pain in the testes. The pain, which usually develops gradually over several hours or days, is followed by sudden redness and swelling of the scrotum. Generally, only one testicle is affected. The affected testicle is hard and sore, and the other testicle may feel tender. The patient has **chills**, a low-grade **fever**, and usually has acute urethritis (inflammation of the urethra).

Sometimes, there is a discharge from the urethra and blood in the semen. Ejaculation can be painful.

Enlarged lymph nodes in the groin cause scrotal pain that intensifies throughout the day and may become so severe that walking normally becomes impossible.

Diagnosis

Doctors test for epididymitis through:

- Urinalysis, which will likely show an elevated white blood-cell count and the presence of bacteria.

- Urine culture, to identify the organism responsible for the infection.

- Examination of discharges from the urethra and prostate gland.

- Blood tests to measure white-cell counts, which will be elevated.

- Ultrasound, which will reveal an enlarged epididymis.

The condition may lead to an **abscess** or cause such complications as **infertility**, so it is best to consult a urologist about the condition and treatment.

Treatment

Conventional treatment involves the use of antibiotics to treat the infection and pain killers to ease the pain. With alternative therapies, the treatment involves increasing circulation to the area. This reduces inflammation, which helps the body heal.

Fasting is recommended for some people, since digestion slows down the body's healing mechanisms. A water fast is best, but if that isn't possible, the patient should confine intake to fruit and vegetable juices. If food must be eaten, a light diet of fresh fruits and vegetables is recommended. Fasting eases pain. Fluids should also be increased.

In **traditional Chinese medicine**, there are formulas of herbs that need to be designed to fit the individual case. Herbs like philodendron (Huang Bai) are used for inflammation in the lower torso area. **Pulsatilla**, which helps with swelling and pain, particularly in the genitals, and podophyllum are the most effective in treating epididymitis. These plants, however, are toxic, and the herb should only be taken under the direct supervision of an experienced herbalist. **Echinacea**, **horsetail**, **saw palmetto** berries, **cranberry** extract, and chimaphilla are also effective.

Hydrotherapy may also help. Sitting in hot water increases circulation to the prostate area, alleviating discomfort and speeding recovery. Patients are advised to sit in a tub for 15 to 30 minutes once or twice a day. The water should be as hot as can be tolerated.

Homeopathy is also an option. Homeopathic physicians may prescribe remedies that are specific to the person.

Since epididymitis is caused by an infection and often involves the urinary tract, the following alternative remedies may also be helpful in treatment of the condition:

- Acupuncture, which may help ward off another infection.

- Aromatherapy. A hot sitz bath with drops of **juniper** berry or sandalwood may relieve symptoms of the infection.

- Chiropractic. Strengthening bladder muscles by adjusting the joints and bones in the pelvic area may keep infection at bay.

Allopathic treatment

Epididymitis is traditionally treated with antibiotic therapy. To prevent reinfection, patients must take their medication exactly as prescribed, even if the patient's symptoms disappear or if he begins to feel better. Over-the-counter anti-inflammatories may be taken to relieve pain. The over-the-counter medicines will have the same effects as herbal anti-inflammatories.

Bed rest is recommended until symptoms subside, and patients are advised to wear athletic supporters when they resume normal activities. If pain is severe, a local anesthetic like lidocaine (Xylocaine) may be injected directly into the spermatic cord. Scrotal ice packs and scrotal elevation are also recommended.

Self-care

A patient who has epididymitis should not drink beverages that contain **caffeine**. To prevent **constipation**, he should use stool softeners or eat plenty of fruit, nuts, whole grain cereals, and other foods with laxative properties.

Strenuous activity should be avoided until symptoms disappear. Sexual activity should not be resumed until a month after symptoms disappear.

If a second course of treatment doesn't eradicate stubborn symptoms, long-term anti-inflammatory therapy may be recommended. In rare instances, chronic symptoms require surgery.

Surgery

There are two surgical procedures used to treat epididymitis, and both of them cause sterility.

Epididymectomy involves removing the inflamed section of the epididymitis through a small incision in the scrotum.

Bilateral vasectomy prevents fluid and sperm from passing through the epididymis. This procedure is usually performed on men who have chronic epididymitis or on elderly patients undergoing prostate surgery.

Before considering surgeries that will lead to infertility, patients may want to try alternative therapies.

Expected results

Herbal preparations are very effective in treating epididymitis. Some sources say that given in medicinal doses, the herbs pulsatilla and podophyllum can treat epididymitis with the same results as conventional medicine.

Pain may begin to subside within 24 hours of treatment, but complete healing may take weeks or even months.

Prevention

Using condoms and not having sex with anyone who has a sexually transmitted disease (STD) can prevent some cases of epididymitis. Also, drinking plenty of

KEY TERMS

. . . .

Acute—Refers to a condition or pain that is sharp and short in course.

Chronic—A condition that has a long duration.

Testicle—One of the two male sex glands, located in the scrotum, where sperm and hormones are produced.

Urethra—Refers to the opening at the end of the penis; drains urine from the bladder.

Vas deferens—The duct that stores sperm and carries it from the testicles to the urethra.

fluids, which will increase urine flow, will help prevent urine retention, which can lead to infection.

Resources

BOOKS

The Alternative Advisor. Alexandria, Virginia: Time-Life Books, 1997.

The Alternative Health and Medicine Encyclopedia. Detroit: Visible Ink Press, 1995.

The Medical Advisor. Alexandria, Virginia: Time-Life Books, 1996.

Shaw, Michael, ed. *Everything You Need to Know About Diseases.* Springhouse, Pennsylvania: Springhouse Corporation, 1996.

PERIODICALS

Baren, Jill M., "The Acute Scrotum: Serious or Benign?" *Emergency Medicine* 28, 8 (August 1996): 24-45.

OTHER

"Epididymitis." *Adam.com.* http://www.adam.com/ency/article/001279.htm (20 June 2000).

"Epididymitis." *AlternativeMedicine.com.* http://www.alternativemedicine.com (20 June 2000).

"Epididymitis." http://www.duj.com/epididymitis.html. (7 June 1998).

"Epididymitis." http://www.thriveonline.com/health/Library/illsymp/illness203.html. (6 June 1998).

Lisa Frick

Epilepsy

Definition

Epilepsy is a condition characterized by recurrent seizures that may include repetitive muscle jerking called convulsions. A seizure is a sudden disruption of the brain's normal electrical activity accompanied by altered consciousness and/or other neurological and behavioral manifestations.

Description

Epilepsy affects 1–2% of the population of the United States. Although epilepsy is as common in adults over 60 as in children under 10, 25% of all cases develop before the age of five. One in every two cases develops before the age of 25. About 125,000 new cases of epilepsy are diagnosed each year, and a significant number of children and adults that have not been diagnosed or treated have epilepsy.

Most seizures are benign, but a seizure that lasts a long time can lead to status epilepticus, a life-threatening condition characterized by continuous seizures, sustained loss of consciousness, and respiratory distress. Nonconvulsive epilepsy can impair physical coordination, vision, and other senses. Undiagnosed seizures can lead to conditions that are more serious and more difficult to manage.

Types of seizures

Generalized epileptic seizures occur when electrical abnormalities exist throughout the brain. A partial seizure does not involve the entire brain. A partial seizure begins in an area called an epileptic focus, but may spread to other parts of the brain and cause a generalized seizure. Some people who have epilepsy have more than one type of seizure.

Motor attacks cause parts of the body to jerk repeatedly. A motor attack usually lasts less than an hour and may last only a few minutes. Sensory seizures begin with numbness or tingling in one area. The sensation may move along one side of the body or the back before subsiding.

Visual seizures that affect the area of the brain that controls sight cause people to hallucinate. Auditory seizures affect the part of the brain that controls hearing and cause the patient to imagine hearing voices, music, and other sounds. Other types of seizures can cause confusion, upset stomach, or emotional distress.

PARTIAL SEIZURES. Simple partial seizures do not spread from the focal area where they arise. Symptoms are determined by the part of the brain affected. The patient usually remains conscious during the seizure and can later describe it in detail.

COMPLEX PARTIAL SEIZURES. A distinctive smell, taste, or other unusual sensation (aura) may signal the start of a complex partial seizure.

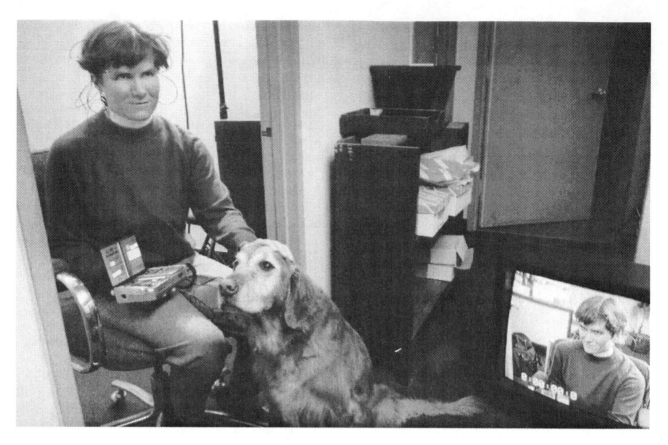

An epilepsy sufferer, hooked to brain-monitoring equipment, sits with her seizure-predicting dog. *(A/P Wide World Photos. Reproduced by permission.)*

Complex partial seizures start as simple partial seizures, but move beyond the focal area and cause loss of consciousness. Complex partial seizures can become major motor seizures. Although a person having a complex partial seizure may not seem to be unconscious, he or she does not know what is happening and may behave inappropriately. He or she will not remember the seizure, but may seem confused or intoxicated for a few minutes after it ends.

Causes & symptoms

The origin of 50–70% of all cases of epilepsy is unknown. Epilepsy sometimes results from trauma at birth. Such causes include insufficient oxygen to the brain; head injury; heavy bleeding or incompatibility between a woman's blood and the blood of her newborn baby; and infection immediately before, after, or at the time of birth.

Other causes of epilepsy include:

• head trauma resulting from a car accident, gunshot wound, or other injury

• alcoholism

• brain **abscess** or inflammation of membranes covering the brain or spinal cord

• phenylketonuria (PKU), a disease that is present at birth, is often characterized by seizures, and can result in mental retardation

• other inherited disorders

• infectious diseases such as **measles**, **mumps**, and diphtheria

• degenerative disease

• lead poisoning, mercury poisoning, carbon monoxide poisoning, or ingestion of some other poisonous substance

• genetic factors

Status epilepticus, a condition in which a person suffers from continuous seizures and may have trouble breathing, can be caused by:

• suddenly discontinuing antiseizure medication

• hypoxic or metabolic encephalopathy (brain disease resulting from lack of oxygen or malfunctioning of other physical or chemical processes)

• acute head injury

• infection spread from blood (for example, **meningitis** or encephalitis) caused by inflammation of the brain or the membranes that cover it

Diagnosis

Personal and family medical history, description of seizure activity, and physical and neurological examinations help primary care physicians, neurologists, and epileptologists diagnose this disorder. Doctors rule out conditions that cause symptoms that resemble epilepsy, including small strokes (transient ischemic attacks, or TIAs), fainting (syncope), pseudoseizures, and sleep attacks (**narcolepsy**).

Neuropsychological testing uncovers learning or memory problems. Neuroimaging provides views of brain areas involved in seizure activity.

The electroencephalogram (EEG) is the main test used to diagnose epilepsy. EEGs use electrodes placed on or within the skull to record the brain's electrical activity and pinpoint the exact location of abnormal discharges.

The patient may be asked to remain motionless during a short-term EEG or to go about his normal activities during extended monitoring. Some patients are deprived of sleep or exposed to seizure triggers, such as rapid, deep breathing (hyperventilation) or flashing lights (photic stimulation). In some cases, people may be hospitalized for EEG monitorings that can last as long as two weeks. Video EEGs also document what the patient was doing when the seizure occurred and how the seizure changed his or her behavior.

Other techniques used to diagnose epilepsy include:

• Magnetic resonance imaging (MRI), which provides clear, detailed images of the brain. Functional MRI (fMRI), performed while the patient does various tasks, can measure shifts in electrical intensity and blood flow and indicate which brain region each activity affects.

• Positron emission tomography (PET) and single photon emission tomography (SPECT) monitor blood flow and chemical activity in the brain area being tested. PET and SPECT are very effective in locating the brain region where metabolic changes take place between seizures.

Treatment

Relaxation techniques

Stress increases seizure activity in 30% of people who have epilepsy. **Relaxation** techniques can provide some sense of control over the disorder, but they should never be used instead of antiseizure medication or without the approval of the patient's doctor. **Yoga**, medita-

tion, and favorite pastimes help some people relax and manage stress more successfully. **Biofeedback** can teach adults and older adolescents how to recognize an aura and what to do to stop its spread. Children under 14 usually are not able to understand and apply principles of biofeedback.

Acupuncture

Acupuncture treatments (acupuncture needles inserted for a few minutes or left in place for as long as 30 minutes) make some people feel pleasantly relaxed.

Acupressure

Acupressure can have the same effect on children or on adults who dislike needles.

Aromatherapy

Aromatherapy involves mixing aromatic plant oils into water or other oils and massaging them into the skin or using a special burner to waft their fragrance throughout the room. Aromatherapy oils affect the body and the brain, and undiluted oils should never be applied directly to the skin. Ylang ylang, **chamomile**, or **lavender** can create a soothing mood. People who have epilepsy should not use **rosemary**, **hyssop**, citrus (such as lemon), **sage**, or sweet **fennel**, which seem to stimulate the brain.

Nutritional therapy

KETOGENIC DIET. A special high-fat, low-protein, low-carbohydrate diet is sometimes used to treat patients whose severe seizures have not responded to other treatment. Calculated according to age, height, and weight, the ketogenic diet induces mild starvation and dehydration. This forces the body to create an excessive supply of ketones, natural chemicals with seizure-suppressing properties.

The goal of this controversial approach is to maintain or improve seizure control while reducing medication. The ketogenic diet works best with children between the ages of one and 10. It is introduced over a period of several days, and most children are hospitalized during the early stages of treatment.

If a child following this diet remains seizure-free for at least six months, increased amounts of carbohydrates and protein are gradually added. If the child shows no improvement after three months, the diet is gradually discontinued. A 2003 study of the diet and its effect on growth noted that if used, clinicians should recommend adequate intake of energy and protein and a higher proportion of unsaturated to saturated dietary fats. The report also recommended use of vitamin and mineral supplements with the diet.

Introduced in the 1920s, the ketogenic diet has had limited, short–term success in controlling seizure activity. Its use exposes patients to such potentially harmful side effects as:

• staphylococcal infections

• stunted or delayed growth

• low blood sugar (hypoglycemia)

• excess fat in the blood (hyperlipidemia)

• disease resulting from **calcium** deposits in the urinary tract (urolithiasis)

• disease of the optic nerve (optic neuropathy)

Homeopathy

Homeopathic therapy also can work for people with seizures, especially constitutional homeopathic treatment that acts at the deepest levels to address the needs of the individual person.

Allopathic treatment

The goal of epilepsy treatment is to eliminate seizures or make the symptoms less frequent and less severe. Long-term anticonvulsant drug therapy is the most common form of epilepsy treatment.

Medication

A combination of drugs may be needed to control some symptoms, but most patients who have epilepsy take one of the following medications:

• Dilantin (phenytoin)

• Tegretol (carbamazepine)

• Barbita (phenobarbital)

• Mysoline (primidone)

• Depakene (valproic acid, **sodium** valproate)

• Klonopin (clonazepam)

• Zarontin (ethosuximide)

Dilantin, Tegretol, Barbita, and Mysoline are used to manage or control generalized tonic-clonic and complex partial seizures. Depakene, Klonopin, and Zarontin are prescribed for patients who have absence seizures.

Neurontin (gabapentin), Lamictal (lamotrigine), and topiramate (Topamax) are among medications more recently approved in the United States to treat adults who have partial seizures or partial and grand mal seizures. Another new medication called Levetiracetam (Keppra) has been approved and shows particularly good results in reducing partial seizures among elderly patients with few side effects. This is important, because elderly patients often have other conditions and must take other medications that might interact with seizure medications. In 2003, Keppra's manufacturer was working on a new antiepilectic drug from the same chemical family as Keppra that should be more potent and effective. Available medications frequently change, and the physician will determine the best treatment for an individual patient. A 2003 report found that monotherapy, or using just one medication rather than a combination, works better for most patients. The less complicated the treatment, the more likely the patient will comply and better manager the seizure disorder.

Even an epileptic patient whose seizures are well controlled should have regular blood tests to measure levels of antiseizure medication in his or her system and to check to see if the medication is causing any changes in his or her blood or liver. A doctor should be notified if any signs of drug toxicity appear, including uncontrolled eye movements; sluggishness, **dizziness**, or hyperactivity; inability to see clearly or speak distinctly; **nausea** or **vomiting**; or sleep problems.

Status epilepticus requires emergency treatment, usually with Valium (Ativan), Dilantin, or Barbita. An intravenous dextrose (sugar) solution is given to a patient whose condition is due low blood sugar, and a vitamin B_1 preparation is administered intravenously when status epilepticus results from chronic alcohol withdrawal. Because dextrose and **thiamine** are essentially harmless and because delay in treatment can be disastrous, these medications are given routinely, as it is usually difficult to obtain an adequate history from a patient suffering from status epilepticus.

Intractable seizures are seizures that cannot be controlled with medication or without sedation or other unacceptable side effects. Surgery may be used to eliminate or control intractable seizures.

Surgery

Surgery can be used to treat patients whose intractable seizures stem from small focal lesions that can be removed without endangering the patient, changing the patient's personality, dulling the patient's senses, or reducing the patient's ability to function.

A physical examination is conducted to verify that a patient's seizures are caused by epilepsy, and surgery is not used to treat patients with severe psychiatric disturbances or medical problems that raise risk factors to unacceptable levels.

Surgery is never recommended unless:

- The best available antiseizure medications have failed to control the patient's symptoms satisfactorily.

- The origin of the patient's seizures has been precisely located.

- There is good reason to believe that surgery will significantly improve the patient's health and quality of life.

Every patient considering epilepsy surgery is carefully evaluated by one or more neurologists, neurosurgeons, neuropsychologists, and/or social workers. A psychiatrist, chaplain, or other spiritual advisor may help the patient and his family cope with the stresses that occur during and after the selection process.

TYPES OF SURGERY. Surgical techniques used to treat intractable epilepsy include:

- Lesionectomy. Removing the lesion (diseased brain tissue) and some surrounding brain tissue is very effective in controlling seizures. Lesionectomy is generally more successful than surgery performed on patients whose seizures are not caused by clearly defined lesions, but removing only part of the lesion lessens the effectiveness of the procedure.

- Temporal resections. Removing part of the temporal lobe and the part of the brain associated with feelings, memory, and emotions (the hippocampus) provides good or excellent seizure control in 75–80% of properly selected patients with appropriate types of temporal lobe epilepsy. Some patients experience post-operative speech and memory problems.

- Extra-temporal resection. This procedure involves removing some or all of the frontal lobe, the part of the brain directly behind the forehead. The frontal lobe helps regulate movement, planning, judgment, and personality. Special care must be taken to prevent post-operative problems with movement and speech. Extra-temporal resection is most successful in patients whose seizures are not widespread.

- Hemispherectomy. This method of removing brain tissue is restricted to patients with severe epilepsy and abnormal discharges that often extend from one side of the brain to the other. Hemispherectomies are most often performed on infants or young children who have had an extensive brain disease or disorder since birth or from a very young age.

- Corpus callosotomy. This procedure, an alternative to hemispherectomy in patients with congenital hemiplegia, removes some or all of the white matter that separates the two halves of the brain. Corpus callosotomy is performed almost exclusively on children who are frequently injured during falls caused by seizures. If removing two–thirds of the corpus callosum does not produce lasting improvement in the patient's condition, the remaining one-third will be removed during another operation.

- Multiple subpial transection. This procedure is used to control the spread of seizures that originate in or affect the "eloquent" cortex, the area of the brain responsible for complex thought and reasoning.

Other forms of treatment

VAGUS NERVE STIMULATION. Approved for adults and adolescents (over 16 years old) with intractable seizures, vagus nerve stimulation (VNS) uses a pacemaker-like device implanted under the skin in the upper left chest, to provide intermittent stimulation to the vagus nerve. Stretching from the side of the neck into the brain, the vagus nerve affects swallowing, speech, breathing, and many other functions, and VNS may prevent or shorten some seizures.

First aid for seizures

A person with epilepsy having a seizure should not be restrained, but sharp or dangerous objects should be moved out of reach. Anyone having a complex partial seizure can be warned away from danger by someone calling his/her name in a clear, calm voice.

A person with epilepsy having a grand mal seizure should be helped to lie down, and those aiding the patient should contact emergency medical personnel. Tight clothing should be loosened. A soft, flat object like a towel or the palm of a hand should be placed under the person's head. Forcing a hard object into the mouth of someone having a grand mal seizure could cause injuries or breathing problems. If the person's mouth is open, placing a folded cloth or other soft object between his or her teeth will protect the tongue. Turning the patient's head to the side will help with breathing. After a grand mal seizure has ended, the person who had the seizure should be told what has happened and reminded of where he or she is.

Expected results

People who have epilepsy have a higher than average rate of suicide; sudden, unexplained death; and drowning and other accidental fatalities.

Benign focal epilepsy of childhood and some absence seizures may disappear in time, but remission is unlikely if seizures occur several times a day, several times in a 48-hour period, or more frequently than in the past.

Epilepsy can be partially or completely controlled if the individual takes antiseizure medication according to directions; avoids seizure-inducing sights, sounds, and other triggers; gets enough sleep; and eats regular, balanced meals.

Anyone who has epilepsy should wear a bracelet or necklace identifying the seizure disorder and listing the medication he or she takes.

Prevention

Eating properly, getting enough sleep, and controlling stress and fevers can help prevent seizures. A person who has epilepsy should be careful not to hyperventilate. Those who experience auras should find a safe place to lie down and stay until the seizure passes. Anticonvulsant medications should not be stopped suddenly and, if other medications are prescribed or discontinued, the doctor treating the seizures should be notified. In some conditions, such as severe head injury, brain surgery, or subarachnoid hemorrhage, anticonvulsant medications may be given to the patient to prevent seizures.

Resources

BOOKS

"Seizures." *Reader's Digest Guide to Medical Cures & Treatments : A Complete A-to-Z Sourcebook of Medical Treatments, Alternative Opinions, and Home Remedies.* Canada: The Reader's Digest Association, Inc., 1996.

Shaw, Michael, ed. *Everything You Need to Know about Diseases.* Springhouse, PA: Springhouse Corporation, 1996.

PERIODICALS

Batchelor, Lori, et al. "An Interdisciplinary Approach to Implementing the Ketogenic Diet for the Treatment of Seizures." *Pediatric Nursing* (September/October 1997): 465–471.

"Data Analysis Shows Keppra Reduced Partial Seizures in Elderly Patients." *Clinical Trials Week* (April 28, 2003): 26.

Dichter, M.A., and M.J. Brodie. "Drug Therapy: New Antiepileptic Drugs." *The New England Journal of Medicine* (15 June 1996): 1583-1588.

Dilorio, Colleen, et al. "The Epilelpsy Medication and Treatment Complexity Index: Reliability and Validity Testing." *Journal of Neuroscience Nursing* (June 2003): 155–158.

"Epilepsy Surgery and Vagus Nerve Stimulation Are Effective When Drugs Fail." *Medical Devices & Surgical Technology Week* (May 4, 2003): 33.

Finn, Robert. "Partial Seizures Double Risk of Sleep Disturbances (Consider in Diagnosis, Management)." *Clinical Psychiatry News* (June 2003): 36–41.

Lannox, Susan L. "Epilepsy Surgery for Partial Seizures." *Pediatric Nursing* (September–October 1997): 453-458.

Liu, Yeou-Mei Christiana, et al. "A Prospetive Study: Growth and Nutritional Status of Children Treated With the Ketogenic Diet." *Journal of the American Dietetic Association* (June 2003): 707.

McDonald, Melori E. "Use of the Ketogenic Diet in Treating Children with Seizures." *Pediatric Nursing* (September-October 1997): 461-463.

> ## KEY TERMS
>
> **Acupressure**—Needleless acupuncture.
>
> **Acupuncture**—An ancient Chinese method of relieving pain or treating illness by piercing specific areas of the body with fine needles.
>
> **Biofeedback**—A learning technique that helps individuals influence automatic body functions.
>
> **Epileptologist**—A physician who specializes in the treatment of epilepsy.

"New Drug Candidate Shows Promise." *Clinical Trials Week* (April 7, 2003): 26.

ORGANIZATIONS

American Epilepsy Society. 638 Prospect Avenue, Hartford, CT 06105-4298. (205) 232-4825.

Epilepsy Concern International Service Group. 1282 Wynnewood Drive, West Palm Beach, FL 33417. (407) 683–0044.

Epilepsy Foundation of America. 4251 Garden City Drive, Landover, MD 20875-2267. (800) 532-1000.

Epilepsy Information Service. (800) 642-0500.

OTHER

Bourgeois, Blaise F.D. *Epilepsy Surgery in Children.* http://www.neuro.wustl.edu/epilepsy/21children.html (3 March 1998).

Cosgrove, G. Rees, and Andrew J. Cole. *Surgical Treatment of Epilepsy.* http://neurosurgery.mgh.harvard.edu/ep–sxtre.htm (3 March 1998).

Epilepsy. http://www.ninds.nih.gov/healinfo/disorder/epilepsy/epilepfs.htm (28 February 1998).

Epilepsy and Dental Health. http://www.epinet.org.au/efv-dent.html (3 March 1998).

Epilepsy Facts and Figures. http://www.efa.org/what/education/FACTS.html (28 February 1998).

Frequently Asked Questions (FAQs) About the Ketogenic Diet. http://www-leland.Stanford.edu/group/ketodiet/FAQ.html (28 February 1998).

Surgery for Epilepsy: NIH Consensus Statement Online. http://neurosurgery.mgh.harvard.edu/epil-nih.htm (3 March 1998).

The USC Vagus Nerve Stimulator Program. http://www.usc.edu/hsc/medicine/neurology/VNS.html (3 March 1998).

Mai Tran
Teresa G. Odle

Epimedium

Description

Epimedium is a genus of 21 species and is a member of the buttercup family. *Epimedium* is a woody, pungent ornamental herb found in western and eastern Asia and the Mediterranean. Various hybrids are grown elsewhere and most often are used as groundcover, particularly in shady areas. The herb also goes by the name horny goat weed and barrenwort. The Chinese call it *Yin Yang Huo*, which means "licentious goat plant."

The plant was named epimedium because it is akin to a plant found in the ancient southwest Asian kingdom of Media, now a part of Iran. Plants used for medicinal purposes include *Epimedium sagittatum*, *Epimedium brevicornum*, *Epimedium wushanense*, *Epimedium koreanum*, and *Epimedium pubescens*.

General use

The use of epimedium as a medicinal herb dates back thousands of years. Shen Nong's *Canon of Medicinal Herbs*, compiled around 400 A.D., mentions its use.

The odorless, bitter herb has been used as a:

- Kidney tonic to help relieve problems of frequent urination and correct problems of lightheadedness and weakness associated with improper body fluid volumes.

- Reproductive system tonic to treat **impotence** and premature ejaculation.

- Rejuvenating tonic, as an aphrodisiac or to relieve fatigue.

The herb, which dilates blood vessels, has also been used to treat coronary **heart disease**, **asthma**, **bronchitis**, and sinusitis. An expectorant, it can be used to control coughing. It can also be used to lower blood pressure.

Studies have shown that epimedium raises adrenaline, noradrenaline, serotonin, and dopamine levels in animals. It is the dopamine that may be responsible for the herb's use as a reproductive tonic. The increased dopamine levels in the body set off a chain reaction that leads to a release of testosterone, the male sex hormone.

Other evidence suggests the herb increases sensitivity in nerve endings, which may explain why it is prescribed as an aphrodisiac.

Preparations

The herb is collected in summer or early autumn, then dried in the sun. Some use it unprepared, while others bake it with sheep fat.

The herb can be ingested as a tea infusion. To make the tea, one ounce of the cut leaves are added to a pint of hot water. The recommended dosage is one to three cups per day. The tea should be taken with food.

KEY TERMS

Expectorant—A preparation that loosens or liquefies thick mucus.

Impotence—Refers to a condition where the penis is unable to get erect or stay erect.

Shen Nong—A legendary emperor, he was called the "Divine Farmer" of China. Shen Nong made many discoveries concerning herbal medicine and cataloged 365 species of medicinal plants. An early herbal text, written around 400 A.D., was named after him.

Sinusitis—An infection of the sinus cavities characterized by pain in the eyes and cheeks, fever, and difficulty breathing through the nose.

Suet—Refers to the hard fat found around cattle and sheep kidneys and loins; it is used in cooking.

A powder form may be made by combining 100 kg of dried epimedium leaves with 20 kg of refined suet, then stir-frying the concoction.

Epimedium may also be combined with **lycium fruit** to make a tea concoction to stimulate the Kidneys and reproductive system. Combine one ounce of epimedium and wolfberries (lycium) with hot water and drink after the concoction has steeped for 10 to 15 minutes. Note that individuals with **allergies** to tomatoes and other vegetables in the nightshade family may also be allergic to lycium berries.

Precautions

When buying epimedium, be sure to pick leaves with a dark color. Those that are yellow or blanched probably sat in the sun too long when drying and won't be as effective.

Also, purchase herbs from reputable companies to ensure their purity.

Side effects

Ingesting an excess amount of the herb can lead to **vomiting**, **dizziness**, thirst, and nosebleed.

Interactions

Just like other drugs, herbs can be hazardous to health both by themselves and particularly in certain combinations. For this reason, consult a knowledgeable herbal therapist before taking epimedium to find out what it can and can't be used with. Also, be aware that herbs can interfere with prescription medication.

Resources

BOOKS

Bown, Deni. *Encyclopedia of Herbs and Their Uses*. New York: Dorling Kindersley, 1995.

Keys, John D. *Chinese Herbs: Their Botany, Chemistry, and Pharmacodynamics*. Rutland, Vt.: Charles E. Tuttle, 1976.

OTHER

"Epimedium." *Herbwalk.com*. http://herbwalk.com/remedy/herb_Epimedium_132.html.

"*Epimedium grandiflorum*." *AdvancedHerbals.com*. http://www.advancedherbals.com/herbs/div/epimedium_grandiflorum.html.

"Traditional Chinese Medicine Herbal Database." *ChinaMed.net*. http://www.china-med.net/unified_site/herb_library/materia_medica.html.

Lisa Frick

Erectile dysfunction *see* **Impotence**

Essential fatty acids

Description

Essential fatty acids (EFAs) are fats that are essential to the diet because the body cannot produce them. Essential fatty acids are extremely important nutrients for health. They are present in every healthy cell in the body, and are critical for the normal growth and functioning of the cells, muscles, nerves, and organs. EFAs are also used by the body to produce a class of hormone-like substances called prostaglandins, which are key to many important processes. Deficiencies of EFAs are linked to a variety of health problems, including major ones such as **heart disease**, **cancer**, and diabetes. It has been estimated that as many as 80% of American people may consume insufficient quantities of EFAs.

Very few health issues have received as much attention during the past several decades as the question of fat in the diet. Sixty-eight percent of deaths in America are related to fat consumption and diet, including heart disease (44% of deaths), cancer (22%) and diabetes (2%). There are several types of dietary fats. Saturated fat is found mainly in animal products, including meat and dairy products, and avocados, and nuts. **Cholesterol** is a dietary fat that is only found in animal products. Cholesterol is also made by the body in small amounts from saturated fats. Heavy consumption of saturated fat and cholesterol has been linked to heart disease and cancer. Unsaturated fats are typically oils from vegetables, nuts, and are present in some fish. These are considered the healthiest dietary fats. Essential fatty acids are unsaturated fats. EFAs are the only fats that may need to be increased in the American diet.

Scientists classify essential fatty acids into two types, **omega-3 fatty acids** and **omega-6 fatty acids**, depending on their chemical composition. Technically, the omega-3 fatty acids are alpha-linolenic acid, stearidonic acid, and two others called EPA and DHA. Alpha-linolenic acid is found mainly in **flaxseed** oil, canola oil, soybeans, walnuts, hemp seeds, and dark green leafy vegetables. Stearidonic acid is found in rarer types of seeds and nuts, including black currant seeds. EPA and DHA are present in cold-water fish, including salmon, trout, sardines, mackerel, and cod. Cod liver oil is a popular nutritional supplement for omega-3 EFAs.

Omega-6 fatty acids are more common in the American diet than the omega-3 EFAs. These include **linoleic acid**, which is found in safflower, olive, almond, sunflower, hemp, soybean, walnut, pumpkin, sesame, and flaxseed oils. Gamma-linolenic acid (GLA) is found in some seeds and *evening primrose oil*. Arachidonic acid (AA) is present in meat and animal products.

Both types of EFAs, omega-3 and omega-6 fatty acids, are necessary in a healthy diet. Deficiencies of EFAs have been brought about by changes in diet and the modern processing of foods and oils. Many nutritionists believe that a major dietary problem is the use of hydrogenated oils, which are present in margarine and many processed foods. Hydrogenated oils are highly refined by industrial processes, and contain toxic by-products and trans-fatty acids. Trans-fatty acids are fat molecules with chemically altered structures, and are believed to have several detrimental effects on the body. Trans-fatty acids interfere with the absorption of healthy EFAs, and may contribute to **atherosclerosis**, or damage to the arteries. Deep-fried foods, which are cooked in oil that is altered by very high temperatures, also contain trans-fatty acids. Many health professionals, including those at the World Heath Organization, have protested against the use of hydrogenated oils in food and the consumption of trans-fatty acids. Health conditions linked to the consumption of trans-fatty acids and hydrogenated oils include cancer, heart disease, high cholesterol, diabetes, **obesity**, immune system disorders, decreased sperm counts, and infant development problems.

Dietary changes that have contributed to EFA deficiency or imbalances include the increased use of oils that contain few or no omega-3 EFAs; the industrial milling of flour that removes the EFA-containing germ;

the increase of sugar and fried foods in the diet that may interfere with the body's absorption of EFAs; and the decreased consumption of fish.

A balance of omega-3 and omega-6 EFAs in the diet is recommended by experts. Americans typically consume higher quantities of omega-6 EFAs, because these are found in meat, animal products, and common cooking oils. Research has shown that too many omega-6 EFAs in the diet can lead to the imbalanced production of prostaglandins, which may contribute to health problems. Experts recommend that omega-3 and omega-6 EFAs be present in the diet in a ratio of around one to three. Americans consume a ratio as high as one to 40. Thus, the need for greater amounts of omega-3 EFAs in the diet has increased.

Symptoms of EFA deficiency or imbalance include dry or scaly skin, excessively dry hair, cracked fingernails, **fatigue**, weakness, frequent **infections**, **allergies**, mood disorders, hyperactivity, **depression**, memory and learning problems, slow wound healing, aching joints, poor digestion, high blood pressure, obesity, and high cholesterol.

General use

EFA supplementation is recommended for more than 60 health conditions. EFAs are used therapeutically to treat and prevent cardiovascular problems, including heart disease, high cholesterol, strokes, and high blood pressure. EFAs also have anti-inflammatory effects in the body, and are used in the nutritional treatment of arthritis, **asthma**, allergies, and skin conditions (e.g., **eczema**). EFAs are used as support for immune system disorders including **AIDS**, **multiple sclerosis**, lupus, and cancer.

Other conditions that may improve with EFA supplementation include **acne** and other skin problems, diabetes, depression, menopausal problems, nervous conditions, obesity, memory and learning disabilities, eye problems, and digestive disorders. EFAs are recommended for weight loss programs, as they may assist fat metabolism in the body. EFA supplementation is a recommended preventative practice, as well.

Preparations

Common EFA supplements are flaxseed oil, **evening primrose oil**, **borage oil**, **black currant seed oil**, hemp seed oil, and cod liver oil. Consumers should search for supplements that contain both omega-3 and omega-6 EFAs, because imbalances of EFAs may occur if either is taken in excess over long periods of time. Flaxseed oil is a recommended supplement, because it contains the highest percentage of omega-3 fatty acids with some omega-6

EFAs, as well. Flaxseed oil is generally the least expensive source of omega-3 EFAs as well, generally much cheaper than **fish oil** supplements. Evening primrose oil is a popular supplement as well, because the GLA it contains has shown benefits in treating **premenstrual syndrome** and other conditions. However, evening primrose oil contains no omega-3 EFAs. Hemp seed oil is a well-balanced source of both EFAs.

Supplements are available from health food stores in liquid and capsule form. The recommended daily dosage is one to two tablespoons (13-26 capsules), taken with meals. EFAs can also be obtained from a diet that includes cold-water fish consumed twice per week, whole grains, dark green leafy vegetables, walnuts, pumpkin seeds, **wheat germ**, soy products, canola oil, and other foods mentioned above. Whole flaxseeds are a wholesome source of EFAs as well, and can be freshly ground and added to salads and other dishes. Supplements that contain the enzyme lipase help the body more efficiently digest the oils.

Precautions

EFA supplements are generally fragile products, and must be produced, packaged and handled properly. Consumers should search for quality EFA supplements produced by reputable manufacturers. Products that are organically grown and certified by a third party are recommended. EFA products should be produced by "cold or modified expeller pressing," which means that they were produced without damaging temperatures or pressure. Products should be packaged in light-resistant containers, because sunlight damages EFAs. Packages should include manufacturing and expiration dates, in order to assure freshness. Stores and consumers should keep EFA products under refrigeration, because heat damages them. Taste can indicate the quality of EFA oils: those that have no flavor usually are overly refined, and those that taste bitter are old or spoiled. Because of their low temperature threshold, nearly all oils that are used as EFA supplements are not suitable for use as cooking oils.

In 2001, The U.S. Food and Drug Administration (FDA) began cautioning pregnant and nursing women and parents of infants and toddlers about the potential dangers of exposure to mercury from fish rich in omega-3 fatty acids, and from fish oil capsules. High levels of mercury can affect brain development in fetuses and young children. The FDA recommends that these groups instead opt for younger species of fish such as canned tuna or farm-raised fish and skip fish oil capsules altogether. Vegetarians can supplement their **diets** with foods high in aplah-linoleic acids, including certain oils, flaxseed, and walnuts.

Side effects

Side effects with most EFA supplements are rare, because EFAs are nontoxic and are used by the body as energy when taken in excess. The exception is cod liver and fish oil supplements, which can cause **vitamin A** and D toxicity when taken in excess. Side effects of vitamin A and D toxicity include headaches, skin discoloration, fatigue, **nausea**, and gastrointestinal problems. Fish oil supplements that have vitamins A and D removed are available.

Interactions

To maximize the benefits of EFA supplements, several recommendations can be followed. EFA users should reduce the amount of fat, particularly saturated fat from animal products, in their diet. The American Heart Association recommends that a healthy diet contains 30% or less of its total calories from fat. For 2000 total calories per day, 600 calories or less should be from fat, including EFA supplements. Consumers should also completely eliminate hydrogenated and partially hydrogenated oils from their diets. This includes eliminating all processed foods that contain them, such as margarine and many packaged foods. Other foods that contain trans-fatty acids, such as deep fried foods, should also be eliminated. Recommended cooking oils are olive, safflower, canola, and sesame oils. EFA effectiveness may be increased by lowering the intake of sugar and alcohol in the diet. Nutrients that assist EFA uptake are the B-complex vitamins, **vitamin C**, **zinc**, and **magnesium**. As with any supplement, EFA effectiveness can be augmented with a nutritious, high fiber diet that emphasizes fresh and natural foods, and the intake of fish two times a week.

Resources

BOOKS

Barilla, Jean. *The Nutrition Superbook: The Good Fats and Oils*. New Canaan, CT: Keats, 1996.

Erasmus, Udo. *Fats That Heal, Fats That Kill*. Burnaby, Canada: Alive Books, 1993.

Finnegan, John. *The Facts about Fats*. Berkeley: Celestial Arts, 1993.

Rudin, Dr. Donald O. and Clara Felix. *The Omega-3 Phenomenon*. New York: Rawson, 1987.

Schmidt, Michael. *Smart Fats*. Berkeley: Frog Press, 1997.

PERIODICALS

"Getting Omega–3 Without the Mercury." *Nutrition Today* (July-August 2002): 142.

"Oil–in–One." *Better Nutrition* (September 2002).

ORGANIZATIONS

Northwest Academy of Preventative Medicine. 15615 Bellevue-Redmond Road, Bellevue, WA 98008. (206) 881-9660.

Nutrition Health Review. 171 Madison Avenue, New York, NY 10016.

Nutrition Science News. 1401 Pearl Street, Boulder, CO 80302. (303) 939-8440.

Omega Nutrition. 720 East Washington St., Sequim, WA 98382. (800) 745-8580.

Douglas Dupler
Teresa G. Odle

Essential oils

Description

Essential oils are the fragrant oils that are present in many plants. Hundreds of plants yield essential oils that are used as perfumes, food flavorings, medicines, and as fragrant and antiseptic additives in many common products.

Essential oils have been used for thousands of years. The ancient civilizations of Mesopotamia, more than 5,000 years ago, had machines for obtaining essential oils from plants. Essential oils were the primary source of perfumes for the ancient civilizations of Egypt, India, Greece, and Rome. Essential oils have been found in 3,000-year-old tombs in the Pyramids, and early Greek physicians, including Hippocrates, mentioned aromatic plant essences and oil massages for their healing and mood-enhancing qualities. The Romans associated essential oils and their fine aromas with wealth and success. **Ayurvedic medicine**, the world's oldest healing system, has long recommended essential oil massage as a health treatment for many conditions.

In modern times, essential oils are used in the manufacture of high quality perfumes, as additives in many common products, and in the healing practice of **aromatherapy**. Aromatherapy was begun in the 1920s by a French chemist named Réné-Maurice Gattefosse, who became convinced of the healing powers of essential oils when he used **lavender** oil to effectively heal a severe burn on his body. Gattefosse also discovered that essential oils could be absorbed into the bloodstream when applied to the skin, and had medicinal effects inside the body. Another Frenchman, Dr. Jean Valnet, used essential oils during World War II to treat soldiers, and wrote a major book on the topic in 1964 called *Aromatherapie*. European biochemist, Marguerite Maury, performed thorough studies of how essential oils influence the body and emotions, and popularized essential oil massages as therapy. In the 1990s, aromatherapy was one of the fastest-growing alternative health treatments.

Essential oils are produced using several techniques. Distillation uses water and steam to remove the oils from dried or fresh plants, and the expression method uses machines to squeeze the oil out of plants. Other techniques may use alcohol or solvents to remove essential oils from plant materials.

Essential oils are extremely concentrated. It would take roughly thirty cups of herbal tea to equal the concentration of plant essence in one drop of essential oil. Some essential oils made from rose plants require 4,000 pounds of rose petals to make one pound of essential oil, and are thus very expensive. Lavender is one of the easiest essential oils to produce, because it only takes one hundred pounds of plant material to produce one pound of essential oil. Essential oils are generally very complex chemically, containing many different substances and compounds. Some experts have theorized that essential oils are the lifeblood of a plant, and contain compounds that the plant uses to fight **infections** and drive away germs and parasites. Scientific research has isolated hundreds of chemicals in essential oils, and has shown many essential oils to have anti-bacterial, anti-fungal, and anti-parasitic properties. Some essential oils contain more than 200 identified chemical substances.

Although there are hundreds of essential oils that are used regularly in healing treatments and perfumes, some of the more commonly used essential oils are lavender, **chamomile**, **peppermint**, **tea tree oil**, **eucalyptus**, geranium, jasmine, rose, lemon, orange, **rosemary**, frankincense, and sandalwood.

General use

Essential oils are used in several healing systems, including aromatherapy, Ayurvedic medicine, and **massage therapy**. Essential oils are used for skin and scalp conditions including **acne**, **athlete's foot**, **burns**, cuts, dandruff, **eczema**, insect bites, parasites, **sunburn**, **warts**, and wrinkles. They are recommended for muscle, joint, and circulation problems such as arthritis, high blood pressure, **cellulite**, aches and pains, and **varicose veins**. For respiratory problems and infections, various essential oils are prescribed for **allergies**, **asthma**, **earache**, sinus infections, congestion, and colds and flu. Essential oils are also used to improve digestion, promote hormonal balance, and tone the nervous system in conditions including **anxiety**, **depression**, **sexual dysfunction**, and exhaustion.

Essential oils can be used as quick and effective mood enhancers, for increasing energy and alertness or reducing **stress** and promoting **relaxation**. Essential oils can be used as perfumes and lotions, and can be used as incense to improve the atmosphere in houses and offices.

In 2002, several reports were made on the benefits of tea tree oil in fighting infections. Although still preliminary, these reports will help pave the way to greater acceptance of essential oils in the mainstream medical community. In the case of tea tree oil, one small study showed its effectiveness in fighting orthopedic (bone, joint, and soft tissue) infections. Another recent study showed promising results for tea tree oil gel in topical treatment of recurrent herpes labialis.

Preparations

Essential oils work by entering the body in two ways, through the nose and through the skin. The nose is a powerful sense organ, and the sense of smell is connected directly to the limbic system of the brain, which helps control emotions, memory, and several functions in the body. Research has shown that aromas and the sense of smell influence memory recall, moods, and bodily responses such as heart rate, respiration, hormone levels, and stress reactions. Essential oils with their potent aromas can be used to enhance moods, promote relaxation, and increase energy levels.

Essential oils are also absorbed by the skin, and act medicinally once they are absorbed into the body. For instance, eucalyptus oil, long used in common **cough** and cold remedies, can be rubbed on the chest to break up congestion and mucus inside the lungs. Some essential oils, such as tea tree oil, lavender, and **thyme**, have natural antiseptics in them, and can be applied to cuts, burns, and sores to disinfect and promote healing.

Because essential oils are very strong and concentrated, they should be diluted with *base oils* before rubbing them directly on the body. Base oils are gentle and inexpensive oils, and common ones include almond, jojoba, grapeseed, sunflower, and **sesame oil**. Mineral oil is not recommended as a base oil. Essential oils should be diluted to make up 1–3% of a base oil solution, which is one to three drops of essential oil per teaspoon of base oil. For larger quantities, 20 to 60 drops can be added per 100 milliliters of base oil. Only a few essential oils can be rubbed directly on the skin without dilution. These are lavender, tea tree oil, eucalyptus, and geranium, although people with sensitive skin should use them with care.

Allergic reactions are possible with essential oils. People with sensitive skin or allergies should perform a simple skin test when using essential oils for the first time. To do a skin test, one drop of essential oil can be added to a teaspoon of base oil, and a small amount of this solution can be rubbed on a sensitive spot on the skin, such as the soft side of the arm or behind the ear. If no irritation occurs after 24 hours, then the essential oil is non-allergenic.

Essential oils can be used in a variety of ways. They can be added to massage oils for therapeutic massages. Essential oil solutions can be used on the skin, scalp and hair as lotions, conditioners, and perfumes. A few drops of essential oils can be added to bath water or used in the sauna. Essential oil diffusers, lamps, and candles are available which use heat and steam to spread (diffuse) the aroma of essential oils in rooms. Essential oils can be added to hot-and-cold compresses for injuries and aches. Some essential oils, like tea tree, **fennel**, and peppermint oil, can be combined with a mixture of water and apple cider vinegar and used as mouthwash. For colds and congestion in the lungs or sinuses, essential oils can be inhaled by adding a few drops to a pot of boiling water, and covering the head with a towel over the pot and breathing the vapors.

Consumers should search for essential oils made by reputable manufacturers. Essential oils should be certified to be 100% pure, without chemical additives or synthetic fragrances. The highest quality oils are generally obtained from distillation and cold pressing methods.

Precautions

Essential oils should not be taken internally, by mouth, rectum or vagina, unless under medical supervision. Essential oils should be kept away from the eyes. If an essential oil gets into the eyes, they should be rinsed immediately with cold water. Essential oils should be used with care on broken or damaged skin.

Some essential oils have not been thoroughly tested and may be toxic. The oils to be avoided include **arnica**, bitter almond, calamus, cinnamon, clove, **mugwort**, **sage**, **wintergreen**, and **wormwood**. Pregnant women should avoid these and basil, fennel, marjoram, **myrrh**, oregano, star **anise**, and tarragon. In general, any essen-

tial oils that have not been tested or lack adequate information should be avoided.

Some essential oils may cause the skin to become photosensitive, or more sensitive to sunlight and more likely to become sunburned. Essential oils that are photosensitizing include bergamot, orange, lemon, lime, grapefruit, and **angelica** root. These oils should be avoided before exposure to sunlight and ultraviolet light such as in tanning beds. People with sun-related skin problems should avoid these oils.

Those with health conditions should use care with essential oils. Steam inhalation of essential oils is not recommended for asthma sufferers. The essential oils of rosemary, fennel and sage should be avoided by those with **epilepsy**.

Pregnant and nursing women should use caution with essential oils, because their skin and bodies are more sensitive and some oils may cause adverse reactions. Essential oils should not be used during the first three months of **pregnancy**, and after that they should only be used when heavily diluted with base oils. Women with histories of miscarriage should not use essential oils during pregnancy at all. Pregnant women should perform skin tests before using essential oils. Essential oils are not recommended for nursing mothers.

Essential oils should be used with care on children. They are not recommended for children under one year of age, and should be heavily diluted with base oils when used as a skin massage or lotion for children.

Essential oils should be stored out of the reach of children. Clean glass containers are the best storage vessels, and should be dark in color to keep sunlight from damaging the oil. Some essential oils can damage wood, varnish, plastic, and clothing, and should be handled with care.

Side effects

Most readily available essential oils are safe if used in small doses, and side effects are generally rare. Possible side effects include **rashes**, **itching**, and irritation on the skin. Allergic reactions include watery eyes, **sneezing**, and inflammation. Some essential oils may cause **nausea**, **dizziness**, or gastrointestinal discomfort when used in excess or by those with allergic reactions. Some essential oils, particularly those derived from citrus fruit plants, can cause increased sensitivity to sunlight and increased risk of sunburn.

Interactions

Essential oils are not recommended for those taking homeopathic remedies, as essential oils are believed to interfere with their effectiveness. Essential oils are often blended together to enhance their healing effects, and mixtures can be tailored to individual preferences and conditions. Aromatherapists specialize in creating essential oil blends for individuals and health conditions.

Resources

BOOKS

Cooksley, Virginia Gennari. *Aromatherapy: A Lifetime Guide to Healing with Essential Oils*. Englewood Cliffs, New Jersey: Prentice Hall, 1996.

Lawless, Julia. *The Illustrated Encyclopedia of Essential Oils*. Rockport, Massachusetts: Element, 1995.

Wildwood, Chrissie. *The Encyclopedia of Aromatherapy*. Rochester, Vermont: Healing Arts Press, 1996.

PERIODICALS

Walsh, Nancy."Tea Tree Oil for Infections." *Internal Medicine News* (July 1, 2002):16–21.

The Aromatic Thymes. 75 Lakeview Parkway, Barrington, Illinois 60010.

ORGANIZATIONS

American Alliance of Aromatherapy. P.O. Box 750428, Petaluma, California 94975.

Douglas Dupler
Teresa G. Odle

Essiac tea

Description

Essiac tea is based on a Canadian Ojibwa Indian formula containing primarily **burdock root** (*Arctium lappa*), Turkish **rhubarb root** (*Rheum palmatum*), **sheep sorrel** (*Rumex acetosella*), and the inner bark of the **slippery elm** (*Ulmus fulva* or *Ulmus rubra*). It is used in alternative medicine mainly as a treatment for **cancer**.

The formula is said to have been first developed by an Ojibwa healer to purify the body and balance the spir-

it. In 1922, the formula came to the attention of Rene Caisse (essiac is Caisse spelled backwards), a nurse in Ontario, Canada, after hearing first-hand accounts of it curing cancer. She began administering the tea to cancer patients and found it to have remarkable healing abilities. She continued treating cancer patients with the tea until she died in 1978. In 1977, Caisse sold the essiac tea formula to the Resperin Corp. of Ontario, Canada.

Caisse reported that hundreds of her patients had been cured of their cancers through the use of her tea, sometimes used as intramuscular injections. Most of the patients came to her after conventional cancer treatments (surgery, chemotherapy, and radiation therapy) failed. Several alternative health care practitioners report essiac tea seems to work best in patients who have had the least amount of radiation therapy or chemotherapy.

The mainstream medical community does not embrace essiac tea. Critics contend that a certain number of cancers deemed incurable spontaneously go into remission without an adequate medical explanation as to why. Others chalk up the successes to the so-called **placebo effect**, where the belief that the treatment is working effects a cure rather than the treatment itself. The treatment is not approved by the American Medical Association or the American Cancer Society.

In 1938, a bill in the Canadian Parliament to legalize essiac tea failed by three votes. It is still not approved for marketing in the United States or Canada. However, the Canadian Health and Welfare Department permits compassionate use of essiac tea on an emergency basis.

In 1975 and again in 1982, the Memorial Sloan-Kettering Cancer Center in New York tested only the sorrel component in the tea. They boiled it which may have neutralized any beneficial compounds in the leftover tea and administered it to mice with cancerous tumors. It determined the formula had no anticancer effects. The National Cancer Institute and Canadian Bureau of Prescription Drugs reached the same conclusion in the 1980s.

General use

Essiac tea is generally used by alternative health care practitioners to treat, and even cure, various forms of cancer and the side effects of conventional cancer therapy. It is also used to treat **AIDS**. It is used to a lesser extent to treat a variety of other medical conditions, including diabetes, skin inflammation, liver and thyroid problems, **diarrhea**, ulcers, and some other degenerative diseases. It is more commonly used in Canada than the United States. Other uses include treating **pain**, purifying the blood, healing **wounds**, lowering **cholesterol**, and increasing energy levels.

Although each of the four main ingredients in essiac tea are used to treat other conditions, only the sorrel is used separately to treat cancer. Only when the four are combined do they effect anti-cancer properties. It is not clear exactly how or why the ingredients work in combination, but it is generally believed they work synergistically to stimulate production of antibodies. Caisse herself said she believed essiac tea purified the blood and carried away damaged tissue and infection related to the cancer. She also believed the tea strengthened the immune system, allowing healthy cells to destroy cancerous cells.

Caisse also maintained that tumors not destroyed by essiac tea would be shrunk and could be surgically removed after six to eight weeks of treatment. To insure any malignant cells that remained after treatment and surgery were destroyed, Caisse recommended at least three months of additional weekly essiac treatments.

One of Caisse's patients was her mother, Friseide Caisse, who was diagnosed with liver cancer at the age of 72. Her mother's physician reportedly said she had only days to live. Rene Caisse began giving her mother daily intramuscular injections of the tea. Friseide began recovering within a few days and after a few months, with less frequent doses of essiac, her cancer was gone. She lived to be 90, finally succumbing to **heart disease**.

Preparations

The four main ingredients of Essiac tea are sold separately and can be combined at home. Essiac tea is also marketed as tea bags and in bottles of the prepared formula. The basic formula for essiac tea is to combine 6.5 c of cut burdock root, 16 oz of powdered sheep sorrel (including stems, seeds, and leaves), 1 oz of powdered Turkish rhubarb root, and 4 oz of powdered slippery elm bark. Mix the ingredients thoroughly. Boil 2 gal of fresh spring water, add 8 oz of the essiac blend, cover, and boil on high heat for 10 minutes. Turn heat off and let sit for six hours. Remove cover and stir. Replace cover and let steep another six hours. Turn on heat and return the mixture to a boil. Remove from heat and strain into another pot. Wash original pot and strain mixture again into it. Then pour liquid into amber bottles, cap, and store in a dark cool location. Refrigerate after opening.

The formula is ready to use immediately. When ready, shake the bottle well to mix the sediments. Blend 4 tsp of the essiac formula with 4 tsp of warm spring water. The usual daily dosage is 2–4 oz of tea for persons weighing 100–150 lb and 2 oz for every 50 lb over 150 lb. Some alternative health practitioners recommend regular doses of essiac to strengthen the immune system and as a preventative for certain diseases, including cancer. The frequency ranges from daily to weekly.

KEY TERMS

Chemotherapy—The use of chemical agents to treat or control diseases, especially cancer.

Cholesterol—A steroid alcohol found in human cells and body fluids, implicated in the onset of heart disease.

Degenerative diseases—A group of diseases characterized by progressive degenerative changes in tissue, including arteriosclerosis, diabetes mellitus, and osteoarthritis.

Diabetes—Any of a variety of abnormal conditions characterized by excessive amounts of urine.

Diabetes mellitus—A degenerative disease characterized by inadequate production or absorption of insulin, excessive urine production, and excessive amounts of sugar in the blood and urine.

Precautions

Essiac tea is not recommended for pregnant or lactating women. The formula should not be prepared or stored in plastic or aluminum containers. Sunlight and freezing temperatures destroys the formula's effectiveness. It is generally recommended that persons consult with their physician before treating any condition with essiac. It is important to remember that essiac is often used in combination with traditional cancer treatments, such as chemotherapy, radiation, and surgery.

Side effects

No major adverse side effect have been associated with essiac tea.

Interactions

Essiac is not known to adversely interact with other medications or nutritional supplements.

Resources

BOOKS

Glum, Gary L. *Calling of an Angel.* Los Angeles: Silent Walker Publishing, 1988.

Olsen, Cynthia and Dr. Jim Chan. *Essiac: A Native Herbal Cancer Remedy.* Pagosa Springs, CO: Kali Press, 1998.

Snow, Sheila and Mali Klein. *Essiac Essentials.* Dublin: Gill & Macmillan, 1999.

Walters, Richard. *Options: The Alternative Cancer Therapy Book.* New York: Avery Publishing Group, 1992.

PERIODICALS

McCutcheon, Lynn. "Essiac: The Not-so-Remarkable Cancer Remedy." *Skeptical Inquirer.* (July/Aug. 1998): 43-46.

Steinberg, Phillip N. "Cat's Claw, Essiac, and Whole-leaf Aloe Vera: Mother Nature's Healers." *Let's Live.* (Sept. 1996): 70-72.

Tyler, Varro E. "Essiac: A Native Herbal Cancer Remedy." *Nutrition Forum.* (May/June 1998): 24.

Ken R. Wells

Eucalyptus

Description

The eucalyptus tree is a large, fast-growing evergreen that is native to Australia and Tasmania. The tree can grow to 375-480 feet (125-160 meters). Eucalyptus belongs to the myrtle (Myrtaceae) family. There are more than 300 species of eucalyptus, and *Eucalyptus globulus* is the most well-known species. One species (*E. amygdalin*) is the tallest tree known in the world. The tree grows best in areas with an average temperature of 60°F (15°C).

Eucalyptus trees constitute over 75% of the tree population of Australia. The eucalyptus tree is also known in Australia as the blue gum tree or malee. Other names for eucalyptus include Australian **fever** tree and stringy bark tree. The name is actually derived from the Greek word "eucalyptos," which means "well covered," and refers to the cuplike membrane that covers the budding flowers of the tree.

The bluish green leaves carry the medicinal properties of the tree and grow to a length of 6-12 inches (15-30 cm). While the leathery leaves are the sole food for koala bears, the leaves also contain a fragrant volatile oil that has antiseptic, expectorant, antibacterial, anti-inflammatory, deodorant, diuretic, and antispasmodic properties. Other constituents of the leaves include tannins, phenolic acids, flavonoids (eucalyptin, hyperin, hyperoside, quercitin, quercitrin, rutin), sesquiterpenes, aldehydes, and ketones.

Eucalyptus oil is obtained through a steam distillation process that removes the oil from the fresh, mature leaves and branch tips of older trees. Approximately 25 species of eucalyptus trees in Australia are grown for their oil.

There are three grades of eucalyptus oil: medicinal, which contains the compound eucalyptol (also called cineol); industrial, in which a component of the oil is used in mining operations; and aromatic, which is used in perfumes and fragrant soap products. These oils vary greatly in character. When choosing an oil for therapeutic use, it is important to know from what species the oil was derived. Species used medicinally include *E. globulus*, which contains up to 70% eucalyptol; *E. polybractea*, which contains 85% eucalyptol; and *E. Smithii. Eucalyptus amygdalina* and *E. dives* contain little eucalyptol and are used to separate metallic sulfides from ores in the mining industry. *Eucalyptus citriodora* contains a lemon-scented oil and is an ingredient in perfumes, as is *E. odorata* and *E. Sturtiana*. Two species, *E. dives* and *E. radiata*, have oils with a strong **peppermint** odor.

The most common species grown for its medicinal oil is *Eucalyptus globulus*. The eucalyptol found in this species is a chief ingredient in many over-the-counter cold and **cough** remedies, such as cough lozenges, chest rubs, and decongestants. It acts to stimulate blood flow and protects against infection and germs. The *British Pharmocopoeia* requires that commercial eucalyptus oils contain 55% eucalyptol by volume.

Origins

The Australian aborigines have used eucalyptus for hundreds of years as a remedy for fever, **wounds**, coughs, **asthma**, and joint **pain**. Australian settlers named the eucalyptus the fever tree because of its disease-fighting properties. Baron Ferdinand von Miller, a German botanist and explorer, was responsible for making the properties of eucalyptus known to the world in the mid-1800s. Likening eucalyptus' scent to that of cajaput oil (a disinfectant), von Miller suggested that eucalyptus might also be used as a disinfectant in fever districts. Seeds of the tree were sent to Algiers, France and planted. The trees thrived and, because of the drying action of the roots, turned one of the marshiest areas of Algiers into a dry and healthy environment, thereby driving away malaria-carrying mosquitoes. Eucalyptus trees were then planted in temperate areas around the world to prevent **malaria**. As a result, eucalyptus trees are now cultivated in China, India, Portugal, Spain, Egypt, South and North Africa, Algeria, South America, and in the southern portion of the United States.

Commercial production of eucalyptus began in Victoria, Australia in 1860. The nineteenth century eclectic doctors adopted eucalyptus as a treatment for fevers, **laryngitis**, asthma, chronic **bronchitis**, **whooping cough**, **gonorrhea**, ulcers, gangrenous tissue, **edema**, and gastrointestinal disturbances. European doctors used eucalyptus oil to sterilize their surgical and medical equipment. Eucalyptus leaves were often made into cigars or cigarettes and smoked to relieve asthma and bronchial congestion.

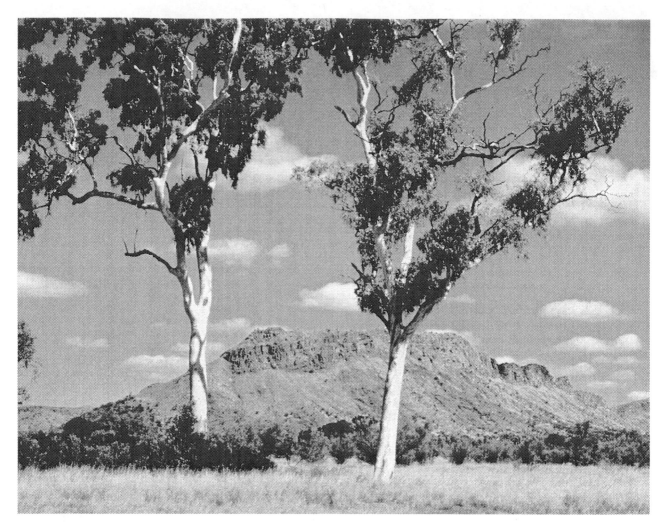

Eucalyptus trees in Australia. *(JLM Visuals. Reproduced by permission.)*

Modern medicines around the world have included eucalyptus in their practices. Indian ayurvedics use eucalyptus to treat headaches resulting from colds. Eucalyptus is listed in the *Indian Pharmacopoeia* as an expectorant and in the *Chinese Pharmacopoeia* as a skin irritant used in nerve pain. In France, eucalyptus leaves are applied topically to relieve congestion from colds and to treat acute bronchial disease. A standardized eucalyptus tea is licensed in Germany to treat bronchitis and throat inflammations. Eucalyptus is also an ingredient in German herbal cough preparations. The German Commission E has approved the internal use of eucalyptus to treat congestion of the respiratory tract, and the external use to treat rheumatic complaints. In the United States, eucalyptus is a component of many decongestant and expectorating cough and cold remedies, such as cough drops, cough syrups, and vapor baths. Eucalyptus is often used in veterinary medicine. It is used to treat horses with flu, dogs with distemper, and to treat parasitic skin conditions.

General use

Eucalyptus is most popular for its ability to clear congestion due to colds, coughs, flu, asthma, and sinusitis. The tannins found in eucalyptus have astringent properties that reduce mucous membrane inflammation of the upper respiratory tract. Eucalyptol, the chemical component of the oil, works to loosen phlegm. Cough drops containing eucalyptus promote saliva production, which increases swallowing and lessens the coughing impulse. Earaches can also be treated with eucalyptus. When inhaled, the eucalyptus fumes open the eustachian tubes, draining fluids and relieving pressure. Eucalyptus enhances breathing, which makes it an effective remedy for asthma, bronchitis, sinusitis, whooping cough, and colds.

Eucalyptus is a component of many topical arthritis creams and analgesic ointments. When applied to the skin, eucalyptus stimulates blood flow and creates a warm feeling to the area, relieving pain in muscles and joints.

The oil extracted from the eucalyptus leaf has powerful antiseptic, deodorizing, and antibacterial properties. It is especially effective in killing several strains of *Staphylococcus* bacteria. A mixture of 2% eucalyptus oil evaporated in an aroma lamp has been shown to destroy 70% of the *Staphylococcus* bacteria in the affected room. When the oil is applied to cuts, scrapes, and other minor wounds, it inhibits **infections** and viruses. A 2002 report out of Australia made researchers around the world take note when two cases of patients with staph infections resistant to traditional antibiotic therapy responded to a mixture of eucalyptus leaf oil abstract. The Australian researchers recommended formal clinical trials to test the therapy, based on an ancient aboriginal remedy. Eucalyptus also fights plaque-forming bacteria and is used to treat **gum disease** and gingivitis.

In large doses, the oil can be a kidney irritant and can induce excretion of bodily fluids and waste products. Eucalyptus oil added to water may be gargled to relieve **sore throat** pain or used as a mouthwash to heal mouth sores or gum disorders. Consequently, eucalyptus is an ingredient in many commercial mouthwashes.

Eucalyptus' pain-relieving properties make it a good remedy for muscle tension. One study showed that a mixture of eucalyptus, peppermint, and ethanol oils successfully relieved headache-related muscle tension.

Eucalyptus may lower blood sugar levels. Placing a drop of the oil on the tongue may reduce **nausea**. The oil has also been used to kill dust mites and fleas.

Eucalyptus oil is one of the most well-known fragrances in **aromatherapy**. Two species of eucalyptus are used in aromatherapy oils: *E. globulus* and *E. citriodora*. The essential oil of eucalyptus is used to relieve cramps, cleanse the blood, heal wounds, disinfect the air, and to treat conditions such as asthma, bronchitis, throat and sinus infections, fevers, **kidney infections**, rheumatism, bladder infections, and sore muscles.

The essential oil can be diluted and added to a massage oil to ease aching muscles. The oil can be added to hot water and inhaled to reduce nasal congestion. It can also be diffused in the room of a sick patient to disinfect the air.

Some believe that inhaling the diffused oil can enhance concentration and thought processes. Studies have shown that inhalation of the cineole compound of eucalyptus stimulates coordination and motor activities in mice. Eucalyptus oil may also uplift the spirit during times of emotional overload or general sluggishness.

Applying a diluted oil to the skin instead of inhaling it increases the rate of absorption into the blood. Often the speed with which it is absorbed is so fast, the odor can be detected on the breath within minutes.

The oil is also an effective febrifuge, and a cold compress with eucalyptus oil added to it has a cooling effect that is useful in helping to reduce a fever. The essential oil of eucalyptus is also used to treat wounds, herpes simplex virus, skin ulcers, and **acne**. Combined with water, the oil makes an effective insect repellant. Because of its skin-moistening properties, the oil is often an ingredient in **dandruff** shampoo.

Eucalyptus oil may be combined with other oils that have similar properties, such as niaouli, pine, Swiss pine, **hyssop**, and **thyme** oils. It also mixes well with lemon, verbena, balm, and **lavender** oils.

Preparations

Eucalyptus is available as a tincture, cream, ointment, essential oil, or lozenge. Many health food stores carry fresh or dried eucalyptus leaf in bulk. Eucalyptus can be ingested through the use of teas or tincture preparations, inhaled, or applied externally.

Eucalyptus infusion is ingested to treat coughs, colds, bronchitis, congestion, and throat infections. To create an infusion, 1 cup of boiling water is poured over 1-2 teaspoons of crushed eucalyptus leaves. The mixture is covered and steeped for 10 minutes and is then strained. Up to 2 cups can be drunk daily.

Inhaling eucalyptus vapors is beneficial for sinus and bronchial congestion that occurs with bronchitis, whooping cough, colds, asthma, **influenza**, and other respiratory illnesses. A drop of eucalyptus oil or two to three fresh or dried leaves are added to a pan of boiling water or to a commercial vaporizer. The pan is removed from the heat, a towel is placed over the pan and the patient's head, and the patient inhales the rising steam. Patients should close their eyes when inhaling the steam to protect them from eucalyptus' strong fumes.

For healing wounds and preventing infection, the wound is washed and then diluted eucalyptus oil or crushed eucalyptus leaves are applied to the affected area.

For relief of muscle aches or arthritis pain, several drops of the diluted oil are rubbed onto the affected area, or a few drops of diluted oil are added to bath water for a healing bath. Adding eucalyptus leaves wrapped in a cloth to running bath water is also effective.

For gum disease, a few drops of diluted oil are placed on a fingertip and massaged into the gums.

Tinctures should contain 5-10% essential oil of eucalyptus. A person can take 1 ml three times daily.

Ointments should contain 5-20% essential oil of eucalyptus. The person should use as directed for chapped hands, joint and muscle pains, and dandruff.

Precautions

Children or infants should not be treated with eucalyptus. Of special note, eucalyptus oil should not be applied to the facial areas (especially the nose or eyes) of small children or infants. Pregnant or breast-feeding women should not use eucalyptus.

People with digestive problems, stomach or intestinal inflammations, biliary duct disorders, or liver disease should not take eucalyptus.

Undiluted eucalyptus oil should never be ingested. Small amounts of undiluted oil (even in amounts as little as one teaspoon) are toxic and may cause circulatory problems, collapse, suffocation, or death. Eucalyptus oil should always be diluted in a carrier oil such as almond, grapeseed, or other vegetable oil before applying to the skin.

Side effects

Nausea, **vomiting**, or **diarrhea** may occur in rare cases. Applying eucalyptus to the skin may cause a rash in those who are sensitive or allergic to eucalyptus.

Interactions

Eucalyptus works to detoxify the body. If it is used simultaneously with other drugs, the effects of those drugs may be weakened.

Resources

BOOKS

Fischer-Rizzi, Susanne. *Medicine of the Earth*. Rudra Press, 1996.

Prevention. *The Complete Book of Natural and Medicinal Cures*. Rodale Press, Inc., 1994.

PERIODICALS

"One Answer to MRSA May be Growing on Trees: Eucalyptus Leaves Show Power over Pathogen." *Hospital Infection Control* 29, no. 1 (January 2002):11.

Jennifer Wurges
Teresa G. Odle

Eucommia bark

Description

Eucommmia bark is the gray, grooved bark of the tree *Eucommia ulmoides*, commonly called the hardy rubber tree or the gutta-percha tree. The Chinese name for eucommia bark is *Du Zhong*. This name refers to a Taoist monk who was said to be immortal, suggesting that the herb provides long life, good health, and vitality. The tree is a member of the rubber family and is native to the mountainous regions of China. It normally grows to about 50 ft (15 m) in height. Small patches of bark are harvested from trees over 10 years old in late summer and early autumn. The outer bark is peeled away and the smooth inner bark is dried. This inner bark contains a pure white, elastic latex that is thought to contain the compounds that account for eucommia bark's healing properties. Older, thicker inner bark with more latex is considered more desirable for the herbalist to use than younger, thinner bark.

Although traditionally only the bark of *E. ulmoides* was used for healing, research in the later half of the 1990s in Japan indicates that the leaves also have healing properties. The green leaves are shiny, narrow, and pointed. The tree's flowers are very small and are not used in healing.

General use

Eucommia bark has been used in **traditional Chinese herbalism** for over 3,000 years. Since the tree does not grow widely outside China, this herb was not used in other cultures until recently.

Eucommia bark is strongly associated with the kidneys and to a lesser extent with the liver. In Chinese medicine, the kidneys store *jing*. *Jing* is an essential life source and associated with whole body growth and development, as well as normal sexual and reproductive functioning. The kidney and liver *jing* also affects the bones, ligaments, and tendons.

In the Chinese system of health, *yin* aspects must be kept in balance with *yang* aspects. Ill health occurs when the energies and elements of the body are out of balance or in disharmony. Health is restored by taking herbs and treatments that restore that balance.

Eucommia bark is the primary herb used to increase *yang* functions in the body. However, it also supports *yin* functions. Eucommia bark helps to build strong bones and a flexible skeleton with strong ligaments and tendons. It is a primary herb used to heal tissues that are slow to mend after an injury or that have weakened through **stress** or age. It is given to treat lower back and leg **pain**, stiffness, arthritis, and knee problems including continual dislocation. Eucommia bark is also believed to have diuretic properties that aid in reducing swelling. Although it can be used alone, eucommia bark is most often used in conjunction with other herbs that support its functions.

In addition to healing tissues, eucommia bark has two other major functions. In pregnant women it is given to calm the fetus, soothe the uterus, and prevent miscarriage. Eucommia bark also has the ability to reduce blood pressure. This property has been investigated since 1974, and may be related to its mild diuretic action. Eucommia bark is used in almost all Chinese formulas to lower blood pressure.

Other modern uses of eucommia bark include treatment of **impotence**, premature ejaculation, and as a mild anti-inflammatory. It is included in tonics that boost the immune system and generally improve wellness. However, there is little rigorous scientific research to support these uses.

In the late 1990s Japanese researchers became interested in eucommia bark. In 2000, researchers at Nihon University in Chiba, Japan, published two studies showing that both the leaves and the bark of *Eucommia ulmoides* contained a compound that encourages the development of collagen in rats. Collagen is an important part of connective tissues such as tendons and ligaments. However, they found that the compound was present in much greater quantities in fresh leaves and fresh bark, and that much of it was destroyed during the drying process.

In modern Japan, eucommia leaves are also believed to help with weight loss by reducing the urge to eat. For this reason, in the late 1990s eucommia leaves became an increasingly popular herb there. However, there are no scientific studies to support this function of the herb.

Preparations

Eucommia bark is harvested and dried. Before boiling, it is sliced to expose the inside of the bark. The bark is then boiled to make a decoction. Generally this decoction is combined with other herbs and extracts to create *yang* enhancing tonics to treat kidney and liver deficiencies and impotence.

Precautions

Eucommia bark has a long history of use with no substantial reported problems.

Side effects

No side effects have been reported with the use of eucommia bark.

KEY TERMS

Collagen—Collagen is a white, fibrous protein that is found in skin, bones, ligaments, tendons, cartilage, and all other connective tissue.

Decoction—Decoctions are made by boiling an herb, then straining the solid material out.

Diuretic—A diuretic is any substance that increases the production of urine.

Yang aspects—Yang aspects are qualities such as warmth, light, and activity.

Yin aspects—Yin aspects are the opposite of yang aspects and are represented by qualities such as cold, stillness, darkness and passiveness.

Interactions

Eucommia bark is often used in conjunction with other herbs with no reported interactions. Since eucommia bark has been used almost exclusively in Chinese medicine, there are no studies of its interactions with Western pharmaceuticals. People who are taking tonics containing eucommia bark should tell their doctors before taking traditional drugs, especially drugs that regulate blood pressure.

Resources

BOOKS

Molony, David. *Complete Guide to Chinese Herbal Medicine.* New York: Berkeley Books, 1998.

Teegaurden, Ron. *The Ancient Wisdom of the Chinese Tonic Herbs.* New York: Warner Books, 1998.

ORGANIZATIONS

American Association of Oriental Medicine (AAOM) 433 Front Street, Catasauqua, PA 18032. (610) 266-2433

Tish Davidson

Euphrasea officinalis see **Eyebright**

Evening primrose oil

Description

Evening primrose (*Oenothera biennis*) is a tall, hardy, native biennial of the Onagraceae family. Its Latin name is derived from the Greek word *oinos* for wine and *thera* for hunt and reflects the folk belief that the herb

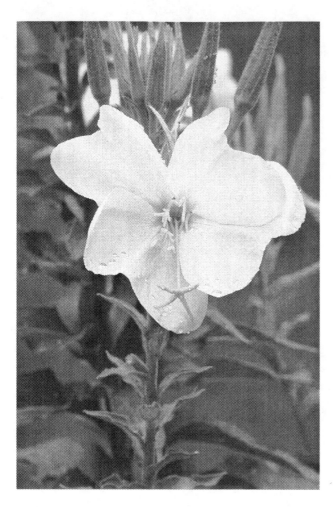

Evening primrose flower. *(Photo Researchers, Inc. Reproduced by permission.)*

fatty acids including gamma **linoleic acid** (GLA). GLA is often deficient in the Western diet and is needed to encourage the production of prostraglandins. Low levels of essential fatty acids may increase the symptoms of **premenstrual syndrome** (PMS), diabetes, etc. Evening primrose oil has been used to treat PMS and menopausal symptoms, **asthma**, and has been shown to reduce high blood **cholesterol** levels.

Research conducted in Great Britain has indicated that evening primrose oil can also be medicinally useful in the treatment of nerve disorders, such as **multiple sclerosis** and **rheumatoid arthritis**. The essential oil does appear to be of some benefit in cases of alcohol poisoning and in alleviating hangovers, and to ease symptoms of alcohol withdrawal. The oil can also help relieve dry eyes, brittle nails, and **acne** when combined with **zinc**. When taken as a supplement, evening primrose has helped to promote weight loss.

Traditionally, Native Americans valued evening primrose as a treatment for **bruises** and cuts. The Flambeau Ojibwe tribe soaked the whole plant in warm water to make a poultice for healing bruises and to overcome skin problems. The mucilaginous juice in the stem and leaf can be applied externally to soothe skin irritations, or may be eaten to relieve digestive discomfort and for its stimulating effect on the liver and spleen. The astringent properties of the plant are helpful to soothe inflamed tissue. The plant has sedative properties and has been used to decrease hyperactivity in children.

The entire plant is edible. The root from the first-year growth is a nutritious pot herb. Boiled roots taste somewhat like parsnips.

Evening primrose oil is valued for its antioxidant properties. **Antioxidants** are substances that counteract the damaging effects of oxidation in living tissue. A team of Canadian researchers has recently identified the specific antioxidant compounds in evening primrose oil; one of them, a yellow substance known as catechin, appears to inhibit the growth of cancerous tumors and to lower the risk of **heart disease**.

could minimize the ill effect of over-indulgence in wine following a hunt.

The plant thrives in dry, sunny meadows, and is abundant in many parts of the world. The leaves of the first-year plant form a bright-green, basal rosette. In the second year, the coarse, erect stalk reaches up to 4 ft (1.2 m) with hairy, alternate, lanceolate leaves with a distinctive mid rib. Leaves grow from 3–6 in (7.6–15.2 cm) long. The blossoms are pale yellow with a slight lemon scent and a cup-like shape. They grow in clusters along the flower stalk, and bloom from June to September, opening at dusk to attract pollinating insects and night-flying moths. These phosphorescent blossoms inspired a common name for the herb: evening star. The seeds grow within an oblong, hairy capsule. The root is large and fleshy.

General use

The medicinal components of evening primrose are found in the seed-extracted oil, which contains **essential**

Preparations

Evening primrose oil is prepared commercially and widely available in health food stores. The extract should be stored in a cool, dry place in order to avoid spoilage. Capsules are also available. Correct dosage should be decided in consultation with a practitioner.

An ointment can be prepared by mixing one part of the diced plant with four parts of heated petroleum jelly. Stored in a tightly closed container and refrigerated, the

Antioxidant—Any of several substances that have been shown to counteract the damaging effects of oxidation in human and animal tissue. Evening primrose oil is rich in antioxidants.

Biennial—A plant that requires two years to complete the cycle from seed to maturity and death.

Catechin—A yellow, slightly bitter antioxidant found in evening primrose oil. Catechin appears to slow tumor growth and to protect against heart disease.

Mucilage—A gelatin-like plant substance found in leaves and stems. Any substance that resembles mucilage in having a thick or sticky texture is said to be mucilaginous.

preparation will maintain its effectiveness. Apply as needed to soothe the skin.

Precautions

Use by persons with **epilepsy** is discouraged because evening primrose oil appears to lower the effectiveness of medications used to treat epilepsy. Physicians should be consulted before using evening primrose oil on children.

Side effects

There have been some reports of **headache, nausea**, loose stools, and skin rash after using evening primrose preparations.

Resources

BOOKS

Lust, John. *The Herb Book*. New York: Batam Books, 1974.

Mabey, Richard. *The New Age Herbalist*. New York: Simon & Schuster, 1988.

McVicar, Jekka. *Herbs for the Home*. New York: Viking Studio Books, 1995.

Phillips, Roger and Nicky Foy. *The Random House Book of Herbs*. New York: Random House, 1990.

PERIODICALS

Wettasinghe, M., F. Shahidi, and R. Amarowicz. "Identification and Quantification of Low Molecular Weight Phenolic Antioxidants in Seeds of Evening Primrose (*Oenothera biennis L.*)." *Journal of Agricultural and Food Chemistry* 50 (February 27, 2002): 1267-1271.

Clare Hanrahan
Rebecca J. Frey, PhD

Evodia fruit

Description

Evodia fruit is the small, reddish fruit of the plant *Evodia rutaecarpa*. This plant is native to northern China and Korea, although it is cultivated as an ornamental landscaping plant in many other places in the world.

E. rutaecarpa is a deciduous tree that grows to a height of about 30 ft (10 m) along the sunny edges of woodlands and in suburban settings as an ornamental. It has long, dark green, shiny leaves and blooms with many small clusters of white flowers in the summer. The fruit, which is the part of the plant used in healing, is reddish when it appears in August and darkens to black by November. The fruit is harvested for medicinal purposes when it is not yet ripe and reddish brown in color. It is then either used fresh or dried. Evodia fruit is also known by its Chinese name *wu zhu yu* and is called *gosyuyu* in Japan.

General use

Evodia fruit has been used since at least the first century A.D. in **traditional Chinese medicine** (TCM). It is characterized as having a warm nature and an acrid, bitter, slightly toxic taste, although the fruit is quite fragrant.

Taken internally, evodia fruit is used to treat symptoms of abdominal distress. These include **nausea, vomiting**, and **diarrhea**. It is said to be especially effective in treating morning diarrhea. Evodia is used to stimulate the appetite and to treat abdominal symptoms associated with lack of interest in food.

Evodia is also used as a painkiller. It is a remedy for headaches, especially headaches associated with nausea and vomiting. Traditional Chinese herbalists also use it to treat **pain** in the upper abdomen and pain associated with abdominal hernias. According to Chinese herbalism, the warm nature of the evodia fruit counteracts cold conditions in the stomach.

There are several other reported uses of evodia fruit. The root bark taken internally is considered useful for expelling parasitic tapeworms and pinworms. The fruit is also believed to have contraceptive properties. Various healers report that the fruit also has anti-inflammatory, anti-tumor, anti-viral, astringent, and diuretic properties. Although evodia fruit has been used for thousands of years in China, its use has recently increased in Japan.

Scientists, primarily from Japan and China, have undertaken laboratory studies of evodia fruit to determine which traditional uses are supported by modern medical findings. Chinese researchers in Taiwan have consistently reported that extracts of evodia fruit interfere with blood clotting. In the future, this finding could be of significance in treating **stroke**.

Japanese researchers have discovered that in test tube studies extracts of evodia fruit strongly inhibit the growth of one specific bacteria (*Helicobacter pylori*, a bacteria usually treated in mainstream medicine with antibiotics). Unlike conventional antibiotics, the extract did not alter the growth patterns of any other intestinal bacteria. This finding supports the traditional use of evodia fruit in digestive disorders.

Other Japanese researchers have found that compounds extracted from dried evodia fruit have anti-inflammatory and pain reducing properties in dogs. Reduction of pain is believed to occur because the compounds interfere with pain receptors.

Preparations

Evodia fruit can be used fresh, or it can be dried and ground into a powder for medicinal use. Powdered evodia fruit is sometimes mixed with vinegar to make a paste that is applied externally to the navel to relieve **indigestion**. A similar paste is applied to the soles of the feet to treat high blood pressure or directly to sores in the mouth. Powdered evodia fruit is also taken internally.

Evodia fruit is often mixed with other herbs, such as **ginger**, **pinellia** root, or **coptis**, in formulas to control vomiting. In addition, evodia fruit is used in the TCM formulas ilex and evodia to treat symptoms of cold and flu, including **fever**, **chills**, swollen glands, and sort throat.

Precautions

Evodia fruit is considered by herbalists to be slightly toxic. They recommend that people not take this herb without supervision to prevent overdose and side effects associated with long-term use. Pregnant women should not use evodia fruit. Women who desire to conceive a child should keep in mind that evodia fruit is thought to have anti-fertility properties.

Side effects

Herbalists consider evodia fruit mildly toxic.

Interactions

Evodia fruit is often used in conjunction with other herbs with no reported interactions. Since evodia fruit has been used almost exclusively in Chinese medicine, there are no studies of its interactions with Western pharmaceuticals.

KEY TERMS

. . . .

Deciduous—A tree or bush that sheds its leaves seasonally.

Diuretic—A diuretic is any substance that increases the production of urine.

Yin—Yin aspects are the opposite of yang aspects and are represented by qualities such as cold, stillness, darkness, and passiveness.

Resources

BOOKS

Chevallier, Andrew. *Encyclopedia of Medicinal Plants.* London: Dorling Kindersley Publishers, 1996.

Molony, David. *Complete Guide to Chinese Herbal Medicine.* New York: Berkeley Books, 1998.

ORGANIZATIONS

American Association of Oriental Medicine (AAOM). 433 Front Street, Catasauqua, PA 18032. (610) 266-2433

OTHER

"Plants for the Future: *Evodia rutaecarpa*." http://www.metalab.unc.edu (January 17, 2001).

Tish Davidson

Exercise

Definition

Exercise is any activity requiring physical exertion done for the sake of health. Activities range from walking and **yoga** to lifting weights and **martial arts**.

Origins

Regular exercise as a way of promoting health can be traced back at least 5,000 years to India, where yoga originated. In China, exercises involving martial arts, such as **t'ai chi**, **qigong**, and kung fu, developed possibly 2,500 years ago. The ancient Greeks also had exercise programs 2,500 years ago, which led to the first Olympic games in 776 B.C. Other exercise routines have been in use throughout Asia for hundreds of years.

Only within the last 100 years have the scientific and medical communities documented the benefits that even light but regular exercise has on physical and mental health.

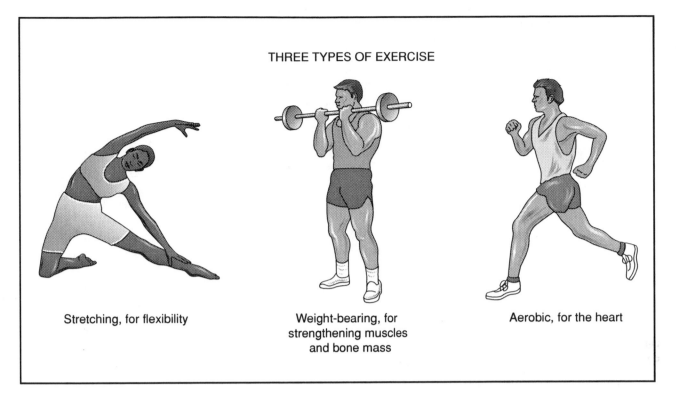

THREE TYPES OF EXERCISE

Stretching, for flexibility

Weight-bearing, for
strengthening muscles
and bone mass

Aerobic, for the heart

Exercise is utilized to improve health, maintain fitness, and is important as a means of physical rehabilitation. *(Illustration by Electronic Illustrators Group. The Gale Group.)*

The earliest forms of exercise stressed activities that involved stretching and light muscle resistance. Next came martial arts that promoted self-defense. In nearly all forms of Asian exercise routines, some type of **meditation** was a major component because the ancients believed physical and mental health went together. The ancient Greek and Roman civilizations advocated vigorous physical activity since exercise was associated with military training. The Greeks also believed that a healthy body would promote a healthy mind.

"Physical culture" was popular in the nineteenth and early twentieth centuries. Medical journals showed exercise machines in the 1800s in Europe and North America. Although weight training became popular with a small number of people in the 1940s, it was not until the 1960s that regular exercise programs began to flourish throughout the United States. Gymnasiums, once used mainly by male weight lifters and boxers as training facilities, now are common throughout the United States. Today's gyms and health clubs offer a wide range of exercise activities for men and women that can fit every lifestyle, age group, and exertion level.

Benefits

The medical community recognizes that regular exercise, along with a proper diet, is one of the two most

important factors in maintaining good physical and mental health, and in preventing and managing many diseases. Most certified physical trainers advocate at least 20 minutes of exercise at least three times a week. But for people who have a sedentary lifestyle, even walking for 10 minutes a day has health benefits. One study of 13,000 people followed for more than eight years showed that people who walk 30 minutes a day have a significantly reduced risk of premature death than people who did not exercise regularly.

Walking and other cardiovascular exercises can reduce the risk of **heart disease**, some cancers, **hypertension** (high blood pressure), arthritis, **osteoporosis**, **stroke**, and **depression**. A study by the Centers for Disease Control and Prevention (CDC) reported in 2001 that running just once a month could help keep bones strong. In addition to physical benefits, a 2001 study showed that exercising just 10 minutes a day can improve mental outlook.

A study released in 2003 reported that exercise combined with **behavioral therapy** may even help manage the symptoms experienced by Gulf War veterans. Specifically, exercise helped improve symptoms related to **fatigue**, distress, cognitive problems, and mental health functioning. In the same year, the American Heart Association released a statement saying that exercise was beneficial even for patients awaiting heart transplants. Another study showed that women who participated in strenuous physical activity over a number of years could reduce their risk of **breast cancer**. Finally, research showed that men and women age 40 to 50 who exercised moderately for 60 to 90 minutes a day were less likely to catch a cold than those who sat around.

Description

Exercise comes in many forms, but there are three basic types: resistance, aerobics, and stretching. Yoga and martial arts are basically muscle stretching routines, walking and running are primarily aerobic, and weight lifting is mainly resistance. However, exercises such as swimming are considered crossover activities since they build muscle and provide a good aerobic, or cardiovascular, workout. Certified physical trainers usually advocate a combination program that involves stretching, aerobics, and at least some resistance activity for 30-60 minutes a day three times a week.

Stretching and meditative exercises

The most common types of alternative health exercises are the ancient disciplines of yoga and the martial arts (such as t'ai chi and qigong).

YOGA. The ancient East Indian discipline of yoga is probably the most widely practiced exercise advocated by alternative health practitioners. This may be because there is a heavy emphasis on mental conditioning as well as physical exertion. Yoga is the practice of incorporating mind, body, and spirit through a series of physical postures, breathing exercises, and meditation. It improves muscle flexibility, strength, and tone while calming the mind and spirit. Most contemporary **stress** reduction techniques are based on yoga principles.

There are a variety of yoga styles, each with its own unique focus. In the United States, **hatha yoga** is the most practiced. The pace is slow and involves a lot of stretching and breathing exercises. Much like the Chinese philosophy of yin and yang, hatha yoga strives to balance the opposite forces of ha (sun) and tha (moon). Astanga, or power yoga, involves more intense yoga postures done in rapid succession. Its vigorous workout is especially good in developing muscle strength. Iyengar yoga promotes body alignment while kripalu yoga develops mind, body, and spirit awareness. Pranayama yoga is a series of breathing exercises designed to increase vitality and energy.

Yoga helps strengthen the heart and slow respiration. Studies have shown it is beneficial in treating a variety of conditions, including heart disease, hypertension, arthritis, depression, fatigue, chronic **pain**, and carpal-tunnel syndrome. A 2001 study at the Cleveland Clinic Foundation in Ohio looked at yoga's effect on people suffering from lower back pain and pain due to conditions like **carpal tunnel syndrome** and arthritis. After a four-week period, investigators noted that yoga helped lessen pain, improve participants' moods and decreased pain medication requirements.

There are four main groups of yoga postures, also called asanas: standing, seated, reclining prone, and reclining supine. Other groups include forward bends, back bends, side bends, twists, inverted, and balancing. Within each group there are dozens of different yoga poses at beginning and advanced levels.

MARTIAL ARTS. While the words "martial arts" may be associated with conflict, they usually are graceful exercise movements that keep the body and mind strong and healthy. They can be performed by young and old. Martial arts range from simple stretching and meditative exercises to complicated and demanding exercises requiring more physical activity and mental concentration.

Probably the most popular among alternative health participants is t'ai chi, derived from the Chinese philosophy of Taoism and based on the concept of yin and yang. T'ai chi has a self-defense aspect based on counteracting an opponent's attack and then counterattacking, all in the same movement. As an exercise to maintain health, t'ai chi strengthens muscles and joints. It requires deep breathing techniques that increase blood circulation, benefiting the heart, lungs, and other organs. New research states that t'ai chi may improve physical functioning, like bending and lifting, in older age.

Another martial art growing in popularity in the United States is qigong (pronounced chee kung), although it has several forms that are more Taoist and Buddhist than martial. Qigong is a gentle exercise program that can increase vitality, enhance the immune system, and relieve stress when performed regularly. In China, there are hospitals that use qigong to treat terminal illnesses, particularly **cancer**.

Cardiovascular and aerobic

Aerobic, also called cardiovascular, exercises use a variety of muscle groups continuously and rhythmically, increasing heart rate and breathing. Specific aerobic activities include walking, jogging, running, bicycling, swimming, tennis, and cross-country skiing. Another popular form is aerobic dance exercise. Routines should last 10-60 minutes and be performed at least three times a week. Aerobic exercise is especially beneficial for losing weight and building endurance.

Aerobic exercises can be done outside a formal setting, with little or no equipment. However, since boredom is a frequent cause for stopping exercise, it often is beneficial to participate in exercise classes or join a gym or health club. Exercising with a group often helps with motivation. Also, health clubs usually offer a variety of stationary aerobic equipment, such as bikes, treadmills, stair climbers, and rowing machines.

Resistance

Resistance exercises generally are accomplished by lifting weights such as barbells and dumbbells, or by using a variety of resistance machines. They can also be done using only the body as resistance, such as doing push-ups, pull-ups, and sit-ups. Resistance exercise is particularly good for building muscles. For patients with kidney disease, weight lifting offers added benefit. Chronic kidney disease can lead to muscle wasting, which is compounded by low-protein **diets** that may be described for these patients. A 2001 study demonstrated that resistance training can improve muscle mass in kidney disease patients.

Unlike aerobics, which can be done daily, weight-lifting exercises require a period for the muscles to rest and rebuild. A total-body workout should be done every other day, or two to three times a week. A more advanced workout would exercise the lower body muscles one day and upper body muscles the next. It is also important to do 5-10 minutes each of warm-up and cool-down exercises, which will help increase flexibility and decrease soreness and fatigue.

Preparations

No advance preparations are required for exercising. However, a trainer can test a person's strength level and outline an appropriate program. Proper shoes are essential, especially for running. Any exercise should start with a warm-up of 5-10 minutes. Anyone considering a regular exercise program should consult first with a doctor, and possibly a sports podiatrist, to avoid strain and injury. Persons with serious health problems, such as heart disease, diabetes, **AIDS**, **asthma**, and arthritis should only begin an exercise regimen with their doctor's approval.

Precautions

In most people, the main exercise precaution is to avoid strain and overexertion. Exercise doesn't need to be strenuous to be beneficial. People with certain chronic health problems should take special precautions. Diabetics should closely monitor their blood sugar levels before and after exercising. Heart disease patients should never exercise to the point of chest pain. Exercise can induce asthma. It is essential for people with asthma to get their doctor's permission before starting an exercise program. It also is important for people to be shown the proper form in any activity to avoid strain and possible injury, especially when using exercise equipment. People also should know what parts of the body might be stressed by a particular exercise. They can then use supplemental exercises or stretches to add balance to the exercise program.

Side effects

The primary adverse effects of exercising can be sore muscles and stiff joints a day or two after beginning an exercise routine. These pains may last for several days. Other minor problems can include headaches, **dizziness**, fatigue, and **nausea**, usually indicating the exercise routine is too strenuous. A person can agitate old injuries or create new ones by improperly using equipment or wearing inadequately cushioned shoes.

Research & general acceptance

There almost is universal acceptance by allopathic and homeopathic health practitioners that exercise can be beneficial to overall good health. Thousands of studies during the past several decades link regular exercise to reduced risks for heart disease, stroke, diabetes, **obesity**, depression, hypertension, and osteoporosis. For example, a 1998 study by Harvard University of more than 11,000 people showed that people who exercise for an hour a day cut their risk of stroke in half over people who do not exercise regularly.

Training & certification

No special training or certification is required for exercising. People who want help in developing an exercise program should consult a certified physical trainer.

Resources

BOOKS

Devi, Nischala Joy, and Dean Ornish. *The Healing Path of Yoga: Time-Honored Wisdom and Scientifically Proven Methods That Alleviate Stress, Open Your Heart, and Enrich Your Life.* New York: Three Rivers Press, 2000.

Feuerstein, Georg, et al. *The Yoga Tradition: Its History, Literature, Philosophy and Practice.* Prescott, AZ: Hohm Press, 1998.

Goldberg, Linn, and Diane L. Elliot. *The Healing Power of Exercise: Your Guide to Preventing and Treating Diabetes, Depression, Heart Disease, High Blood Pressure, Arthritis, and More.* New York: John Wiley & Sons, 2000.

McArdle, William D., et al. *Essentials of Exercise Physiology.* Philadelphia: Lippincott, Williams & Wilkins, 1999.

Norris, Christopher M. *The Complete Guide to Stretching.* London: A & C Black, 2000.

KEY TERMS

Aerobic—Any cardiovascular exercise that increases heart rate and breathing, such as jogging, bicycling, and swimming.

Cardiovascular—Relating to the heart and blood vessels.

Kung fu—Another name for qigong; today it more commonly means a Chinese martial arts practice.

Osteoporosis—A bone disease that causes a loss in bone density; occurs most often in post-menopausal women.

Qigong—A Chinese exercise system (similar to t'ai chi) where people learn how to control the flow and distribution of qi (life energy); thought to improve health and harmony of mind and body.

T'ai chi—A slow, relaxed, stylized form of exercise developed by the Chinese; can be called an "inner" martial art.

Taoism—A philosophy of life based on the writings of Chinese philosopher Lao-tse who lived about 500 B.C.

Yin and yang—A Taoist concept that the universe is split into two separate but complementary aspects. Balance is sought between the passive force of yin (female) and the active force of yang (male). The idea of balance between yin and yang is important in traditional Chinese medicine and is the object of various healing arts.

PERIODICALS

Castaneda, Carmen, et al. "Resistance Training to Counteract the Catabolism of a Low-protein Diet in Patients with Chronic Renal Insufficiency." *Annals of Internal Medicine* (December 4, 2001): 965–912.

"Cognitive Behavioral Therapy Plus Exercise May Alleviate Symptoms." *Mental Health Weekly Digest* (March 31, 2003): 3.

"Exercise May Help Patients." *Heart Disease Weekly* (March 30, 2003): 44.

"Fast Facts." *Runner's World* (November 2001): 24.

Mooney, Linda, and Shelly Reese. "I Fought My Cancer Comeback in the Gym." *Prevention* (June 1999): 177.

"Stay Active to Stay Cold-Free: A Recent Study Found that You can Ward Off the Sniffle with a Little Exercise." *Natural Health* (March 2003): 30.

Sternberg, Steve. "Exercise Helps Some Cancer." *Science News* (May 3, 1997): 269.

"Strenuous Physical Activity Throughout Life can Decrease Risk ." *Cancer Weekly* (March 18, 2003): 32.

"Study is First to Confirm Link Between Exercise and Changes in Brain." *Obesity, Fitness and Wellness Week* (February 22, 2003): 13.

"Yoga Provides a Fresh Twist on Pain Relief." *Tufts University Health and Nutrition Letter* (November 2001): 2.

ORGANIZATIONS

Aerobic and Fitness Association of America. 15250 Ventura Blvd., Suite 200, Sherman Oaks, CA 91403. (877) 968-2639. http://www.afaa.com

American Council on Exercise. 5820 Oberlin Dr., Suite 102, San Diego, CA 92121-0378. (858) 535-8227. http://www.acefitness.org

American Society of Exercise Physiologists. Department of Exercise Physiology, The College of St. Scholastica, 1200 Kenwood Ave., Duluth, MN 55811. (218) 723-6297. http://www.css.edu/asep

National Council of Strength & Fitness. P.O. Box 557486, Miami, FL 33255. (800) 772-6273. http://www.ncsf.org

Ken R. Wells
Teresa G. Odle

Eyebright

Description

Eyebright (*Euphrasia officinalis*) is an annual plant that grows wild in meadows, grassy areas, heaths, and pastures of Britain, northern and western Asia, North America, and Europe. It belongs to the Scrophulariaceae plant family, which also includes the **foxglove** plant.

Eyebright grows to a height of 4-8 inches (10-20 cm) and has small white or purple flowers with red spots. These petals resemble bloodshot eyes, suggesting the plant's name and its eye-clearing action. Downy hairs cover the stems, which produce toothed leaves.

Eyebright is a semiparasitic plant. This means that it is nourished by the roots of other plants. Generally, it does not grow well if transplanted from the wild. The plant is harvested during the late summer or fall when the flowers are in bloom. The whole plant is cut off just above the root and then dried.

Eyebright contains vitamins A, C, D, and B complex; **iron**; silicon; and traces of **iodine**, **copper**, and **zinc**. Other components of eyebright include tannins, iridoid glycosides, the flavonoids rutin and quercetin, **essential fatty acids**, glycoside aucuboside, caffeic and ferulic acids, sterols, choline, and a volatile oil.

History

The Latin name *Euphrasia* is derived from the Greek word "Euphrosyne," meaning gladness. Euphrosyne was the name of one of three Graces known for her joy and happiness. The ancient Greeks used eyebright to treat eye **infections**, thereby creating happiness.

Eyebright has been used as a folk medicine to treat eye inflammations and infections, coughs, and poor memory since the Middle Ages. The poet Milton mentions eyebright in his book *Paradise Lost*, in which the archangel Michael gives eyebright to Adam to cure an eye infection. In 1485, eyebright was listed in a German book on medicinal herbs. Many sixteenth century herbalists championed eyebright as a treatment for various eye diseases. During the time of Queen Elizabeth, an eyebright ale was popular. Dried eyebright was often combined with tobacco and smoked to provide relief for bronchial colds.

General use

Modern herbalists still prescribe eyebright as a popular remedy for eye irritations and disorders, such as **conjunctivitis** and blepharitis. Icelanders use the juice from the pressed plant to treat most eye afflictions. Scottish people make an infusion in milk for inflamed or weak eyes. Eyebright is used to treat poor vision, eye strain, eye infections, sensitivity to light, and eye ulcers. Eyebright's antiseptic properties are highly regarded in soothing and cooling eyes that itch, burn, weep, and are red.

Eyebright is beneficial in the treatment of coughs, colds, **allergies**, sinusitis, **hay fever**, earaches, headaches, **jaundice**, throat and bronchial congestion, hoarseness, flu, and sinus inflammation. The flavonoids in eyebright act as anti-inflammatory agents that can help relieve inflamed mucous membranes of the eyes, sinuses, and upper respiratory tract. Eyebright's astringent properties also help reduce inflammation and mucous drainage, making the plant a popular remedy for many allergy, cold, and sinus symptoms.

Preparations

The stems, leaves, and flowers of the plant are collected and dried for medicinal use. Eyebright is often combined with **goldenseal** to treat eye afflictions. Eyebright may also be combined with **goldenrod**, **elder** flower, and/or goldenseal to provide relief from congestion.

In **homeopathy**, *Euphrasia officinalis* is a remedy used to treat colds accompanied by a nonirritating, watery nasal discharge and frequent burning tears. Conjunctivitis with symptoms of red eyes and lips, and acrid, watery tears may also be treated with this remedy. *Euphrasia officinalis* is also used as a remedy for **measles** and allergies.

KEY TERMS

. . . .

Annual—A plant that grows every year.

Blepharitis—A condition where the eyelids become red, irritated, and scaly. The eyes are painful, red, and inflamed.

Conjunctivitis—An inflammation of the mucous membranes that cover the outer eyeball and line the eyelids. The eye appears red or pink and is itchy or sore.

Infusion—An herbal tea created by steeping herbs in hot water. Generally, leaves and flowers are used in infusions.

Tincture—The concentrated solution of an herbal extract made with alcohol.

Eyebright is available in bulk form for teas or compresses, and in capsule and tincture forms. Capsules and tinctures should be used as directed on the commercial package.

To make a tea, 1 cup of boiling water is poured over 2-3 teaspoons of dried eyebright and steeped for 5-10 minutes. One cup should be drunk three times daily to maintain eyesight, relieve nasal congestion, and soothe coughs. This infusion can also be used as an eye bath to treat inflamed or painful eyes. The mixture is cooled, and then the eyes are bathed with the warm liquid three to four times daily.

To make a compress, 1-2 tablespoons of dried eyebright are simmered in 1 pint (0.4 l) of water for 10 minutes. The mixture is cooled and then strained. A clean cloth is dipped in the mixture, wrung out, and then placed over the eyes for 15 minutes several times daily. Caution should be used when applying compresses. An unsterilized, homemade compress of eyebright may contain bacteria that could lead to an eye infection.

Precautions

A qualified herbalist should be consulted before administering eyebright to children. Although herbalists maintain the benefits of eyebright, there are no known scientific studies or research to validate these claims.

Side effects

If a tincture solution of eyebright is placed on the eyes, tearing, **itching**, reddening, and swelling of the eyelids may develop because of the alcohol in the tincture. Eyebright may also cause a skin rash or **nausea**.

Interactions

There are no known interactions.

Resources

BOOKS

Pahlow, Mannfried. *Healing Plants.* Barron's Educational Series, Inc., 1993.

Jennifer Wurges

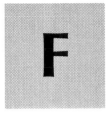

Facial massage

Definition

Facial massage is a very popular Western beauty treatment to slow down the **aging** process and achieve younger-looking and healthier skin. It is also used to relieve **stress**, **migraine headache**, **premenstrual syndrome** (PMS) and sinus congestion. It may involve a whole massage session, a portion of a whole-body massage or a part of a facial treatment. Facial massage can be done by a professional massage therapist, an esthetician, or a cosmetologist. Simple massage can also be done at home. Massage of the face is usually done with the hands; however, mechanical massaging devices are also used in beauty salons or spas. A small amount of oil or lotion is often applied to facilitate movement over the delicate facial areas.

In Eastern therapies, facial massage is part of a full-body treatment in which pressure points on the face and neck are stimulated in order to release blockages in the flow of qi, or vital energy. Lotions or oils are not used on the face in **acupressure**, **shiatsu**, or **yoga** techniques of facial massage.

Origins

Massage has been used for **pain** relief, healing and cosmetic improvement by people of all cultures since ancient times. The first written record of **massage therapy** is a Chinese medical text dating from the third century B.C. The ancient Greeks, Persians, Japanese, and Indians also recorded the use of massage treatment in great detail in their early medical literature.

The Western version of facial massage as a cosmetic treatment is a relatively recent twentieth-century innovation. It has become especially popular in Europe. Many of the best-known European practitioners have set up shop in the United States and taught others. This form of facial massage has generally been regarded as belonging more to estheticians and makeup artists than to massage therapists.

Benefits

Western-style facial massage may offer the following potential benefits:

• improvement of facial skin and muscle tone.

• relaxation of facial and eye muscles

• relief from tension headaches and facial pain

• alleviation of stress and anxiety

• overall physical and mental relaxation

Facial massage as part of Eastern therapies may offer the following potential benefits:

• stimulation of meridian points on the face

• relief from eyestrain

• correction of liver and gall bladder imbalances

• relief of neck tension

• alleviation of nervous disorders

• relief of premenstrual water retention

Description

Western-style facial massage

In Western massage, a facial massage as part of a full-body treatment is different from a full facial treatment, which includes masks, steaming, and similar techniques. A regular massage simply includes massage of the face, usually at the beginning or the end of the massage session.

For a Western facial massage, a gentle effleurage (gliding) movement is most often used. To perform the facial massage, the strokes must be gentle as well as stimulating, in order not to stretch the skin. Pressure strokes should move upward to give the muscles of the face a lift rather than dragging them down. A typical facial massage includes the following steps:

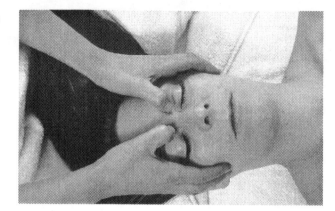

Massage therapist performing a facial massage. (Custom Medical Stock Photo. Reproduced by permission.)

- Before the massage, wash hands with soap and clean water. If the person to be massaged wears contact lens, ask her or him to remove them.

- Position: The most comfortable position has the client lying down on a massage table or sitting in a chair. Facial massage can be done, however, on any flat surface like a clean floor.

- Using a small amount of cleanser, gently wash the client's face. Wet cotton pads or facial sponges or wedges can be used to apply the cleanser. Then remove the cleanser, using fresh damp cotton pads.

- Apply the massage cream or lotion and begin massaging the face and neck areas in small symmetrical circles. The strokes should move up the neck and along the contour of the face. Do not leave out any facial muscles.

- Next, gently glide the back of the hands across the forehead with light pressure. Placing the thumbs side by side on the center of the forehead with the hands cradling the face, draw the thumbs outward towards the temples and make a gentle sweeping movement around the temple. Repeat the movement several times to relieve tension in the temples.

- Apply pressure in the hollow areas under the eyebrows by placing the hands along the sides of the face; use the thumb to press gently under the ridge one spot at a time. Move the pressure point from the inner to the outer edge of the brows and repeat the thumb pressure. This technique can help relieve tension **headache**.

- Position the thumbs alongside the nose bridge with hands **cupping** the face. Firmly slide the thumbs downward to the nostrils and outwards along the contour of the cheeks applying pressure along the way. Gently release the pressure when the thumbs reach the hairline. Then pull both hands up alongside the face towards the top of the head and away from the face. Repeat this motion two more times.

- Position fingertips in the cheek muscles and gently make circling movements counter-clockwise for a few times moving along the cheek muscles. This motion alleviates tension in the cheek area.

- Gently **stroke** the ears with the index fingers and thumbs while moving along the rims of the ears. This technique is very relaxing and enjoyable.

- Position the fingers just behind the neck while pressing with a thumb pad on a spot in the jaw area and circling this spot before moving to the next one. Holding the chin with the fingers, stroke the chin with the thumbs using circular motions downward. Finish the jaw massage with gentle strokes alongside the chin. This movement releases tension in the mouth and jaw.

- Make circular motions on the scalp and comb the fingers through the hair to release tension from the face and the head and to stimulate the scalp.

- Finally, remove the massage cream or lotion with fresh and damp cotton pads. Most facials end with a special lotion applied to the face.

Facial massage in Eastern therapies

In shiatsu, acupressure, and similar Eastern therapies, pressure is applied to points on the face in order to stimulate or unblock the flow of vital energy in specific meridians. The pressure points located on the face, along with the conditions that they are used to treat, are as follows:

- Stomach 1, under the center of the eye along the nasal bone: Tension and eyestrain.

- Stomach 3, about 4 cm below stomach 1 at the level of the base of the nose: Sinus and nasal congestion.

- Stomach 4, at the corners of the mouth: General stress and tension.

- Stomach 6, about 2 cm in front of the base of the ear lobe: Toothache.

- Conception vessel (end), between the lower lip and chin: Tension in the face and mouth.

- Bladder 1, at the inside corner of the eye: Headache and eyestrain.

- Gall bladder 1, a hollow about 2 cm from the outside corner of the eye: Headaches.

- Gall bladder 2, the hollow directly above and in front of the ear lobe: Ringing in the ears, swollen eyes, and dizziness.

Some yoga techniques include self-treatment for eye problems or tension by pressing the palms or knuckles against the pressure points surrounding the eyes.

Preparations

Western-style facial massage may require the following items:

- Towel to drape over the shoulders of the person to be massaged.
- Mild cleansing lotion to cleanse the face before massage.
- Moistened cotton pads, cotton-tipped swaps and facial tissues to remove cosmetics, cleansers and massage cream.
- Facial lotion or cream to facilitate the massage.

Facial massage as part of Eastern therapies does not require any specific preparation.

Precautions

Facial massage should not be done if any of the following conditions are present:

- Wearing contact lenses. The client should remove contact lenses before the procedure.
- Open sores, **boils** or cuts on the face.
- Inflamed or bruised skin.
- Recent scar tissue.
- **Acne, psoriasis** or **eczema**. Facial massage can worsen these conditions.

Side effects

Facial massage may irritate and worsen such skin conditions as acne, psoriasis or eczema.

Research & general acceptance

Western-style facial massage is a popular cosmetic procedure for many women and some men to improve the way the skin looks and feels. There is also evidence that massage can reduce stress, headache and facial pain.

Training & certification

Training requirements for cosmetologists and estheticians vary from state to state, ranging from a hair-care license to passing a required licensing examination. In addition to the techniques of facial massage, these beauticians may also be knowledgeable regarding clinical cosmetology and skin care.

Facial massage can also be performed by massage therapists as part of a full-body massage. Certified therapists are graduates of accredited massage programs who have passed the national certification examination in ther-

---

apeutic massage. They are also required to participate in continuing education programs to keep their skills current.

Practitioners of shiatsu, acupressure, and similar Eastern therapies may be certified or licensed by institutions in the United States and abroad that offer instruction in these forms of treatment.

Resources

BOOKS

Beck, Mark F. *Milady's Theory and Practice of Therapeutic Massage,* 3rd ed. Albany, NY: Milady Publishing.

Gach, Michael Reed, with Carolyn Marco. *Acu-Yoga: Self-Help Techniques to Relieve Tension.* New York: Japan Publications, Inc., 1998.

Novick, Nelson Lee. *You Can Look Younger at Any Age: A Leading Dermatologist's Guide.* New York: Henry Holt and Company, 1996.

Price, Shirley. *Practical Aromatherapy,* Chapter Four, "Yin, Yang, and Shiatsu." London: Thorsons, 1994.

Tourles, Stephanie. *Naturally Healthy Skin.* Pownal, VT: Schoolhouse Road, 1999.

ORGANIZATIONS

American Massage Therapy Association. 820 Davis St., Suite 100. Evanston, IL 60201. (847) 864-0123. Fax: (847) 864-1178. E-mail: info@inet.amtamassage.org. http://www.amtamassage.org

National Association of Nurse Massage Therapists. 1710 East Linden St. Tucson, AZ 85719.

National Certification Board of Therapeutic Massage and Bodywork. 8201 Greensboro Dr., Suite 300. McLean, VA 22102. (703) 610-9015 or (800) 296-0664.

Mai Tran

Faith healing *see* **Prayer and spirituality**

Farsightedness *see* **Hyperopia**

Fasting

Definition

Fasting is voluntarily not eating food for varying lengths of time. Fasting is used as a medical therapy

---

for many conditions. It is also a spiritual practice in many religions.

Origins

Used for thousands of years, fasting is one of the oldest therapies in medicine. Many of the great doctors of ancient times and many of the oldest healing systems have recommended it as an integral method of healing and prevention. Hippocrates, the father of Western medicine, believed fasting enabled the body to heal itself. Paracelsus, another great healer in the Western tradition, wrote 500 years ago that "fasting is the greatest remedy, the physician within." **Ayurvedic medicine**, the world's oldest healing system, has long advocated fasting as a major treatment.

Fasting has also been used in nearly every religion in the world, including Christianity, Judaism, Buddhism, and Islam. Many of history's great spiritual leaders fasted for mental and spiritual clarity, including Jesus, Buddha, and Mohammed. In one of the famous political acts of the last century, the Indian leader Mahatma Gandhi fasted for 21 days to promote peace.

Fasting has been used in Europe as a medical treatment for years. Many spas and treatment centers, particularly those in Germany, Sweden, and Russia, use medically supervised fasting. Fasting has gained popularity in American alternative medicine over the past several decades, and many doctors feel it is beneficial. Fasting is a central therapy in **detoxification**, a healing method founded on the principle that the build up of toxic substances in the body is responsible for many illnesses and conditions.

Benefits

Fasting can be used for nearly every chronic condition, including **allergies**, **anxiety**, arthritis, **asthma**, **depression**, diabetes, headaches, **heart disease**, high **cholesterol**, low blood sugar, digestive disorders, mental illness, and **obesity**. Fasting is an effective and safe weight loss method. It is frequently prescribed as a detoxification treatment for those with conditions that may be influenced by environmental factors, such as **cancer** and **multiple chemical sensitivity**. Fasting has been used successfully to help treat people who have been exposed to high levels of toxic materials due to accident or occupation. Fasting is thought to be beneficial as a preventative measure to increase overall health, vitality, and resistance to disease. Fasting is also used as a method of mental and spiritual rejuvenation.

Description

The principle of fasting is simple. When the intake of food is temporarily stopped, many systems of the body are given a break from the hard work of digestion. The extra energy gives the body the chance to heal and restore itself, and burning stored calories gets rid of toxic substances stored in the body.

The digestive tract is the part of the body most exposed to environmental threats, including bacteria, viruses, parasites, and toxins. It requires the most immune system support. When food is broken down in the intestines, it travels through the blood to the liver, the largest organ of the body's natural detoxification system. The liver breaks down and removes the toxic by-products produced by digestion, including natural ones and the chemicals now present in the food supply. During fasting, the liver and immune system are essentially freed to detoxify and heal other parts of the body.

Many healers claim that fasting is a particularly useful therapy for Americans and for the modern lifestyle, subjected to heavy **diets**, overeating, and constant exposure to food additives and chemicals. Some alternative practitioners have gone so far as to estimate that the average American is carrying 5-10 pounds of toxic substances in their bodies, for which fasting is the quickest and most effective means of removal.

Physiology of fasting

Through evolution, the body became very efficient at storing energy and handling situations when no food was available. For many centuries, fasting was probably a normal occurrence for most people, and the body adapted to it. It is estimated that even very thin people can survive for 40 days or more without food. The body has a special mechanism that is initiated when no food is eaten. Fasting is not starvation, but rather the body's burning of stored energy. Starvation occurs when the body no longer has any stored energy and begins using essential tissues such as organs for an energy source. Therapeutic fasts are stopped long before this happens.

Many physiological changes occur in the body during fasting. During the first day or so, the body uses its glycogen reserves, the sugars that are the basic energy supply. After these are depleted, the body begins using fat. However, the brain, which has high fuel requirements, still needs glucose (sugars converted from glycogen). To obtain glucose for the brain, the body begins to break down muscle tissue during the second day of the fast. Thus, during fasting some muscle loss will occur. To fuel the brain, the body would need to burn over a pound of muscle a day, but the body has developed another way to create energy that saves important muscle mass. This protein-sparing process is called ketosis, which occurs during the third day of a fast for men and the second day for women. In this highly efficient state, the liver begins converting stored fat and other nonessential tissues into ketones, which can be used by the brain, muscles, and heart as energy. It is at this point in the fast that sensations of hunger generally go away, and many people experience normal or even increased energy levels. Hormone levels and certain functions become more stable in this state as well. The goal of most fasts is to allow the body to reach the ketosis state in order to burn excess fat and unneeded or damaged tissue. Thus, fasts longer than three days are generally recommended as therapy.

Weight loss occurs most rapidly during the first few days of a fast, up to 2 pounds per day. In following days, the figure drops to around 0.5 pound per day. An average weight loss of a pound a day for an entire fast can be expected. Studies show that cutting back just once a month can jump-start healthier eating and help rid one's body of a lifetime of extra calories.

Performing a fast

Fasts can be performed for varying lengths of time, depending on the person and his or her health requirements. For chronic conditions, therapists recommend from two to four weeks to get the most benefits. Seven-day fasts are also commonly performed. A popular fasting program for prevention and general health is a three-day fast taken four times per year, at the change of each season. These can be easily performed over long weekends. Preventative fasts of one day per week are used by many people as well.

Juice fasts are also used by many people, although these are not technically fasts. Juice fasts are less intensive than water fasts because the body doesn't reach the ketosis stage. The advantage of juice fasts is that fruit and vegetable drinks can supply extra energy and nutrients. People can fit a few days of juice fasting into their normal schedules without significant drops in energy. Juice fasts are also said to have cleansing and detoxifying effects. The disadvantage of juice fasts is that the body never gets to the ketosis stage, so these fasters are thought to lack the deep detoxification and healing effects of the water fast.

Medical supervision is recommended for any fast over three days. Most alternative medicine practitioners, such as homeopaths, naturopathic doctors, and ayurvedic doctors, can supervise and monitor patients during fasts. Those performing extended fasts and those with health conditions may require blood, urine, and other tests during fasting. There are many alternative health clinics that perform medically supervised fasts as well. Some conventional medical doctors may also supervise patients during fasts. Costs and insurance coverage vary, depending on the doctor, clinic, and requirements of the patient.

Preparations

Fasts must be entered and exited with care. To enter a fast, the diet should be gradually lightened over a few days. First, heavy foods such as meats and dairy products should be eliminated for a day or two. Grains, nuts, and beans should then be reduced for several days. The day before a fast, only easily digested foods like fruits, light salads, and soups should be eaten. During the fast, only pure water and occasional herbal teas should be drunk. If you **exercise**, keep your workouts during fasting light and relatively brief, stopping immediately if you feel dizzy, lightheaded or short of breath.

Fasts should be ended as gradually as they are entered, going from lighter to heavier foods progressively. The diet after a fast should emphasize fresh, wholesome foods. Fasters should particularly take care not to overeat when they complete a fast.

Precautions

Fasting isn't appropriate for everyone and, in some cases, could be harmful. Any person undertaking a first fast longer than three days should seek medical supervision.

Those with health conditions should always have medical support during fasting. Plenty of water should be taken by fasters since dehydration can occur. Saunas and sweating therapies are sometimes recommended to assist detoxification, but should be used sparingly. Those fasting should significantly slow down their lifestyles. Taking time off of work is helpful, or at least reducing the work load. Fasters should also get plenty of rest. Exercise should be kept light, such as walking and gentle stretching.

Side effects

Those fasting may experience side effects of **fatigue**, malaise, aches and pains, emotional duress, **acne**, headaches, allergies, swelling, **vomiting**, **bad breath**, and symptoms of colds and flu. These reactions are sometimes called *healing crises*, which are caused by temporarily increased levels of toxins in the body due to elimination and cleansing. Lower energy levels should be expected during a fast.

Research & general acceptance

The physiology of fasting has been widely studied and documented by medical science. Beneficial effects such as lowered cholesterol and improved general functioning have been shown. Fasting as a treatment for illness and disease has been studied less, although some studies around the world have shown beneficial results. A 1984 study showed that workers in Taiwan who had severe **chemical poisoning** had dramatic improvement after a ten-day fast. In Russia and Japan, studies have demonstrated fasting to be an effective treatment for mental illness. A few years ago, fasting was featured on the cover of the *New England Journal of Medicine*, although mainstream medicine has generally ignored fasting and detoxification treatments as valid medical procedures.

The majority of research that exists on fasting is testimonial, consisting of individual personal accounts of healing without statistics or controlled scientific experiments. In the alternative medical community, fasting is an essential and widely accepted treatment for many illnesses and chronic conditions.

Training & certification

The International Association of Professional Natural Hygienists (IAPNH) is an organization of healthcare professionals who specialize in therapeutic fasting. It certifies doctors who have completed approved residencies in therapeutic fasting, including conventional medical doctors, naturopaths, and osteopathic doctors.

Resources

BOOKS

Cott, Alan. *Fasting: The Ultimate Diet*. Chicago: Hastings House, 1997.

Fuhrman, Joel, M.D. *Fasting and Eating for Health*. New York: St. Martin's, 1995.

Page, Linda, N.D. *Healthy Healing*. CA: Healthy Healing Publications, 1998.

PERIODICALS

Kallen, Ben."The Slow Fast: Fasting May Not be for You, but a Few 1,000–Calorie Days can Launch You into Better Health." *Men's Fitness* (April 2002): 34.

ORGANIZATIONS

Fasting Center International. 32 West Anapurna St., #360, Santa Barbara, CA 93101. http://www.fasting.com.

Douglas Dupler
Teresa G. Odle

Fatigue

Definition

Fatigue is physical and/or mental exhaustion that can be triggered by **stress**, medication, overwork, or mental and physical illness or disease.

Description

Everyone experiences fatigue occasionally. It is the body's way of signaling its need for rest and sleep. But when fatigue becomes a persistent feeling of tiredness or exhaustion that goes beyond normal sleepiness, it is usually a sign that something more serious is amiss.

Physically, fatigue is characterized by a profound lack of energy, feelings of muscle weakness, and slowed movements or central nervous system reactions. Fatigue can also trigger serious mental exhaustion. Persistent fatigue can cause a lack of mental clarity (or feeling of mental "fuzziness"), difficulty concentrating, and in some cases, **memory loss**.

Causes & symptoms

Fatigue may be the result of one or more environmental causes such as inadequate rest, improper diet, work and home stressors, or poor physical conditioning, or one symptom of a chronic medical condition or disease process in the body. **Heart disease**, low blood pressure, diabetes, end-stage renal disease, iron-deficiency **anemia**, **narcolepsy**, and **cancer** can cause long-term, ongoing fatigue symptoms. Acute illnesses such as viral and bacterial **infections** can also trigger temporary feelings of exhaustion. In addition, mental disorders such as **depression** can also cause fatigue. A 2002 report suggests that a disorder called hypocalcaemia may be a frequent cause of fatigue.

A number of medications, including antihistamines, antibiotics, and blood pressure medications, may cause drowsiness as a side effect. Individuals already suffering from fatigue who are prescribed one of these medications may wish to check with their healthcare providers about alternative treatments.

Extreme fatigue which persists, unabated, for at least six months, is not the result of a diagnosed disease or illness, and is characterized by flu-like symptoms such as swollen lymph nodes, **sore throat**, and muscle weakness and/or **pain** may indicate a diagnosis of **chronic fatigue syndrome**. Chronic fatigue syndrome (or CFS, sometimes called chronic fatigue immune deficiency syndrome), is a debilitating illness that causes overwhelming exhaustion and a number of neurological and immunological symptoms. Between 1.5 and 2 million Americans are estimated to suffer from the disorder. In late 2001, a panel of experts convened and announced that CFS is definitely associated with the immune system, and likely caused by a virus or bacteria, though no single cause has been identified.

Diagnosis

Because fatigue is a symptom of a number of different disorders, diseases, and lifestyle choices, diagnosis may be difficult. A thorough examination and patient history by a qualified healthcare provider is the first step in determining the cause of the fatigue. A physician can rule out physical conditions and diseases that feature fatigue as a symptom, and can also determine if prescription drugs, poor dietary habits, work environment, or other external stressors could be triggering the exhaustion. Several diagnostic tests may also be required to rule out common physical causes of exhaustion, such as blood tests to check for iron-deficiency anemia.

Diagnosis of chronic fatigue syndrome is significantly more difficult. Because there is no specific biological marker or conclusive blood test to check for the disorder, healthcare providers must rely on the patient's presentation and severity of symptoms to make a diagnosis. In many cases, individuals with chronic fatigue syndrome go through a battery of invasive diagnostic tests and several years of consultation with medical professionals before receiving a correct diagnosis.

Treatment

The treatment of fatigue depends on its direct cause, but there are several commonly prescribed treatments for non-specific fatigue, including dietary and lifestyle changes, the use of **essential oils** and herbal therapies, deep breathing exercises, **traditional Chinese medicine**, and **color therapy**.

Dietary changes

Inadequate or inappropriate nutritional intake can cause fatigue symptoms. To maintain an adequate energy supply and promote overall physical well-being, individuals should eat a balanced diet and observe the following nutritional guidelines:

- Drinking plenty of water. Individuals should try to drink 9 to 12 glasses of water a day. Dehydration can reduce blood volume, which leads to feelings of fatigue.

- Eating iron-rich foods (i.e., liver, raisins, spinach, apricots). **Iron** enables the blood to transport oxygen throughout the tissues, organs, and muscles, and diminished oxygenation of the blood can result in fatigue.

- Avoiding high-fat meals and snacks. High-fat foods take longer to digest, reducing blood flow to the brain, heart, and rest of the body while blood flow is increased to the stomach.

- Eating unrefined carbohydrates and proteins together for sustained energy.

- Balancing proteins. Limiting protein to 15-20 grams per meal and two snacks of 15 grams is recommended. Not getting enough protein adds to fatigue. Pregnant or breastfeeding women should eat more protein.

- Getting the recommended daily allowance of B complex vitamins (specifically, **pantothenic acid**, **folic acid**, **thiamine**, and **vitamin B_{12}**). Deficiencies in these vitamins can trigger fatigue.

- Getting the recommended daily allowance of **selenium**, **riboflavin**, and **niacin**. These are all essential nutritional elements in metabolizing food energy.

- A 2002 report suggested that **calcium** and **Vitamin D** supplementation can lessen fatigue symptoms in person with hypocalcaemia-caused fatigue.

• Controlling portions. Individuals should only eat when they're hungry, and stop when they're full. An over-stuffed stomach can cause short-term fatigue, and individuals who are overweight are much more likely to regularly experience fatigue symptoms.

Lifestyle changes

Lifestyle factors such as a high-stress job, erratic work hours, lack of social or family support, or erratic sleep patterns can all cause prolonged fatigue. If stress is an issue, a number of **relaxation** therapies and techniques are available to help alleviate tension, including massage, **yoga**, **aromatherapy**, **hydrotherapy**, progressive relaxation exercises, **meditation**, and **guided imagery**. Some may also benefit from individual or family counseling or **psychotherapy** sessions to work through stress-related fatigue that is a result of family or social issues.

Maintaining healthy sleep patterns is critical to proper rest. Having a set "bedtime" helps to keep sleep on schedule. A calm and restful sleeping environment is also important to healthy sleep. Above all, the bedroom should be quiet and comfortable, away from loud noises and with adequate window treatments to keep sunlight and street-lights out. Removing distractions from the bedroom such as televisions and telephones can also be helpful.

Essential oils

Aromatherapists, hydrotherapists, and other holistic healthcare providers may recommend the use of essential oils of **rosemary** (*Rosmarinus officinalis*), **eucalyptus** blue gum (*Eucalyptus globulus*), **peppermint**, (*Mentha x piperata*), or scots pine oil (*Pinus sylvestris*) to stimulate the nervous system and reduce fatigue. These oils can be added to bathwater or massage oil as a topical application. Citrus oils such as lemon, orange, grapefruit, and lime have a similar effect, and can be added to a steam bath or vaporizer for inhalation.

Herbal remedies

Herbal remedies that act as circulatory stimulants can offset the symptoms of fatigue in some individuals. An herbalist may recommend an infusion of **ginger** (*Zingiber officinale*) root or treatment with **cayenne** (*Capsicum annuum*), balmony (*Chelone glabra*), **damiana** (*Turnera diffusa*), ginseng (*Panax ginseng*), or rosemary (*Rosmarinus officinalis*) to treat ongoing fatigue.

An infusion is prepared by mixing the herb with boiling water, steeping it for several minutes, and then removing the herb from the infusion before drinking. A strainer, tea ball, or infuser can be used to immerse loose herb in the boiling water before steeping and separating it. A second method of infusion is to mix the loose herbal preparation with cold water first, bringing the mixture to a boil in a pan or teapot, and then separating the tea from the infusion with a strainer before drinking.

Caffeine-containing central nervous system stimulants such as tea (*Camellia senensis*) and cola (*Cola nitida*) can provide temporary, short-term relief of fatigue symptoms. However, long-term use of **caffeine** can cause restlessness, irritability, and other unwanted side effects, and in some cases may actually work to increase fatigue after the stimulating effects of the caffeine wear off. To avoid these problems, caffeine intake should be limited to 300 mg or less a day (the equivalent of 4-8 cups of brewed, hot tea).

Traditional Chinese medicine

Chinese medicine regards fatigue as a blockage or misalignment of *qi*, or energy flow, inside the human body. The practitioner of Chinese medicine chooses **acupuncture** and/or herbal therapy to rebalance the entire system. The Chinese formula Minot Bupleurum soup (or Xiao Chia Hu Tang) has been used for nearly 2,000 years for the type of chronic fatigue that comes after the flu. In this condition, the person has low-grade **fever**, **nausea**, and fatigue. There are other formulas that are helpful in other cases. Acupuncture involves the placement of a series of thin needles into the skin at targeted locations on the body known as acupoints in order to harmonize the energy flow within the human body.

Deep breathing exercises

Individuals under stress often experience fast, shallow breathing. This type of breathing, known as chest breathing, can lead to shortness of breath, increased muscle tension, inadequate oxygenation of blood, and fatigue. Breathing exercises can both improve respiratory function and relieve stress and fatigue.

Deep breathing exercises are best performed while lying flat on the back on a hard surface, usually the floor. The knees are bent, and the body (particularly the mouth, nose, and face) is relaxed. One hand should be placed on the chest and one on the abdomen to monitor breathing technique. With proper breathing techniques, the abdomen will rise further than the chest. The individual takes a series of long, deep breaths through the nose, attempting to raise the abdomen instead of the chest. Air is exhaled through the relaxed mouth. Deep breathing can be continued for up to 20 minutes. After the **exercise** is complete, the individual checks again for body tension and relaxation. Once deep breathing techniques have been mastered, an individual can use deep breathing at any time or place as a quick method of relieving tension and preventing fatigue.

Color therapy

Color therapy, also known as chromatherapy, is based on the premise that certain colors are infused with healing energies. The therapy uses the seven colors of the rainbow to promote balance and healing in the mind and body. Red promotes energy, empowerment, and stimulation. Physically, it is thought to improve circulation and stimulate red blood cell production. Red is associated with the seventh chakra, located at the root, or base of the spine. In yoga, the chakras are specific spiritual energy centers of the body.

Therapeutic color can be administered in a number of ways. Practitioners of Ayurvedic, or traditional Indian medicine, wrap their patients in colored cloth chosen for its therapeutic hue. Individuals suffering from fatigue would be wrapped in reds and oranges chosen for their uplifting and energizing properties. Patients may also be bathed in light from a color filtered light source to enhance the healing effects of the treatment.

Individuals may also be treated with color-infused water. This is achieved by placing translucent red colored paper or colored plastic wrap over and around a glass of water and placing the glass in direct sunlight so the water can soak up the healing properties and vibrations of the color. Environmental color sources may also be used to promote feelings of stimulation and energy. Red wall and window treatments, furniture, clothing, and even food may be recommended for their energizing healing properties.

Color therapy can be used in conjunction with both hydrotherapy and aromatherapy to heighten the therapeutic effect. Spas and holistic healthcare providers may recommend red color baths or soaks, which combine the benefits of a warm or hot water soak with energizing essential oils and the fatigue-fighting effects of bright red hues used in color therapy.

Allopathic treatment

Conventional medicine recommends the dietary and lifestyle changes outlined above as a first line of defense against fatigue. Individuals who experience occasional fatigue symptoms may benefit from short-term use of caffeine-containing central nervous stimulants, which make people more alert, less drowsy, and improve coordination. However, these should be prescribed with extreme caution, as overuse of the drug can lead to serious **sleep disorders**, like **insomnia**.

Another reason to avoid extended use of caffeine is its associated withdrawal symptoms. People who use large amounts of caffeine over long periods build up a tolerance to it. When that happens, they have to use more

and more caffeine to get the same effects. Heavy caffeine use can also lead to dependence. If an individual stops using caffeine abruptly, withdrawal symptoms may occur, including **headache**, fatigue, drowsiness, yawning, irritability, restlessness, **vomiting**, or runny nose. These symptoms can go on for as long as a week.

KEY TERMS

Aromatherapy—The therapeutic use of plant-derived, aromatic essential oils to promote physical and psychological well-being.

Guided imagery—The use of relaxation and mental visualization to improve mood and/or physical well-being.

Hydrotherapy—Hydrotherapy, or water therapy, is use of water (hot, cold, steam, or ice) to relieve discomfort and promote physical well-being.

Expected results

Fatigue related to a chronic disease or condition may last indefinitely, but can be alleviated to a degree through some of the treatment options outlined here. Exhaustion that can be linked to environmental stressors is usually easily alleviated when those stressors are dealt with properly.

There is no known cure for chronic fatigue syndrome, but steps can be taken to lessen symptoms and improve quality of life for these individuals while researchers continue to seek a cure.

Prevention

Many of the treatments outlined above are also recommended to prevent the onset of fatigue. Getting adequate rest and maintaining a consistent bedtime schedule are the most effective ways to combat fatigue. A balanced diet and moderate exercise program are also important to maintaining a consistent energy level.

Resources

BOOKS

Davis, Martha et al. *The Relaxation & Stress Reduction Workbook*. 4th edition. Oakland, CA: New Harbinger Publications, Inc., 1995.

Hoffman, David. *The Complete Illustrated Herbal*. New York: Barnes & Noble Books, 1999.

Johnson, Hillary. *Osler's Web: Inside the Labyrinth of the Chronic Fatigue Syndrome Epidemic*. New York: Crown Publishers, 1996.

Lawless, Julia. *The Complete Illustrated Guide to Aromatherapy*. Boston, MA: Element Books, 1997.

Medical Economics Corporation. *The PDR for Herbal Medicines*. Montvale, NJ: Medical Economics Corporation, 1998.

PERIODICALS

de Vries, ACH, and Oudesluys-Murphy, AM. "Fatigue Due to Hypocalcaemia." *The Lancet* (February 2, 2002): 443.

"Immune System Dysfunction May Play a Key Role." *Medical Letter on the CDC & FDA* (January 20, 2002): 5.

Paula Ford-Martin
Teresa G. Odle

Feldenkrais

Definition

The Feldenkrais method is an educational system that allows the body to move and function more efficiently and comfortably. Its goal is to re-educate the nervous system and improve motor ability. The system can accomplish much more, relieving pressure on joints and weak points, and allowing the body to heal repetitive strain injuries. Continued use of the method can relieve **pain** and lead to higher standards of achievement in sports, the **martial arts**, dancing and other physical disciplines.

Pupils are taught to become aware of their movements and to become aware of how they use their bodies, thus discovering possible areas of **stress** and strain. The goal of Feldenkrais is to take the individual from merely functioning, to functioning well, free of pain and restriction of movement. Feldenkrais himself stated that his goal was, "To make the impossible possible, the possible easy, and the easy, elegant."

Origins

Moshe Feldenkrais (1904–1984) was a Russian-born Israeli physicist and engineer who was also an active soccer player and judo master. He devised his system in response to his own recurring knee injury, which had restricted his movement and caused him great pain over a long period of time. Feldenkrais believed that repeated muscle patterns cause the parts of the brain controlling those muscles to stay in a fixed pattern as well. He thought that the more the muscles are used, the more parts of the brain can be activated. He devised a method of re-educating the neuromuscular system and re-evaluating movement to increase efficiency and reduce stress, using his knowledge of mechanics and engineering, and applying some of his martial arts training.

MOSHE FELDENKRAIS 1904–1984

Moshe Feldenkrais was born on the border between Russia and Poland. When he was only a boy of 13, he traveled to Palestine on foot. The journey took a year, and once there, young Feldenkrais worked as a laborer and cartographer, also tutoring others in mathematics. Moving to France in 1933, he graduated in mechanical and electrical engineering from the Ecole des Travaux Publiques de Paris.

Feldenkrais became the first person to open a Judo center in Paris after meeting with Jigaro Kano. He was also one of the first Europeans to become a black belt in Judo, in 1936.

Obtaining his Ph.D. at the Sorbonne, he went on to assist Nobel Prize laureate, Frédéric Joliot-Curie at the Curie Institute. During World War II in England, he worked on the new sonar anti-submarine research.

Prompted by a recurring leg injury, he applied his knowledge of the martial arts and his training as an engineer to devise a method of re-integrating the body. The concept was that more efficient movement would allow for the treatment of pain or disability, and the better-functioning of the body as a whole. Later on, he would begin to teach what he had learned to others in Tel Aviv.

In addition to many books about judo, including *Higher Judo*, he wrote six books on his method.

Patricia Skinner

Benefits

This method of re-educating the nervous system can be beneficial to a wide range of people, including athletes, children, the elderly, martial artists, those who are handicapped, people with special needs, and those suffering from degenerative diseases. It has also proved popular with artists, particularly musicians, a number of whom have used Feldenkrais to improve their performance.

The Feldenkrais Guild of North America (FGNA) states that over half of the those who turn to Feldenkrais practitioners are seeking relief from pain. Many people who have pain from an injury compensate by changing their movements to limit pain. Often these changed movements remain after the pain from the original injury is gone, and new pain may occur. Feldenkrais helps students become aware of the changed movements and allows them to learn new movements that relieve their pain. Apart from the obvious physical benefits of more efficient movement and freedom from pain and restriction, Feldenkrais practitioners assert that there are other positive benefits for overall physical and mental health. Feldenkrais can result in increased awareness, flexibility, and coordination, and better **relaxation**. Feldenkrais practitioners have also noted other benefits in their students, including improvements in awareness, flexibility, coordination, breathing, digestion, sleep, mood, mental alertness, energy, and range of motion, as well as reduced stress and **hypertension**, and fewer headaches and backaches.

Musicians and athletes can improve their performance in many ways when they learn to use their bodies more efficiently. Feldenkrais can also help injured athletes regain lost potential and free them from pain and restriction of movement.

There are numerous accounts of the remarkable results obtained when Feldenkrais is taught to handicapped children so that they can learn to function despite their limitations. Handicapped people can learn to make full use of whatever potential they have, and to have more confidence in their abilities. Practitioners who specialize in teaching Feldenkrais to those who have handicaps have in many cases allowed the patient to discover ways of performing tasks which were previously thought to be impossible for them.

The elderly, whose movements are often restricted by pain and stiffness, can learn to overcome these obstacles with Feldenkrais instruction. In some instances even severe cases of arthritis have been conquered. Theoretically, Feldenkrais can make possible renewed levels of energy and freedom from restriction.

Description

Feldenkrais is described a being a dual system, with two components: "Awareness Through Movement" and "Functional Integration." The system aims to re-educate the body so that habitual movements that cause strain or pain can be relearned to improve efficiency and eliminate dangerous or painful action.

Feldenkrais helps to translate intention into action. In practice, an individual can learn to achieve his or her highest potential, while at the same time learning to avoid and eliminate stresses, strains, and the possibility of injury.

Functional integration

During this session, the patient wears comfortable clothing, and may sit, stand, walk, or lie on a low padded table. The practitioner helps the pupil by guiding him or her through a number of movements. The practitioner may use touch to communicate with the student, but touch is not used to correct any movements. The purpose of this session is to increase a student's awareness of his or her own movement and become open to different pos-

sibilities for movement. The instruction can be focused on a particular activity that the student does every day, or that causes him or her pain. The student can learn to alter habitual movements and re-educate the neuromuscular system. This type of session is particularly useful for those who suffer from limitations originating from misuse, stress, illness, or accident. It can also help athletes and musicians perform to the best of their ability by increasing their possibilities for movement. It offers students the potential for improving their physical and mental performance in addition to heightening the sense of well-being.

Awareness through movement

Feldenkrais's martial arts background can be clearly identified in many of the aspects of Awareness Through Movement (ATM). During group sessions, pupils are taught to become acutely aware of all their movements and to imagine them, so that they can improve the efficiency of their actions in their minds, and put them into practice. Pupils are encouraged to be disciplined about practicing their exercises, to achieve maximum benefit.

Awareness through movement is described as an exploratory, nonjudgmental process through which pupils are encouraged to observe and learn about themselves and their movements. The range of this therapy is wide, and there are thousands of different lessons designed to help specific areas.

Preparations

No preparation is necessary for the practice of Feldenkrais, and all are encouraged to seek help from this system. No condition is considered a preclusion to the benefits of Feldenkrais.

Precautions

As with any therapy or treatment, care should be taken to choose a qualified practitioner. Feldenkrais practitioners stress that the body must not be forced to do anything, and if any movement is painful, or even uncomfortable, it should be discontinued immediately and the patient should seek professional help.

Side effects

No known side effects are associated with the practice of Feldenkrais.

Research & general acceptance

Since Moshe Feldenkrais began to teach his method, it has gradually gained acceptance as an education system. Published research using the method can be found in U.S. and foreign publications.

Training & certification

Guild-accredited Feldenkrais training courses leading to certification for the practice or teaching of the method are available throughout the United States and in other countries. Guild-certified Feldenkrais practitioners undergo a four-year training course (800 hours) that includes studying numerous movements and becoming aware of the smallest details in movement. After two years of formal training, practitioners may become authorized. The FGNA can be contacted to find a certified Feldenkrais practitioner.

Resources

BOOKS

Alon, Ruthy. *Mindful Spontaneity: Lessons in the Feldenkrais Method.* 2d ed. Berkeley: North Atlantic Books, 1996.

Bratman, Steven. *The Alternative Medicine Sourcebook.* 2d ed. Chicago: Lowell House, 1999.

Feldenkrais, Moshe. *Awareness Through Movement.* New York: HarperSanFrancisco, 1991.

Rywerant, Yochanan. *The Feldenkrais Method.* Chicago: Keats Publishing, 1991.

Shafarman, Steven. *Awareness Heals: the Feldenkrais Method for Dynamic Health.* Cambridge, Mass.: Perseus Publishing, 1997.

Somerville, Robert. *Alternative Medicine: the definitive guide.* Tiburon, Calif.: Future Medicine Publishing, Inc., 1999.

Stillerman, Elaine. *The Encyclopedia of Bodywork.* New York: Facts On File, Inc., 1996.

Thomas, Richard, and C. Norman Shealy, eds. *The Complete Family Guide to Alternative Medicine.* Dorset, U.K.: Element Books Ltd., 1996.

Zemach-Bersin, David and Kaethe, and Mark Reese. *Relaxercise.* New York: HarperSanFrancisco, 1990.

ORGANIZATIONS

Feldenkrais Guild of North America. 3611 SW Hood Ave., Suite 100, Portland, OR 97201. (800) 775-2118. (503) 221-6612. Fax: (503) 221-6616. <http://www.feldenkrais.com/>

Patricia Skinner

Feng shui

Definition

Feng shui, pronounced "foong swee" (Cantonese) or "fong shway" (Mandarin) is the Chinese art of arranging buildings, objects, and space in the environment in order to achieve energy, harmony, and balance. The English translation of Feng shui is "the way of Wind (feng) and Water (shui)" or "the natural forces of the universe."

Origins

Feng shui, derived from the Chinese concept of yin and yang, has been practiced for thousands of years. Evidence of the existence of this practice can be found in the alignment and organization of graves in the Yangshao villages from 6000 B.C. In fact, there is compelling evidence that suggests that feng shui was not strictly an Asian entity. In prehistoric Europe, the practice of arranging objects and structures to be in harmony with the universe was a relatively common practice.

A popular theory regarding the origins of feng shui suggests that the practice stemmed from ancient shaman who understood the vital importance of strategically placing a village. Areas which possessed mild winds would generate plentiful harvests while harsh winds would stunt crop growth or destroy the harvest altogether. In addition, the placement of a village in close proximity to flowing water and fresh springs would stimulate growth and ensure health, while stagnant water would foster disease and disharmony within the community. As the centuries passed, these shaman correlated their thoughts on wind and water with the teachings of Daoism, thus creating the practice of feng shui.

Benefits

As a design philosophy, "good" feng shui is believed to promote health, prosperity, creativity, positive social relationships, self-confidence, contemplation, and respect for others.

Description

An ancient Daoist Chinese theory of design and placement, feng shui grew from observations that an individual's surroundings elicit positive and negative effects. According to Daoism, everything that exists contains qi (chi), the energy or life force. This qi possesses two properties, yin (receptive) and yang (active)—they are opposites and cannot exist without the other. Within the qi, eight constituents compose the universe (the Lake, the Mountain, Fire, Water, Heaven, Thunder,

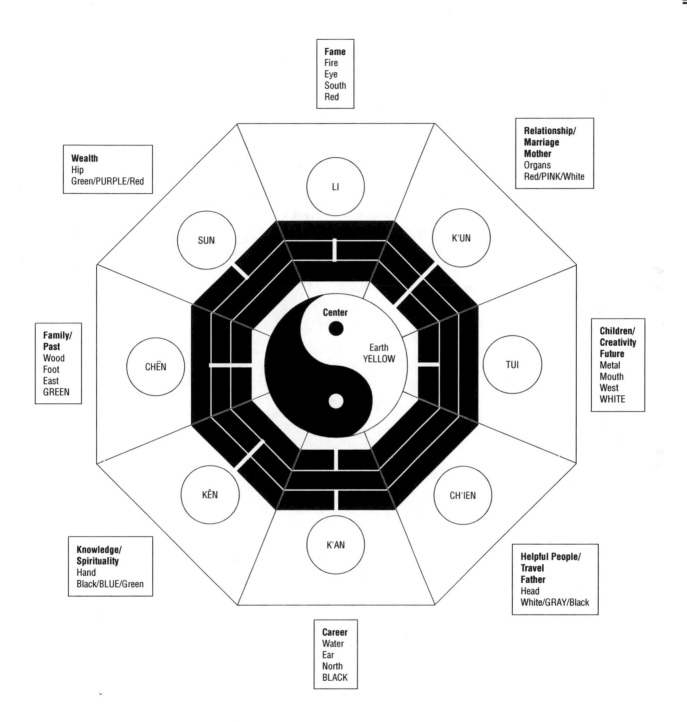

Fame
Fire
Eye
South
Red

Relationship/
Marriage
Mother
Organs
Red/PINK/White

Wealth
Hip
Green/PURPLE/Red

LI

SUN

K'UN

Center

Earth
YELLOW

Family/
Past
Wood
Foot
East
GREEN

CHÊN

TUI

Children/
Creativity
Future
Metal
Mouth
West
WHITE

KÊN

CH'IEN

Knowledge/
Spirituality
Hand
Black/BLUE/Green

K'AN

Helpful People/
Travel
Father
Head
White/GRAY/Black

Career
Water
Ear
North
BLACK

(Illustration by GGS Information Services, Inc. The Gale Group.)

Wind, and Earth). Each trigram, or combination of three yin/yang elements, represents a particular quality and pattern of energy. In turn, the proper arrangement of these energetic qualities would affect not only the qi of the environment, but that of the individual within the environment as well. With feng shui, the goal is to bring both into harmony so as to foster prosperity, health, and well-being with the Wind (feng) dispersing the qi throughout the universe and Water (shui).

The *ba gua,* or "Sequence of the Later Heaven," is the arrangement of the energy trigrams so that they exist in harmony and balance. Each trigram has a balancing partner that contributes to universal harmony. For example, Earth is balanced by the Mountain, Fire is balanced by the Water, Wind is balanced by Heaven, and Thunder is balanced by Lake. The *ba gau* is laid in a circular pattern with Fire at the top, followed by Earth, the Lake, Heaven, Water, the Mountain, Thunder, and Wind (clockwise). The Taiji (or yin-yang symbol) is located in the center of the trigrams, and represents the unifying force of the universe.

Practitioners of feng shui use the ba gua to determine the energy flow throughout the home and in other living spaces. By corresponding the trigram pattern to the different parts of a room, a practitioner determines whether the room is in harmony with the universe. For example, when analyzing a home office or workspace of a writer or artist, a feng shui specialist would pay particular attention to the portion of the room that corresponds to the Lake of the *ba gua,* because the Lake represents creative energy. If there is clutter or disorganization in the section of the room that corresponds to the Lake, or if the room is partitioned so that the Lake section is actually occupied by a bookcase or closet, then the environment would be considered to stifle creativity. A feng shui specialist might recommend moving the office to a more hospitable room in the house, or reconstructing the storage space to free up the creative energy in the Lake section of the room. Good health is said to be located in the Wind trigram of the *ba gua,* so maintaining this space and using it effectively is critical to practitioners of feng shui.

There are many other design tenets of feng shui, but some of the most commonly used and basic concepts include:

• Energy, or qi, enters and exits rooms through doorways. Doors facing each other encourage qi to move too quickly through and out of the room. Doors on adjoining walls encourage a circular movement of qi that is considered relaxing and "good" feng shui.

• Arranging chairs, beds, chaises, sofas, or other seating with their backs to the door and/or windows is not recommended in feng shui. It is considered "bad" feng shui to leave the back exposed to possible attack through the door.

• Homes located at the end of a cul-de-sac, across from a church or other spiritual center, at the end of a bridge, or near a freeway are not desirable to feng shui practitioners because these locations all have either too fast or not enough energy flow.

• When choosing a home site to build on, the ideal location according to feng shui principles is a rectangular plot of land, on a hill, with open space in front of the home.

• The front door of a home should be in proportion to the size of the house. Too large or too small an entrance will not facilitate proper qi flow through the home.

• Mirrors used in the home should not face chairs or beds.

• Windows should face only pleasing, natural views when at all possible. If a view is dreary, the feng shui of the room can be improved by using window treatments inside and/or window box plantings outside.

Precautions

Individuals should observe basic building code and fire safety rules when redesigning a home according to feng shui principles.

Feng shui adjustments to living space should not be relied upon as a sole source of treatment for individuals with health problems. Although feng shui principles can be employed as an adjunct, or complementary, treatment, proper diagnosis and treatment from a qualified healthcare professional is necessary in treating any chronic or acute physical disorder.

Research & general acceptance

Feng shui has been practiced throughout Asia for thousands of years, and has recently grown in popularity in the United States as a tool for home design. Although considered part of **traditional Chinese medicine** in Asia, it is not largely regarded as a healthcare tool in the United States, preventative or otherwise.

Training & certification

Certification and/or licensing is not required to practice feng shui in the United States. However, there are some national organizations that offer training and certification programs.

Resources

BOOKS

Henwood, Belinda. *Feng Shui: How to create harmony and balance in your living and working environment.* Pownal, VT: Storey Books, 1999.

Williams, Tom. *The Complete Illustrated Guide to Chinese Medicine.* Boston, MA: Element Books, 1996.

KEY TERMS

Daoism—Also called Taoism, Dao means "the way." Daoism is a holistic spiritual philosophy of the universe that is based on the idea that all elements in the universe are interactive and interdependent with each other and that the universe and natural world are in a constant state of change, or flux.

ORGANIZATIONS

Geomancy, the Feng Shui Education Association. 2939 Ulloa Street, San Francisco, CA 94116. (415) 753-6408. http://www.geofengshui.com.

Paula Ford-Martin

Fennel

Description

Fennel (*Foeniculum vulgare*), also known as *F. officinale*, is a member of the Umbelliferae (Apiaceae) or carrot family, along with dill (*Anethum graveolens*), caraway (*Carum carvi*), and **anise** (*Pimpinella anisum*). Fennel has a thick, spindle-shaped taproot that produces a pithy, smooth or finely-fluted round stem that may reach to 6 ft (1.8 m) in height. The finely divided leaves, with numerous thread-like segments, grow from a sheath surrounding the stalk at the base of the leaf stem. The delicate, blue-green filiform leaf segments have a pungent scent, somewhat similar to **licorice**, and an anise-like flavor. This characteristic is due to the presence of the phytochemical anethol, also a primary constituent of anise oil. Fennel's tiny yellow flowers form in large, compound umbells. The blossoms are frequently visited by bees, wasps, and other insects, and fennel leaf is a favorite food of the swallowtail-butterfly.

This perennial native of the Mediterranean is called marathon in Greece, a name derived from the word *maraino*, meaning to grow thin. Fennel was recommended as an herb for weight reduction, "to make people more lean that are too fat," according to the seventeenth century herbalist and astrologer Nicholas Culpeper. He considered fennel to be an herb of Mercury, under the sign of Virgo. In Chinese and Hindu cultures fennel was ingested to speed the elimination of poisons from the system, particularly after snakebite and scorpion stings. As one of the ancient Saxon people's nine sacred herbs, fennel was credited with the power to cure what were then believed to be the nine causes of disease. Fennel was also valued as a magic herb. In the Middle Ages it was draped over doorways on Midsummer's Eve to protect the household from evil spirits. As an added measure of protection, the tiny seeds were stuffed into keyholes to keep ghosts from entering the room.

Fennel was introduced to North America by Spanish missionaries for cultivation in their medicinal gardens. Fennel escaped cultivation from the mission gardens, and is now known in California as wild anise. English settlers brought the herb with them to the New England colonies where it became part of their kitchen gardens. In Puritan folk medicine fennel was taken as a digestive aid. The herb is still found growing on the sites of these early English settlements. This attractive, aromatic and sun-loving herb thrives on roadsides, embankments, sea cliffs, and in dry, stony fields.

There are several different species and varieties of fennel that may be annual, biennial, or perennial. *F. vulgare var. dulce*, known as sweet fennel, or *finocchio*, is cultivated for the fleshy basal stalks. The stalks may be eaten fresh, like celery, or boiled and baked as a vegetable. This delicacy is known in Italy as *carosella*. Fennel has naturalized in most temperate areas of the world, and is extensively cultivated for medicinal, ornamental, and culinary uses.

General use

The seeds, leaves, and roots of fennel are safe and edible. The essential oil, extracted from the seeds, is toxic even in small amounts. Fennel has been widely used in culinary and medicinal preparations for centuries. The herb acts as a carminative, and was traditionally employed as a digestive aid and remedy for flatulence. An infusion or decoction of the dried seeds is antispasmodic and will ease stomach pains and speed up the digestion of fatty foods. Fennel is a proven remedy for **colic** in infants, and is safe when administered as a mild infusion of the leaf and seed. It is also used for coughs and colds. Fennel exerts a calming influence on the bronchial tissues. The seeds contain large amounts of the phytochemical alpha-pinene, which acts as an expectorant and helps to loosen phlegm in the lungs. An eyewash, prepared from a decoction of the crushed seeds, is said to improve eyesight and reduce irritation and eyestrain. Fennel has a long history of use as a galactagogue. The seed, when boiled in barley **water**, acts to increase the flow of breast milk in nursing mothers. A poultice of the herb may be helpful to relieve swelling of the breasts during lactation. A leaf and seed tea has been used to expel hookworm and kill intestinal bacteria. Fen-

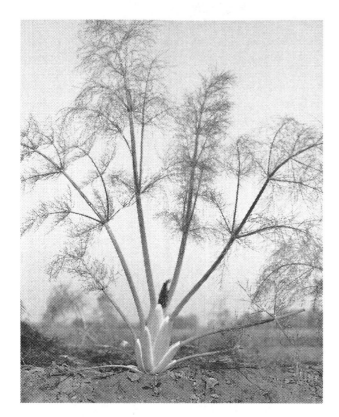

Fennel plant. *(National Audubon Society Collection/Photo Researchers, Inc. Reproduced with permission.)*

nel has also been used to promote appetite. The entire herb is used in culinary dishes, and the fleshy sheaths surrounding the base of the leaf stems are a staple in Italian cuisine. The foliage, known as fennel weed, is used to flavor eggs, fish, stews, and vegetables. The root is sometimes grated fresh and added to salads. The licorice-flavored seeds are traditionally served after meals in India to cleanse the breath. The flowers produce a yellow tint and the leaves a light brown hue as a natural dye for wool fabrics.

Fennel seed contains volatile oil, most of which is identified as trans-anethole, with a much smaller amount identified as fenchone. Other components of the essential oil include limonene, camphene, and alpha-pinene.

Preparations

Harvest fennel leaf from time to time throughout the growing season. Use the fresh leaf when possible as the herb may lose much of the flavor when dried. The leaves may also be frozen for later use. Harvest the seeds in autumn. Seeds are fully ripe just as the color fades and the seed-bearing umbells turn from yellow-green to a light brown. Cut the brown umbell from the stalk and place it in a paper bag to dry in a warm room. Shake the dried

seeds from the umbell and store them in tightly sealed, clearly labelled, dark-glass containers. Harvest the root late in the fall at the same time the stems are harvested as a vegetable. The root is generally less medicinally potent than the seeds.

Seed infusion: Crush 1 tsp–1 tbsp of the dried seed, add to 1 cup of unchlorinated water, fresh milk, or barley water, in a non-metallic pot. Bring to a boil; then steep, covered, for about 10 minutes. A standard dosage of the tea is two to three cups per day.

Root decoction: Add one ounce of the clean, thinly-sliced dry root, or 2 oz of thinly-sliced fresh root, to 1 pt of unchlorinated water in a non-metallic pot. Bring to a boil and simmer for about 10 minutes. Strain and cover. A decoction may be refrigerated for up to two days and retain its healing qualities.

Tincture: Combine half a cup of dried fennel seeds with 1 pt of brandy or vodka in a glass container. Seal the container with an airtight lid. Leave to macerate in a darkened place for two weeks. Shake daily. Strain the mixture through a cheesecloth or muslin bag and pour into a dark bottle for storage up to two years. Dosage is 2–4 ml of the tincture two times a day.

Precautions

Pregnant women should not use the herb, seeds, tincture, or essential oil of fennel in medicinal remedies. Small amounts used as a culinary spice are considered safe. In large doses fennel acts as a uterine stimulant. The essential oil of fennel is toxic in doses as small as 5 ml, and may cause skin irritation, **vomiting**, seizure, and respiratory problems. The volatile oil should not be ingested. The herb and seed oil may cause **contact dermatitis** in sensitive individuals.

Interactions

None reported.

Resources

BOOKS

Elias, Jason, and Shelagh Ryan Masline. *The A to Z Guide to Healing Herbal Remedies.* New York: Random House Value Publishing, Inc., 1996.

McIntyre, Anne. *The Medicinal Garden.* New York: Henry Holt and Company, LLC, 1997.

Ody, Penelope. *The Complete Medicinal Herbal.* New York: Dorling Kindersley, 1993.

PDR for Herbal Medicines. Montvale, NJ: Medical Economics Company, 1998.

Prevention's 200 Herbal Remedies. Emmaus, PA: Rodale Press, Inc., 1997.

Tierra, Lesley. *The Herbs of Life, Health & Healing Using Western & Chinese Techniques*. Santa Cruz, CA: The Crossing Press, Inc., 1997.

Tyler, Varro E., Ph.D. *Herbs Of Choice, The Therapeutic Use of Phytomedicinals*. New York: The Haworth Press, Inc., 1994.

Tyler, Varro E., Ph.D. *The Honest Herbal*. New York: Pharmaceutical Products Press, 1993.

Weiss, Gaea and Shandor. *Growing & Using The Healing Herbs*. New York: Wings Books, 1992.

PERIODICALS

Diana Erney. "Healing Garden: Fennel's Not Just for Cooking." *Organic Gardening* (September/October 1999): 20.

Clare Hanrahan

Fenugreek

Description

Fenugreek is an herb native to southeastern Europe, northern Africa, and western Asia, but is widely cultivated in other parts of the world. Its botanical name is *Trigonella foenum-graecum*; its English name comes from two Latin words meaning Greek hay. Fenugreek is an annual plant that grows 2–3 ft (0.6–0.9 m) tall, with a strong odor and small pale yellow flowers. The seed of the fenugreek plant contains many active compounds with pharmaceutical applications. The seeds are collected in the autumn. The chemical components of fenugreek seed include **iron**, **vitamin A**, vitamin B_1, **vitamin C**, phosphates, flavonoids, saponins, trigonelline, and other alkaloids. The seed is also high in fiber and protein.

General use

Quite apart from its therapeutic value, fenugreek is used as a seasoning and flavoring agent in foods, particularly in Egypt, India, and the Middle East. The maple smell and flavor of fenugreek have led to its use as a spice in foods, beverages, confections, tobacco, and imitation maple syrup. In some countries, the seeds are eaten raw or boiled, or the greens are enjoyed as a fresh salad. Extracts of fenugreek are used in some cosmetic products as well.

In addition to its use in flavoring foods, the antifungal and antibacterial properties of fenugreek are now being applied to food preservation. In June 2002, a high school student from Maryland was awarded a Lemelson-MIT Invention Apprenticeship for her invention of a food packaging paper made from fenugreek seeds.

The best-documented medical use of fenugreek is to control blood sugar in both insulin-dependent (type 1) and noninsulin-dependent (type 2) diabetics. Some studies also show that serum **cholesterol** levels in diabetics, and perhaps in others, are reduced by fenugreek. Doses as low as 15 mg per day may produce beneficial effects on **fasting** blood sugar, elevation of blood sugar after a meal, and overall glycemic control. The use of fenugreek is likely to alter the diabetic patient's need for insulin or other medications used to control blood sugar. This treatment should be supervised by a health care provider familiar with the use of herbal therapies for diabetes. The recommended doses of fenugreek can vary rather widely.

The seeds of fenugreek can also act as a bulk laxative as a result of their fiber and mucilage content. These portions of the seed swell up from being in contact with **water**, filling the bowel and stimulating peristaltic activity. For laxative purposes, 0.5–1 tsp of freshly powdered herb per cup of water, followed by an additional 8 oz water, can be taken one to three times daily. Patients should begin with the lowest effective dose of fenugreek; they should also avoid taking oral medications or vitamins at the same time as the herb.

Capsules of fenugreek seed are sometimes recommended as a galactogogue, or agent to increase milk production in the lactating mother. This use of the herb should be undertaken cautiously, since the evidence of safety for the nursing infant is only anecdotal. Some commercial teas promoted for the purpose of increasing lactation use fenugreek as an ingredient, but herbal concentration in teas can vary widely and are generally somewhat low.

There is some evidence that internal use of fenugreek seed can decrease some stone-forming substances in the kidney, particularly **calcium** oxalate. Patients who are prone to this type of kidney stone may wish to consult a health care provider about the advisability and dose of fenugreek seed for this use.

Fenugreek may encourage a flagging appetite, and is sometimes given during convalescence from illnesses to improve food intake, weight gain, and speed of recuperation.

Cancer researchers are also studying fenugreek for its potential effectiveness as a cancer chemopreventive. It is thought that fenugreek may help to prevent cancer by raising the levels of vitamin C, **vitamin E**, and other **antioxidants** in the bloodstream.

Historically, fenugreek has been used as a topical treatment for abscesses, **boils**, **burns**, **eczema**, **gout**, and ulceration of the skin as it has an anti-inflammatory effect. It is also reputedly useful for a number of digestive complaints, including **gastritis** and gastric ulcers. A study published in 2002 found that both an aqueous solution and a gel fraction derived from fenugreek have anti-ulcer effects comparable to those of omeprazole, a standard medication given to reduce gastric secretions. The researchers found that the fenugreek solution protected the gastric mucosa from injury as well as reducing the secretion of gastric acid.

Fenugreek reportedly can be helpful in the induction of **childbirth**, as it is known to stimulate uterine contractions. For this reason it should not be taken during **pregnancy**. As a gargle, fenugreek may relieve sore throats and coughing. Arthritis, **bronchitis**, fevers, and male reproductive conditions are other traditional but unsubstantiated indications for this herb.

Preparations

Fenugreek may be purchased as bulk seeds, capsules, tinctures, or in teas. Due to the strong, bitter taste, capsules are used most often. The dose is variable, depending on the form of the herb that is used. The seeds may also be soaked to make a tea. For topical use, powdered fenugreek seed is mixed with water to form a paste. Herbal supplements should be stored in a cool, dry place, away from direct light and out of the reach of children.

Precautions

Fenugreek may, when taken in larger amounts than are used to season foods, cause contractions of the uterus. For this reason, women who are pregnant should avoid therapeutic doses. Frequent topical use of fenugreek preparations may cause skin irritation and sensitization. Symptoms of allergic reaction include swelling, numbness, and **wheezing**. This herb should not be used by anyone with sensitivity to fenugreek. Large doses (over 100 g per day) may cause intestinal symptoms, including **diarrhea**, **nausea**, and **gas**. Blood sugar can also drop to abnormally low levels. Fenugreek is generally recognized as safe, but its safety is not well-documented for use in small children, lactating women, or persons with liver or kidney disease.

Side effects

Depending on the dose used, fenugreek may cause a maple syrup odor in the patient's sweat and urine.

Interactions

Fenugreek can enhance anticoagulant activity, and should not be used with other herbs or medications (heparin, warfarin, ticlopidine) that have this effect due to increased risk of bleeding. It can lower blood sugar to a marked degree; blood sugar levels should be monitored closely, particularly in people who are taking insulin, glipizide, or other hypoglycemic agents. Medications that are being taken to control diabetes may need to have dosages adjusted, which should be done under medical supervision. In theory, since fenugreek is high in mucilage, it can alter the absorption of any oral medication. Corticosteroid and other hormone treatments may be less effective. Monoamine oxidase inhibitors (MAOIs) may have increased activity when used in conjunction with fenugreek.

Resources

BOOKS

Bratman, Steven, and David Kroll. *Natural Health Bible.* Rocklin, CA: Prima Publishing, 1999.

Griffith, H. Winter. *Vitamins, Herbs, Minerals & Supplements: The Complete Guide.* Tucson, AZ: Fisher Books, 1998.

Jellin, Jeff, Forrest Batz, and Kathy Hitchens. *Pharmacist's Letter/Prescriber's Letter Natural Medicines Comprehensive Database.* Stockton, CA: Therapeutic Research Faculty, 1999.

Leninger, Skye. *The Natural Pharmacy.* Rocklin, CA: Prima Health, 1998.

Pelletier, Kenneth R., MD. *The Best Alternative Medicine,* Part I: Naturopathic Medicine. New York: Simon & Schuster, 2002.

PERIODICALS

Devasena, T., and V. P. Menon. "Enhancement of Circulatory Antioxidants by Fenugreek During 1,2-Dimethylhydrazine-Induced Rat Colon Carcinogenesis." *Journal of Biochemistry, Molecular Biology, and Biophysics* 6 (August 2002): 289-292.

Gabay, M. P. "Galactogogues: Medications That Induce Lactation." *Journal of Human Lactation* 18 (August 2002): 274-279.

Genet, S., R. K. Kale, and N. Z. Baquer. "Alterations in Antioxidant Enzymes and Oxidative Damage in Experimental Diabetic Rat Tissues: Effect of Vanadate and Fenugreek (*Trigonellafoenum graecum*)." *Molecular and Cellular Biochemistry* 236 (July 2002): 7-12.

Ohr, Linda M. "Catching Up with Diabetes." *Food Technology* 56 (September 2002): 87-92.

Pandian, R. S., C. V. Anuradha, and P. Viswanathan. "Gastroprotective Effect of Fenugreek Seeds (*Trigonella foenum graecum*) on Experimental Gastric Ulcer in Rats." *Journal of Ethnopharmacology* 81 (August 2002): 393-397.

ORGANIZATIONS

American Botanical Council. PO Box 144345. Austin, TX 78714-4345.

Centre for International Ethnomedicinal Education and Research (CIEER). <www.cieer.org>.

Herb Research Foundation. 1007 Pearl St., Suite 200, Boulder, CO 80302. (303) 449-2265. <www.herbs.org>.

OTHER

MIT News. "Lemelson-MIT Program Awards 2002 High School Apprenticeship to Inventive Maryland Student." <web.mit.edu/invent>.

Judith Turner
Rebecca J. Frey, PhD

Ferrum phosphoricum

Description

Ferrum phosphoricum, abbreviated as *ferrum phos.,* is a homeopathic remedy compound made from **iron** and **phosphorus**. Its name is Latin for iron phosphate. The homeopathic formula of iron phosphate is derived from mixing iron sulfate, phosphate, and **sodium** acetate.

General use

Based on the homeopathic "law of similars," which states that any substance that can cause certain symptoms when given to healthy people can cure sick people with similar symptoms, *ferrum phos.* is the remedy of choice for patients in the early stages of **fever** or other inflammatory conditions. It may also be given to patients suffering from low energy or **anemia**. Of the 2,000–3,000 homeopathic remedies that are available, *ferrum phos.* is one that often appears on "short lists" of those recommended for a home medicine chest.

It is important to note, however, that homeopaths do not prescribe a given remedy on the basis of a few physical symptoms. They try to match the remedy to the totality of the patient's symptoms, including emotional characteristics and personality traits. Thus a classically trained homeopath would not give *ferrum phos.* automatically to every patient who walked into the office complaining of fever or a viral illness. A contemporary American practitioner of **homeopathy** recommends giving *ferrum phos.* when the person does not have clear and distinct symptoms that would point to another remedy. The profile of the *ferrum phos.* person is that he or she has a lower fever and is more alert than one who needs **belladonna** but less upset and fearful than one who needs **aconite**. Where a patient with the belladonna profile may have a face that is flushed all over with fever, the *ferrum phos.* patient has clearly defined pink or red patches on the cheeks. The *ferrum phos.* patient is not focused solely on his or her discomfort and may have conversations with others as if he or she were not ill.

Other characteristics of *ferrum phos.* patients include a tendency to tire easily. They are nervous, sensitive people, disturbed by anxiety-provoking dreams. They may be restless sleepers, even though their illnesses are often brought on by overexertion. In addition, ferrum phos. patients often bleed easily; they are more prone to **nosebleeds** or minor bleeding from the gums at the onset of an illness. If they **cough** up mucus, it is likely to be streaked with blood.

The homeopathic definition of "symptom" is broader than the standard medical understanding. To a homeopath, symptoms represent the body's attempts to deal with an internal or external ailment. They are guides to choosing the correct remedy rather than problems to be suppressed. A homeopathic practitioner who is asking a patient about symptoms will inquire about the circumstances (e.g., light or dark, heat or cold, rest or activity, etc.) that make the patient feel better or worse. These factors are called modalities in homeopathy. In terms of modalities, gentle motion and applications of cold make ferrum phos. patients feel better, while cold air, nighttime, standing up, and heavy exertion make them feel worse.

A homeopathic practitioner might prescribe ferrum phos. for any of the following conditions:

• tickling coughs accompanied by chest pain

• laryngitis

- red and swollen tonsils
- fevers that start slowly
- ear **infections** that have not yet produced pus
- incontinence, involuntary urination with coughing, bedwetting
- rheumatic joints
- menstrual periods that begin with headaches
- anemia
- fatigue
- nosebleeds
- sore throats, especially in singers
- vomiting
- diarrhea
- heart palpitations

Preparations

Ferrum phos. is available in the United States in both liquid and tablet form. It can be purchased from homeopathic pharmacies or over the internet. Common potencies of *ferrum phos.* are 30C and 6X. The abbreviation 30C stands for a centesimal potency. This indicates that a process of dilution, along with vigorous shaking (succussion) of the remedy, has been repeated 30 times to achieve the desired potency. The abbreviation 6X indicates a decimal potency, and means that this decimal dilution has been repeated six times. In homeopathic practice, the strength of the remedy is in inverse proportion to the amount of chemical or plant extract in the alcohol or water; thus a 30C preparation of *ferrum phos.* is considered a much higher potency than a 6X preparation. People using homeopathic remedies at home are generally encouraged to use the lower potencies such as 6X or 12X.

Precautions

The precautions recommended by homeopaths reflect concerns about proper administration of the remedies rather than specifying categories of patients who should not receive a given remedy. The quantity of a homeopathic remedy, for example, is less critical than the frequency of dosing. Homeopathy follows the principle of minimal dosing, which means in practice that the patient is not given a second dose of a remedy (or a dose of a different remedy) until the first has completed its action. Minimal dosing is based on the homeopathic belief that remedies work by stimulating or "jump-starting" the body's own natural defenses against illness rather than by killing germs. In general, however, the more severe the patient's acute symptoms, the more often he or she

would be given the remedy. A *ferrum phos.* patient with a bad cold might be given a dose of the remedy every three to six hours, while one with a milder illness might be given only one or two doses a day.

Precautions regarding homeopathic remedies also include avoiding contamination of the medicine. The patient should not touch the medicine; it should be dispensed into a cup and tipped directly into the patient's mouth. Homeopathic remedies are not taken with water but allowed to dissolve in the mouth. Patients are asked not to eat or drink for about twenty minutes before and after each dose.

Side effects

Homeopathic remedies rarely have side effects in the usual sense of the phrase because they are so dilute. On the other hand, a homeopathic remedy may sometimes appear to be making a patient's symptoms temporarily worse as part of the healing process. This temporary aggravation of the symptoms would be regarded by homeopaths as an indication that the remedy is effectively stimulating the patient's body to heal itself.

Interactions

Homeopathic practitioners are not as a rule concerned with drug interactions, in part because homeopathic remedies are so dilute that there is little of the original substance to interact with a prescription given by an allopathic physician. In addition, the homeopathic "single medicine" principle, according to which a patient is given only one homeopathic remedy at a time for a given illness, also minimizes potential interactions among different remedies. For example, a *ferrum phos.* patient would not be given a different cold or cough remedy unless the homeopath determined that the patient's symptoms were changing and required a remedy with a different symptom profile. There is, however, an ongoing debate among homeopathic practitioners about the legitimacy of combination remedies. Many homeopathic pharmacies sell preparations that are low-potency combinations of the most commonly used remedies for use at home. Conservative homeopaths maintain that the possibility of interactions among the different ingredients makes it difficult to evaluate the effectiveness of these combinations.

Homeopaths are, however, concerned about the effect of other substances on homeopathic preparations. They believe that remedies can lose potency through interaction with heat, light, or other substances. Guidelines for proper storage of homeopathic remedies include keeping them away from strong sunlight and high temperatures, keeping them in their original containers, and not storing them

KEY TERMS

Antidote—Any substance that slows or stops the effects of a homeopathic remedy. Coffee and camphor are considered to be particularly powerful antidotes.

Law of similars—A principle of homeopathic treatment according to which substances that cause specific symptoms in healthy people are given to sick people with similar symptoms.

Modality—A factor or circumstance that makes a patient's symptoms better or worse. Modalities include such factors as time of day, room temperature, the patient's level of activity, sleep patterns, etc.

Potency—The number of times that a homeopathic remedy has been diluted and succussed (shaken). In centesimal potencies, one part of the medicinal substance has been diluted with 99 parts of water or alcohol; in decimal potencies, the ratio is 1:9.

Succussion—A part of the process of making homeopathic remedies, in which the medicinal substance is diluted in distilled water and then shaken vigorously.

Symptom—In homeopathy, a positive sign of the body's self-defense and self-healing that assists the practitioner to choose the correct remedy. Symptoms include the patient's emotional state and psychological characteristics as well as physical symptoms in the narrow sense.

near perfumes, bleach, or other strong-smelling substances. In addition, patients under the care of a homeopath are instructed to avoid coffee or products containing camphor (lip balms, chest rubs, etc.) during a period of homeopathic treatment and for two days after the last dose. Homeopaths believe that these substances counteract or "antidote" the effects of homeopathic remedies.

Resources

BOOKS

Cummings, Stephen, and Dana Ullman. *Everybody's Guide to Homeopathic Medicines.* New York: G. P. Putnam's Sons, 1991.

MacEoin, Beth. *Homeopathy.* New York: HarperCollins Publishers, 1994.

Stein, Diane. "Homeopathy." In *All Women Are Healers: A Comprehensive Guide to Natural Healing.* Freedom, CA: The Crossing Press, 1996.

ORGANIZATIONS

Boiron Research Foundation. 1208 Amosland Road, Norwood, PA 19074.

Homeopathic Educational Services. 2124 Kittredge Street, Berkeley, CA 94704. (510) 649-0294. (800) 359-9051.

International Foundation for the Promotion of Homeopathy. 2366 Eastlake Avenue East, Suite 301, Seattle, WA 98102. (206) 324-8230.

National Center for Homeopathy (NCH). 801 North Fairfax Street, Suite 306, Alexandria, VA 22314. (703) 548-7790. Fax: (703) 548-7792.

Rebecca J. Frey, PhD

Fever

Definition

A fever is a rise in body temperature to greater than 100°F (37.8°C).

Description

A healthy person's body temperature fluctuates between 97°F (36.1°C) and 100°F (37.8°C), with the average being 98.6°F (37°C). The body maintains stability within this range by balancing the heat produced by the metabolism with the heat lost to the environment. The "thermostat" that controls this process is located in the hypothalamus, a small structure located deep within the brain. The nervous system constantly relays information about the body's temperature to the thermostat. In turn, the thermostat activates different physical responses designed to cool or warm the body, depending on the circumstances. These responses include:

- decreasing or increasing the flow of blood from the body's core, where it is warmed, to the surface, where it is cooled

- slowing down or speeding up the rate at which the body turns food into energy (metabolic rate)

- inducing shivering, which generates heat through muscle contraction

- inducing sweating, which cools the body through evaporation

A fever occurs when the body's thermostat resets at a higher temperature, which primarily happens in response to an infection. To reach the higher temperature, the body moves blood to the warmer interior, increases the metabolic rate, and induces shivering. The chills that often accompany a fever are caused by the movement of blood to the body's core, which leaves the surface and extremities cold. Once the body reaches the higher temperature, the shivering and chills stop. When the infection has been overcome or drugs such as aspirin or acetaminophen (Tylenol) have

A dramatic rise in body temperature often includes the following symptoms: A. Loss of fluid results in dehydration. B. The hypothalamic set-point is increased, raising metabolism. C. Blood vessels in skin dilate. D. Sweat glands produce excess perspiration. E. Increased pulse rate. F. Increased hypothalmic set-point may introduce chills **and shivering to promote heat production from muscles. G. Skin becomes more heat-sensitive.** *(Illustration by Electronic Illustrators Group. The Gale Group)*

been taken, the thermostat resets to normal. When this happens, the body's cooling mechanisms switch on. The blood moves to the surface and sweating occurs.

Fever is an important component of the immune response, though its role is not completely understood. Physicians believe that an elevated body temperature has several effects. Certain chemicals in the immune system react with the fever-inducing agent and trigger the resetting of the thermostat. These immune system chemicals also increase the production of cells that fight off the invading bacteria or viruses. Higher temperatures also inhibit the growth of some bacteria and speed up the chemical reactions that help the body's cells repair themselves. Changes in blood circulation may cause the heart rate to increase, which speeds the arrival of white blood cells to the sites of infection.

Causes & symptoms

Fevers are primarily caused by viral or bacterial **infections**, such as **pneumonia** or **influenza**. However, other conditions can induce a fever, including these:

- allergic reactions
- autoimmune diseases
- trauma, such as breaking a bone
- cancer
- excessive exposure to the sun
- intense **exercise**
- hormonal imbalances
- certain drugs
- damage to the hypothalamus

When an infection occurs, fever-inducing agents called pyrogens are released, either by the body's immune system or by the invading cells themselves. These pyrogens trigger the resetting of the thermostat. In other circumstances, an uncontrolled release of pyrogens may occur when the immune system overreacts due to an allergic reaction or becomes damaged due to an autoimmune disease. A **stroke** or tumor can damage the hypothalamus, causing the body's thermostat to malfunction.

Excessive exposure to the sun or intense exercise in hot weather can result in heat stroke, a condition in which the body's cooling mechanisms fail. Malignant **hyperthermia** is a rare, inherited condition in which a person develops a very high fever when given certain anesthetics or muscle relaxants in preparation for surgery.

A recent study showed that most parents have misconceptions about fever and view it as a disease rather than a symptom. How long a fever lasts and how high it may go depend on several factors, including its cause and the patient's age and overall health. Most fevers caused by infections are acute, appearing suddenly and then dissipating as the immune system defeats the infectious agent. An infectious fever may also rise and fall throughout the day, reaching its peak in the late afternoon or early evening. A low-grade fever that lasts for several weeks is associated with autoimmune diseases such as lupus or with some cancers, particularly **leukemia** and lymphoma.

Diagnosis

A fever is usually diagnosed using a thermometer. A variety of different thermometers are available, including traditional oral and rectal thermometers made of glass and mercury, and more sophisticated electronic ones that can be inserted in the ear. For adults and older children, temperature readings are usually taken orally. Younger children who cannot or will not hold a thermometer in their mouths can have their temperatures taken by placing an oral thermometer under their armpits. Infants generally have their temperature taken rectally using a rectal thermometer.

As important as registering a patient's temperature is determining the underlying cause of the fever. The physician can make a diagnosis by checking for accompanying symptoms and by reviewing the patient's medical history, any recent trips he or she has taken, what he or she may have ingested, or any illnesses he or she has been exposed to. Blood tests hold additional clues. Antibodies in the blood point to the presence of an infectious agent, which can be verified by growing the organism in a culture. Blood tests can also provide the doctor with white blood cell counts. Ultrasound tests, magnetic resonance imaging (MRI) tests, or computed tomography (CT) scans may be ordered if the doctor cannot readily determine the cause of a fever.

Treatment

Often, doctors must remind patients, especially parents, not to "overtreat" low fevers but to remember that they are symptoms of an underlying disease or condition. Alternative therapies for treatment of fever focus not only on reducing fever but also on boosting the immune function to help the body fight infections more effectively. They include nutritional therapy, herbal therapy and **traditional Chinese medicine**.

Nutritional therapy

Naturopaths often recommend that patients take high doses of **vitamin C** to ward off diseases and prevent fever. In addition to vitamin C, other **antioxidants** such as **vitamin A** and **zinc** also boost the immune function. Naturopaths may also suggest reducing sugar intake (even fruit juices) because sugar depresses the immune system. To replace fluid that is lost during fever, patients are advised to drink vegetable juices and eat soups.

Herbal therapy

Western herbalists use tea preparations containing herbs such as bupleurum root or **boneset** to reduce fever. Mild herbs such as **peppermint**, elderflower, or **yarrow** can provide comfort to the child who has a mild fever. Others believe in sweating a fever out, literally. They often recommend that patients take hot baths to induce sweating. This helps induce or increase fever, which is believed to help the body get rid of infections.

Chinese medicine (TCM) offers many herbs and formulas for fevers. There are many distinct kinds of fevers, also called heat syndromes. For example, an excess-heat syndrome is characterized by a high fever, great thirst, and lots of sweating. Deficiency heat syndrome is characterized by a low-grade fever with afternoon fevers or night sweats. For excess heat, herbs that are dispersing and cold in nature are used. For chronic and low-grade fevers, herbs that tonify the yin (cooling aspect) are used as well as herbs that get rid of heat. There are even herbs such as bupleurum root (called *Chai Hu* in TCM) that are used for intermittent fevers or conditions alternating between fever and chills. Alternating fevers and chills occur in **malaria**, conditions connected to **AIDS**, **chronic fatigue syndrome**, and Epstein-Barr virus. The individual pattern should be diagnosed by a trained practitioner.

Aromatherapy

Patients can reduce feverish symptoms by inhaling **essential oils** of camphor, **eucalyptus**, lemon, and **hyssop**. These oils can also be mixed with an unscented body lotion or a vegetable oil for **aromatherapy** massage.

Homeopathy

Homeopathic doctors may prescribe herbal remedies based on the patient's overall personality profile as well as specific symptoms.

Allopathic treatment

Physicians agree that the most effective treatment for a fever is to address its underlying cause. Also, because a fever helps the immune system fight infection, some clinicians suggest it be allowed to run its course. Drugs to lower fever (antipyretics) can be given if a patient (particularly a child) is uncomfortable. These include aspirin, acetaminophen (Tylenol), and ibuprofen (Advil). Aspirin, however, should not be given to a child or adolescent with a fever since this drug has been linked to an increased risk of Reye's syndrome. Sponging a child or infant with tepid (lukewarm) water can also help reduce mild fevers.

A fever requires emergency treatment under the following circumstances:

- Newborn (three months or younger) with a fever above 100.5°F (38°C).

- Infant or child with a fever above 103°F (39.4°C). A very high fever in a small child can trigger seizures (febrile seizures) and therefore should be treated immediately.

- Fever accompanied by severe **headache**, neck stiffness, mental confusion, or severe swelling of the throat. A fever accompanied by these symptoms can indicate the presence of a serious infection, such as **meningitis**, and should be brought to the immediate attention of a physician.

Expected results

Most fevers caused by infection end as soon as the immune system rids the body of the pathogen. Most fevers do not produce any lasting effects. The prognosis for fevers associated with more chronic conditions, such as autoimmune disease, depends upon the overall outcome of the disorder.

Resources

BOOKS

Bennett, J. Claude, and Fred Plum, eds. *Cecil Textbook of Medicine*. Philadelphia: W. B. Saunders, 1996.

"Children's Health." In *Alternative Medicine: The Definitive Guide*, compiled by The Burton Goldberg Group. Tiburon, CA: Future Medicine Publishing, 1999.

"Fever and Chills." In *Reader's Digest Guide to Medical Cures and Treatment*. New York: Reader's Digest Association, 1996.

Gelfand, Jeffrey, et al. "Fever, Including Fever of Unknown Origin." In *Harrison's Principles of Internal Medicine*, edited by Kurt Isselbacher, et al. New York: McGraw-Hill, 1997.

Tierney, Lawrence M., M.D., et al., eds. *Current Medical Diagnosis and Treatment*. Stamford, CT: Appleton & Lange, 1996.

KEY TERMS

Antipyretic—A drug that lowers fever, like aspirin or acetaminophen.

Autoimmune disease—Condition in which a person's immune system attacks the body's own cells, causing tissue destruction.

Epstein-Barr virus—A common herpes virus that is responsible for causing infectious mononucleosis. This virus is problematic in people who have a compromised immune system.

Febrile seizure—Convulsions brought on by fever.

Malignant hyperthermia—A rare, inherited condition in which a person develops a very high fever when given certain anesthetics or muscle relaxants in preparation for surgery.

Meningitis—A potentially fatal inflammation of the thin membrane covering the brain and spinal cord.

Metabolism—The chemical process by which the body turns food into energy, which can be given off as heat.

Pyrogen—A chemical circulating in the blood that causes a rise in body temperature.

Reye's syndrome—A disorder principally affecting the liver and brain, marked by the rapid development of life-threatening neurological symptoms.

PERIODICALS

Bernath, Vivienne F. "Tepid Sponging and Paracetamol for Reduction of Body Temperature in Febrile Children." *The Medical Journal of Australia* (February 4, 2002):130.

Huffman, Grace B. "Parental Misconceptions about Fever in Children." *American Family Physician* (February 1, 2002):482.

Mai Tran
Teresa G. Odle

Fever blister *see* **Cold sores**

Feverfew

Description

Feverfew (*Chrysanthemum parthenium* or *Tanacetum parthenium*) is named for one of the herb's traditional medicinal uses as a febrifuge, from the Latin *febrifu-*

gia, indicating its fever-reducing action. This European native of the Compositae (Asteraceae) or aster family has naturalized throughout North and South America, escaping from cultivation. It can be found along roadsides and along the borders of wooded areas. Other common names include featherfew, febrifuge plant, featherfoil, mid-summer daisy, and wild **chamomile**.

Feverfew is a bushy and herbaceous perennial that grows from a branched and tapering root to produce erect, round and slightly grooved stems. The feathery, aromatic and bitter-tasting leaves are arranged alternately along the length of the many-branched stem. They are a yellow-green, stalked, and bipinnate with deeply cut, toothed segments in an oval shape. Flowers bloom in mid to late-summer in flat-topped clusters at the end of stems that may reach to a height of three feet. Smaller than daisies, and without the protruding central disk of chamomile, feverfew blossoms have yellow centers consisting of tightly-bunched tubular florets surrounded by creamy white rays. Bees seem to avoid feverfew, deterred by its pungent aroma. The plant self-seeds freely, and thrives in full sun or partial shade in most soil.

General use

Feverfew leaves and flowers are used medicinally. Among its many uses, the herb has become a popular and proven herbal remedy for the treatment of migraine headaches. This important use of the plant was recorded as far back as 1633 by the British herbalist Gerard. With frequent use, over time, feverfew can reduce the frequency, severity, and duration of migraine headaches and allay **nausea** and **vomiting**. It is most effective when used as a preventive. It acts to inhibit serotonin and histamine, substances that dilate blood vessels, and helps to prevent the spasms in blood vessels that trigger migraine headaches. This much-researched herb has been shown to inhibit production of leukotines and other inflammatory substances. It is an effective remedy for relieving the **pain** and inflammation of arthritis and alleviating **hay fever**, **asthma** and other allergy symptoms.

Other traditional uses of feverfew dating back to ancient Greece and Rome include its use as an emmenagogue, which is an infusion taken in cases of sluggish **menstruation** to relieve congestion and promote periodic flow. The herb has also been used after **childbirth** to help expel the placenta.

Feverfew was valued in past centuries for its believed protection against the plague and the bite of mad dogs. In the seventeenth century the herbalist John Parkinson recommended feverfew as a remedy to speed recovery from opium overdose. It has also been used in treating alcoholic delirium tremens, and to expel intesti-

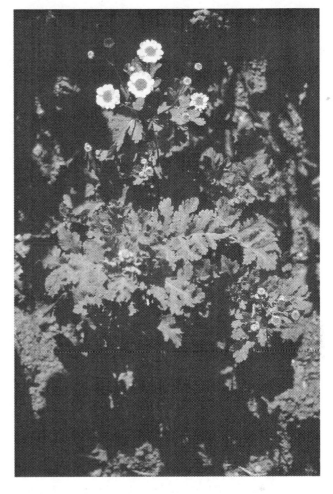

Feverfew (*Tanacetum parthenium*). *(Photo by Henriette Kress. Reproduced by permission.)*

nal **worms**. The English physician Culpeper recommended an external application of the fresh herb to treat ague, as the disease **malaria** was once called. Feverfew is a bitter digestive and liver tonic. A hot infusion may reduce **fever** and congestion from colds. The infusion, taken cold, has tonic properties. Feverfew may relieve mild **depression**, promote restful sleep, and ease the nerve pain of **sciatica** and **shingles**. Externally the strong infusion is an antiseptic skin wash for treatment of insect stings and bites. The wash may also be used as an insect repellent. Feverfew leaves and stems, gathered fresh, may be used as a dye plant, with a chrome mordant, to produce a light green-yellow color in natural fibres such as wool. Feverfew flowers have a purgative action if ingested, and if the blossom heads are carried into areas where bees are located, the insects will fly away.

The active compounds in feverfew include sesquiterpene lactones, predominantly parthenolide. Other phytochemicals include pyrethrin, volatile oils, tannins, bitter resin, and flavonoids.

Preparations

Feverfew should be harvested just as the plant comes into flower and before the blossoms are fully open. Leaves are removed from the stalks and dried on paper-lined trays in a light, airy room, away from direct sunlight. The dried herb should be stored in clearly-labeled, tightly-sealed, dark glass containers.

Capsules: Feverfew leaf in capsule form, at a 250 mg daily dose, is recommended for medicinal use. It may take four to six weeks before the herb provides noticeable relief. Studies of some commercially-prepared capsules revealed that many did not contain a sufficient quantity of the active ingredient to be medicinally effective. Feverfew may be more medicinally potent when gathered fresh. Three to four fresh leaves, taken daily over a period of time are medicinally effective. A certified practitioner can help determine the most effective and safest levels for individual cases.

Syrup: Fresh feverfew leaf can be added to honey, or to a simple sugar syrup. The honey will act as a preservative and mask the bitter taste of the herb.

Infusion: Two to three teaspoons of chopped, fresh feverfew leaves are placed in a warmed container. One cup of fresh, nonchlorinated boiled water is added to the herbs and the mixture is covered. The tea is infused for about 15 minutes, then strained. A stronger infusion, using double the amount of leaf and steeping twice as long, is useful as a skin wash for repelling insects, or soothing inflammations and **wounds**. The strong infusion has also been used as a mouthwash following tooth extraction. The prepared tea will store for about two days in the refrigerator in an airtight container. Dosage: Feverfew may be enjoyed by the cupful three times a day.

Tincture: Combine four ounces of finely-cut fresh, or powdered dry herb with one pint of brandy, gin, or vodka, in a glass container. The alcohol should be enough to cover the plant parts. Place the mixture away from light for about two weeks, shaking several times each day. Strain and store in a tightly capped, dark glass bottle. A standard dose is 30 drops of the tincture three times a day.

Precautions

Since herbal preparations are not regulated by the Food and Drug Administration (FDA), consumers in the United States should check the labels of commercial products carefully for dosage instructions and the part(s) of the plant used for or contained in the product. A 2002 study of commercial feverfew preparations found wide variations in the recommended dosages and parthenolide contents of the products that were tested. The researchers found that ".. intake of parthenolide would range from 0.06 to 9.7 mg/day, a 160-fold variation." Any adverse effects from feverfew preparations or any other herbal products sold as dietary supplements should be reported to the FDA's Center for Food Safety and Applied **Nutrition**, listed under Resources.

Feverfew should not be used by pregnant or lactating women. Children under two years of age should not be given feverfew. Chewing the fresh leaves may irritate the mucous membranes in the mouth causing mouth ulcers in some persons. Traditionally the fresh herb was enclosed between slices of bread to minimize the irritation and mask the bitter taste of the fresh leaves. Persons on prescribed blood-thinning drugs should not ingest feverfew as it might interfere with the rate of blood clotting.

Side effects

Feverfew is a safe herb of proven medicinal value. No side effects are reported when taken in designated therapeutic doses. Some cases of **contact dermatitis** and airborne **dermatitis**, however, have been reported by researchers in Denmark and the United States.

Interactions

According to the *PDR For Herbal Medicines*, feverfew may interact with anti-thrombotic medications, including aspirin and warfarin. The tannins in feverfew have been reported to interfere with **iron** absorption in persons who take supplemental iron.

Taking NSAIDs together with feverfew will decrease the beneficial effects of the herb.

Resources

BOOKS

Duke, James A., Ph.D. *The Green Pharmacy*. Emmaus, PA: Rodale Press, 1997.

Hoffmann, David. *The New Holistic Herbal*. 3rd ed. Boston: Element Books, Inc., 1991.

McIntyre, Anne. *The Medicinal Garden*. New York: Henry Holt and Company, Inc., 1997.

PDR for Herbal Medicines. Montvale, NJ: Medical Economics Company, 1998.

Pelletier, Kenneth R., MD. *The Best Alternative Medicine*, Part I: Western Herbal Medicine. New York: Simon & Schuster, 2002.

Prevention's 200 Herbal Remedies. Emmaus, PA: Rodale Press, Inc., 1997.

Schar, Douglas. *The Backyard Medicine Chest, An Herbal Primer*. Washington, DC: Elliott & Clark Publishing, 1995.

Tyler, Varro E., Ph.D. *Herbs Of Choice, The Therapeutic Use of Phytomedicinals*. New York: The Haworth Press, Inc., 1994.

KEY TERMS

Antispasmodic—A substance that relieves spasms in blood vessels or cramping in muscles. Feverfew has antispasmodic properties.

Delirium tremens—A potentially fatal withdrawal syndrome in persons who have become physically dependent on alcohol, characterized by shaking, sweating, hallucinations, nausea, and agitation.

Emmenagogue—A substance or medication given to bring on a woman's menstrual period.

Flavonoids—Plant pigments that have a variety of effects on human physiology.

Histamine—A substance released from cells that causes some of the symptoms of an allergic reaction.

Nonsteroidal anti-inflammatory drugs (NSAIDs)—A term used for a group of pain-relieving medications that also reduce inflammation when used over a period of time. NSAIDs are often given to patients with osteoarthritis.

Parthenolide—A sesquiterpene lactone isolated from feverfew that is thought to be responsible for most of its medical effectiveness.

Volatile oil—A concentrated oil that has been distilled from a plant; "volatile" means that the oil evaporates at room temperature.

Weiss, Gaea and Shandor. *Growing & Using The Healing Herbs.* New York: Wings Books, 1992.

PERIODICALS

Craig, Winston J. "Feverfew: For the Relief of Migraines." *Vibrant Life* 18 (July-August 2002): 40-41.

Nelson, M. H., S. E. Cobb, and J. Shelton. "Variations in Parthenolide Content and Daily Dose of Feverfew Products." *American Journal of Health-System Pharmacy* 59 (August 15, 2002): 1527-1531.

Paulsen, E., L. P. Christensen, and K. E. Andersen. "Do Monoterpenes Released from Feverfew (*Tanacetum parthenium*) Plants Cause Airborne Compositae Dermatitis?" *Contact Dermatitis* 47 (July 2002): 14-18.

Pfaffenrath, V., H. C. Diener, M. Fischer, et al. "The Efficacy and Safety of *Tanacetum parthenium* (Feverfew) in Migraine Prophylaxis— A Double-Blind, Multicentre, Randomized Placebo-Controlled Dose-Response Study." *Cephalalgia* 22 (September 2002): 523-532.

ORGANIZATIONS

American Botanical Council. 6200 Manor Road, Austin, TX 78714-4345. (512) 926-4900. <www.herbalgram.org>.

Herb Research Foundation. 1007 Pearl St., Suite 200, Boulder, CO 80302. (303) 449-2265. <www.herbs.org>.

United States Food and Drug Administration (FDA), Center for Food Safety and Applied Nutrition. 5100 Paint Branch Parkway, College Park, MD 20740. (888) SAFEFOOD. <www.cfsan.fda.gov>.

OTHER

"Feverfew." HolisticOnLine. http://www.holistic-online.com/Herbal-Med.

Clare Hanrahan
Rebecca J. Frey, PhD

Feverwort *see* **Boneset**

Fibrocystic breast disease

Definition

Fibrocystic breast disease is a general term that refers to a variety of symptoms and diagnoses, including breast lumpiness, tenderness, and a wide range of vaguely-defined benign breast conditions. The term is also used diagnostically to describe the appearance of breast tissues viewed under the microscope, on x-ray film, or on ultrasound equipment.

Description

There is no such thing as a typical or normal female breast. Breasts come in all shapes and sizes, with varying textures from smooth to extremely lumpy. The tissues of the female breast change in response to hormone levels, normal **aging**, nursing (lactation), weight shifts, and injury. To further complicate matters, the breast has several types of tissue, each of which may respond differently to changes in body chemistry.

Fibrocystic breast disease is clearly not a single, specific disease process. Variations or changes in the way the breast feels or looks on an x ray may cause the condition to be called "fibrocystic change." Other names have been used to refer to this imprecise and ill-defined term: mammary dysplasia, mastopathy, chronic cystic mastitis, indurative mastopathy, mastalgia, lumpy breasts, or physiologic nodularity.

Estimates vary, but 40–90% of all women have some evidence of fibrocystic condition, change, or disease. It is most common among women ages 30–50, but may be seen at other ages.

Causes & symptoms

Fibrocystic condition refers to technical findings. This discussion will focus on symptoms a woman expe-

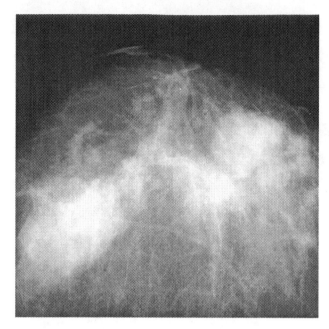

A mammogram of a female breast, indicating multiple cysts.
(Custom Medical Stock photo. Reproduced by permission.)

riences, which may fall under the general category of the fibrocystic condition.

The breast is not a soft, smooth, pulpy organ. It is actually a type of sweat gland. Milk, the breasts' version of sweat, is secreted when the breast receives appropriate hormonal and environmental stimulation.

The normal breast contains milk glands, with their accompanying ducts, or pipelines, for transporting the milk. These complex structures may not only alter in size, but can increase or decrease in number as needed. Fibrous connective tissue, fatty tissue, nerves, blood and lymph vessels, and lymph nodes, with their different shapes and textures, lie among the ever-changing milk glands. This explains why a woman's breasts may not feel uniform in texture, and why "lumpiness" may wax and wane.

Fibrocystic condition is the tenderness, enlargement, and/or changing lumpiness that many women encounter just before or during their menstrual periods. At this time, female hormones are preparing the breasts for **pregnancy**, by stimulating the milk-producing cells and storing fluid. Each breast may contain as much as three to six teaspoons of excess liquid. Swelling, with increased sensitivity or **pain**, may result. If pregnancy does not occur, the body reabsorbs the fluid, and the engorgement and discomfort are relieved.

These symptoms range from mildly annoying in some women to extremely painful in others. The severity of the sensations may vary from month to month in the same woman. Although sometimes distressing, this ex-

perience is the body's normal response to routine hormonal changes.

This cycle of breast sensitivity, pain, and/or enlargement can also result from medications. Some hormone replacement therapies used for post-menopausal women can produce these effects. Other medications, primarily, but not exclusively, those with hormones, may also provoke these symptoms.

Breast pain unrelated to hormone shifts is called "noncyclic" pain. This area-specific pain is also called "trigger-zone breast pain," and it may be continuous, or may be felt intermittently. Trauma, such as a blow to the area, or a breast biopsy performed several years before, or sensitivity to certain medications may also underlie this type of pain. Fibrocystic condition may be cited as the cause of otherwise unexplained breast pain.

Lumps, apart from those clearly associated with hormone cycles, may also be placed under the heading of fibrocystic condition. These lumps stand out from enlarged general breast tissue. The obvious concern with such lumps is **cancer**, although noncancerous lumps also occur. Two noncancerous types, fibroadenomas and cysts, are discussed here.

Fibroadenomas are tumors which form in the tissues outside the milk ducts. The cause of fibroadenomas is unknown. They generally feel smooth and firm, with a somewhat rubber-like texture. Typically a fibroadenoma is not attached to surrounding tissue, and will move slightly when touched. They are most commonly found in adolescents and women in their early 20s but can arise at any age.

Cysts are fluid-filled sacs in the breast. They probably develop as ducts become clogged with old cells in the process of normal emptying and filling. Cysts usually feel soft and round or oval. However, a cyst deep within the breast may feel hard, as it pushes up against firmer breast tissue. A woman with a cyst may experience pain, especially if it increases in size before her menstrual cycle, as many do. Women age 30–50 are most likely to develop cysts.

Sometimes one area of breast tissue persistently feels thicker or more prominent than the rest of the breast. This may be caused by hardened scar tissue and/or dead fat tissue from surgery or trauma. Often the cause of such tissue is unknown.

A number of other breast problems which are benign or noncancerous may be placed under the heading of fibrocystic condition. These include disorders which may lead to breast inflammation (mastitis), infection, nipple discharge, dilated milk ducts, milk-filled cyst, wart-like growth in the duct, and excess growth of fibrous tissue around the glands.

Diagnosis

Breast cancer is the concern in most cases of an abnormal breast symptom. A newly discovered breast lump should be brought to the attention of a family physician or an obstetrician-gynecologist. A physical examination of the area is usually performed. Depending on the findings, the patient may be referred for tests.

The most common tests are mammography and breast ultrasound. A cyst may be definitively diagnosed by ultrasound. To relieve the discomfort, the patient may choose to have the cyst suctioned, or drained. If there is any question as to the fluid diagnosis, the fluid is sent for analysis.

If a lump cannot be proven benign by mammography and ultrasound, a breast biopsy may be considered. Tissue is removed through a needle to obtain a sample of the lump. The sample is examined under the microscope by a pathologist, and a detailed diagnosis regarding the type of benign lesion or cancer is established.

A ductogram evaluates nipple discharge. A very fine tube is threaded into the duct, dye is injected, and the area is looked at for diagnosis. Other breast conditions such as inflammation or infection are usually recognized on the basis of suspicious history, such as breast-feeding and characteristic symptoms such as pain, redness, and swelling. A positive response to appropriate therapies will support the diagnosis.

Treatment

Warm soaks, heating pads, or ice packs may provide comfort. A well-fitted support bra worn day and night can minimize physical movement and do much to relieve breast discomfort. Breast massage may promote removal of excess fluid from tissues and alleviate symptoms. Massaging the breast with **castor oil**, straight or infused with herbs or diluted **essential oils**, can help reduce and dissipate fibroadenomas as well as keep women in touch with changes in their breasts.

Many women have reported relief of symptoms when **caffeine** was reduced or eliminated from their **diets**. Decreasing salt intake before and during the period when breasts are most sensitive may also ease swelling and discomfort. Vitamins A, B complex, and E and **selenium** supplements have been reported to be helpful. Because fat promotes estrogen production, and estrogen is thought to be linked to breast tenderness, low-fat diets and elimination of dairy products also seem to decrease soreness for some women. Restricting salt intake may also help reduce fluid retention and lessen

breast pain. It may take several months to realize the effects of these various treatments.

Evening primrose oil (*Oenothera biennis*), flax oil, and fish oils have been reported to be effective in relieving cyclic breast pain for some women. In addition, a focus on liver cleansing is important to assist the body in conjugation and elimination of excess estrogens. The herb chaste tree (*Vitex angus-castus*) can be used to help relieve symptoms of **premenstrual syndrome** (PMS), including breast tenderness.

A Chinese herbalist may recommend Herba cum Radice Asari with Radix Angelicae Sinensis and Flos Carthami Tinctorii for painful breast lumps, or Rhizoma Cyperi Rotundi with Radix Bupleuri and Fructus Trichosanthis for breast masses that swell around the time of **menstruation**.

Allopathic treatment

A lump that has been proven benign can be left in the breast. Some women may choose to have a lump such as a fibroadenoma surgically removed, especially if it is large. **Infections** are treated with warm compresses and antibiotics. Lactating women are encouraged to continue breastfeeding, as it promotes drainage and healing. A serious infection may progress to form an **abscess** which may need surgical drainage.

Once a specific disorder within the broad category of fibrocystic condition is identified, treatment can be prescribed. Symptoms of cyclical breast sensitivity and engorgement may be treated with diet, medication, and/or physical modifications.

Over-the-counter analgesics (pain relievers) such as acetaminophen (Tylenol) or ibuprofen (Advil) may be recommended. In some cases, treatment with hormones or hormone blockers may prove successful. Birth control pills may be prescribed.

Expected results

Most benign breast conditions carry no increased risk for the development of breast cancer. However, a small percentage of biopsies will uncover overgrowth of tissue in a particular pattern in some women that indicates a 15–20% risk of developing breast cancer over the next 20 years. Strict attention to early detection measures, such as annual mammograms, is especially important for these women.

Prevention

No way has yet been proven to prevent the various manifestations of fibrocystic condition from occurring.

Some alternative practitioners believe that elimination of foods high in methylxanthines (primarily coffee and chocolate) can decrease or reverse fibrocystic breast changes.

Resources

BOOKS

Kneece, Judy C. *Finding a Lump In Your Breast.* Columbia, SC: EduCare Publishing, 1996.

Love, Susan M., with Karen Lindsey. *Dr. Susan Love's Breast Book.* 2nd ed. Reading, MA: Addison-Wesley, 1995.

PERIODICALS

"Benign Conditions." *Harvard Women's Health Watch* 5 (May 1998): 4–5.

Paula Ford-Martin

Fibroids *see* **Uterine fibroids**

Fibromyalgia

Definition

Fibromyalgia is described as inflammation of the fibrous or connective tissue of the body. Widespread muscle **pain**, **fatigue**, and multiple tender points characterize these conditions. Many individuals with fibromyalgia describe the symptoms as similar to the aches and pains of a severe case of the flu. Fibrositis, fibromyalgia, and fibromyositis are names given to a set of symptoms believed to be caused by the same general problem.

Description

Fibromyalgia is more common than previously thought, with as many as 3-6% of the population affected by the disorder. Fibromyalgia is more prevalent in adults than children, with more women affected than men, particularly women of childbearing age.

Causes & symptoms

The exact cause of fibromyalgia is not known. Sometimes it occurs in several members of a family, suggesting that it may be an inherited disorder. People with fibromyalgia are most likely to complain of three primary symptoms: muscle and joint pain, stiffness, and fatigue.

Pain is the major symptom with aches, tenderness, and stiffness of multiple muscles, joints, and soft tissues. The pain also tends to move from one part of the body to another. It is most common in the neck, shoulders, chest, arms, legs, hips, and back. Although the pain is present most of the time and may last for years, the severity of the pain may fluctuate.

Symptoms of fatigue may result from the individual's chronic pain coupled with **anxiety** about the problem and how to find relief. The inflammatory process also produces chemicals that are known to cause fatigue. Other common symptoms are tension headaches, difficulty swallowing, recurrent abdominal pain, **diarrhea**, and numbness or tingling of the extremities. **Stress**, anxiety, **depression**, or lack of sleep can increase symptoms. Intensity of symptoms is variable ranging from gradual improvement to episodes of recurrent symptoms.

Diagnosis

Diagnosis is difficult and frequently missed because symptoms of fibromyalgia are vague and generalized. Coexisting nerve and muscle disorders such as **rheumatoid arthritis**, spinal arthritis, or **Lyme disease** may further complicate the diagnostic process. Presently, there are no tests available to specifically diagnose fibromyalgia. The diagnosis is usually made after ruling out other medical conditions with similar symptoms.

Because of the emotional distress experienced by people with this condition and the influence of stress on the symptoms themselves, fibromyalgia has often been labeled a psychological problem. Recognition of the underlying inflammatory process involved in fibromyalgia has helped promote the validity of this disease.

The American College of Rheumatology has developed standards for fibromyalgia that health care practitioners can use to diagnose this condition. According to these standards, a person is thought to have fibromyalgia if he or she has widespread pain in combination with tenderness in at least 11 of the 18 sites known as trigger points. Trigger point sites include the base of the neck, along the backbone, in front of the hip and elbow, and at the rear of the knee and shoulder.

Treatment

There is no known cure for fibromyalgia. Therefore, the goal of treatment is successful symptom management. Treatment usually requires a combination of therapies, **exercise**, and lifestyle adjustments. Adequate rest is essential in the treatment of fibromyalgia. The diet should include a large variety of fruits and vegetables, which provide the body with trace elements and minerals that are necessary for healthy muscles. Avoidance of stimulating foods or drinks (such as coffee) and medications like decongestants prior to bedtime is advised. A patient's clear understanding of his or her role in the recovery process is imperative for successful management of this condition.

Treatments found to be helpful include heat and occasionally cold compress applications. A regular stretching program is often useful. Aerobic activities focusing on increasing the heart rate are the preferred forms of exercise over most other forms of exertion. Exercise programs need to include good warm-up and cool-down sessions, with special attention given to avoiding exercises causing joint pain. **Hydrotherapy** exercises (exercises in a pool or tub) may be useful in providing a low impact exercise environment while soothing muscle and joint pain.

Massage therapy can be helpful, especially when a family member is instructed on specific massage techniques to manage episodes of increased symptoms. Short sessions are most helpful as repetitious movement can aggravate the condition. Specific attention to mental health, including psychological consultation, may also be important, since depression may precede or accompany fibromyalgia. **Relaxation** exercises, **yoga**, **aromatherapy**, **guided imagery**, and other relaxation therapies can be useful in easing stress and promoting overall well-being. **Acupuncture** can be very helpful for symptom relief and in easing the general condition.

Herbalists and aromatherapists may recommend tub soaks or compresses with **lavender** (*Lavandula angustifolia*), **chamomile** (*Chamaemelum nobilis*), or **juniper** (*Juniperus communis*) to soothe muscle and joint pain.

Allopathic treatment

People with fibromyalgia often need a rheumatology consultation (a meeting with a doctor who specializes in disorders of the joints, muscles, and soft tissue) to decide the cause of various rheumatic symptoms, to be educated about fibromyalgia and its treatment, and to exclude other rheumatic diseases. A treatment program must be individualized to meet the patient's needs. The rheumatologist, as the team leader, enlists and coordinates the expertise of other health professionals in the care of the patient.

If diet, exercise, and adequate rest do not relieve the symptoms of fibromyalgia, medications may be pre-

---

KEY TERMS

Connective tissue—Tissue that supports and binds other body tissue and parts.

Lyme disease—An acute recurrent inflammatory disease involving one or a few joints, believed to be transmitted by a tickborne virus. The condition was originally described in the community of Lyme, Connecticut, but has also been reported in other parts of the United States and other countries. Knees and other large joints are most commonly involved with local inflammation and swelling.

Rheumatology—The study of disorders characterized by inflammation, degeneration of connective tissue, and related structures of the body. These disorders are sometimes collectively referred to as rheumatism.

---

scribed. Medications prescribed and found to have some benefit include antidepressant drugs, muscle relaxants, and anti-inflammatory drugs.

Expected results

Fibromyalgia is a chronic health problem. The symptoms sometimes improve and at other times worsen, but they often continue for months to years.

Prevention

There is no known or specific prevention for fibromyalgia. However, similar to many other medical conditions, remaining as healthy as possible with a good diet, safe exercise, and adequate rest is the best prevention.

Resources

BOOKS

Skelly, Mari et al. *Alternative Treatments for Fibromyalgia & Chronic Fatigue Syndrome: Insights from Practitioners and Patients.* Alameda, CA: Hunter House, 1999.

ORGANIZATIONS

The American College of Rheumatology. 60 Executive Park S., Ste. 150, Atlanta, GA 30329. (404) 633-3777. http://www.rheumatology.org.

Arthritis Foundation. 1330 W. Peachtree Street, Atlanta, GA 30309. (800) 283-7800. http://www.arthritis.org.

Paula Ford-Martin

Fish oil

Description

Fish oils are derived from such cold-water fish as salmon, cod, tuna, or mackerel. They have recently acquired a new visibility as dietary supplements because they are high in **omega-3 fatty acids**. Omega-3 fatty acids, together with the **omega-6 fatty acids**, are important components of a healthful diet. The body cannot manufacture them, therefore they must be obtained from grains, fruits, vegetable oils, and other foods. In addition, people should consume a balanced ratio of omega-6 and omega-3 fatty acids. Some researchers believe that these two types of fatty acids should be consumed in a 1:1 ratio, while others maintain that people should obtain several times more omega-3 than omega-6 fatty acids from their diet. In either case, the fact that fish oils are high in omega-3 fatty acids may help people to maintain a good balance between the two types of fatty acids. The most important types of omega-3 fatty acids found in fish oils are eicosapentanoic acid (EPA) and docosahexaenoic acid (DHA). The body needs EPA to produce prostaglandins, which are hormone-like substances that help to protect the heart and the cell membranes. DHA is required for the normal development of the brain, the eyes, and the reproductive system.

General use

In general, fish oils are recommended as dietary supplements to lower the levels of triglycerides in the blood, counteract inflammation in various parts of the body, and thin the blood.

Heart disease and stroke

The omega-3 fatty acids in fish oils increase the concentrations of good **cholesterol** (high density lipoproteins, HDL) in the blood while decreasing the concentrations of bad cholesterol (triglycerides). They also lower the total cholesterol level. Furthermore, these omega-3 oils protect the heart by preventing the formation of **blood clots** and fatty deposits (plaque) on the arterial walls. In people with coronary **heart disease**, fish oils may help to reduce the risk of blood clots in the brain or in the lungs; **pain** associated with **angina**; and the risk of cardiac arrythmias.

The benefits of omega-3 fatty acids have been shown in clinical studies. Investigation of the possible benefits of fish oils began when researchers discovered that Eskimos rarely suffer from heart attacks or **rheumatoid arthritis** (RA) even though their diet is high in fat from fish, seals, and whales. Because these sources of fat

have a high omega-3 fatty acid content, it was assumed that the type of fatty acid that they contained helped to protect the Eskimos from the usual consequences of high-fat **diets**. Later studies confirmed that diets high in omega-3 fatty acids decrease the risk of heart attacks, strokes, and abnormal heart rhythms. In one study of 20,551 doctors, those who ate at least one fish meal per week cut their risk of heart attacks in half compared to those who ate fish once a month or less. In the five-year Lyon study, men who followed a **Mediterranean diet** with emphasis on omega-3-rich oils, fish, fruits, and vegetables had their **heart attack** rates reduced by 70% compared to subjects in the control group. One question, however, is whether fish oil used by itself as a dietary supplement is as effective as a diet high in fish, since the two are not the same. One open trial of 11,324 people who were followed for three to five years found that fish oil did reduce the risk of death from heart attack. This study, however, was not a double-blind study, and its results cannot be taken as conclusive.

High blood pressure

Fish oils may help to control high blood pressure. Several studies have shown that taking fish oil can lower blood pressure. On the other hand, a 1997 study involving 2,000 subjects found no significant effect.

Rheumatoid arthritis

Fish oil may be useful in managing the symptoms of early rheumatoid arthritis (RA). A significant reduction in joint tenderness, morning stiffness, and **fatigue**, coupled with an increase in grip strength, has been observed in patients taking fish oil capsules. Fish oil appears to reduce the symptoms of RA without side effects, and to increase the effectiveness of standard medications for it. Fish oil does not, however, appear to slow the progress of RA.

Asthma

It has been claimed that fish oils reduce inflammation of the airways and may prevent **asthma** attacks. According to one author, allergic disorders such as asthma may be triggered by too much omega-6 and too little omega-3 fats in the diet. Two studies undertaken in 1994 and 1996 respectively, however, found no benefits from using fish oil in the management of asthma.

Psoriasis and autoimmune disorders

Several small studies indicate that fish oil may be helpful in treating **psoriasis**, which is an inflammatory disorder of the skin; in lupus; and in Raynaud's phenomenon, an autoimmune disorder in which the patient's hands and feet are abnormally sensitive to cold and emotional **stress**. With respect to the Raynaud's patients, small double-blind studies showed that very high doses of fish oil reduce their responses to cold. It appears, however, that doses as high as 12 g of fish oil daily are necessary to provide this effect. With respect to lupus, a small study of 30 subjects found that 14 out of 17 patients given daily doses of 20 g of EPA derived from fish oil had significant improvement. Subjects given a placebo either showed no improvement or got worse.

Osteoporosis

When taken together with **calcium, essential fatty acids** may help to protect women from **osteoporosis**. One 18-month study of 65 postmenopausal women found that those who were given a combination of omega-6 fatty acids (GLA) and omega-3 fatty acids from fish oil together with calcium had higher bone density and fewer **fractures** than those who were given the calcium and a placebo.

Gynecological problems

Fish oil supplements may be helpful in alleviating the symptoms of **premenstrual syndrome** (PMS) and painful periods. A number of different substances that are high in fatty acids, including **flaxseed** oil and GLA as well as fish oil, have been recommended for painful menstrual periods. One four-month study of adolescents suggests that fish oil is useful in treating this condition. Forty-two young women were divided into two groups; half received a daily dose of 6 g of fish oil for two months, followed by two months of placebo. The other half received the placebo and fish oil in reverse order. The results indicated that the subjects had significantly less menstrual pain while taking the fish oil.

Bipolar disorder and depression

Fish oil does appear to offer considerable benefits to people with **bipolar disorder**. A four-month double-blind study of 30 subjects indicated that fish oil improves emotional stability and helps to prevent relapses. Of the 14 persons who took fish oil, 11 stayed well or improved, while only six out of 16 subjects given placebos stayed well. A 2001 report looked at the effects of fish oil on mood and **depression**. Two large studies showed a strong connection between rates of depression and bipolar disorder in countries with high amounts of fish in diets. Although researchers cannot say that fish oil is the only reason for the difference, evidence continues to mount that omega-3 and omega-6 fatty acids may work as mood stabilizers.

Other conditions

Fish oil has been touted as a useful treatment for diabetic neuropathy, **allergies**, migraine headaches, **Crohn's disease**, **gout**, and ulcerative colitis, but there has been little systematic research involving these applications. In addition, health food manufacturers list **hair loss**, memory problems, muscle strain, failing eyesight, liver complaints, rickets, and dental problems as ailments that can be treated with fish oil. No clinical studies have been cited in support of these claims.

Early studies in laboratories indicate that fish oils might prolong life in people with autoimmune disorders like diabetes. Early results show that a diet high in fish oils helped improve immune system function in these patients.

Preparations

There is no minimum daily requirement of fish oil as such, but a healthy diet should supply at least 5 g of essential fatty acids every day. Typical doses of fish oil are 3–9 g daily, although some participants in research studies have taken much higher doses. If fish oil is taken as a dietary supplement, it should be taken in large enough doses to supply about 1.8 g of EPA and 0.9 g of DHA on a daily basis. Fish oil capsules are available in health food stores as over-the-counter items; prices range from $7 for 180 capsules of Norwegian cod liver oil to $14 for 180 capsules of salmon oil. Capsules of tuna oil and halibut liver oil are also available from several commercial suppliers.

Precautions

Fish oil can easily become rancid. The capsules can be stored in the refrigerator to slow the rate of oxidation. Another option is to purchase capsules that have added **vitamin E**.

The type of fish oil may make a difference. Although cod liver oil is the easiest form to obtain, it can cause a buildup of **vitamin A** and **vitamin D** in the body because these two vitamins are fat-soluble. Pregnant women should not take more than 2,500 IU of vitamin A per day because higher amounts can cause birth defects. Other adults should not consume more than 5,000 IU of vitamin A per day. Vitamin D can produce toxicity when taken at levels above 1,000 IU daily for long periods of time. Persons who obtain their fish oil from cod liver oil should check the label to see how much vitamin A and vitamin D it contains. It may be prudent to take salmon oil, mackerel oil, or oil from other coldwater fish.

Women who are pregnant or breast-feeding should talk to their physicians before taking fish oil supplements or any other medications.

Because fish oil can thin the blood, it should not be taken together with aspirin and other nonsteroidal anti-inflammatory drugs (NSAIDs, or over-the-counter pain killers), Coumadin (warfarin), or other anti-clotting medications. Fish oil does not seem to cause problems with bleeding when it is taken by itself, however.

Side effects

Fish oil generally appears to be safe when taken as a dietary supplement. The most common side effects are mild **indigestion** or a fishy taste in the mouth.

Interactions

Fish oil supplements may interact with nonsteroidal anti-inflammatory drugs (NSAIDs), warfarin, or other anti-clotting medications to cause excessive bleeding.

Resources

BOOKS

Murray, Michael, ND, and Joseph Pizzorno, ND. *Encyclopedia of Natural Medicine.* 2nd ed. Rocklin, CA: Prima Publishing, 1998.

Sears, Barry. *The Omega Rx Zone: The Miracle of the New High-Dose Fish Oil.* Regan Books, 2002.

PERIODICALS

Nichols, Sonia. "Fish Oil Diets Extend Survival in Autoimmune-Prone Mice." *Diabetes Week* (November 26, 2001): 3.

"Omega-3 Fatty Acids in the Treatment of Depression." *Harvard Mental Health Letter* (October 2001).

ORGANIZATIONS

American Association of Naturopathic Physicians (AANP). 8201 Greensboro Drive, Suite 300, McLean, VA 22102. (703) 610-9037. <http://www.naturopathic.org>.

Mai Tran
Teresa G. Odle

5-HTP

Description

The acronym for 5-hydroxytryptophan (or 5-hydroxy-L-tryptophan) is 5-HTP, a compound found primarily in the brain. This compound is made from tryptophan, a natural amino acid inherent in foods. Tryptophan is an essential amino acid, which means that it cannot be made by the body. It must be obtained from food, particularly proteins. In the liver and brain, 5-HTP is converted to an important monoamine neurotransmitter called serotonin. Neurotransmitters are chemical messengers that transmit signals between neurons (nerve cells) in the brain.

Taking 5-HTP increases the body's supply of the compound, which leads to higher serotonin levels in the brain. Serotonin, also called 5-hydroxytryptamine or 5-HT, plays an important role in controlling behavior and moods. It influences many normal brain activities and also regulates the activity of other neurotransmitters. Having adequate levels of serotonin instills a feeling of **relaxation**, calmness, and mild euphoria (extreme happiness). Low levels of serotonin, serotonin deficiency syndrome, leads to **depression, anxiety**, irritability, **insomnia**, and many other problems.

Conditions associated with low levels of serotonin include:

- anxiety
- attention deficit hyperactivity disorder (ADHD)
- bulimia
- depression
- **epilepsy**
- **fibromyalgia**
- headaches
- hyperactivity
- insomnia
- **obesity**
- obsessive compulsive disorder (OCD)
- panic attacks

• **premenstrual syndrome** (PMS)

• schizophrenia

• seasonal affective disorder (SAD)

This compound has other effects on the body. It is an antioxidant that protects the body from damage by substances called free radicals (unstable, toxic molecules). In this role, 5-HTP may help slow the **aging** process and protect the body from illness. Because serotonin is used to make **melatonin**, taking 5-HTP may help achieve some of the same benefits as melatonin, such as treating **jet lag**, depression, and insomnia. There is some evidence that 5-HTP can replenish the supply of the pain-relieving molecules called endorphins. Studies have shown that low levels of endorphins are associated with **chronic fatigue syndrome**, fibromyalgia, **stress**, and depression. In addition, 5-HTP affects other neurotransmitters, including norepinephrine and dopamine.

General use

In studies, 5-HTP has been proven effective in the treatment of carbohydrate cravings and binge eating, chronic headaches, depression, fibromyalgia, insomnia, anxiety, and panic disorders.

Most of the clinical research with 5-HTP focuses on the treatment of depression. In 15 separate studies, 5-HTP was tested on a total of 511 patients with different kinds of depression. Over half (56%) of these patients had significant improvement in depression while taking 5-HTP. The compound was found to be as effective as the selective serotonin reuptake inhibitor (SSRI) fluvoxamine and the tricyclic antidepressants, chloripramine and imipramine. Most of these studies used relatively high doses ranging from 50–3,250 mg daily.

Three clinical studies have found that 5-HTP can significantly improve the **pain**, anxiety, morning stiffness, and **fatigue** associated with fibromyalgia. The doses ranged from 300–400 mg daily. In one study, 5-HTP treatment was as effective as a tricyclic antidepressant (amitriptyline) and monamine oxidase inhibitors (MAOI; pargilyne or phenelzine).

Three clinical studies have found that 5-HTP use led to decreased intake of food, and subsequent weight loss in obese patients. The dose used in one study was 900 mg daily, which initially caused **nausea** in 80% of the patients.

A few clinical trials have found that 5-HTP can effectively prevent chronic headaches, including **migraine headache** and tension **headache**. In addition, 5-HTP compared favorably with propranolol and methysergide, drugs commonly used to prevent migraines.

In treating insomnia, 5-HTP is effective because it increases the length of rapid eye movement (REM) sleep, which improves sleep quality.

The symptoms of anxiety may be significantly reduced by 5-HTP. In studies, it instilled a sense of relief in patients with panic disorders.

Other conditions that may be treated with 5-HTP, but for which no studies exist, include chronic fatigue syndrome, premenstrual syndrome, **Parkinson's disease**, and seizure disorders (such as epilepsy).

Although 5-HTP may be a useful alternative to conventional antidepressant drugs, one study indicated that it may be of no value for patients who have failed to respond to traditional drugs. In this study, patients who failed to respond to tricyclic antidepressants were treated with either 5-HTP or a monoamine oxidase inhibitor (MAO-I). Half of the patients improved with the MAO-I treatment, while none showed any benefit from 5-HTP treatment.

Preparations

The 5-HTP preparation that is available commercially is isolated from the seed of an African plant called *Griffonia simplicifolia*. It is available as an enteric coated tablet, which does not break down until it reaches the intestine.

The recommended starting dose for headaches, weight loss, depression, and fibromyalgia is 50 mg three times daily. It can be taken with food. However, for weight loss it should be taken 20 minutes before eating. If it is not effective after two weeks, the dose may be increased to 100 mg three times daily, but only with the recommendation of a physician. Insomnia is treated with 25 mg (which may be increased to 100 mg after a few days) taken 30-45 minutes before bedtime.

Precautions

The Mayo Clinic detected, and the U. S. Federal Drug Administration (FDA) confirmed, the presence of a contaminant (peak X) in 5-HTP produced by six different manufacturers. This contaminant is similar to one found in L-tryptophan, which in 1989 caused the potentially fatal eosinophilia myalgia syndrome (EMS) in some persons. The L-tryptophan supplements were subsequently banned by the FDA. There have been 10 reports of EMS associated with 5-HTP use. The 5-HTP contaminant was not at levels high enough to cause illness. However, taking excessive doses of 5-HTP may lead to toxic levels of peak X.

Long term studies on the safety of 5-HTP use have not been conducted. To be safe, 5-HTP should be considered a short-term remedy.

Pregnant women should not take 5-HTP because there are no clinical studies on the compound's use among this population.

Side effects

Side effects associated with 5-HTP are rare but may include headaches, mild **stomachaches**, nausea, nasal congestion, and **constipation**. There are anecdotal reports that taking high doses of 5-HTP causes nightmares or vivid dreams. Side effects may be minimized by starting with a low dose of 5-HTP and taking it with food.

Interactions

It is theorized that the effectiveness of 5-HTP may be enhanced by taking vitamin B_6 and niacinamide. The action of 5-HTP may be enhanced by extracts of **ginger**, **passionflower** (*Passiflora incarnata*), St. John's wort, and *Ginkgo biloba*.

Dopa-decarbolylase inhibitors, such as carbidopa or benserazide block the enzyme that is responsible for the destruction of dopamine. However, a study by the Massachusetts College of Pharmacy and Health Sciences demonstrated that 5-HTP reaches the brain without the use of a dopa-decarboxylase inhibitor, and will produce the benefits of stress reduction and reduced food intake even when used alone.

There is a chance of developing serotonin syndrome when taking 5-HTP with an antidepressant drug. Serotonin syndrome was seen in patients taking high doses (greater than 1,200 mg daily) of L-tryptophan and MAO inhibitors. Combining 5-HTP with an MAOI or selective serotonin reuptake inhibitor antidepressant should be done with caution, under the supervision of a physician.

Resources

BOOKS

Murray, Michael T. *5-HTP: The Natural Way to Boost Serotonin and Overcome Depression, Obesity, and Insomnia*. New York: Bantam Books, 1998.

PERIODICALS

Amer, A., J. Breu, J. McDermott, R. J. Wurtman, and T. J. Maher. "5-Hydroxy-L-tryptophan suppresses food intake in food-deprived and stressed rats." *Pharmacol Biochem Behav.* 77 (January 2004): 137–43.

Birdsall, Timothy C. "5-Hydroxytryptophan: A Clinically-Effective Serotonin Precursor." *Alternative Medicine Review* 3 (1998): 271–80.

Juhl, John H. "Fibromyalgia and the Serotonin Pathway." *Alternative Medicine Review* 3 (1998): 367–75.

Morgenthaler, John. "5-HTP: The Natural Alternative to Prozac." *Total Health* 19 (July/August 1997): 48+.

KEY TERMS

Eosinophilia myalgia syndrome (EMS)—A chronic, painful disease of the immune system that causes joint pain, fatigue, shortness of breath, and swelling of the arms and legs. EMS can be fatal.

Monoamine oxidase inhibitor (MAOI)—An antidepressant drug that prevents the breakdown of monoamine neurotransmitters (such as serotonin) in the gaps between nerve cells. Nardil and Parnate are common MAOI brands.

Neurotransmitter—A chemical messenger that transmits signals between adjacent nerve cells in the brain.

Selective serotonin reuptake inhibitor (SSRI)—A family of antidepressant drugs that block the reabsorption of serotonin by nerve cells. Prozac, Zoloft, and Paxil are common brand names for these drugs.

Serotonin syndrome—A syndrome characterized by agitation, confusion, delirium, and perspiration, which is caused by high levels of serotonin in the brain.

Tricyclic antidepressant (TCA)—A group of antidepressant drugs that all have three rings in their chemical structure. Their mechanism of action is not fully understood, but they appear to extend the duration of action of some neurohormones, including serotonin and norepinephrine. They have also been used to treat some forms of chronic pain. Common brand names are Aventyl, Elavil, Surmontil, and Vivactil.

Murray, Michael T. "5-HTP and NADH." *Better Nutrition* 60 (September 1998): 20+.

Myers, Stephen. "Use of Neurotransmitter Precursors for Treatment of Depression." *Alternative Medicine Review* 5 (2000): 64–71.

ORGANIZATIONS

Serotonin Deficiency Foundation (SDF). P.O. Box 751390, Petaluma, CA 94975-1390. (800) 976-2783.

Belinda Rowland
Samuel Uretsky, Pharm.D.

5-Hydroxytryptophan *see* **5-HTP**

Flatulence *see* **Gas**

Flavonoids *see* **Bioflavonoids**

Flaxseed

Description

Flaxseed (also called linseed) comes from the flax plant (*Linum usitatissimum*), which belongs to the Linaceae plant family. The flax plant is a small, single-stemmed annual that grows to about 2 ft (0.6 m) tall and has grayish green leaves and sky-blue flowers. Historically, flax has been cultivated for thousands of years. Linen made from flax has been found in the tombs of Egyptian pharaohs and is referred to in the Bible and in Homer's *Odyssey*. The Roman naturalist Pliny wrote about the laxative and therapeutic powers of flax in the first century A.D., and many authorities believe it has been used as a folk remedy since ancient times. Flax is believed to be native to Egypt, but its origins are questionable since it has been used widely around the world. It is cultivated in many places, including Europe, South America, Asia, and parts of the United States. Only the seeds (flaxseed) and oil of the flax plant (flaxseed oil) are used medicinally. Linseed oil is the term usually used for the oil found in polishes, varnishes, and paints.

Flaxseed oil is derived from the flax plant's crushed seeds, which resemble common sesame seeds but are darker. The amber oil is very rich in a type of fat called alpha-linolenic acid (ALA), an omega-3 fatty acid that is good for the heart and found in certain plants. High amounts of **omega-3 fatty acids** are found in fish and smaller amounts are found in green leafy vegetables, soy-derived foods, and nuts. Many doctors consider these acids important for cardiovascular health. Studies suggest that they can lower triglyceride levels and reduce blood pressure. Omega-3 fatty acids may also decrease the risk of heart attacks and strokes by preventing the formation of dangerous **blood clots** within arteries. In high dosages, the fatty acids may help to alleviate arthritis, though flaxseed products have not yet been shown to be effective for this purpose.

In addition to omega-3 fatty acids, flaxseed products also contain potentially therapeutic chemicals called lignans. Lignans are believed to have antioxidant properties and may also act as phytoestrogens, very weak forms of estrogen found in fruits, vegetables, whole grains, and beans. Unlike human estrogen, phytoestrogens have dual properties: they can mimic the effects of the hormone in some parts of the body while blocking its effects in others. Many herbalists believe that phytoestrogens can be useful in the prevention or treatment of a variety of diseases, including **cancer**, cardiovascular disease, and **osteoporosis**. The estrogen-blocking effects of phytoestrogens may be particularly effective at combating certain cancers that depend on hormones, such as cancers of the breast or uterus. Women who consume large amounts of lignans appear to have lower rates of **breast cancer**. The fact that **heart disease** and certain cancers occur less frequently in Asian countries is sometimes attributed to a diet rich in plant foods containing phytoestrogens.

General use

While not approved by the United States Food and Drug Administration (FDA), flaxseed products are reputed to have a number of beneficial effects. Flaxseed is sometimes referred to as a nutraceutical, a recently coined term that includes any food or food ingredient thought to confer health benefits, including preventing and treating disease. Several studies, some conducted in people, suggest that flaxseed products (or agents contained in them) may help to keep the heart and cardiovascular system healthy. Flaxseed products may lower **cholesterol** levels, help control blood pressure, and may reduce the buildup of plaque in arteries. Test tube and rat studies suggest that chemicals in flaxseed may help to prevent or shrink cancerous tumors. Due to its estrogen-like effects, some women use flaxseed oil to ease breast tenderness, alleviate symptoms of **premenstrual syndrome** (PMS), and help control menopausal symptoms. Flaxseed oil has also been recommended to treat skin conditions, inflammation, and arthritis. It is usually taken internally for all the purposes mentioned above. The oil may be used externally to help the healing of scalds and **burns**.

More recently, flaxseed has been shown to be beneficial for people suffering from digestive disorders. It is now recommended as an "effective herbal agent" for treating **irritable bowel syndrome** (IBS).

The link between flaxseed and heart disease has been examined in a number of published studies. One of these studies published in the journal *Atherosclerosis* in 1997, observed the effects of adding flaxseed to the diet of rabbits with **atherosclerosis**. Researchers found that flaxseed reduced the development of plaque build-up by almost 50%. The authors concluded that flaxseed may help to prevent heart attacks and strokes related to high cholesterol levels. A study involving several dozen men with mild high blood pressure, which was published in the *Journal of Human Hypertension* in 1990, suggests that flaxseed oil may slightly lower blood pressure.

Research also suggests that flaxseed products may have potential as cancer fighters. One study, published in *Cancer Letters* in 1998, investigated how dietary flaxseed affects the development of cancer. Mice were fed a diet supplemented with 2.5%, 5%, or 10% flaxseed for several weeks before and after being injected with cancerous cells. The more flaxseed the mice received, the fewer tumors they developed. Depending on how much flaxseed they received, mice who were fed the herb developed fewer tumors than the mice who did not receive the flaxseed. Additionally, the tumors that developed in flaxseed-fed mice were smaller than those found in mice who did not receive flaxseed. The authors of the study concluded that flaxseed may be a useful nutritional aid in preventing the spread of cancer in people. In another study, which focused on breast cancer in rats, flaxseed flour was associated with a reduction in tumor size. In the study, which was published in *Nutrition and Cancer* in 1992, flaxseed flour also reduced the number of tumors that developed. However, researchers noted that more studies were needed in this area.

While the cancer-inhibiting effects of flaxseed have not been thoroughly studied in people, some practitioners of alternative medicine are already recommending the herb as a potential anticancer agent. Prominent herbalists maintain that the lignans found in flaxseed may help to control cancer of the breast or uterus. Some also recommend the herb for the prevention and treatment of **endometriosis**.

The therapeutic effects of flaxseed are not limited to people, according to some authorities. It is sometimes used as a purgative in horses and sheep. In addition, flaxseed is included in a rapidly expanding list of nutraceutical products for dogs, cats, and other domestic pets.

Preparations

Flaxseed products are commercially available as whole or ground seeds, gelatin capsules, and oil. Some herbalists recommend adding the ground or whole seeds to the diet to get the maximum benefit from the herb. Whole seeds can be stored in a cool, dry place for up to one year. Crushed seeds should be used immediately or frozen for future use. No standard guidelines have been established on how much of these forms should be consumed. Research subjects have been given as much as 1/4 cup of ground flaxseed per day, but a Canadian **nutrition** expert suggests that 1–2 tablespoons per day is enough for most adults.

Several nutraceutical companies are marketing a flaxseed ingredient as of 2002. The flaxseed ingredient is a fine-milled flour with 5% lignan content, intended for addition to commercial baked goods, snack foods, cereals, dry pet foods, and similar products.

Capsules can be taken according to package directions. Some herbalists feel that the capsules available are highly processed, contain fewer beneficial properties, and may be an expensive alternative to flaxseed oil.

The optimum daily dosage of flaxseed oil has not been established. Usually, 1 tablespoon daily of the oil

can be taken for general health. As a remedy, 1-3 tablespoons may be taken daily based on the person's weight and health needs. Some people consume the oil as an ingredient in salad dressing. The oil is often combined with limewater when used to treat burns and scalds.

Precautions

Flaxseed products are not known to be harmful when taken in recommended dosages, though it is important to remember that the long-term effects of taking flax-derived remedies (in any amount) have not been studied. Due to lack of sufficient medical study, flaxseed products should be used with caution in children, women who are pregnant or breast-feeding, and people with liver or kidney disease.

Because flaxseed oil tends to become rancid relatively quickly, it should be kept in the refrigerator. While the oil may be added to cooked food, it should not be used during cooking because heat can destroy the effectiveness of the oil.

Persons who are adding ground flaxseed to their diet for its fiber content are advised to start off with small amounts and increase them gradually, and to drink plenty of water. Otherwise the high fiber content of flaxseed can produce intestinal cramping and **diarrhea**.

Consumers should read the labels of all flaxseed products to insure that the product is for medicinal or nutritional purposes.

Side effects

When taken in recommended dosages, flaxseed products are not associated with any significant side effects.

Interactions

Consumers should consult their healthcare professional for information on flaxseed products and interactions with medications and other remedies. More specifically, the omega-3 fatty acids in flaxseed may increase the blood-thinning effects of such medications as aspirin or warfarin. Flaxseed may help a group of medications known as statins (lovastatin, simvastatin, etc.), which are given to lower blood cholesterol, to work more effectively.

Flaxseed may help to reduce the toxic side effects (kidney damage and high blood pressure) of cyclosporine, which is a drug given to organ transplant patients to prevent rejection of the new organ.

Flaxseed appears to reduce the risk of ulcers from high doses of NSAIDs.

In general, flaxseed oil should not be taken at the same time of day as prescription medications or other di-

KEY TERMS

Antioxidant—An agent that helps to protect cells from damage caused by free radicals, the destructive fragments of oxygen produced as a byproduct during normal metabolic processes.

Atherosclerosis—Narrowing and hardening of the arteries due to plaque buildup.

Nonsteroidal anti-inflammatory drugs (NSAIDs)—A term used for a group of pain-relieving medications that also reduce inflammation when used over a period of time. NSAIDs are often given to patients with osteoarthritis.

Nutraceutical—Any food or food ingredient that is thought to provide health benefits, including the prevention and treatment of disease. Flaxseed is considered a nutraceutical.

Osteoporosis—An age-related disease in which bones become fragile and prone to debilitating fractures.

Purgative—A substance that encourages bowel movements.

Triglyceride—A term referring to the total amount of fat in the blood. Triglyceride should not be confused with cholesterol, which is technically classified as a steroid and not as a fat.

etary supplements, as it will slow down the body's absorption of them.

Resources

BOOKS

Gruenwald, Joerg. *PDR for Herbal Medicines.* Montvale, NJ: Medical Economics, 1998.

Pelletier, Kenneth R., MD. *The Best Alternative Medicine,* Part I: Food for Thought. New York: Simon & Schuster, 2002.

PERIODICALS

Aubertin, Amy. "Flaxseed Comes of Age: Good Nutrition in a Small Package." *Environmental Nutrition* 25 (August 2002): 2.

"Flaxseed Ingredient." (Suppliers' Corner) *Nutraceuticals World* 5 (September 2002): 95.

Greenberg, Michael, Heather Amitrone, and Edward M. Galiczynski, Jr. "A Contemporary Review of Irritable Bowel Syndrome.(Recertification Series)." *Physician Assistant* 26 (August 2002): 26-33.

"Is There Flaxseed in Your Fridge Yet?" *Tufts University Health and Nutrition Letter* 20 (September 2002): 3.

Lemay, A., S. Dodin, N. Kadri, et al. "Flaxseed Dietary Supplement Versus Hormone Replacement Therapy in Hyper-

cholesterolemic Menopausal Women." *Obstetrics and Gynecology* 100 (September 2002): 495-504.

Prasad, K. "Dietary Flax Seed in Prevention of Hypercholesterolemic Atherosclerosis." *Atherosclerosis* 132, no. 1 (1997): 69-76.

Yan, L., J.A.Yee, D. Li, et al. "Dietary Flaxseed Supplementation and Experimental Metastasis of Melanoma Cells in Mice." *Cancer Letters* 124, no. 2 (1998): 181-186.

ORGANIZATIONS

American Botanical Council. P.O. Box 144345, Austin, TX 78714-4345. http://www.herbalgram.org.

United States Food and Drug Administration (FDA), Center for Food Safety and Applied Nutrition. 5100 Paint Branch Parkway, College Park, MD 20740. (888) SAFEFOOD. <www.cfsan.fda.gov>.

Greg Annussek
Rebecca J. Frey, PhD

Flower remedies

Definition

Flower remedies are specially prepared flower essences, containing the healing energy of plants. They are prescribed according to a patient's emotional disposition, as ascertained by the therapist, doctor, or patients themselves.

Origins

Perhaps the most famous and widely used system is the Bach flower remedies. This system originated in the 1920s when British physician and bacteriologist, Dr. Edward Bach (1886–1936), noticed that patients with physical complaints often seemed to be suffering from anxiety or some kind of negative emotion. He concluded that assessing a patient's emotional disposition and prescribing an appropriate flower essence could treat the physical illness. Bach was a qualified medical doctor, but he also practiced **homeopathy**.

As a result of his own serious illness in 1917, Bach began a search for a new and simple system of medicine that would treat the whole person. In 1930, he gave up his flourishing practice on Harley Street at the Royal London Homeopathic Hospital and moved to the countryside to devote his life to this research. It is known that at this point, he ceased to dispense the mixture of homeopathy and allopathic medicine that he had been using. Instead, he began investigating the healing properties of plant essences and discovered that he possessed an "intu-

BACH FLOWER REMEDIES

Name	Remedy
Agrimony	Upset by arguments, nonconfrontational, conceals worry and pain
Aspen	Fear of the unknown, anxiety, prone to nightmares, and apprehension
Beech	Critical, intolerant, and negative
Centaury	Submissive and weak-willed
Cerato	Self doubting and overly dependent
Cherry plum	Emotional thoughts and desperation
Chestnut	Repeats mistakes and has no hindsight
Chicory	Selfish, controlling, attention-seeking, and possessive
Clematis	Absorbed, impractical, and indifferent
Crab apple	Shame and self-loathing
Elm	Overwhelmed and feelings of inadequacy
Gentian	Negative, doubt, and depression
Gorse	Pessimism, hopelessness, and despair
Heather	Self-centered and self-absorbed
Holly	Jealousy, hatred, suspicion, and envy
Honeysuckle	Homesick, living in the past, and nostalgic
Hornbeam	Procrastination, fatigue, and mental exhaustion
Impatiens	Impatience, irritability, and impulsive
Larch	No confidence, inferiority complex, and despondency
Mimulus	Timid, shy, and fear of the unknown
Mustard	Sadness and depression of unknown origin
Oak	Obstinate, inflexible, and overachieving
Olive	Exhaustion
Pine	Guilt and self blame
Red chesnut	Fear and anxiety for loved ones
Rock rose	Nightmares, hysteria, terror, and panic
Rock water	Obsessive, repression, perfectionism, and self denial
Scleranthus	Indecision, low mental clarity, and confusion
Star-of-Bethlehem	Grief and distress
Sweet chesnut	Despair and hopelessness
Vervain	Overbearing and fanatical
Vine	Arrogant, ruthless, and inflexible
Walnut	Difficulty accepting change
Water violet	Pride and aloofness
White chestnut	Worry, preoccupation, and unwanted thoughts
Wild oat	Dissatisfaction
Wild rose	Apathy and resignation
Willow	Self pity and bitterness

ition" for judging the properties of each flower. Accordingly, he developed the system of treatment that bears his name, and is also the foundation for all other flower-remedy systems.

The Bach Flower Remedies were ostensibly the only system of significance from the 1920s until the 1970s, when there was a renewed interest in the subject by doctors working in the field of natural medicine. Perhaps the most notable was Dr. Richard Katz, who was seeking new methods of dealing with modern **stress** and the resulting ailments. He focused on the concept of a psychic, psychological effect and chose to pursue this line of research.

In 1979, Katz founded the Flower Essence Society in California, (FES). This society pledged to further the research and development of Bach's principles. As of 2000, FES hosts a database of over 100 flower essences from more than 50 countries. FES is now an international organization of health practitioners, researchers, students, and others concerned with flower essence therapy.

The Society has connections with an estimated 50,000 active practitioners from around the world, who use flower essence therapy as part of their treatment. FES encourages the study of the plants themselves to determine the characteristics of flower essences. They are compiling an extensive database of case studies and practitioner reports of the use of essences therapeutically, allowing verification and development of the original definitions. They are also engaged in the scientific study of flower essence therapy.

FES says they have developed the theories of Paracelsus and Goethe who researched the "signatures" and "gestures" of botanical specimens, on the premise that the human body and soul are a reflection of the system of nature. FES plant research interprets the therapeutic properties of flower essences according to these insights.

In this regard, they have devised 12 "windows of perception" for monitoring the attributes of plants. Each of these windows reveals an aspect of the plant's qualities, although they maintain that what they are seeking is a "whole which is greater than the sum of its parts." The 12 windows are not considered independent classifications, but more of a blended tapestry of views of the qualities that each plant possesses.

The first window is concerned with the "form" of a plant—its shape classification. The second focuses on its "gesture" or spatial relationship. The third window is a plant's botanical classification; the Flower Essence Society maintains that considering a plant's botanical family is essential to obtaining an overview of its properties as a flower essence. The fourth window concerns the time orientation of a particular specimen regarding the daily and

EDWARD BACH 1886–1936

Edward Bach was a graduate of University College Hospital (M.B., B.S., M.R.C.S.) in England. He left his flourishing Harley Street practice in favor of homeopathy, seeking a more natural system of healing than allopathic medicine. He concluded that healing should be as simple and natural as the development of plants, which were nourished and given healing properties by earth, air, water, and sun.

Bach believed that he could sense the individual healing properties of flowers by placing his hands over the petals. His remedies were prepared by floating summer flowers in a bowl of clear stream water exposed to sunlight for three hours.

He developed 38 remedies, one for each of the negative states of mind suffered by human beings, which he classified under seven group headings: fear, uncertainty, insufficient interest in present circumstances, loneliness, over sensitivity to influences and ideas, despondency or despair, and overcare for the welfare of others. The Bach remedies can be prescribed for plants, animals, and other living creatures as well as human beings.

Joan Matthews

seasonal cycles. Why do some flowers bloom at different times of the day, while others, such as the evening primrose, respond to the moon? The fifth window observes a plant's relationship to its environment. Where a plant chooses to grow, and where it cannot survive, reveals much about its qualities. The sixth window observes a plant's relationship to the Four Elements and the Four Ethers, as FES maintains that plants exist in one of the elemental or etheric forces in addition to their physical life. "Elements" refers to those developed by the Greeks, as opposed to the modern concept of "molecular building blocks." It seems that commonly, two elements predominate in a plant, indicating a polarity of qualities, while two can be said to be recessive. The seventh window relates to a plant's relationship with the other kingdoms of nature: mineral, animal and human, while the eighth relates to the color and color variations of a plant. Katz explains how the language of color tells us so much about the "soul qualities" of a plant. The ninth window concerns all other sensory perceptions of a plant, such as fragrance, texture, and taste. The tenth window involves assessing the chemical substances and properties; the eleventh studies medicinal and herbal uses, as by studying the physical healing properties of plants, we can also understand something of their more subtle effects on the soul. Finally, the twelfth window involves the study of the lore, mythology, folk wisdom, and spiritual and ritual qualities associated with a particular plant. Katz relates how in the past, human beings were more in touch with the natural world, and the remnants of this unconscious plant wisdom live on in the form of folklore, mythology, and so on.

Benefits

Flower remedies are more homeopathic than herbal in the way they work, effecting energy levels rather than chemical balances. They have been described as "liquid energy." The theory is that they encapsulate the flowers' healing energy, and are said to deal with and overcome negative emotions, and so relieve blockages in the flow of human energy that can cause illness.

Description

Because flower remedies operate on approximately the same principles as homeopathy, practitioners quite often prescribe the two therapies in conjunction with each other. They can also be used concurrently with allopathic medicine.

The system consists of 38 remedies, each for a different disposition. The basic theory is that if the remedy for the correct disposition is chosen, the physical illness resulting from the present emotional state can then be cured. There is a **rescue remedy** made up of five of the essences—cherry plum, clematis, impatiens, rock star, and star of Bethlehem—that is recommended for the treatment of any kind of physical or emotional shock. Therapists recommended that rescue remedy be kept on hand to help with all emergencies.

The 38 Bach Remedies are:

- agrimony: puts on a cheerful front, hides true feelings, and worries or problems
- aspen: feelings of apprehension, dark foreboding, and premonitions
- beech: critical, intolerant, picky
- centaury: easily comes under the influence of others, weak-willed
- cerato: unsure, no confidence in own judgement, intuition, and seeks approval from others
- cherry plum: phobic, fear of being out of control, and tension
- chestnut bud: repeats mistakes, does not learn from experience
- chicory: self-centered, possessive, clingy, demanding, self pity
- clematis: absent minded, dreamy, apathetic, and lack of connection with reality

- crab apple: a "cleanser" for prudishness, self–disgust, feeling unclean
- elm: a sense of being temporarily overwhelmed in people who are usually capable and in control
- gentian: discouraged, doubting, despondent
- gorse: feelings of pessimism, accepting defeat
- heather: need for company, talks about self, and concentrates on own problems
- holly: jealousy, envy, suspicion, anger, and hatred
- honeysuckle: reluctance to enter the present and let the past go
- hornbeam: reluctant to face a new day, weary, can't cope (mental fatigue)
- impatiens: impatience, always in a hurry, and resentful of constraints
- larch: feelings of inadequacy and apprehension, lack of confidence and will to succeed
- mimulus: fearful of specific things, shy, and timid
- mustard: beset by "dark cloud" and gloom for no apparent reason
- oak: courageous, persevering, naturally strong but temporarily overcome by difficulties
- olive: for physical and mental renewal, to overcome exhaustion from problems of long–standing
- pine: for self–reproach, always apologizing, assuming guilt
- red chestnut: constant worry and concern for others
- rock rose: panic, intense alarm, dread, horror
- rock water: rigid–minded, self–denial, restriction
- scleranthus: indecision, uncertainty, fluctuating moods
- star of Bethlehem: consoling, following shock or grief or serious news
- sweet chestnut: desolation, despair, bleak outlook
- vervain: insistent, fanatical, over–enthusiastic
- vine: dominating, overbearing, autocratic, tyrannical
- walnut: protects during a period of adjustment or vulnerability
- water violet: proud, aloof, reserved, enjoys being alone
- white chestnut: preoccupation with worry, unwanted thoughts
- wild oat: drifting, lack of direction in life
- wild rose: apathy, resignation, no point in life
- willow bitter: resentful, dissatisfied, feeling life is unfair

Originally, Bach collected the dew from chosen flowers by hand to provide his patients with the required remedy. This became impractical when his treatment became so popular that production could not keep up with demand. He then set about finding a way to manufacture the remedies, and found that floating the freshly picked petals on the surface of spring water in a glass bowl and leaving them in strong sunlight for three hours produced the desired effect. Therapists explain that the water is "potentized" by the essence of the flowers. The potentized water can then be bottled and sold. For more woody specimens, the procedure is to boil them in a sterilized pan of water for 30 minutes. These two methods produce "mother tinctures" and the same two methods devised by Bach are still used today. Flower essences do not contain any artificial chemical substances, except for alcohol preservative.

Bach remedies cost around $10 each, and there is no set time limit for treatment. It may take days, weeks, or in some cases months. Flower essences cost around $6 each, and there is also no set time for the length of treatment, or the amount of essences that may be taken. These treatments are not generally covered by medical insurance.

Precautions

Bach remedies and flower essences are not difficult to understand, and are considered suitable for self administration. The only difficulty may be in finding the correct remedy, as it can sometimes be tricky to pinpoint an individual's emotional disposition. They are even safe for babies, children, and animals. An important aspect of treatment with flower remedies, is that if you feel instinctively that you need a particular remedy, you are encouraged to act on that instinct. However, it is advisable not to continue a particular remedy once you feel you no longer need it, and to try a different one if you feel that progress is not being made.

The remedies are administered from a stoppered bottle and need to be diluted. Individuals sensitive to alcohol can apply the concentrate directly to temples, wrists, behind the ears, or underarms. They should be kept in a cool dark place; like this they should last indefinitely. However, a diluted remedy should not be kept longer than three weeks. Two drops of each diluted remedy should be taken four times a day, including first thing in the morning and last thing at night. If the rescue remedy is being used, four drops should be used instead. Most therapists recommend that they be taken in spring water, but the remedy can be taken directly from the bottle, if care is taken that the dropper does not touch the tongue, as this would introduce bacteria that would spoil the remedy.

It is not recommended that more than six or seven Bach remedies be used at any one time. Instead, it is preferable to divide a larger amount up into two lots to ensure the optimum effectiveness of the remedies. No combination, or amount of combinations of the remedies can cause any harm, rather they become less effective.

Unlike FES, the Bach Centre does not encourage research to "prove" that the remedies work, preferring that people find out for themselves. They strive to keep the use of the Bach remedies as simple as possible, and to this end they do not keep case records. Bach warned before he died that others would try to change his work and make it more complicated. He was determined to keep it simple so that anyone could use it, and that is why he limited the system to only 38 remedies. The Centre points out that many who have used Bach's research as a starting point have added other remedies to the list, even some that Bach himself rejected.

Side effects

Flower remedies or essences are generally regarded as being totally safe, and there are no known side effects apart from the rare appearance of a slight rash, which is not a reason to discontinue treatment, says the Bach Centre.

Research & general acceptance

Bach flower remedies and flower essences have not yet officially won the support of allopathic medicine, despite the fact that more and more medical doctors are referring patients for such treatments on the strength of personal conviction. However, it is difficult to discount the scores of testimonials. Some practitioners refer skeptics to the research that has been done regarding the "auras" of living things. Theoretically, the stronger the aura, the more alive an organism is. Flower essences have very strong auras.

Among mainstream medical practitioners, psychiatrists and family practitioners appear to be more willing to study flower essences than physicians in other specialties. One pilot study at Penn State Hershey Medical Center found that the Bach flower essences were effective in reducing the symptoms of **attention-deficit hyperactivity disorder** (ADHD) in children as measured by two standard assessment instruments for ADHD.

Another area of medicine in which acceptance of Bach flower essences is growing is small-animal veterinary practice. Two full-length books on the use of flower essences for behavioral problems in animals were published in 1999, and some schools of veterinary medicine now include flower essences as part of elective courses in holistic or complementary veterinary treatments.

Training & certification

The official Bach International Education Program training courses are all recognized by the Dr. Edward

Bach Foundation, and taught by accredited Bach trainers. These qualifications are not recognized by the medical authorities.

Bach therapy may be self-administered, but for those who would prefer the advice of a practitioner, look for a registered Bach practitioner, or a homeopath or herbalist who also deals with the Bach flower remedies.

Resources

BOOKS

Bach, Edward. *Heal Thyself.* Essex, UK: C.W. Daniel Company, Ltd., 1931.

Graham, Helen, and Gregory Vlamis. *Bach Flower Remedies for Animals.* Tallahassee, FL: Findhorn Press, Inc., 1999.

Howard, Judy, Stefan Ball, and Kate Aldous (illustrator). *Bach Flower Remedies for Animals.* London, UK: The C. W. Daniel Co., Ltd., 1999.

Kaslof, Leslie. *The Traditional Flower Remedies of Dr. Edward Bach.* New Canaan, CT: Keats, 1993

Somerville, R. *Flower Remedies* New York: Time-Life Books.

Vlannis, Gregory. *Flowers to the Rescue.* New York: Thorras, 1986.

PERIODICALS

Downey, R. P. "Healing with Flower Essences." *Beginnings* 22 (July-August 2002): 11-12.

"Flowers to the Rescue." *Women's Health Letter* 8 (July 2002): 3-4.

Mehta, Satwant K. "Oral Flower Essences for ADHD." (Letters to the Editor.) *Journal of the American Academy of Child and Adolescent Psychiatry* 41 (August 2002): 895-896.

ORGANIZATIONS

The Dr. Edward Bach Centre, Mount. Vernon, Bakers Lane, Sotwell, Oxon, OX10 OPX, UK. centre@bachcentre.com. http://www.bachcentre.com.

The Flower Essence Society. P.O. Box 459, Nevada City, CA 95959. (800) 736-9222 (US & Canada). (53) 265-9163. Fax: (530) 265-0584. mail@flowersociety.org. http://www.flowersociety.org.

National Center for Complementary and Alternative Medicine Clearinghouse. P. O. Box 7923, Gaithersburg, MD 20898. (888) 644-6226. <www.nccam.nci.nih.gov>.

Patricia Skinner
Rebecca J. Frey, PhD

Flu *see* **Influenza**

Fluid retention *see* **Edema**

Fo ti

Description

Fo ti is the American name for the herb *Polygonum multiflorum*. Polygonum is a member of the Polygonaceae family of plants. In Chinese herbalism, fo ti is called *he shou wu* or *ho shou wu*. Other names are fleeceflower and Chinese cornbind. In Japan the herb is called *kashuu*. It is one of the most popular herbs in Oriental medicine, used as an overall health tonic, as a tincture to increase longevity, and as a remedy for various health conditions.

Fo ti is a perennial flowering vine that reaches heights of 3–6 ft (0.97–1.8 m). It is native to southwestern China, Japan and Taiwan, but can be cultivated in many regions, including parts of North America.

The root of the plant is the part most frequently used for medicinal purposes, although Chinese herbalists occasionally use the stems for different applications. The root has a sweet and slightly bitter taste. Chinese herbalists claim it has slightly warming effects in the body, and works by increasing levels of blood and vital essence. These are two of three essential substances in the body, according to Chinese medicine. Chinese herbalists also maintain that fo ti strengthens the liver and kidneys. Fo ti root is used in conjunction with other herbs in many medicinal tonics.

Research in the West has shown that fo ti has antitumor and antibacterial properties. It also lowers blood pressure (hypotensive effects) and increases circulation (vasodilatory effects). Fo ti contains emodin and rhein, two laxative agents that have shown promising anti-cancer activity as well. Fo ti also contains **lecithin**, a B vitamin that aids in fat metabolism and lowers **cholesterol**. Researchers have isolated a flavonoid in fo ti called catachin, which is also found in **green tea**. Catachin inhibits tumor cells and has antioxidant effects, which may be the source of the anti-aging properties that the herb is known for in China.

General use

Fo ti is recommended for many conditions. It is used as an overall health strengthener, and to prevent premature aging and graying hair. Chinese medicine recommends it to increase sperm quality in men and fertility in women. It is used for diseases associated with weakness in the liver and kidneys. These illnesses are characterized by blurred vision, **dizziness**, weakness in the knees and lower back, intermittent fevers, dull complexion, swollen lymph glands, and sores and **boils** on the skin. Fo ti has also been used traditionally in Chinese medicine for non-acute **malaria**, for lowering cholesterol, and for nervous disorders. As it has both laxative and tonic effects, it is good for **constipation** in the elderly. It is also used to treat vaginal discharges, and its slightly sedative effect makes it a treatment for **insomnia**. In Chinese medicine, the vine part of polygonum, which is called *ye jiao teng*, is used to treat insomnia as well as irritability and numb or **itching** sensations in the limbs. In the West, fo ti is showing promise as an adjunctive form of herbal therapy in **cancer** treatment.

Preparations

Fo ti can be purchased as whole or sliced roots, in tablets, and as a tincture. It is available in health food stores as well as Chinese herb stores and markets. The reader should note that the Chinese don't recognize fo ti as the herb's proper name; in Chinese markets it should be referred to as *he shou wu* or as polygonum.

Fo ti root usually comes in slices. The older and larger the root, the higher quality and more expensive. In addition, dark roots are considered a higher grade than roots that have white streaks in them. The root can be eaten or prepared as a tea or tincture. To make tea, the root should be boiled for 30 minutes or more to extract all the active ingredients. For one serving of the root or tea, 5–15 g are recommended. For a tincture, chopped roots can be soaked in alcohol for one month or longer, and 30 drops of the tincture can be taken daily. Tinctures can also be purchased; daily dosages vary according to the concentration.

For sedative purposes, fo ti vine is generally taken with the evening meal or before bedtime. Fo ti can be taken continuously for up to one month; the patient should then wait one month before using it again.

Fo ti is used in many herbal tonics. For longevity and overall health, it is combined with Asian ginseng. Chinese herbalists recommend combining fo ti with Asian ginseng, **dong quai,** and **tangerine peel** as a tonic for non-acute malaria or for recovery from a long illness. For sore knees and lower back problems, herbalists combine fo ti with **cuscuta**, psorolea fruit, and **lycium fruit**. As part of a program of cancer treatment, fo ti is combined with other tonic and immune-enhancing herbs, including **Korean ginseng**, **astragalus**, milletia, and codonopsis. Experienced herbalists can assist consumers with special preparations and applications.

KEY TERMS

Catachin—A flavonoid found in fo ti that has antioxidant and tumor-inhibiting qualities.

Flavonoids—Pigments found in plants that protect plants against environmental stress. In humans, they appear to have anti-aging effects.

Tonic—Any substance that strengthens and tones the entire system.

Sedative—A substance or medication that calms and lowers bodily activity.

Precautions

Fo ti is generally a safe herb, but it is not recommended for patients with **diarrhea** or heavy phlegm in the respiratory tract.

Side effects

Reported side effects with fo ti are generally rare. They include diarrhea, abdominal **pain**, **nausea**, numbness in the extremities, flushing of the face, and skin **rashes**.

Interactions

Some herbalists advise patients to reduce their intake of onions, **garlic**, and chives while taking fo ti for extended periods.

Resources

BOOKS

Foster, S., and Y. Chongxi. *Herbal Emissaries.* Rochester, VT: Healing Arts Press, 1992.

Reid, Daniel P. *Chinese Herbal Medicine.* Boston: Shambhala, 1993.

Yance, Donald R. *Herbal Medicine, Healing and Cancer.* Chicago: Keats, 1999.

PERIODICALS

HerbalGram (a quarterly journal of the American Botanical Council and Herb Research Foundation). P.O. Box 144345, Austin, TX 78714-4345. (800) 373-7105. http://www.herbalgram.org.

Qi: The Journal of Traditional Eastern Health and Fitness. P.O. Box 18476, Anaheim Hills, CA 92817. http://www.qi-journal.com.

Douglas Dupler

Folate *see* **Folic acid**

Folic acid

Description

Folic acid is a water-soluable vitamin belonging to the B-complex group of vitamins. These vitamins help the body break down complex carbohydrates into simple sugars that can be readily used for energy. Excess B vitamins are excreted from the body rather than stored for later use. This is why sufficient daily intake of folic acid is necessary.

Folic acid is also known as folate, or folacin. It is one of the nutrients most often found to be deficient in the Western diet, and there is evidence that deficiency is a problem worldwide. Folic acid is found in leafy green vegetables, beans, peas and lentils, liver, beets, Brussels sprouts, poultry, nutritional yeast, tuna, **wheat germ**, mushrooms, oranges, asparagus, broccoli, spinach, bananas, strawberries, and cantaloupes. In 1998, the U.S. Food and Drug Administration (FDA) required food manufacturers to add folic acid to enriched bread and grain products, to boost intake and to help prevent neural tube defects (NTD) in the fetus during **pregnancy**.

General use

Folic acid works together with **vitamin B$_{12}$** and **vitamin C** to metabolize protein. It is important for the formation of red and white blood cells. Folic acid is necessary for the proper differentiation and growth of cells, and for the development of the fetus. It is also used to form the nucleic acid of DNA and RNA. It increases the appetite, stimulates the production of stomach acid for digestion, and aids in maintaining a healthy liver. A folic acid deficiency may lead to megaloblastic **anemia**, in which there is decreased production of red blood cells, and the cells that are produced are abnormally large. This reduces the amounts of oxygen and nutrients that are able to reach the tissues. Symptoms may include **fatigue**, reduced secretion of digestive acids, confusion, and forgetfulness. During pregnancy, a folic acid deficiency may lead to preeclampsia, premature birth, and increased bleeding after birth.

People who are at high risk for strokes and **heart disease** may benefit from folic acid supplements. An elevated blood level of the amino acid homocysteine has been identified as a risk factor for some of these diseases. High levels of homocysteine have also been found to contribute to problems with **osteoporosis**. Folic acid, together with vitamins B$_6$ and B$_{12}$, aids in the breakdown of homocysteine, and may help reverse the problems associated with elevated levels.

Pregnant women have an increased need for folic acid, both for themselves and their unborn child. Folic acid is necessary for the proper growth and development of the fetus. Adequate intake of folic acid is vital for the prevention of several types of birth defects, particularly neural tube defects (NTDs). The neural tube of the embryo develops into the brain, spinal cord, spinal column, and the skull. If this tube forms incompletely during the first few months of pregnancy, a serious—and often fatal— defect such as spina bifida or anencephaly, may occur. Folic acid, taken from one year to one month before conception through the first four months of pregnancy, can reduce the risk of NTDs by 50–70%. It also helps prevent cleft lip and palate.

Research shows that folic acid can be used to successfully treat **cervical dysplasia**, a condition that is diagnosed by a Pap smear, and consists of abnormal cells in the cervix. This condition is considered to be a possible precursor to cervical **cancer**. Daily consumption of 1,000 micrograms (mcg) of folic acid for three or more months has resulted in improved cervical cells upon repeat Pap smears.

Studies suggest that long-term use of folic acid supplements may also help prevent lung and colon cancers. Researchers have also found that alcoholics who have low folic acid levels face a greatly increased chance of developing colon cancer.

Preparations

Supplements are taken to correct a folic acid deficiency. Since the functioning of the B vitamins is interrelated, it is generally recommended that the appropriate dose of B-complex vitamins be taken in place of single B vitamin supplements. The Recommended Dietary Allowance (RDA) for folate is 400 mcg per day for adults, 600 mcg per day for pregnant women, and 500 mcg daily for nursing women. Medicinal dosages of up to 1,000 to 2,000 mcg per day may be prescribed.

Precautions

Folic acid is not stable. It is easily destroyed by exposure to light, air, water, and cooking. Therefore, the supplement should be stored inside a dark container in a cold, dry place, such as a refrigerator. Many medications interfere with the body's absorption and ability to use folic acid. These medications include sulfa drugs, sleeping pills, estrogen, anti-convulsants, birth control pills, antacids, quinine, and some antibiotics.

The anemia caused by folic acid deficiency is identical to that caused by lack of vitamin B$_{12}$. Using large amounts of folic acid (e.g., over 5,000 mcg per day) can mask a vitamin B$_{12}$ deficiency, since the anemia will improve but the other effects of vitamin B$_{12}$ deficiency will continue. This can lead to irreversible nerve damage.

KEY TERMS

Homocysteine—An amino acid involved in the breakdown and absorption of protein in the body.

Preeclampsia—A serious disorder of late pregnancy, in which the blood pressure rises, there is a large amount of retained fluids, and the kidneys become less effective and excrete proteins directly into the urine.

Raynaud's disease—A symptom of various underlying conditions affecting blood circulation in the fingers and toes, and causing them to be sensitive to cold.

Recommended Daily Allowance (RDA)—Guidelines for the amounts of vitamins and minerals necessary for proper health and nutrition. The RDA was established by the National Academy of Sciences in 1989.

Water-soluble vitamins—Vitamins that are not stored in the body and are easily excreted. These vitamins must be consumed regularly as foods or supplements to maintain health.

Therefore, people with megaloblastic anemia should be treated under medical supervision, since regular testing may be required.

Side effects

Folic acid is generally considered safe at levels of 5,000 mcg or less. Side effects are uncommon. However, large doses may cause **nausea**, decreased appetite, bloating, **gas**, decreased ability to concentrate, and **insomnia**. Large doses may also decrease the effects of phenytoin (Dilantin), a seizure medication.

Interactions

As with all B-complex vitamins, it is best to take folic acid with the other B vitamins. Vitamin C is important to the absorption and functioning of folic acid in the body.

Resources

BOOKS

Braverman, Eric R., M.D., Carl C. Pfeiffer, M.D., Ph.D., Ken Blum, Ph.D., and Richard Smayda, D.O. *The Healing Nutrients Within.* New Canaan, CT: Keats Publishing, 1997.

PERIODICALS

Fallest-Strobl, Patricia, Ph.D., David Koch, James Stein, and Patrick McBride. "Homocysteine: A New Risk Factor for Atherosclerosis." *American Family Physician* (October 15, 1997): 1607-14.

ORGANIZATIONS

Centers for Disease Control and Prevention. 4770 Buford Highway NE, MSF-45, Atlanta, GA 30341-3724. (888)232-6789. Flo@cdc.gov. <http://www.cdc.gov/nceh/ programs/cddh/folic/folicfaqs.htm>.

OTHER

Adams, Suzanne L. *The Art of Cytology: Folic Acid/ B-12 Deficiency* [cited June 6, 2004]. <http://www.concentric.net/ ~Suza2/page22.htm>.

"Folic Acid." Cybervitamins [cited June 6, 2004]. <http://www. cybervitamins.com/folicacid.htm>.

"Folic Acid: Coming to A Grocery Store Near You" [cited June 6, 2004]. <http://www.mayohealth.org/mayo/9710/htm/ folic.htm>.

"Folic acid (oral/injectible)." Dr. Koop.com. Inc. 700 N. Mopac, Suite 400, Austin, TX 78731. <http://www. drkoop.com/hcr/drugstore/ pharmacy/leaflets/english/d00241a1.asp>.

Pregnancy and Nutrition Update. MayoHealth [cited June 6, 2004]. <http://www.mayohealth.org/mayo/9601/htm/ pregvit.htm>.

Food poisoning

Definition

Food poisoning is a general term for health problems arising from eating food contaminated by viruses, chemicals, or bacterial toxins. Types of food poisoning include bacterial food poisoning, shellfish poisoning, and mushroom poisoning. The medical term for food poisoning is **gastroenteritis**.

Description

The Centers for Disease Control and Prevention (CDC) estimates that there are up to 33 million cases of food poisoning in the United States each year. Many cases are mild, and they pass so rapidly that they are never diagnosed. Occasionally, a severe outbreak creates a newsworthy public health hazard, but these instances are rare. Anyone can get food poisoning, but the very young, the very old, and those with compromised immune systems have the most severe and life-threatening cases.

Causes & symptoms

General indications of food poisoning include diarrhea, stomach **pain** or cramps, gurgling sounds in the stomach, **fever**, **nausea**, and **vomiting**. Dehydration is a common complication, since fluids and electrolytes are lost through vomiting and diarrhea. Dehydration is more

SAFE SEAFOOD
Abalone
Arctic char
Crawfish
Dungeness crab
Fish sticks
Flounder
Grouper
Haddock
Halibut
Mahi mahi
Marlin
Octopus
Orange roughy
Red snapper
Scallops
Sea bass
Shrimp
Sole
Squid
Talapia
Tuna
Wahoo
Whiting
Wild Pacific salmon
Yellowtail

likely to happen in the very young, the elderly, and people who are taking diuretics.

Bacterial sources of food poisoning

Bacteria are major causes of food poisoning. Symptoms of bacterial food poisoning occur because foodborne bacteria release enterotoxins, or poisons, as a byproduct of their growth in the body. These toxins often diminish the absorptive ability of the intestines and cause the secretion of water and electrolytes that leads to dehydration. The severity of symptoms depends on the type of bacteria, the amount of bacteria and food consumed, and the individual's health and sensitivity to the bacteria's toxin.

SALMONELLA. Symptoms of poisoning begin 12–72 hours after eating food contaminated with *Salmonella*.

Classic food poisoning symptoms, including fever, occur for about two to five days. *Salmonella* is usually transmitted through the consumption of food contaminated by human or other animal feces. This contamination is mostly due to lack of hand washing by food handlers.

ESCHERICHIA COLI (E. COLI). Symptoms of food poisoning from *E. coli* 0157:H7 and similar strains of *E. coli* are slower to appear than those caused by some of the other foodborne bacteria. One to three days after eating contaminated food, the victim begins to have severe abdominal cramps and watery diarrhea that usually becomes bloody. The diarrhea may consist mostly of blood and very little stool, so the condition is sometimes called hemorrhagic colitis. There is little or no fever, the bloody diarrhea lasts from one to eight days, and the condition usually resolves by itself. Food contamination from *E. coli* O157:H7 has mostly been found in raw or undercooked ground beef. Raw milk has also been a source of food poisoning by *E. coli*.

CAMPYLOBACTER JEJUNI. *C. jejuni* **infections** are most often caused by contaminated chicken, but unchlorinated water and raw milk may also be sources of infection. Classic symptoms of food poisoning, including fever and diarrhea, begin two to five days after consuming food or water contaminated with *C. jejuni*. The diarrhea may be watery and may contain blood. Symptoms last from seven to 10 days, and relapses occur in about one quarter of the people who are infected.

***STAPHYLOCOCCUS AUREUS* (STAPH).** *Staph* is spread primarily by food handlers with *Staph* infections on their skin. However, contaminated equipment and food preparation surfaces may also be at fault. Almost any food can be contaminated, but salad dressings, milk products, cream pastries, and food kept at room temperature, rather than hot or cold, are likely candidates. Classic symptoms of food poisoning appear rapidly, usually two to eight hours after the contaminated food is eaten. Such symptoms usually last only three to six hours and rarely more than two days. Most cases are mild and the victim recovers without any assistance.

SHIGELLA. Symptoms of food poisoning by *Shigella* appear 36–72 hours after eating contaminated food. These symptoms are slightly different from those associated with most foodborne bacteria. In addition to the familiar symptoms of food poisoning, up to 40% of children with severe infections show neurological symptoms. These include seizures, confusion, **headache**, lethargy, and a stiff, sore neck. The disease runs its course in two to three days.

CLOSTRIDIUM BOTULINUM. *C. botulinum* (commonly known as botulism) is the deadliest of the bacterial foodborne illnesses. Sources for adult botulism are

SEAFOOD WITH EVIDENCE OF CHEMICALS AND TOXINS	
Fish	**Chemicals/Toxins**
Bass	Dioxin, chlordane, DDT, PCBs
Catfish	Chlordane, DDT, dioxin, PCBs, etc.
Caviar	Chlordane, DDT, PCBs
Cod	DDT, PCBs
Maine lobster	PCBs
Shark	DDT, PCBs, mercury
Striped bass	PCBs, chlordane, DDT, mercury, etc.
Sturgeon	Chlordane, DDT, dieldrin, mercury, etc.
Swordfish	Mercury, DDT, PCBs
Whitefish	Dioxin

often improperly canned or preserved food. Symptoms of adult botulism appear about 18 to 36 hours after the contaminated food is eaten, although there are documented times of onset ranging from four hours to eight days. Unlike other foodborne illnesses, there is no vomiting and diarrhea associated with botulism. Initially, a person suffering from botulism feels weakness, **dizziness**, and double vision. Symptoms progress to difficulty with speaking and swallowing. The toxins from *C. botulinum* are neurotoxins—they poison the nervous system, causing paralysis. If the disease proceeds unchecked, paralysis will move throughout the body. Eventually, without medical intervention, the respiratory muscles will become paralyzed and the victim will suffocate.

With infant botulism, the spores of *C. botulinum* lodge in the infant's intestinal tract. Honey, especially when consumed by infants younger than 12 months, is sometimes the source of these spores. Onset of the symptoms is gradual. The infant initially has **constipation**, followed by poor feeding, lethargy, weakness, drooling, and a distinctive wailing cry. Eventually the baby loses the ability to control its head muscles. Paralysis then progresses to the rest of the body.

Fish-associated food poisoning

Ciguatera fish poisoning is caused by toxins accumulated in the tissues of certain tropical fish, including groupers, barracudas, snappers, and mackerel. Signs of poisoning occur about six hours after eating the fish. Around the mouth, there may be numbness and tingling, which may spread to other places including the hands and feet. There is often muscle pain and weakness, headache, dizziness, joint pain, sensitivity to temperature, heart ar-

rhythmias, dramatic changes in heart rate, and reduced blood pressure. Reef fish contaminated with ciguatoxin are being exported all over the world, occurrence of ciguatera is becoming more likely in colder climates.

Pufferfish, or *fugu*, is a traditional gourmet dish served mostly in Japan. The skin and other organs of the pufferfish contain a strong poison called tetradotoxin. The first stage of tetradotoxin poisoning is indicated by numbness of the lips and tongue, which may occur 20–180 minutes after eating the fish. This is followed by tingling and numbness of the face, hands, and feet. Classic symptoms of food poisoning are accompanied by other neurological symptoms such as light-headedness, headache, and unsteady gait. The second stage of tetradotoxin poisoning brings on a progressive paralysis. Breathing, talking, and other movement becomes difficult. Cyanosis (bluish or purplish skin discoloration), low blood pressure, and arrhythmias may occur. Convulsions and mental impairment may happen right before death, or the person may be completely lucid, though unmoving. Death usually occurs four to six hours after ingestion of the fish if there is no proper intervention; that time, however, has been known to be as little as 20 minutes.

Shellfish poisoning is caused by toxins made by certain algae eaten by shellfish. The toxins are then accumulated in the bodies of the shellfish. Cockles, mussels, clams, oysters, and scallops are most often affected. Sometimes the toxin-producing algae multiply to such an extent that they cause the waters they live in to take on the reddish color of their bodies. This phenomenon is known as a red tide. Warnings are often given against eating shellfish from such areas. Symptoms of food poisoning show up within a half an hour to two hours of eating the

TYPES OF FOOD POISONING	
Type	**Cause**
Traveler's diarrhea	Usually caused by *E. coli* bacteria found in contaminated food and water.
Salmonella	Caused by bacteria in contaminated poultry, eggs, meat, and dairy products. Although it can be fatal, most cases are mild.
Botulism	Caused by anaerobic bacteria that is found in home canned products and honey.
Viral	Caused most often by contaminated raw seafood.
Chemical	Caused by pesticides.

shellfish, depending on the amount and type eaten. There may be burning and tingling in the face and mouth, numbness, drowsiness, muscular pain, dizziness, diarrhea, stomachache, confusion, nausea, vomiting, odd temperature sensations, difficulty breathing, and possibly coma. The symptoms may last from a few hours to a few days.

Histamine poisoning can occur from eating fish whose body tissues have begun to produce high levels of histamine. Mackerel, tuna, and mahi mahi are most often the sources. After consumption of the fish, immediate facial flushing and **hives** may occur, as well as classic symptoms of food poisoning becoming evident a few minutes later. Symptoms usually last less than 24 hours.

Mushroom poisoning

Mushroom poisoning is classified by the effects of the poisons. Protoplasmic poisons result in cell destruction, often in the liver, which progresses to complete organ failure. Neurotoxins cause neurological symptoms such as sweating, convulsions, hallucinations, excitement, **depression**, coma, and colon spasms. Gastrointestinal (G/I) irritants rapidly bring on the classic symptoms of food poisoning and then resolve just as quickly. Disulfiram-like poisons are generally nontoxic, except when alcohol is consumed within 72 hours of eating them. In these cases, the poisons cause headache, nausea, vomiting, flushing, and cardiac disturbances for two to three hours.

Other possible sources

Other possible sources of food poisoning include ingestion of green or sprouting raw potatoes, ingestion of

fava beans by susceptible persons, and ergot poisoning from ingestion of contaminated grain. Chemical contaminant food poisoning may result from the ingestion of unwashed produce sprayed with arsenic, lead, or insecticides. Food served or stored in lead-glazed pottery cadmium-lined containers may also lead to food poisoning.

Diagnosis

An important aspect of diagnosing food poisoning is the clinical interview. A history of the illness should be thoroughly traced to include ingestion of food, recent travel, and contact with those showing similar symptoms of illness. Because it may take 30 minutes to three days for symptoms to develop, it is not necessarily the most recent food eaten that is the cause of the symptoms. Diagnosis is confirmed with a stool culture. Other laboratory tests may be used to examine vomitus, blood, or the contaminated food. A blood chemistry panel may be performed to determine the extent of any tissue damage or electrolyte imbalances. Many cases of food poisoning go undiagnosed, and treatment focuses on the short-lived G/I symptoms.

Botulism is usually diagnosed from its distinctive neurological symptoms, since rapid treatment is essential to save the patient's life. Electromyography, a test analyzing the electrical activity of muscles, may later be done to further confirm diagnosis. The test shows abnormal muscle activity in most cases of botulism.

Treatment

Those suffering from food poisoning should reduce all sugar and normal food for eight to 24 hours, and increase fluids to avoid dehydration. Charcoal tablets, *Lactobacillus acidophilus*, *Lactobacillus bulgaricus*, and citrus seed extract are all recommended. For mild cases of food poisoning, the homeopathic remedies *Arsenicum album, Veratrum album, Podophyllum,* or *Nux vomica* are recommended. The remedy should be given in 12c potency every three to four hours until symptoms subside. If a ready-made electrolyte replacement is not available, a homemade one can be made by dissolving exactly 1 tsp (5 ml) of salt and 4 tsp (20 ml) of sugar in 1 qt (1 l) of water.

Cinnamon (*Cinnamonum zeylanicum*), cloves (*Syzigium aromaticum*), oregano (*Origanum vulgare*), and **sage** (*Salvia officinalis*) are food herbs that are also strong inhibitors of bacteria. Liberal amounts can be added to foods, especially when traveling. **Grapefruit seed extract** has a natural antibiotic effect and may be of help. Large amounts of **garlic**, in food and in supplement form, are also recommended for the same reason.

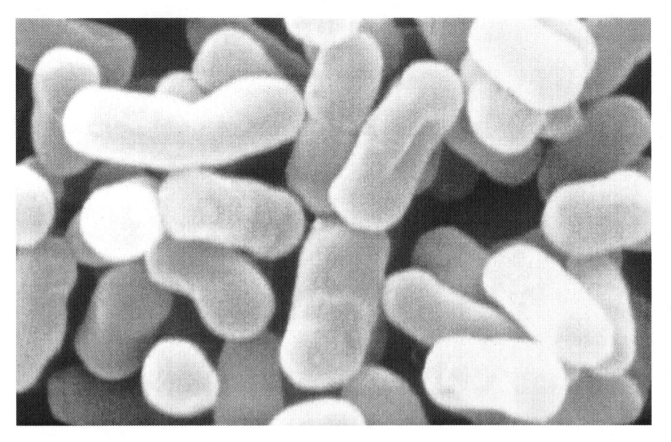

Magnified image of *Escherichia coli (E. coli)*. *(Custom Medical Stock Photo. Reproduced by permission.)*

Allopathic treatment

In serious cases of food poisoning, medications may be given to stop abdominal cramping and vomiting. Medications are not usually given for the diarrhea, since stopping it might keep toxins in the body longer and prolong the illness. Severe bacterial food poisonings are sometimes treated with antibiotics, but their use is controversial. Washing out the stomach contents to remove the toxic substances may be required. This procedure is called gastric lavage, familiarly known as having the stomach pumped. Neurotoxins often interfere with the breathing process. If the ability to breathe is affected, patients may have to be put on a mechanical ventilator to assist their breathing and are fed intravenously until the paralysis passes.

People who show any signs of botulism poisoning must receive immediate emergency medical care. Both infants and adults suffering from food poisoning by *C. botulinum* require hospitalization, often in the intensive care unit. A botulism antitoxin is given to adults, if it can be administered within 72 hours after symptoms are first observed. If given later, it provides no benefit. Nasogastric intubation is recommended for the feeding of infants with active botulism. As well as supplying **nutrition**, it will stimulate peristalsis, helping in the elimination of *C. botulinum*.

Treatment of food poisoning that is usually not an emergency situation may include drugs such as **ipecac** syrup to induce vomiting or laxatives to empty the intestines. Intravenous fluids containing salts and dextrose may be given to correct dehydration and electrolyte imbalances. Pain medications are given for severe stomach pain. Atropine is given for muscarine-type mushroom poisoning. If illness comes on after eating unidentified mushrooms, vomiting should be induced immediately, and the vomitus saved for laboratory testing. Intravenous mannitol is sometimes used to treat severe ciguatera poisoning. Antihistamines may be effective in reducing the symptoms of histamine fish poisoning. In 2001, Japanese scientists made a synthetic version of ciguatoxin, an important step in developing an antibody to help diagnose ciguatera.

In mild cases of food poisoning, dietary modifications are often the only treatment necessary. During periods of active vomiting and diarrhea, people with food poisoning should avoid solid food for eight to 24 hours, and should increase fluids. Clear liquids should be consumed in small quantities. Once active symptoms stop, a diet of bland, easily digested foods such as broth, eggs, rice and other cooked grains, and toast is recommended

COMMON PATHOGENS CAUSING FOOD POISONING	
Pathogen	**Common Host(s)**
Campylobacter	Poultry
E.coli 0157:H7	Undercooked, contaminated ground beef
Listeria	Found in a variety of raw foods, such as uncooked meats and vegetables, and in processed foods that become contaminated after processing
Salmonella	Poultry, eggs, meat, and milk
Shigella	This bacteria is transmitted through direct contact with an infected person or from food or water that become contaminated by an infected person
Vibrio	Contaminated seafood

Source: Food Safety and Inspection Service, U.S. Department of Agriculture. *(Stanley Publishing. Reproduced by permission.)*

for two to three days. Milk products, spicy food, alcohol, sweets, raw vegetables, and fresh fruit should be avoided.

Expected results

Many cases of food poisoning clear up on their own within a week without medical assistance. There are usually few complications once possible dehydration has been addressed. **Fatigue** may continue for a few days after active symptoms stop, however. In the more severe types of poisoning, especially those involving neurotoxins, the respiratory muscles may become paralyzed. In such cases, death will result from asphyxiation unless there is medical intervention. Deaths due to food poisoning are rare and tend to occur in the very young, the very old, and in people whose immune systems are already weakened.

C. botulinum, is likely to cause serious illness or fatalities, even when ingested in very small quantities. Children affected by food poisoning from *E. coli* often need to be hospitalized. In some cases, *E. coli* toxins may be absorbed into the blood stream where they destroy red blood cells and platelets, which are important in blood clotting. About 5% of victims, regardless of age, develop hemolytic uremia syndrome, which results in kidney failure.

Prevention

Eighty-four percent of adults surveyed in 2001 were unaware that feces on beef and poultry was the main carrier of salmonella, campylobacter, and *E. coli*. Other

than informing the public, food poisoning prevention efforts include:

- hot foods should be kept hot, and cold foods should be kept cold
- meat should be cooked to the recommended internal temperature; eggs should be cooked until no longer runny
- leftovers should be refrigerated promptly and food should never be left to stand at room temperature
- contact of utensils and surfaces with the juices of raw meats should be avoided
- fruits and vegetables should be washed before using
- unpasteurized dairy products and fruit juices should be avoided
- bulging or leaking canned foods or any food that smells spoiled should be discarded
- hands should be washed with soap before food preparation and after using the bathroom
- food preparation surfaces should be sanitized regularly
- infants under 12 months should not be fed honey, which may contain spores of *C. botulinum*
- proper canning and adequate heating of home-canned food before serving are essential (boiling for three minutes is recommended)

Taking *Lactobacillus acidophilus* or *L. bulgaricus* may help prevent food poisoning, especially when traveling. Populating the intestines with these bacteria will make it less likely that harmful bacteria are able to gain a foothold.

KEY TERMS

Arrhythmia—A disrupted heartbeat pattern.

Disulfiram-like poison—Disulfiram is a chemical compound that causes a severe physiological reaction to alcohol. This poison behaves like disulfiram.

Electrolytes—Salts and minerals in the body that are important because they control body fluid balance and support all major body reactions.

Nasogastric intubation—Insertion of a tube through the nose and mouth for delivery of food and oxygen.

Neurotoxin—A poison that acts on the central nervous system.

Peristalsis—Waves of contractions, such as through the intestines, forcing the contents onward.

Resources

PERIODICALS

"Chicken and Beef are Often Contaminated with Feces." *Health and Medicine Week* (October 1, 2001).

Ramsay, Sarah. "Organic Chemistry Takes on Tropical Seafood Poisoning." *The Lancet* (December 1, 2001): 1878.

OTHER

FDA Center for Food Safety & Applied Nutrition. *Foodborne Pathogenic Microorganisms and Natural Toxins Handbook.* [cited October 2002]. <http://vm.cfsan.fda.gov/~mow/intro.html>.

Merck & Co., Inc. "*E. coli* O157:H7 Infection." *The Merck Manual Online.* [cited October 2002]. <http://www.merck.com/pubs/mmanual/section3/chapter28/28b.htm>.

Merck & Co., Inc. "Gastroenteritis." *The Merck Manual Online.* [cited October 2002]. <http://www.merck.com/pubs/mmanual_home/sec9/106.htm>.

Patience Paradox
Teresa G. Odle

Foxglove

Description

Foxglove, also called *Digitalis purpurea*, is a common biennial garden plant that contains digitoxin, digoxin, and other cardiac glycosides. These are chemicals that affect the heart. Digitalis is poisonous; it can be fatal even in small doses. It was the original source of the drug called digitalis.

Foxglove is a native of Europe. It was first known by the Anglo-Saxon name *foxes glofa* (the glove of the fox), because its flowers look like the fingers of a glove. This name is also thought to be related to a northern legend that bad fairies gave the blossoms to the fox to put on his toes, so that he could muffle his footfalls while he hunted for prey. The legend may account in part for some of the common names of digitalis: dead man's bells, fairy finger, fairy bells, fairy thimbles, fairy cap, ladies' thimble, lady-finger, rabbit's flower, throatwort, flapdock, flopdock, lion's mouth, and Scotch mercury.

Foxglove was first introduced to the United States as an ornamental garden plant. During the first year, foxglove produces only leaves. In its second season it produces a tall, leafy flowering stalk that grows 3–4 ft (0.9–1.2 m) tall. In early summer, many tubular, bell-shaped flowers bloom; they are about 2 in (5.08 cm) long and vary in color from white to lavender and purple.

Foxglove was originally used for congestive heart failure and atrial fibrillation (chaotic contractions across the atrium of the heart). Foxglove helps the muscles of the heart to contract, reduces the frequency of heartbeats, and lowers the amount of oxygen the heart needs to work. The cardiac glycosides in foxglove block an enzyme that regulates the heart's electrical activity. The dried leaves, ripe dried seeds, and fresh leaves of the one-year-old plant, or the leaves of the two-year old plant are the parts that were used in medicine.

In spite of its use in the past, foxglove has been largely replaced as a heart medicine by standardized pharmaceutical preparations because it is one of the most dangerous medicinal plants in the world. Foxglove is, in fact, a useful example of the importance of standardization in testing the efficacy and possible toxicity of present-day popular herbal medicines. Its sap, flowers, seeds, and leaves are all poisonous; the leaves, even when dried, contain the largest amount of cardiac glycosides. The upper leaves of the stem are more dangerous than the lower leaves. Foxglove is most toxic just before the seeds ripen. It tastes spicy hot or bitter and smells slightly bad.

In folk medicine, foxglove was first used in Ireland. Its use spread to Scotland, England, and then to central Europe. It was taken to treat abscesses, **boils**, headaches, paralysis, and stomach ulcers. It was also applied to the body to help **wounds** heal and to cure ulcers. It has not been proven to be an effective treatment for any of these ailments.

In 1775, William Withering, an English doctor, first discovered the accepted medicinal use of foxglove. He identified digitalis as a treatment for swelling or **edema**

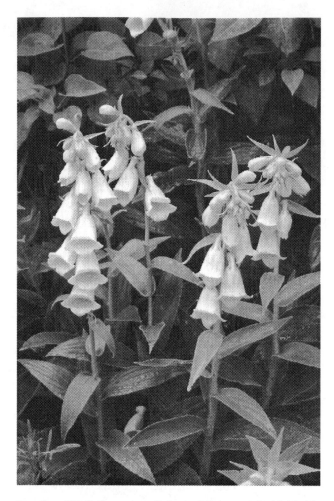

Foxglove (*Digitalis purpurea*) plant. *(Photograph by Michael P. Gadomski. Photo Researchers, Inc. Reproduced by permission.)*

associated with congestive heart failure. Withering published a paper in 1785 that is considered a classic in the medical literature. Foxglove was used to treat **heart disease** during the eighteenth and nineteenth centuries.

General use

Foxglove is no longer used as a heart medicine because the therapeutic dose and the lethal dose are very close. Seasonal variations in the level of cardiac glycosides in the plant make the safe dose impossible to estimate except by an experienced physician and prescriber of the herb who monitors the patient on an hourly basis for signs of overdose. Few living doctors and herbalists can safely use digitalis as a plant extract. Specific standardized doses of pharmaceutical digoxin are used instead. Even so, patients receiving the drug must be closely monitored.

Preparations

In present-day usage, foxglove is used as an ingredient in a class of heart drugs called digitalis. Digoxin (Lanoxin) is the most common drug made from digitalis. Digitalis is usually taken orally, as capsules, as an elixir, or as tablets. It can also be given in an injection.

Precautions

Used improperly, foxglove is deadly; it can make the heart stop or cause a person to suffocate. Eating any part of the plant can be fatal. The therapeutic dose of foxglove is very close to the lethal dose. Foxglove should therefore not be used.

An overdose of foxglove interferes with the heart's normal electrical rhythms; it can make the heart beat too slowly or cause extra heartbeats. An overdose of foxglove may also cause **diarrhea**, **headache**, loss of appetite, and **vomiting**. More serious and potentially deadly reactions to an overdose affect the heart and the central nervous system. Foxglove can disrupt the heart's rhythm, including life-threatening ventricular tachycardia, or atrial tachycardia with atrioventricular block. In the central nervous system, foxglove can cause confusion, **depression**, drowsiness, hallucinations, psychoses, and visual disturbances.

Poisoning from foxglove occasionally occurs from the misuse of such herbal preparations as dried foxglove leaves used in a tea, or from overdoses of prescribed digitalis. It can also occur when foxglove is confused with **comfrey**, a plant used for tea that belongs to the borage family. The two herbs look very much alike.

Side effects

Some patients who take pharmaceutical preparations of digitalis may experience such side effects as too much muscle tone in the stomach and intestines, diarrhea, headache, loss of appetite, and vomiting. These side effects are the same as some symptoms of a foxglove overdose. Digitalis preparations can have toxic side effects due to overdose or other conditions. The most serious are arrhythmias, abnormal heart rhythms that can be life-threatening.

Interactions

The use of digitalis can increase the toxicity of other cardioactive drugs. Hypersensitivity to digitalis, dehydration, or the use of diuretics that cause people to lose fluids and salts may increase the risk of side effects from digoxin. The risk of cardiac arrhythmias is increased when people taking digitalis also take amphetamines or diet pills; medicine for **asthma** or other breathing problems; or medicine for colds, sinus problems, **hay fever**, or other **allergies**. Taking any of these drugs with digitalis also affects how much digitalis is in the body and how effective it will be.

Resources

BOOKS

PDR for Herbal Medicines. Montvale, NJ: Medical Economics Company, 1998.

PERIODICALS

Dickson, C. "Mountain Healing: Medicinal Plants of the Southern Appalachians." *Mother Earth News* 173 (1999): 18.

Goldman, Peter. "Herbal Medicines Today and the Roots of Modern Pharmacology." *Annals of Internal Medicine* 135 (October 16, 2001): 594–600.

OTHER

Sievers, A. F. "Foxglove." *The Herb Hunters Guide.* Washington, DC: Miscellaneous Publication, No. 77. 1930 [cited December 2002]. <http://newcrop.hort.purdue.edu/newcrop/herbhunters/foxglove.html>.

Lori De Milto
Rebecca J. Frey, PhD

Fractures

Definition

A fracture is a crack or break in a bone. It results from the application of excessive force through injuries, such as a fall or a hard blow.

Description

Up to the age of 50, more men suffer from fractures than women because of occupational hazards. However, after the age of 50, more women suffer fractures than men because of osteoperosis. Simple, or closed, fractures are not obvious on the surface because the skin remains intact. Compound, or open, fractures break through the skin, exposing bone. They are generally more serious than closed fractures. When bones are broken, there may be an accompanying soft tissue injury or an infection either in the surrounding tissue or the bone itself. If an artery is damaged, there can be a significant loss of blood. Single and multiple fractures refer to the number of breaks in the same bone. Fractures are termed complete if the break is completely through the bone, and described as incomplete, or greenstick, if the fracture occurs partly across a bone shaft. This latter type of fracture is often the result of bending or crushing on the bone. A stress fracture is usually a small break in the bone due to repeated or prolonged force.

Causes & symptoms

Fractures usually result from an injury to a bone that causes the bone tissue or cartilage to be disrupted or broken. Bones weakened by disease or misuse will be more likely to break. In some women who have gone through **menopause**, the bones fracture easily due to osteoperosis. This is because the body produces less estrogen at that time of life, and estrogen is a major regulator of bone density through its effects on **calcium** in the body. Moderate **exercise** and weight training is helpful in building and maintaining strong bones; so, the bones of an inactive person may also tend to fracture easier than those who are moderately active. However, individuals with a very high activity level have a greater risk of fractures. This group includes children and athletes participating in contact sports. Because bones start to thin out with the **aging** process, the elderly are also at a high risk of sustaining a fracture. Diseases that may lead to an increased risk of fractures include Paget's disease, rickets, osteogenesis imperfecta, **osteoporosis**, tumors, deficiencies of vitamins A or D, and **stroke** induced paralysis.

Fractures usually begin with intense **pain** and swelling at the site of injury. Obvious deformities, such as a crooked or otherwise misshapen limb, point to a possible fracture. Pain that prevents the use of a limb may also indicate a break. In severe fractures, there may be a loss of pulses below the fracture site and a resultant numbness, tingling, or paralysis in the feet, hands, fingers, or toes below the site. An open fracture is often accompanied by bleeding or bruising. If a leg is fractured, there will usually be difficulty bearing weight on it. If there is **dizziness**, sweating, disorientation, or thirst, the onset of shock may be indicated.

Diagnosis

Diagnosis begins immediately with the individual's own observation of symptoms. A thorough medical his-

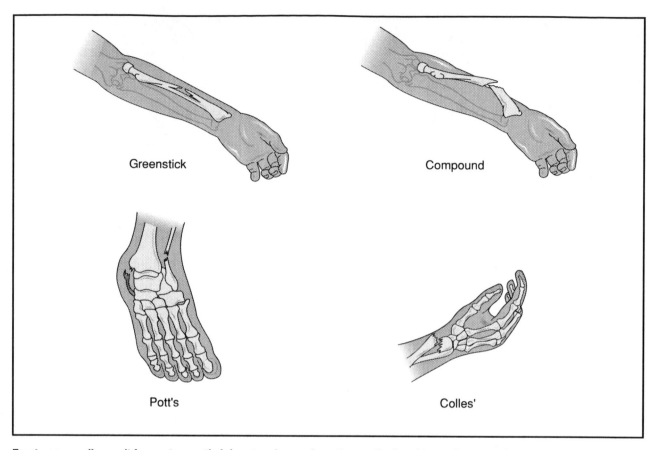

Fractures usually result from a traumatic injury to a bone where the continuity of bone tissues or bony cartilage are disrupted or broken. The illustrations above feature common sites where fractures occur. *(Illustration by Electronic Illustrators Group. The Gale Group)*

tory and physical exam completed by a physician often provides enough information to determine if further testing is necessary. An x ray of the injured area is most commonly used to determine the presence of a bone fracture. However, it is important to note that not all fractures are apparent on an initial x ray. Rib fractures are often difficult to diagnose and may require several views at different angles. If the fracture is open and occurs in conjunction with soft tissue injury, further laboratory studies may have to be done.

In the event of stress fractures, a tuning fork can provide a simple, inexpensive test. The tuning fork is a metal instrument with a stem and two prongs that vibrate when struck. If a patient has increased pain when the tuning fork is placed on the bone, such as the lower leg bone or shinbone, the likelihood of a stress fracture is high. Bone scans also are helpful in detecting stress fractures or other difficult-to-detect fractures.

Treatment

Prevention is the most effective way to avoid fractures. Wearing protective gear, such as a helmet, or using protective equipment, such as safety gear, while playing sports may greatly reduce the risk of a fracture.

A daily multivitamin and mineral supplement (for instance, containing calcium, **magnesium**, **boron**, strontium) is recommended to help build and maintain a healthy, resilient skeleton. These, together with an adequate protein intake, will also help rebuild the bone and surrounding tissue. Some physical therapists use electrostimulation over a fractured site to promote and expedite healing. Chinese traditional medicine seeks to reconnect the qi through the meridian lines along the line of a fracture. **Homeopathy** can enhance the body's healing process. A particularly useful homeopathic remedy for soft tissue is *Arnica* 12c, taken every 10 minutes for the first two hours after injury, and then once every eight hours for two to three days. *Symphytum officinalis* is also a good remedy to help heal the fractured bone.

Calming herbs are often useful for relief of pain and tension. Cups of **chamomile** (*Matricaria recutitca*), **catnip** (*Nepeta cataria*), or **lemon balm** (*Melissa officinalis*) tea can be given freely for a calming effect. Fifteen drops of **skullcap** (*Scutellaria lateriflora*), **St. John's wort**

(*Hypericum perforatum*), or **valerian** (*Valeriana officinalis*) tincture can be given every half hour as needed. A tea to encourage the bone tissue to knit and heal can be made by mixing together one ounce each of **comfrey** leaves (*Symphytum officinale*), nettles (*Urtica dioica*), and oatstraw (*Avena sativa*), plus half an ounce each of **horsetail**, skullcap, and **marsh mallow** root (*Althaea officinalis*). One quarter ounce each of **fennel** seeds (*Foeniculum officinalis*) and **peppermint** leaves (*Mentha piperita*) should also be added. A strong tea should be made of one ounce of the mixture in one quart of boiling water, which should steep for at least a half hour. The dosage is two cups taken daily. Frequent soaks or compresses with comfrey root in the water is recommended if there is no broken skin. *Arnica montana*, *Calendula officinalis*, St. John's wort, or comfrey salves or ointments can improve healing when applied externally, as well.

After initial treatments, the application of contrast **hydrotherapy** to a hand or foot below the area of the fracture can be used to assist healing by enhancing circulation. Contrast hydrotherapy uses an alternating series of hot and cold water applications. Either compresses or basins of water may be used. First, hot compress is applied for three minutes. It is followed by cold water for 30 seconds. These applications are repeated three times each, ending with the cold water.

Allopathic treatment

Broken bones need to be treated as soon as possible by a physician. Temporary measures include applying ice packs to injured areas, and the use of aspirin or nonsteroidal anti-inflammatories (NSAIDS) to reduce pain and swelling. Initial first aid for a fracture may include splinting, control of blood loss, and monitoring of vital signs, such as breathing and circulation. Medical treatment will depend on the location of the fracture, its type and severity, and the individual's age and general health status. If an open fracture is accompanied by serious soft tissue injury, it may be necessary to control bleeding and the shock that can accompany it.

Immobilization of the fracture site can be done internally or externally. The primary goal of immobilization is to maintain the realignment of the bone long enough for healing to start and progress. Immobilization by external fixation uses splints, casts, or braces; this may be the primary and only procedure for fracture treatment. Splinting to immobilize a fracture can be done with or without traction. In emergency situations, splinting is a useful form of fracture management, if medical care is not immediately available. It should be done without causing additional pain and without moving the bone segments. In a clinical environment, plaster of Paris casts are used for immobilization. Braces are useful as they often allow movement above and below the fracture site.

Open reduction is surgery that is usually performed by an orthopedist. It allows the surgeon to examine and correct soft tissue damage while the bones are being repositioned into their normal alignment. Internal fixation devices, such as metal screws, plates, and pins, hold the bones in place as they heal. Fragments are often held together with metal rods. Later, the physician may or may not elect to remove these devices when healing is complete. Open reduction is most often used for open, severe, or comminuted fractures. Fractures with little or no displacement of the bones do not usually require such surgery.

Closed reduction refers to realigning the bones without using surgery. It is accomplished by manually adjusting the bones or using traction, and often requires the use of an anesthetic. Traction is a form of closed reduction that works by applying a steady force to the bones, pulling on them with weights until the proper alignment is achieved. The traction device can also be used to immobilize the affected area while the bone heals. Since traction restricts movement, this treatment means that the patient will be confined to bed rest for an extended period of time.

In external fixation, pins or screws are attached to the bone directly above and below the site of the fracture. They are then connected to a device of metal bars fixed over the skin. These act as a frame, keeping the bones aligned so they can heal properly. With any type of treatment for a fracture, muscle and joint strength and flexibility should be maintained through proper exercises done as the bone tissue heals.

Healing time for fractures varies from person to person, with the elderly generally needing more time to heal completely. Recovery is complete when there is no bone motion at the fracture site, and x rays indicate complete healing.

Expected results

Fractures can normally be cured with proper first aid and after care. Proper realignment of the bones is much more difficult if the break has occurred more than six hours in the past. If broken bones are not properly treated, deformities may occur as the bones heal, and strength and flexibility may be affected.

Prevention

Adequate calcium intake, as well as intakes of other minerals like magnesium, boron, strontium, and others, is necessary for strong bones and can help decrease the risk of fractures. Foods rich in calcium should be eaten. These include fish, dairy products, sardines, broccoli, en-

KEY TERMS

Bone scan—A diagnostic procedure in which radioactive tracer is injected and images are taken of specific areas or the entire skeleton.

Osteoporosis—Literally meaning "porous bones," this condition occurs when bones lose an excessive amount of their protein and mineral content, particularly calcium. Over time, bone mass and strength are reduced leading to the increased risk of fractures.

Paget's disease—A common disease of the bone of unknown cause usually affecting middle-aged and elderly people, characterized by excessive bone destruction and unorganized bone repair.

Rickets—A condition caused by the deficiency of vitamin D, calcium, and usually phosphorus, seen primarily in infancy and childhood, and characterized by abnormal bone formation.

riched soymilk, seaweed, tahini, and other sesame seed foods, nuts, molasses, and dark leafy green vegetables. Calcium supplements may be also be useful; however, those with bone meal or oyster shell have been found to often contain toxic heavy metals. Adequate stores of **vitamin D** are needed to help use calcium, therefore, some time should be spent in the sun, as this will activate vitamin D and help decrease fractures. Safety measures to avoid accidents that may bring on fractures include wearing seat belts and protective sports gear, when appropriate. Estrogen replacement combined with exercise and weight training for women past the age of 50 has been shown to help prevent osteoporosis and the fractures that may result from this condition.

Resources

BOOKS

American Red Cross Editors. *First Aid and Safety.* St. Louis: Mosby, 1993.

The Editors of Time-Life Books. *The Medical Advisor: The Complete Guide to Alternative and Conventional Treatments.* Alexandria, VA: Time-Life, Inc., 1996.

Romm, Aviva Jill. *Natural Healing for Babies and Children.* Freedom, CA: The Crossing Press, 1996.

OTHER

American Academy of Orthopedic Surgeons. http://orthoinfo. aaos.org/brochure/.

drkoop.com. http://www.drkoop.com/conditions/ency/article/ 000001.htm.

Patience Paradox

French green clay

Description

French green clay is a substance that is used for external cosmetic treatments as well as some internal applications by practitioners of alternative medicine. It was used in ancient Egypt, Greece, and Rome to treat a variety of skin problems and digestive disorders.

From the standpoint of mineralogy, French green clay belongs to a subcategory of clay minerals known as illite clays, the other two major groups being kaolinite and smectite clays. Clay minerals in general are important because they make up about 40 percent of such common rocks as shale, and they are the main components of soil. Illite clays are usually formed by weathering or by changes produced in aluminum-rich minerals by heat and acidic ground water. They often occur intermixed with kaolinite clays—which are typically used in the ceramics industry. Illite clays have been used successfully by environmental managers to remove such heavy metals as lead, cadmium, and **chromium** from industrial wastewater.

French green clay takes its name from the fact that rock quarries located in southern France enjoyed a virtual monopoly on its production until similar deposits of illite clays were identified in China, Montana, and Wyoming. The clay's green color comes from a combination of **iron** oxides and decomposed plant matter, mostly **kelp** seaweed and other algae. Grey-green clays are considered less valuable than those with a brighter color. The other components of French green clay include a mineral known as montmorillonite, as well as **dolomite, magnesium, calcium, potassium, manganese, phosphorus, zinc,** aluminum, silicon, **copper, selenium,** and cobalt.

French green clay is prepared for the commercial market by a process of sun-drying and crushing. After the clay has been mined, it is spread in the sun to remove excess water. It is then ground by large hydraulic crushers and micronized, or finely pulverized. The last stage in the process is a final period of sun-drying to remove the last traces of water. French green clay is available in a dry powdered form for a variety of uses as well as in premixed soaps, scrubs, facial powders, and masks for cosmetic purposes. Prices for an eight-ounce jar of powdered clay range between $4.50 and $11.00 in health food stores. Soaps made with French green clay are priced at about $4.50 a bar.

General use

External

French green clay is most commonly used in the United States and Canada for cosmetic purposes, as distinct from medicinal treatments. It is regarded as a useful treatment for stimulating the skin and removing impurities from the epidermis (outermost layer of skin cells). The clay works by adsorbing impurities from the skin cells, by causing dead cells to slough off, and by stimulating the flow of blood to the epidermis. As the clay dries on the skin, it causes the pores to tighten and the skin to feel firm.

Other external uses for French green clay include poultices to treat arthritis, sore muscles, and sprains; ready-to-use pastes for application to cuts, **bruises**, insect bites, stings, and minor **burns**; and mineral baths for **stress** relief. Some practitioners maintain that the plant matter in French green clay has anti-inflammatory as well as antiseptic or bactericidal properties. It is interesting that a group of Italian researchers reported in 2002 that French green clay powder is as effective as salicylic sugar powder in preventing infection of the umbilical stump in newborns. The clay powder was found to be superior to powders containing **colloidal silver**, antibiotics, or fuchsine.

Internal

Internal uses of French green clay are more popular in Europe than in North America, although some American alternative healers recommend drinking or gargling with solutions of French green clay to cleanse the digestive tract, treat **nausea** or other gastric disorders, ease menstrual cramps, or relieve sore throats. It is claimed that French green clay absorbs toxins from the stomach and intestines as well as neutralizing radioactivity in the body. A French naturopath states that the copper in the clay fights **infections**, the cobalt helps to prevent **anemia**, the selenium aids liver function and slows down the **aging** process, and the other minerals restore the body's overall equilibrium.

Preparations

External

Facial masks: Commercial prepackaged clay masks are generally spread on the face directly from the jar or tube, care being taken to avoid the eye area. After the clay dries—usually about 10–15 minutes— the mask is washed off with warm running water. To make a facial mask from powdered clay, combine 1/2 to 1 tbsp of the powder with 1–2 tbsp of water and apply to the skin; rinse with warm water after 10 minutes. Some users add a few drops of **aloe** vera gel to the clay mixture. A recipe for a facial mask for oily skin consists of mixing 1 tbsp of powdered clay with 5 drops of **jojoba oil**.

A recipe for a "gourmet spa facial mask" calls for mixing 1/4-cup of French green clay powder with 1/4-cup water. After the clay and water have been well blended, 2 tbsp of honey and 1/4-cup of mashed banana or avocado are added to the mixture. The mask is applied to the face, allowed to remain for 10 min, and rinsed off with warm water.

Deodorizing foot treatment: A half-cup of powdered French green clay is mixed with 1/2-cup of water and 2–3 drops of tea tree essential oil. The mixture is applied to the feet, covered loosely with plastic wrap, and rinsed off after 15 min with cool water. The feet may then be rubbed with a moisturizing cream.

Poultice: One poultice recipe calls for mixing several tablespoons of powdered clay with enough water to form a thick paste and allowing it to stand in a glass bowl for two hours. The paste is then applied in a layer about 1/4-in thick to a piece of gauze. The poultice is applied to the injured area with the gauze uppermost and held in place with adhesive tape. It can be left in place as long as two hours, but the clay should not be allowed to dry. Up to 6 drops of essential oil of **lavender**, Roman **chamomile**, **ginger**, or **rosemary** may be added if desired. Poultices should not be reused but discarded after use.

Mineral bath: A half-cup of powdered French green clay can be added to a tub of warm water to soothe sunburned or irritated skin, or relieve arthritis or muscle pains.

Internal

To cleanse the digestive system, mix 1 tsp of powdered clay in an 8–10-ounce glass of mineral water and allow to stand overnight. The mixture may be taken the next morning either as the clear liquid that has risen to the top or after stirring to recombine the clay and water. It is to be taken every morning for 21 days. The treatment should not be repeated until a week after the last dose. The clay mixture can also be used to relieve menstrual cramps; it is taken each morning during the first three weeks of the woman's cycle. After the flow begins, a warm clay poultice can be applied to the abdomen in the morning and evening.

A recipe for a **sore throat** gargle consists of 1–2 tsp of clay added to a glass of salt water with 1–2 drops of essential oil of rosemary or lavender. The gargle can be used several times a day until the symptoms are relieved.

A European regimen for treating **hemorrhoids** consists of drinking three glasses of powdered clay in water each day for three weeks, alternating with three weeks without the mixture over a total period of three months. The clay-and-mineral water mixture can also be combined with tinctures of Indian vine and **witch hazel**. In addition, poultices made with green clay can be applied to the affected areas in the morning, followed by a cold bath. The poultices may also be applied at night.

Precautions

Alternative healers state that French green clay should never be mixed with metal spoons or stored in metal containers; the only materials that should be used in preparation or storage are wooden spoons or glass stirrers, and either glass or ceramic containers. It is thought that the clay loses its beneficial qualities through contact with metal. This belief has some scientific basis in the fact that illite clays have been found to be highly effective in removing heavy metals in the wastewater produced by various industries.

External

As a rule, French green clay masks should be used only once a week because the clay tends to dry the skin. In addition, cosmetics containing French green clay are not recommended for naturally dry or sensitive skins, as the mineral content of the clay is an irritant. Soaps made with French green clay should be used only for oily skin.

Internal

French green clay may cause **constipation** when taken internally. Some practitioners recommend drinking only the water without the clay at the bottom of the glass in the morning for this reason.

Side effects

French green clay may cause skin **rashes** or patches of dry flaky skin when used on the face. It may cause constipation when taken internally. No side effects from mineral baths or poultices have been reported.

A group of American toxicologists reported in 2003 that illite clays as a group appear to be safe for short-term internal use in humans as well as external cosmetic applications. There have, however, been isolated reports of lung damage caused in workers exposed to particles of montmorillonite—one of the major components of French green clay—in spray paints and primers.

Interactions

No interactions with prescription drugs or herbal remedies have been reported for French green clay as of 2004. However, because of the adsorptive qualities of French green clay, it may interfere with absorption of medications.

Resources

BOOKS

Dextreit, Raymond. *L'argile qui guérit. Memento de médecine naturelle* . Paris: éditions de la revue Vivre en harmonie,

---

KEY TERMS

Adsorption—A process in which an extremely thin layer of one substance (liquid, gas, or solid) forms on the surface of another substance. French green clay works as a cosmetic treatment by adsorbing toxic substances from the skin.

Epidermis—The outermost layer of skin cells.

Illite—A family of hydrous potassium aluminosilicate clays, characterized by a three-layer structure and a gray, light green, or yellow-brown color. The name is derived from Illinois, where these clays were first classified in 1937. French green clay belongs to this group of clays.

Poultice—A soft cloth filled with a warm moist mass of grains, herbs, or other medications applied to sores or injured parts of the body.

1976. Translated into English as *The Healing Power of Clay* . Geneva, Switzerland: Editions Aquarius, S. A., 1987.

Pough, Frederick H. *A Field Guide to Rocks and Minerals.* Boston: Houghton Mifflin Company, 1988.

PERIODICALS

Elmore, A. R.; Cosmetic Ingredient Review Expert Panel. "Final report on the safety assessment of aluminum silicate, calcium silicate, magnesium aluminum silicate, magnesium silicate, magnesium trisilicate, sodium magnesium silicate, zirconium silicate, attapulgite, bentonite, Fuller's earth, hectorite, kaolin, lithium magnesium silicate, lithium magnesium sodium silicate, montmorillonite, pyrophyllite, and zeolite." *International Journal of Toxicology* 22 (2003, Supplement 1): 37–102.

Katsumata, H., S. Kaneco, K. Inomata, et al. "Removal of Heavy Metals in Rinsing Wastewater from Plating Factory by Adsorption with Economical Viable Materials." *Journal of Environmental Management* 69 (October 2003): 187–191.

Pezzati, M., E. C. Biagioli, E. Martelli, et al. "Umbilical Cord Care: The Effect of Eight Different Cord-Care Regimens on Cord Separation Time and Other Outcomes." *Biology of the Neonate* 81 (January 2002): 38–44.

ORGANIZATIONS

Cosmetic Ingredient Review (CIR). 1101 17th Street NW, Suite 310, Washington, DC 20036. (202) 331-0651. Fax: (202) 331-0088. <http://www.cir-safety.org>.

Society of Cosmetic Chemists (SCC). 120 Wall Street, Suite 2400, New York, NY 10005-4088. (212) 668-1500. Fax: (202) 668-1504. <http://www.scconline.org>.

U. S. Food and Drug Administration (FDA). 5600 Fishers Lane, Rockville, MD 20857-0001. (888) INFO-FDA. <http://www.fda.gov>.

Rebecca J. Frey, PhD

Fritillaria

Description

Fritillaria is the processed bulb of *Fritillaria cirrhosa*, a flowering plant in the Liliaceae family. A perennial temperate herb, it grows in mountain slope and subalpine meadows, usually on open, stony, and moist hillsides. In the West, fritillaria is most commonly regarded as an ornamental garden plant. By contrast, it is traditionally valued as an herbal remedy in Nepal and China, where it grows in the Gansu, Qinghai, Sichuan, Xizang, and Yunnan provinces. Two related species, *F. thunbergii* and *F. hupehensis*, are also used medicinally, and in some regions, *F. unibracteata, F. przewalski,* and *F. delavayi* are used as botanical substitutes.

In **traditional Chinese medicine**, fritillaria is called *chuan bei mu* which translates as "Shell mother from Sichuan." English common names include fritillary, tendrilled fritillary bulb, and Sichuan fritillary bulb. Its pharmaceutical name, used to distinguish it as a medicine, is Bulbus Fritillariae Cirrhosae and it is one of more than 500 plants recognized as official drugs in traditional Chinese medicine.

General use

Practitioners of Chinese medicine believe that fritillaria affects the heart and lung meridians, or energy pathways in the body, and use it primarily to treat various lung conditions, including **asthma**, **bronchitis**, **tuberculosis**, and coughs of any type. In the traditional Chinese medical system, the white color of fritillaria is thought to indicate its usefulness for ailments of the lungs, which are associated with the color white. Fritillaria's medicinal properties are considered bitter, sweet, and mildly cold.

Fritillaria is used for many types of **cough**, particularly chronic cough, cough associated with difficult expectoration, and cough with blood-streaked sputum. Chinese practitioners prescribe it to moisten dry mucous membranes, resolve phlegm, and control coughing. It is thought to be most effective for coughs accompanied by reduced appetite and a stifling sensation in the chest and upper abdomen, symptoms that indicate suppressed qi, or vital energy.

Fritillaria's secondary use is as a lymphatic decongestant to reduce swellings, nodules, fibrocystic breasts, goiter, and swollen lymph glands. In China, it also is used for thyroid and **lung cancer**.

Research on *F. cirrhosa* and its botanical relatives has generally been conducted in China and has focused on pharmacological investigation. These studies show that *F. cirrhosa* and other related species contain compounds that have antitussive and expectorant activity because they inhibit contraction of bronchial smooth muscle and decrease secretion of mucus. Compounds responsible for this activity, as defined in Western chemistry, include several bioactive isosteroidal alkaloids (verticine, verticinone, isoverticine, imperialine, hupehenine, ebeiedine, ebeienine, and ebeiedinone) and two nucleosides (thymidine and adenosine). The discovery of a new diterpenoid ester in fritillaria was reported in 2002.

Animal research has also demonstrated central nervous-system inhibition, including prolonged decrease in blood pressure, stimulation of the heart muscle, and dysfunction of breathing.

Preparations

Fritillaria is not generally available in American health food stores but processed forms are available at Chinese pharmacies and Asian groceries. Chinese patent medicines containing fritillaria can be purchased over the Internet; typical prices are $13–$15 for a 4-oz bottle. As medicine, fritillaria is graded into four categories, based on shape and the location in which it was grown: *song-pei, lu-pei, ching-pei,* and *ming-pei.* Because the raw bulb is toxic, all medicinal forms are processed. Good quality processed powder is white and has a fine consistency. Small, white, lobed bulbs that have been boiled or steamed and dried also may be available.

The standard dose ranges from 3–12 grams daily as a decoction (strong tea) or 1–1.5 grams as powder. Pills in equivalent doses are also available, and the herb also may be applied externally as either a powder or cream.

Practitioners of Chinese medicine commonly combine fritillaria in patent formulas along with other Chinese herbs such as ma huang (*Ephedra sinica*) and ballanflower (*Platycodon grandiflorum*). It is in many cough medicine formulas in liquid form. The following are the major herbs with which it is combined and the symptoms for which the combinations are prescribed:

- bitter apricot kernel (*Prunus armeniaca; xing ren*) for cough and **wheezing** with copious sputum

- loquat leaf (*Eriobotrya japonica; pi pa ye*), dwarf lilyturf root (*Ophiopogon japonicus; mai men dong*) and Solomon's seal root (*Polygonatum odoratum; yu zhu*) for chronic cough with **fatigue**, irritability, and lack of appetite

- thin-leaf milkwort root (*Polygala tenuifolia; yuan zhi*), hoelen fungus (*Poria cocos; fu ling*), and snakegourd fruit (*Trichosanthes* spp.; *gua lou*) for painful obstruction of the chest with palpitations and insommnia

- Zhejiang fritillary bulb (*F. thunbergii; zhe bei mu*) for scrofula (a form of tuberculosis affecting the lymph nodes) and abscess

Precautions

The unprocessed bulb of fritillaria is toxic, although commercial sources are generally processed. Pregnant women should not use fritillaria unless under the advice of a practitioner trained in the use of the herb. Fritillaria should never be given to children. It is also contraindicated for patients with digestive weakness.

Australian authorities recommend that products containing *F. cirrhosa* include the following label caution: "Warning: Do not exceed the stated dose." Canadian regulations list *F. thunbergii*, a close relative of *F. cirrhosa*, as unacceptable for inclusion in non-medicinal oral products.

A general precaution to observe when using any Chinese patent medicine is to purchase only well-known brands recommended by a practitioner of traditional Chinese medicine. Cases have been reported of incorrect labeling, contamination with heavy metals, and substitution of Western pharmaceuticals for the Chinese ingredients. Any of these occurrences can present a serious health hazard.

Side effects

Side effects from fritillaria extracts used in Chinese patent medicines are rare, but this is partly because fritillaria is usually a minor ingredient in these formulae, often only 10% of the formula by weight. Even in medicines that list fritillaria as a major ingredient, it is never more than 28% of the compound. Tests of fritillaria extract in human subjects reported no side effects when the extract was taken by mouth. On the other hand, high-dosage intravenous injections of alkaloids isolated from fritillaria produced pupil dilation, tremor, slowing of the heart rate, and lowered blood pressure in human subjects.

Interactions

No interactions with standard pharmaceuticals have been described in the literature, but the absence of reported interactions may again be due to the fact that fritillaria extract is not the sole ingredient in any Chinese medicine.

Tradition dictates not to combine fritillaria with **aconite** root (*wu tou*) or *qin jiao (Gentiana macrophylla)*.

Resources

BOOKS

Bensky, D. and Andrew Gamble. *Chinese Herbal Medicine: Materia Medica.* Revised ed. Seattle, WA: Eastland Press, 1993.

Fan, W. *A Manual of Chinese Herbal Medicine: Principles and Practice for Easy Reference.* East Lansing, MI: Shambala, 1996.

KEY TERMS

Alkaloids—A diverse group of nitrogen-containing substances that typically taste bitter. Most alkaloids are toxic, although a minority of them are medicinally beneficial.

Cold—In Chinese pathology, the term defines a condition that has insufficient warmth, either objective (hypothermia) or subjective (feeling cold).

Decoction—A strong tea brewed for twenty to thirty minutes; generally used for woodier herbs.

Meridians—Energetic pathways inside the body through which qi flows.

Nucleosides—Any of various compounds consisting of a sugar and a purine or pyrimidine base, especially a compound obtained by hydrolysis of a nucleic acid

Patent formulas—Chinese herbal formulas that were patented centuries ago and are believed to be proven over centuries of use and study

Qi—The Chinese medical term for physiological energy or more generally for the life force.

Sputum—Matter coughed up from the respiratory tract, including saliva, mucus, or phlegm.

Holmes, P. *Jade Remedies: A Chinese Herbal Reference for the West.* Boulder, CO: Snow Lotus Press, 1997.

Reid, Daniel. *Chinese Herbal Medicine.* Boston, MA: Shambhala, 1996.

PERIODICALS

Atta-Ur-Rahman, Akhtar M. N., M. I. Choudhary, Y. Tsuda et al. "New Steroidal Alkaloids from *Fritillaria imperialis* and Their Cholinesterase Inhibiting Activities." *Chemical and Pharmaceutical Bulletin (Tokyo)* 50 (August 2002): 1013-1016.

Ruan, H., Y. Zhang, J. Wu et al. "Structure of a Novel Diterpenoid Ester, Fritillahupehin from Bulbs of *Fritillaria hupehensis Hsiao and K.C. Hsia.*" *Fitoterapia* 73 (July 2002): 288-291.

ORGANIZATIONS

American Association of Oriental Medicine. 5530 Wisconsin Avenue, Suite 1210, Chevy Chase, MD 20815. (301) 941-1064. <www.aaom.org>.

Institute of Traditional Medicine. 2017 SE Hawthorne Blvd., Portland, OR 97214. (503) 233-4907. <www.itmonline.org>.

Erika Lenz
Rebecca J. Frey, PhD

Frostbite and frostnip

Definition

Frostbite is localized tissue injury that occurs because of exposure to freezing or near freezing temperatures. Frostnip is a milder cold injury that does not cause tissue loss.

Description

In North America, frostbite is largely confined to Alaska, Canada, and the northern states. In recent years, there has been a substantial decline in the number of cases. This is probably for several reasons, including better winter clothing and footwear and greater public understanding of how to avoid cold-weather dangers. At the same time, the nature of the at-risk population has changed. Rising numbers of homeless people have made frostbite an urban as well as a rural public health concern. The growing popularity of outdoor winter activities has also expanded the at-risk population.

Causes & symptoms

Frostbite

Skin exposed to temperatures a little below the freezing mark can take hours to freeze, but very cold skin can freeze in minutes or seconds. Air temperature, wind speed, and moisture all affect how cold the skin becomes. A strong wind can lower skin temperature considerably by dispersing the thin protective layer of warm air that surrounds our bodies. Wet clothing readily draws heat away from the skin. The evaporation of moisture on the skin also produces cooling. For these reasons, wet skin or clothing on a windy day can lead to frostbite even if the air temperature is above the freezing mark.

The extent of permanent injury, however, is determined more by the length of time the skin is frozen than by how cold the skin and the underlying tissues become. Thus, homeless people and others whose self-preservation instincts may be clouded by alcohol or psychiatric illness face a greater risk of frostbite-related amputation. They are more likely to stay out in the cold when prudence dictates seeking shelter or medical attention. Alcohol also affects blood circulation in the extremities in a way that can increase the severity of injury, as does **smoking**. A review of 125 Saskatchewan frostbite cases found a tie to alcohol in 46% and to psychiatric illness in 17%. Driving in poor weather can also be dangerous: vehicular failure was a predisposing factor in 15% of the Saskatchewan cases.

Frostbite is classified by degree of injury (first, second, third, or fourth), or simply divided into two types, superficial (corresponding to first- or second-degree in-

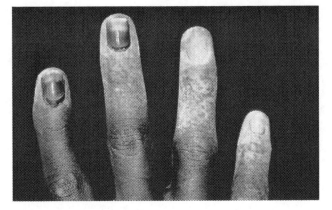

Human hand with frostbite. *(Photo Researchers, Inc. Reproduced by permission.)*

jury) and deep (corresponding to third- or fourth-degree injury). Most frostbite injuries affect the feet or hands. The remaining 10% of cases typically involve the ears, nose, cheeks, or penis. Once frostbite sets in, the affected part begins to feel cold and, usually, numb; this is followed by a feeling of clumsiness. The skin turns white or yellowish. Many patients experience severe **pain** in the affected part during rewarming treatment and an intense throbbing pain that arises two or three days later and can last days or weeks. As the skin begins to thaw during treatment, **edema** often occurs, causing swelling in the area. In second- and higher-degree frostbite, **blisters** appear. Third-degree cases produce deep, blood-filled blisters and, during the second week, a hard black eschar (scab). Fourth-degree frostbite penetrates below the skin to the muscles, tendons, nerves, and bones. In severe cases of frostbite, the dead tissue can mummify and drop off. Affected areas are also more prone to infection.

Frostnip

Like frostbite, frostnip is associated with ice crystal formation in the tissues, but no tissue destruction occurs and the crystals dissolve as soon as the skin is warmed. Frostnip affects areas such as the earlobes, cheeks, nose, fingers, and toes. The skin turns pale and numb or tingly until warming begins.

Diagnosis

Frostbite diagnosis relies on a physical examination and may also include conventional radiography (x rays), angiography (x-ray examination of the blood vessels using an injected dye to provide contrast), thermography (use of a heat-sensitive device for measuring blood flow), and other techniques for predicting the course of injury and identifying tissue that requires surgical removal. During the initial treatment period, however, severity is difficult to judge. Diagnostic tests only become useful 3-5 days after rewarming, once the blood vessels have stabilized.

Treatment

Mechanical treatment

Frostnipped fingers are helped by blowing warm air on them or holding them under one's armpits. Other frostnipped areas can be covered with warm hands. The injured areas should never be rubbed.

By contrast, emergency medical help should always be sought whenever frostbite is suspected. While waiting for help to arrive, one should, if possible, remove wet or tight clothing and put on dry, loose clothing or wraps. A splint and padding are used to protect the injured area. Rubbing the area with snow or anything else is dangerous. The key to prehospital treatment is to avoid partial thawing and refreezing, which releases more mediators of inflammation and makes the injury substantially worse. For this reason, the affected part must be kept away from heat sources such as campfires and car heaters. Experts advise rewarming in the field only when emergency help will take more than two hours to arrive and refreezing can be prevented.

Because the outcome of a frostbite injury cannot be predicted at first, all hospital treatment follows the same route. Treatment begins by rewarming the affected part for 15-30 minutes in water at a temperature of 104-108°F (40-42.2°C). This rapid rewarming halts ice crystal formation and dilates narrowed blood vessels. **Aloe** vera (which acts against inflammatory mediators) is applied to the affected part, which is then splinted, elevated, and wrapped in a dressing. Milky blisters are debrided (cleaned by removing foreign material), and hemorrhagic (blood-filled) blisters are simply covered with aloe vera.

Hydrotherapy

Alternative practitioners suggest several kinds of treatment to speed recovery from frostbite after leaving the hospital. Bathing the affected part in warm water or using contrast **hydrotherapy** can enhance circulation. Contrast hydrotherapy involves a series of hot and cold water applications. A hot compress (as hot as the patient can stand) is applied to the affected area for three minutes followed by an ice-cold compress for 30 seconds. These applications are repeated three times each, ending with the cold compress. For patients who have been hospitalized with frostbite, hydrotherapy should only be performed after checking with a physician to ensure it is done correctly and does not aggravate the condition.

Homeopathy

Homeopathic *Hypericum* (*Hypericum perforatum*) is recommended when nerve endings are affected (espe-

cially in the fingers and toes) and *Arnica* (*Arnica montana*) is prescribed for shock and if there is accompanying blunt trauma to the frostbitten area.

Nutritional supplements

Cayenne pepper (*Capsicum frutescens*) can enhance circulation and relieve pain. Drinking hot **ginger** (*Zingiber officinale*) tea also aids circulation.

Other complementary therapies

Other possible approaches include **acupuncture** to avoid permanent nerve damage and oxygen therapy.

Allopathic treatment

In addition to the necessary rewarming and debridement described above, a **tetanus** shot and antibiotics may be used to prevent infection. The patient is given ibuprofen to combat inflammation. Narcotics are needed in most cases to reduce the excruciating pain that occurs as sensation returns during rewarming. Except when injury is minimal, treatment generally requires a hospital stay of several days, during which hydrotherapy and physical therapy are used to restore the affected part to health. Experts recommend a cautious approach to tissue removal, and advise that 22–45 days must pass before a decision on amputation can safely be made.

Expected results

The rapid rewarming approach to frostbite treatment, pioneered in the 1980s, has proved to be much more effective than older methods in preventing tissue loss and amputation. The extreme, throbbing pain that many frostbite sufferers endure for days or weeks after rewarming is not the only prolonged symptom of frostbite. During the first weeks or months, people often experience tingling, a burning sensation, or a sensation resembling shocks from an electric current. Other possible consequences of frostbite include changes of skin color, nail deformation or loss, joint stiffness and pain, hyperhidrosis (excessive sweating), and heightened sensitivity to cold. For everyone, a degree of sensory loss lasting at least four years—and sometimes a lifetime—is inevitable.

Prevention

With the appropriate knowledge and precautions, frostbite can be prevented even in the coldest and most challenging environments. Appropriate clothing and footwear are essential. To prevent heat loss and keep the blood circulating properly, clothing should be worn loosely and in layers. Covering the hands, feet, and head is also crucial for preventing heat loss. Outer garments need to be wind and water resistant, and wet clothing and footwear must be replaced as quickly as possible. Alcohol and drugs should be avoided because of their harmful effects on judgment and reasoning. Experts also warn against alcohol use and smoking in the cold because of the circulatory changes they produce. Paying close attention to the weather report before venturing outdoors and avoiding unnecessary risks such as driving in isolated areas during a blizzard are also important.

Resources

BOOKS

The Burton Goldberg Group. *Alternative Medicine: The Definitive Guide.* Tiburon, CA: Future Medicine Publishing,1993.

Danzl, Daniel F. "Disturbances Due to Cold." In *Conn's Current Therapy,* edited by Robert E. Rakel. Philadelphia: W.B. Saunders,1998.

McCauley, Robert L., et al. "Frostbite and Other Cold-Induced Injuries." In *Wilderness Medicine: Management of Wilderness and Environmental Emergencies,* edited by Paul S. Auerbach. St. Louis: Mosby, 1995.

PERIODICALS

Gill, Paul G., Jr. "Winning the Cold War." *Outdoor Life* (February 1993): 62+.

Phillips, David. "How Frostbite Performs Its Misery." *Canadian Geographic* (January-February 1995): 20+.

Reamy, Brian V. "Frostbite: Review and Current Concepts." *Journal of the American Board of Family Practice* (January-February 1998): 34-40. http://www.medscape.com/ ABFP/JABFP/1998/v11.n01/fp1101.05.ream/fp1101.05.r eam.html. (6 June 1998).

Winkelmann, Terry. "The Cold Facts about Frostbite." *Stride* (Winter 1997). http://www.stridemag.com/db_area/ archives/1997/v2n4/frost.html. (6 June 1998).

Judith Turner

Fungal infections

Definition

Fungi are types of parasitic plants that include molds, mildew, and yeast. A fungal infection is an in-

flammatory condition in which fungi multiply and invade the skin, the digestive tract, the genitals, and other body tissues, particularly, the lungs and liver. Fungal infections of the skin are often called ringworm or tinea.

Description

Microscopic fungi, which are called dermatophytes, often live exclusively on such dead body tissues as hair, the outer layer of the skin, and the nails. The fungus grows best in moist, damp, dark places with poor ventilation and on skin that is irritated, weakened, or continuously moist. Superficial fungal infections include tinea capitis, an infection of the neck and scalp; tinea barbae, also called barber's itch, along the beard area in adult males; tinea corporis on parts of the body, such as the arms, shoulders, or face; tinea cruris, or **jock itch**, involving the groin; tinea pedis, or **athlete's foot**; tinea versicolor; and tinea unguium, or infection of the nails. The term tinea gladiatorum is sometimes used to describe ringworm infections in atheletes. Tinea gladiatorum is most common in swimmers, wrestlers, and athletes involved in other contact sports. Fungal infections of the skin and nails are very common in children, but they can affect all age groups.

Systemic fungal infections occur when spores are touched or inhaled, or there is an overgrowth of fungi in or on the body. Such infections are most often a serious problem in those with suppressed immune systems. Candidiasis is a rather common fungal infection. When it occurs in the mouth, it is called thrush. Less often, it occurs in the mucous membranes of other parts of the digestive system, or in the vagina, heart valves, urinary tract, eyes, or blood. Other systemic fungal infections include aspergillosis, which mostly affects the lungs and may also spread to the brain and kidneys; blastomycosis, a lung infection that may spread through the bloodstream; coccidioidomycosis, also known as San Joaquin or valley **fever;** mucormycosis, which can develop into a very serious, life-threatening infection; and histoplasmosis.

Causes & symptoms

Fungi are widespread in the environment, so it is not unusual that a certain amount of fungi and their spores end up being inhaled into the lungs or landing on the skin. Under conditions of moisture, warmth, irritation, or injury, these fungi grow rapidly and may cause illness. Superficial fungal infections may be due to an overgrowth of fungi already present, or the infection may be the result of contact with an infected person or with contaminated surfaces, bed sheets, towels, or clothing. Fungal infections can be spread from one part of the body to another by scratching or touching. Additionally, tinea unguium infec-

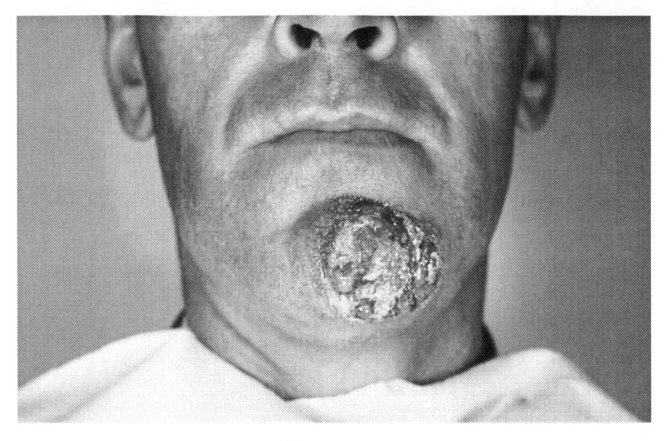

Ringworm on a man's chin. These infections are most common on the feet, scalp, or in toenails, but they can infect any part of the skin. *(Custom Medical Stock Photo. Reproduced by permission.)*

tions have been linked to the use of methyl methacrylate, a glue used for attaching acrylic fingernails.

Fungal spores are often present in soil and are likely to be inhaled when the soil is dug up or otherwise disturbed. Systemic fungal infections are commonly contracted in this way. In addition, fungi that normally inhabit the intestines, such as *Candida albicans*, may multiply, causing an infection due to an overgrowth of the fungi.

Tinea infections usually cause itchy, red, scaly, ring-shaped patches on the skin that spread easily. Hairs in the area of infection often fall out or break off, and the skin may crack. The skin may also develop a secondary bacterial infection. In tinea unguium, the nails discolor, crack, and thicken. Tinea versicolor may cause pigment changes in the skin that persist for up to a year.

Systemic fungal infections develop slowly. Symptoms often may be nonexistent, or there may be only the feeling of having a cold or the flu. Coughing, a fever, chest **pain**, **chills**, weight loss, and difficulty with breathing may become evident. Additional symptoms depend on the type and site of the infection.

Fungal infections are more common and more severe in people taking antibiotics, corticosteroids, immunosuppressant drugs, and contraceptives. This is also the case in people with endocrine disorders, immune diseases, and other conditions such as **obesity, AIDS, tuberculosis,** major **burns, leukemia,** and **diabetes mellitus.** Fungal infections often occur due to the use of antibiotic drugs for other conditions, because antibiotics kill off the bacteria that normally keep fungi at bay.

Diagnosis

Fungal infections of the skin, hair, and nails often can be diagnosed based on the characteristic appearance of affected areas. A KOH (**potassium** hydroxide) prep is a simple laboratory test to confirm the diagnosis. The test uses tissue samples treated with a 20% potassium hydroxide solution to detect fungi. Examining the skin with a Wood's ultraviolet lamp is another easy and convenient method to determine the presence of a fungus. Culture and sensitivity testing can be used if a more definitive diagnosis is required. Systemic fungal infections may be initially diagnosed from blood tests. Confirmation is determined by cultures made from sputum, blood, urine, bone marrow, or infected tissue samples.

Treatment

Among the herbs that slow down or halt the growth of fungus are **goldenseal** (*Hydrastis canadensis*), **myrrh** (*Commiphora molmol*), **garlic** (*Allium sativa*), **pau d'arco** (*Tabeebuia impestiginosa*), **turmeric** (*Curcuma longa*), oregano (*Origanum vulgare*), cinnamon (*Cinnamonum zeylanicum*), jewelweed, **sage** (*Salvia officinalis*), *Impatiens aurea*, **yellow dock** (*Rumex crispus*), the lichen known as old man's beard (*Usnea barbata*), **black walnut** husks and bark (*Juglans nigra*), **licorice** (*Glycyrrhiza glabra*), and *Calendula officinalis*. These herbs can be applied to external fungus as infusions, salves, powders, or vinegars. Many of them can also be taken internally as capsules or tinctures. Antifungal herbs can be quite strong, however, and care should be taken that a given remedy is suitable for internal use.

When an infusion is used, the affected area should be washed or soaked in the herbal water for at least 15 minutes twice daily. Store-bought or homemade tea bags can be soaked in water or vinegar for about 10 minutes and then used as a poultice for the same effect. Herbal vinegars make excellent remedies for fungus, as vinegar is in itself antifungal. "Gourmet" vinegars with such antifungal ingredients as oregano and garlic are often readily available at grocery stores. The vinegar can be applied a few times daily with cotton or compresses. In addition, a bentonite clay dusting powder can be useful for drying out the environment of moist skin in which fungus thrives. It works best when mixed with powdered antifungal herbs such as myrrh or goldenseal. Dusting powder is especially helpful for athlete's foot.

Many herbs high in **essential oils** also have antifungal action, particularly tea tree (*Melaleuca alternifolia*), oregano, **lavender** (*Lavandula officinalis*), *Eucalyptus* spp., rose geranium (*Pelargonium graveolens*), **peppermint** (*Mentha piperita*), **chamomile** (*Matricaria recutita*), and myrrh. Peppermint oil is especially helpful in relieving the **itching** associated with many fungal infections. The simplest way to use **aromatherapy** to fight fungal infections is to add several drops of any single essential oil or combination of oils to bathwater. Essential oil can also be added to mixtures for soaking or compresses. Tea tree is the herb most frequently recommended for the treatment of superficial fungal infections. As with all essential oils, the full-strength oil should be diluted in a carrier. A dilution of **tea tree oil** can be made by adding the essential oil to a carrier oil. This mixture can be added directly to the site of a skin infection.

A healthy diet should be maintained. Foods that are high in yeast, such as beer and wine, breads, and baked goods should be avoided. Fermented foods and sugary foods, including honey and fruit juices, should also be avoided until symptoms have cleared. Antifungal culinary herbs such as garlic, tumeric, oregano, sage, and cinnamon should be used liberally in foods. Yogurt containing live cultures can be incorporated into the diet to supply needed gut bacteria, and help reduce digestive infections such as candidiasis and thrush. *Lactobacillus acidophilus* and *Lactobacillus bulgaricus* can also be taken directly as supplements.

Supplements that can be taken for fungal infections include vitamins A, B complex, C, and E. Caprylic acid, an extract of the coconut plant, is also recommended as an antifungal, as well as **grapefruit seed extract**. **Essential fatty acids**, contained in **evening primrose oil**, fish liver oil, or **flaxseed** oil, can help reduce the inflammation of systemic or superficial fungal infections. A dose of one of these oils is recommended as a daily supplement.

Allopathic treatment

Superficial fungal infections are usually treated with such antifungal creams or sprays as tolnaftate (Aftate or Tinactin), clotrimazole, miconazole nitrate (Micatin products), econazole, ketoconazole, ciclopirox, naftifine, itraconazole, terbinafine, fluconazole, or Whitfield's tincture made of salicylic acid and benzoic acid. If the infection is resistant, a doctor may prescribe an oral antifungal drug such as ketoconazole or griseofulvin. Drugs used for systemic infections include amphotericin B, which is highly toxic and is used for severe or life-threatening infections; the azoles, particularly fluconazole and itraconazole, which have been found to be the least toxic of these medications; and flucytosine alone or in combination with other antifungal medications. Fungal infections that become inflamed may be treated with a combination antifungal/steroid medication. Certain infections may require surgery.

Expected results

Infections usually respond to treatment within several weeks. However, many fungal infections are resistant to treatment, and it may take an extended time and repeated treatments to effect a cure. Infections may spread, and secondary bacterial infections may develop. Medications for fungal infections are often strong, and their use may cause such undesirable side effects as **headache, dizziness, nausea, vomiting,** or abdominal pain. Fungal infections are usually not serious in otherwise healthy individuals. However, a systemic fungal infection may be severe and life-threatening for those with compromised immune systems.

Prevention

Good personal hygiene should be maintained. In the case of superficial infections, the skin should be kept

Journal of Dermatologic Treatment 13 (June 2002): 73-76.

KEY TERMS

Azole—Any member of a group of chemical compounds with five-membered rings containing one or more nitrogen atoms. Several azoles are used as antifungal medications.

Bentonite clay—A green clay of aluminum silicate containing magnesium and trace minerals. The clay can draw out agents of infection.

Dermatophyte—A type of fungus that is parasitic on skin and causes a skin disease.

Tinea—A term that refers to any of several fungal infections of the skin, especially ringworm.

clean and dry, and care should be taken to avoid contact with other parts of the body. If someone in the household has a superficial fungal infection, bed sheets, towels, floors, shower stalls, and other contact surfaces should be washed with hot water and disinfected after use.

Resources

BOOKS

Duke, James A., Michael Castleman, and Alice Feinstein. *The Green Pharmacy.* Emmaus, PA: Rodale Press, 1997.

PERIODICALS

Farschian, M., R. Yaghoobi, and K. Samadi. "Fluconazole Versus Ketoconazole in the Treatment of Tinea Versicolor."

Kohl, T. D., et al. "Tinea gladiatorum: Pennsylvania's Experience." *Clinical Journal of Sports Medicine* 12 (May 2002): 165-171.

Lipozencic J., M. Skerlev, R. Orofino-Costa et al. "A Randomized, Double-Blind, Parallel-Group, Duration-Finding Study of Oral Terbinafine and Open-Label, High-Dose Griseofulvin in Children with Tinea Capitis Due to *Microsporum* Species." *British Journal of Dermatology* 146 (May 2002): 816-823.

Weinstein, A., and B. Berman. "Topical Treatment of Common Superficial Tinea Infections." *American Family Physician* 65 (May 15, 2002): 2095-2102.

ORGANIZATIONS

American Academy of Dermatology. 930 East Woodfield Rd., PO Box 4014, Schaumburg, IL 60168. (847) 330-0230. <www.aad.org>.

OTHER

drkoop.com Medical Encyclopedia. "Ringworm." http://www.drkoop.com/conditions/ency/article/001439.htm.

Merck & Co., Inc. *The Merck Manual of Diagnosis and Therapy.* http://www.merck.com/pubs/mmanual/section10/chapter113/113a.htm.

Merck & Co., Inc. *The Merck Manual of Diagnosis and Therapy.* http://www.merck.com/pubs/mmanual/section13/chapter158/158a.htm.

Patience Paradox
Rebecca J. Frey, PhD

Furuncles *see* **Boils**

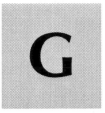

Gallstones

Definition

Gallstones are solid crystal deposits that form in the gallbladder, a pear-shaped organ that stores bile until it is needed to help digest fatty foods. These crystals can migrate to other parts of the digestive tract, causing severe **pain** and life-threatening complications. Gallstones vary in size and chemical structure. They may be as tiny as a grain of sand, or as large as a golf ball.

Description

Gallstones usually develop in adults between the ages of 20 and 50. The risk of developing gallstones increases with age. Young women are up to six times more likely to develop gallstones than men in the same age group. In patients over 50, however, the condition affects men and women with equal frequency. Native Americans develop gallstones more often than any other segment of the population, and Mexican Americans have the second highest incidence of this disease. Gallstones tend to be passed down genetically in families.

Eighty percent of gallstones are composed of **cholesterol**. They are formed when the liver produces more cholesterol than the digestive juices can liquefy. The remaining 20% of gallstones are composed of **calcium** and an orange-yellow waste product called bilirubin, which gives urine its characteristic color and sometimes causes **jaundice**.

People who have gallstones may remain without symptoms for an extended period, especially if the stones remain in the gallbladder. In most cases, medical treatment is only deemed necessary if the individual is experiencing symptoms. When symptoms do appear, it is usually because the stones have left the gallbladder and are stuck somewhere else within the biliary system, blocking the flow of bile. If gallstones remain stuck in the biliary system, there can be damage to the liver, pancreas, or the gallbladder itself.

Gallstones bring on several disorders including:

• Cholelithiasis: Gallstones within the gallbladder itself. Pain is caused by the contractions of the gallbladder around the stone.

• Choledocholithiasis: The presence of gallstones within the common bile duct, which is the passage between that empties into the small intestine. Once discovered, common duct stones need to be removed in order to avoid further problems.

• Cholecystitis: A disorder marked by inflammation of the gallbladder. It is usually caused by the passage of a stone from the gallbladder into the cystic duct, which connects the gallbladder to the common bile duct. Cholecystitis causes painful enlargement of the gallbladder and is responsible for 10–25% of all gallbladder surgery.

Causes & symptoms

Gallstones are caused by an alteration in the chemical composition of bile, which is a fluid that helps the body break down and absorb fats. It is widely held that a diet high in fats and processed foods, and low in fiber and whole foods, is a strong contributor to gallstone formation. High levels of estrogen, insulin, or cholesterol can increase a person's risk of developing gallstones. If left untreated, the risk of developing **anemia** is also increased.

Gallbladder attacks usually follow a meal of rich foods, typically high in fat. The attacks often occur in the middle of the night, sometimes waking the patient with such intense pain that the episode ends in a visit to the emergency room. Pain often occurs on the right side of the body. The pain of a gallbladder attack begins in the abdomen and may radiate to the chest, back, or the area between the shoulders. Other symptoms of gallstones include inability to digest fats, low **fever**, **chills** and sweating, **nausea** and **vomiting**, **indigestion**, **gas**, belching, and clay-colored bowel movements.

Pregnancy or the use of birth control pills slow down gallbladder activity and increase the risk of gall-

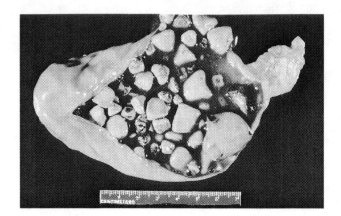

A specimen of a gallbladder with stones. *(Custom Medical Stock Photo. Reproduced by permission.)*

stones, as do diabetes, **pancreatitis**, and **celiac disease**. This is due to an individual's higher levels of cholesterol, insulin, or estrogen from oral contraceptives. Other factors that may encourage gallstone formation are:

• infection

• anemia

• obesity

• intestinal disorders

• coronary artery disease

• multiple pregnancies

• a high-fat, low-fiber diet

• smoking

• heavy drinking

• rapid weight loss

Diagnosis

When gallstones are suspected, blood tests for liver enzyme levels are often given. The levels are usually elevated when the stone cannot pass through the cystic duct or bile duct. Test results, taken together with symptom history (see above) and a physical exam, are simple and relatively inexpensive for diagnosing the presence of gallstones. However, ultrasound is the method of choice for a definite diagnosis. It has a high degree of accuracy, except in diagnosing cholecystitis (a stone in the cystic duct). Cholescintigraphy is an alternative method of diagnosis, in which radioactive dye is injected and photographed as it passes through the biliary system.

Treatment

An allergic reaction to certain foods may contribute to gallbladder attacks. These foods should be identified and removed from the diet, or at least seriously limited. Foods that might possibly bring on allergic reactions include eggs, pork, onions, chicken, milk, coffee, citrus, corn, nuts, and beans.

Other dietary changes may help relieve the symptoms of gallstones. Generally, a vegetarian diet is protective against the formation of gallstones. Recurrent attacks can be diminished by maintaining a healthy weight and a healthy diet.

Choleretic herbs encourage the liver to secrete bile. They help maintain the appropriate chemical composition of bile so that it does not form stones. These herbs include:

• A tincture of **dandelion** (*Taraxacum officinale*), 2–6 ml once daily.

• Milk thistle seeds (*Sylibum marianum*), a dose equivalent to 70–210 mg of silymarin.

• Artichoke leaves (*Cynara scolymus*), 150 mg three times per day.

• Turmeric (*Curcuma longa*), used as a spice; 150 mg three times per day.

Use of the above herbs cause some possible reactions, such as gas, **diarrhea**, nausea, and indigestion.

Other therapeutic approaches that have been found to be helpful in treating gallstones include **homeopathy**, traditional Chinese herbal medicine, and **acupuncture**. Knowledgeable practitioners should be consulted.

Allopathic treatment

Watchful waiting

One-third of all patients with gallstones never experience a second attack. For this reason, many doctors advise an attitude of "wait and see" after the first episode. Changing the diet or following a sensible weight loss plan may be the only treatments required. A person having only occasional mild gallstone attacks may be able to manage them by using non-prescription forms of acetaminophen, such as Tylenol or Anacin. A doctor should be notified if pain intensifies or lasts for more than three hours; if the fever rises above 101°F (38.3°C); or if the skin or whites of the eyes have a yellowish cast.

Surgery

Surgical removal of the gallbladder, called cholecystectomy, is the most common conventional treatment for recurrent or worsening gallstone attacks. However, surgery is unecessary in most cases where the gallstones remain without symptoms. Laparoscopic cholecystectomy is the technique most widely used. It has mostly replaced traditional open surgery because of a shorter recovery time, decreased pain, and reduced scarring. However, the open surgery procedure is still used in about 5% of cases because of various complications.

Nonsurgical therapy

If surgery is considered inappropriate, gallstones can be dissolved in 30–40% of patients by taking bile acids in tablet form. Dissolution of gallstones by this method may take many months or years depending on the size. Unfortunately, though, recurrence of stones is common after cessation of the medication.

Lithotripsy uses high-frequency sound waves directed through the skin to break up the stones. The process can be combined with the use of bile acid tablets. However, lithotripsy requires special equipment and is not always readily available.

Direct cholangiography can be used to remove gallstones by contact dissolution. The procedure is used to insert a catheter to inject medication into the gallbladder. Stones are often dissolved within a few hours by this method.

Expected results

Forty percent of all patients with gallstones have "silent gallstones" that do not require treatment. If symptoms develop, however, medical intervention may become necessary. Gallstone problems requiring treatment may also develop **infections** that require antibiotics. In rare instances, severe inflammation can cause the gallbladder to burst, causing a potentially fatal situation. The gallbladder is not an organ that is required to retain health. It can be successfully removed, with no recurrence of stones. Fat digestion, however, becomes more difficult after surgery, since the gallbladder is no longer there to store and release bile as needed.

Prevention

It is easier, in general, to prevent gallstones than to reverse the process. The best way to prevent gallstones is to minimize risk factors. Since gallstones seem to develop more often in people who are obese, eating a balanced diet, exercising, and losing weight may help keep gallstones from forming. In addition, a diet high in dietary fiber and low in fats, especially saturated fats, is recommended. Processed foods should be replaced by complex carbohydrates, such as whole grains.

Increased intake of fluids will dilute the bile and inhibit gallstone formation. Six to eight glasses of water should be consumed daily, along with plenty of herbal teas and diluted juices.

KEY TERMS

Bile—A bitter, greenish liquid secreted by the liver that aids in the digestion and absorption of fats.

Cholecystectomy—Surgical removal of the gallbladder.

Common bile duct—The passage through which bile travels from the cystic duct to the small intestine.

Lithotripsy—A nonsurgical technique for removing gallstones by breaking them apart with high-frequency sound waves.

Recent studies indicate that consumption of about two tablespoons of olive oil per day, which can be mixed with food, helps reduce cholesterol levels in the bloodstream and the gallbladder. However, large amounts of olive oil, taken as a so-called liver flush, should be avoided. This method can stress the gallbladder and lead to an emergency situation.

Resources

BOOKS

The Editors of Time-Life Books. *The Medical Advisor: The Complete Guide to Alternative and Conventional Treatments.* Alexandria, VA: Time-Life, Inc., 1996.

Gottlieb, Bill, ed. *New Choices in Natural Healing.* Emmaus, PA: Rodale Press, Inc., 1995.

Murray, Michael, N.D., and Joseph Pizzorno. *Encyclopedia of Natural Medicine.* Rocklin, CA: Prima Publishing, 1991.

Shaw, Michael, ed. *Everything You Need to Know About Diseases.* Springhouse, PA: Springhouse Corporation, 1995.

PERIODICALS

"Exercise Prevents Gallstone Disease." *Journal Watch*

ORGANIZATIONS

National Digestive Diseases Clearinghouse (NDDIC). 2 Information Way, Bethesda, MD 20892-3570. http://www.niddk.nih.gov/health/digest/nddic.htm.

National Institute of Diabetes and Digestive and Kidney Disorders of the National Institutes of Health. Bethesda, MD 20892. http://www.niddk.nih/gov/.

OTHER

Gallbladder Problems. http://www.sleh.com/fact-d04-gall.html.

http://www.thriveonline.com/health/Library/illsymp/illness229.html.

WebMD/Lycos. "How Are Gallstones and Gallbladder Disease Diagnosed?" http://webmd.lycos.com/content/dmk/dmk_article_3961803.

Patience Paradox

Gamma-linoleic acid

Description

Gamma-linoleic acid (GLA) is an omega-6 polyunsaturated fatty acid made in the body from linolenic acid, an essential fatty acid (EFA). GLA is the product of the body's first biochemical step in the transformation of a major essential fatty acid, linolenic acid (LA), into important prostaglandins. Prostaglandins are essential to the proper functioning of each cell. Every cell's structure in the human body depends on fatty acids formed from GLA.

General use

Evening primrose oil, very high in GLA, has been used for decades to treat medical conditions. Native American women chewed evening primrose seeds to relieve menstrual problems. Evening primrose was also used by Native Americans and early American settlers from Europe to treat coughs and stomach problems. In the 1800s, the leaves of the plant were used to treat several skin conditions.

EPO was imported to Europe during the 1600s and 1700s, and used to treat **gout, rheumatoid arthritis**, headaches, and skin conditions.

In animal studies gamma-linoleic acid has been shown to reduce certain inflammations and reduce joint tissue injury. Human studies showed similar findings in its anti-inflammatory effects.

GLA has also been used as a treatment option for a number of conditions, including **alcoholism, asthma**, attention deficit/hyperactivity disorder (ADHD), high **cholesterol**, diabetic neuropathy, certain cancers, **eczema** (a skin inflammation), **hypertension** (high blood pressure), **premenstrual syndrome** (PMS), rheumatoid arthritis, and scleroderma (a skin disease.)

There is also research data that indicates GLA in combination with other measures may help in treating people with Sjögren's syndrome— a chronic inflammatory disease of the immune system that effects mostly older women.

Other animal studies suggest GLA may enhance **calcium** absorption, helping to reduce calcium loss and osteporosis. Osteoporosis is a disease occurring primarily in women after **menopause** in which the bones become very porous, break easily, and heal slowly. It may lead to curvature of the spine after vertebrae collapse.

Among the conditions GLA is most often used for are:

• Rheumatoid arthritis. GLA has been studied for many years for its possible effects in treating arthritis and other inflammatory conditions . GLA has been shown to be most promising in treating people with this crippling condition, due to its anti-inflammatory properties. At least three studies have shown GLA reduces inflammation and joint tissue injury, thereby reducing the **pain** associated with this condition. In one study, GLA reduced the incidence of tender jointsby 36%, and swollen joints by 28%.

• ADHD. Studies suggest that GLA may be helpful (combined with other therapies) for helping to alleviate ADHD symptoms in children.

• Diabetes. Some studies show that GLA can help improve nerve function and help reduce **peripheral neuropathy**, which causes numbness, tingling, pain, or burning in the feet, legs, and toes and hands, in diabetics.

• High cholesterol. Research indicates that high doses of GLA may improve blood lipid levels in people with high cholesterol. A late 1990 study showed that oral intake of 2 grams of GLA daily for six weeks lowered total cholesterol levels by 13% and triglycerides by 37%.

• Skin conditions. A number of studies have been done regarding GLA and eczema with contradicting results. Several studies showed GLA relieved the symptoms such as **itching**, redness, and scaling of the skin, to varying degrees. It has also been shown to be helpful in reducing the symptoms of scleroderma and skin inflammations, such as dermatitis.

• **Cancer**. Studies have shown GLA effectively killed 40 types of human cancer cells in vitro without damaging normal cells This sentence is very misleading and makes GLA sound like a cure for cancer. Other in vitro or test tube studies have also shown GLA has potential to suppress tumor growth and metastasis, the spreading of cancer from the original site to other parts of the body. Several studies have shown it may be helpful specifically in treating pancreatic, bladder, and colon cancer. It has shown promising results as a cancer therapy when combined with the anticancer drugs tamoxifen and paclitaxol. Research into its effects on cancer are in the earliest stages and there is no evidence that GLA prevents or cures any type of cancer.

• Hypertension. Several studies suggest GLA may help reduce blood pressure in some people with hypertension and thereby decrease the risk of heart attacks. Results of these studies are not considered conclusive.

• PMS. Studies show GLA is remarkably helpful in treating some PMS symptoms. One study showed that of the women who took the drug Efamol, which contains 9% GLA, 61% experienced complete relief from symptoms while 23% had partial relief. These symptoms included breast tenderness, **depression**, irritability, swelling, and bloating.

Gamma-linolenic acid, in combination with eicosapentaenoic acid (EPA), in the form of borage seed and fish oils, significantly reduced the need for breathing support in patients with the lung condition acute respiratory distress syndrome. It cut the average number of days a patient is in a hospital's intensive care unit from 17.5 to 12.8, according to a study published in the August 1999 issue of *Critical Care Medicine*.

"The consumption of GLA may offer new strategies for treatment and prevention of certain chronic diseases. Potential candidates [such as] rheumatoid arthritis patients, will have to take GLA supplements in order to meet the beneficial dosages used in clinical studies, because GLA is not readily found in common foods," wrote Yang-Yi Fan and Robert S. Chapkin, scientists from Texas A&M University, in the September 1998 issue of *The Journal of Nutrition*.

Preparations

Gammalinoleic acid is found naturally in fish, animal organs such as liver, and certain plant seed oils. The major sources of GLA are **borage oil** (18–27% GLA), black currant oil (15–20% GLA), and evening primrose oil (7–14% GLA.) GLA is not available as a pure extract, but only as an ingredient in combination formulas.

Dosage varies by condition it is used to treat:

• skin conditions: 360–750 milligrams (mg) daily

• PMS: 240–320 mg daily

• rheumatoid arthritis: 750 mg–2.8 g daily for six to 12 months

• diabetic neuropathy: 480 mg daily

• high blood pressure: 1.3 g daily

• high cholesterol: Up to 2 g daily

The United States Food and Drug Administration (FDA) has not established recommended daily allowances (RDA) for gamma-linoleic acid.

Patients should consult with a heathcare professional regarding the proper dosage.

Several forms of GLA supplements are available, including a concentrated form. It is also available as evening primrose oil, borage oil, and **black currant seed oil**. It is also available in multi-nutrient formulas that often contain any combination of **fish oil**, flax seed oil, **omega-6 fatty acids**, and **essential fatty acids**. The usual amount of GLA in these is from 200–400 milligrams per capsule. The cost of a bottle of 30 capsules ranges from $8 to $15. The concentrations of GLA in these oils varies and the number of capsules needed depends on the amount of GLA.

Precautions

Gamma-linoleic acid should not be used by women who are pregnant or breastfeeding without consulting a physician. Hemophiliacs and people who take the blood-thinning drug warfarin (Coumadin) should consult a physician before taking GLA. It should also not be taken before surgery because it may increase bleeding. Persons with high blood pressure or heart or blood vessel conditions should consult a physician before taking GLA.

Side effects

There is no evidence that GLA is toxic in daily doses of up to 2.8 grams. There have been no reports of serious side effects by people taking GLA supplements. It is generally well tolerated by most people. Possible minor side effects include upset stomach, **diarrhea**, soft stool, bloating, and **gas**. Persons who take GLA and experience difficulty breathing, chest or throat tightness, chest pain, **hives**, rash, or itchy or swollen skin may be allergic to it. They should stop taking it and consult a physician immediately.

Interactions

No adverse interactions between gamma-linoleic acid and other medications, vitamins, or nutritional supplements have been reported.

Resources

BOOKS

Editors of Prevention Health Books. *Outsmart Arthritis* New York, NY: St. Martin's Press, 2003.

Graedon, Teresa, and Joe Graedon. *The People's Pharmacy Guide to Home and Herbal Remedies* New York, NY: St. Martin's Press, 2002.

Murray, Frank, and Len Saputo. *Natural Supplements for Diabetes: Reduce Your Risk and Lower Your Insulin Dependency With Natural Remedies* Charlottesville, VA: Hampton Roads Publishing Co., 2003.

Newman, Rosemary K., and C. W. Newman. *Gamma-Linolenic Acid: What You Need to Know* Garden City Park, NY: Avery Penguin Putnam, 2001.

Reinagel, Monica. *Secrets of Evening Primrose Oil* New York, NY: St. Martin's Press, 2000.

Werbach, M. R. *Nutritional Influences on Illness, Third Edition*. Tarzana, CA: Third Line Press, 1999.

PERIODICALS

Baumann, Leslie S. "Cosmeceutical Critique: Evening Primrose Oil." *Skin & Allergy News* (March 2004): 46–47.

Belch, Jill J.F., and Alexander Hill. "Evening Primrose Oil and Borage Oil in Rheumatologic Conditions." *American Journal of Clinical Nutrition* (January 2000): 352S.

KEY TERMS

Attention deficit/hyperactivity disorder (ADHD)— A condition, occurring mainly in children, characterized by hyperactivity, inability to concentrate, and impulsive or inappropriate behavior.

Corticosteroids— Drugs used to treat inflammation.

Dermatitis— Inflammation of the skin resulting in redness, swelling, itching, or blistering.

Eczema— An inflammation of the skin characterized by redness, itching, and scaly or crusty patches.

Eicosapeniaenoic acid— A type of acid derived from gamma-linoleic acid.

Essential Fatty Acids— A group of necessary fats that the human body cannot produce on its own and must be obtained through diet.

Femur— The main bone in the human thigh and the strongest bone in the body.

Gout— A painful disease, mainly of the toes and feet, that causes swollen joints.

Hypertension— High blood pressure, which if untreated, can lead to heart disease and stroke.

Lipids— A group of organic compounds consisting of fats, oils, and related substances that, along with proteins and carbohydrates, are the structural components of living cells.

Lumbar vertebrae— Five bones in the lower spine.

Metastasis— The spreading of cancer from the original site to other parts of the body.

Nonsteroidal anti-inflammatory drugs (NSAIDS)— A class of drugs used to treat inflammation and pain.

Omega-6 fatty acids— A group of essential fatty acids that the humans body cannot produce on its own and must be obtained through diet.

Osteoporosis— A disease occurring most commonly in women after menopause in which the bones become very porous, break easily, and heal slowly. It may lead to curvature of the spine after vertebrae collapse.

Paclitaxol— A drug used to treat some forms of cancer.

Peripheral neuropathy— A nerve disease associated with diabetes that causes numbness, tingling, pain, or burning in the feet, legs, and toes.

Polyunsaturated— A group of fats that are less likely to be converted into cholesterol in the body than other fats.

Premenstrual syndrome (PMS)— A group of symptoms, including nervous tension, irritability, tender breasts, and headache, experienced by some women in the days before menstruation caused by changes in hormone levels.

Prostaglandin— An unsaturated fatty acid in humans that helps to control smooth muscle contraction, blood pressure, inflammation, and body temperature.

Rheumatoid arthritis— Inflammation of joints which causes stiffness and damage to joints.

Scleroderma— A skin disease.

Sjögren's syndrome— A chronic inflammatory disease that effects mostly older women, causing dry eyes and mouth.

Tamoxifen— A drug used to treat cancer.

Triglycerides— A chemical compound in many of the fats and oils of animal and vegetable tissues and, like cholesterol, can have an adverse effect on human health in excessive amounts.

Vasodilatation— A widening of the blood vessels.

Deineka, V. I. "Triglyceride Composition Seed Oils from Certain Plants." *Chemistry of Natural Compounds* (November 2003): 523–527.

Essig, Maria G. "Evening Primrose Oil Reverses Some Diabetes Induced Vasodilatation Deficiencies in Rat Model." *Heart Disease Weekly* (November 17, 2002): 24.

Fan, Yang-Yi, and Robert S. Chapkin. "Importance of Dietary Gamma-Linolenic Acid in Human Health and Nutrition." *The Journal of Nutrition* (September 1998): 1411–1414.

"Gamma-Linolenic Acid (GLA)." *Alternative Medicine Review* (March 2004): 70–79.

Ken R. Wells

Gangrene

Definition

Gangrene is a term used to describe the decay or death of an organ, tissue, or bone caused by a lack of oxygen and nutrients. It is a complication resulting from tissue injuries (such as frostbite), the obstruction of blood flow, or the processes of chronic diseases such as **diabetes mellitus**. Externally, the hands and feet are the areas most often affected by gangrene; internally, it is most likely to affect the gallbladder and the intestines.

Gangrene is referred to as wet, or moist, if a bacterial infection is involved. In dry gangrene, there is no infection.

Description

Gangrene is often characterized by **pain** followed by numbness. The infection may first go unnoticed, especially in the elderly or those individuals with a loss of sensation. The area affected by gangrene may be cold and pale, especially early in the disease. **Blisters** may be apparent and the patient may experience an increased heart rate and profuse sweating. As the tissue dies, the skin begins to darken. The dead tissue gradually separates and falls away from the healthy tissue.

Dry gangrene is often seen in advanced cases of diabetes and arteriosclerosis. The tissue doesn't become infected, rather it dries out and shrivels over a period of weeks or months. Wet gangrene progresses much more rapidly. The affected area becomes swollen and gives off a foul smelling discharge. Death may occur within a matter of hours or days. **Fever**, rapid heart rate, rapid breathing, altered mental state, loss of appetite, **diarrhea**, **vomiting**, and vascular collapse may occur as the infection progresses.

Causes & symptoms

The primary cause of gangrene is often an injury to the blood vessels, causing either an interruption of blood flow, the introduction of a bacterial infection, or both. Such injuries may include **burns**, infected **bedsores**, **boils**, frostbite, compound **fractures**, deep cuts, or gunshot **wounds**. Gangrene can also develop due to the poor circulation and obstructions in the blood vessels associated with abnormal **blood clots**, torsion of organs, and diseases such as diabetes, **heart disease**, and Raynaud's disease. Gangrene of the internal organs may be attributed to a ruptured appendix, internal wounds, or the complications of surgery.

The bloodstream is the body's main transport system. When blood flow is diminished, the flow of the oxygen and nutrients needed to keep tissues healthy is greatly decreased. The white blood cells needed to fight infection are not readily available. In such an environment, invading bacteria thrive and multiply quickly. *Streptococcus* spp. and *Staphylococcus* spp. are the most common agents of external skin infection.

Gas gangrene, also called progressive or clostridial myonecrosis, is a type of moist gangrene most commonly caused by an infection of *Clostridium perfringens*, or other species that are capable of thriving under conditions where there is little oxygen. These bacteria produce gases and poisonous toxins as they grow in the tissues. Gas gangrene

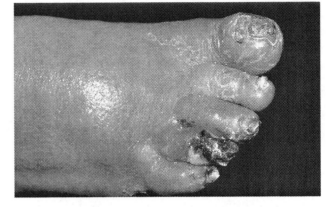

A close-up of gangrene in the toes of a diabetic patient. *(Photo Researchers, Inc. Reproduced by permission.)*

causes the death of tissue, the destruction of red blood cells, and the damaging of the walls of the blood vessels and parts of the kidneys. Early symptoms include sweating, fear, and **anxiety**. Gas gangrene is a life-threatening condition and should receive prompt medical attention.

Diagnosis

A diagnosis of gangrene will be based on a combination of patient history, a physical examination, blood test results, and other laboratory findings. A physician will look for a history of recent trauma, surgery, **cancer**, or chronic disease. Blood tests will be used to determine whether infection is present and to determine how much the infection has spread. A sample of drainage from a wound or obtained through surgery may be tested to identify the bacteria causing the infection and to aid in determining treatment. In the case of gas gangrene, the gas produced by the bacteria may be detected beneath the skin by pressing into the swollen areas. The crackling sounds of gas bubbles may also be heard in the affected area and the surrounding tissues.

X-ray studies and other imaging techniques, such as computed tomography (CT) scans or magnetic resonance imaging (MRI), may be helpful in making a diagnosis by showing evidence of gas accumulation or muscle tissue death. These techniques, however, are not sufficient alone to provide an accurate diagnosis of gangrene. Precise diagnosis often requires surgical exploration of the wound.

Treatment

Chelation therapy is a treatment that uses an intravenous solution containing the drug ethylenediamine tetra-acetic acid (EDTA), among other substances. In the bloodstream, EDTA binds and removes toxins and plaque formation on arterial walls. It promotes circulation throughout the body, and is reportedly, although not proven, able to reverse the processes leading to gangrene. Early intervention is necessary, however.

Other alternative and complementary treatments are used to treat gangrene. Herbal remedies such as **goldenseal** can be applied topically. **Biofeedback** and hypnosis can increase blood flow. Diabetics will receive herbal and **traditional Chinese medicine** remedies and nutritional supplements to help prevent gangrene.

Allopathic treatment

Pain medications and large amounts of intravenous antibiotics are given. Prompt surgical removal of infected and destroyed tissue is required for healing to take place. Gas gangrene is often treated with the antitoxin for clostridium as well. In a number of cases, amputation may have to be used to keep the infection under control.

In hyperbaric oxygen (HBO) therapy the patient is placed in a pressurized chamber and receives 100% pure oxygen to breathe. This has been shown useful in inhibiting the production of toxins in gas gangrene and for getting oxygen quickly to tissues, especially following a crushing injury that might lead to gangrene. HBO therapy must be carried out early in the process and used before any surgical removal. The therapy, though useful, does have adverse side effects. It requires skilled technicians and may not be widely available.

Expected results

The outcomes for gangrene are generally favorable if the infection is recognized and treated early in the progression of the disease. Left untreated, gas gangrene will result in a decrease in blood pressure, kidney failure, and coma. Overall, about 20% of those infected with gas gangrene die from the disease, and another 20% require an amputation. Gangrene is most dangerous to the elderly, those who are immuno-compromised, and those who have internal **infections** and chronic conditions such as diabetes. Individuals suffering from dry gangrene often have multiple health problems that complicate recovery and may prove fatal.

Prevention

Infections and injuries should be thoroughly cleaned and monitored; medical attention should be pursued if symptoms worsen or remain unresolved. Gastrointestinal wounds should be surgically explored, drained, and repaired. Use of antibiotic therapy prior to and directly following surgery has been shown to reduce the rates of infection.

Patients with diabetes or severe arteriosclerosis should take particular care of their hands and feet to avoid the de-

---

KEY TERMS

Amputation—The surgical removal of a part of the body.

Antitoxin—A vaccine used to stimulate immunity against a specific disease.

Arteriosclerosis—A disease characterized by build-up on the artery walls that can lead to the obstruction of blood flow.

Debridement—The surgical removal of dead tissue.

Raynaud's disease—A condition in which there is poor circulation and decreased oxygen in the hands and feet particularly.

Torsion—The accidental twisting of tissues in the body that may decrease the blood and oxygen supply to the affected area.

---

creased circulation and unchecked infection that may lead to gangrene. Any injury or infection, however slight, should be cared for promptly. There should be a focus on proper foot care, including keeping the feet clean, dry, and warm, wearing well-fitting shoes and not going barefoot. It is important to avoid **smoking**, since tobacco use constricts the blood vessels of the hands and feet, decreasing circulation.

Resources

BOOKS

Bunch, Bryan, ed. *The Family Encyclopedia of Diseases: a Complete and Concise Guide to Illnesses and Symptoms.* New York: Scientific Publishing, Inc., 1999.

The Burton Goldberg Group *Alternative Medicine: The Definitive Guide.* Tiburon, CA: Future Medicine Publishing, 1993.

OTHER

drkoop.com http://www.drkoop.com/conditions/foot_care/library/ gangrene.asp.

drkoop.com http://www.drkoop.com/conditions/ency/article/000620.htm.

The Merck Manual http://www.merck.com/pubs/mmanual/section21/chapter292/292a.htm.

Patience Paradox

Ganoderma

Description

Ganoderma is the name of the fungus *Ganoderma lucidum*. It is also called the **reishi mushroom** or in Chinese *ling zhi*. It is one of the most popular medicinal mushrooms in China, Japan, and the United States.

Ganoderma grows on logs or tree stumps. It has a shiny, hard, asymmetrical cap that ranges in color from yellow to black. The cap, spores, and mycelium are all used medicinally. Wild ganoderma is rare in Asia.

In ancient China, ganoderma was so rare and so highly prized that it was reserved for the emperors and called the "Elixir of Life." In 1972, Japanese researchers successfully cultivated the mushroom. There are six different colors of cap: red, green, white, black, yellow, and purple. These researchers showed that all colors are the same species, and that the color variations are the result of differences in environmental conditions. Despite this, some herbalists insist that certain colors of reishi mushroom are more potent or effective in healing certain conditions than others.

General use

Ganoderma is considered one of the most important herbs in Asian healing. Its use extends to almost every system of the body. Not only is it believed to heal physical ailments, it is said to bring about a peaceful state of mind, and to increase spiritual potency energy for Taoists and other Asian spiritual seekers.

Ganoderma has been used in China for over 4,000 years. It is the primary shen tonic in Chinese herbalism. In a broad sense, it is used to help a person adapt both physically and mentally to the world. It is used to strengthen and calm the nerves, improve memory, and prevent or delay senility.

Herbalists consider ganoderma an adaptogen, or natural regulator, suppressing the immune system if it is overactive and boosting it if it is underactive. Many health claims are made on the effect that ganoderma has on the immune system. These claims are based primarily on the presence of high molecular weight polysaccharides and free radical **antioxidants** in ganoderma extracts. Ganoderma also contains the elements **potassium** (K), **magnesium** (Mg), **calcium** (Ca), and germanium (Ge).

Ganoderma is used in Japan and China to treat **cancer** and to stimulate the immune system after radiation or chemotherapy. It is also used to treat myasthenia gravis and **systemic lupus erythematosus** (SLE), both autoimmune diseases. In Japan and China, ganoderma is also used to treat symptoms of viral diseases such as colds, **influenza**, **canker sores**, and **hepatitis**.

Quite a few research studies on ganoderma extracts have been done at universities in Japan, China, and South Korea. Many of these are test-tube or animal studies. The results are not clear-cut, but they seem to indicate that at least in these non-human systems, ganoderma has an effect on the immune system, some anti-tumor properties, and some anti-viral activity. One group of researchers reported in 2002 that ganoderma appears to protect the liver from inflammation caused by infection.

More recent research in Asian universities has investigated the effects of ganoderma on human cells or tissues. A recent study done in Taiwan indicates that ganoderma inhibits apoptosis (cell self-destruction) in human white blood cells. This finding may help to explain ganoderma's beneficial effects on the immune system.

Ganoderma has recently attracted the attention of Western cancer researchers. A case study report from Columbia University indicates that a Japanese dietary supplement containing ganoderma as well as genistein, a soybean derivative, may be useful in the prevention and treatment of **prostate cancer**.

Ganoderma is also used in treating conditions of the nervous system. It is used to calm the nerves, cure **insomnia**, reduce **stress**, eliminate nervous exhaustion, and increase determination and focus. Laboratory studies show fairly conclusively that ganoderma does act as a sedative on cells of the central nervous system and possibly has painkilling and anti-convulsive properties.

Ganoderma is frequently used to treat **allergies**, **hay fever**, bronchial **asthma**, and to reduce skin inflammation. Laboratory studies support these uses and show that some components of ganoderma have a strong antihistaminic effect that interrupts the development of allergic reactions.

Many conditions of the blood and circulatory system are treated with ganoderma. These include:

• altitude sickness

• **atherosclerosis**

• cardiac arrhythmia

• coronary heart disease

• high blood pressure

• high blood sugar

• high cholesterol

• low blood pressure

• **stroke**

Scientific research shows that compounds found in ganoderma do lower blood sugar and also interfere with the clotting of blood platelets. This reduction in clotting may account for ganoderma's effectiveness against stroke and atherosclerosis.

Ganoderma is also used to treat a variety of other diseases. These uses are generally backed up by little or no scientific evidence. They include:

- gastroenteritis
- **diarrhea**
- constipation
- gallstones
- ulcer
- acne
- hair loss
- inflammation of the kidneys
- menstrual cramps
- erectile dysfunction
- low sex drive

Preparations

Virtually all ganoderma available commercially are from cultivated mushrooms. Different preparations are made using the cap, the spores, and the mycelium. These preparations are available in the form of fresh and dried whole mushrooms, capsules, concentrated drips, extracts, tablets, tea bags, tea granules, and tinctures. A common dose is 1,800–2,400 mg in capsule form per day. However, doses vary hugely depending on the condition being treated and the strength and part of the mushroom being used.

Precautions

Although no toxic reactions to ganoderma have been reported, people with allergies to other mushrooms may also experience allergic reactions to ganoderma.

Side effects

Large doses (2–9 g) of ganoderma taken regularly over the course of 3–6 months may result in diarrhea, upset stomach, and **dizziness**. **Nosebleeds** from high doses of ganoderma have also been reported. Some herbalists claim that large doses of **vitamin C** taken with this herb will control the symptoms of diarrhea.

Interactions

Ganoderma and other Chinese herbs are often used together with no reported interactions; in fact, a new health food supplement is made from reishi mushrooms grown on herbs, in the belief that the mushrooms absorb some of the properties of the herbs on which they're grown.

KEY TERMS

Adaptogen—A substance that regulates, either by stimulating or suppressing, a system to bring it back within its normal, healthy range.

Apoptosis—A type of cell death in which a damaged cell shuts down and in effect commits suicide. Ganoderma appears to inhibit apoptosis in human white blood cells.

Atherosclerosis—In this disease, deposits of fatty materials build up on the walls of arterial blood vessels, causing them to narrow or become obstructed. Blood pressure increases, leading to heart disease.

Myasthenia gravis—A muscle weakness that occurs because the body makes antibodies to the natural chemical that facilitates transmission of impulses between the nerve and the muscle.

Mycelium—The part of the fungus that grows into the log and supports the fruiting body or cap. It is analogous to the roots of a plant.

Reishi mushroom—Another name for ganoderma.

Shen—One of the five body energies. It influences mental, spiritual, and creative energy. Shen tonics address deficiencies in this type of energy.

Spores—Fine powder-like reproductive bodies of the mushroom.

Systemic lupus erythematosus (SLE)—A multi-symptom disease caused by failure of the immune system to regulate itself.

With regard to Western pharmaceuticals, ganoderma has been reported to produce negative interactions with warfarin, a blood-thinning medication. Because ganoderma extract may cause a drop in blood pressure, persons who are taking prescription antihypertensives (medications to lower blood pressure) should use ganoderma only if they are being monitored by a physician.

Resources

BOOKS

Peirce, Andrea. *The American Pharmaceutical Association Practical Guide to Natural Medicines.* New York: William Morrow and Company, 1999.

Teegaurden, Ron. *The Ancient Wisdom of the Chinese Tonic Herbs.* New York: Warner Books, 1998.

PERIODICALS

Fuchs, Nan Kathryn. "A Brand New Super Nutrient!" *Women's Health Letter* 8 (August 2002): 1-3.

Ghafar, M. A., E. Golliday, J. Bingham, et al. "Regression of Prostate Cancer Following Administration of Genistein Combined Polysaccharide (GCP), a Nutritional Supplement: A Case Report." *Journal of Alternative and Complementary Medicine* 8 (August 2002): 493-497.

Hsu, M. J., S. S. Lee, and W. W. Lin. "Polysaccharide Purified from *Ganoderma lucidum* Inhibits Spontaneous and Fas-Mediated Apoptosis in Human Neutrophils through Activation of the Phosphatidylinositol 3 Kinase/Akt Signaling Pathway." *Journal of Leukocyte Biology* 72 (July 2002): 207-216.

Liu, X., J. P. Yuan, C. K. Chung, and X. J. Chen. "Antitumor Activity of the Sporoderm-Broken Germinating Spores of *Ganoderma lucidum*." *Cancer Letter* 182 (August 28, 2002): 155-161.

Zhang, G. L., Y. H. Wang, W. Ni, et al. "Hepatoprotective Role of *Ganoderma lucidum* Polysaccharide Against BCG-Induced Immune Liver Injury in Mice." *World Journal of Gastroenterology* 8 (August 2002): 728-733.

ORGANIZATIONS

American Association of Oriental Medicine. 5530 Wisconsin Avenue, Suite 1210, Chevy Chase, MD 20815. (301) 941-1064. <www.aaom.org>.

Centre for International Ethnomedicinal Education and Research (CIEER). <www.cieer.org>.

Tish Davidson
Rebecca J. Frey, PhD

Garden mint *see* **Spearmint**

Gardenia

Description

Gardenias are members of the madder, or Rubiaceae, family. Though not native to either North or South America, they were named for an eighteenth-century American physician and naturalist, Alexander Garden. Gardenias were originally found only in China and Japan, but today there are over 200 different species of gardenia, mostly hybrid, in existence throughout the world. Gardenias are most prevalent in China, Japan, tropical regions of Southeast Asia and the Pacific islands, and South Africa. With proper conditions, gardenias grow into shrub-like bushes or small trees that can reach 5 ft (1.5 m) in height.

Most species of gardenia, however, are very tender plants that require an average temperature of at least 60°F (28.9°C), sunlight with some protection, and just the right amount of humidity. They often survive far better in greenhouses than outside. Gardenias are often rambling plants that form mounds of glossy dark green foliage. The leaves are oval in shape and very shiny. The flowers vary in color from pale yellow with purple markings to creamy white, and they have a classic, heavy, sweet scent reminiscent of green apple. All gardenia blossoms have an almost wax-like appearance and can be either single or double, depending on the species. Most gardenias flower in the winter or early spring, and the blossom is followed by the appearance of a large, yellowish-red, bitter-tasting berry that contains a crystalline compound called acrocetin.

The most commonly listed botanical species of gardenia include:

- *Gardenia jasminoides*. This species is easily the most common of these rare, fragile plants. It reaches heights of 2 ft (61 cm) and grows into a tall bushy green shrub that produces white, highly fragrant flowers. *G. jasminoides* is a native of China, and the gardenia most commonly used in Chinese herbal medicine. Its name comes from the fact that it was first introduced to the Western world from Cape Colony in Africa, and the aroma of its large white flowers was said to be very like the scent of jasmine.

- *Gardenia jasminoides fortunata*. This plant is a hybrid version of *G. jasminoides* that is somewhat more hardy.

- *Gardenia nitida*. This gardenia is a slightly taller plant that grows up to 3 ft (93 cm) and also produces white blossoms.

- *Gardenia radicans floreplena*. This plant is a low spreading dwarf variety from Japan that grows only to heights of 18 in (46 cm), and has double-blossomed flowers.

- *Gardenia thunbergia*. This gardenia grows to 4 ft (1.2 m) and is often cultivated in American greenhouses. It is found as both tree and shrub, and has white flowers with long tube-like necks.

- *Gardenia rothmania*. This plant is also a particular favorite of American botanists, but does not survive well in North America outside of a greenhouse. It also exists as both tree and shrub, and has pale yellow flowers with short, tube-like necks and purple markings.

General use

Gardenias are widely used as exotic ornamental flowers in corsages, as houseplants, and in some regions, as outdoor plants. A yellow silk dye has been made for centuries from the chemical compound acrocetin extracted from the gardenia berry.

Chinese herbal medicine, however, makes the most extensive use of the gardenia. Its Chinese name is *zhi zi*. The traditional medicinal actions attributed to gardenia include calming irritability; cooling blood and clearing away heat (a yin/yang imbalance often characterized by deficient yin); reducing swelling; and moving stagnant blood that has congealed in one place, usually following trauma. Gardenia is considered to be very effective as a hemostatic agent, which means that it stops bleeding; and also effective in treating injuries to the muscles, joints, and tendons. Gardenia is commonly used in Chinese herbal formulas to treat **infections**, particularly bladder infections; abscesses; **jaundice**; and blood in the urine, sputum, or stool. Because of its perceived ability to ease agitation or irritability, it is also used in formulas to treat **anxiety** or **insomnia**. It is also helpful in correcting menopausal imbalances reflected in insomnia and **depression**, nervous tension, **headache**, and **dizziness**.

The United States Department of Agriculture Agricultural Research Service phytochemical and ethnobotanical database lists the following species of gardenia as having specific medicinal properties:

- *Gardenia gummifera*. This species can be helpful in treating digestive problems, including dyspepsia and **diarrhea**; or used as an astringent and expectorant for nervous conditions and spasms.

- *Gardenia storckii*. This variety can be used in treating constipation.

- *Gardenia lucida*. This gardenia has antiseptic properties that can kill both bacteria and insects.

- *Gardenia pseudopsidium*. This species has been used to treat smallpox.

- *Gardenia jasminoides*. This gardenia has been found to be helpful in the treatment of **pain**, nose bleeds, **fever**, and **influenza**; in healing **wounds** and reducing swelling; and in treating mastitis, **hepatitis** and the hematuria that accompanies bladder infection.

- *Gardenia augusta*. This variety has shown effectiveness in the treatment of headaches, fever, delirium, mastitis, and jaundice related to liver problems.

- *Gardenia campanulata*. This plant is used in healing wounds, **burns**, and scalds; in reducing swelling; as a treatment for fever and influenza; in treating jaundice associated with liver problems; and in stopping bleeding.

- *Gardenia labifolia*. This gardenia has been found effective in treating the bites of certain snakes.

Preparations

The kernel within the gardenia berry is often removed for use in herbal poultices put on sports injuries such as sprains, pulled muscles, or inflammation of nerves. The use of gardenia poultices is particularly

---

KEY TERMS

Astringent—Any substance or medication that causes soft tissue to contract or constrict. Some types of gardenia have astringent properties.

Cold-deficiency diarrhea—In Chinese herbal medicine, this condition is described as cold settling in the abdomen when resistance is low, causing cramping, some gas, and loose, watery stools without any burning sensations.

Expectorant—A substance or medication that promotes the coughing up of phlegm.

Hematuria—A condition in which red blood cells are present in the urine. Blood in the urine may be readily visible or small amounts may give the urine a smoky appearance.

Hemostatic—A drug or medication that stops bleeding. Gardenia is used as a hemostatic agent in traditional Chinese medicine.

---

common in Chinese medicine. Traditional Chinese practitioners make a paste of the herb with flour and wine. The powdered berry is given in both decoctions and capsules. When gardenia is used to stop bleeding it is usually burned before it is simmered in water.

Precautions

Chinese herbalists state that gardenia should not be used when there is cold deficiency (watery) diarrhea present.

It is important to remember that Chinese herbal medicine is based upon individual prescriptions developed for each patient and their unique symptoms. Chinese herbs should not be taken, either individually or in formulas, unless a practitioner of Chinese herbal medicine is first consulted.

Side effects

Gardenia has laxative properties, and can cause loose stools when taken frequently or in large amounts.

Resources

BOOKS

Molony, David, and Ming Ming Pan Molony. *The American Association of Oriental Medicine's Complete Guide to Chinese Herbal Medicine.* New York: Berkley Publishing, 1999.

Phillips, Ellen, and C. Colston Burrell. *Rodale's Illustrated Encyclopedia of Perennials.* Emmaus, PA: Rodale Press, Inc., 1993.

Reid, Daniel P. *Chinese Herbal Medicine*. Boston: Shambhala, 1993.

OTHER

Dr. Duke's Phytochemical and Ethnobotanical Databases. http://www.ars-grm.gov/cgibm/duke/ethnobot.htm

Joan Schonbeck

Garlic

Description

Garlic (*Allium sativa*), is a plant with long, flat grasslike leaves and a papery hood around the flowers. The greenish white or pink flowers are found grouped together at the end of a long stalk. The stalk rises directly from the flower bulb, which is the part of the plant used as food and medicine. The bulb is made up of many smaller bulbs covered with a papery skin known as cloves. Although garlic is known as the "stinking rose" it is actually a member of the lily family.

The most active components of fresh garlic are an amino acid called alliin and an enzyme called allinase. When a clove of garlic is chewed, chopped, bruised, or cut, these compounds mix to form allicin, which is responsible for garlic's strong smell. Allicin, in turn, breaks down into other **sulfur** compounds within a few hours. These compounds have a variety of overlapping healing properties.

Garlic also contains a wide range of trace minerals. These include **copper**, **iron**, **zinc**, **magnesium**, germanium, and **selenium**. The integrity of the growers and suppliers of garlic are important to the integrity of the garlic used. A soil rich with the presence of trace minerals will produce a healthful bulb of garlic, full of those minerals. Depleted soils produce a depleted product. In addition, garlic contains many sulfur compounds, vitamins A and C, and various **amino acids**.

General use

The ancient Indians, Chinese, Egyptians, Greeks, Romans, and other peoples have used garlic for thousands of years, as food and as medicine. One of the most famed usages of garlic was during the Middle Ages, when it was reputed to have been highly effective against the plague.

As early as 1858, Louis Pasteur formally studied and recorded garlic's antibiotic properties. Dr. Albert Schweitzer used the herb to successfully treat cholera,

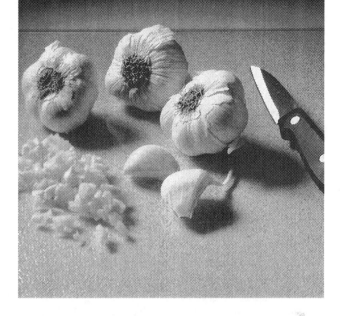

Whole, cloved, and minced garlic. *(Photograph by Robert J. Huffman. Field Mark Publications. Reproduced by permission.)*

typhus, and dysentery in Africa in the 1950s. Before antibiotics were widely available, garlic was used as a treatment for battle **wounds** during both World Wars.

Garlic can be used in the treatment of a variety of bacterial, viral, and **fungal infections**. It has been shown to be effective against staph, strep, *E. coli*, *Salmonella*, Vibrio cholera, *H. pylori*, *Candida albicans*, and other microorganisms. Garlic also helps prevent against **heart disease** and strokes. Current studies show that garlic can improve immune function and may even help in the prevention of **cancer**. To be of benefit in chronic conditions, garlic should be used daily over an extended period of time.

Heart disease

One of the main causes of heart disease is the buildup of plaque on the walls of the blood vessels. This plaque is mostly made up of **cholesterol** and other fatty substances found in the blood. When large amounts of plaque get stuck on artery walls, they block the flow of blood and cause **blood clots** to form. Parts of the artery wall may even be destroyed completely.

In arteriosclerosis, otherwise known as "hardening of the arteries," the major arteries may become so stiff and clogged, that the heart cannot get necessary nutrients and oxygen. This usually causes a **heart attack**. High serum cholesterol levels are a major risk factor for having a heart attack.

Studies show that people who eat garlic regularly have improved serum cholesterol levels. Some people with high cholesterol have been able to get within normal levels by eating 1–2 cloves per day. In addition, low-density lipoprotein (LDL) and triglyceride levels are decreased and high-density lipoprotein (HDL) levels are increased. This correlates with an overall reduced cholesterol level. These benefits are significant in preventing heart disease as well as strokes. While garlic's contribution to reducing levels of harmful plaques has been known for some time, a 2003 study found that garlic also lowered levels of homocysteine, a type of amino acid that is now considered a major risk factor for heart attacks. Manufactured garlic supplements appear to be equally as beneficial as eating the fresh cloves. It takes at least one month of using garlic for laboratory results to be seen.

Hypertension

Hypertension, or high blood pressure, is also a significant cause of heart problems. It is one of the leading causes of disability and death due to **stroke**, heart attack, heart failure, and kidney failure. Garlic can help reduce blood pressure through the actions of its sulfur compounds and its ability to reduce the fatty substances, such as cholesterol, found in the bloodstream. Use of garlic also can help normalize low blood pressure.

Platelet aggregation

Platelets clot the blood in order to repair breaks in the blood vessel walls. When there is an injury, platelets are attracted to the damaged area and become attached to the wall and to other platelets. Platelet aggregation, as this process is called, plugs up the break and prevents further blood loss while the injury is being repaired. This is a good and necessary part of healing an injury.

However, if there are serious problems with the heart and blood vessels and there is too much injury and clotting, the vessels may become clogged with platelets. This can lead to strokes and heart disease. The sulfur compounds in garlic—particularly ajoene—give the platelets a slippery quality. They are less able to clump together, thus slowing down platelet aggregation. Garlic can be used effectively in the same way as a daily dose of aspirin to reduce or prevent platelet aggregation over an extended time.

Cancer

Studies have found that garlic blocks the formation of powerful carcinogens, called nitrosamines, which may be formed during the digestion of food. This may be why in populations where people consume a large amount of garlic, there is a decreased incidence of all types of cancer. The **antioxidants** found in garlic may also contribute to this effect by protecting against the cell dam-age by cancer-causing free radicals. Studies show that use of garlic may also inhibit the growth of a variety of tumors. However, cancer-related studies are not conclusive and relate to consumption of raw or cooked garlic, not garlic supplements.

Infectious conditions

Eating garlic is good for helping the body's immune system resist **infections**. While garlic is not as strong as modern antibiotics, it is believed to kill some strains of bacteria that have become resistant to antibiotics. Studies have shown garlic treats yeast infections, and it can kill many of the viruses responsible for colds and flu. While daily consumption of garlic was once highly recommended for HIV-positive individuals, the National Institutes of Health (NIH) reported in 2002 that garlic supplements greatly reduced levels of saquinavir, an HIV protease inhibitor, in patients' blood. The NIH began cautioning patients who used garlic to control cholesterol levels who also used saquinavir or combination therapies, since garlic might interfere with their effectiveness.

Modern doctors have been reconsidering the causes of many diseases. They have discovered that bacteria and viruses may be the cause of sicknesses that were formerly not thought to be caused by infections. This includes gastric ulcers, colitis, and **Kaposi's sarcoma**. Garlic may be useful in treating or preventing these due to its antimicrobial properties.

Diabetes

Garlic has the ability to lower and help keep blood sugar stable by helping to increase the amount of insulin available in the bloodstream. This action, together with garlic's ability to lower cholesterol and blood pressure, make it an excellent daily supplement for people with diabetes. A 2003 report showed that long-term use of garlic helped improve the blood vessel systems of diabetic rats.

Other health conditions

Garlic is effective in the treatment of numerous other conditions. For example:

- The consumption of 1–3 cloves per day is useful for immune support and as a preventive against diseases and infection.

- Warmed garlic oil in the ear canal can be used to treat ear infections.

- Garlic can be used to treat respiratory complaints such as **asthma** and chronic **bronchitis**.

- Garlic helps increase the body's ability to handle the digestion of meat and fats.

- Garlic can be used to help kill and expel intestinal **worms** in both animals and humans.

- When added to a pet's food, garlic helps repel fleas.

- Garlic is helpful in getting rid of athlete's foot.

- Garlic relieves **gas** and other stomach complaints.

- The sulfur compounds found in garlic can bind to heavy metals and other toxins and help remove them from the body.

- Garlic can be used externally for cuts, wounds, and skin eruptions.

- The taste of garlic in mother's milk stimulates improved nursing. Infants eat more and nurse longer. They appear to relish the taste of slightly garlicky milk. The components of garlic that reach the infant through the mother's milk also may be helpful in relieving **colic** and infections.

Preparations

Used internally

Garlic can be eaten raw or cooked, taken as tablets or capsules, and used as a tincture or syrup. The raw cloves can be directly applied externally.

The suggested dosage for fresh whole garlic is one to three cloves per day. The cloves can be chewed and held in the mouth or swallowed. Consuming raw garlic can actually be a pleasure if the herb is crushed or grated and mixed with food or a tablespoon of honey. The dosage for tinctures is 2–4 ml or 15–40 drops taken twice daily. One tablespoon of the syrup should be taken three times a day, or as needed to relieve coughing. Garlic oil should be slightly warmed, and 1–3 drops should be put in the affected ear 1–3 times per day.

Tablets and capsules are often more convenient to use than raw garlic, and they are more likely to be tolerated by garlic-sensitive individuals. Garlic pills also minimize the garlic taste and odor. Manufacturers vary on which components of the herb are emphasized.

In general, the following dosages are appropriate, but product labels also should be consulted:

- 400–500 mg of allicin, twice daily

- a dose equaling approximately 4,000 mcg of allicin potential, once or twice daily

- 400–1,200 mg of dried garlic powder

- 1,000–7,200 mg of aged garlic

- a dose equivalent to 0.03–0.12 ml of garlic oil, three times per day

Manufactured garlic pills come in a variety of forms, and a great deal of controversy continues about what type is best. Studying the manufacturers' literature and other information is important to make a good decision about which preparation to use. The types of garlic preparations include:

- garlic oil capsules

- encapsulated powdered garlic

- odorless garlic pills

- allicin-stabilized pills

- aged garlic extract

Used externally

A poultice can be made using grated or crushed fresh garlic. The herb material should be placed directly on the site of injury or eruption, either "as is" or mixed with enough honey to make a paste. The poultice can be held in place with a cloth or bandage.

A compress of garlic is less messy than a poultice and may be less irritating to the site of the injury. It is made by wrapping grated or crushed fresh garlic in a single piece of cheesecloth. As with the poultice, the compress is placed directly on the affected area.

Garlic oil can be made by putting a whole bulb of grated or finely chopped garlic into a pint jar of olive oil, and letting it sit undisturbed in a warm place, away from direct sunlight, for at least two weeks. Then it can be strained and refrigerated. The garlic oil will stay fresh in the refrigerator for up to two years.

A garlic suppository can be used to treat vaginal yeast or mild bacterial infections. A clove of fresh garlic should be peeled and slightly crushed or bruised. If crushed garlic irritates the vaginal tissue, an alternative that might lessen the desired antimicrobial effect is to use the whole, uncrushed garlic clove. The clove should be wrapped in a single layer of cheesecloth and inserted into the vaginal canal overnight for 5-10 days. Dental floss or a length of the cheesecloth can be used to make the suppository easier to retrieve. If the garlic causes a burning sensation, this can be eased with the insertion of plain yogurt into the vagina.

Precautions

Consumers will find a wide variety of garlic preparations on the market. Therefore, it is important to study manufacturers' claims, talk to knowledgeable practitioners, and find out which formulations are most effective for a given condition.

Due to the high concentration of sulfur compounds in garlic, it should be avoided by those allergic to sulfur. Garlic inhibits clotting, thereby causing increased bleeding times. Hemophiliacs and those on anticoagulant medication should consult a physician before taking garlic on a daily basis. This also applies to individuals who are preparing to undergo surgery. Medicinal use of garlic should be discontinued for at least 1–2 weeks before surgery. HIV patients receiving protease inhibitor or combination therapy should check with their physicians before using garlic supplements, as garlic may interfere with the therapy's effectiveness.

Side effects

Raw garlic can be very irritating to the digestive system. Excessive intake (usually, more than three or four cloves a day) can cause bloating, gas, cramping, **diarrhea**, and may even damage the red blood cells. When applied to the skin, garlic may cause **itching**, redness and swelling. Garlic that is cooked, aged, or made into pills is not nearly as harsh on the system. However, these forms may not be as suitable as raw garlic in treating some conditions, particularly infections.

Garlic travels through the lungs and the bloodstream, giving a pungent garlic odor to the breath, skin, and perspiration. The odor will be present for at least 4–18 hours, sometimes even when so-called odorless garlic pills are used.

Interactions

Garlic does well when combined with **coltsfoot** or **lobelia** for treating asthma and bronchitis. Although onion is not as potent as garlic, it has similar actions, and the two often are combined. Use of garlic is contraindicated in individuals using the anticoagulant drug warfarin or certain HIV therapies.

Resources

BOOKS

Green, James *The Male Herbal*. Freedom, CA: The Crossing Press, 1991.

Murray, N.D., Michael T. *The Healing Power of Herbs: The Enlightened Person's Guide to the Wonders of Medicinal Plants*. Roseville, CA: Prima Publishing, 1992, 1995.

Romm, Aviva Jill. *Natural Healing for Babies and Children*. Freedom, CA: The Crossing Press, 1996.

Weed, Susun. *Menopausal Years: The Wise Woman Way, Alternative Approaches for Women*. Woodstock, NY: Ash Tree Publishing, 2000.

PERIODICALS

Gangel, Elaine Kierl."Garlic Supplements and HIV Medication." *American Family Physician* (March 15, 2002):1225.

"Garlic Attenuates Time-dependent Changes in Reactivity of Isolated Aorta." *Cardiovascular Week* (October 27, 2003):8.

KEY TERMS

Anticoagulant—Reduces or prevents the blood's tendency to clot in order to prevent blockages in the arteries.

Antimicrobial—Having the ability to help the immune system resist or destroy a wide spectrum of disease-causing organisms.

Carcinogens—Chemical substances that cause cell mutations, and ultimately, cancer.

Cholesterol—A fatty substance found only in animals; used in the body to build cell walls and in the forming of bile and sex hormones.

Free radicals—Highly reactive toxins in the body that can bind to cells and damage them. Antioxidants are useful in neutralizing these compounds.

HDL—Beneficial lipoprotein molecules that transport cholesterol to the liver to be processed and excreted, thereby lowering cholesterol levels.

LDL—Lipoproteins that transport cholesterol to body tissues for storage and thereby raise cholesterol levels.

Plaque—A buildup of fats, cholesterol, calcium, and fibrous tissue in the blood that tends to attach to and weaken artery walls.

Stroke—A condition caused by the blockage of blood flow and oxygen to the brain. Paralysis, coma, and death may result.

Suppository—A herbal treatment prepared to be inserted into the vagina or the rectum.

Novick, Jeff."Garlic and Cancer." *Health Science* 25, no. 1(Winter 2002):6.

"UCLA Researchers Find Garlic Has Ability to Reduce Heart Disease Risk Factors." *Townsend Letter for Doctors and Patients* (July 2003):22.

OTHER

"Garlic." Herb Directory by Name. http://www.holisticonline. com/w_holisticonline.htm

"Garlic." http://www.botanical.com/botanical/mgmh/g/ garlic06.html

"Garlic and Cancer Prevention." http://www.mayohealth.org/ mayo/askdiet/htm/new/qd000223.htm

"Garlic's Breath of Health." http://www.usaweekend.com/ health/carper_archive/950402eat_smart_garlic.html

Patience Paradox
Teresa G. Odle

Gas

Definition

Gas, or flatus, is produced when naturally occurring bacteria in the gastrointestinal tract begin to break down, or digest, food. When an excess of air builds up in the tract from swallowing air or a disorder that prevents digestion, it is released as gas. Gastrointestinal gases include methane, carbon dioxide, nitrogen, and hydrogen.

Description

Gas production is an essential, normal function of the gastrointesinal tract, and most healthy individuals pass up to 1,200 cc (over 40 oz) of gas each day. However, when gas causes excessive pain and cramping (**colic**) then evaluation and treatment are appropriate.

Causes & symptoms

Gastrointestinal gas production can be increased by certain foods, illnesses, and some medications. Common causes of excessive gas include:

- Gas-producing foods. Onions, beans, the cabbage family, and other fibrous foods can cause excessive gas or intestinal spasms in some individuals.

- Gastrointestinal diseases and disorders. Increased flatulence is a defining symptom of **irritable bowel syndrome**, **diverticulitis**, lactose intolerance, malabsorption problems, dysbiosis (digestive problems), and other gastrointestinal disorders.

- Air swallowing. Swallowing too much air while eating or chewing gum can introduce extra gas to the gastrointestinal tract.

- Medications. Certain prescription and over-the-counter medications may cause gas as a side-effect.

- Stress and food **allergies** can also cause gas.

Symptoms of excessive gas production include:

- flatulence
- belching, or burping
- abdominal cramping, or colic
- abdominal pain

Diagnosis

A thorough medical and dietary history and physical examination performed by a healthcare professional can usually identify the cause of gas pains resulting from changes to diet or medication. Gas problems triggered by gastrointestinal disease may be harder to diagnose, and will typically require additional medical testing such

COMMON REMEDIES FOR GAS	
Remedy	**Description**
Acupressure	Press inward at the point three finger widths below the navel known as Conception Vessel 6.
Exercise	Exercise after meals and regularly to increase digestion and expel gas.
Herbal medicine	Anise water, peppermint or chamomile tea, and fennel may relieve gas.
Homeopathy	Carbo vegetabilis is used to relieve gas. Nux vomica is used to treat gas that accompanies constipation. Chamomilla is used to treat gas in infants.
Diet	Increase fiber intake. Do not mix carbohydrates with proteins at the same meal. Avoid beans, peas, cheese, sodas, and alcohol. Do not overeat. Chew food well and eat slowly.
Hydrotherapy	Alternate a warm compress with a vigorous cold friction rub on the abdomen.
Yoga	The Boat, Bow, Cobra, and Pigeon positions all encourage digestion and help relieve gas pain.

as colonoscopy, barium enema, or an upper and/or lower gastrointestinal (GI) series.

Treatment

For excessive gas caused by a particular food or beverage, adjustments to diet can relieve most symptoms. Gas caused by air swallowing can be alleviated by eating more slowly and avoiding gum chewing.

An herbalist or naturopathic healthcare professional may recommend a preparation of a carminative (gas reducing) herb such as **valerian** (*Valeriana officinalis*), or peppermint (*Mentha piperita*), which may be helpful in eliminating discomfort and gas-related bloating.

Homeopathic remedies for excessive intestinal gas include *Carbo vegetabilis*, *Nux vomica*, and *Chamomilla*. The prescription of a specific homeopathic remedy will depend on an individual's overall symptom picture, mood, and temperament, and should only be prescribed by a qualified homeopathic physician.

Hydrotherapy, acupressure, **acupuncture**, yoga, **reflexology**, and mild exercise can also help to relieve the pain and discomfort of excessive gas.

Allopathic treatment

Over-the-counter preparations of the enzyme alpha-D-galactosidase (Beano) can alleviate gas symptoms caused by ingestion of certain foods in some individuals. These preparations are typically available in liquid or tablet form. Other non-prescription medications such as Gas-X, Phazyme, and Mylanta contain the ingredient simethicone, which can reduce gas bubbles within the gastrointestinal tract.

Expected results

Mild excess gas is typically easy to treat, especially that triggered by dietary causes. Gas caused by gastrointestinal disease may be more difficult to manage, and successful treatment depends on the type and severity of the disorder.

Prevention

Avoiding fermented foods, drastic increases in fiber intake, and excessive air intake can prevent gas in some individuals. Lactose intolerant individuals should avoid dairy products.

Resources

BOOKS

Hoffman, David. *The Complete Illustrated Herbal.* New York: Barnes & Noble Books, 1999.

PERIODICALS

Wu, Olivia. "Miss the Bloat: How to Avoid Bloating." *Vegetarian Times* (June 2000): 80.

ORGANIZATIONS

The National Institute of Diabetes & Digestive & Kidney Diseases (NIDDK). Office of Communications and Public Liaison. NIDDK, National Institutes of Health, 31 Center Drive, MSC 2560, Bethesda, MD 20892-2560. http://www.niddk.nih.gov/index.htm.

Paula Ford-Martin

Gastritis

Definition

Gastritis commonly refers to inflammation of the lining of the stomach, but the term is often used to cover a variety of symptoms resulting from this inflammation, as well as symptoms of burning or discomfort. True gastritis comes in several forms and is diagnosed using a combination of tests. In the 1990s, scientists discovered that the main cause of most gastritis is infection by a bacterium called *Helicobacter pylori*.

Description

Gastritis should not be confused with common symptoms of upper abdominal discomfort. It has been associated with ulcers, particularly peptic ulcers, and in some cases, chronic gastritis can lead to more serious complications.

Nonerosive H. pylori gastritis

Under current theory, the main cause of true gastritis is *H. pylori* infection, which is found in an average of 90% of patients with chronic gastritis. *H. pylori* is a bacterium whose outer layer is resistant to the normal effects of stomach acid in breaking down bacteria. The resistance of *H. pylori* means that the bacterium may remain in the stomach for long periods of times, even years, and eventually cause symptoms of gastritis or ulcers when other factors are introduced, such as the presence of specific genes or the use of nonsteroidal anti-inflammatory drugs (NSAIDs). Studies of the role of *H. pylori* in the development of gastritis and peptic ulcers have disproved the former belief that **stress** leads to most stomach and duodenal ulcers. The newer findings have resulted in improved treatment and reduction of stomach ulcers. *H. pylori* is most likely transmitted between humans, although the specific routes of transmission are still under study. Studies were also underway to determine the role of *H. pylori* and resulting chronic gastritis in the development of gastric cancers.

Erosive and hemorrhagic gastritis

After *H. pylori*, the second most common cause of chronic gastritis is the use of NSAIDs. These commonly used **pain** killers, including aspirin, fenoprofen, ibuprofen and naproxen, can lead to gastritis and peptic ulcers. Other forms of erosive gastritis are caused by alcohol or corrosive agents, or by injuries to the stomach tissues from the ingestion of foreign bodies.

Other forms of gastritis

Clinicians differ on the classification of the less common and specific forms of gastritis, particularly since there is so much overlap with *H. pylori* in development of chronic gastritis and complications of gastritis. Other types of gastritis that may be diagnosed include:

• Acute stress gastritis. This is the most serious form of gastritis. It usually occurs in critically ill patients, such as those in intensive care. Stress erosions may develop suddenly as a result of severe trauma or stresses on the stomach lining.

• Atrophic gastritis. This form of gastritis results from chronic gastritis. It is characterized by atrophy, or a decrease in size and wasting away of the gastric lining. Gastric atrophy is the final stage of chronic gastritis and may be a precursor of gastric **cancer**.

• Superficial gastritis. This term is often used to describe the initial stages of chronic gastritis.

• Uncommon specific forms of gastritis include granulomatous, eosiniphilic, and lymphocytic gastritis.

Causes & symptoms

Nonerosive H. pylori gastritis

H. pylori gastritis is caused by infection from the *H. pylori* bacterium. It is believed that most infection occurs in childhood. Clinicians think that there may be more than one route for the bacterium. Its prevalence and distribution differs in nations around the world. The presence of *H. pylori* has been detected in 86–99% of patients with chronic superficial gastritis. Physicians are still learning about the link of *H. pylori* to chronic gastritis and peptic ulcers, since many patients with *H. pylori* infection do not develop symptoms or peptic ulcers. *H. pylori* is also seen in 90–100% of patients with duodenal ulcers.

The symptoms of *H. pylori* gastritis include abdominal pain and reduced acid secretion in the stomach. The majority of patients with *H. pylori* infection, however, suffer no symptoms, even though the infection may lead to ulcers and resulting symptoms. Ulcer symptoms include dull, gnawing pain, often two to three hours after meals; and pain in the middle of the night when the stomach is empty.

Erosive and hemorrhagic gastritis

The most common cause of this form of gastritis is the use of NSAIDs. Other causes may be **alcoholism** or stress from surgery or critical illness. The role of NSAIDs in development of gastritis and peptic ulcers depends on the dose level. Although even low doses of aspirin or other nonsteroidal anti-inflammatory drugs may cause some gastric upset, low doses generally will not lead to gastritis. However, as many as 10–30% of patients on higher and more frequent doses of NSAIDs, such as those with chronic arthritis, may develop gastric ulcers. Patients with *H. pylori* already present in the stomach who are treated with NSAIDs are much more susceptible to ulcers and other gastrointestinal effects of these pain killers.

Patients with erosive gastritis may also show no symptoms. When symptoms do occur, they may include **anorexia nervosa**, gastric pain, **nausea**, and **vomiting**.

Other forms of gastritis

Less common forms of gastritis may result from a number of generalized diseases or from complications of chronic gastritis. Any number of mechanisms may cause various less common forms of gastritis and they may differ slightly in their symptoms and clinical signs. However, they all have inflammation of the gastric mucosa in common. Research recently found that severe gastritis may occur rarely as a result of infectious **mononucleosis**.

Diagnosis

Nonerosive H. pylori gastritis

H. pylori gastritis is easily diagnosed through the use of the urea breath test. This test detects active presence of *H. pylori* infection. Other serological tests, which may be readily available in a physician's office, may be used to detect *H. pylori* infection. Newly developed versions offer rapid diagnosis. New stool antigen tests were developed and made available in 2002. The choice of test will depend on cost, availability and the physician's experience, since nearly all of the available tests have an accuracy rate of 90% or better. Endoscopy, or the examination of the stomach area using a hollow tube inserted through the mouth, may be ordered to confirm the diagnosis. A biopsy of the gastric lining also may be ordered.

Erosive or hemorrhagic gastritis

The patient's clinical history may be particularly important in the diagnosis of this type of gastritis, since its cause is most often the result of chronic use of NSAIDs, alcoholism, or abuse of other substances.

Other forms of gastritis

Gastritis that has developed to the stage of duodenal or gastric ulcers usually requires endoscopy for diagnosis. It allows the physician to perform a biopsy for possible malignancy and for *H. pylori*. Sometimes, an upper gastrointestinal x-ray study with barium is ordered. Some diseases such as Zollinger-Ellison syndrome, an ulcer disease of the upper gastrointestinal tract, may show large mucosal folds in the stomach and duodenum on radiographs or in endoscopy. Other tests check for changes in gastric function.

Treatment

Some alternative treatments for gastritis follow mainstream medical practice in distinguishing between gastritis and other digestive disorders; others treat all disorders originating in the stomach in similar fashion.

Dietary supplements

Of all the alternative treatments for gastritis, dietary supplements of various types are the most likely to have been tested in clinical research. Some alternative practitioners have used the following supplements:

- Capsaicin. Capsaicin is the active ingredient in chili peppers. One study in human subjects indicates that capsaicin offers some protection against gastritis caused by aspirin.

- Antioxidants. **Vitamin C** and beta-carotene given in combination appear to be beneficial to most patients with chronic atrophic gastritis.

- Amino acids. Several studies indicate that cysteine speeds healing in bleeding gastritis related to NSAIDs and in atrophic gastritis. **Glutamine** appears to protect against the development of stress-related gastritis.

- Vitamins. Preliminary research suggests that large doses of **vitamin A** may reduce or eliminate erosive gastritis. **Vitamin B$_{12}$** is helpful for patients with prenicious **anemia** related to atrophic gastritis.

- Gamma oryzanol. In one study, 87% of patients with various types of gastritis reported at least some improvement from a daily dose of 300 mg of gamma oryzanol.

Herbal therapy

Herbs that have been recommended for gastritis include:

- **Licorice**. Licorice is a traditional remedy for stomach inflammation. It also appears to inhibit the growth of *H. pylori*. People who gain water weight or develop high blood pressure as side effects of taking licorice can be treated with licorice that has had the glycyrrhizin removed.

- Goldenseal. This herb contains berberine, a compound with antibiotic properties. There is some evidence that berberine is active against *H. pylori*.

- **Chamomile**. Chamomile contains apigenin, a bioflavonoid that inhibits *H. pylori*, and chamazulene, a compound that counteracts free radicals.

- Marsh mallow and **slippery elm**. These herbs have demulcent properties, which means that they soothe irritated mucous membranes.

- Echinacea and geranium. These herbs are recommended by some practitioners for their antiseptic and analgesic (pain-relieving) properties.

Naturopathic practitioners also advise patients with gastritis to eat certain categories of food separately. Patients are advised to eat protein foods by themselves or with green leafy vegetables; to eat fruits alone; and to avoid combining proteins and starches.

Acupuncture/acupressure

One source recommends applying gentle pressure to a point on the abdomen known as CV (conception vessel) 12, midway between the navel and the breastbone. Pressure should be applied when the stomach is empty. Trained acupuncturists treat stomach problems by releasing energy from the spleen and from other energy points associated with digestion.

Yoga

The Bow Pose is recommended by some teachers of **yoga** for stomach disorders because it puts pressure on a number of acupoints on the abdomen associated with the digestive process and with the stomach meridian.

Chinese herbal medicine

The Chinese traditionally use a tea made from **ginger** (*Zingiber officinale*) as a stomachic, to improve digestive functions.

Reflexology

A trained reflexologist will gently massage the stomach reflexes located on the hands and feet. On the hands, the stomach reflexes are on the palms, below the pads of the middle and index fingers. On the feet, the stomach reflexes are located on the sole just below the pad of the big toe.

Allopathic treatment

H. pylori gastritis

The discovery of *H. pylori*'s role in the development of gastritis and ulcers has led to improved treatment of chronic gastritis. Since the infection can be treated with antibiotics, the bacterium can be completely eliminated up to 90% of the time. The treatment, however, may be uncomfortable for patients and relies heavily on patient compliance. No single antibiotic has been found that would eliminate *H. pylori* on its own, so various combinations of antibiotics have been prescribed to treat the infection.

TRIPLE THERAPY. As of early 1998, triple therapy was the preferred treatment for patients with *H. pylori* gastritis. This treatment regimen usually involves a two-week course of three drugs. An antibiotic such as amoxicillin or tetracycline, and another antibiotic such as clarithromycin or metronidazole are used in combination with bismuth subsalicylate, a substance that helps protect the lining of the stomach from acid. However, this treatment often fails due to poor patient compliance and quadruple therapy is required.

DUAL THERAPY. Dual therapy involves the use of an antibiotic and a proton pump inhibitor. Proton pump inhibitors help reduce stomach acid by halting the mechanism that pumps acid into the stomach. Dual therapy has not been proven to be as effective as triple therapy, but may be ordered for some patients who can more comfortably handle the use of fewer drugs.

OTHER TREATMENTS. Scientists have experimented with quadruple therapy, which adds an antisecretory drug, or one that suppresses gastric secretion, to the standard triple therapy. One study showed this therapy to be effective with only a week's course of treatment in more than 90% of patients. The goal is to develop the most effective therapy combination that can work in one week of treatment or less.

Treatment of erosive gastritis

Patients with erosive gastritis may be given treatments similar to those for *H. pylori*, especially since some studies have demonstrated a link between *H. pylori* and NSAIDs in causing ulcers. The patient will most likely be advised to avoid NSAIDs.

Other forms of gastritis

Specific treatment will depend on the cause and type of gastritis. These may include prednisone or antibiotics. Critically ill patients at high risk for bleeding may be treated with preventive drugs to reduce the risk of acute stress gastritis. Sometimes surgery is recommended, but is weighed against the possibility of surgical complications or death. Once heavy bleeding occurs in acute stress gastritis, mortality is as high as 60%.

Expected results

The results expected from alternative treatments for gastritis include accelerated healing from some of the dietary therapies, and some symptomatic relief from **acupressure**, yoga, and **reflexology**.

The discovery of *H. pylori* has improved the prognosis for patients with gastritis and ulcers. Since treatment exists to eradicate the infection, recurrence is much less common. The prognosis for patients with acute stress gastritis is much poorer, with a 60% or higher mortality rate among those bleeding heavily. Recent studies have shown that infection with *H. pylori* and resulting gastritis may lead to such complications as chronic gastritis or as serious as gastric adenoma, a form of stomach cancer.

Prevention

The widespread detection and treatment of *H. pylori* as a preventive measure in gastritis has been discussed but not resolved. Until more is known about the routes through which *H.pylori* is spread, specific prevention recommendations are not available. It was estimated in late 2002 that the organism was present in 80% of middle-aged adults in developing countries and about 20% of those in industrialized countries. Erosive gastritis from NSAIDs can be prevented with cessation of use of these drugs. An education campaign was launched in 1998 to educate patients, particularly an **aging** population of arthritis sufferers, about the risk of developing ulcers from NSAIDs and alternative drugs.

Resources

BOOK

Burton Goldberg Group. *Alternative Medicine: The Definitive Guide.* Puyallup, WA: Future Medicine Publishing, Inc., 1994.

Gach, Michael Reed and Carolyn Marco. *Acu-Yoga: Self Help Techniques to Relieve Tension.* Tokyo and New York: Japan Publications, Inc., 1998.

LaMont, J. Thomas. *Gastrointestinal Infections, Diagnosis and Management.* New York: Marcel Dekker, Inc. 1997.

Murray, Michael, N.D., and Joseph Pizzorno, N.D. *Encyclopedia of Natural Medicine.* Rocklin, CA: Prima Publishing, 1991.

PERIODICALS

Graham, David Y. "NSAIDs, Helicobacter Pylori, and Pandora's Box." *The New England Journal of Medicine* (December 26, 2002):2162.

"Helicobacter Pylori Infection." *Internal Medicine Alert* (December 15, 2002):179–182.

"Severe Gastritis May Occasionally Result from Infectious Mononucleosis." *Gastroenterology Week* (June 23, 2003):20.

ORGANIZATION

National Digestive Diseases Information Clearinghouse (NDDIC). 2 Information Way, Bethesda, MD 20892-3570. http://www.niddk.nih.gov.

KEY TERMS

Apigenin—A bioflavonoid contained in chamomile that appears to inhibit *H. pylori*.

Atrophic—Characterized by a wasting away of a part of the body.

Capsaicin—A crystalline, bitter compound found in peppers. It may be helpful in treating some forms of gastritis.

Demulcent—A medication or substance that is used to soothe irritated mucosa. Some of the herbs recommended to treat gastritis have demulcent properties.

Helicobacter pylori—The bacterium that is implicated in most cases of nonerosive gastritis.

NSAIDs—An abbreviation for nonsteroidal anti-inflammatory drugs. Heavy use of NSAIDs is the most common cause of erosive gastritis.

OTHER

American College of Gastroenterology. http://www.acg.org.

Rebecca J. Frey, PhD
Teresa G. Odle

Gastrodia

Description

Gastrodia is a preparation made from the rhizome or tuber of an orchid, *Gastrodia elata*. It is a member of the Orchidaceae family. *Gastrodia elata* is a native of the Far East; its natural areas of distribution include Tibet, western China, Korea, and Japan. While gastrodia appears in the oldest lists of Chinese medicinal herbs, it was not known to Western herbalists.

Gastrodia is first mentioned in the *Shennong Bencao Jing*, which was compiled around A.D. 100. A later Chinese herbalist named Tao Hong placed gastrodia in the category of superior herbs, which meant that it could be taken for long periods of time, and that it could be used to promote longevity as well as to treat illnesses. It was originally called *chiqian*, which means "red arrow" in Chinese, because its stem is red and arrow-shaped. Later it was named *tian ma*, or "heavenly hemp," which is the name that it still bears in Chinese herbal formularies.

Like other wild orchids, *Gastrodia elata* has been placed on the list of endangered species. The increasing difficulty of finding wild gastrodia in the 1970s led to an interesting discovery about this plant. Chinese herbalists tried to cultivate gastrodia, but failed until biologists discovered that the plant needs two fungi in order to survive and reproduce. It needs the *Armillaria mellea* mushroom on its tuber in order to grow and mature; and it requires a second fungus called *Mycena osmundicola* to help its seeds to sprout. After this complicated relationship was understood, herbalists were able to grow gastrodia.

Another aspect of this discovery was the finding that most of the medicinal benefits associated with gastrodia are actually produced by the *Armillaria* mushroom. Many growers then decided to cultivate the mushroom by itself without the gastrodia tuber. Some herbalists now use the *Armillaria* mushroom in their preparations instead of wild or cultivated gastrodia.

General use

In the categories of Chinese herbal medicine, gastrodia is classified as having a sweet and slightly warm nature with a neutral taste. Its traditional uses are to calm the liver and to clear the meridians by invigorating the patient's circulation. In the categories of Western medicine, gastrodia is said to have sedative and analgesic properties. The specific conditions that were treated by gastrodia include migraine headaches, **dizziness** or vertigo due to liver inflammations, convulsions caused by heat excess, paralysis, general **fatigue**, numbness in the hands or feet, and **pain** in the joints. More recently, gastrodia has been used to relieve nervous headaches, pain in the trigeminal nerve, nocturnal emissions, difficult breathing, **insomnia** due to **stress**, and **hypertension**.

Chemical analysis of gastrodia indicates that it contains significant amounts of **calcium**, **magnesium**, and **potassium**. Its active ingredients include gastrodioside, vanillin (from the rhizome), and vanillyl alcohol (from the tuber). These last two compounds are related to vanilla flavoring, which comes from another orchid called *Vanilla plantifolia*. Research indicates that vanillin has anticonvulsive properties. Other research suggests that the gastrodia tuber has analgesic and sedative effects because the compounds in it decrease the level of dopamine in the brain. Most of the other traditional Chinese uses for gastrodia have not been corroborated by research.

Preparations

Single-herb preparations

Gastrodia preparations are made from the tubers and rhizomes, or underground stems, of the plant. The rhizomes are dug in winter or spring. The bark is then removed and the rhizomes are cleaned and boiled, or steamed and baked. They are soaked in water a second time and sliced. In traditional Chinese herbal medicine, gastrodia is given as a decoction (concentration of herb after boiling down), in doses of 3–10 g per day.

The *Armillaria* mushroom that is necessary for the growth of the gastrodia tuber has been given the Chinese name of *tian ma mihuanjun*. It is more potent than the gastrodia tuber because it is the source of the tuber's active compounds. Although exact comparisons have not yet been determined, most Chinese practitioners use about half the customary dosage of gastrodia when they are replacing it with *Armillaria*. The mushroom or the gastrodia tuber are given in powdered form, in doses of 1.0–1.5 g, two or three times per day.

Herbal formulas

Gastrodia has been a favorite herb to use in combination formulas to treat specific conditions. Most of these formulas are made up as tablets or capsules. A Chinese pharmacology textbook lists the following herbal mixtures containing gastrodia:

- For dizziness and **headache** caused by a hyperactive liver: gastrodia combined with uncaria and haliotis.

- For disturbances caused by wind-phlegm: gastrodia with **pinellia** and atractylodes.

- For migraine: gastrodia combined with cnidium.

- For convulsions caused by liver heat: gastrodia with antelope horn and uncaria.

- To clear the meridians and relieve pain or numbness in the limbs: gastrodia combined with achyranthes, *chin-chiu*, and *chiang-huo*.

Precautions

Gastrodia is considered a mild herb by the Chinese, and therefore generally safe to use. It is best, however, to consult an experienced practitioner of Chinese herbal medicine before using gastrodia either as a single herb or in formulas.

Side effects

One source reports that the side effects of gastrodia include skin **allergies**, **hair loss**, and other allergic reactions.

Interactions

Because gastrodia has not been used by Western herbalists, its potential interactions with standard pharmaceutical preparations have not been studied.

KEY TERMS

Analgesic—A substance or medication given to relieve pain.

Meridians—In Chinese medicine, pathways of subtle energy that link and regulate the various structures, organs, and substances in the human body. Gastrodia is recommended to clear the meridians of obstructions caused by dampness and wind.

Rhizome—A root-like underground plant stem, often horizontal in position.

Sedative—A substance or medication given to calm and soothe. In traditional Chinese herbal medicine, gastrodia is used as a sedative to the liver.

Tuber—The thick, fleshy, underground stem of a plant.

Resources

BOOKS
Reid, Daniel P. *Chinese Herbal Medicine*. Boston: Shambhala, 1993.

ORGANIZATIONS
American Association of Oriental Medicine (AAOM). 433 Front Street, Catasauqua, PA 18032. (610) 266-2433.

American Foundation of Traditional Chinese Medicine (AFTCM). 505 Beach Street, San Francisco, CA 94133. (415) 776-0502. Fax: (415) 392-7003. aftcm@earthlink.net.

OTHER
Dr. James A. Duke. Phytochemical and Ethnobotanical Databases. United States Department of Agriculture, Agricultural Research Service. Beltsville Agricultural Research Center. Beltsville, MD.

Rebecca J. Frey, PhD

Gastroenteritis

Definition

Gastroenteritis is a general term for infection or irritation of the digestive tract, particularly the stomach and intestine. It is frequently referred to as stomach or intestinal flu, although the **influenza** virus does not cause this illness. Major symptoms include **nausea, vomiting, diarrhea**, and abdominal cramps. **Fever** and overall weakness sometimes accompany these symptoms. Gastroenteritis typically lasts about three days. Adults usually recover without problem, but children, the elderly, and persons with an underlying disease are more vulnerable to complications such as dehydration.

Description

Gastroenteritis is an uncomfortable and inconvenient ailment, but it is rarely life-threatening in the United States and other developed nations. However, in the United States an estimated 220,000 children younger than age five are hospitalized annually with gastroenteritis symptoms. Of these children, 300 die as a result of severe diarrhea and dehydration. In developing nations, diarrhea-related illnesses are a major source of mortality. In 1990, approximately three million deaths occurred worldwide as a result of diarrheal illness.

Viral gastroenteritis

Gastroenteritis is usually caused by infection with one of these viruses: rotavirus, adenovirus, astrovirus, calicivirus, and small round-structured viruses (SRSVs). These viruses are found all over the world and are particularly problematic where sanitation is poor. Typical exposure to these viruses occurs through the fecal-to-oral route, by ingesting food that is contaminated with fecal material or by coming in contact with an infected person's vomit or diarrhea and then inadvertently bringing the contaminant to the mouth. Other routes of transmission are quite likely, because exposure to as few as 100 virus particles can cause an infection.

Typically, children are more vulnerable to rotaviruses—the most common cause of acute watery diarrhea. It is estimated that each year rotaviruses cause 800,000 deaths worldwide in children younger than age five. For this reason, much research has gone into developing a vaccine to protect children from this virus. Adults can be infected with rotaviruses, but these **infections** typically have minimal or no symptoms.

Adenoviruses and astroviruses are minor causes of childhood gastroenteritis, and children may become infected with caliciviruses and SRSVs. Adults experience illness from astroviruses as well, but the major causes of adult viral gastroenteritis are the caliciviruses and SRSVs. The SRSVs are a type of calicivirus and include the Norwalk, Southhampton, and Lonsdale viruses. SRSVs are the most likely to produce vomiting as a major symptom.

Bacterial gastroenteritis

Bacterial gastroenteritis is frequently a result of poor sanitation, the lack of safe drinking water, or contaminat-

ed food—conditions that are common in developing nations. Natural or man-made disasters can worsen underlying sanitation and food-safety problems. In developed nations, modern food production, handling, and distribution systems and methods may expose millions of people to disease-causing bacteria. Common types of bacterial gastroenteritis can be linked to *Salmonella* and *Campylobacter* bacteria; however, *Escherichia coli* 0157 and *Listeria monocytogenes* are creating increased concern in developed nations. Cholera and shigella remain two diseases of great concern in developing countries, and research to develop long-term vaccines against them is underway.

Causes & symptoms

Gastroenteritis arises from ingestion of viruses, certain bacteria, or parasites. Spoiled food may also cause illness. Certain medications and excessive alcohol can irritate the digestive tract to the point of inducing gastroenteritis. Regardless of the cause, the symptoms of gastroenteritis include diarrhea, nausea, vomiting, abdominal **pain**, and cramps. Sufferers may also experience bloating, low fever, and overall tiredness. Typically, the symptoms last only two to three days, but some viruses may last up to a week.

A typical bout of gastroenteritis should not require a visit to the doctor. However, medical treatment is essential if symptoms worsen or if there are complications. Infants, young children, the elderly, and persons with underlying disease require special attention in this regard.

Dehydration is the greatest danger presented by gastroenteritis. The loss of fluids through diarrhea and vomiting can upset the body's electrolyte balance, leading to potentially life-threatening problems, such as heart beat abnormalities (arrhythmia). The risk of dehydration increases the longer that symptoms are present. Signs of dehydration include a **dry mouth**, increased or excessive thirst, or scanty urination.

Symptoms that do not clear up within a week may point to an infection or disorder more serious than gastroenteritis. Symptoms of great concern include a fever of 102°F (38.9°C) or above, blood or mucus in the diarrhea, blood in the vomit, and severe abdominal pain or swelling. Persons experiencing these symptoms should seek prompt medical attention.

Diagnosis

The symptoms of gastroenteritis are usually sufficient for identifying the illness. Unless there are complications or there is an outbreak that affects several people, identifying the specific cause of the illness is not a priority. However, if it is necessary to identify the infectious agent, a stool sample will be collected and analyzed for the presence of viruses, disease-causing (pathogenic) bacteria, or parasites.

Treatment

Gastroenteritis is a self-limiting illness that will resolve by itself. Symptoms of uncomplicated gastroenteritis can be relieved with adjustments in diet, herbal remedies, and **homeopathy**. An infusion of meadowsweet (*Filipendula ulmaria*) may be effective in reducing nausea and stomach acidity. Once the worst symptoms are relieved, **slippery elm** (*Ulmus fulva*) can be used to calm the digestive tract.

The homeopathic remedies *Arsenicum album*, **ipecac**, and *Nux vomica* are also believed to relieve the symptoms of gastroenteritis. In Chinese herbal medicine, the patent remedies Po Chai and Pill Curing can be effective for relieving nausea and diarrhea.

Supplementing the bacteria that are beneficial to a person's health (**probiotics**) is recommended during the recovery phase of gastroenteritis. Specifically, live cultures of *Lactobacillus acidophilus* are said to be effective in soothing the digestive tract and returning the intestinal flora to normal. In fact, in 2002, a new study found it was reasonably effective in treating children with acute infectious diarrhea. *L. acidophilus* is found in live-culture yogurt and in capsule or powder form at health food stores. **Castor oil** packs applied to the abdomen can reduce inflammation, spasms, and discomfort.

It is important to stay hydrated and nourished during a bout of gastroenteritis. In the absence of dehydration, it should be sufficient to drink generous amounts of nonalcoholic fluids, such as water or juice. **Caffeine** should be avoided, since it increases urine output.

The traditional BRAT diet—bananas, rice, applesauce, and toast—is tolerated by the tender gastrointestinal system, but it is not particularly nutritious. Many, but not all, medical researchers recommend a diet that includes complex carbohydrates (rice, wheat, potatoes, bread, and cereal, for example), lean meats, yogurt, fruit, and vegetables. Milk and other dairy products shouldn't create problems if they are part of the normal diet. Fatty foods or foods with a lot of sugar should be avoided. These recommendations are based on clinical experience and controlled trials, but are not universally accepted.

Allopathic treatment

Over-the-counter medications such as Pepto Bismol are useful in relieving the symptoms of gastroenteritis. These medications work by altering the intestine's ability to move or secrete spontaneously, by absorbing toxins and water, or by altering intestinal microflora. Some over-the-counter medicines use more than one element to treat symptoms, and this information should be included on the label.

If over-the-counter medications are ineffective, a doctor may prescribe a more powerful anti-diarrheal drug, such as motofen or lomotil. If pathogenic bacteria or parasites are found in the patient's stool sample, medications such as antibiotics will be prescribed.

Minimal to moderate dehydration is treated with oral rehydrating solutions that contain glucose and electrolytes. These solutions are commercially available under names such as Naturalyte, Pedialyte, Infalyte, and Rehydralyte. If vomiting prevents the patient from taking a full dose of solution, he or she may better tolerate fluid taken in small, frequent amounts. Should oral rehydration fail or severe dehydration occur, medical treatment in the form of intravenous (IV) therapy is required. IV therapy can be followed with oral rehydration as the patient's condition improves. Once normal hydration is achieved, the patient can return to a regular diet.

Sometimes, a child's dehydration is so severe that it requires hospitalization with IV therapy. However, a study published in 2002 informed pediatricians that often, rapid intravenous rehydration and rapid nasogastric hydration in the emergency department are safe and effective alternatives to hospitalization for many children with viral gastroenteritis. Not only does this save money, it also saves a child the more frightening experience of being in a hospital overnight and the routine laboratory testing he or she would endure in the hospital setting.

Expected results

Gastroenteritis usually clears up within two to three days and there are no long-term effects. If dehydration occurs, recovery is extended by a few days.

Prevention

Gastroenteritis can be avoided by practicing good hygiene, which includes washing hands thoroughly after using the bathroom or coming in contact with an infected person, using disinfectants to clean areas the infected person has come in contact with, and washing infected linens in hot water. Making sure that food is well-cooked and unspoiled can prevent bacterial gastroenteritis, but may not be effective against viral gastroenteritis.

Resources

BOOKS

Hoffman, David. *The Complete Illustrated Herbal.* New York: Barnes & Noble, 1999.

Midthun, Karen, and Albert Z. Kapikian. "Viral Gastroenteritis." In *Gastrointestinal and Hepatic Infections,* edited by

Christina Surawicz and Robert L. Owen. Philadelphia: W.B. Saunders, 1995.

PERIODICALS

Burke, Michael G."For Gastroenteritis, Rehydration But no Hospitalization." *Contemporary Pediatrics* (June 2002): 125.

Gorbach, Sherwood L. "Efficacy of Lactobacillus in Treatment of Acute Diarrhea." *Nutrition Today* 31, no. 6 (December 1996): 195.

Hart, C. Anthony, and Nigel A. Cunliffe. "Viral Gastroenteritis." *Current Opinion in Infectious Diseases* 10 (1997): 408.

Moss, Peter J., and Michael W. McKendrick. "Bacterial Gastroenteritis." *Current Opinion in Infectious Diseases* 10 (1997): 402.

Van Niel, Cornelius W., and others. "Lactobacillus Therapy for Acute Infectious Diarrhea in Children: A Meta-analysis." *Pediatrics* (April 2002): 678.

Paula Ford-Martin
Teresa G. Odle

Gelsemium

Description

Gelsemium sempervirens is also known as yellow jasmine, false jasmine, wild woodbine, and Carolina jasmine. It is a woody, climbing vine with dark leaves and groups of yellow, bell-shaped flowers that bloom in early spring. The flowers are very fragrant. It is native to the coastal areas extending from Virginia to Florida, and in Mexico, and is the state flower of South Carolina.

Gelsemium contains extremely toxic alkaloid components, and is not in current medical use. Even very small doses may prove lethal. It was reportedly discovered in the nineteenth century as a result of mistaken identity for another herb. A sick farmer took it for an attack of "bilious fever," and became quite ill. When the symptoms resolved, he discovered that his prior illness had also disappeared. It came into use as an agent to treat **fever**, spasmodic disorders, and the **pain** of **neuralgia**.

General use

The herb form of gelsemium has historically been used for migraines resulting from excessive cerebral blood flow, severe **wheezing** attacks of **asthma**, **insomnia**, and nerve pain, particularly trigeminal neuralgia. The latter condition is a disorder of the trigeminal nerve, which causes shooting pain in the area of the lips, gums, cheek, chin, and occasionally around the eye. Use of the herb form has not been recommended for some time due to the extremely toxic potential of the alkaloids this plant contains.

Homeopathic remedies incorporating gelsemium have specific indications. As with other homeopathic treatments, they contain infinitesimal amounts of the active ingredient, so that toxicity is highly unlikely. Some of the recommendations for the use of homeopathic gelsemium include **migraine headache**, **anxiety**, chemotherapy support, dental support, **influenza**, **nausea**, and recovery from surgery.

Homeopathic gelsemium is thought to relieve anxiety in the form of apprehension about particular events, as well as generalized anxiety. The 30C formulation is recommended for this purpose, taken as needed up to three or four times daily, for no longer than one week. The 6C formulation may be used two or three times prior to undergoing chemotherapy treatment. Similar dosing is recommended prior to a visit to the dentist.

True influenza is a respiratory ailment, although symptoms also include aches, fever, **chills**, and **headache**. Homeopathic recommendations for gelsemium due to flu symptoms include mild fever, dull headache at the nape of the neck, and **dizziness**. Gelsemium 6C can be used for as long as five days, once every three to four hours, during the illness.

Migraine headaches that are felt primarily in the back of the head or as constrictive pain may be helped by homeopathic preparations of gelsemium. Visual aura and aching of the neck and shoulders may accompany this type of headache. For best results, gelsemium 30C is taken as soon as symptoms begin, every 30 minutes, for up to three doses if needed.

Homeopathic gelsemium is also recommended to support surgical recovery, particularly for those who are quite apprehensive and restless. The 6C formulation may be taken for a few days preceding the surgery, up to four doses per day.

Consult a practitioner of **homeopathy** to determine the best indicated doses and combinations of remedies for a particular health issue.

Preparations

The dried root, harvested in autumn, is the usable portion of the plant. Gelsemium is currently unavailable in medicinal formulations due to the narrow safety margins and dangerous toxicity.

Precautions

Gelsemium is an extremely toxic herb because of the alkaloid component, related to strychnine, which exists in all parts of the plant. Symptoms can include sweating, nausea, muscular weakness, dilated pupils, lowered temperature, and convulsions. It can excessively depress the nervous system, and can cause death due to respiratory failure. A lethal dose is approximately 2–3 grams for an adult, and 500 mg for a child. Ingestion of as little as a single flower has reportedly resulted in the fatality of a child. Accidental ingestion of the plant under any circumstances warrants emergency treatment.

The safety margin of gelsemium is extremely small. It should never be used, especially in children, or in women who are pregnant or lactating. Oral use of preparations from the rhizome or root are also considered unsafe. It is particularly dangerous for people with any sort of **heart disease**.

Side effects

There are no reported side effects, although individual aggravations may occur.

Interactions

The effects of aspirin and phenacetin may be increased by gelsemium.

Resources

BOOKS

Lininger, Schuyler W., Alan R. Gaby, Skye W. Lininger, and Jamie Miller. *The Natural Pharmacy.* Roseville, California: Prima Health, 1998.

KEY TERMS

Alkaloid—One of a group of organic compounds which are generally toxic.

Neuralgia—Severe nerve pain.

Phenacetin—A compound formerly used to ease pain or fever, but withdrawn because of its serious side effects.

Rhizome—A horizontal, underground stem that sends out roots.

OTHER

Grieve, M. *Gelsemium.* http://www.botanical.com/botanical/mgmh/g/gelsem07.html. (1995).

Judith Turner

Gelsemium sempervirons see **Gelsemium**
Gem healing *see* **Crystal healing**

Genital herpes
Definition

Genital herpes is a sexually transmitted disease caused by the herpes simplex virus. The disease is characterized by the formation of fluid-filled, painful **blisters** in the genital area.

Description

Genital herpes is a sexually transmitted disease spread by vaginal, anal, and oral contact. The first herpes infection a person has is called a primary infection. It develops about four to seven days after contact with the disease. Once a person has been infected with the herpes virus, it cannot be completely cured. Instead, the virus can lay latent in the sensory nerve ganglia for days, months, or even years between outbreaks. When the virus becomes activated there is a recurrent infection of the skin. An active herpes infection is then obvious because of the sores that develop. However, an active infection may occur without visible sores. Up to 75% of people with herpes may not know they have the infection.

Newborn babies who are infected with herpes virus experience a very severe, and possibly fatal, disease called neonatal herpes. In the United States, one in 3,000–5,000 babies born will be infected with herpes

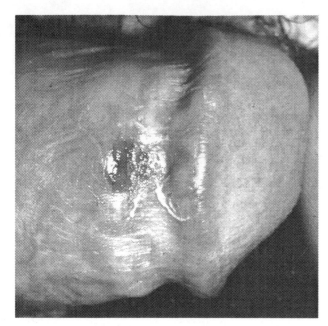

A close-up view of a penis with a blister (center of image) caused by the herpes simplex virus. *(Photograph by Dr. P. Marazzi, Custom Medical Stock Photo. Reproduced by permission.)*

virus. Babies usually become infected during passage through the birth canal, but they also can become infected during **pregnancy** if the membranes rupture early.

Causes & symptoms

Genital herpes results from an infection by herpes simplex virus. There are several different kinds of human herpes viruses. Only two of these, herpes simplex type 1 (HSV-1) and type 2 (HSV-2), can cause herpes. HSV-2 is most often responsible for genital **infections**. HSV-1 usually causes oral herpes, but it can also cause genital herpes about 10-30% of the time. While the herpes virus can infect anyone, not everyone will show symptoms. Risk factors include early age at first sexual activity, multiple sexual partners, and a medical history of other sexually transmitted diseases (STDs).

The first symptoms of a primary herpes infection usually occur within two to seven days after contact with an infected person but may take up to two weeks. Symptoms of a primary infection are usually more severe than those of recurrent infections. For up to 70% of people, a primary infection causes general symptoms such as tiredness, **headache, fever, chills**, muscle aches, loss of appetite, and painful, swollen lymph nodes. These symptoms are greatest during the first three to four days of the infection and disappear within a week.

Most people with genital herpes experience prodromes, or symptoms of the oncoming disease. This might entail **pain**, burning, **itching**, or tingling at the site on the genital area, legs, or buttocks where blisters will form. The prodrome stage may occur anywhere from a few hours, to one or two days before an outbreak of the infection. Following that, small red bumps appear. These bumps quickly become fluid-filled blisters that may also fill with pus, and become covered with a scab. The blisters may burst and become painful sores. Blisters may continue to erupt for a week or longer. Pain usually subsides within two weeks, and the blisters and sores heal without scarring by three to four weeks. It is possible to pass the virus to other parts of the body by touching an open sore and then bringing the fingers into contact with the mouth, the eyes, or a break in the skin. The highest risk for spreading the herpes virus is the time during the appearance of blisters up to the formation of scabs. However, an infected person can spread herpes virus to other people even in the absence of sores.

Women can experience a very severe and painful primary herpes infection. In addition to the vaginal area, blisters often appear on the clitoris, at the urinary opening, in the rectum and around the anus, and on the buttocks and thighs. The cervix is almost always involved, causing a watery discharge. About one in 10 women get a vaginal **yeast infection** as a complication of herpes. In men, the herpes blisters usually form on the penis but can also appear on the scrotum, thighs, around the anus, and in the rectum. Men may also have a urinary discharge with a genital herpes infection. Both men and women may experience painful or difficult urination, swelling of the urethra, **meningitis**, and throat infections, with women experiencing these symptoms more often than men.

It is unknown exactly what triggers a latent herpes virus to activate, but several conditions seem to be connected with the onset of an active infection. These include illness, **stress**, tiredness, sunlight, **menstruation**, skin damage, food **allergies**, and extreme hot or cold temperatures. Most people with genital herpes experience one or more outbreaks per year. About 40% experience six or more outbreaks per year. Active recurrences of herpes are usually less severe than the primary infection. There are fewer blisters, less pain, and the time period from the beginning of symptoms to healing is shorter than the primary infection.

Diagnosis

Because genital herpes is so common, it can be initially diagnosed by symptoms. A Tzanck test can also be used for a quick initial diagnosis. It is performed using a sample scraped from the base of an active blister. A confirmation of the diagnosis can be done by making a tissue culture of material scraped from the skin lesions, testing the blood for herpes antibodies, or examining fluid and scrapings from the lesions by a method called direct immunofluorescent assay. Since most infants infected with the herpes virus are born to mothers with no symptoms of infection, newborns and pregnant women are often routinely given blood tests called the TORCH antibody panel, which includes a test for herpes. Babies also need to be checked for signs of herpes infection in their eyes. Skin sores and sores in the mouth should be sampled for the presence of herpes simplex.

Treatment

An imbalance in the **amino acids lysine** and **arginine** is thought to be one contributing factor in herpes virus outbreaks. Supplementation with lysine may help maintain the correct balance and prevent recurrences of herpes. Patients may take 500 mg of lysine daily and increase to 1,000 mg three times a day during an outbreak. Intake of foods that are rich in the amino acid arginine should be avoided, including chocolate, peanuts, almonds, and other nuts and seeds.

Clinical experience indicates a connection between high stress and herpes outbreaks. Many people respond well to stress reduction and **relaxation** techniques. **Acupressure** and massage may relieve tiredness and stress. **Meditation, yoga, t'ai chi, acupuncture** and **hypnotherapy** can also help relieve stress and promote relaxation. Counseling and support groups are often recommended to deal with the emotional and psychological stress of the disease.

An extract of bovine thymus gland can be taken to improve immune function and help the body fight against viral infections such as herpes. Some herbs are also able to serve as antivirals. They include **echinacea** and **garlic**, *Allium sativum.* **Siberian ginseng**, *Eleutherococcus senticosus,* is useful to relieve the stress response that can bring on recurrent herpes outbreaks. Supplementation with beta-carotene and **vitamin E** is recommended during an outbreak. Homeopathic remedies that may be helpful treatments for genital herpes include *Rhus tox* 6c and *Apis mellifica* 6c.

There are **traditional Chinese medicine** combinations that are useful for herpes outbreaks. One, called Zhi Bai Lui Wai Di Huang, is a mixture of philodendron and other remedies. Another is Long Dan Xie Gan Tang, a soup made to drain the liver. A traditional Chinese medicine practitioner can help create the right combination specific to the outbreak.

Red marine algae, both taken internally and applied topically, is thought to be effective in treating herpes. Other topical treatments may be helpful in inhibiting the growth of the herpes virus, in minimizing the damage it causes, or in helping the sores heal. **Zinc** may also be used both internally and externally. Oral supplementation coupled with an application of zinc sulfate ointment may help heal sores and fight recurrent outbreaks. Lithium succinate ointment may interfere with viral replication. An ointment made with glycyrrhizinic acid, a component of **licorice**, *Glycyrrhiza glabra*, seems to inactivate the virus. Topical applications of vitamin E oil or **tea tree oil** (*Melaleuca* spp.) help dry up the sores.

Allopathic treatment

There is no cure for a herpes infection. Aspirin may be used to reduce pain and inflammation. Antiviral drugs are available that may lessen the symptoms and decrease the length of outbreaks. There is evidence that some may also help prevent the spreading of the disease and reduce recurrence of future outbreaks. For the best results, treatment with antiviral drugs has to begin during the prodrome stage, before blisters are visible. Depending on the length of the outbreak, drug treatment may continue for up to 10 days.

Acyclovir (Zovirax) is the drug of choice for herpes infection and can be given intravenously, taken by mouth, or applied directly to sores as an ointment. Intravenous acyclovir is given to patients who require hospitalization, usually due to severe primary infections or complications of herpes such as aseptic meningitis or sacral ganglionitis, an inflammation of nerve bundles. Acyclovir reduces the virus shedding period, the duration of the blisters, and the healing time. Patients with herpes outbreaks happening more often than six to eight per year may be given a long-term course of treatment with acyclovir. This is referred to as suppressive therapy. Patients on suppressive therapy have longer periods between herpes outbreaks. Alternatively, patients may use short-term suppressive therapy to lessen the chance of developing an active infection during special occasions such as weddings or holidays. Side effects of acyclovir include **nausea, vomiting**, itchy rash, and **hives**. Other drugs that may be used include famciclovir (Famvir), valacyclovir (Valtrex), vidarabine (Vira-A), idoxuridine (Herplex Liquifilm, Stoxil), trifluorothymidine (Viroptic), and penciclovir (Denavir).

Neonatal herpes is a serious condition. Even with treatment, babies may not survive or they may suffer serious damage to the nervous system. Newborns with herpes infections are normally treated with intravenous acyclovir or vidarabine for 10 days. However, infected babies may have to be treated with long-term suppressive therapy. These drugs have greatly reduced deaths and have also increased the number of babies who are relatively healthy by one year of age.

Expected results

Genital herpes is usually not a serious disease, with several major exceptions. Sometimes, a primary infection can be severe and may require hospitalization for treatment. Complications that may arise include aseptic meningitis and nervous system damage. There may also be **constipation**, **impotence**, and difficulty with urination. In addition, people who are immunosuppressed due to disease or medication are at risk for a very severe, and possibly fatal, herpes infection. And even with antiviral treatment, neonatal herpes infections can be fatal or cause permanent nervous system damage.

Prevention

The only way to definitely prevent a genital herpes infection is to avoid contact with infected people. This is not an easy solution because many people aren't aware that they are infected. Use of condoms and spermicidal jellies or foams with nonoxynol-9 is recommended with all partners whose disease status is questionable or unknown. However, condoms may not protect against herpes when there is skin contact with someone with an open sore that cannot be covered by a condom. Use of dental dams or squares of non-microwaveable plastic wrap is also recommended. Sexual contact should be avoided altogether during a herpes outbreak. Touching affected areas should be avoided, since this can spread the infection to other sites. In order to prevent a child from contracting a herpes infection through contact in the birth canal, doctors usually perform Caesarean sec-

tions on women who have active herpes sores when they go into labor.

Resources

BOOKS

Ebel, Charles. *Managing Herpes: How to Live and Love With a Chronic STD*. Durham, NC: American Social Health Association, 1998.

Sacks, Stephen L. *The Truth About Herpes*. Seattle: Gordon Soules Book Publisher, 1997.

PERIODICALS

Murray, N.D., Michael T. "Natural Help for Herpes and Cold Sores." *Let's Live* (April 1997).

OTHER

drkoop.com, Inc. http://www.drkoop.com/conditions/sexual_health/page_59_277.asp.

Merck & Co., Inc. *The Merck Manual Online*. http://www.merck.com/pubs/mmanual/section13/chapter164/164k.htm.

Mother Nature.com. http://www.mothernature.com/ ency/ homeo/ herpes_simplex_hm.asp.

Patience Paradox

Genital warts

Definition

Genital warts, or condylomata acuminata, are also called venereal warts. These warts are painless, pink or grayish growths on the skin and mucous membranes of the genitals and anal area. They are usually found in clusters. Genital warts are very contagious and spread through sexual contact with an infected person.

Description

Genital warts are the most common sexually transmitted disease (STD) in the general population of the United States. It is estimated that 1% of sexually active people between the ages of 18 and 45 have genital warts; however, studies indicate that as many as 40% of sexually active adults may carry the virus that causes genital warts. Certain strains of the virus that cause genital warts may also cause cervical changes and **cancer**.

Causes & symptoms

Genital warts are caused by several subtypes of HPV, the same virus that causes warts on other parts of the body. Symptoms develop about one to six months after being exposed to the virus. Once contracted, the virus remains in the infected person's body. This is true even if the warts are not visible. In addition to the visible warts, symptoms may include bleeding, **pain**, odor, **itching**, and redness in affected areas. These symptoms may appear without the warts, and the warts may appear without other symptoms. **Stress** may contribute to recurrent outbreaks.

Genital warts may be difficult to detect. At any given time, at least a quarter of all HPV **infections** are in a state of regression, in which the infection remains dormant in the body and there are no outbreaks of warts or other readily detected symptoms. In addition, warts that occur deep inside the vagina, on the cervix, or within the anus may go undetected.

HPV can be transmitted through oral, anal, or genital contact with an infected person, even if warts are not visible. Care must be taken, because the virus may also be transmitted via objects that have been recently exposed to the virus. These may include unwashed or improperly cleaned medical equipment, as well as underwear, tanning beds, and sex toys.

Risk factors for contracting genital warts include:

• multiple sex partners

• infection with another sexually transmitted disease (STD)

• pregnancy

• anal intercourse

• poor personal hygiene

• heavy perspiration

Genital warts vary somewhat in appearance. They may either be flat or resemble raspberries in appearance. The warts begin as small, red or pinkish growths. They may grow in clusters as large as four inches across, and may interfere with intercourse and **childbirth**. The warts grow on warm, moist tissue. In women, they occur on the external genitalia, the cervix, and the walls of the vagina. In men, they develop in the urethra and on the shaft of the penis. The warts may also spread to the area surrounding the anus.

Diagnosis

Genital warts are usually identified and diagnosed by their characteristic appearance. A sexual history should be taken, and tests for other STDs may be administered. If cervical warts are suspected, a colposcopy exam to view the cervix is necessary for diagnosis. A Papanicolaou (pap) smear may be performed, and the doctor may order a biopsy of the warts to rule out cancer.

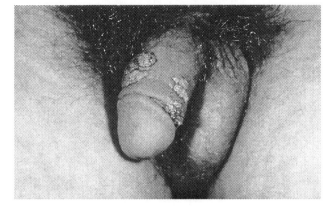

Man with genital warts. (*Custom Medical Stock Photo. Reproduced by permission.*)

Treatment

Genital warts are contagious, and should be assessed and treated under the supervision of a healthcare practitioner. A **traditional Chinese medicine** practitioner or an acupuncturist will probably recommend treatments to cleanse the liver and enhance immune functioning. A generally recommended homeopathic remedy is the application of a tincture of *Thuja occidentalis* (common names **thuja**, northern white cedar, and arborvitae, or tree-of-life) directly to the warts. A homeopathic physician should be consulted for a work-up for further treatment.

The direct topical application of **vitamin A**, thuja, **lomatium** (*Lomatium dissectum*) isolate, or **tea tree oil** (*Melaleuca alternifolia*) helps resolve warts and prevent recurrence of outbreaks. With the exception of the tea tree oil, these herbs should also be taken internally in addition to direct application. It has also been noted that deficiencies of **folic acid** and vitamins A and C contribute to this condition. Such deficiencies may be risk factors for a progression to abnormal cervical cells and cancer; therefore, supplementation is recommended. It should be noted that beta-carotene is often suggested as an alternative to taking high dosages of vitamin A.

Treatments that focus on emotional and psychological factors have been shown to be effective in reducing or eliminating outbreaks of warts. **Hypnotherapy** and techniques of stress reduction and **relaxation** are highly recommended.

Allopathic treatment

There is no cure for genital warts, as the virus cannot be destroyed once it enters the body. The warts themselves may be burned off with electrocautery or lasers;

KEY TERMS

Cervix—The entrance of the uterus, which protrudes into the vagina.

Electrocautery—An instrument that uses heat from an electric current to remove small growths on the skin.

Mucous membranes—Thin sheets of tissue that cover and protect body passages that open to the outside. These membranes secrete mucus and absorb water and various salts.

Papanicolau (pap) smear—A diagnostic test using a sampling of tissue from the cervix.

Papilloma—A benign growth on the skin or mucous membrane.

frozen with liquid nitrogen for easy removal; or surgically removed. Podophyllum resin, trichloroacetic acid, interferon inducers, 5-fluorouracil cream, bichloroacetic acid, or trichloroacetic acid can be used as a topical treatment. These medications require several weeks of treatment and may irritate the skin. Pregnant women should be sure to inform their health care provider of this condition, as some of the medications for warts may cause fetal abnormalities. Genital warts can also be treated with injections of interferon, either into muscle tissue or directly into the lesions.

Unfortunately, regardless of the treatment regime, genital warts have a high rate of recurrence. Several courses of treatment may be required. Sexual partners should be diagnosed and treated as well. Because of the connection between certain strains of HPV and cervical cancer, infected women should also have yearly pap smears.

Expected results

As with many warts, genital warts may spontaneously disappear over time. Although the warts are not cancerous by themselves, HPV infection in women appears to increase the risk of later cervical cancer. Recurrence is common with all methods of treatment.

Prevention

The only reliable method of prevention is sexual abstinence. The use of condoms is often recommended; however, condoms protect only a limited area and should not be relied upon for complete protection from genital warts. Circumcision may sometimes prevent recurrence of the visible warts.

Resources

BOOKS

Editors of Time-Life Books. *The Medical Advisor: The Complete Guide to Alternative and Conventional Treatments.* Alexandria, VA: Time-Life Books, 1996.

Rakel, Robert E., ed. *Conn's Current Therapy.* Philadelphia: W. B. Saunders, 1998.

Tierney, Lawrence M., M.D., et al., eds. *Current Medical Diagnosis and Treatment.* Stamford, CT: Appleton & Lange, 1998.

OTHER

"Genital warts." The Merck Manual Online. http://www.merck.com/pubs/mmanual/section13/chapter164/164l.htm.

Patience Paradox

Gentiana

Description

Gentiana is a plant extract made from gentians, which are a group of perennial plants belonging to the Gentianaceae family. There are about 180 species of gentians worldwide. They have a long history of use in healing both in Asian and **Western herbalism**. In the West, the common gentian used in healing is *Gentiana lutea*, or yellow gentian. In China, two different gentians are used in healing, *Gentiana macrophylla*, known in Chinese as *qin jiao*; and *Gentiana scabra*, known in Chinese as *long dan cao*.

G. lutea grows wild or cultivated in many places from Europe to India. It is also cultivated in North America. It grows to a height of about 4 ft (1.2 m), primarily in temperate alpine and subalpine meadows. The plant produces a spike of showy yellow-orange flowers. *G. macrophylla* grows in China and Siberia, and *G. scabra* grows in China and Japan.

There are some differences in height, leaf size, and flower among these three gentians, but the roots and rhizomes (underground stems) used to make gentiana are very similar. Gentians have a single long, strong taproot that can extend as far as 3 ft (1 m) into the earth. The top of the taproot can be as thick as a child's arm and is surrounded by a cluster of rhizomes. The root has an extremely bitter taste. Other names for gentiana include bitter root, bitterwort, and gall weed.

General use

Gentiana has been used for centuries. It gets its name from Gentius, King of Illyria (a part of Greece) from 180–167 B.C., who is said to have discovered the medicinal value of these plants. Gentian is one of the most intensely bitter herbs ever discovered. It is an ingredient in Angostura™ **bitters**. At one time it was used as a substitute for **hops** in making beer. Gentiana is also used in small amounts as a food flavoring, and is added to many anti-smoking products.

In Western herbalism, gentiana is used for digestive problems. It is an ingredient in aperitifs that are drunk a half-hour or so before eating to stimulate the appetite and digestion. Liqueurs made using fresh gentiana have been used for generations in Europe; in the eighteenth century gentian wine was served before eating as a stomachic, or aid to digestion.

In addition to stimulating digestion and appetite, gentiana is used to relieve **heartburn** and stomach ache, and to treat **vomiting**, **diarrhea**, abdominal fullness, and intestinal **gas**. Western herbalists also use gentiana for treating **fever**, **sore throat**, **jaundice**, and arthritis. It is used externally to treat **wounds**.

In **traditional Chinese medicine**, *G. macrophylla*, or *qin jiao*, is considered to have a neutral nature and a bitter, pungent taste. It is associated with the liver, stomach, and gallbladder. It is used as a tonic for the digestive system, and to treat arthritis; chronic low-grade fever; jaundice; **hepatitis**; and **constipation**. It is also an ingredient of several common formulas.

According to Chinese herbalists, another gentian, *Gentiana scabra*, or *long dan cao*, has a cold nature and a bitter taste. It is associated with the liver, stomach, gallbladder, and bladder. *Long dan cao* is used in formulas to treat pink eye (**conjunctivitis**); high blood pressure; acute urinary **infections**; testicular **pain**; leucorrhea (whitish vaginal discharge); vaginal pain; tantrums in children; fever; and balance problems.

A long history of folk use coupled with modern scientific investigation shows that gentiana works well as a stomach tonic and digestive stimulant. The German Federal Health Agency's Commission E, established in 1978 to independently review and evaluate scientific literature and case studies pertaining to herb and plant medications, has approved gentiana for use in Germany. It is considered safe and effective in treating such digestive complaints as loss of appetite, abdominal bloating, and gas.

In laboratory studies gentiana was found to contain a substance called amargogentin, which is possibly the bitterest compound ever found. It can be tasted at dilutions of 1:50,000. Its bitterness triggers the secretion of saliva, thus stimulating the production of gastric juice and bile and preparing the digestive system to process food. This reaction makes gentiana effective in treating almost all conditions related to sluggish digestion.

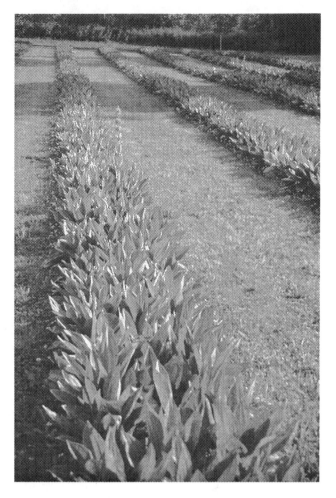

Gentian (**Gentiana lutea**). (Photo by Henriette Kress. Reproduced by permission.)

Other research shows that gentiana has selective antifungal, anti-inflammatory, and antispasmodic activity in laboratory experiments. There is much less scientific evidence to support such other traditional uses as treating pain and fever.

Preparations

Gentian roots are harvested in the autumn. They are used fresh in the production of liqueurs, but are dried for medicinal use. The better roots are dried quickly and remain whitish for several months before they darken. Roots that are dried too slowly will ferment.

Gentiana is available in many forms including an extract, dried powdered rhizome, tea, tincture, and decoction. The liquid remedies are very bitter, and sweetening is often added to make them more palatable. Gentian tea can be made by adding 1 tsp of powdered dried rhizome to every 3 cups (750 ml) of water. One tablespoon of this tea is taken about half an hour before eating. Smaller amounts of tincture and decoction can also be taken before eating.

In traditional Chinese medicine, gentiana is used in a formula (*long dan xie gan wan*) to treat chronic bladder infections, herpes, **blisters** in the mouth, and **dizziness**.

Precautions

German health authorities recommend that gentiana not be used by people who have stomach (gastric) or intestinal (duodenal) ulcers. In a few sensitive people, gentiana can cause stomach irritation and **headache**. Chinese herbalists recommend that gentiana not be used when there is frequent urination and chronic pain with weight loss.

Side effects

Overdoses of gentiana may cause **nausea** and vomiting.

Interactions

A long history of use in both East and West suggests that there are no interactions with either herbs or modern pharmaceuticals. Few studies, however, have been done to verify these observations.

Resources

BOOKS

Chevallier, Andrew. *Encyclopedia of Medicinal Plants*. New York: DK Publishers, Inc., 1996.

PDR for Herbal Medicines. Montvale, NJ: Medical Economics Company, 1999.

Peirce, Andrea. *The American Pharmaceutical Association Practical Guide to Natural Medicines*. New York: William Morrow and Company, 1999.

ORGANIZATIONS

American Association of Oriental Medicine (AAOM). 433 Front Street, Catasauqua, PA 18032. (610) 266-2433

OTHER

Plants for a Future: Gentiana. http://www.pfaf.org.

Tish Davidson

Gentiana lutea see **Gentiana**

Geriatric massage

Definition

Geriatric massage is a form of massage designed to meet the specific needs of the elderly population. It involves the use of hands to manipulate the soft tissues of the body to improve blood circulation, relieve **pain**, and increase range of motion. Active or passive movement of the joints may also be part of geriatric massage.

Old people often suffer from a variety of such age-related diseases as **Parkinson's disease**, arthritis, diabetes, or **heart disease**. As a result, they have poor blood circulation and limited physical activity. Many of them are also anxious, depressed, and lonely. Geriatric massage can help them maintain and improve their overall health, as well as regain certain physical functions that have been reduced or lost due to **aging**. In addition, it can relieve **anxiety** and **depression** and provide comfort to touch-deprived elderly patients.

Origins

Modern massage techniques were brought into the United States from Sweden in the 1850s by two brothers, Dr. Charles and Dr. George Taylor. Their massage technique was invented by a Swedish fencing instructor named Per Henrik Ling in the 1830s. When he was injured in the elbows, he reportedly cured himself using tapping movements around the affected area. He later developed the technique currently known as **Swedish massage**. This massage technique involves the application of long gliding strokes, friction, kneading and tapping movements on the soft tissues of the body. Passive or active joint movements are also used.

Benefits

Geriatric massage offers the following benefits:

• Increase in blood circulation, thus preventing such complications of diabetes as leg ulcers or gangrene.

• Improvement in lymphatic flow, which increases the excretion of toxic substances from the body.

- Alleviation of **headache** and pain.
- Speeding up of healing from injury and illness.
- Partial restoration of mobility lost due to Parkinson's disease or arthritis.
- Mental and physical relaxation.
- Improvement in length and quality of sleep.
- Relief of **stress**, anxiety, depression, and loneliness.
- Improvement of the patient's quality of life and self-esteem.

Description

Geriatric massage uses the same basic massage techniques as general massage. It is, however, tailored to the specific health conditions and needs of the elderly population. Geriatric massage has the following characteristics:

- Short sessions. A geriatric massage session usually lasts no longer than 30 minutes, as a longer session may be too much for an elderly person.
- Use of gentle hand motions. These motions are comfortable and soothing to the body. They are designed to improve blood circulation and heart function, prevent diabetic complications, relieve muscle tension, and relax the body and the mind.
- Passive movement and gentle stretching of shoulders, legs and feet to improve joint mobility and flexibility.
- Gentle massaging of the hands and feet (if the joints are not inflamed) to prevent stiffness and relieve pain.
- Occasional use of stronger movements such as friction and pressure strokes. These are sometimes used to massage such areas as the shoulders to improve flexibility.

Precautions

Geriatric massage should not be used as a replacement for **exercise** programs or medical treatment in nursing homes. In addition, it should not be given to elderly patients with the following conditions:

- broken bones or body areas that are inflamed, swollen or bruised
- open or unhealed bed sores
- varicose veins
- recent surgery
- severe acute pain
- certain heart conditions
- certain kinds of cancer
- a history of **blood clots** (The blood clots may become dislodged and travel to the lungs as a result of massage.)

- drug treatment with blood thinners (These medications increase the risk of bleeding under the skin.)

Side effects

Geriatric massage is very gentle and rarely causes adverse effects. More vigorous forms of massage, however, have been associated with bleeding in such vital organs as the liver or with the formation of blood clots.

Research & general acceptance

Geriatric massage is gaining acceptance in the medical community. It is being prescribed to elderly patients to improve blood circulation and relieve arthritic symptoms. It is sometimes prescribed for Parkinson's disease patients to help improve mobility. While most patients have to pay for this service, some insurance companies do reimburse prescribed massage treatment. As of 2000, however, Medicare and Medicaid do not pay for this treatment.

Training & certification

There are 58 school programs accredited by the Commission for **Massage Therapy** Accreditation/Approval in the United States. The schools provide a minimum of 500 hours of massage training. Certified therapists are graduates of these programs who have passed the national certification examination in therapeutic massage. They are also required to participate in continuing education programs to keep their skills current.

Resources

BOOKS

Beck, Mark F. *Milady's Theory and Practice of Therapeutic Massage*, 3rd ed. Albany, NY: Milady Publishing.

Maxwell-Hudson, Clare. *Massage: The Ultimate Illustrated Guide*. New York: DK Publishing, Inc., 1999.

ORGANIZATIONS

American Massage Therapy Association. 820 Davis St., Suite 100, Evanston, IL 60201. (847) 864-0123. Fax: (847) 864-1178. info@inet.amtamassage.org. http://wwww.amta-massage.org.

Day-Break Geriatric Massage Project. P.O. Box 1815, Sebastopol, CA 95473.

National Association of Nurse Massage Therapists. 1710 East Linden St., Tucson, AZ 85719.

National Certification Board of Therapeutic Massage and Bodywork. 8201 Greensboro Dr., Suite 300, McLean, VA 22102. (703) 610-9015 or (800) 296-0664.

Mai Tran

German chamomile *see* **Chamomile**

German measles *see* **Rubella**

Gerson therapy

Definition

Gerson therapy aims to treat the whole person, not just symptoms. It is a general cleansing therapy for the entire body. The therapy can achieve the following: **detoxification**, restoration of metabolic functions, enabling the digestion and elimination of **cancer** masses through the blood stream, and recovery of the organs, especially the liver.

Origins

Max Gerson was a pioneer in the world of alternative medicine. His therapy proved itself by providing a cure for just about every degenerative disease that plagues modern society, at a time when the first rumblings of disenchantment with so-called "modern medicine" were being heard. Among his initial successes was a 99% cure rate at a sanitarium for **tuberculosis**, unheard of with allopathic medicine. Beginning his work in the 1920s in Germany, he later immigrated to the United States, where in 1938 he was licensed to practice in New York. In 1946 he became the first physician to demonstrate recovered cancer patients before a U.S. Congressional Committee. Gerson had a 50% success rate even with terminal cancer patients that allopathic medicine had given up on. Albert Schweitzer referred to him as "a medical genius that walked among us."

Gerson first began to develop his therapy when he discovered that he could cure himself from terrible migraines by eating nothing but fresh fruit and vegetables.

Benefits

Gerson therapy has reported successes with the following: cancer, migraine, ulcers, **asthma**, **glaucoma**, edemas, **eczema**, diabetes, **schizophrenia**, **emphysema**, **epilepsy**, **allergies**, **psoriasis**, tuberculosis, arteriosclerosis, heart diseases, **rheumatoid arthritis**, kidney diseases, lupus erythematosus, **multiple sclerosis**, and high blood pressure; all of them common diseases and conditions. Gerson demonstrated that dramatic initial improvements can be expected within one week of starting his therapy, which involves taking nothing but absolutely fresh fruit and vegetable juices, coffee, **chamomile** and **castor oil** enemas, and additional nutrients according to the prescription of a practitioner who is conversant with the principles of the Gerson therapy.

Description

Gerson described how our food has been affected by the lowering of the quality of soil with the use of artificial fertilizers and pesticides. He went on to describe the growing of fruits and vegetables as the human being's "external metabolism." He lists numerous examples in his book of people from around the world who were living the same existence that they have lived for centuries, untouched by "civilization." These people, he noted, were living free of the diseases that modern societies considered commonplace.

It is essential that the juices for this therapy are organic; any traces of pesticides will prevent success with diseases such as cancer, for it is only when complete detoxification can be achieved that the body will be able to overcome such scourges.

The length of therapy will probably be between two weeks and two months, depending on the illness. But for cancer patients, it may be necessary to follow with an easier form of the diet in order to prevent a recurrence. The cost of therapy varies. If carried out at home under the supervision of a physician, the major expenses will be doctor's visits and organic fruit and vegetables. If clinic treatment is preferred, the Gerson Institute can help and advise.

Preparations

The central theory of the Gerson therapy is fresh juices, which should be drunk immediately after they are prepared. When they are left for longer than 20 minutes, the vital enzymes begin to oxidize, and after about 40 minutes, will no longer be suitable for the therapy. The following should also be observed:

• A press-type juicer should be used; centrifuges do not produce satisfactory juice for this treatment.

• Fresh veal liver should be juiced (under 4 lb) and the juice drunk raw (Gerson could find nothing better for replacing vital enzymes necessary for repairing the human organism).

- Cooking and enema water should be free of chemicals.
- Salt, tobacco, alcohol, and black tea are forbidden.
- No drugs should be taken except aspirin. Gerson's prescription for **pain** relief consisted of the following: coffee enemas (given every two hours if necessary), 5 g of aspirin, 100 mg of **vitamin C** and 50 mg of **niacin**, up to four times in the course of 24 hours. He noted that this also produced restful sleep in even the worst cases.
- Toothpaste or anything containing fluoride should be eliminated.
- Aerosol sprays, air fresheners, insecticides, paint fumes etc., should be avoided completely.
- Deodorants, hair dye, perms, cosmetics and aluminum cooking pans should be eliminated.
- Proteins fats and oils must be eliminated, along with all smoked, canned and processed foods.
- The diet should be strictly adhered to, along with all medication, and the prescribed enemas.
- Chemotherapy, radiation therapy etc., must be avoided as they damage the immune system and hinder healing.

Precautions

The Gerson therapy is a powerful tool for detoxification, and can produce healing crises. Most patients suffer from **nausea** and fevers when the initial flush of toxins is released into the bloodstream. Enemas are designed to help with this, and **peppermint** tea is also recommended. In the case of seriously ill patients, it is advisable to have an understanding practitioner on hand to help with this difficult process. Some of the methods used in Gerson therapy have produced bad outcomes. Coffee enemas have been known to cause deaths and patients undergoing Gerson therapy have been admitted to the hospital with bacterial **infections** most likely caused by ingesting raw calf's liver.

Side effects

Patients are warned that after detoxification by the Gerson therapy, the body becomes hypersensitive to drugs, particularly anesthetic. Dentists should be advised of this, and no drugs should be taken without the advice of a physician.

Research & general acceptance

In 1946 Gerson's therapy was out-voted in congress by four votes in favor of surgery, radiation, and chemicals. This situation remains today, despite increased popularity of alternative and complementary medicine. In 1990, two agencies reviewing patient records could find no evidence that the method was effective in treating cancer. However,

KEY TERMS

Healing crisis—When the body is supplied with nutrients it needs to heal itself, the first thing it does is to flush out toxins from the cells. When these toxins are circulating in the blood stream, they produce symptoms such as nausea, fevers, and extreme sensitivity.

Metabolic—Pertaining to chemical processes within the body that result in growth, production of energy and elimination of waste.

Toxification—When the body is unable to eliminate poisonous substances, they remain clogged in the system and eventually cause a breakdown of normal function.

Oxidize—When oxygen reacts with a substance, it causes a decomposition of its living elements.

many alternative practitioners have shown that detoxification can improve the effectiveness of healing techniques.

Training & certification

The Gerson Institute maintains a list of practitioners specializing in the Gerson method.

Resources

BOOKS

Gerson, Max. *A Cancer Therapy, Results of Fifty Cases.* Bonita, CA: Gerson Inst., 1958.

PERIODICALS

"Gerson Method." *Cancer* (July-August 1990): 252-255.

Hunter, Beatric Trum. "Improving the Quality of One's Life (Book Corners)." *Townsend Letter for Doctors and Patients* (July 2002): 131.

ORGANIZATIONS

The Gerson Institute. P.O. Box 430, Bonita, CA 92002. (619) 585-7600. Fax: (619) 585-7610. http://www.gerson.org.

Patricia Skinner
Teresa G. Odle

Ginger

Description

Ginger (*Zingiber officinale*) belongs to the Zingiberaceae plant family, which also includes **turmeric** and

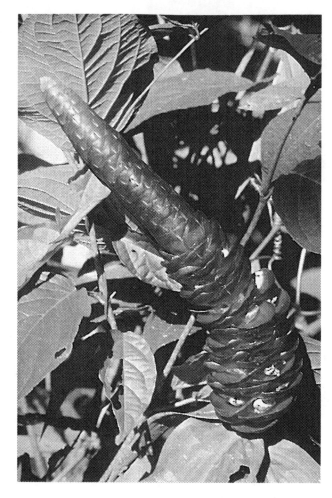

Ginger plant. *(JLM Visuals. Reproduced with permission.)*

cardamom. Ginger comes from the Sanskrit word "horn-root." It grows in Jamaica, India, Haiti, Hawaii, and Nigeria. This perennial plant grows 3–4 ft (0.9–1.2 m) tall. It has thin, sharp leaves 6–12 in (15–30 cm) long. The tangled, beige root is used medicinally, and can be 1–6 in (2.5–15 cm) in length. The root has a sharp, pungent taste and aroma.

Ginger contains several chemical components as outlined by Michael Murray, N.D. in *The Healing Power of Herbs*:

- starch (50%)

- protein (9%)

- lipids (including glycerides, phosphatidic acid, lecithins, and fatty acids; 6-8%)

- protease (2.26%)

- volatile oils (including gingerol, shogoal, zingiberene, and zingiberol; 1-3%)

- pungent principles

- vitamins A and B$_3$ (niacin)

The pungent principles (including the volatile oil gingerol) are the most medicinally potent because they inhibit prostaglandin and leukotriene formations (products in the body that influence blood flow and inflammation). They also give ginger its pungent aroma.

General use

Historically, ginger has been used to aid digestion. According to Michael Castleman in *The Healing Herbs*, ancient Greeks wrapped ginger inside their bread and ate it as an after-dinner digestive. This practice led to their invention of gingerbread. English society concocted ginger beer to soothe the stomach. In the 1800s, the Eclectics used ginger powder and tea for several digestive complaints, including **indigestion**, **gas**, **nausea**, and infant **diarrhea**.

Beginning in the 1980s, several studies have shown that ginger is useful in aiding digestion. A 1999 German study reported the results from 12 volunteers who took 100 mg twice daily of ginger extract when **fasting** and then with a meal. In both instances, ginger was linked to increased digestive movement through the stomach and duodenum.

A study in India published in 2000 reported the effects of ginger (in combination with other spices including cumin, **fenugreek**, and mustard) on pancreatic action in rats. During the eight-week study, the combination of spices in more than a single dose stimulated several **digestive enzymes** in the pancreas.

The Japanese use ginger as an antidote for fish poisoning, especially with sushi. Ginger is thought to fight harmful intestinal bacteria (like *E. coli*, *Staphylococcus*, and *Streptococcus*) without killing beneficial bacteria. Ginger aids *Lactobacillus* growth in the intestines while killing the *Schistosoma* and *Anisakis* parasites.

Because ginger is an antibacterial, it can work against ulcers caused by *Helicobacter pylori*. Ginger creates an anti-ulcer environment by multiplying the stomach's protective components. Ginger's anti-inflammatory abilities have also been shown to help reduce hip and **knee pain** in some **osteoarthritis** patients.

According to a 1998 report that reviewed the results from 10 clinical studies, ginger also helps to suppress the nausea and **vomiting** associated with **pregnancy**. However, a 2002 conference presentation cautions family physicians to reconsider recommending ginger to their pregnant patients because of the possibility for miscarriage.

Ginger lowers **cholesterol** levels by impairing cholesterol absorption, helping it convert to bile acids and then increasing bile elimination. In a 1998 study, rabbits were fed both cholesterol and 200 mg of ginger extract. The rabbits had a smaller amount of **atherosclerosis**. Ginger also enhances blood circulation and acts as a blood thinner.

Coughs can be relieved by drinking ginger tea made from dried or powdered ginger. It is ginger's pungent taste that releases secretions to help throat congestion.

Preliminary studies also show ginger may have potential cancer-fighting properties. No definitive results have been reported and research continues.

Preparations

Ginger is used in teas, ginger ale, ginger beer, capsules, broths, and as a spice when cooking Asian and Jamaican dishes. Ginger tea for coughs, nausea, digestion, and arthritis can be made by adding 2 tsp (10 ml) of freshly grated root or powdered root to 1 cup (250 ml) of boiling water and steeping for 10 minutes. A cup of the ginger tea, while still warm, should be sipped every 2-2.5 hours.

A compress for arthritic **pain** can be made by grating an unpeeled ginger root in a clockwise direction, then tying it in a moistened muslin cloth, dropping it in a pot of boiling water, and letting it simmer. When the broth is removed from the stove, a cotton cloth is dipped into the broth and the excess moisture squeezed into the pot. While lying flat on the back, the person places the cloth on the aching body part. The broth can also be added to the bath for soaking.

Ginger comes in 250–500 mg capsules of dried ginger root. One to 2 grams of dry powered ginger equals about 1/3 oz of fresh ginger (10 g). A cup of ginger tea contains 250 mg; an 8 oz glass of ginger ale contains 1,000 mg, and a spiced dish contains 500 mg. To prevent **motion sickness**, German health authorities recommend 2–4 g of powdered ginger daily. Another recommended dose is 250 mg four to six times a day.

To bring more blood circulation to arthritic joints, one to two capsules (250 mg each) per day are recommended initially. If results are good, the amount can be increased to six per day, taken between meals.

Ginger can be taken with onions and **garlic**. These agents work in harmony to stimulate the pancreas and decrease cholesterol.

As a blood thinner, two 250 mg capsules of ginger can be taken between meals up to three times a day.

Precautions

Despite studies showing ginger's aid for pregnancy nausea, the German Commission E has recommended

KEY TERMS

Atherosclerosis—Artery disorder where plaque forms on the arteries. The plaque is usually made up of cholesterol and lipids.

Duodenum—The beginning of the small intestine.

Eclectics—Nineteenth century herbal scientists in the United States who founded the Reformed Medical School. Their outlook was based on herbal medicines of Europe, Asia, and Indian.

Lactobacillus—The healthy bacteria found in the intestine.

Lipids—Groups of oily substances, such as fatty acids, stored in the body as energy reserves.

Perennial—A plant that lives for many years; comes back yearly without replanting.

Protease—The enzyme that digests proteins.

Protein—Complex groups of substances (including nitrogen, carbon, oxygen, iron, and hydrogen) that contain amino acids. Protein is vital to all animals because it makes up the hormones and enzymes controlling the body's actions.

Starch—Complex carbohydrates.

that pregnant women not use ginger. Some studies indicate that high amounts of ginger might cause miscarriages. Researchers cannot follow up their suspicions with human clinical trials because of the danger posed to unborn fetuses. Dosages over 6 g could cause gastric problems and possibly ulcers. Ginger may slow down blood clotting time. Before taking ginger, consumers should check dosages with a healthcare provider.

Consumers should not ingest the whole ginger plant; it has been found to damage the liver in animals. Ginger root is not recommended for people with **gallstones**.

Side effects

Ginger may cause **heartburn**.

Interactions

Ginger can interfere with the digestion of iron- and fat-soluble vitamins. Ginger also interacts with several medications. The herb can inhibit warfarin **sodium**, which is a blood thinner. Ginger can also interfere with absorption of tetracycline, digoxin, sulfa drugs, and phenothiazines. Consumers should check with their healthcare provider for drug or other interactions.

Resources

BOOKS

Castleman, Michael. *The Healing Herbs.* Emmaus, PA: Rodale Press, 1991.

Heinerman, John. *Heinerman's Encyclopedia of Healing, Herbs & Spices.* Upper Saddle River, NJ: Prentice Hall, 1996.

Landis, Robyn, with Karta Pukh Singh Khalsa. *Herbal Defense.* New York: Warner Books, Inc. 1997.

Murray, Michael, N.D. *The Healing Power of Herbs.* 2nd ed. Roseville, CA: Prima Publishing, 1995.

PERIODICALS

Jancin, Bruce. "Ginger for Nausea in Pregancy: Use Caution. (Good Efficacy, Lingering Safety Issues)." *Family Practice News* (January 15, 2002):16.

Tyler, Varro E., Ph.D., Sc.D. "Honest Herbalist: Spotlight on Ginger." *Prevention Magazine* (February 1998): 82-85.

Sharon Crawford
Teresa G. Odle

Gingivitis *see* **Gum disease**

Ginkgo biloba

Description

Ginkgo biloba, known as the maidenhair tree, is one of the oldest trees on Earth, once part of the flora of the Mesozoic period. The ginkgo tree is the only surviving species of the Ginkgoaceae family. This ancient deciduous tree may live for thousands of years. Ginkgo is indigenous to China, Japan, and Korea, but also thrived in North America and Europe prior to the Ice Age. This drastic climate change destroyed the wild ginkgo tree throughout much of the world. In China, ginkgo was cultivated in temple gardens as a sacred tree known as *bai gou*, thus assuring its survival there for more than 200 million years. Ginkgo fossils found from the Permian period are identical to the living tree, which is sometimes called a living fossil.

Ginkgo trees may grow to 122 ft (37.2 m) tall and measure 4 ft (1.2 m) in girth. The female trees have a somewhat pointed shape at the top, like a pyramid. The male trees are broader at the crown. The bark of the ornamental ginkgo tree is rough and fissured and may be ash to dark-brown in color. Distinctive, fan-shaped leaves with long stalks emerge from a sheath on the stem. Leaves are bright green in spring and summer, and turn to golden yellow in the fall. Ginkgo trees may take as long as 30 years to flower. Ginkgo is dioecious, with male and female flowers blooming on separate trees. Blossoms grow singly from the axils of the leaf. The female flowers appear at the end of a leafless branch. The yellow, plum-shaped fruits develop an unpleasant scent as they ripen. They contain an edible inner seed that is available in Asian country marketplaces. Ginkgo's longevity may be due, in part, to its remarkable resistance to disease, pollution, and insect damage. Ginkgo trees are part of the landscape plan in many urban areas throughout the world. Millions of ginkgo trees, grown for harvest of the medicinal leaves, are raised on plantations in the United States, France, South Korea, and Japan, and are exported to Europe for pharmaceutical processing.

General use

Ginkgo leaves, fresh or dry, and seeds, separated from the outer layer of the fruit, are used medicinally. Ginkgo has remarkable healing virtues that have been recorded as far back as 2800 B.C. in the oldest Chinese materia medica. Ginkgo seeds were traditionally served to guests along with alcohol drinks in Japan. An enzyme present in the ginkgo seed has been shown in clinical research to speed up alcohol metabolism in the body, underscoring the wisdom of this folk custom. The leaf extract has been used in Asia for thousands of years to treat **allergies**, **asthma**, and **bronchitis**. It is also valued in Chinese medicine as a heart tonic, helpful in the treatment of cardiac arrhythmia. Ginkgo was first introduced to Europe in 1730, and to North America in 1784 where it was planted as an exotic garden ornamental near Philadelphia. Ginkgo medicinal extracts are the primary prescription medicines used in France and Germany.

Ginkgo acts to increase blood flow throughout the body, particularly cerebral blood flow. It acts as a circulatory system tonic, stimulating greater tone in the venous system. The herb is a useful and proven remedy for numerous diseases caused by restricted blood flow. European physicians prescribe the extract for treatment of Raynaud's disease, a condition of impaired circulation to the fingers. It is also recommended to treat intermittent claudication, a circulatory condition that results in painful cramping of the calf muscles in the leg that impairs the ability to walk. German herbalists recommend ingesting the extract for treatment of leg ulcers, and large doses are used to treat **varicose veins**. Ginkgo is widely recommended in Europe for the treatment of **stroke**. The dried leaf extract may also act to prevent hemmorrhagic stroke by strengthening the blood capillaries throughout the body. In studies of patients with atherosclerotic clogging of the penile artery, long-term therapy with ginkgo extract has provided significant improvement in erectile function. Ginkgo extract also acts to eliminate damaging free radicals in the body, and has been shown to be effective in treatment of **premenstrual syndrome**, relieving tender or painful breasts.

Ginkgo extract is believed to benefit the elderly. This ancient herb is believed by some to enhance oxygen utilization and thus improve memory, concentration, and other mental faculties. In 2002, studies suggested that although gingko does have positive effects on **dementia**, its effects on age-related **memory loss** and **tinnitus** (ringing in the ears) are not scientifically proven. The herbal extract has also been shown to improve long-distance vision and may reverse damage to the retina of the eye. Studies have also demonstrated its value in the treatment of **depression** in elderly persons. The ginkgo extract may provide relief for persons with **headache**, sinusitis, and vertigo.

The active constituents in the ginkgo tree, known as ginkgolides, interfere with a blood protein known as the platelet activating factor, or PAF. Other phytochemicals in ginkgo include flavonoids, **bioflavonoids**, proanthocyanidins, trilactonic diterpenes (including the ginkgolides A, B, C, and M), and bilabolide, a trilactonic sesquiterpene. The therapeutic effects of this herb have not been attributed to a single chemical constituent; rather, the medicinal benefits are due to the synergy between the various chemical constituents. The standardized extract of ginkgo must be taken consistently to be effective. A period of at least 12 weeks of use may be required before the beneficial results are evident.

Preparations

Ginkgo's active principles are diluted in the leaves. The herb must be processed to extract the active phytochemicals before it is medicinally useful. It would take an estimated 50 fresh ginkgo leaves to yield one standard dose of the extract. Dry extracts of the leaf, standardized to a potency of 24% flavone glycosides and 6% terpenes, are commercially available. A standard dose is 40 mg, three times daily, though dosages as high as 240 mg daily are sometimes indicated.

Ginkgo extracts are widely used in Europe where they are sold in prescription form or over the counter as an approved drug. This is not the case in the United States, where ginkgo extract is sold as a food supplement in tablet and capsule form.

Precautions

Ginkgo is generally safe and non-toxic in therapeutic dosages. Exceeding a daily dose of 240 mg of the dried extract may result in restlessness, **diarrhea**, and mild gastrointestinal disorders. Those on anticoagulants should have their doctor adjust their dose or should avoid ginkgo

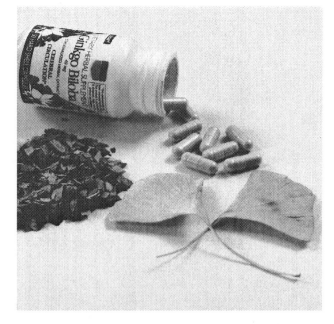

Various forms of ginko biloba. *(Photograph by Robert J. Huffman. Field Mark Publications. Reproduced by permission.)*

in order to avoid over-thinning their blood and hemorrhaging. Ginkgo should be avoided two days before and one to two weeks after surgery to avoid bleeding complications. Pregnant women should avoid ginkgo supplements because scientists have discovered a compound called colchicine in the placental blood of women who took ginkgo biloba. A 2002 report cautioned that the compound could cause problems for the growing fetus.

In 2002, a case of ginkgo seed poisoning was reported in a toddler in Japan, but she had ingested 50 or more pieces of roasted ginkgo seeds. She experienced severe **vomiting** and seizures.

Side effects

Severe allergic skin reactions, similar to those caused by poison ivy, have been reported after contact with the fruit pulp of ginkgo. Eating even a small amount of the fruit has caused severe gastrointestinal irritation in some persons. People with persistent headaches should stop taking ginkgo. Some patients on medications for nervous system disease should avoid ginkgo. It can interact with some other medicines, but clinical information is still emerging.

Interactions

The chemically active ginkgolides present in the extract, specifically the ginkgolide B component, act to reduce the clotting time of blood and may interact with antithrombotic medicines, including aspirin.

Resources

BOOKS

Duke, James A., Ph.D. *The Green Pharmacy.* Emmaus, PA: Rodale Press, 1997.

Elias, Jason, and Shelagh Ryan Masline. *The A to Z Guide to Healing Herbal Remedies.* New York: Lynn Sonberg Book Associates, 1996.

Murray, Michael T. *The Healing Power of Herbs.* 2nd ed. Roseville, CA: Prima Publications, Inc., 1995.

Ody, Penelope. *The Complete Medicinal Herbal.* New York: DK Publishing, Inc., 1993.

PDR for Herbal Medicines. Montvale, NJ: Medical Economics Company, 1998.

Prevention's 200 Herbal Remedies. Emmaus, PA: Rodale Press, Inc., 1997.

Tyler, Varro E., Ph.D. *Herbs Of Choice, The Therapeutic Use of Phytomedicinals.* Binghamton, NY: Haworth Press, Inc., 1994.

Tyler, Varro E., Ph.D. *The Honest Herbal.* Binghamton, NY: Haworth Press, Inc., 1993.

Weiss, Gaea and Shandor. *Growing & Using The Healing Herbs.* New York: Random House Value Pub., Inc., 1992.

PERIODICALS

Ernst, Edzard."The Risk-Benefit Profile of Commonly Used Herbal Therapies: Ginkgo, St. John's Wort, Ginseng, Echinacea, Saw Palmetto, and Kava." *Annals of Internal Medicine* (January 1, 2002):42.

Roan, Shari."Prenatal: Forget Ginkgo Biloba. (Small Packages)." *Fit Pregnancy* (February – March 2002):34.

Kajiyama, Yo, Kenichi Fujii, Hajime Takeuchi, Yutaka Manabe."Ginkgo Seed Poisoning." *Pediatrics* (February 2002):325.

Clare Hanrahan
Teresa G. Odle

Ginseng, American

Description

American ginseng, scientific name *Panax quinquefolius*, is a close relative of **Korean ginseng** (*Panax ginseng*), and belongs to the Araliaceae family, which is the same as **Siberian ginseng** (*Eleutherococcus senticosus*). It is a perennial herb, distinguished by its dark green leaves and clusters of red berries, that grows wild in eastern North America. The root of the plant is used medicinally, particularly in China, where **traditional Chinese medicine** places a high value on it.

Of the traditional ginsengs, American ginseng is probably the least used and researched variety. Americans have never been large consumers of American ginseng. In the past, American ginseng was an uncommon folk remedy used as a mild stimulant, tonic, and digestive aid. Most of this herb was exported to China, where most ginseng is consumed. American ginseng is considered a less potent member of the ginseng family, but it is a highly prized tonic and herbal remedy.

American ginseng was used medicinally by many Native American tribes as a health stimulant and sexual tonic and for various health problems including headaches, female **infertility**, digestive problems, **fever**, and **earache**. American ginseng was introduced by Native Americans to European settlers in North America in the early 1700s. A French Jesuit priest named Jartoux had traveled through China and was convinced of the medicinal powers of Korean ginseng. In 1714, he published a paper in Britain about Korean ginseng and its healing powers, and theorized that the plant may grow wild in the favorable climate of North America. Another Jesuit missionary in Canada, Joseph Lafitau (1681-1746), read the article and began searching the woods near his dwelling. Lafitau found American ginseng plants, which bear a close resemblance to their Asian cousins, and sent samples of them to China. A thriving trade of American ginseng began around 1718, it was sent to the Orient, gathered by Native Americans, French fur traders, and early frontiersmen including Daniel Boone.

American ginseng grows wild in the forests of the eastern United States and southeastern Canada. It grows in shady, moist and hilly regions, but the plant is becoming increasingly scarce due to over-harvesting and logging practices. In Kentucky, Tennessee, Virginia, and Illinois, American ginseng holds status as a threatened or an endangered species. Some botanists believe that pollution and a thinning ozone layer are contributing to its decline. Efforts at protecting wild American ginseng have not been successful, as the demand for it in the Far East makes it a lucrative crop for poachers. It sometimes sells for as much as $600-800 per pound.

The majority of American ginseng on the market is now cultivated, although it is a sensitive plant and difficult to farm. In the United States, Wisconsin grows 80% of the American ginseng crop. Canada grows more American ginseng than any country, and is second only to China in total ginseng production.

Scientific research

The majority of research performed on ginseng has been done on the Korean and Siberian varieties. Clinical and chemical research on American ginseng is yet to be done. One reason for this is the American medical establishment's skepticism of herbal remedies.

American ginseng is classified as an adaptogen, which is a substance that helps the body adapt to **stress**

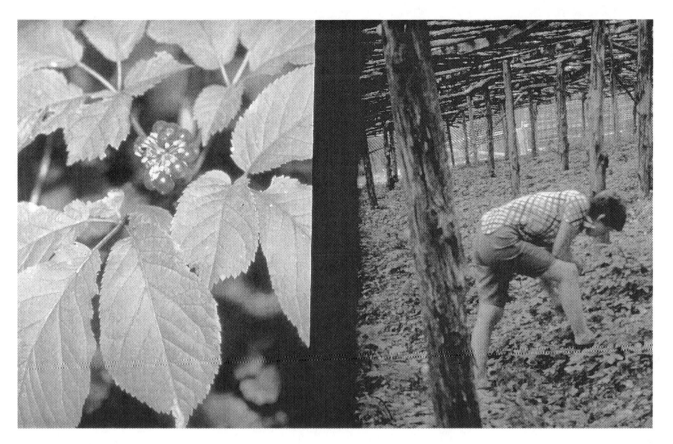

Cultivated American ginseng. *(JLM Visuals. Reproduced with permission.)*

and improves immune response. Adaptogens must also be non-toxic and cause no major physiological changes or side effects. American ginseng root has an array of complex chemicals, and scientists have determined that the active ingredients are saponin triterpenoid glycosides, or chemicals commonly called ginsenocides. American ginseng contains nearly 30 ginsenocides. However, American ginseng has been found to contain higher levels of ginsenocide Rb1, which has a sedative effect on the central nervous system, than other species of ginseng. Thus, scientific research has been consistent with Chinese herbalists' claims that American ginseng is less stimulating than Korean ginseng. The research implies that American ginseng can provide the strengthening and immune-enhancing effects of other ginseng without overstimulation to those people with high levels of stress and mental stimulation. American ginseng may be the best ginseng for Americans, whose fast-paced and energetic lifestyles may call for more calming and balancing herbs.

General use

American ginseng can be used by those people who seek the adaptogenic effects (toning, strengthening, and immune enhancing effects) of *Panax ginseng* without the highly stimulating aspects. Chinese herbalists consider American ginseng to be a cooling herb, so it can be used as a tonic and immune strengthener for people who are over-stressed or suffer from hot conditions like high blood pressure, excess nervous energy, or ulcers. American ginseng, according to Chinese herbalists, is more suitable and balancing for women and children than *Panax ginseng*, and is more applicable for the elderly who wish to avoid stimulants. American ginseng is also used in Chinese medicine for chronic fevers; to aid in the recovery of infectious diseases; for strengthening the lungs in cases of **tuberculosis, bronchitis** and **asthma**; and for the loss of the voice associated with respiratory disorders.

Preparations

American ginseng can be purchased as whole roots, powder, capsules, or a liquid tincture. For whole roots, wild ginseng is the highest quality and also the most expensive. Also available are organically grown cultivated roots, which are free from pesticides and chemicals. The easiest way to prepare ginseng roots is to make a tea from them. Ginseng roots are very hard and brittle. They should be sliced and simmered in water for 45 minutes or longer to extract the majority of ginsenocides. Experts recommend avoiding metal pots, which can reduce its antioxidant properties. Some herbalists recommend boiling **ginger** or **licorice** root with American ginseng to increase its effectiveness. For each serving of tea, two or more teaspoons of ginseng root are recommended.

Ginseng root can also be made into a tincture using alcohol, as ginsenocides are soluble and well-preserved in alcohol. Vodka or clear alcohol can be used, and the ginseng roots should be chopped finely or put in a blender with the alcohol. Enough alcohol should be used to completely saturate and cover the roots, and the solution should be kept in a sealed glass bottle for a month or longer. The solution should be shaken frequently to promote the extraction process. The liquid can be strained from the roots after distilling, and kept for up to three years. Half a teaspoon or more of the solution can be taken as a daily serving.

Ginseng powder is also available and can be made into tea or taken with water or juice. One half to one teaspoon is recommended per serving. Extracts of American ginseng are also available, in liquid or tablet form, some of which offer standardized quantities of ginsenocides. Packages of standardized products should be labeled with the appropriate dosage.

American ginseng is usually taken two to three times per day between meals. It should not be taken continuously for long periods of time, unless prescribed by a doctor.

Precautions

Pregnant women should use American ginseng only under a doctor's orders and avoid any products that contain *Panax ginseng.*

Consumers should assure that the American ginseng product they purchase is a reputable one. Because of the high price and demand of American ginseng, some questionable products are on the market. Generally, wild American ginseng is of higher quality than the cultivated plant, and the older and larger the root, the higher the quantity of ginsenocides present. In addition, consumers should be careful not to confuse American ginseng with *Panax ginseng,* which has been shown to produce more serious adverse side effects. A 2002 report stated that the effects of *Panax ginseng* seemed more likely when the herb was used in combination with other products than when it was used alone.

Side effects

In general, American ginseng is gentle and side effects are rare. Side effects may occur with American ginseng when taken in the wrong dosages, over too long a time, or by people whose constitutions, **allergies,** or

---

KEY TERMS

Adaptogen—Substance that helps the body adapt to any stress.

Ginseng intoxication—Possible side effects of taking *Panax ginseng* products.

Ginsenocides—Active chemicals found in American ginseng.

---

health conditions disagree with the herb. Also, products combining Korean ginseng with American ginseng may increase the chances for side effects.

Interactions

Due to the lack of research done on American ginseng, no known interactions are reported.

Resources

BOOKS

Duke, J.A. *Ginseng: A Concise Handbook.* Algonac, MI: Reference Publications, 1989.

Foster, S. and Y. Chongxi. *Herbal Emissaries.* Rochester, VT: Healing Arts Press, 1992.

Fulder, Stephan. *The Book of Ginseng and Other Chinese Herbs for Vitality.* Rochester, VT: Healing Arts Press, 1993.

Hobbs, Christopher. *Ginseng: The Energy Herb.* Loveland, CO: Botanica Press, 1996.

PERIODICALS

Walsh, Nancy. "Adverse Events Seen with Ginseng Combinations. (Post Menopausal Bleeding, Agracnulocytosis)." *OB GYN News* (March 1, 2002):24.

ORGANIZATIONS

American Botanical Council and Herb Research Foundation. *HerbalGram.* P.O. Box 144345, Austin, TX 78714-4345. (800) 373-7105. http://www.herbalgram.org.

New York Ginseng Association. P.O. Box 127, Roxbury, NY 12474. (607) 326-3005.

Douglas Dupler
Teresa G. Odle

Ginseng, Korean

Description

Korean ginseng is one of the most widely used and acclaimed herbs in the world. Its scientific name is

---

Panax ginseng, which is the species from which Chinese, Korean, red, and white ginseng are produced. Chinese and Korean ginseng are the same plant cultivated in different regions, and have slightly different properties according to Chinese medicine. White ginseng is simply the dried or powdered root of Korean ginseng, while red ginseng is the same root that is steamed and dried in heat or sunlight. Red ginseng is said to be slightly stronger and more stimulating in the body than white, according to Chinese herbalism.

Korean ginseng has had a long and illustrious history as an herb for health, and has been used for thousands of years throughout the Orient as a medicine and tonic. Early Chinese medicine texts written in the first century A.D. mention ginseng, and ginseng has long been classified by Chinese medicine as a "superior" herb. This means it is said to promote longevity and vitality. Legends around the world have touted ginseng as an aphrodisiac and sexual tonic. Researchers have found a slight connection between sex drive and consuming ginseng, although a direct link and the mechanism of action are still researched and disputed.

Korean ginseng grows on moist, shaded mountainsides in China, Korea, and Russia. It is a perennial herb that reaches heights of two or more feet, and is distinguished by its dark green leaves and red clusters of berries. The root of the plant is the part valued for its medicinal properties. The root is long and slender and sometimes resembles the shape of the human body. Asian legends claim that this "man-root" has magical powers for those lucky enough to afford or find it, and the roots bearing the closest resemblance to the human body are still the most valuable ones. The word *ren shen* in Chinese means roughly "the essence of the earth in the shape of a man."

Korean ginseng has historically been one of the most expensive of herbs, as it has been highly in demand in China and the Far East for centuries. Wars have been fought in Asia over lands where it grew wild. Wild Korean ginseng is now nearly extinct from many regions. Single roots of wild plants have recently been auctioned in China and New York City for sums approaching $50,000. Most of the world's supply of Korean ginseng is cultivated by farmers in Korea and China.

Because of the number of herbs sold under the name of ginseng, there can be some confusion for the consumer. Korean ginseng is a member of the *Araliaceae* family of plants, which also includes closely related **American ginseng** (*Panax quinquefolius*) and **Siberian ginseng** (*Eleutherococcus senticosus*). Both American and Siberian ginseng are considered by Chinese herbalists to be different herbs than Korean ginseng, and are said to have different effects and healing properties in the body. To add more confusion, there are eight herbs in Chinese medicine which are sometimes called ginseng, including black ginseng, purple ginseng, and prince's ginseng, some of which are not at all botanically related to *Panax ginseng*, so consumers should choose ginseng products with awareness.

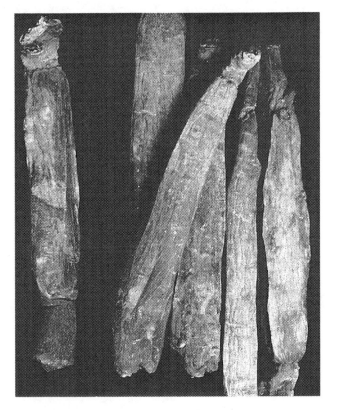

Dried Korean ginseng. *(Custom Medical Stock Photo. Reproduced by permission.)*

General use

The word *panax* is formed from Greek roots meaning "cure-all," and *Panax ginseng* has long been considered to be one of the great healing and strengthening herbs in natural medicine. Ginseng is classified as an *adaptogen*, which is a substance that helps the body adapt to **stress** and balance itself without causing major side effects. Korean ginseng is used as a tonic for improving overall health and stamina, and Chinese herbalists particularly recommend it for the ill, weak, or elderly. Korean ginseng has long been asserted to have longevity, anti-senility, and memory improvement effects in the aged population. As it helps the body to adapt to stress, athletes may use ginseng as herbal support during rigorous training. Korean ginseng generally increases physical and mental energy. It is a good tonic for the adrenal glands, and is used by those suffering from exhaustion, burnout, or debilitation from chronic illness.

Traditional Chinese medicine also prescribes Korean ginseng to treat diabetes, and research has shown that it enhances the release of insulin from the pancreas and lowers blood sugar levels. Korean ginseng has been demonstrated to lower blood **cholesterol** levels. It has also been shown to have antioxidant effects and to increase immune system activity, which makes it a good herbal support for those suffering from **cancer** and **AIDS** and other chronic conditions that impair the immune system. Further uses of Korean ginseng in Chinese medicine include treatment of **impotence**, **asthma**, and digestive weakness.

Research

Scientists have isolated what they believe are the primary active ingredients in ginseng, chemicals termed *saponin triterpenoid glycosides*, or commonly called *ginsenocides*. There are nearly 30 ginsenocides in Korean ginseng. Much research on Korean ginseng has been conducted in China, but controlled human experiments with it have not been easily accessible to the English-speaking world. Recent research in China was summarized by Dr. C. Lui in the February 1992 issue of the *Journal of Ethnopharmacology*, where he wrote that *Panax ginseng* was found to contain 28 ginsenocides that "act on the central nervous system, cardiovascular system and endocrine secretion, promote immune function, and have effects on anti-aging and relieving stress."

To summarize other research, Korean ginseng has been shown in studies to have significant effects for the following.

- Physical improvement and performance enhancement for athletes: A study performed over three years in Germany showed athletes given ginseng had favorable improvement in several categories over a control group who took a placebo. Another 1982 study showed that athletes given ginseng had improved oxygen intake and faster recovery time than those given placebos.
- Mental performance improvement and mood enhancement: In general, studies show that ginseng enhances mental performance, learning time, and memory. One study of sixteen volunteers showed improvement on a wide variety of mental tests, including mathematics. Another study showed that those performing intricate and mentally demanding tasks improved performance when given Korean ginseng. Finally, a study has shown improvement of mood in **depression** sufferers with the use of ginseng.
- Antifatigue and antistress actions: Patients with chronic **fatigue** who were given ginseng showed a statistically significant improvement in physical tests and in mental attention and concentration, when compared with those given placebos.

- Lowering blood sugar: Animal studies have shown that ginseng can facilitate the release of insulin from the pancreas and increase the number of insulin receptors in the body.
- Antioxidant properties: Scientific analysis of ginseng has shown that it has antioxidant effects, similar to the effects of vitamins A, C, and E. Thus, ginseng could be beneficial in combating the negative effects of pollution, radiation, and aging.
- Cholesterol reduction: Some studies have shown that Korean ginseng reduces total cholesterol and increases levels of good cholesterol in the body.
- Anticancer effects and immune system stimulation: Several tests have shown that Korean ginseng increases immune cell activity in the body, including the activity of T-cells and lymphocytes, which are instrumental in fighting cancer and other immune system disorders like AIDS. A Korean study indicates that taking ginseng may reduce the chances of getting cancer, as a survey of more than 1,800 patients in a hospital in Seoul showed that those who did not have cancer were more likely to have taken ginseng regularly than those patients who had contracted cancer.
- Physical and mental improvement in the elderly: One study showed significant improvement in an elderly test group in visual and auditory reaction time and cardiopulmonary function when given controlled amounts of Korean ginseng. Korean ginseng has also been shown to alleviate symptoms of menopause.
- Impotence: Studies of human sexual function and Korean ginseng have been generally inconclusive, despite the wide acclaim of ginseng as a sexual tonic. Tests with lab animals and ginseng have shown some interesting results, indicating that Korean ginseng promotes the growth of male reproductive organs, increases sperm and testoterone levels, and increases sexual activity in laboratory animals. In general, scientists believe the link between ginseng and sex drive is due to ginseng's effect of strengthening overall health and balancing the hormonal system.

Preparations

Korean ginseng can be purchased as whole roots, powder, liquid extracts, and tea. Roots should be sliced and boiled in water for up to 45 minutes to extract all the beneficial nutrients. One to five grams of dry root is the recommended amount for one serving of tea. Herbalists recommend that ginseng not be boiled in metal pots, to protect its antioxidant properties. Ginseng should be taken between meals for best assimilation.

Some high quality Korean ginseng extracts and products are standardized to contain a specified amount of ginsenosides. The recommended dosage for extracts containing four to eight percent of ginsenosides is 100 mg once or twice daily. The recommended dosage for non-standardized root powder or extracts is 1–2 g daily, taken in capsules or as a tea. It is recommended that ginseng be taken in cycles and not continuously; after each week of taking ginseng, a few days without ingesting the herb should be observed. Likewise, Korean ginseng should not be taken longer than two months at a time, after which one month's rest period should be allowed before resuming the cycle again. Chinese herbalists recommend that ginseng be taken primarily in the autumn and winter months.

Precautions

Consumers should be aware of the different kinds of ginseng, and which type is best suited for them. Red Korean ginseng is considered stronger and more stimulating than white, wild ginseng is stronger than cultivated, and Korean ginseng is generally believed to be slightly stronger than Chinese. Furthermore, American and Siberian ginseng have slightly different properties than Korean ginseng, and consumers should make an informed choice as to which herb is best suited for them. Chinese herbalists do not recommend Korean ginseng for those people who have "heat" disorders in their bodies, such as ulcers, high blood pressure, tension headaches, and symptoms associated with high stress levels. Korean ginseng is generally not recommended for those with symptoms of nervousness, mental imbalance, inflammation, or **fever**. Korean ginseng is not recommended for pregnant or lactating women, and women of childbearing age should use ginseng sparingly, as some studies imply that it can influence estrogen levels. Also, Chinese herbalists typically only prescribe ginseng to older people or the weak, as they believe that younger and stronger people do not benefit as much from it and ginseng is "wasted on the young."

Because of the number of and demand for ginseng products on the market, consumers should search for a reputable brand, preferably with a standardized percentage of active ingredients. To illustrate the mislabeling found with some ginseng products, *Consumer Reports* magazine analyzed 10 nationally-distributed ginseng products in 1995. They found that several of them lacked significant amounts of ginsenocides, despite claims on the packaging to the contrary. Ginseng fraud has led the American Botanical Council, publisher of *HerbalGram* magazine, to initiate the Ginseng Evaluation Program, a comprehensive study and standardization of ginseng products on the American market. This study and its labeling standards are still under development, and consumers should watch for it.

KEY TERMS

Adaptogen—Substance that improves the body's ability to adapt to stress.

Ginsenocide—Active substances found in ginseng.

Side effects

Korean ginseng acts as a slight stimulant in the body, and in some cases can cause overstimulation, irritability, nervousness, and **insomnia**, although strong side effects are generally rare. Taking too high a dosage of ginseng, or taking ginseng for too long without a break, can cause *ginseng intoxication*, for which symptoms might include headaches, insomnia, seeing spots, **dizziness**, shortage of breath and gastrointestinal discomfort. Long-term use may cause menstrual abnormalities and breast tenderness in some women.

Interactions

Those taking hormonal drugs should use ginseng with care. Ginseng should not be taken with **caffeine** or other stimulants as these may increase its stimulatory effects and cause uncomfortable side effects. In early 2002, researchers reported that adverse effects and drug interactions from ginseng were more likely to occur when it was used in combination with other products than when ginseng was used alone.

Resources

BOOKS

Duke, J.A. *Ginseng: A Concise Handbook.* Algonac, MI: Reference Publications, 1989.

Foster, S. and Chongxi, Y. *Herbal Emissaries.* Rochester, VT: Healing Arts Press, 1992.

Fulder, Stephan. *The Book of Ginseng and Other Chinese Herbs for Vitality.* Rochester, VT: Healing Arts Press, 1993.

Hobbs, Christopher. *Ginseng: The Energy Herb.* Loveland, CO: Botanica Press, 1996.

PERIODICALS

HerbalGram (a quarterly journal of the American Botanical Council and Herb Research Foundation). P.O. Box 144345, Austin, TX 78714-4345. (800) 373-7105.

Walsh, Nancy. "Adverse Events Seen with Ginseng Combinations (Effects Reversible and Mild)." *Internal Medicine News* (January 15, 2002):17.

Douglas Dupler
Teresa G. Odle

Ginseng, Siberian

Description

Siberian ginseng, *Eleutherococcus senticosus*, is also known as eleuthero ginseng or eleuthero. It is in the same botanical family as **Korean ginseng** (*Panax ginseng*) and **American ginseng** (*Panax quinquefolius*). Siberian ginseng is one of the most widely used herbs in the world.

Siberian ginseng is a thin, thorny shrub that grows up to 15 ft (4.6 m) high. It is native to forests in southeastern Russia, northern China, Japan, and Korea. The root of the plant is used medicinally.

The family of ginseng plants has historically been used for medicinal purposes. Korean ginseng, also called Asian, red, or white ginseng, has been used in China for thousands of years. In China, it is a celebrated herb known to promote strength, energy, and longevity. American ginseng was discovered in North America in the early 1700s, and has since been used as a medicine and tonic. Siberian ginseng has been used in Chinese medicine for more than 2,000 years, to increase energy and vitality and to treat respiratory and other **infections**, although Chinese herbalists use Korean and American ginseng much more frequently. Siberian ginseng was used in Eastern Europe as a folk remedy for hundreds of years, but it was not until the 1940s that it became a popular herb in Russia and Europe.

The Russian physician I. I. Brekhman is credited with making Siberian ginseng popular. Brekhman had studied Korean ginseng in the 1940s and documented some of its effects on the body. He determined that ginseng was an *adaptogen*. To be classified as an adaptogen, an agent must be shown to help the body adapt to **stress**, improve balance and overall immune function, be nontoxic and cause minimal side effects. Brekhman searched his native Russian forests for an alternative to expensive Korean ginseng, and concentrated on Siberian ginseng. Brekhman discovered that Siberian ginseng was also an adaptogen, offering some of the same benefits of Korean ginseng, although containing a different chemical composition.

During the next 30 years in the Soviet Union, Siberian ginseng became the focus of many studies. It was found to increase endurance and performance of athletes, and many famous Soviet Olympic champions included Siberian ginseng as part of their training programs. Siberian ginseng was so touted that Soviet astronauts carried it into space with them, as opposed to the amphetamines carried by American astronauts. Soviet scientists found that Siberian ginseng strengthened the immune system, and gave Siberian ginseng to highly stressed workers as herbal support. After the Chernobyl nuclear accident, Siberian ginseng was given to people who had been exposed to radiation.

Research

Siberian ginseng's active ingredients are a complex group of chemicals called *eleutherosides*. Eleutherosides are different than the ginsenocides found in the *Panax* varieties of ginseng, which is consistent with Chinese herbalists' claims that Siberian ginseng acts differently in the body than Korean or American ginseng. There has been some debate among herbalists whether Siberian ginseng should be considered a true ginseng at all, due to this difference in active ingredients.

Much of the research done on Siberian ginseng was performed by Soviet scientists in the former Soviet Union. Many of the study results are still unavailable in English. Those that have been translated and more recent studies have corroborated the benefits of Siberian ginseng.

- Siberian ginseng has been documented in many studies to improve physical endurance, oxygen uptake, recovery, and overall performance in athletes, ranging from runners to weightlifters. A 1986 study in Japan showed that eleuthero ginseng improves oxygen uptake in exercising muscle.

- Siberian ginseng normalized blood pressure in patients with high and low blood pressure. Siberian ginseng has been shown to reduce stress symptoms in general. A 1996 study in Japan concluded that Siberian ginseng can protect against gastric ulcers.

- Animal studies showed Siberian ginseng helped fight against toxic chemicals and exposure to harmful levels of radiation. A 1992 Russian study showed that Siberian ginseng reduced the occurrence of tumors in rats when exposed to radiation. Another Russian study showed that women undergoing radiation for **breast cancer** had a significant reduction of side effects when given Siberian ginseng.

- A 1987 German study, using human subjects in a double-blind test, demonstrated that eleuthero ginseng boosts immune system response and enhances the body's overall resistance to infection. Other studies have shown that Siberian ginseng increases activity of lymphocytes and killer cells in the immune system.

General use

Siberian ginseng can be used as an overall strengthener for the body and immune system. It is an effective herbal support for stress, **fatigue**, and exhaustion; for athletes in training; for prevention of colds and flus; for those undergoing chemotherapy or radiation treatment; and for people suffering from chronic diseases such as chronic fatigue, **fibromyalgia**, or **AIDS**. Siberian ginseng is also used to aid recovery from nervous conditions like **depression**, **anxiety**, or nervous breakdown.

A group of Armenian researchers reported in 2003 that a compound containing Siberian ginseng is safe and effective in treating familial Mediterranean **fever**, an inherited disorder characterized by recurrent attacks of fever and severe abdominal **pain**.

Preparations

Siberian ginseng is available as a fresh root or dried root powder, tea, liquid extract, or capsule/tablet form. The recommended dosage for root powder is 1–2 g daily, taken in capsules or mixed with water or juice. Dosages should be divided and taken two or three times per day, between meals. The dosage for the liquid extract is 1–2 ml twice daily. Recently, Siberian ginseng products have been made available that contain standardized percentages of eleutherosides. Siberian ginseng can be taken continuously, but it is generally recommended that for every three months of ginseng use, two- to four-week rest periods should be observed. Siberian ginseng is sometimes combined with other adaptogens, like Korean or American ginseng, **astragalus**, or **schisandra**, to increase its effectiveness.

Precautions

Pregnant women and children should use Siberian ginseng with caution, consulting a practitioner prior to use. Those taking hormonal drugs should use ginseng with care. Furthermore, consumers should be aware of the different medicinal properties of Korean, American, and Siberian ginseng, in order to choose the herb best suited for their constitution and health conditions.

Consumers should choose only high-quality ginseng products made by reputable manufacturers. In a 1995 *Consumer Reports* magazine analysis of 10 nationally distributed ginseng products, several brands were lacking in active ingredients. Ginseng product fraud has led the American Botanical Council, publisher of *Herbal-Gram* magazine, to initiate the Ginseng Evaluation Program. Started in 1993, this program provides a comprehensive study of ginseng products and has enacted measures to reduce mislabeling and increase consumer confidence in ginseng products. In 1999, however, the Center for Food Safety and Applied Nutrition of the Food and Drug Administration (FDA) reported several instances of Siberian ginseng products that contained pieces of the roots and leaves of a hazardous plant, *Periploca sepium*.

Side effects

In general, side effects with Siberian ginseng are rare and more mild than those that occur with American and Korean ginseng. Mild **diarrhea** has been reported with its use, and **insomnia** may occur if it is taken too close to bedtime.

Siberian ginseng appears to be less likely than most herbs to interact with other medications. Researchers in South Carolina reported in 2003 that Siberian ginseng did not affect the body's metabolism of such drugs as dextromethorphan and benzodiazepine tranquilizers when the ginseng was taken in recommended dosages.

Resources

BOOKS

Duke, J.A. *Ginseng: A Concise Handbook*. Algonac, MI: Reference Publications, 1989.

Foster, S., and Y. Chongxi. *Herbal Emissaries*. Rochester, VT: Healing Arts Press, 1992.

Fulder, Stephan. *The Book of Ginseng and Other Chinese Herbs for Vitality*. Rochester, VT: Healing Arts Press, 1993.

Hobbs, Christopher. *Ginseng: The Energy Herb*. Loveland, CO: Botanica Press, 1996.

Pelletier, Kenneth R., MD. *The Best Alternative Medicine*, Part I: Western Herbalism. New York: Simon & Schuster, 2002.

PERIODICALS

Amaryan, G., V. Astvatsatryan, E. Gabrielyan, et al. "Double-Blind, Placebo-Controlled, Randomized, Pilot Clinical Trial of ImmunoGuard—A Standardized Fixed Combination of *Andrographis paniculata Nees*, with *Eleuterococcus senticosus Maxim*, *Schizandra chinensis Bail.* and *Glycyrrhiza glabra L.* Extracts in Patients with Familial Mediterranean Fever." *Phytomedicine* 10 (May 2003): 271–285.

Donovan, J. L., C. L. DeVane, K. D. Chavin, et al. "Siberian Ginseng (*Eleuteroccus senticosus*) Effects on CYP2D6 and CYP3A4 Activity in Normal Volunteers." *Drug Metabolism and Disposition* 31 (May 2003): 519–522.

ORGANIZATIONS

American Botanical Council. P.O. Box 144345, Austin, TX 78714-4345. (800) 373-7105. <http://www.herbalgram.org.>

National Center for Complementary and Alternative Medicine (NCCAM) Clearinghouse. P.O. Box 7923, Gaithersburg, MD 20898-7923. (888) 644-6226. <http://nccam.nih.gov>.

New York Ginseng Association. P.O. Box 127, Roxbury, NY 12474. (607) 326-3005.

U. S. Food and Drug Administration (FDA). 5600 Fishers Lane, Rockville, MD 20857. (888) 463-6332. <http://www.fda.gov>.

OTHER

HerbalGram (a quarterly journal of the American Botanical Council and Herb Research Foundation). P.O. Box 144345, Austin, TX 78714-4345. (800) 373-7105.

Douglas Dupler
Teresa G. Odle
Rebecca J. Frey, PhD

Glaucoma

Definition

Glaucoma is a slowly progressive eye condition that causes damage to the optic nerve. It is the leading cause of blindness among African-Americans and older adults in the United States. Because there are usually no symptoms early on in the disease, about half of the people with glaucoma do not even know they have it.

Description

Over two million people in the United States have glaucoma, and 80,000 of those are legally blind as a result of the disease. Glaucoma can strike any age group, even newborn infants. Susceptibility to the disease increases with age. African-Americans are at a three times higher risk of glaucoma than the rest of the population.

There are at least 20 different types of glaucoma. These can be divided into four main types:

- Open-angle glaucoma. Accounts for over 60–70% of all cases. It is usually chronic and often bilateral.

- Closed-angle glaucoma. Usually an acute condition, as opposed to open-angle glaucoma that is chronic.

- Congenital glaucoma occurs in infants, usually under the age of one.

- Secondary glaucoma may be associated with eye diseases, other diseases, and certain types of medications.

Causes & symptoms

Glaucoma is the result of disruptions of normal processes to maintain pressure within the eye tissue. The iris, cornea, and lens of the eye are bathed in a nutritive liquid called the aqueous humor, which is made by cells within the eye. Excess fluid is continually removed by a spongy meshwork of drainage canals. Glaucoma occurs if there is a build up of the aqueous humor due to poor drainage or overproduction. As the fluid builds up there is increased pressure on the retina at the back of the eye. This increases the pressure, reducing the blood supply to the nerves of the retina, causing the nerves to die. This may distort and destroy the optic nerve. As nerve cells are destroyed, blind spots develop, and there is a progressive loss of vision. A change in the production and strength of collagen may also contribute to the onset of the disease. Collagen is a protein that helps maintain the structure and function of eye tissue. **Stress** and **allergies** may aggravate glaucoma symptoms.

It is probable that most cases of glaucoma are partially due to a genetic predisposition. At least 10 defective genes have been identified that may cause glaucoma. Although there are still many unknown factors that trigger the disease, a number of processes have been implicated. They include age-related changes, congenital abnormalities, injuries to the eye tissue, and problems related to other eye diseases. Vision loss in all forms of glaucoma is caused by damage to the optic nerve, the retina, and the collagen protein that makes up eye tissue. Use of certain medications, including antihypertensives, antihistamines, anticholinergics, and antidepressants may also contribute to the development of glaucoma. Corticosteroid eye drops, which are often used for other eye disorders, may destroy the integrity of eye tissue. Other types of eye drops may cause the pupils to dilate, increasing intraocular eye pressure (IOP), which may also lead to glaucoma in those who have a tendency to the disease.

Chronic open-angle glaucoma at first develops without noticeable symptoms. The pressure buildup is gradual and it does not bring on discomfort. Moreover, the vision loss is too gradual to be noticed at first, and the brain will compensate for blind spots. Over an extended period of time, the elevated pressure pushes against and damages the optic nerve and the retina. If glaucoma is left untreated, vision loss becomes evident and the condition becomes painful.

Acute closed-angle glaucoma is obvious from the beginning. The symptoms are blurred vision, severe eye **pain**, sensitivity to light, **nausea** and **vomiting**, dilated pupils, reddened eyes, and halos visualized around lights. The corneas may become hazy-looking. Acute closed-angle glaucoma is an emergency situation. It needs to be treated immediately. Congenital glaucoma is evident at birth. Symptoms are bulging eyes, cloudy corneas, enlarged corneas, excessive teariness, and sensitivity to light.

Risk factors that increase the probability of developing glaucoma include:

- ocular **hypertension**, a slightly increased IOP
- age over 40
- diabetic
- high blood pressure
- migraine headaches
- nearsightedness, farsightedness, and other visual disturbances
- a family history of glaucoma
- being of African-American ethnicity

Diagnosis

Sometimes glaucoma can be diagnosed with a routine eye exam by an opthamologist, who can make a definitive diagnosis of glaucoma. IOP, defects in the field of vision, and the appearance of the optic nerve, are all considered in the diagnosis of glaucoma. Visual field tests can detect blind spots in a patient's field of vision before the patient is aware of them. An instrument, known as a tonometer, is used to measure eye pressure. Since IOP can vary throughout the day, a person may have to return for several visits to measure eye pressure at different times of the day. An ophthalmoscope is used to examine the inner aspects and the back of the eyes, including the optic nerve, for changes and damage. A slit lamp may be used to allow the doctor further examination of the eye. Another test, gonioscopy, can distinguish between narrow-angle and open-angle glaucoma. A gonioscope allows visualization of the angle between the iris and the cornea.

Treatment

Vitamin C, taken in dosages up to bowel tolerance, is reported to reduce pressure within the eye and restore collagen balance. A vitamin C supplement with **bioflavonoids**, especially rutin and **lutein**, are particularly recommended. There is evidence that **marijuana** (*Cannabis sativa*) lowers IOP, as well. Although it is a controlled substance, marijuana can often be prescribed by a professional licensed to treat glaucoma. **Bilberry** (*Vaccinium* sp.) helps maintain collagen balance and prevents the breakdown of vitamin C. Many people with glaucoma have been shown to have deficiencies of **chromium** and **zinc**. Supplementation with these two minerals may, therefore, deter the onset or progression of the disease. Alpha lipoic acid and other **antioxidants** may improve visual functioning.

A naturopathic approach called contrast **hydrotherapy** can be used to stimulate circulation in the eyes.

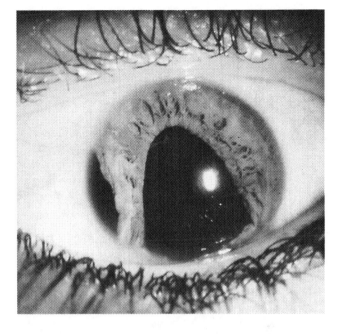

A close-up view of an inflamed eye in acute glaucoma, with an irregularly enlarged pupil. *(Custom Medical Stock Photo. Reproduced by permission.)*

Compresses can be applied over the eyes, alternating three minutes with hot water and one minute with cold water, always ending with the cold. **Biofeedback** can be used to reduce the pressure in the eyes by increasing **relaxation**. **Meditation**, stress reduction, **t'ai chi**, **yoga**, **exercise**, and **acupuncture** also may lower IOP. Remedies used to lower IOP must be taken continually to avoid optic nerve damage. In addition to other treatments, a glaucoma patient should always remain under the care of an ophthalmologist or optometrist who is licensed to treat glaucoma, so that IOP and optic nerve damage can be monitored.

Allopathic treatment

The objective of glaucoma treatment is usually to decrease IOP. When glaucoma is diagnosed, drugs, typically given as eye drops, are usually tried before surgery. Several classes of medications are effective at lowering IOP and thus, at preventing optic nerve damage in chronic and neonatal glaucoma. These inlcude beta-blockers, such as Timoptic, and carbonic anhydrase inhibitors, such as acetazolamide. Alpha-2 agonists, such as Alphagan, inhibit the production of aqueous humor. Miotics, such as pilocarpine, and prostaglandin analogues, like Xalatan, increase the drainage of aqueous humor. Different medications lower IOP different amounts, and a combination of medications may be necessary. Attacks of acute closed-angle glaucoma are medical emergencies. In such cases, IOP is rapidly lowered by use of acetazolamide, hyperosmotic agents, a topical beta-blocker, and pilocarpine. All of these drugs have side effects, some of which are rare, but serious and potentially life threatening. Patients taking them should be monitored closely, especially for cardiovascular, pulmonary, and behavioral symptoms. IOP should also be monitored and measured three to four times per year.

Laser peripheral iridiotomy or other microsurgery is used to open the drainage canals or to make an opening in the iris to increase the outflow of aqueous humor. These surgeries are usually successful, but effects often last less than a year. Nevertheless, they are an effective treatment for patients whose IOP is not sufficiently lowered by drugs or for those who cannot tolerate the drugs. Surgery is usually used in cases of congenital glaucoma, since the medications are often too harsh for children. Youngsters often respond to surgery better than adults, and have an excellent chance for preserving lifelong good vision.

Expected results

If glaucoma is left untreated, optic nerve damage will result in a progressive loss of vision. Once blindness develops due to glaucoma, it cannot be reversed. With early treatment and monitoring, however, serious vision loss can usually be prevented.

Prevention

While glaucoma is not preventable, early detection and treatment can help to prevent serious damage to vision. Those with risk factors should have regular eye exams and avoid medicines that tend to be implicated in the development of glaucoma, including some over-the-counter cold and allergy medications. All medications should be checked for their ingredients. Alternatives for drugs that aggravate glaucoma should be discussed with a healthcare provider.

Resources

BOOKS

The Editors of Time-Life Books. *The Medical Advisor: The Complete Guide to Alternative and Conventional Treatments*. Alexandria, VA: Time-Life, Inc., 1996.

Epstein, David L., R. Rand Allingham, and Joel S. Schuman. *Chandler and Grant's Glaucoma*. 4th ed. Baltimore: Williams & Wilkins, 1997.

Marks, Edith and Rita Montauredes. *Coping with Glaucoma*. New York: Avery, 1997.

ORGANIZATIONS

American Academy of Ophthalmology. P.O. Box 7424, San Francisco, CA 94120-7424. <http://www.eyenet.org/aao_index.html.>

KEY TERMS

Alpha-2 agonist—A class of drugs that bind to and stimulate alpha-2 adrenergic receptors, causing responses similar to those of adrenaline and noradrenaline, by inhibiting aqueous humor production.

Beta-blocker—A class of drugs that bind beta-adrenergic receptors and thereby decrease the ability of the body's own natural epinephrine to bind to those receptors, leading to the reduction of aqueous humor secretion.

Cornea—The clear, bowl-shaped structure at the front of the eye located in front of the colored part of the eye. The cornea lets light into the eye and partially focuses it.

Gonioscope—An instrument that consists of a magnifier and a lens equipped with mirrors and sits on the patient's cornea.

Miotic—A drug that causes pupils to contract.

Ophthalmoscope—An instrument, with special lighting, designed to view structures in the eye.

Optic nerve—The nerve that carries visual messages from the retina to the brain.

Retina—The light-sensitive layer of the eye.

OTHER

drkoop.com. http://www.drkoop.com/conditions/ency/article/001620.htm.

Patience Paradox

Glucosamine

Description

Glucosamine is an amino sugar that occurs naturally in the body. This one-molecule substance consists of glucose and a hydrogen and nitrogen amine. Amino sugars are different from other body sugars, as they form part of carbohydrates. Their function is also different as they are not a source of energy, but rather are included in body tissue structure. Therefore, glucosamine plays a role in forming and maintaining the body's tissues— for example, constructing nails, skin, eyes, bones, ligaments, tendons, heart valves, discharging mucus from the respiratory system, digestive system, and urinary tract. Glucosamine helps blend **sulfur** into the cartilage. When people grow older, their bodies may lose the capacity to make enough glucosamine, so the cartilage in such weight-bearing joints as the hips, knees, and hands is destroyed. The remaining cartilage then hardens and forms **bone spurs**, causing **pain**, deformed joints, and limited joint movement.

Glucosamine is not readily available from any primary food source. Commercial preparations of glucosamine are derived from chitin, which is a substance found in the outer covering of such shellfish as lobster, crab, and shrimp, as well as in such animal connective tissues as the marrow of chicken bones. Commercially prepared glucosamine comes in three formats: glucosamine sulfate, glucosamine hydrochloride, and N-acetyl-glucosamine (NAG).

General use

Glucosamine works to stimulate joint function and repair. It is most effective in treating **osteoarthritis** (OA), the most prevalent type of arthritis. A number of studies over the last 20 years have shown that glucosamine is helpful in relieving arthritis symptoms. For example, a 1982 clinical study compared usage of the NSAID ibuprofen with glucosamine sulfate, for osteoarthritis of the knee. During the first two weeks, ibuprofen decreased pain faster, but by the fourth week the glucosamine group was well ahead in pain relief. The overall results showed 44% of the glucosamine group had pain relief compared to 15% for ibuprofen. A British study published in 2002 reported similar findings regarding the effectiveness of glucosamine in relieving pain associated with arthritis. A team of Japanese researchers has suggested that glucosamine relieves the pain of arthritis by suppressing the functions of neutrophils, which are white blood cells that contribute to the joint inflammation found in arthritis. Other researchers think that the sulfur content of glucosamine contributes to its healing properties.

Several studies have concluded that over-the-counter preparations of glucosamine sulfate are safe for long-term treatment of osteoarthritis. These are readily available in the dietary supplement sections of most pharmacies. Glucosamine preparations are sometimes classified as nutraceuticals, a term used to refer to foods or food ingredients that are thought to provide medical or health benefits.

Harvard Medical School recently conducted a somewhat unorthodox study in which patients scheduled for hip surgery were given ground chicken bone supplements. After two weeks of taking these supplements, their pain was reduced considerably.

Glucosamine supplements can also aid in treating sports injuries, **bursitis**, food and respiratory **allergies**, **asthma**, **osteoporosis**, **tendinitis**, **vaginitis**, some skin problems, and candidiasis.

As of 2002, however, updated guidelines issued by the American College of Rheumatology for the treatment of osteoarthritis continued to list glucosamine along with **acupuncture** and electromagnetic therapy as treatments that are still under investigation for treating OA.

Preparations

Although commercially prepared glucosamine comes in three formats: glucosamine sulfate, glucosamine hydrochloride, and N-acetyl-glucosamine (NAG), not all three work the same. There are also differing opinions on which is better.

One claim states that glucosamine hydrochloride works 50% better than glucosamine sulfate because hydrocholoride is the main stomach acid helping the digestive system to put more active ingredients into the body. Another prefers glucosamine sulfate because of its high absorption rate of 98% documented in human studies and its sulfur content. Studies as far back as the 1930s show that people with arthritis usually have low levels of sulfur.

N-acetyl-glucosamine (NAG) can be beneficial to individuals with **Crohn's disease** or ulcerative colitis. Individuals with these diseases cannot change glucosamine to NAG as fast as those without the diseases. In one study, cells from patients' intestines were soaked in a solution with a 10:1 ratio of radioactive NAG to glucosamine. These cells consolidated more NAG than did the cells from the intestines of patients without Crohn's disease or ulcerative colitis.

Glucosamine is also sold mixed in formulas with **devil's claw**, pregnenolone, **methylsulfonylmethane** (**MSM**), and **chondroitin** sulfate. Chondroitin sulfate is one of the main glycosaminoglycans (GAGs) that is contained in shark cartilage and sea cucumber. Although studies show that chondroitin sulfate has benefits, it is hard to absorb because it contains large molecules.

Further confusion can arise because glucosamine is classified and sold as a dietary supplement, meaning it has not gone through the FDA approval process. As with any dietary supplement, patients with arthritis who are considering glucosamine formulations should consult their healthcare practitioner.

The standard dosage is 500 mg three times daily. Obese people may need to take higher dosages based on their weight.

Precautions

Persons on potassium-reduced **diets**, with **heart disease**, renal diseases, or high blood pressure related to salt intake should avoid either the regular or salt-free glucosamine supplements.

Diabetics should be aware that glucosamine contains the sugar glucose, and can raise blood sugar and insulin levels. A 2000 study of 15 nondiabetic patients at the Los Angeles College of Chiropractic and MetaResponse Science showed that those who took 1,500 mg of glucosamine a day for 12 weeks had raised insulin levels. The conclusion was that the insulin rise would probably be more in diabetics. However, researchers cautioned diabetics there is no need to discard their glucosamine supplements as more controlled studies are required.

Despite the concern regarding the use of glucosamine sulfate in persons with allergies to the sulfa drugs or the sulfite additives in food, sulfur itself is a necessary mineral and human blood contains large amounts of sulfur's sulfate form. Studies show that glucosamine sulfate is safe for long term use to treat osteoarthritis, with the exception of medical conditions listed above and below.

Side effects

High dosages of glucosamine may cause gastric problems, **nausea**, **diarrhea**, **indigestion**, and **heartburn**. Glucosamine should be taken with meals to help avoid these problems

Interactions

Glucosamine should not be taken with heart medications or insulin. Those taking diuretics may require higher amounts of glucosamine on a daily basis.

Resources

BOOKS

Ali, Elvis, et al. *The All-In-One Guide to Natural Remedies and Supplements.* Niagara Falls: AGES Publications, 2000.

Balch, James F., M.D. and Phyllis A. Balch, C.N.C. *Prescription for Nutritional Healing.* 2nd ed. New York: Penguin Putnam, 1997.

Murray, Michael, N.D. *Encyclopedia of Nutritional Supplements.* Roseville, CA: Prima Publishing, 1996.

Rothenberg, Mikel, M.D. and Charles Chapman. *Dictionary of Medical Terms.* 3rd ed. Hauppauge, NY: Barron's Educational Series, 1994.

PERIODICALS

Hua, J., K. Sakamoto, and I. Nagaoka. "Inhibitory Actions of Glucosamine, a Therapeutic Agent for Osteoarthritis, on the Functions of Neutrophils." *Journal of Leukocyte Biology* 71 (April 2002): 632-640.

> ## KEY TERMS
>
> **Amino acids**—Organic acids containing nitrogen that are the building blocks of proteins.
>
> **Carbohydrates**—Organic substances, usually from plant sources. They are made up of carbon, hydrogen, and oxygen, and are the diet's major source of energy.
>
> **Chitin**—A transparent horny substance found in the outer coverings of shellfish. Chitin is used to make commercial preparations of glucosamine.
>
> **Glucose**—Simple sugar that serves as cells' main energy source.
>
> **NSAIDs**—Nonsteroidal anti-inflammatory drugs given to suppress inflammation. Ibuprofen is a typical NSAID.
>
> **Nutraceutical**—A food or food ingredient that is thought to provide medical or health benefits. Glucosamine preparations are classified as nutraceuticals.
>
> **Osteoarthritis**—Degenerative joint disease that affects the hip, knee, or spine. Pain occurs after exercise and the joints can become stiff and swell. This is the most common type of arthritis and occurs in 80% of people over 50.
>
> **Rheumatology**—The medical specialty that studies and treats disorders of the joints and muscles.
>
> **Tendinitis**—Inflammation of tissues that connect muscles to bones. Tendinitis is usually caused by strain or an injury.

"Joint Remedies." *Consumer Reports* 67 (January 2002): 18-21.

Parcell, S. "Sulfur in Human Nutrition and Applications in Medicine." *Alternative Medicine Review* 7 (February 2002): 22-44.

Phoon, S., and N. Manolios. "Glucosamine. A Nutraceutical in Osteoarthritis." *Australian Family Physician* 31 (June 2002): 539-541.

Ruane, R., and P. Griffiths. "Glucosamine Therapy Compared to Ibuprofen for Joint Pain." *British Journal of Community Nursing* 7 (March 2002): 148-152.

Schnitzer, T. J., and the American College of Rheumatology. "Update of ACR Guidelines for Osteoarthritis: Role of the Coxibs." *Journal of Pain and Symptom Management* 23 (April 2002)(Supplement 4): S24-S30.

ORGANIZATIONS

American College of Rheumatology. 1800 Century Place, Suite 250, Atlanta, GA 30345. (404)633-3777. <www.rheumatology.org>.

OTHER

"Glucosamine: Is it a beneficial arthritis treatment?" <http://www.onhealth.com>.

Sharon Crawford
Rebecca J. Frey, PhD

Glutamine

Description

In healthy individuals, glutamine is a neutral, nonessential amino acid. **Amino acids** are critical to humans, since they form the proteins that are the building blocks for many body tissues, including muscles. Glutamine is the most abundant amino acid in our bodies. It performs several important functions in the body, particularly in those that are stressed because of certain diseases or conditions. Glutamine can be added to the body medically by physicians or through dietary supplements that people purchase without prescriptions.

General use

Researchers continue to study glutamine's properties and effects. It is the most plentiful amino acid in the bloodstream and the body continues to produce it unless some sort of stress occurs. **Cancer, burns** or trauma, excessive **exercise**, and certain other stressful situations to the body may cause glutamine levels to drop.

Research suggests that when glutamine levels fall and are not replaced, several body functions are affected, particularly within the digestive tract. Glutamine also is considered important to overall immunity, or ability to fight off diseases and **infections**. In the past few decades, interest has grown for use of glutamine in helping cancer patients. Research continues on using glutamine therapy to help patients with sepsis, burns, trauma, **inflammatory bowel disease**, acquired immune deficiency syndrome (**AIDS**), bone marrow transplants, and other potential diseases and conditions.

Some clinical research has reported glutamine aided patients with multiple trauma and burns by helping them fight off infections. It may help AIDS patients put on weight at a much lower cost, and with fewer complications, than human growth hormone. Athletes who overtrain have higher rates of infectious diseases and **allergies**; it is thought a diet high in glutamine can help improve these athletes' immune functions.

As more people have begun looking for ways to enhance fitness, they have turned to protein supplements. In 2003, it was reported that more than 1.2 million athletes used some type of performance-boosting supplement. Glutamine is used in the fitness industry as a supplement for bodybuilders who want to reduce muscle breakdown, or for recreational athletes on vigorous training schedules who feel the supplement fuels their immune systems.

Preparations

As a protein, glutamine occurs naturally in some foods, including meat, fish, legumes, peanuts, eggs, tofu, and dairy products. It also is highly concentrated in raw cabbage and beets. Cooking can destroy glutamine, particularly in vegetables. Much of a person's glutamine needs, even when exercising hard, can come from food sources. A 3–oz serving of meat contains about 3–4 grams of glutamine.

Glutamine supplements come in several forms. Some manufacturers sell tablets that also contain **antioxidants** (vitamins). The most common forms of glutamine supplements are protein powders that can be added to liquids and prepared protein drinks and shakes. Another amino acid called alanine may be combined with glutamine. The combined protein supplement is called alanylglutamine. The powder form is probably the most convenient and least expensive form of the supplement. When glutamine is used for medical purposes in a hospital setting, it may be administered via an enteral route, or through a tube directly into the intestine.

In 2002, the powder cost about 10 cents a gram, while the capsules cost between 12 and 23 cents per gram. Capsules deliver fewer grams of glutamine than the powder and the glutamine in capsules does not absorb as quickly as that in powder. The powder reportedly tastes mild and is not noticeable when added to favorite drinks.

Recommended doses of glutamine for fitness uses such as bodybuilding vary, but generally are 8–20 grams (g) a day and average about 15 g a day. Cancer patients on glutamine therapy may take a higher dose, about 30 g a day. An average daily therapeutic dose for the general public is 1.5–6 g.

Precautions

The powdered form of glutamine should be dissolved in a liquid and consumed quickly before it breaks down. Some literature recommends taking glutamine immediately before or after meals, or at the same time as eating protein, usually twice per day.

Glutamine is marketed as a dietary supplement, and therefore, the products are not regulated the same as prescription drugs. Those who take glutamine must be cautioned to carefully read labels; some supplements are not what they appear to be. In 2004, the U.S. Food and Drug Administration (FDA) outlined a new process to try to work toward better safety of the 29,000 dietary supplements on the American market. However, consumers still need to be cautious of contents and claims of dietary supplements. It also is important to follow dosage directions and/or to check with a physician or other certified medical or complementary medicine practitioner to ensure the correct dose is being taken. Finally, while many fitness promoters tout glutamine's effects, some researchers disagree with the science behind the claims. In time, more and larger clinical trails may be able to clear up the controversy over glutamine's ability to increase muscle size and strength in recreational athletes.

Side effects

No noticeable negative side effects of glutamine at recommended dosage and preparations had been reported as of May 2004. However, long-term research is ongoing.

Interactions

As of May 2004, glutamine has not been shown to interact with any particular drugs or with other supplements. However, research on glutamine supplements is limited and ongoing. Consumption of cabbage can worsen goiters and a condition called **hypothyroidism**. Since glutamine is not a regulated substance, it is best to consult a physician when adding the supplement to the diet and to mention regular glutamine supplementation to a health professional when he or she is treating a patient for a new disease or condition, or adding or changing drug therapy.

Resources

PERIODICALS

"Advanced Nutrition: Absorbing Stuff from Team FLEX." *Flex* (February 2003): 183–191.

Krenkel, Jessica A. "Glutamine Supplementation in Bone Marrow Transplantation (BMT)." *Topics in Clinical Nutrition* (September 2002): 83–91.

Nick, Gina L. "Impact of Glutamine–rich Foods on Immune Function (Medicinal Properties in Whole Foods." *Townsend Letter for Doctors and Nurses* (April 2002): 148–157.

"Protein Supplements of Little Use, Says Trial." *Nutraceuticals International* (May 2001).

Rowley, Brian. "Glutamine Facts. (Hotline: Nutrition and Supplements)." *Muscle & Fitness* (January 2002): 38–42.

Rowley, Brian. "Amino Acids Essential for Muscle Growth. (Stack of the Month)." *Muscle & Fitness* (August 2003): 184–185.

Yeager, Selene. "Take a Powder. (Fitness Chick)." *Bicycling* (August 2003): 77–78.

ORGANIZATIONS

Center for Science in the Public Interest. 1875 Connecticut Avenue NW, Suite 300, Washington, DC, 20009. 202-332-9110. <http://www.cspinet.org>.

OTHER

Bird, Patrick J. *Glutamine Supplements and Exercise* University of Florida. [cited June 6, 2004]. <http://www.hhp.ufl.edu/keepingfit/ARTICLE/glutamine.htm>.

"Glutamine." QFAC Bodybuilding [cited June 6, 2004]. <http://www.qfac.com/glutamine.html>.

"Report Offers Science-based Process and Guidelines to Evaluate Safety of Dietary Supplements." The National Academies Press Release. <http://www4.nationalacademies.org>.

Teresa G. Odle

Glutathione

Description

Glutathione is produced in the human liver and plays a key role in intermediary metabolism, immune response and health, though many of its mechanisms and much of its behavior await further medical understanding. It is also known as gamma-Glutamylcysteineglycine and GHS. It is a small protein composed of three **amino acids**, *cysteine*, *glutamic acid* and *glyceine*. Glutatione is found in two forms, a monomer that is a single molecule of the protein, and a dimmer that is two of the single

PHOTO GALLERY

Entries with this symbol ❧ *in the main body have corresponding
photographs in this alphabetically arranged color section.*

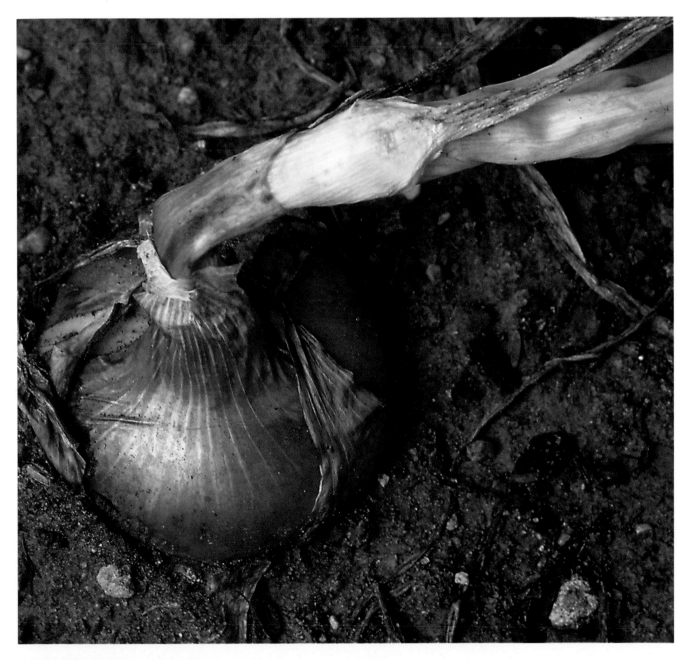

Onion plant *(Allium cepa)*. *(PlantaPhile Germany. Reproduced by permission.)*

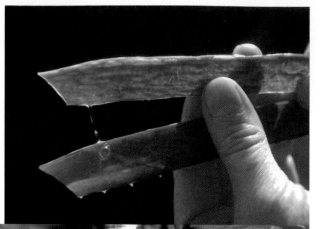

TOP ROW Leaves of an aloe plant.
(Photograph by Robert J. Huffman. Field Mark Publications. Reproduced by permission.)
MIDDLE ROW Ashwaganda *(Withiana somnifera).*
(PlantaPhile Germany. Reproduced by permission.)
Barberry plant *(Berberis vulgaris).*
(PlantaPhile Germany. Reproduced by permission.)

BOTTOM ROW Belladonna plant.
(Photo Researchers, Inc. Reproduced by permission.)
Black cohosh plant *(Cimicifuga racemosa).*
(PlantaPhile Germany. Reproduced by permission.)

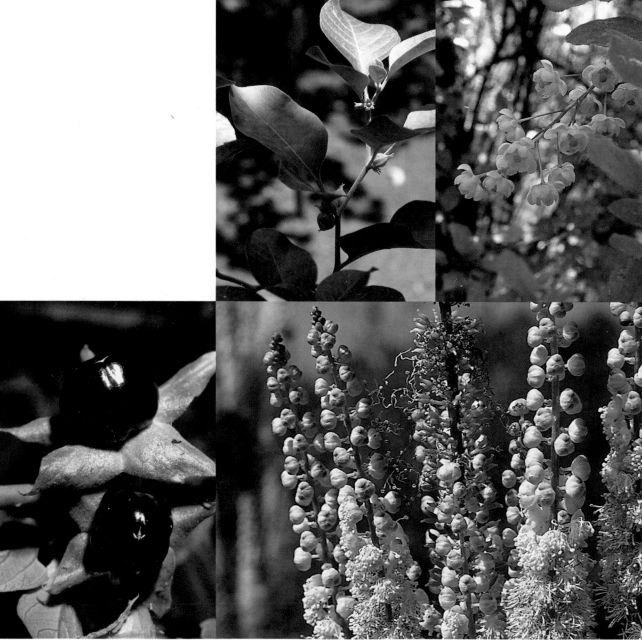

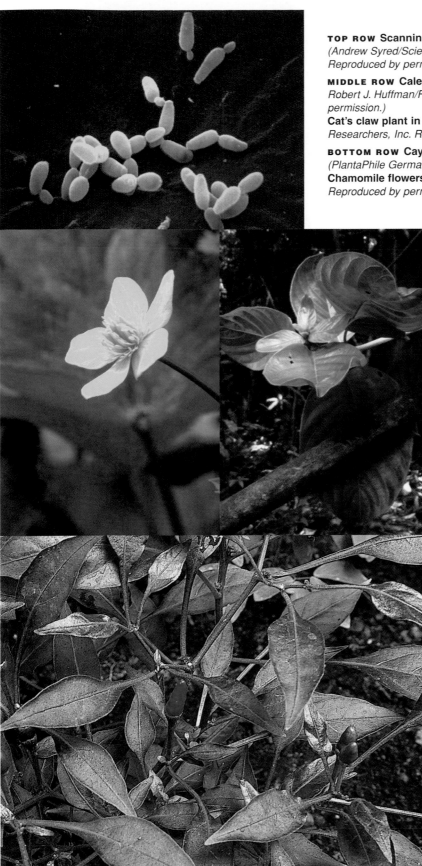

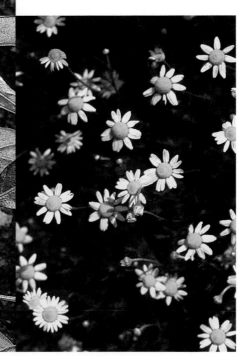

TOP ROW Scanning electron micrograph of brewer's yeast. *(Andrew Syred/Science Photo Library/Photo Researchers, Inc. Reproduced by permission.)*

MIDDLE ROW Calendula (marigold) flowers. *(Photograph by Robert J. Huffman/Field Mark Publications. Reproduced by permission.)*
Cat's claw plant in the Amazon rainforest. *(Photo Researchers, Inc. Reproduced by permission.)*

BOTTOM ROW Cayenne pepper *(Capsicum frutescens).* *(PlantaPhile Germany. Reproduced by permission.)*
Chamomile flowers. *(Scott Camazine/Photo Researchers, Inc. Reproduced by permission.)*

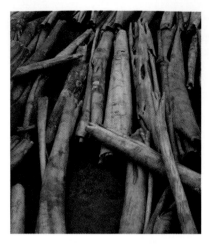

Cinnamon bark drying by a road in Sumatra. *(Photo Researchers, Inc. Reproduced by permission.)*

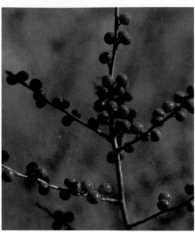

High-bush cranberry in Michigan. *(Photograph by Robert J. Huffman/Field Mark Publications. Reproduced by permission.)*

A dandelion plant with flower. *(Photograph by Robert J. Huffman/Field Mark Publications. Reproduced by permission.)*

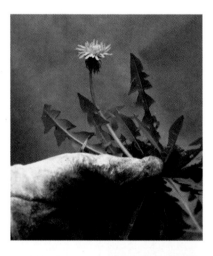

Echinacea flowers, also called purple coneflowers. *(Photo Researchers, Inc. Reproduced by permission.)*

Elder *(Sambuccus nigra).* *(PlantaPhile Germany. Reproduced by permission.)*

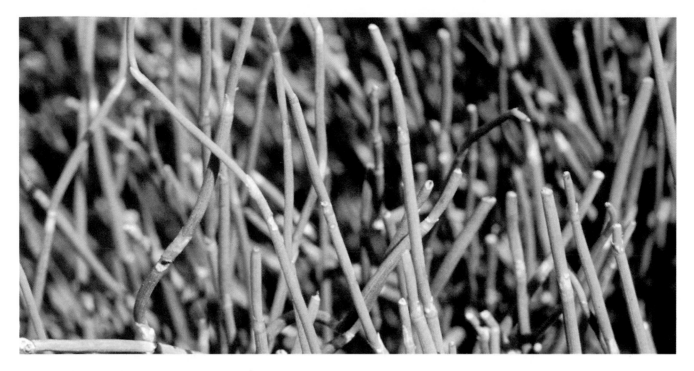

Ephedra *(Ephedra sinica).* (PlantaPhile Germany. Reproduced by permission.)

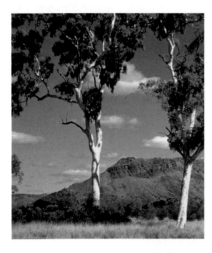

Eucalyptus trees in Australia. *(JLM Visuals. Reproduced by permission.)*

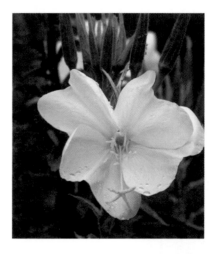

Evening primose flower. *(Photo Researchers, Inc. Reproduced by permission.)*

Whole, cloved, and minced garlic. *(Photograph by Robert J. Huffman. Field Mark Publications. Reproduced by permission.)*

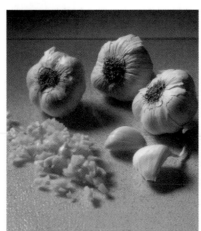

Ginger plant. *(JLM Visuals. Reproduced with permission.)*

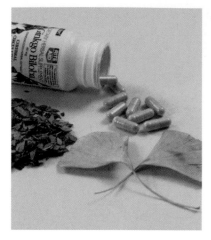

Various forms of ginko biloba. *(Photograph by Robert J. Huffman. Field Mark Publications. Reproduced by permission.)*

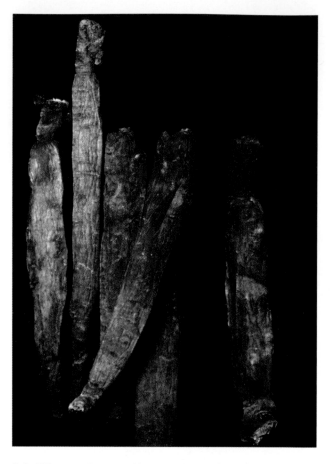

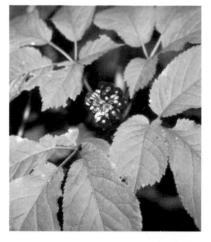

Cultivated American ginseng. *(JLM Visuals. Reproduced with permission.)*

Dried Korean ginseng. *(Custom Medical Stock Photo. Reproduced by permission.)*

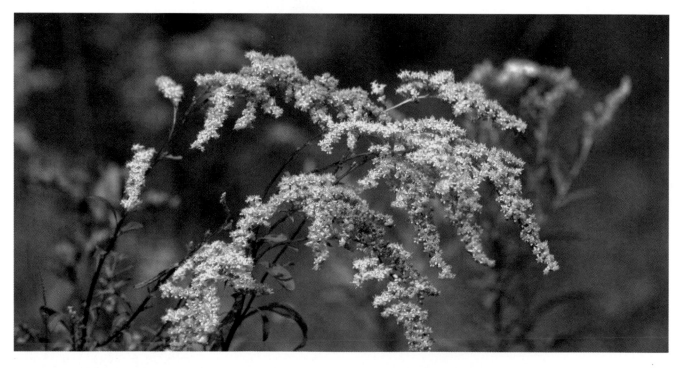

Flowering goldenrod plant. *(John Dudak/Phototake NYC. Reproduced with permission.)*

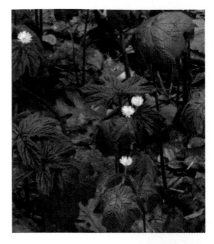

Cluster of goldenseal plants. *(Photo Researchers, Inc. Reproduced by permission.)*

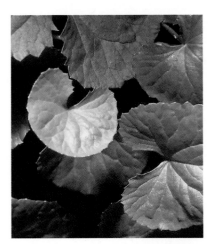

Gotu kola (*Centella asiatica*). *(PlantaPhile Germany. Reproduced by permission.)*

Purple grapes. *(Photograph by James Lee Sikkema. Reproduced by permission.)*

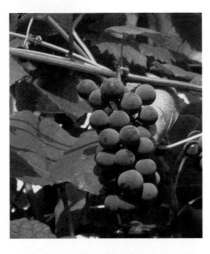

Green tea plant (*Camellia sinensis*). *(PlantaPhile Germany. Reproduced by permission.)*

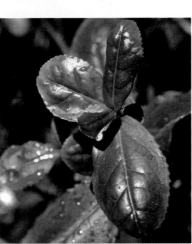

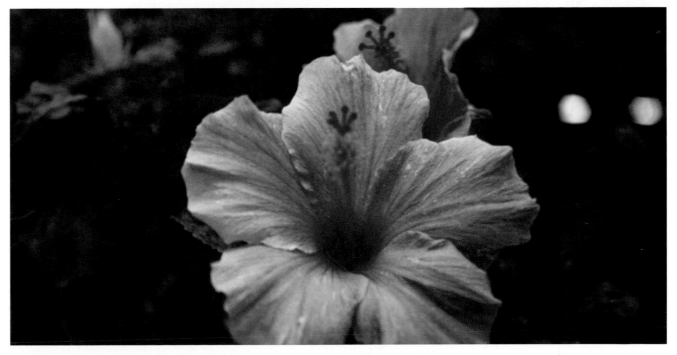

Hibiscus flower. *(Photo by Kelly Quinn. Reproduced by permission.)*

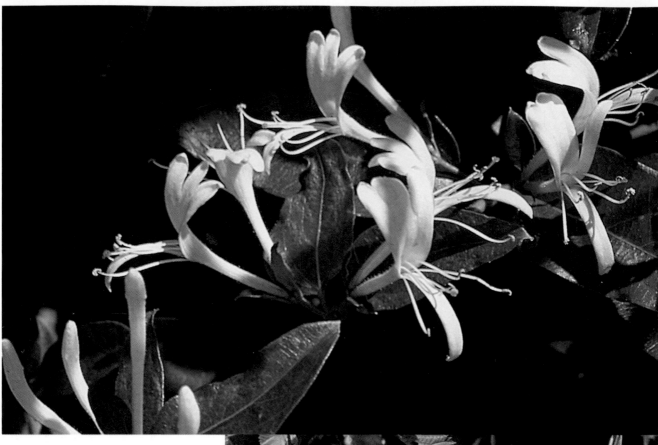

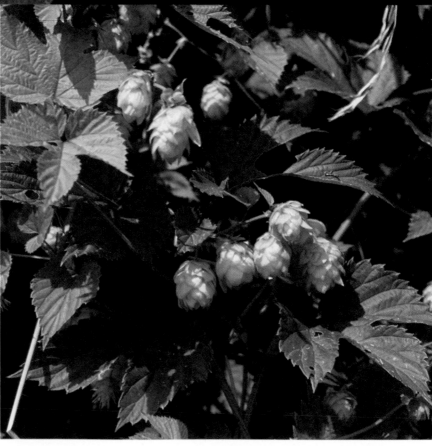

ABOVE Honeysuckle plant *(Lonicera caprifolia).* *(PlantaPhile Germany. Reproduced by permission.)*

RIGHT Hops plants. *(Photograph by Bill Howes. Frank Lane Picture Agency/Corbis-Bettmann. Reproduced by permission.)*

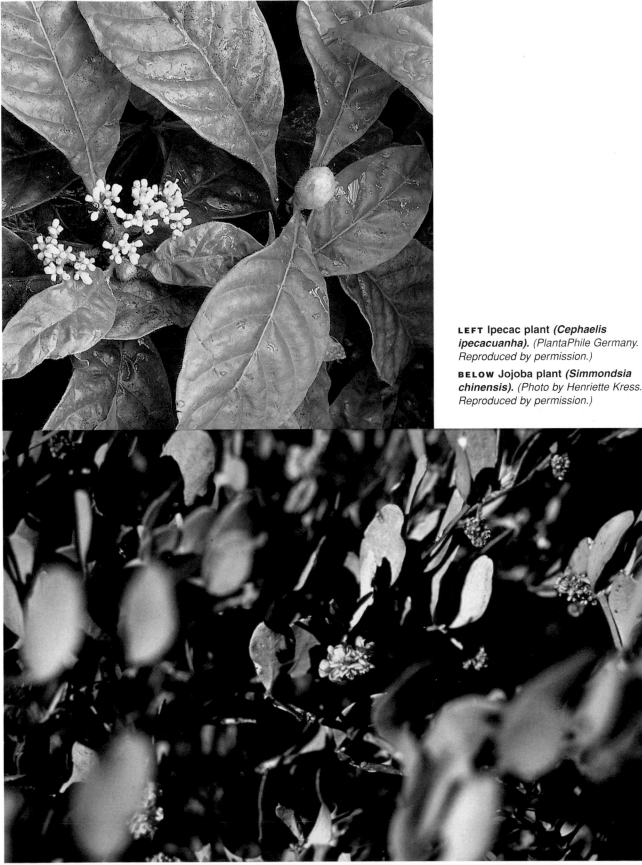

LEFT Ipecac plant *(Cephaelis ipecacuanha).* (PlantaPhile Germany. Reproduced by permission.)

BELOW Jojoba plant *(Simmondsia chinensis).* (Photo by Henriette Kress. Reproduced by permission.)

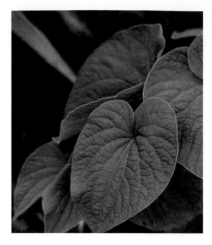

Kava kava leaves. *(Photo Researchers, Inc. Reproduced by permission.)*

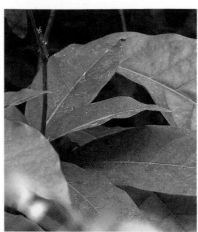

Kola nut *(Cola acuminata).* *(PlantaPhile Germany. Reproduced by permission.)*

Lavender *(Lavendula officinalis).* *(Photo by Henriette Kress. Reproduced by permission.)*

Lemongrass plant *(Cymbopogon citratus).* *(PlantaPhile Germany. Reproduced by permission.)*

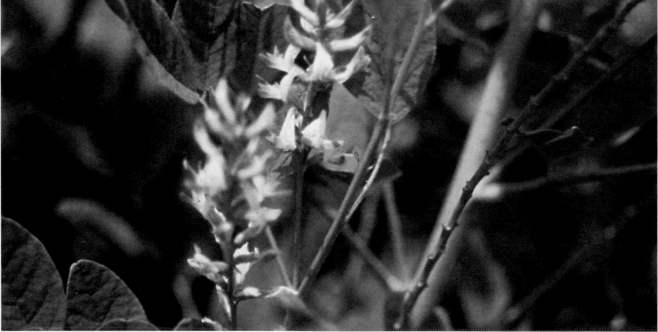

Licorice plant *(Glycyrrhiza glabra).* *(Photo by Henriette Kress. Reproduced by permission.)*

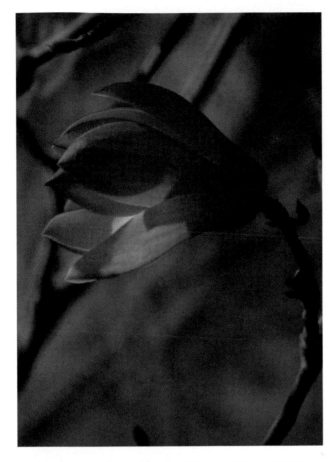

Magnolia flower. *(Photograph by Robert J. Huffman. Field Mark Publications. Reproduced by permission.)*

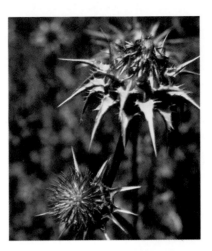

Milk thistle *(Silybum marianum)*. *(Photo by Henriette Kress. Reproduced by permission.)*

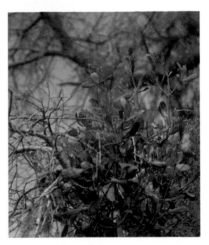

Mistletoe plant on a tree. *(JLM Visuals. Reproduced by permission.)*

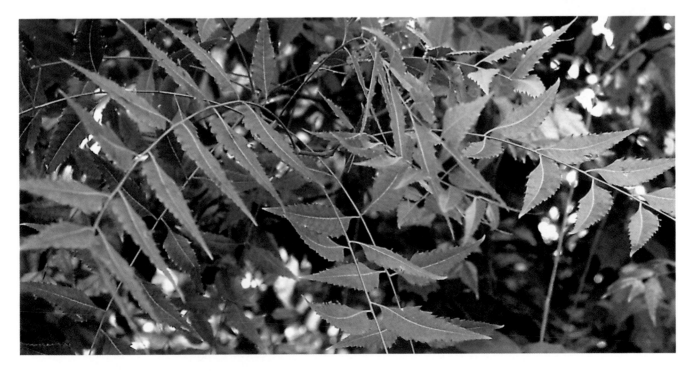

Neem *(Antelaea azadirachtu)*. *(PlantaPhile Germany. Reproduced by permission.)*

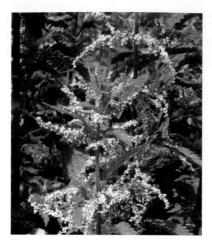

Nettles *(Urtica diocia).* (PlantaPhile Germany. Reproduced by permission.)

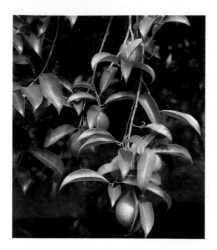

Nutmeg *(Myristica fragrans).* (PlantaPhile Germany. Reproduced by permission.)

Passionflower *(Passiflora incarnata).* (PlantaPhile Germany. Reproduced by permission.)

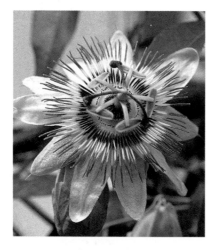

Peppermint plants in Oregon. *(Photo Researchers, Inc. Reproduced by permission.)*

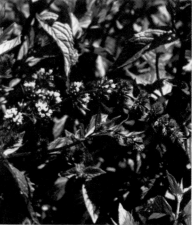

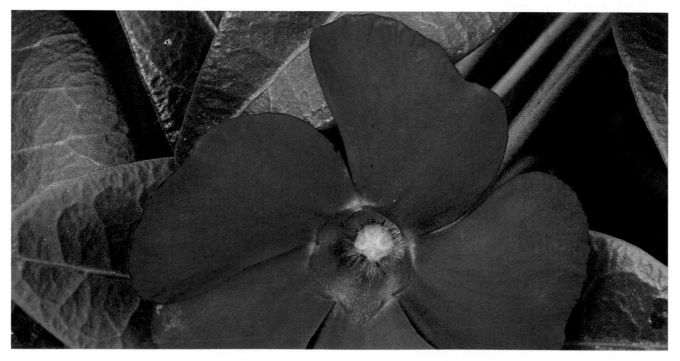

Periwinkle *(Vinca minor).* (PlantaPhile Germany. Reproduced by permission.)

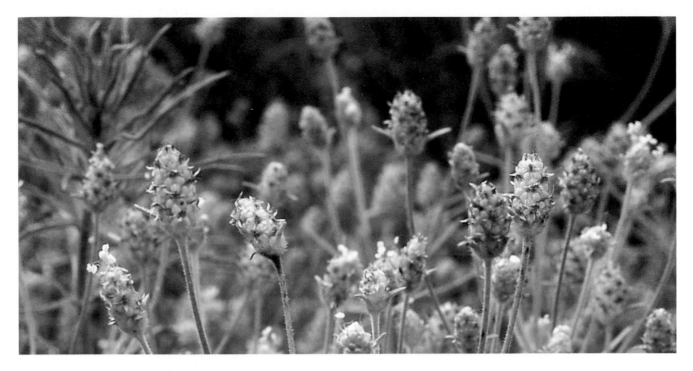

Psyllium *(Plantago afra)*. *(PlantaPhile Germany. Reproduced by permission.)*

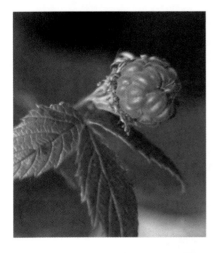

Raspberry on a bush. *(Photograph by Robert J. Huffman. Field Mark Publications. Reproduced by permission.)*

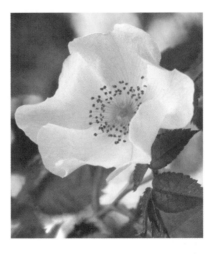

Rose hip plant *(Rosa canina)*. *(PlantaPhile Germany. Reproduced by permission.)*

Rosemary *(Rosmarinus officinalis)*. *(Photo by Henriette Kress. Reproduced by permission.)*

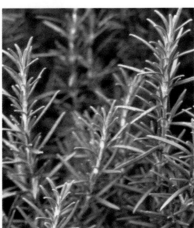

Saffron *(Crocus sativus)*. *(PlantaPhile Germany. Reproduced by permission.)*

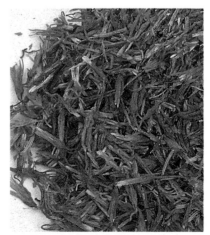

TOP ROW Saw palmetto leaves. *(Photo Researchers, Inc. Reproduced by permission.)*
MIDDLE ROW Fresh Shiitake mushrooms. *(Photo by Kelly Quinn. Reproduced by permission.)*
St. John's wort flowers. *(Photo Researchers, Inc. Reproduced by permission.)*
BOTTOM ROW Turmeric *(Curcuma longa).* *(PlantaPhile Germany. Reproduced by permission.)*
Uva ursi plant *(Arctostaphylos uva-ursi).* *(PlantaPhile Germany. Reproduced by permission.)*

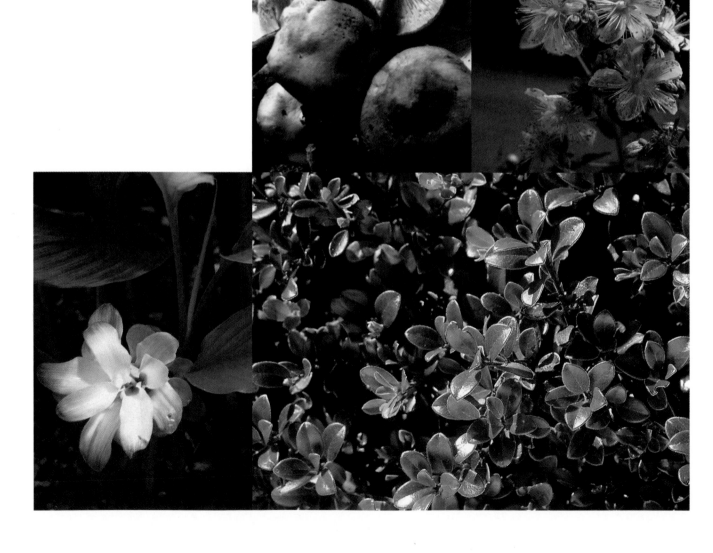

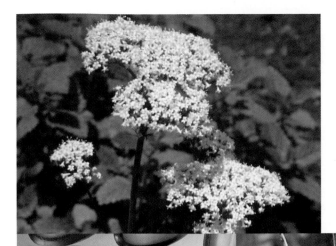

TOP ROW Valerian flowers. *(Photo Researchers, Inc. Reproduced by permission.)*

MIDDLE ROW Vitamin E capsules. *(David Doody/FPG International Corp. Reproduced by permission.)*
Wheat plant *(Triticum aestivum).* *(PlantaPhile Germany. Reproduced by permission.)*

BOTTOM ROW Witch hazel blooming in Great Smoky Mountains National Park. *(Photo Researchers, Inc. Reproduced by permission.)*
Yarrow *(Achillea millefolium).* *(Photo by Henriette Kress. Reproduced by permission.)*

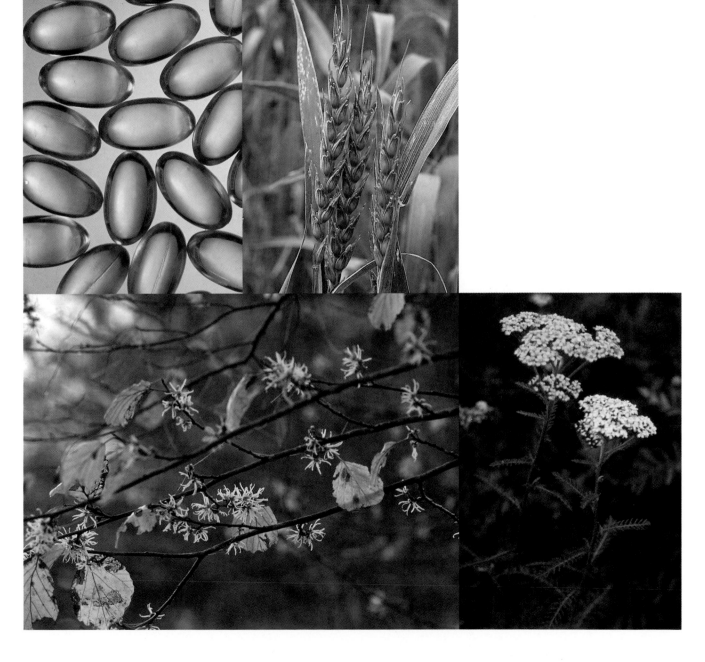

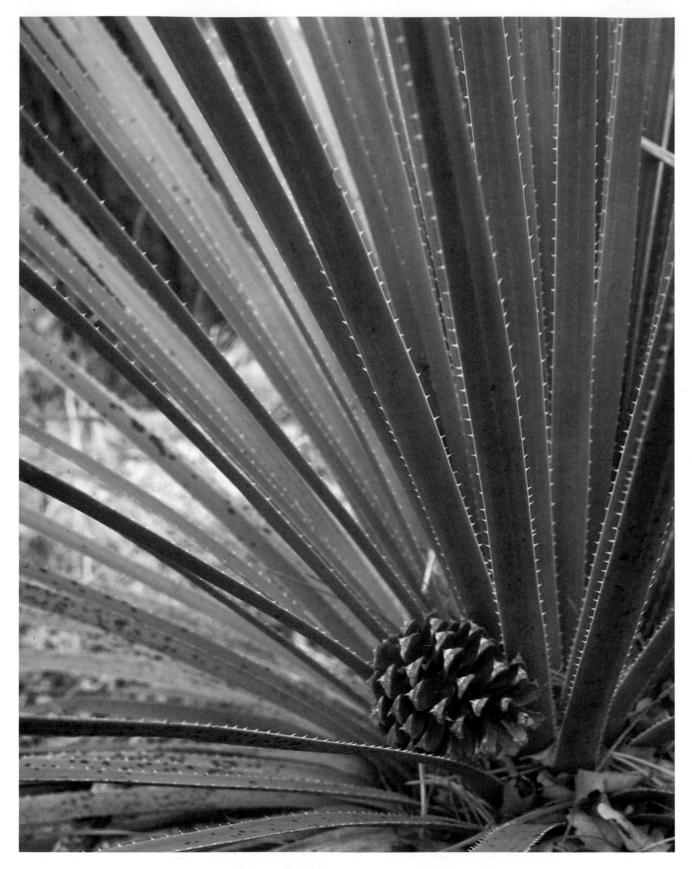

Leaves of a yucca plant. *(Photograph by Robert J. Huffman. Field Mark Publications. Reproduced by permission.)*

molecules joined together. The monomer is sometimes called reduced glutathione, while the dimmer is also called oxidized glutathione. The monomer is the active form of glutathione. Oxidized glutathione is broken down to the single molecule by an enzyme called glutathione reductase.

Glutathione, in purified extracted form, is a white powder that is soluble in water and in alcohol. It is found naturally in many fruits, vegetables, and meats. However, absorption rates of glutathione from food sources in the human gastrointestinal tract are low.

General use

Glutathione was first isolated in yeast in 1929. Its metabolism in the body was described in 1984, and its role in **cancer** treatment dates from 1984.

Glutathione is a major antioxidant highly active in human lungs and many other organ systems and tissues. It has many reported uses. It has a critical role in protecting cells from oxidative **stress** and maintaining the immune system. Higher blood levels of glutathione have been associated with better health in elderly people, but the exact association between glutathione and the **aging** process has not been determined.

Among the uses that have been reported for glutathione are:

• treatment of poisoning, particularly heavy metal poisons

• treatment of idiopathic pulmonary firbosis

• increasing the effectiveness and reducing the toxicity of *cis-platinum*, a chemo drug used to treat breast cancer

• treating Parkinson's disease

• lowering blood pressure in patients with diabetes

• increasing male sperm counts in humans and animals

• treatment of liver cancer

• treatment of sickle cell anemia

Claims made about glutathione have included that it will increase energy, improve concentration, slow aging, and protect the skin.

The importance of glutathione is generally recognized, although its specific functions and appropriate clinical use remain under study. Similarly, because ingested glutathione has little or no effect on intracellular glutathione levels, there are questions regarding the optimal method for raising the intracellular levels.

In addition to ongoing studies of the role of glutathione in cancer and cancer therapy, there are currently clinical trials of glutathione in Amyotrophic lateral sclerosis (ALS). The U. S. National Cancer Institute has included glutathione in a study to determine whether nutritional factors could inhibit development of some types of cancer.

European researchers, with support from the Cystic Fibrosis Foundation, are examining the potential uses of inhaled glutathione in cystic fibrosis. Some physicians also use inhaled glutathione in treating airway restriction and **asthma**. Other studies are investigating whether administration of alpha-lipoic acid, a material that can elevate intracellular glutathione, may be beneficial in restoring the immune system in **AIDS** patients.

Preparations

Although glutathione is marketed as a nutritional supplement, it does not appear that glutathione supplements actually increase the levels of glutathione inside cells. In human studies, oral doses of glutathione had little effect in raising blood levels . Further, glutathione is so widely distributed in common foods that supplements are not normally required. Supplements of **vitamin C** are more effective at increasing intracellular glutathione than taking oral glutathione supplements. Oral supplements of whey protein and of alpha-lipoic acid appear to help restore intracellular levels of glutathione.

Glutathione is available as capsules of 50, 100, and 250 milligrams. It is also included in many multivitamin and multi-nutrient formulations.

Precautions

At this time, the only established precautions are sensitivity to any of the inactive ingredients in the preparations of glutathione or the products used to stimulate glutathione levels. This is a discussion of glutathione, not C and whey. There is some new literature that suggests supplementing it may be helpful to some cancer patients, but detrimental to others.

Side effects

There are no established side effects to glutathione or to the substances used to elevate glutathione levels.

Training & certification

Glutathione has been classified as an orphan drug for treatment of AIDS. For this purpose, medical licensure is required. Glutathione has been given intravenously for amelioration of the side effects of cisplatin therapy. Specific training is required to order, prepare, start, and monitor intravenous therapy. No specific training is required to use glutathione or the compounds which have been reported to raise glutathione levels for other purposes.

Resources

BOOKS

Pressman, A. H. *Glutathione: the Ultimate Antioxidant.* New York: St. Martin's Press, 1997.

Rozzorno J. E., J. T. Murray, eds. *Textbook of Natural Medicine, 2nd ed.* Edinborough, Scotland: Churchill Livingston, 1999.

PERIODICALS

Carlo, M. D. Jr, and R. F. Loeser. "Increased oxidative stress with aging reduces chondrocyte survival: correlation with intracellular glutathione levels." *Arthritis Rheum* (December 2003): 3419–30.

Hamilton D., and G. Batist. "Glutathione analogues in cancer treatment." *Curr Oncol Rep* (March 2004): 116–22.

Wessner, B., E. M. Strasser, A. Spittler, and E. Roth. "Effect of single and combined supply of glutamine, glycine, N-acetylcysteine, and R,S-alpha-lipoic acid on glutathione content of myelomonocytic cells." *Clin Nutr* (December 2003): 515–22.

Witschi A., S. Reddy, B. Stofer, and B. H. Lauterburg. "The systemic availability of oral glutathione." *Eur J Clin Pharmacol*

Wu, G., Y. Z. Fang, S. Yang, J. R. Lupton, and N. D. Turner. "Glutathione metabolism and its implications for health." *J Nutr* (March 2004): 489–92.

Zenger, F., S. Russmann, E. Junker, C. Wuthrich, M. H. Bui, and B. H. Lauterburg. "Decreased glutathione in patients with anorexia nervosa. Risk factor for toxic liver injury?" *Eur J Clin Nutr.* (February 2004): 238–43.

ORGANIZATIONS

ALS Therapy Development Foundation. 215 First Street, Cambridge Mass. 02142.

Cystic Fibrosis Foundation. 6931 Arlington Road, Bethesda MD 20814.

NCCAM Clearinghouse. P.O. Box 7923 Gaithersburg, MD 20898.

Samuel Uretsky, Pharm.D.

Goatweed *see* **St. John's wort**

Goldenrod

Description

Averaging about 4 ft (1.2 m) in height, goldenrod is a perennial with clusters of bright yellow flowers. It has been used for centuries in the treatment of **kidney stones**, urinary tract **infections**, and a variety of other medical conditions. One legend has it that a 10-year-old boy who received an infusion of goldenrod for several months in the late eighteenth century passed 50 gravel stones larger than a pea. Native Americans used goldenrod to alleviate **sore throat**, and blue mountain tea made from goldenrod leaves is sometimes used to combat **fatigue** in the Appalachian Mountains. Goldenrod varieties belong to the plant family Asteraceae. While European goldenrod (*Solidago virgaurea*) is perhaps the most well known variety, other species of the plant (there are over 100 and counting) appear to have roughly equivalent medicinal properties—in particular, the ability to increase the flow of urine. In Europe, *Solidago virgaurea* is often used interchangeably with other species of goldenrod such as *Solidago serotina* and *Solidago canadensis* in the drug of commerce. Only the aboveground parts of the plant, mainly the flowers and leaves, are considered to have medicinal value.

Goldenrod grows in Europe, Asia, northern Africa, and North America, but most medicinal goldenrod originates in Bulgaria, Hungary, Poland, and other eastern European countries. It thrives in a wide variety of habitats, including hills, woods, meadows, and rocky terrain. Contrary to popular belief, goldenrod does not play a significant role in triggering **hay fever** reactions. This myth probably developed due to the fact that goldenrod blooms around the same time and in the same places as the ragweed responsible for most seasonal **allergies**. Studies of goldenrod pollen indicate that it is not a potent allergen for most people. However, it is in some. Goldenrod is also a very potent anti-allergic herb for sufferers of hay **fever**.

The genus name *Solidago* is derived from the Latin verb *solidare*, which can be translated "to make whole." Goldenrod received this appellation due to its reputation through the ages as a wound-healing drug. This also ex-

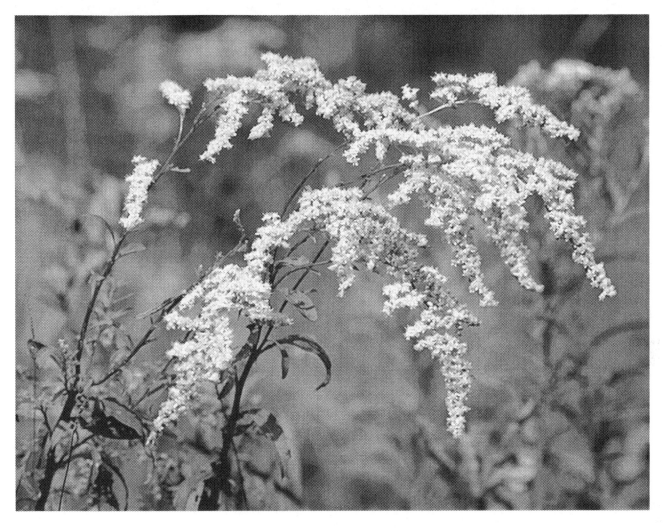

Flowering goldenrod plant. *(John Dudak/Phototake NYC. Reproduced with permission.)*

plains why goldenrod has sometimes been referred to as "woundwort" during its long history as a folk remedy. While not valued much today as a wound healer, goldenrod has been approved by the authoritative German Commission E as a diuretic, anti-inflammatory, and antispasmodic for the treatment of urinary tract disorders. Research suggests that goldenrod can increase the production of urine, which is often helpful in cases of urinary tract infection or kidney stones, without reducing levels of important electrolytes, such as **sodium** and chloride, the way that some man-made diuretics do. While it is not known exactly how goldenrod produces its therapeutic effects, researchers have focused on several naturally occurring chemicals in the plant. Most experts believe that goldenrod's ability to increase urine production is due to the presence of flavonoids and saponins, which stimulate the kidneys to release fluid. Another chemical in goldenrod, a phenolic glycoside called leiocarposide, may be responsible for goldenrod's anti-inflammatory effects. In one study of *Solidago virgaurea* involving rodents, researchers from Cairo University found that the anti-inflammatory activity of goldenrod was comparable to that of diclofenac, a nonsteroidal anti-inflammatory drug (NSAID) prescribed for conditions such as **rheumatoid arthritis**. The tannins in goldenrod have been associated with astringent properties. The herb also contains a small amount of essential oil.

General use

While not yet popular in the United States or approved for use by the United States Food and Drug Administration (FDA), goldenrod is used widely in Europe to treat urinary tract infections and help eliminate kidney or bladder stones. The Commission E has approved goldenrod as flushing-out therapy for inflammatory diseases of the lower urinary tract and for helping to eliminate and prevent stones. Goldenrod is considered useful in treating these disorders for several reasons. The herb can help to eliminate bacteria and stones by increasing the flow of urine and thereby "washing" them out. As an anti-inflammatory and antispasmodic, goldenrod may help to soothe irritated tissue in the urinary tract and prevent muscle spasms.

Goldenrod is not used as a cure for any of these disorders—for example, antibiotics are considered the primary therapy in cases of urinary tract infections—but it can be a helpful component of treatment. In Germany, where goldenrod has government approval as an aid in treating urinary tract disorders, the plant is often combined with java tea leaf, birch leaf, or **uva ursi** leaf. Compared to other herbal diuretics, goldenrod is considered well tolerated due to its lack of side effects and contraindications.

Throughout its history, goldenrod has been used to treat a variety of other medical problems. These include **hemorrhoids**, diabetes, **tuberculosis**, liver enlargement, **gout**, internal bleeding, **diarrhea**, **asthma**, rheumatism, enlarged prostate, infections of the mouth and throat, and external **wounds**. In the Appalachian Mountain region of the United States, goldenrod leaves have been used to prepare blue mountain tea, which is recommended by folk practitioners there to combat fatigue and physical exhaustion. As of early 2000, sufficient scientific evidence to support these additional uses is lacking.

Preparations

Dosage of goldenrod generally ranges from 6–12 g of cut herb per day. The drug, which is recommended for internal use only, can be taken as a tea, liquid extract, or tincture. No matter which preparation is used, it is important to drink plenty of fluids (6–8 glasses a day) while using goldenrod in order to increase its effectiveness as a diuretic.

Goldenrod tea can be prepared by steeping 3–5 g (1 or 2 teaspoonfuls) of the herb in 150 ml of simmering water. The mixture should be strained after about 15 minutes. Dosage is two to four cups of tea a day, taken between meals. The liquid extract preparation is usually taken two to three times a day in doses of 0.5–2.0 ml. Dosage for the tincture is 0.5–1.0 ml two to three times a day.

Precautions

While self-care measures such as goldenrod may be an effective component of treatment for disorders of the urinary tract, these medical conditions can be serious and require consultation with a doctor. People who suffer from **edema** due to reduced heart or kidney function should not use goldenrod without medical supervision.

KEY TERMS

Antispasmodic—An agent with the ability to prevent or relieve convulsions or muscle spasms.

Astringent—An agent that helps to contract tissue and prevent the secretion of internal body fluids such as blood or mucus. Astringents are typically used to treat external wounds or to prevent bleeding from the nose or throat.

Diuretic—An agent that increases the production of urine.

Edema—Abnormal swelling of tissue due to fluid buildup. Edema, which typically occurs in the legs, liver, and lungs, is often a complication of heart or kidney problems.

Electrolytes—Substances in the blood, such as sodium and potassium, that help to regulate fluid balance in the body.

Due to lack of sufficient medical study, goldenrod should be used with caution in children, women who are pregnant or breast-feeding, and people with kidney disease. To ensure optimum effectiveness, protect goldenrod from direct sunlight and moisture during storage.

Most studies of goldenrod's effects as a diuretic, anti-inflammatory, and antispasmodic have been conducted in the test tube or in rodents. Goldenrod's effectiveness in humans is not well demonstrated as of early 2000.

Side effects

When taken in recommended dosages, goldenrod has not been associated with any significant or bothersome side effects. Allergic reactions may occur in some people.

Interactions

No drugs are known to interact adversely with goldenrod. In Germany, goldenrod has been combined with java tea leaf, birch leaf, and uva ursi leaf without apparent harm.

Resources

BOOKS

Gruenwald, Joerg. *PDR for Herbal Medicines*. Montvale, NJ: Medical Economics, 1998.

Sifton, David W. *PDR Family Guide to Natural Medicines and Healing Therapies*. New York: Three Rivers Press, 1999.

Tyler, Varro E. *Herbs of Choice*. Binghamton, NY: Haworth Press, Inc., 1994.

PERIODICALS

el-Ghazaly, M., M.T. Khayyal, S.N. Okpanyi, et al. "Study of the anti-inflammatory activity of *Populus tremula, Solidago virgaurea* and *Fraxinus excelsior.*" *Arzneimittelforschung* 42, no. 3 (1992): 333-6.

Leuschner, J. "Anti-inflammatory, spasmolytic and diuretic effects of a commercially available *Solidago gigantea* Herb Extract." *Arzneimittelforschung* 45, no. 2 (1995): 165–8.

ORGANIZATIONS

American Botanical Council. P.O. Box 144345, Austin, TX 78714-4345.

Herb Research Foundation. 1007 Pearl Street, Suite 200, Boulder, CO 80302.

OTHER

Herb Research Foundation. http://www.herbs.org (January 17, 2001).

OnHealth. http://www.onhealth.com (January 17, 2001).

Discovery Health. http://www.discoveryhealth.com (January 17, 2001).

Greg Annussek

Goldenseal

Description

Goldenseal (*Hydrastis canadensis*) is a perennial North American native plant found wild in eastern deciduous woodlands and damp meadows as far north as Vermont and Minnesota, and south to Georgia and Arkansas. This versatile herb is sought for its valuable rootstock and inner twig bark. Goldenseal is a member of the Ranunculaceae, or buttercup family. It is a mainstay of **Native American medicine**, and a popular folk remedy. Goldenseal has multiple uses, both internally and externally. It is sometimes called poor man's ginseng. This traditional medicinal herb has been known by many names, including yellow paint root, orange root, eye root, Indian plant, tumeric root, eye balm, **jaundice** root, yellow puccoon, and ground **raspberry**. Native American tribes valued this natural antiseptic herb for many medicinal uses and as a clothing dye. Early colonists soon came to appreciate its infection-fighting action. The Native American use of goldenseal as a **cancer** treatment was first mentioned in the herbal, *Essays Toward a Materia Medica of the United States* first published by Benjamin Smith Barton in 1798.

The yellow rootstock is the main, known medicinal part of the herb. In cultivation, goldenseal requires up to four years growth before the rootstock is ready for harvest. The thick and knotty rhizome produces a hairy stem

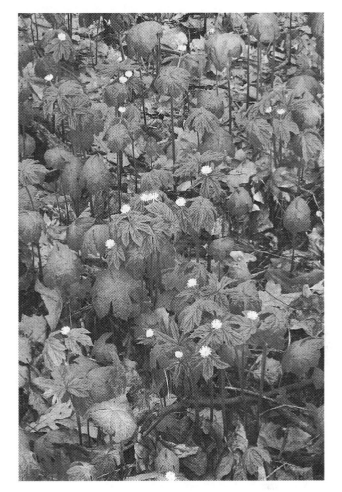

Cluster of goldenseal plants. *(Photo Researchers, Inc. Reproduced by permission.)*

that grows to 2 ft (61 cm) high. Goldenseal has only two large leaves, each five-lobed with double-toothed edges growing atop a forked stem. Leaves are serrated at the top edges. A single flower with greenish-white sepals crowns the hairy stem. The fruit looks like a raspberry, hence one of the plant's common names. Pharmaceutical companies harvest goldenseal root in large quantities for use. The herb is fully endangered on extinction risk lists in the wild due to over-collection of the rhizome. An estimated 250,000 pounds of rootstock of this popular herbal remedy are sold each year, and most of this has been collected in the wild.

General use

The underground portion of the stem, called the rhizome, as well as the inner twig bark, are the medicinal part of this multiple-use native remedy. The goldenseal rhizome is rich in alkaloids: hydrastine, berberine, and canadine, in addition to other phytochemicals, oils, and resin. Goldenseal has been considered a cure-all medicinal herb because of its wide variety of medicinal applications. It is a bitter herb that is effective when taken internally to promote digestion. The herb is particularly helpful when used to treat inflammation and infection of the mucous membranes lining the upper respiratory tract, and the digestive and genitourinary tract. Its anti-bacterial properties improve all catarrhal conditions, and it is helpful against amoebic infection. Goldenseal potentiates insulin and stimulates liver, kidney, and lung function. The astringent herb may also be used to help control bleeding, so it is helpful in circumstances of excessive and painful **menstruation** or postpartum hemorrhage. It is antiseptic, diuretic, and acts as a mild laxative and internal body cleanser. Goldenseal is used in treatment of peptic ulcers, and stimulates the flow of bile. Applied externally as rhizome bark powder or tincture, the herbal preparations can help treat **gum disease**, vaginal infection, **eczema**, **impetigo**, **conjunctivitis**, inflammations of the ear, and possibly ringworm. Its diuretic and anti-inflammatory effects can help lower blood pressure. The berberine alkaloid in goldenseal stimulates uterine contractions, and the herb is useful to treat **pelvic inflammatory disease** (PID). Goldenseal is high in **iron**, **manganese**, silicon, and other minerals. Goldenseal was once considered a good substitute for quinine. The herb has been used as a remedy for diphtheria, **tonsillitis**, chronic catarrh of the intestines, typhoid **fever**, **gonorrhea**, leucorrea, and **syphilis**. It is no wonder that with all these medicinal benefits, this wonderful herb is disappearing in the wild.

Preparations

The rootstock of goldenseal, harvested in spring or fall in the third or fourth year of growth, can be used in decoction, liquid extract, tablet, and tincture. When purchasing commercially prepared remedies, avoid the wild-crafted sources to help protect this valuable herb in its wild habitat.

To prepare an eyewash of goldenseal, mix equal parts of powdered rootstock and boric acid with boiling hot water. Stir well and allow to cool. Strain the mixture and store in a dark glass container. For one dosage, retrieve one teaspoon of the resulting liquid per one half cup water as a soothing eyewash solution. It is important to keep all equipment totally sterile, apply with a sterilized eyedropper, and discard old liquid eyewash (over one or two days).

For an infusion, use one teaspoon of powdered rootstock to a pint of boiling water. Let stand until cold. Dosage is 1–2 teaspoons, three to six times per day, for up to seven days. The infusion may also be used as a gargle.

To prepare a tincture, combine one part fresh herb to three parts alcohol (50% alcohol/water solution) in glass container. Set aside in dark place. Shake daily for two weeks. Strain through muslin or cheesecloth, and store in dark bottle. The tincture should maintain potency for two years. Standard dosage, unless otherwise prescribed, is one teaspoon, three times daily, for short periods (one or two weeks).

To make capsules, pulverize the dried root into a fine powder. Place in gelatin capsules. Dosage is two capsules, three times daily for three weeks, then discontinue for the next three weeks.

Precautions

Pregnant and breast-feeding women should not use this herb as it may stimulate uterine contraction. Patients with high blood pressure should also avoid goldenseal. The herb should be taken only for very limited periods, as it builds up in the mucosa of the system and its strong alkaloids are neurotoxic over an extended time (i.e., several months of daily use). Three weeks on and three weeks off is a good routine for dosage. Do not eat the plant fresh, as it can irritate mucous tissues.

Side effects

Goldenseal use can destroy organisms that are beneficial to the body, as well as those that are pathological. It should be used only for limited periods of time.

Interactions

Goldenseal is often combined with other herbs in preparations. **Myrrh** gum (*Commiphora myrrha*) and **echinacea** (*Echinacea augustifolia*) extract may be added to goldenseal in salve preparations. Goldenseal combines well with **mullein** (*Verbascum thapus*) for **earache**, and with **chamomile** (*Matricaria chamomilla*) and meadowsweet (*Filipendula ulmaria*) for stomach aches. Combine in infusion with **gotu kola** (*Centella asiatica*) for a brain tonic.

Resources

BOOKS

Balch, James F., M.D., and Phyllis A. Balch, C.N.C. *Prescription for Nutritional Healing.* New York: Penguin Putnam, Inc., 2000.
Bown, Deni. *The Herb Society of America, Encyclopedia of Herbs & Their Uses.* New York: DK Publishing, Inc., 1995.
Hoffmann, David. *The New Holistic Herbal.* Boston: Element, 1991.
Lust, John. *The Herb Book.* New York: Bantam Books, 1982.
Werbach, Melvyn R., M.D., and Michael T. Murray, N.D. *Botanical Influences on Illness.* Tarzana, CA: Third Line Press, 2000.

OTHER

Foster, Steven. *Goldenseal's Future.* http://www.stevenfoster. com/education/monograph/goldenseal.html.

Clare Hanrahan

Gonorrhea

Definition

Gonorrhea is a highly contagious sexually transmitted disease (STD) caused by the *Neisseria gonorrhoeae* bacterium. The genitourinary tract is the main system that is usually affected, but gonorrhea can also spread to the rectum, the throat, and the eyes. Left untreated, gonorrhea can spread through the bloodstream and infect the brain, heart valves, joints, and the reproductive system. Exposure to an infected mother during birth may cause permanent blindness in the newborn.

Description

Gonorrhea, commonly referred to as "the clap," is the most prevalent reportable disease in the United States. Adolescents and young adults are in the highest risk category, with more than 80% of gonorrhea cases affecting the 15–29 year-old age group. Individuals living in urban areas who have multiple sex partners have the highest risk of contracting the disease. Still, the incidence of gonorrhea has been steadily declining since 1987. This appears to be largely due to increased public awareness about the risks and prevention of contracting STDs such as herpes and HIV. However, in 2002, the Centers for Disease Control (CDC) expressed concern about rising rates of gonorrhea in certain urban areas during 1999 and 2000. About 650,000 new cases of gonorrhea occur every year in the United States. In particular, rates of gonorrhea were increasing substantially among men who have sex with men.

Causes & symptoms

Gonorrhea is transmitted very efficiently. It can be spread by merely contacting the fluids of an infected person as well as by sexual contact. A person runs a 60–90% chance of contracting the disease after just one sexual encounter with an infected person. The symptoms usually begin between one day and two weeks after the initial encounter with the infection.

People who are infected with gonorrhea commonly experience increasingly frequent and painful urination, and

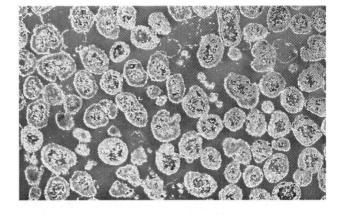

A transmission electron microscopy (TEM) of *Neisseria gonorrhoeae.* (*Custom Medical Stock Photo. Reproduced by permission.*)

the urethra may be painful and swollen. There may be a thick white, yellowish, or bloody discharge from the penis or vagina. Other symptoms may include **nausea**, **vomiting**, **fever**, **chills**, and **pain** during intercourse. In the case of oral infection, there may be a **sore throat** or pain during swallowing. An anal infection may cause rectal **itching**, rectal discharge, and a constant urge to move the bowels. Women who show symptoms of gonorrhea often have abdominal pain and breakthrough bleeding (spotting) between menstrual periods. However, many women who have gonorrhea do not experience any symptoms.

In infants and children, irritation, redness, swelling with a pus-like discharge, and possibly pain and a change in urination may point to a gonorrhea infection. The infection may be due to child abuse or exposure to infected materials. An in-depth history should be taken if gonorrhea is suspected.

Diagnosis

The initial diagnosis of gonorrhea will be based on symptoms, sexual history, and at-risk behavior. One laboratory test for diagnosis involves the observation of a gram-stained sample of the discharge under a microscope. In the gram stain test, the sample is dyed, washed with various solutions, and dyed with a different color. The final color identifies the class of bacteria present in the sample. The advantage of this test is that results can be obtained very quickly so that treatment can commence at the initial visit. In the vast majority of men, it is quite accurate; however, the test is not very accurate for women.

For all women and for men with a questionable gram-stain reading, samples of the discharge from the infected area can be collected and cultured. The sample is incubated for up to two days, which provides enough time for the bacteria to multiply and be accurately identified. This test is very accurate and specific for gonorrhea, but improper handling can lead to a false-negative reading. Other tests coming into favor include the ELISA (enzyme-linked immunosorbent assay) antibody test and DNA probe testing of genetic material from the discharge, both of which are quite accurate in identifying *Neisseria gonorrhoeae*.

Treatment

Although there is nothing that can totally replace antibiotics in the treatment of gonorrhea, certain herbs and minerals may be used to supplement the treatment. These may be used to improve the body's immune function: **zinc**, multivitamins and mineral complexes, **vitamin C**, and **garlic** (*Allium sativum*). *Lactobacillus acidophilus* in supplements and live-culture yogurts help replenish gastrointestinal flora that may be destroyed by the intake of antibiotics.

Several herbs may reduce symptoms and help speed healing. These include **kelp** (*Macrocystis pyrifera* and related species), *Calendula officinalis*, **myrrh** (*Commiphora molmol*), and *Thuja occidentalis*. These herbs can be taken by the mouth or used as a douche. The Chinese herb *Coptis chinensis*, used for damp-heat **infections**, is helpful in treating the genitourinary tract, especially if **pelvic inflammatory disease** (PID) develops. An herbalist should be consulted to make recommendations for further complications. Some recommend a three-day cleansing fast to quicken and support healing. **Fasting** should be done only with the approval and supervision of a physician. Referral to an acupuncturist is also recommended, as there may be **acupressure** and **acupuncture** points that will help with system cleansing.

Allopathic treatment

The typical treatment for gonorrhea is penicillin or a penicillin derivative, given orally or by injection. If the patient is pregnant or allergic to penicillin, erythromycin may be substituted. Gonorrhea has become more difficult and expensive to treat since the 1970s because it has become increasingly resistant to certain antibiotics. In fact, according to projections from the Centers for Disease Control and Prevention, 30% of the strains of gonorrhea were resistant to routine antibiotics in 1994, and resistance has been increasing steadily. Because of this, the doctor may also prescribe probenecid, which will increase the antibiotic activity.

In 2002, the Centers for Disease Control (CDC) updated guidelines concerning antibiotics for treating gonorrhea. Resistance of the infection has increased to certain classes of drugs, particularly when gonorrhea was contracted in certain states, particularly California. Guidelines had already warned against use of these drugs, called fluoroquinolones, in Hawaii, other Pacific islands, and Asia.

Since other STDs, such as **chlamydia** and **syphilis**, often occur with gonorrhea, patients may also be tested and treated for these related infections. Patients should refrain from sexual intercourse until treatment is complete and should return for follow-up testing. Anyone the patient has had sexual contact with during the time of infection should be notified and treated, even if those persons do not show symptoms. Doctors are required to report this disease to public health officials.

More than one health care provider may have to be consulted. Physicians trained in obstetrics or gynecology may be involved if gynecological complications occur. Men who experience complications may be referred to a urologist. There are also infectious disease doctors who specialize in the treatment of infectious diseases, including STDs.

Expected results

The prognosis for patients with gonorrhea varies based on how early the disease is detected and treated. Patients who are treated early and properly can be entirely cured of the disease. The most common complication is PID. PID can occur in up to 40% of women with gonorrhea and may result in damage to the fallopian tubes, an ectopic **pregnancy**, or sterility. If an infected woman is pregnant, gonorrhea can be passed on to the eyes of the newborn during delivery. This can lead to infection and blindness.

Although the risk of **infertility** due to gonorrhea is higher in women than in men, men may also become sterile if urethritis (inflammation of the urethra) develops. Complications of gonorrhea can affect the prostate, testicles, and surrounding glands as well. In either gender, inflammation, abscesses, and scarring can occur. In approximately 2% of patients with untreated gonorrhea, the infection may spread throughout the body and can cause fever, arthritis-like joint pain, and skin lesions.

Prevention

Currently, there is no vaccine for gonorrhea. The best prevention is to abstain from having sex, or to engage in sex only when in a mutually monogamous relationship in which both partners have been tested for STDs. The next line of defense against gonorrhea is the use of condoms, which have been shown to be highly effective in preventing disease. The use of a diaphragm can

KEY TERMS

. . . .

Chlamydia—The most common bacterial sexually transmitted disease in the United States.

Ectopic pregnancy—A pregnancy that occurs outside the uterus, often in the fallopian tubes. The fetus will not survive and in some cases, the pregnancy can result in the death of the mother.

False-negative—A laboratory result that does not detect the presence of a disease that is actually present.

Pelvic inflammatory disease (PID)—An infection of the upper genital tract.

Sexually transmitted diseases (STDs)—A group of diseases that are transmitted by sexual contact. In addition to gonorrhea, this group generally includes chlamydia, HIV (AIDS), genital herpes, syphilis, and genital warts.

Urethra—The canal leading from the bladder, and in men, also a path for semen.

Urethritis—Inflammation of the urethra.

also reduce the risk of infection. Since the risk of contracting gonorrhea increases with the number of sexual partners, those who have sexual contact with more than one partner are advised to be tested regularly for gonorrhea and other STDs.

Resources

BOOKS

Burton Goldberg Group, comp. *Alternative Medicine: The Definitive Guide*. Tiburon, CA: Future Medicine Publishing, 1995.

Editors of Time-Life Books. *The Medical Advisor: The Complete Guide to Alternative and Conventional Treatments*. Alexandria, VA: Time-Life Books, 1996.

Segen, Joseph, M.D., and Joseph Stauffer. *The Patient's Guide to Medical Tests: Everything You Need to Know About the Tests Your Doctor Prescribes*. New York: Facts On File, 1998.

PERIODICALS

"Gonorrhea Rates Rising Among Hardest Hit: HIV Infection Implications are Ominous." *TB Monitor* (May 2002):57.

Mahoney, Diana. "STD Guide Urges Rescreening After Chlamydia Therapy: CDC Also Updates Its Recommendations on Gonorrhea, Genital Herpes, and Nonoxydnol-9." *Family Practice News* (June 15, 2002):1.

ORGANIZATIONS

American Foundation for the Prevention of Venereal Disease, Inc. 799 Broadway, Suite 638, New York, NY 10003. (212) 759-2069.

American Social Health Association. P.O. Box 13827, Research Triangle Park, NC 27709. (919) 361-8400. Fax: (919) 361-8425. http://www.ashastd.org.

National Institute of Allergy and Infectious Diseases, Office of Communications and Public Liaison. Building 31, Room 7A-50, 31 Center Drive MSC 2520, Bethesda, MD 20892-2520. http://www.niaid.nih.gov.

OTHER

"Gonorrhea." *The Merck Manual Online*. http://www.merck.com/pubs/mmanual/section13/chapter164/164b.htm.

Patience Paradox
Teresa G. Odle

Gotu kola

Description

Gotu kola (*Centella asiatica*) is a member of the Apiaceae carrot family. It is also called pennywort, marsh penny, water pennywort, and sheep rot. The name sheep rot comes from the erroneous belief in Europe that gotu kola caused foot rot in sheep. Gotu kola is often mistaken for the **kola nut** plant (*Cola nitida*). However, the two are not related and gotu kola, unlike the kola nut, contains no **caffeine**. Gotu kola is noted in India as a very powerful spiritual herb, and **Ayurvedic medicine** refers to it as *Brahmi* because it helps obtain knowledge of the spiritual being.

Gotu kola, a perennial, grows in India, Sri Lanka, Madagascar, South Africa, China, Indonesia, Australia, and North America. It can grow like a weed, but its description depends on its location. For example, in shallow water, the leaves float; but in dry areas, the plant develops many roots and thin, tiny leaves. The fan-shaped leaves may be smooth or lobed. Red flowers turn into fruit with a diameter of about 0.2 in (5 mm).

Gotu kola's main active components are triterpenoids, although the gotu kola found in India, Sri Lanka, and Madagascar doesn't have the same properties. Gotu kola's triterpenes can have a concentration from 1.1-8%, with most concentrations in the middle range.

Gotu kola from Madagascar is used for most standardized extracts, and its four main triterpene properties are:

• asiatic acid (29-30%)

• madecassic acid (29-30%)

• asiaticoside (40%)

• madecassoside (1-2%)

Gotu kola also contains the following.

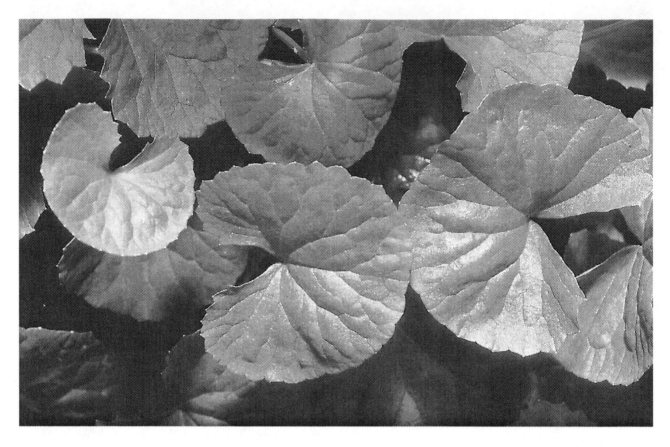

Gotu kola. (*© PlantaPhile, Germany. Reproduced by permission.*)

- volatile oil of a terpene acetate (36% of all the volatile oil)
- camphor
- cineole
- glycerides of some fatty acids
- plant sterols (campesterol, stigmasterol, sitosterol)
- polyacetylene compounds
- flavonoids (kampferol, quercetin)
- myo-inositol (glycoside from the flavonoids)
- sugars
- vellarin
- amino acids
- resins

General use

Traditional use of gotu kola in India and Indonesia included wound treatment. In the 1800s, it became part of Indian medicine practice and was used to treat many skin conditions including leprosy, varicose ulcers, and **eczema**, as well as **fever**, **diarrhea**, and absence of menses.

Chinese medicine uses various parts of the plant. The leaves are used for leukorrhea and fevers that are toxic, while other types of fevers and **boils** are treated with gotu kola shoots. Gotu kola used for longevity has become very popular. Chinese herbalist, Li Ching Yun, is supposed to have lived 256 years from drinking a herbal mixture containing gotu kola. An ancient Sinhalese saying, "Two leaves a day will keep old age away," also illustrates gotu kola's popularity as an agent for longevity.

The plant enhances brain and peripheral circulation, and is said to enhance memory. In the 1880s, the French began using gotu kola as part of regular pharmaceutical medicines.

Many current uses are similar to traditional uses of the plant. In a 1992 study at Kasturba Medical College, researchers fed rats gotu kola extract. After 14 days, the gotu kola-treated rats showed 3-60 times better retention of learned behavior than did rats who didn't receive the extract.

Gotu kola may also play a role in fighting **Alzheimer's disease**, which affects over four million people in the United States. People with this dementia-causing disease have unusual amounts of the protein beta-amyloid (also called plaque) in the brain. A 1999 study conducted by pathology professor Alan Snow at Seattle's University of Washington showed gotu kola's potential for treatment. Snow first mixed a compound from **cat's claw** and tested it in rats and in test tubes. Results showed that cat's claw intervenes with plaque formation. When other extracts were added to the test tubes, including gotu kola and **rosemary**, the results were more pronounced.

Besides its use as a general memory aid, gotu kola has become popular in the Western world for its calming effects as well as for improving concentration. This duality occurs because gotu kola affects both the central nervous system and the brain. It relaxes the nervous system while stimulating the brain to focus better. In a 1999 study at the West Palm Beach Veterans Affairs Medical Center, researchers tested several dietary supplements, including gotu kola, for use in **depression**, **anxiety**, and **sleep disorders**. Researchers found little difference in the results of the natural supplements and low- and high-dose antidepressants. However, the studies indicated patients switch to natural supplements because they think they are safer. The research served as a guideline for healthcare professionals to aid their patients' choice of treatment.

Studies have also shown that gotu kola has positive effects on **varicose veins**, poor blood circulation in the legs and the rest of the circulatory system, leg cramps, and leg swelling. The circulatory improvement occurs because gotu kola decreases vein hardening, improves the connective tissue around veins, and helps the blood to flow through veins. These circulatory and leg benefits were evident in 80% of patients tested in studies conducted in the late 1980s.

Gotu kola also has positive effects on various skin problems. Animal research has shown that tripenoid asiaticoside may help **wounds** heal quicker. Other studies showed that gotu kola helped in healing surgical wounds of the ear, nose, and throat, and promoted healing of episiotomies, **gangrene**, skin grafts, and some skin ulcers. Asiaticoside can also toughen skin, hair, and nails. Research has shown that asiaticoside may provide treatment for leprosy. Leprosy-causing bacteria are coated in a wax-like substance that the immune system can't penetrate. However, gota kola disintegrates this substance, allowing the immune system to attack the bateria.

Clinical trials also show that gotu kola's tripenoids, when purified, can lessen the ravages of scleroderma. Gotu kola can reduce hardening of the skin, decrease joint **pain**, and increase finger movement.

Gotu kola extracts can heal second- and third-degree **burns** from boiling water or gas explosions if the burn is treated immediately. Either topical application or intra-muscular injections can stop the effects of skin **infections** from burns and can stop or reduce skin shrinkage, inflation, and scarring.

Gotu kola extract might be effective in fighting tumors. However, researchers are cautious because animal and human studies need to be completed.

Preparations

Today, gotu kola is often eaten in a salad. It can also be made into a tea by using 0.5–1 tsp (2.5–5 ml) of gotu kola in 1 cup (250 ml) of boiling water. The plant is steeped for 10–15 minutes and the tea is then drunk. This amount can be drunk up to three times a day. Because of its bitter taste, the tea can be enhanced with honey or lemon to taste.

For a poultice on wounds or skin problems, gotu kola leaves can be crushed and applied, or a tincture may be used. A poultice can also be made from gotu kola tea.

For scleroderma, suggestions include 70 mg twice a day. The usual dosage is 0.5–1 g three times daily, a standardized extract dosage is 60–120 mg a day, and a liquid extract approximately 0.5–1 teaspoon can be taken daily.

Precautions

Children under two years old, pregnant women, and people with **epilepsy** should avoid gotu kola. Fair-skinned people and others who have had an allergic reaction to sunlight or other ultraviolet light sources should avoid these sources if they take gotu kola.

Side effects

A rash is the most common side effect when gotu kola is taken internally or applied topically. If injected, some pain and bruising may occur at the injection sight. The asiaticoside component could be a mild skin carcinogen. It is not wise to apply gotu kola topically over a long period of time. The plant may also cause mild headaches or **nausea**. As with any supplement, consultation with a healthcare professional should occur before beginning treatment.

Interactions

Gotu kola should not be mixed with oral diabetes medication or drugs such as Lipitor, Lopid, Mevacor, and Zocor, all of which lower **cholesterol**. Gotu kola can raise cholesterol. It is also best not to mix gotu kola with alcohol or sedatives.

Resources

BOOKS

Castleman, Michael. *The Healing Herbs*. Emmaus, PA: Rodale Press, 1991.

Duke, James A., Ph.D. *The Green Pharmacy.* Emmaus, PA: Rodale Press, 1997.

Murray, Michael, N.D. *Encyclopedia of Nutritional Supplements.* Roseville, CA: Prima Publishing, 1996.

Murray, Michael, N.D. *The Healing Power of Herbs.* 2nd ed. Roseville, CA: Prima Publishing, 1995.

Rothenberg, Mikel, M.D., and Charles Chapman. *Dictionary of Medical terms.* 3rd ed. Hauppauge, NY: Barron's Educational Series, 1994.

PERIODICALS

Schar, Douglas, M.C.P.P. Dip.Phyt. "5 Cutting-edge Superherbs—The Happy-Skin Herb Gotu Kola." *Prevention Magazine* (December 1999).

OTHER

Herbal Information Center. http:/www.kcweb.com/herb/gotu.htm.

The People's Pharmacy Guide to Home and Herbal Remedies. http://www.healthcentral.com.

Sharon Crawford

Gout

Definition

Gout is a form of acute arthritis that causes severe pain and swelling in the joints. It most commonly affects the big toe, but may also affect the heel, ankle, hand, wrist, or elbow. It affects the spine often enough to be a factor in lower back pain. Gout is often a recurring condition. An attack usually comes on suddenly and goes away after 5–10 days. Gout occurs when there are high levels of uric acid circulating in the blood, and the acid crystallizes and settles in the body. According to the National Institutes of Health (NIH), gout accounts for about 5% of all cases of arthritis reported in the United States.

Gout appears to be on the increase in the American population. According to a study published in November 2002, there was a twofold increase in the incidence of gout over the 20 years between 1977 and 1997. It is not yet known whether this increase is the result of improved diagnosis or whether it is associated with risk factors that have not yet been identified.

Description

Uric acid is formed in the bloodstream when the body breaks down waste products, mainly those containing purines. Purines can be produced naturally by the body, and they can be ingested from such high-purine foods as meat. Normally, the kidneys filter uric acid particles out of the blood and excrete it into the urine. If the body produces too much uric acid or the kidneys aren't able to filter enough of it out, there is a buildup of uric acid in the bloodstream. This condition is known as hyperuricemia.

Uric acid does not tend to remain dissolved in the bloodstream. Over the course of years, or even decades, hyperuricemia may cause deposits of crystallized uric acid throughout the body. Joints, tendons, ear tips, and kidneys are favored sites. When the immune system becomes alerted to the urate crystals, it mounts an inflammatory response that includes the pain, redness, swelling, and damage to joint tissue that are the hallmarks of an acute gout attack.

The body's uric acid production tends to increase in males during puberty. Therefore, it should come as no surprise that nine out of ten of those suffering from gout are men. Since it can take up to 20 years of hyperuricemia to have gout symptoms, men don't commonly develop gout until reaching their late 30s or early 40s. If a woman does develop gout, typically, it will be later in her life. According to some medical experts, this is because estrogen protects against hyperuricemia. It is not until estrogen levels begin to fall during **menopause** that urate crystals can begin to accumulate.

Hyperuricemia does not necessarily lead to gout. The tendency to accumulate urate crystals may be due to genetic factors, excess weight, or overindulgence in the wrong kinds of food. In addition, regular use of alcohol to excess, the use of diuretics, and the existence of high levels of **cholesterol** and triglycerides in the blood can increase the risk of developing the disease. In some cases, an underlying disease such as lymphoma, **leukemia**, or hemolytic **anemia** may also lead to gout.

Causes & symptoms

An acute episode of gout often starts without warning. The needle-like urate crystals may be present in the joints for a long time without causing symptoms. Then, there may be a triggering event such as a stubbed toe, an infection, surgery, **stress**, **fatigue**, or even a heavy drinking binge. Patients in intensive care units (ICUs) may have an acute flare-up of gout. In addition, it is now known that chronic occupational exposure to lead leads to decreased excretion of urates and an increased risk of developing gout.

In many cases, the gout attack begins in the middle of the night. There is intense pain, which usually involves only one joint. Often it is the first joint of the big toe. The inflamed skin over the joint is warm, shiny, and red or purplish, and the pain is often so excruciating that the sufferer cannot tolerate the pressure of bedcovers. The inflammation may be accompanied by a **fever**.

Acute symptoms of gout usually resolve in about a week, and then disappear altogether for months or years at a time. Eventually, however, the attacks may occur more frequently, last longer, and do more damage. The urate crystals may eventually settle into hard lumps under the skin around the joints, leading to joint deformity and decreased range of motion. These hard lumps, called tophi, may also develop in the kidneys and other internal organs, under the skin of the ears, or at the elbow. People with gout also face a heightened risk of kidney disease, and almost 20% of people with gout develop **kidney stones**. As of 2002, however, the relationship between gout and kidney stone formation is still not completely understood.

Diagnosis

Doctors can diagnose gout based on a physical examination and the patient's description of symptoms. In order to detect hyperuricemia, doctors can administer a blood test to measure serum urate levels. However, high urate levels merely point to the possibility of gout. Many people with hyperuricemia don't have urate crystal deposits. Also, it has been shown that up to 30% of gout

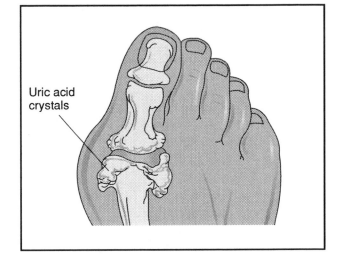

Gout, a form of acute arthritis, most commonly occurs in the big toe. It is caused by high levels of uric acid in the blood, in which urate crystals settle in the tissues of the joints and produce severe pain and swelling. *(Illustration by Electronic Illustrators Group. The Gale Group.)*

sufferers have normal serum urate levels, even at the time of an acute gout attack. The most definitive way to diagnose gout is to take a sample of fluid from an affected joint and test it for the presence of the urate crystals.

Treatment

The symptoms of gout will stop completely a week or so after an acute attack without any intervention. It is important, however, to be diagnosed and treated by a health care practitioner in order to avoid attacks of increasing severity in the future and to prevent permanent damage to the joints, kidneys, and other organs. During an acute attack, treatment should focus on relieving pain and inflammation. On an ongoing basis, the focus is on maintaining normal uric acid levels, repairing tissue damage, and promoting tissue healing.

Diet

Generally, gout is unheard of in vegetarians. It is a condition that responds favorably to improvements in diet and **nutrition**. Recurrent attacks can be avoided by maintaining a healthy weight and limiting the intake of purine-rich foods. A diet high in fiber and low in fat is also recommended. Processed foods should be replaced by complex carbohydrates, such as whole grains. Protein intake should be limited to under 0.8g/kg of body weight per day.

Nutritional supplements

Vitamin E and **selenium** are recommended to decrease the inflammation and tissue damage caused by the accumulation of urates.

Folic acid has been shown to inhibit xanthine oxidase, the main enzyme in uric acid production. The drug allopurinol (see below) is used for this same purpose in the treatment of gout. The therapeutic use of folic acid for this condition should be prescribed and monitored under the supervision of a heath care practitioner. The recommended dosage range is 400–800 micrograms per day.

The **amino acids** alanine, aspartic acid, glutamic acid, and glycine taken daily improve the kidneys' ability to excrete uric acid. **Bromelain**, an enzyme found in pineapples, is an effective anti-inflammatory. It can be used as an alternative to NSAIDs and other prescription anti-inflammatory drugs. It should be taken between meals at a dosage of 200–300 mg, three times per day.

The bioflavonoid quercetin helps the body absorb bromelain. It also helps decrease uric acid production and prevents the inflammation that leads to the acute symptoms of gout and the resulting tissue destruction. Quercetin should be taken at the same time and dosage as bromelain: 200–400 mg, between meals at a three times per day.

Herbs

Dark reddish-blue berries such as cherries, blackberries, **hawthorn** berries, and elderberries are very good sources of flavonoid compounds that have been found to help lower uric acid levels in the body. Flavonoids are effective in decreasing inflammation and preventing and repairing the destruction of joint tissue. An amount of the fresh, frozen, dried, juiced, or otherwise extracted berries equal to half a pound (about 1 cup) fresh should be consumed daily.

Devil's claw, *Harpagophytum procumbens,* has been shown to be of benefit. It can be used to reduce uric acid levels and to relieve joint pain.

Gout represents a serious strain on the kidneys. The dried leaves of nettles, *Urtica dioica,* can be made into a pleasant tea and consumed throughout the day to increase fluid intake and to support kidney functions. However, some people are allergic to nettles.

Therapy

Colchicum is a general homeopathic remedy that can be used for pain relief during a gout attack. It is formulated from the same plant, Autumn crocus, as the drug colchicine, used in the conventional treatment of gout. Gout may be improved by having a constitutional remedy prescribed that is based on the tendency to develop the disease and its symptoms.

During the acute phase of gout, **acupuncture** can be helpful with pain relief.

Applications of ice or cold water can reduce pain and inflammation during acute attacks.

Allopathic treatment

Standard medical treatment of acute attacks of gout includes nonsteroidal anti-inflammatory drugs (NSAIDs) such as naproxen **sodium** (Aleve), ibuprofen (Advil), or indomethacin (Indocin). Daily doses until the symptoms have subsided are recommended. Colchicine(Colbenemid), is also used. Corticosteroids such as prednisone (Deltasone, prednisolone, and corticotropin [ACTH]) may be given orally or may be injected directly into the joint for a more concentrated effect. Because these drugs can cause undesirable side effects, they are used for only about 48 hours so as not to cause major problems. Aspirin and other salicylates should be avoided, because they can impair uric acid excretion and may interfere with the actions of other gout medications.

Once an acute attack has been successfully treated, doctors try to prevent future attacks of gout and long-term joint damage by lowering uric acid levels in the blood. Colchicine is the drug of choice to deter recurrence. This medication can be very hard on the vascular system and the kidneys, however, and it is incompatible with a number of antidepressants, tranquilizers, and antihistamines. It should be avoided by pregnant women and the elderly.

There are two types of drugs used for lowering uric acid levels. Sometimes these drugs resolve the problem completely. However, the use of low-level amounts may be required for a lifetime. Uricosuric drugs, such as probenecid (Benemid) and sulfinpyrazone (Anturane), decrease urates in the blood by increasing their excretion. These drugs may also promote the formation of kidney stones, and they are contraindicated for patients with kidney disease. Xanthine oxidase inhibitors block the production of urates in the body. They can dissolve kidney stones as well as treat gout. Allopurinol is the drug most used in this respect. Its adverse effects include reactions with other medications, and the aggravation of existing skin, vascular, kidney, and liver dysfunction.

Expected results

Gout cannot be cured, but it can be managed successfully. Prompt attention to diet and reducing uric acid levels will rectify many of the problems associated with gout. Kidney problems can also be reversed or improved. Tophi can be dissolved or surgically removed, and with the tophi gone, joint mobility generally improves. Gout is generally more severe in those whose initial symptoms appear before age 30. The coexistence of **hypertension**, diabetes, or kidney disease can make for a much more serious condition.

Prevention

For centuries, gout has been known as the "rich man's disease," a disease of overindulgence in food and drink. While this view is perhaps oversimplified, lifestyle factors clearly influence a person's risk of developing gout. For example, losing weight and limiting alcohol intake can help ward off gout. Since purines are broken down into urates by the body, consumption of foods high in purine should be limited. Foods that are especially high in purines are red meat, organ meats, meat gravies, shellfish, sardines, anchovies, mushrooms, cooked spinach, rhubarb, yeast, asparagus, beer, and wine.

Dehydration promotes the formation of urate crystals, so people taking diuretics, or "water pills," may be better off switching to another type of blood pressure medication. Increased intake of fluids will dilute the urine and encourage excretion of uric acid. Therefore, six to eight glasses of water should be consumed daily, along with plenty of herbal teas and diluted fruit juices.

Consumption of saturated fats impedes uric acid excretion, and consumption of refined carbohydrates, such as sugar and white bread and pasta, increases uric acid production. Both should be seriously limited.

The use of **vitamin C** should be avoided by people with gout, due to the high levels of acidity.

Resources

BOOKS

Parker, James N., M.D., and Philip M. Parker, Ph. D. *The 2002 Official Patient's Sourcebook on Gout*. San Diego, CA: ICON Health Publications, 2002.

PERIODICALS

Arromdee, E., C. J. Michet, C. S. Crowson, et al. "Epidemiology of Gout: Is the Incidence Rising?" *Journal of Rheumatology* 29 (November 2002): 2403–2406.

Conos, Juan J., and Robert Kalish. "Gout: Effective Drug Therapy for Acute Attacks and for the Long Term." *Consultant* (August 1996): 1752– 55.

Emmerson, Bryan T. "The Management of Gout." *New England Journal of Medicine* (February 15, 1996): 445–451.

Hsu, C. Y., T. T. Shih, K. M. Huang, et al. "Tophaceous Gout of the Spine: MR Imaging Features." *Clinical Radiology* 57 (October 2002): 919–925.

Lin, J. L., D. T. Tan, H. H. Ho, and C. C. Yu. "Environmental Lead Exposure and Urate Excretion in the General Population." *American Journal of Medicine* 113 (November 2002): 563–568.

Perez-Ruiz, F., M. Calabozo, G. G. Erauskin, et al. "Renal Underexcretion of Uric Acid is Present in Patients with Apparent High Urinary Uric Acid Output." *Arthritis and Rheumatism* 47 (December 15, 2002): 610–613.

Raj, J. M., S. Sudhakar, K. Sems, and R. W. Carlson. "Arthritis in the Intensive Care Unit." *Critical Care Clinics* 18 (October 2002): 767–780.

Shekarriz, B., and M. L. Stoller. "Uric Acid Nephrolithiasis: Current Concepts and Controversies." *Journal of Urology* 168 (October 2002) (4 Pt 1): 1307–1314.

ORGANIZATIONS

Arthritis Foundation. 1330 W. Peachtree Street, P.O. Box 7669, Atlanta, GA 30357-0669. (800) 283-7800. http://www.arthritis.org.

National Institute of Arthritis and Musculoskeletal and Skin Diseases (NIAMS). National Institutes of Health (NIH), 1 AMS Circle, Bethesda, MD 20892-3675. <www.niams.nih/gov>.

OTHER

National Institute of Arthritis and Musculoskeletal and Skin Diseases (NIAMS). *Questions and Answers About Gout*. Bethesda, MD: NIAMS, 2002. NIH Publication No. 02-5027. <www.niams.nih.gov/hi/topics/gout/gout/htm>.

Patience Paradox
Rebecca J. Frey, PhD

KEY TERMS

Allopurinol—A drug that corrects hyperuricemia by inhibiting urate production.

Colchicine—A drug used to treat painful flare-ups of gout.

Constitutional remedy—A homeopathic medicine prescribed according to each person's character and temperament as well as symptoms.

Corticosteroids—Medications related to a natural body hormone called hydrocortisone, which are used to treat inflammation.

Hyperuricemia—High levels of uric acid in the bloodstream.

Kidney stones—Hard lumpy masses of mineral wastes that are formed in the kidneys and may cause blockages.

Purine—A substance found in foods that is broken down into urate and may contribute to hyperuricemia and gout.

Synovial fluid—Fluid surrounding the joints which acts as a lubricant, reducing the friction between the joints.

Tophus (plural, tophi)—A chalky deposit of a uric acid compound found in gout. Tophi occur most frequently around joints and in the external ear.

Grains-of-paradise fruit

Description

Grains-of-paradise fruit is a member of the Zingiberaceae family (**ginger** group), which is a major family of tropical and subtropical fruits. It is also known as Guinea grains, Melegueta pepper, Piper melegueta and *Aframomum melegueta roscoe,* which is its botanical name.

Aframomum melegueta roscoe is a perennial herb that produces a spicy edible fruit commonly found in the tropical regions, particularly of western Africa. It is somewhat palm-like in appearance, forming dense clumps and growing to a height of 4-5 ft (1.2-1.5 m), with divided smooth leaves that can be up to 9 in (23 cm) long.

There are two types of grains-of-paradise fruit. They resemble the spice cardamom in appearance and pungency, and the commercial variety is perhaps even closer in appearance and scent. True grains-of-paradise fruit tends to be less pungent than cardamom once cooked or heated, however.

The seeds are approximately oval in shape, hard, shiny, and reddish-brown color, whereas cardamom is pale buff-colored. Powdered grains-of-paradise fruit are pale gray. This spice is aromatic and can be distinguished by its hot peppery taste.

General use

In Africa and throughout the tropics, grains-of-paradise fruit (*Aframomum melegueta*) is a cultivated crop and is used as a remedy for a variety of ailments, although it is now rarely used outside these areas. It is one of the plants extensively made use of by African ethnomedicine.

Some confusion surrounds the identity of the true grains-of-paradise fruit, as approximately seven species of fruit are also sometimes mistakenly referred to as grains-of-paradise fruit, particularly *Malabar cardamom, Cardamomum malabaricum,* and *Cardamomum minus,* also the Zanzibar pepper. Grains-of-paradise fruit have even been confused with *Nux vomica,* which is used as a homeopathic remedy. In fact, it is now recognized that *Aframomum melegueta roscoe* is the authentic species. The name "grains-of-paradise fruit" dates from the Middle Ages, and denotes the fact that it was once a highly valued commodity. The west African coast became known as the Grain Coast because grains-of-paradise fruit was traded there.

Considered to be spicy, hot, and slightly bitter, the active constituents of grains-of-paradise fruit include **essential oils** such as gingerol, paradol, and shagaol. It also contains **manganese**, gum, tannin, starch, and a brown resin. It has been proven to be an effective antifungal and antimicrobial agent.

Like cardamom, it is also used as a condiment, due to its pleasant taste, which is pungent without being intensely bitter. It is mainly used nowadays to flavor wines, spirits, and particularly beer, although during the Middle Ages it was a favorite spice in Europe and other parts of the world. This spice, despite its popular beginnings, is hardly known outside of Africa today. Nevertheless, it remains popular as a spice in Arab cuisine, particularly Morocco and Tunisia. It has also been used as a pepper substitute, and may be chewed in cold weather to warm the body. In addition, it is a common addition to veterinary remedies.

The essential oil of grains-of-paradise is available, though not easy to find. Its properties are similar to those of the fruit, but it is often chosen for its fragrance. Grains-of-paradise fruit is used in African countries as an aphrodisiac as well as a treatment for **measles** and leprosy. Interestingly, extract of *Aframomum melegueta* has been shown in laboratory studies to increase sexual arousal and behavior in male rats. It is also used to reduce hemorrhage, particularly associated with **childbirth**.

Other phytomedicinal uses of grains-of-paradise include as a purgative (strong laxative), galactogogue (to increase production of breastmilk), anthelmintic (antiparasitic—it is effective against **worms**, etc.), and hemostatic agent (purifies the blood). It has even been found to be effective against the dreaded schistosomiasis, which is a major problem to the medical authorities on the African continent.

Grains-of-paradise fruit is also effective against intestinal **infections** and infestations, and is also used to calm **indigestion** and **heartburn**. Interestingly, grains-of-paradise fruit is one of the plants presently being researched as a possible alternative to allopathic medicines in tropical countries, where they are attempting to find cheaper and more readily available local phyto-medicinal alternatives to their common health problems, which are chiefly the effects of tropical diseases. Phyto-medicines have often proved to be more effective than synthetic agents. In addition they have a more sympathetic effect on the body, and their production is compatible with current environmental concerns.

Grains of paradise are also used in Chinese herbal medicine, their use being interchangeable with the more readily available cardamom. It is taken for **nausea** and **vomiting**, intestinal discomfort, and **pain** and discomfort during **pregnancy**.

KEY TERMS

Antifungal—A drug or compound effective in treating fungal infections.

Antimicrobial—A drug or medication effective against disease-causing micro-organisms.

Aphrodisiac—A food or drug that stimulates sexual desire.

Ethnomedicine—Medicine pertaining to a particular ethnic group.

Phytomedicinals—Medicinal substances derived from plants.

Schistosomiasis—Also called bilharziasis, this is a disease caused by bodily infestation of blood flukes.

Preparations

The fruit is exclusively the part of the plant used, dried, whole, or powdered. The essential oil can also be obtained. The whole grains may be chewed or can be ground and incorporated into mixtures.

Precautions

As grains-of-paradise fruit is a name given to so many other spices, it is advisable to ensure that the correct species is obtained.

Aframomum melegueta roscoe is included in the FDA's list of botanicals that are generally recognized as safe.

Side effects

No side effects have been reported from grains-of-paradise fruit as of 2002; however, this spice is not frequently used in the United States. People who are allergic to cardamom or ginger should use grains-of-paradise fruit with caution.

Interactions

As of 2002, no interactions have been reported with standard prescription medications.

Resources

BOOKS

Grieve, Mrs. M. F.R.H.S *A Modern Herbal.* London: Tiger Books International, 1992.

PERIODICALS

Kamtchouing, P., G. Y. Mbongue, T. Dimo, et al. "Effects of *Aframomum melegueta* and *Piper guineense* on Sexual Behaviour of Male Rats." *Behavioral Pharmacology* 13 (May 2002): 243-247.

ORGANIZATIONS

Centre for Economic Botany, Royal Botanic Gardens, Kew; Richmond, Surrey; TW9 3AE, United Kingdom. Fax: +44 (0)20 8332 5768. <www.rbgkew.org.uk>.

Centre for International Ethnomedicinal Education and Research (CIEER). <www.cieer.org>.

Patricia Skinner
Rebecca J. Frey, PhD

Grapefruit seed extract

Description

Grapefruit seed is prepared in extract form from the seeds, pulp, and white membranes of grapefruits from grapefruit trees (*Citrus paradisi*). The grapefruit tree, first discovered on the Caribbean island of Barbados in the seventeenth century, was brought to Florida in 1823 for commercial cultivation. The plant was probably named grapefruit because its fruits grow in bunches or clusters. Grapefruit seed extract (GSE) is used as a broad spectrum, non-toxic, antimicrobial compound. The extract comes in two forms, liquid and powder.

GSE was developed by Dr. Jacob Harich, a physicist who was born in Yugoslavia in 1919 and educated in Germany. His education in nuclear physics was interrupted by Word War II. After witnessing the horror of war as a fighter pilot, Harich decided to devote the rest of his life to improving the human condition. He then expanded his educational pursuits to include medicine, including gynecology and immunology. He came to the United States in 1957 to study at Long Island University in New York. As an immunologist, he was interested in studying natural substances that might help protect the body from undesirable microorganisms. In 1963, he moved to Florida, the heart of grapefruit country, and began research on the use of grapefruit seeds as a biocide. By 1990, holistic health practitioners began to recommend the use of GSE to their patients. In 1995, Harich was invited to the Pasteur Institute of France, a leading **AIDS** research center. Researchers at the Center have been investigating the potential of GSE as a prophylactic against the HIV virus as well as against some of the secondary **infections** associated with AIDS. He was also honored by farmers in Europe who use a powdered form of GSE in fish and poultry feed to control *Salmonella* and *Escherichia coli*. In 1996, Harich passed away.

General use

GSE is a broad spectrum bactericide, fungicide, antiviral, and antiparasitic compound. When used in vitro, GSE has been shown to be highly effective against a broad spectrum of bacteria, including *Staphyloccus aureus*, *Streptococcus pyogenes*, *Salmonella typhi*, *Escherichia coli*, *Pseudomonas aeruginosa*, *Klebsiella pneumoniae*, *Shigella dysenteriae*, *Legionella pneumoniae*, *Clostridium tetani*, *Diploccus pneumoniae*, and many others. GSE also strongly inhibits many types of pathogenic fungi and yeast.

Examples of external uses of GSE include:

- mouth and lips: mouthwash, mouth ulcers, thrush, **bad breath**, cracked lips, sunburned lips, and cold sores
- teeth and gums: plaque, tooth decay, toothaches, tooth extraction, gingivitis, and toothbrush cleaner
- nose and sinuses: sinusitis, runny nose (**rhinitis**), and nasal ulcer
- throat: **sore throat**, **tonsillitis**, coughs, hoarseness, and laryngitis
- ears: ear cleaning, earaches, and inflammation of the middle ear (otitis media) in conjunction with internal use
- face: **acne** and shaving
- scalp and hair: shampoo, **dandruff**, **itching** scalp, and head lice
- skin: small cuts, skin abrasions, scratches, minor **burns**, **rashes**, **dermatitis**, **psoriasis**, **shingles**, **eczema**, **nettle** rash, insect **bites and stings**, tick and leech bites, leg ulcers, **warts**, and skin fungi
- feet: **athlete's foot**, sweaty feet, calluses, corns, **blisters**, nail fungi, and cuticular infections
- vagina and genitals: **vaginitis**, yeast infections, vaginal parasites, feminine hygiene, and fungal and parasitic diseases in the male genital area

Examples of internal uses include:

- acute and chronic inflammations in general
- colds and flu
- gastrointestinal infections
- vastritis and gastric and duodenal ulcers
- *Candida albicans* and other fungal diseases
- parasitic diseases
- allergies

Preparations

Grapefruit seeds and pulp contain a combination of **bioflavonoids** and polyphenolic compounds. The polyphenols are unstable but are chemically converted during the GSE synthesis process into more stable substances that belong to a class of compounds called quaternary ammonium compounds. The active quaternary ammonium compound in GSE believed to be responsible for its antimicrobial properties is a diphenol hydroxybenzene complex. The antimicrobial activity appears to develop in the cytoplasmic membrane of the microorganisms. The active ingredients disorganize the cytoplasmic membrane so that the uptake of **amino acids** is prevented. At the same time there is a leakage of low molecular weight cellular contents through the cytoplasmic membrane. Studies have also shown that GSE inhibits cellular respiration.

The extract is prepared by grinding grapefruit seeds and pulp into a fine powder. The powder is dissolved into purified water and distilled to remove fiber and pectin. The distilled slurry is spray dried at low temperatures forming a concentrated grapefruit bioflavonoid powder. This concentrated powder is dissolved in vegetable glycerin and heated. Food grade ammonium chloride and ascorbic acid are added. This mixture is heated under pressure where it undergoes catalytic conversion using natural catalysts, including hydrochloric acid and natural enzymes. The slurry is then cooled, filtered, and treated with ultraviolet light. Residual ammonium chloride in the final product is between 15 and 18%; residual ascorbic acid is between 25 and 35 mg/kg. There is no residue of hydrochloric acid in the final product. In the United States, standardized GSE contains 60% grapefruit extract materials and 40% vegetable glycerin. A powdered form of GSE is also available that contains 50% grapefruit extract materials, 30% silicon dioxide, and 20% vegetable glycerine.

To treat infections, 15 drops in 8 oz of water is used. For diaper yeast infections and as a vaginal douche, 10–15 drops of grapefruit seed extract is used in 4 oz of water.

Precautions

GSE has been shown to be non-toxic at levels many times greater than the recommended dosages. Even when taken daily, GSE seldom produces a significant allergic reaction. However, people who are allergic to citrus fruits should exercise caution in the use of GSE.

Citricidal®, the brand name of a GSE product in the United States containing 60% grapefruit seed extract in an aqueous, vegetable glycerine solution, has, in the United States, been labeled as GRAS (Generally Recognized as Safe) in the Code of Regulations. The Food and Drug Administration (FDA) has approved Citricidal® for cosmetic preparations. In addition, Citricidal® has also been approved by the FDA for the disinfection of foods.

Generally, GSE should never be used at full strength. GSE is extremely irritating to the eyes. If it gets into the eyes, a person should wash the eyes with large amounts of warm water and consult a physician, if necessary.

After an excessive ingestion of GSE, an individual should drink large amounts of water and take up to 3 tsp of **psyllium** husks (or up to 6 psyllium capsules). A doctor should be consulted, if necessary.

Side effects

Since GSE is quite acidic, if it is not properly diluted, it may further irritate already irritated tissues, such as a stomach or intestinal lining.

Interactions

Over 75 different combination herbal preparations containing GSE are available, based on the assumption of Chinese herbal medicine that combinations of substances are more beneficial than single remedies. In addition, the antimicrobial properties of GSE make it an excellent preservative, thus enabling the herbs it accompanies to retain their potency.

Resources

BOOKS

Sachs, Allan. *The Authoritative Guide to Grapefruit Seed Extract.* Mendocino, CA: Life Rhythm, 1997.

Sharamon, Shalila and Bodo J. Baginski. *The Healing Power of Grapefruit Seed.* Twin Lakes, WI: Lotus Light Publications, 1995.

Judith Sims

Grape seed extract

Description

Grape seed extract is the primary commercial source of a group of powerful **antioxidants** known as oligomeric proanthocyanidins (OPCs), also generically called pycnogenol, a class of flavonoids. Laboratory studies have indicated OPCs are much more effective than **vitamin C** and **vitamin E** in neutralizing free oxygen radicals, which contribute to organ degeneration and **aging** in humans. The primary sources of OPCs are **pine bark extract** and grape seed extract. However, the grape seed extract is more widely recommended for its lower cost and because it contains an antioxidant not found in pine bark.

General use

Grape seed extract is a mixture of complex compounds. It has a wide range of therapeutic uses, from preventing **cancer** and cardiovascular disease to alleviating symptoms of **allergies**, ulcers, and **cataracts**. Its antioxidant properties are believed to help slow the aging process. Procyanidins, a group of compounds found in the extract, are thought to increase the effectiveness of other antioxidants, especially vitamin C and vitamin E, by helping them regenerate after neutralizing free radicals in the blood and tissue. OPCs in the extract are water-soluble, making them easily absorbed by the body. They also are able to cross the stubborn blood-brain barrier, providing antioxidant protection to the brain and nervous system. Most of the research on grape seed extract has been done in Europe, so many of its reported benefits have not been reviewed or approved by the U.S. Food and Drug Administration. It is available as an over-the-counter supplement. According to Varro E. Tyler, dean emeritus of the Purdue University School of Pharmacy and Pharmacal Sciences, the procyanidin compounds found in grape seed extract are useful in treating vascular disorders They also are antioxidants, or free-radical scavengers, that help prevent some age-related cancers and **atherosclerosis**. Grape seed extract is a relatively new supplement in the United States, although it has been used in Europe for several decades. Its antioxidant properties were realized in the 1980s with the so-called French paradox, in which researchers discovered that the French had low rates of **heart disease** even though their diet was high in **cholesterol**. This was credited to their widespread consumption of red wine. Further research led to the OPCs concentrated in grape seeds. More recent research suggests that grape seed extract may work at the genetic level, activating a gene that stops oxidation of bad cholesterol. A 2003 study found that grape seed extract worked well in replacing estrogen and blunting **hypertension** in postmenopausal women.

Cardiovascular disease

European studies have shown procyanidins to be useful in treating blood vessel disorders, such as fragile capillaries and poor circulation in the veins. Components bind to the walls of the capillaries, making them less likely to break down with the effects of aging. In one European study, researchers found that treatment with grape seed extract quickly relieved a chronic condition of poor circulation in the veins. Grape seed extract also has been beneficial in treating **edema**, an excessive accumulation of fluid in tissue. Another use of grape seed extract is reducing blood pressure in people with hypertension. A study published in 1998 by cardiovascular researchers at the University of California, Davis, found that flavonoids in the extract helped increase flow in blood vessels, contributing to better regulation of blood pressure.

Cancer

A study published in 1998 by a team of researchers at Creighton University, Georgetown University Medical

Center, and the University of Nebraska at Omaha, reported that grape seed extract significantly inhibited and sometimes killed human cancer cells, while promoting the growth of normal healthy cells. The extract was effective in killing 34–48% of breast, lung, and stomach cancer cells. It was not effective in destroying **leukemia** cells. Other studies have shown grape seed extract, combined with other antioxidants, can reduce the overall risk of developing cancer.

Respiratory conditions

Grape seed extract has been found to be beneficial in treating several respiratory conditions, including **asthma**, **emphysema**, allergies, and sinusitis. Pycnogenol helps inhibit the production of histamines, which decreases sensitivity to pollens and food allergens, thereby reducing allergic reactions.

Other conditions

OPCs in grape seed extract have shown effectiveness in treating a variety of other conditions. As an anti-inflammatory, it helps prevent swelling of joints, heals damaged tissue, and eases **pain** in people with arthritis. Studies have shown OPCs can stop cataract progression, treat and prevent **glaucoma**, and aid in treating several types of retinal disease. One of the extract's most popular uses is in treating the effects of aging, including preventing wrinkles by protecting the skin against ultraviolet radiation damage from **sunburn**, improving skin elasticity and tone, and helping reduce the appearance of scars and stretch marks. A wide range of anecdotal reports tell of grape seed extract helping treat or reduce the effects of headaches, **hemorrhoids**, diabetes, **prostate enlargement**, and **cellulite**, although no clinical research supports these claims.

Preparations

Grape seed extract generally is available in 50 mg (milligram) and 100 mg capsules. The acceptable adult daily dosage has been estimated at up to 150-200 mg, or 50 mg per 50 lb (22.7 kg) of body weight. In Europe, OPCs usually are prescribed at 300 mg a day to treat medical conditions such as **varicose veins**, edema, allergies, inflammation, and skin aging. The extract contains varying amounts of proanthocyanics, although the label should indicate about 75–80% proanthocyanidins to be effective. Research in the United States and Europe has shown it is most effective when used in combination with other antioxidants, especially vitamin C and vitamin E. Grape seed extract is fully absorbed by the body within one hour after consumption. One-half the original dose is still functional within the body after seven hours.

In 2003, a liquid grape seed extract was made available in the United States. This version can be used in a number of beverages, including bottled water, without changing their taste. A 2003 trial at Ohio State University found that lotions made with grape seed extract helped cuts heal more quickly than they would on their own. The lotion helped improve blood flow to the wound site.

Precautions

There are no known precautions associated with grape seed extract. However, persons with serious conditions such as cancer, diabetes, and cardiovascular disease should not substitute grape seed extract for their existing treatments without first consulting with their doctor. There is no clinical evidence that grape seed extract can cure any of these conditions. Since grape seed extract is water-soluble, any excess intake that is not used by the body is eliminated in the urine. Studies have shown it is not carcinogenic, does not cause birth defects, and does not cause cells to mutate. Pregnant women and those with autoimmune conditions should probably avoid grape seed extracts. It is best to check with a clinician to ensure the safest dosage is being taken, as reports may vary on the latest research.

Side effects

Nausea and upset stomach have been reported on occasion. More rarely, allergic reactions in the form of temporary skin **rashes** have occurred in persons sensitive to grape products. There are no reported serious side effects associated with taking grape seed extract. It is non-toxic, even at high dosages.

Interactions

There are no reported negative interactions associated with grape seed extract. However, several studies done in the United States and Europe show the extract has a positive reaction with vitamin C and vitamin E. Studies have shown that OPCs in grape seed extract are as much as 50 times more potent than those in vitamin E and up to 20 times more potent than OPCs in vitamin C.

Resources

BOOKS

Balch, James F. *The Super Antioxidants.* New York: M. Evans and Co., 1998.

Schwitters, Bert. *OPC in Practice, 3rd edition.* Rome: Alfa Omega Editrice, 1995.

PERIODICALS

Dolby, Victoria. "Grape Seeds Pack a Healthy 'Punch' of Proanthocyanidins." *Better Nutrition* (March 1997): 32.

Good, Brian. "A Grape Way to Recover." *Men's Health* (May 2003): 44.

"Grape Seed Antioxidant Extract." *Nutraceuticals World* (June 2003): 93.

"Grape Seed Extract May Be Useful Supplement in Postmenopausal Women." *Heart Disease Weekly* (May 11, 2003): 66.

Langer, Stephen. "Antioxidants: Our Knights in Shining Armor." *Better Nutrition* (May 1997): 46-50.

Sarubin Fragakis, Allison. "Heart Protection After Menopause: Grape Seed's Antioxidant Effect." *Prevention* (October 2003): 55.

Smith, Elizabeth A. "Purple Power." *Drug Topics* (June 1, 1998): 40.

Tyler, Varro E. "Grape Expectations." *Prevention* (June 1997): 80-83.

Tyler, Varro E. "The Miracle of Anti-Aging Herbs." *Prevention* (Nov. 1999): 105.

Ken R. Wells
Teresa G. Odle

Grape skin

Description

Appearance

Grape skin, the outer layer of the grape (*Vitis vinifera*), is either green, red, or purplish-black in color. The skin, stem, seeds, and juice of the grape are used in making wine. Although the skin, stem, and seeds are often used in making the nutritional supplement, grape skin extract, the extract sometimes contains grape skin only. Generally, the skin of red grapes is used in making nutritional supplements.

History

In 1535, sailors on Jacques Cartier's expedition to Canada became seriously ill with scurvy, a vitamin deficiency. This degenerative disease of connective tissues was caused by the lack of vitamins in the typical seafarer's diet—a menu of dried meat and biscuits. The crew was saved by the advice of a Native American, who recommended drinking tea made from the bark of a particular species of pine tree. In the 1930s, researchers discovered that the ascorbic acid (**vitamin C**) in fruits and vegetables prevented scurvy.

The pine extract, however, contained very little vitamin C. For more than 50 years, European biochemists have been researching the seafarers' more likely rescuer—a family of antioxidant polyphenols (acid compounds) called pycnogenols, whose primary active compounds are pigments called oligomeric proanthocyanidins (OPCs). French chemist Jack Masquelier isolated OPCs from peanut skins in 1947 and coined the term "pycnogenols" to describe the unique class of polyphenols to which OPCs belong.

Although people have been drinking wine for centuries, scientific research into the health benefits of products derived from red grapes began in Europe in the mid to late twentieth century. Supplemental OPCs have been used in Europe since 1950 to treat weak blood capillaries, postsurgical **edema** (swelling), **cirrhosis** (liver disease), **varicose veins**, and diabetic **retinopathy** (eye disease resulting from diabetes). Early identification of OPCs as useful for treating capillary fragility gave researchers some indication of their potential value in connective tissue disorders. However, this limited focus tended to overlook the additional therapeutic possibilities of OPCs and, until the latter part of the twentieth century, distracted scientists from investigating broader uses for OPCs.

Aside from pine bark, OPCs are concentrated in grape seeds and skins, wine, green and black teas, beans, and the skins of many fruits. Generally, the more intense the color, the more OPCs in the food, which explains why red wine has a greater health benefit than white wine. When red wine is made, the "must" is used—the skins, seeds, and stems. The must is left in the mixture for a long period of time as the wine ferments and the OPCs emerge, giving red wine its characteristic flavor and color.

In the case of white wine, however, the must is taken out early, so the wine neither darkens nor absorbs as many OPCs. Grape juice also contains OPCs. However,

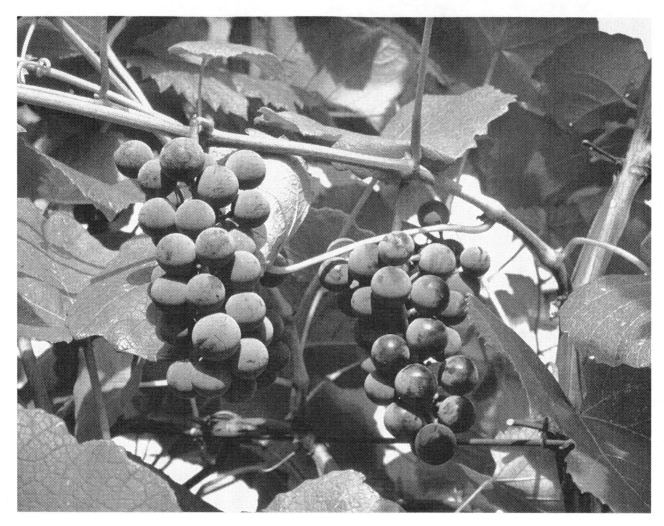

Purple grapes. *(Photograph by James Lee Sikkema. Reproduced by permission.)*

researchers have found that grape juice may not confer the same health benefits as red wine.

Biologic components

Red grape skins contain an array of **bioflavonoids** (quercetin, catechins, flavonols, and anthocyanidins) and nonbioflavonoid polyphenols (acid derivatives). One important nonbioflavonoid in grape skin is called resveratrol. Resveratrol is a plant-specific enzyme that exists in 72 plant species, such as grapes, peanuts, and pine trees. Grapes are the most abundant source of this health-promoting enzyme.

Resveratrol's presence in the plant is induced by **stress**, injury, infection or ultraviolet irradiation. It is thought that the injury to the grape skin, produced during the wine-making process, significantly increases resveratrol levels. The relatively high quantities of the enzyme in the grape skins are thought to help the plant resist **fun-gal infections**, diseases, adverse weather, and insect or animal attack.

General use

There are many possible therapeutic applications of the resveratrol in red grape skin. In clinical studies, resveratrol demonstrated equivalent or better anti-inflammatory effects compared to the well-established anti-inflammatory drugs phenylbutazone and indomethacin. In animal studies, resveratrol inhibited both the acute and chronic phases of inflammation.

In humans, some researchers have found that resveratrol thins the blood more effectively than aspirin, which is often used to decrease the risk of a **heart attack**. In fact, the phrase "French paradox" refers to the idea that although French men consume a high-fat diet, they have one-third as many heart attacks as American men. Moreover, French men have high **cholesterol** and blood pressure levels similar to their American counterparts. Researchers have discovered that the main reason for this phenomenon is the OPCs from the grape skin, not the alcohol content, in the red wine that the French drink.

Preliminary tests in animals also indicate that resveratrol may interfere with the development of **cancer** in three ways: by blocking the action of cancer-causing agents, by inhibiting the development and growth of tumors, and by causing precancerous cells to revert to normal.

Although researchers are uncertain about how much resveratrol is needed to produce beneficial effects in humans, supplementation with red grape skin extract or consuming a glass or two of red wine may prevent or alleviate the following conditions:

- aging
- bruising (capillary fragility)
- cancer (cancer-inhibiting effects)
- diabetes
- fungal infection
- heart disease (hardening of the arteries and high cholesterol)
- inflammation (including **bursitis** and tendonitis)
- Raynaud's syndrome (a blood vessel disorder)
- varicose veins
- vision problems (including **cataracts** and glaucoma)
- wound healing

Preparations

Red grape skin extract is prepared in capsule form as a nutritional supplement. For adult maintenance, the therapeutic range is thought to be 200–600 mg at 30% anthocyanins (OPCs), although guidelines have not been definitively established.

The resveratrol found in red grape skin and its extract is also found in red wine and concord grape juice. However, grape juice has been found to have fewer benefits than red wine, due to the technique for processing the grapes. For example, grape juice has only one-third the anti-clotting properties of red wine.

Precautions

Although research is limited, scientific investigators have not issued any precautions regarding the use of grape skin or grape skin extract. However, people should be aware of the known side effects of red wine and resveratrol.

Side effects

There are many potential side effects to consuming excessive quantities of red wine (such as allergic reactions to sulfites, intoxication, and liver damage) in order to obtain the health benefits of resveratrol. Each individual must weigh the risks versus the benefits of consuming alcohol.

However, resveratrol itself is also a phytoestrogen (plant estrogen). The estrogenic properties of this chemical may play a role in the beneficial cardiovascular effects in red wine. These positive effects include increasing high-density lipoprotein (HDL), the "good cholesterol." On the other hand, it has been noted that drinking red wine may support the proliferation of certain **breast cancer** cells that require estrogen for growth. Thus, resveratrol may have undesirable side effects in some people, including those women with a history of breast cancer or postmenopausal women taking hormone replacement therapy.

Interactions

Scientific investigation on the interactions of grape skin or grape skin extract with drugs, foods, or diseases is very limited and inconclusive. However, if the resveratrol in grape skin is consumed in red wine, a wide range of adverse interactions with drugs and foods may result. It is advisable to consult a physician before consuming alcohol in combination with any type of prescription or over-the-counter medication.

Resources

PERIODICALS

Broiher, Kitty. "Red Wine's Health Benefits May Be Due in Part to 'Estrogen' in Red Wine." *Food Processing* (April 1999): 58.

Fine, Anne Marie. "Oligomeric Pranthocyanidin Complexes: History, Structure, and Phytopharmaceutical Applications." *Alternative Medicine Review* 5 no. 2 (2000): 144–151.

"Grape Compound May Inhibit Cancer." *Cancer Weekly Plus* (January 1994): 13–15.

Maxwell, Simon, Alison Cruikshank, and Gary Thorpe. "Red Wine and Antioxidant Activity in Serum." *The Lancet* (July 1994): 193–194.

Tyler, Varro E. "Grape Expectations." *Prevention* (June 1997): 80–84.

Whitehead, Tom P. et al. "Effect of Red Wine Ingestion on the Antioxidant Capacity of Serum." *Clinical Chemistry* 41 (Jan. 1995): 32–35.

ORGANIZATIONS

American Heart Association, National Center. 7272 Greenville Avenue, Dallas, TX 75231. http://www.americanheart.org.

National Cancer Institute. Public Inquiries Office, Building 31, Room 10A03, 31 Center Drive, MSC 2580, Bethesda, MD 20892. http://www.nci.nih.gov.

Genevieve Slomski

Graves' disease *see* **Hyperthyroidism**

Green tea

Description

Green tea is produced from the leaves of the *Camellia sinensis*, or tea plant. Oolong and black tea are also produced from the plant, but are processed and oxidized in different manners. Of the three, green tea contains the highest levels of polyphenols, the antioxidant substance that is believed to be beneficial in protecting against both **cancer** and **atherosclerosis**.

The tea plant is actually a variation of evergreen bush, with glossy green leaves and small white to pink flowers. The plants can reach a height of 30–40 ft (9–12 m) or taller in the wild, but are generally kept to a height of 6 ft (1.2 m) or less on the tea plantations and gardens where they are grown in China, Argentina, Japan, India, Indonesia, Kenya, Malawi, Sri Lanka, Turkey, Pakistan, Bangladesh, and Tanzania. Tea plants are cultivated in countries where warm, rainy growing conditions are abundant, and are also frequently grown in high altitude areas.

When tea plants reach maturity at three or four years of age, the young leaves and leaf buds—the parts of the plant highest in polyphenols—are harvested. Green tea is produced by steaming or roasting the leaves as soon as they are picked, and then rolling and drying the tea leaves to remove any moisture.

General use

Approximately 2.5 million tons of tea are grown and produced worldwide on an annual basis. Written records date the use of the plant as a beverage since at least the tenth century B.C. in China, and it is thought to be close to 5,000 years old. Tea is the most consumed beverage worldwide (after water). It is also one of the most popular herbal infusions in existence—drunk regularly by over half the world population.

The polyphenols in green tea that act as **antioxidants** may actually inhibit the growth of existing cancer cells. In some animal studies, injections of tea extracts reduced the size of cancerous tumors in animals. The active agent that is thought to have this effect is an antioxidant, epigallocatechin-3-gallate (EGCG).

Recent clinical studies have also indicated that regular use of green tea may reduce the risk of certain types of cancer, including oral, skin, prostate, colon, stomach, and rectal. In one clinical trial, patients with pre-cancerous mouth lesions who were treated with green and black tea extracts achieved a 38% decrease in the number of pre-cancerous cells. Late in 2001, researchers acknowledged one reason for green tea's anticancer effect, but further human studies are needed to clearly define its role in cancer prevention.

The antioxidants in green tea may also be helpful in lowering **cholesterol** and preventing hardening of the arteries and ischemic **heart disease**. Low flavonoid intake has been linked to atherosclerosis in several studies. The data from one 1999 study, which followed more than 3,400 tea-drinking residents of Rotterdam, the Netherlands, concluded that regular, long-term tea consumption can have a protective effect against severe atherosclerosis.

Another preliminary study published in 1999 in the *American Journal of Clinical Nutrition* found that green tea extract may increase energy levels and promote fat oxidation, and consequently, may be a useful tool in weight control. A recent study, reported on in early 2002, showed that topically applied green tea extracts can reduce harmful effects of radiation from the sun. Further study might show that green tea polyphenol applications can help prevent sunburns.

In addition to polyphenols, green tea contains several minerals, including fluoride and aluminum. The fluoride in green tea may be useful in fighting tooth decay. Green tea is also an antibacterial agent, and can help to prevent gingivitis and periodontal disease by killing *E. coli* and streptococcus bacteria. This antibacterial action can also be effective in treating halitosis, or **bad breath**, by killing odor-causing bacteria.

As an herbal remedy, green tea is often recommended to ease stomach discomfort, **vomiting**, and to stop **diarrhea**. The antibacterial action of tea is useful in treating **infections** and **wounds**.

Preparations

Green tea leaves and tea bags can be purchased at most grocery, drug, and health food stores. It is graded by leaf size, with tea containing whole leaves and leaf tips considered the highest quality tea. Tea grades include Broken Orange, Pekoe, Broken Pekoe Souchong, Broken Orange Pekoe, Fannings, and Dust.

Although green tea is grown from a single plant, slight variations in tea processing (usually in the way the tea is rolled) have created a number of varieties of green tea. Popular green tea varieties include Gunpowder, Hyson, Dragonwell, Sencha, and Matcha.

Tea leaves should be kept in an air-tight container to retain flavor and prevent odors and moisture from being absorbed by the tea. It should also be stored in a cool place for no longer than six months before use.

The most common method of preparing green tea is as an infusion. The tea is mixed with boiling water, steeped for several minutes, and then strained or removed from the infusion before drinking. Approximately two teaspoons of loose tea, or a single tea bag, should be used for each cup of boiling water. A strainer, tea ball, or infuser can be used to immerse loose tea in the boiling water before steeping and separating it.

A second method of infusion is to mix loose tea with cold water first, bring the mixture to a boil in a pan or teapot, and then separate the tea from the infusion with a strainer before drinking.

Flavonoids—polyphenols with antioxidative properties—are released into the infusion as the tea steeps. The longer the steeping time, the more flavonoids are released by the tea leaves, although most will infuse into the water during the first five minutes of brewing. Longer steeping time also results in a higher **caffeine** content in the brewed tea.

Green tea leaves can be used in a poultice for treating insect bites and other skin irritations. Green tea leaves are chopped and boiled in water for two to three minutes. After the excess water is squeezed from the leaves, the green tea is applied to the area to be treated and wrapped in a bandage. Green tea also makes an effective astringent, and tea-soaked cloth or tea leaf poultice may help renew tired and puffy eyes.

The antibacterial activity of green tea also makes it appropriate for use in compresses for cuts and abrasions. A quick compress can be made by soaking a pad or ban-

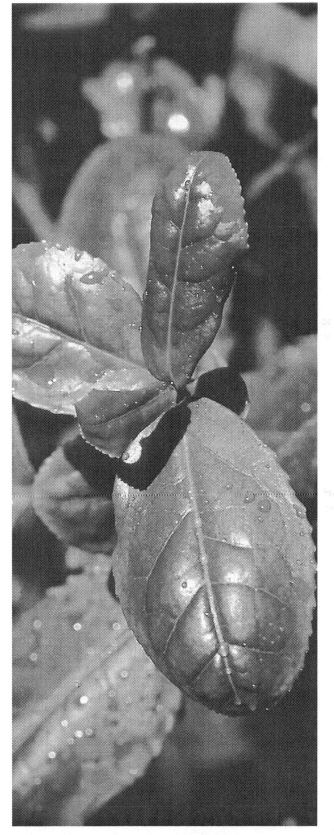

Green tea plant. (© *PlantaPhile, Germany. Reproduced by permission.*)

dage in hot tea, wringing out the excess fluid, and holding the pad firmly against the wound. Once the compress cools, the process can be repeated.

Precautions

The U.S. Food and Drug Administration (FDA) includes tea on their list of "Generally Recognized As Safe" substances. However, pregnant women and women who breast feed should consider limiting their intake of green tea because of its caffeine content. Tea can pass into breast milk and cause **sleep disorders** in nursing infants. Decaffeinated green tea is available that contains only trace amounts (5 mg or less) of caffeine. Women should check with their healthcare professional about drinking tea when pregnant or nursing.

Tea can stimulate the production of gastric acid, and individuals with ulcers may want to avoid drinking green tea for this reason. Those taking warfarin or any blood-thinning drugs should first consult with the physicians before consuming green tea, as it may counter the effects of the drug.

Side effects

Green tea contains caffeine, a central nervous system (CNS) stimulant that can cause restlessness, irritability, difficulty sleeping, tremor, heart palpitations, loss of appetite, and upset stomach. To avoid side effects, caffeine intake should be limited to 300 mg or less a day (the equivalent of 4–8 cups of brewed hot tea). Caffeine-free green tea preparations are available commercially.

The tannin in tea can cause **nausea** when drunk on an empty stomach and inhibit the absorption of non-heme **iron**. Individuals with iron-deficiency **anemia** who take iron supplements should avoid drinking green tea several hours before and after taking supplements. Iron absorption with tea can be increased by consuming foods rich in **vitamin C** with tea, such as a slice of lemon.

Resources

BOOKS

Mitscher, Lester A., and Victoria Dolby. *The Green Tea Book.* New York: Penguin Putnam, 1998.

Rosen, Diana. *The Book of Green Tea.* Pownal, VT: Storey, 1998.

PERIODICALS

"Anticancer Mechanism of Green Tea Identified." *Cancer Weekly* (January 1, 2002): 16.

Bates, Betsy. "Green Tea Extract May Help Prevent Sun Damage (Potential Chemopreventive Agents)." *Skin and Allergy News* (January 2002): 30.

Dulloo, Abdul G., et al. "Efficacy of a Green Tea Extract Rich in Catechin Polyphenols and Caffeine in Increasing 24-h

---

KEY TERMS

Antioxidants—Enzymes that bind with free radicals to neutralize their harmful effects.

Atherosclerosis—A type of arteriosclerosis, or hardening of the arteries, caused by fatty deposits of cholesterol and calcium that build up on the interior walls of the blood vessels and arteries.

Chemopreventative—A chemical or drug that is thought to prevent a disease.

Flavonoids—Polyphenol substances in tea that act as antioxidants.

Free radicals—Reactive molecules created during cell metabolism that can cause tissue and cell damage like that which occurs in aging and with disease processes such as cancer.

Gingivitis—Inflamed and bleeding gums caused by poor dental hygiene, respiratory diseases, and other disease processes.

Infusion—An herbal preparation made by mixing boiling water with an herb, letting the brew steep for 10 minutes, and then straining the herb out of the mixture.

Non-heme iron—Dietary or supplemental iron that is less efficiently absorbed by the body than heme iron (ferrous iron).

Periodontal disease—Disease of the gums and teeth. Symptoms include bleeding and receding gums, gingivitis, abscesses, and loose teeth.

Phytochemical—A naturally occurring chemical substance in a plant.

Polyphenols—Phytochemicals that act as an antioxidant, protecting cells against damaging free radicals.

Energy Expenditure and Fat Oxidation in Humans." *American Journal of Clinical Nutrition* (December 1999): 1040–1045.

Geleijnse, Johanna M., et al. "Tea Flavonoids May Protect Against Atherosclerosis: The Rotterdam Study." *Archives of Internal Medicine* 159 (October 11, 1999): 2170–2174.

Hertli, Peter. "Green Tea and Blood Thinners Don't Mix (Mailbag)." *Prevention* (March 2002): 24.

Mukhtar, H., and N. Ahmad. "Green Tea in Chemoprevention of Cancer." *Toxicological Sciences* 52 (December 1999): 111–7.

Paula Ford-Martin
Teresa G. Odle

Grippe *see* **Influenza**

Guggul

Description

The mukul **myrrh** tree, or *Commiphora mukul*, is small, thorny, and usually devoid of foliage. It grows naturally throughout India and Arabia. Guggul is the gum resin that comes from this tree, which belongs to the same genus as myrrh and has some similar components and actions. Guggul resin contains steroids, diterpenoids, alipathic esters, and carbohydrates. These factors appear to work together to exert the beneficial effects of this botanical.

Guggul has been traditionally used in **Ayurvedic medicine** to treat arthritis, inflammation, bone **fractures**, overweight, and disorders of lipid metabolism. One ancient Ayurvedic reference describes the power of guggul to treat "coating and obstruction of channels." This description stimulated further research into the properties of this **botanical medicine** for preventing and treating **atherosclerosis**, as well as other conditions resulting from high levels of lipids in the body.

General use

Guggul has been recommended for the treatment of arthritis, hypercholesterolemia, nodulocystic **acne**, and overweight. It is one of the primary therapeutic substances used in Ayurvedic medicine to prevent atherosclerosis, as well as one of the most promising herbs or supplements for the prevention and treatment of this condition. Studies in animals have documented not only the protective effects of guggul against atherosclerosis, but have shown actual regression of the condition in animals that already had it.

The active portion of the plant is the gum resin, which contains guggulsterone, a steroid compound. It appears to be effective in lowering blood levels of both total **cholesterol** and low-density lipoprotein (LDL) cholesterol. In trials lasting one to three months, cholesterol levels were reduced by 14–27% and triglycerides by 22–30%. These results are equal to or better than those of some conventional medications used to lower cholesterol, but with fewer side effects. There are several hypotheses to account for the effectiveness of guggul in decreasing serum lipids. It may decrease the production of cholesterol in the liver. Excretion of cholesterol and bile acids are increased, so that less fat and cholesterol are absorbed. Guggul also increases the production of thyroid hormones, which lower the levels of serum lipids. The lowering of serum lipids is what consequently decreases the risk of atherosclerosis. One of the most important ways that gugulipid lowers cholesterol may be by stimulating the liver to remove LDLs from the bloodstream. The effect on high-density lipoprotein (HDL) cholesterol is undetermined, as two studies yielded different conclusions. To lower cholesterol, one recommended dose of gugulipid is 100–500 mg taken daily. This dosage contains 25 mg of guggulsterone. It may take a month or so for the full effect to be experienced. Similar doses of gugulipid are used to promote weight loss.

The thyroid gland is stimulated by guggulsterone. This effect may play a role both in the ability of the substance to decrease cholesterol levels and to promote weight loss by increasing the body's rate of metabolism.

Guggulsterone has significant anti-inflammatory properties, although they are somewhat overshadowed by its effects on lipid metabolism. This finding supports its traditional use in the treatment of **rheumatoid arthritis** and other inflammatory conditions. Studies have shown guggulsterone to be at least as effective as the conventional medications phenylbutazone and ibuprofen (Advil, Motrin) for both acute and chronic types of inflammation in animal models.

Platelet stickiness appears to be reduced by guggul, which is desirable for decreasing the risk of coronary artery disease. Guggul may also promote fibrinolysis (dissolving the fibrin in **blood clots**) and act as an antioxidant. More research is warranted for these properties. They have potential benefits in the prevention of strokes and embolisms.

Studies have shown guggulsterone to have approximately the same effectiveness as the antibiotic tetracycline for the treatment of nodulocystic acne. It decreases inflammation and lowers the risk of recurrence of the condition. Guggul is also thought to have astringent, antiseptic, and antisuppurative (preventing pus formation) qualities that lend themselves to the treatment of this severe, and sometimes scarring, form of acne.

Preparations

In India, guggul has been a standard and approved treatment for high cholesterol since 1986. Guggul is most often available in tablet or capsule form, as a purified extract. Formulations should have a standardized concentration of guggulsterone. Most extracts contain from 5–10% guggulsterone. It is readily available in the United States, but available only by prescription, if at all, in the United Kingdom.

Gugulipid is also a component of some combination nutritional products that are being promoted for the support of normal metabolism of cholesterol and triglycerides. Other components may include inositol hexaniacinate, **chromium**, and vitamin **antioxidants**.

Precautions

Studies in both humans and animals have demonstrated a wide margin of safety and negligible toxicity for guggul, although some cases of liver toxicity have been reported for very high doses. Although it is apparently not toxic to the embryo or fetus either, guggul gum resin should not be used during **pregnancy** or lactation as it is thought to be a uterine stimulant.

Patients who are taking prescribed medications for **heart disease** should use caution in taking this herb.

Side effects

Crude extracts of guggul are more likely to produce side effects than purer products. In the past, effects included loss of appetite, abdominal **pain**, **diarrhea**, and **rashes**. In studies using purer extracts, significant adverse effects have not occurred. **Headache** and mild **nausea** are sometimes reported.

Interactions

Guggul can be problematic for people being treated for thyroid conditions. Since guggul stimulates production of thyroid hormone, it may alter the dosage requirements for thyroid replacement medication. It can also reduce the availability and effectiveness of the heart medications propranolol (Inderal) and diltiazem (Cardizem). Patients should consult a health care practitioner before taking guggul along with any other herbs or medications.

Resources

BOOKS

Bratman, Steven, and David Kroll. *The Natural Health Bible.* Rocklin, CA: Prima Publishing, 1999.

Chevallier, Andrew. *The Encyclopedia of Medicinal Plants.* New York: DK Publishing Inc., 1996.

Lininger, Skye, et. al. *The Natural Pharmacy.* Rocklin, CA: Prima Publishing, 1998.

Murray, Michael T. *The Healing Power of Herbs.* Rocklin, CA: Prima Publishing, 1995.

OTHER

Schauss, Alexander, and Suzanne Munson. *Guggul (Commiphora mukul): Chemistry, Toxicology, and Efficacy of a Hypolipidemic and Hypocholesterolemic Agent.* http://www.nat-med.com/archives/guggul.htm (2000).

Judith Turner

Guided imagery

Definition

Guided imagery is the use of **relaxation** and mental visualization to improve mood and/or physical well-being.

Benefits

The connection between the mind and physical health has been well documented and extensively studied. Positive mental imagery can promote relaxation and reduce **stress**, improve mood, control high blood pressure, alleviate **pain**, boost the immune system, and lower **cholesterol** and blood sugar levels. Through guided imagery techniques, patients can learn to control functions normally controlled by the autonomic nervous system, such as heart rate, blood pressure, respiratory rate, and body temperature.

One of the biggest benefits of using guided imagery as a therapeutic tool is its availability. Imagery can be used virtually anywhere, anytime. It is also an equal opportunity therapy. Although some initial training in the technique may be required, guided imagery is accessible to virtually everyone regardless of economic status, education, or geographical location.

Guided imagery also gives individuals a sense of empowerment, or control. The technique is induced by a therapist who guides the patient. The resulting mental imagery used is solely a product of the individual's imagination. Some individuals have difficulty imagining. They may not get actual clear images but perhaps vague feelings about the guided journey. However, these individuals' brains and nervous systems responses seem to be the same as those with more detailed imaginings.

Patients who feel uncomfortable "opening up" in a traditional therapist-patient session may feel more at ease with a self-directed therapy like guided imagery.

Description

Guided imagery is simply the use of one's imagination to promote mental and physical health. It can be self-directed, where the individual puts himself into a relaxed state and creates his own images, or directed by others. When directed by others, an individual listens to a therapist, video, or audiotaped exercise that leads him through a relaxation and imagery exercise. Some therapists also use guided imagery in group settings.

Guided imagery is a two-part process. The first component involves reaching a state of deep relaxation through breathing and muscle relaxation techniques. During the relaxation phase, the person closes her eyes and focuses on the slow, in and out sensation of breathing. Or, she might focus on releasing the feelings of tension from her muscles, starting with the toes and working up to the top of the head. Relaxation tapes often feature soft music or tranquil, natural sounds such as rolling waves and chirping birds in order to promote feelings of relaxation.

Once complete relaxation is achieved, the second component of the exercise is the imagery, or visualization, itself. There are a number of different types of guided imagery techniques, limited only by the imagination. Some commonly used types include relaxation imagery, healing imagery, pain control imagery, and mental rehearsal.

Relaxation imagery

Relaxation imagery involves conjuring up pleasant, relaxing images that rest the mind and body. These may be experiences that have already happened, or new situations.

Healing imagery

Patients coping with diseases and injuries can imagine **cancer** cells dying, **wounds** healing, and the body mending itself. Or, patients may picture themselves healthy, happy, and symptom-free. Another healing imagery technique is based on the idea of *qi*, or energy flow, an idea borrowed from **traditional Chinese medicine**. Chinese medicine practitioners believe that illness is the result of a blockage or slowing of energy flow in the body. Individuals may use guided imagery to imagine energy moving freely throughout the body as a metaphor for good health.

Pain control imagery

Individuals can control pain through several imagery techniques. One method is to produce a mental image of the pain and then transform that image into something less frightening and more manageable. Another is to imagine the pain disappearing, and the patient as completely pain-free. Or, one may imagine the pain as

MARTIN L. ROSSMAN 1945–

Martin L. Rossman received his B.A. and M.D. degrees from the University of Michigan in Ann Arbor. The Colorado native then set up practice in San Francisco, where he is a Clinical Associate in the Department of Medicine at the University of California Medical Center as well as director and founder of the Collaborative Medicine Center in Mill Valley, and Co-Director of the Academy for Guided Imagery, also in Mill Valley. Dr. Rossman has been a Diplomat of Acupuncture for the National Commission for the Certification of Acupuncturists since 1986, and, since 1989, has been certified for Interactive Guided Imagery through the Academy for Guided Imagery. He also serves as a member of various medical-related associations throughout the United States.

According to Rossman, imagination is the key to understanding the self, and can be used to resolve many issues of mind and body fitness, including stress. Rossman prefers the term complementary medicine to alternative medicine, noting that so many of the therapies have moved into the medical mainstream that they all play a crucial role in health. Rossman's book, *Healing Yourself: A Step-by-Step Program for Better Health Through Imagery*, is one of many writings he has done on imagery. Rossman is a popular speaker in both professional and public settings, and a television and radio personality discussing the virtues of imagery, acupuncture, and other holistic treatments.

He can be reached through The Collaborative Medicine Center, Mill Valley, California at (415)383-3197 or through the Academy for Guided Imagery in Mill Valley at (800)726- 2070.

Jane Spear

something over which he has complete control. For example, patients with back problems may imagine their pain as a high voltage electric current surging through their spine. As they use guided imagery techniques, they can picture themselves reaching for an electrical switch and turning down the power on the current to alleviate the pain.

Mental rehearsal

Mental rehearsal involves imagining a situation or scenario and its ideal outcome. It can be used to reduce **anxiety** about an upcoming situation, such as labor and delivery, surgery, or even a critical life event such as an important competition or a job interview. Individuals picture themselves going through each step of the anxiety-producing event and then successfully completing it.

Preparations

For a successful guided imagery session, individuals should select a quiet, relaxing location where there is a comfortable place to sit or recline. If the guided imagery session is to be prompted with an audiotape or videotape, a stereo, VCR, or portable tape player should be available. Some people find that quiet background music improves their imagery sessions.

The session, which can last anywhere from a few minutes to an hour, should be uninterrupted. Taking the phone off the hook and asking family members for solitude can ensure a more successful and relaxing session.

Imagery combined with other relaxation techniques such as **yoga**, massage, or **aromatherapy** can greatly enhance the effects of these therapies. It can be done virtually anywhere.

Precautions

Because of the state of extreme relaxation involved in guided imagery, individuals should never attempt to use guided imagery while driving or operating heavy machinery.

Side effects

Guided imagery can induce sleepiness, and some individuals may fall asleep during a session. Other than this, there are no known adverse side effects to guided imagery.

Research & general acceptance

Use of guided imagery is a widely accepted practice among mental healthcare providers and is gaining acceptance as a powerful pain control tool across a number of medical disciplines. Results of a study conducted at The Cleveland Clinic Foundation and published in 1999 found that cardiac surgery patients who used a guided imagery tape prior to surgery experienced less pain and anxiety. These patients also left the hospital earlier following surgery than patients who used pain medication only.

Another study conducted by Harvard Medical School researchers found that for more than 200 patients undergoing invasive vascular or renal surgery, guided imagery controlled pain and anxiety more effectively than medication alone.

Training & certification

Guided imagery is used by many licensed therapists, counselors, psychologists, and psychiatrists. There are

KEY TERMS

Aromatherapy—The therapeutic use of plant-derived, aromatic essential oils to promote physical and psychological well-being.

Autonomic nervous system—The part of the nervous system that controls so-called involuntary functions such as heart rate, salivary gland secretion, respiratory function, and pupil dilation.

many self-help books, audiotapes, and videos available that offer instruction in guided imagery techniques.

Resources

BOOKS

Battino, Rubin. *Guided Imagery and Other Approaches to Healing.* Carmarthen, United Kingdom: Crown House Publishing, 2000.

PERIODICALS

Lang, Elvira, et al. "Adjunctive non-pharmacological analgesia for invasive medical procedures: a randomized trial." *The Lancet.* 355, no. 9214, (April 2000): 1486-1490.

ORGANIZATIONS

The Academy for Guided Imagery. P.O. Box 2070, Mill Valley, CA 94942. (800) 726-2070.

OTHER

Brennan, Patricia. "Stress First Aid Kit." (Guided imagery audiotape set.) Available from Inside Out Publishing at (888) 727-3296 or http://www.facingthedawn.com.

Paula Ford-Martin

Gulf War syndrome

Definition

Gulf War syndrome describes a wide spectrum of illnesses and symptoms ranging from **asthma** to **sexual dysfunction** that have been reported by U.S. and U.S. allied soldiers who served in the Persian Gulf War in 1990–91.

Description

Between 1994 and 1999, 145 federally funded research studies on Gulf War-related illnesses were undertaken at a cost of over $133 million. Despite this investment, and the data collected from over 100,000 veterans who have registered with the Department of Defense and/or Veterans Administration as having Gulf War-related illnesses, there is still much debate over the cause and nature of Gulf War Syndrome. Veterans who have the illness experience a wide range of debilitating symptoms that elude a single diagnosis. They are tired, have trouble breathing, have headaches, sleep poorly, are forgetful, and cannot concentrate. Similar experiences among Gulf War veterans have been reported in the United Kingdom and Canada.

Causes & symptoms

There is much current debate over a possible causative agent for Gulf War Syndrome other than the **stress** of warfare. Intensive efforts by the Veterans Administration and other public and private institutions have investigated a wide range of potential factors. These include chemical and biological weapons, the immunizations and preventive treatments used to protect against them, smoke from oil well fires, exposure to depleted uranium, and diseases endemic to the Arabian peninsula. So far investigators have not approached a consensus. They even disagree on the likelihood that a specific agent is responsible, as a combination of these risk factors may have negative health consequences. There is, however, a likelihood that sarin and/or cyclosarin (nerve gases) were released during the destruction of Iraqi munitions at Kharnisiyah, Iraq, and that these chemicals might be linked to the syndrome.

In October 1999, the U.S. Pentagon released a report that hypothesized that an experimental drug known as pyriostigmine bromide, or PB, might be linked to the physical symptoms manifested in Gulf War Syndrome. The experimental drug was given to U.S. and Canadian troops during the war to protect soldiers against the effects of the chemical nerve agent soman.

Statistical analysis shows that the following symptoms are about twice as likely to appear in Gulf War veterans than in their non-combat peers: **depression**, post-traumatic stress disorder (PTSD), chronic **fatigue**, cognitive dysfunction (diminished ability to calculate, order thoughts, evaluate, learn, and remember), **bronchitis**, asthma, **fibromyalgia**, alcohol abuse, **anxiety**, and sexual dysfunction. PTSD is the modern equivalent of shell shock (term used in World War I) and battle fatigue (World War II). It encompasses most of the psychological symptoms of war veterans, not excluding nightmares, panic at sudden loud noises, and inability to adjust to peacetime living.

Chronic fatigue syndrome has a specific medical definition that attempts to separate common fatigue from a more disabling illness in hope of finding a specific cause. Fibromyalgia is another newly defined syndrome, and as such it has arbitrarily rigid defining characteristics. These include a certain duration of illness, a specified minimum number of joint and muscle pains located in designated areas of the body, sleep disturbances, and other associated symptoms and signs. One study comparing unexplained symptoms in Gulf War veterans with symptoms in control subjects found that over half the veterans with unexplained muscle **pain** met the criteria for fibromyalgia, and a significant portion of the veterans with unexplained fatigue met the criteria for chronic fatigue syndrome.

As of 2001, amyotrophic lateral sclerosis (ALS), which is also known as **Lou Gehrig's disease**, has been added to the list of illnesses that occur more frequently in veterans of the Gulf War. Gulf War veterans are twice as likely as other veterans to develop ALS, which is a disease that causes wasting of muscle tissue and kills its victims within three to five years. About 40 Gulf War veterans have been diagnosed with ALS; most have already died.

Researchers have identified three distinct syndromes and several variations in Gulf War veterans. Type one patients suffer primarily from impaired thinking. Type two patients have a greater degree of confusion and ataxia (loss of coordination). Type three patients are the most affected by joint pains, muscle pains, and extremity paresthesias (unnatural sensations like burning or tingling in the arms and legs). In each of the three types, researchers found different but measurable impairments on objective testing of neurological function. The functioning of the nervous system is much more complex and subtle than other body systems. Measuring it requires an equally complex effort. The tests used in this study carefully measured and compared localized nerve performance at several different tasks against the same values in normal subjects. Brain wave response to noise and touch, eye muscle response to spinning, and caloric testing (stimulation of the ear with warm and cold water, which causes vertigo) were clearly different between the normal and the test subjects. The researchers concluded that there was "a generalized injury to the nervous system." Another research group concluded their study by stating that there was "a spectrum of neurologic injury involving the central, peripheral, and autonomic nervous systems."

Diagnosis

Until there is a clear definition of the disease, diagnosis is primarily an exercise in identifying those Gulf War veterans who have an undefined illness in an effort to learn more about them and their symptoms. Both the Department of Defense (DoD) and the Veterans Administration (VA) currently have programs devoted to this problem. Both the DoD's Comprehensive Clinical Evaluation Program and the VA's Persian Gulf Registry provide free, in-depth medical evaluations to Gulf War veterans and their families. In addition to providing individual veterans with critical medical care, these organizations use the cumulative data from these programs to advance research on Gulf War syndrome itself.

Treatment

Specific treatment awaits specific diagnosis and identification of a causative agent. Meanwhile, veterans can benefit from the wide variety of supportive and nonspecific approaches to this and similar problems. The key to working successfully with people living their lives with Gulf War syndrome is long-term, ongoing care, whether it be **hypnotherapy**, **acupuncture**, **homeopathy**, **nutrition**, vitamin/mineral therapy, or bodywork.

Allopathic treatment

There are many drugs available for symptomatic relief. Psychological counseling by those specializing in this area can be immensely beneficial, even life-saving, for those contemplating suicide. Veterans' benefits are available for those who are impaired by their symptoms.

Expected results

The outlook for war veterans is unclear, but will hopefully improve as more information is gathered about the illness. Gradual return to a functioning life may take many years of work and much help. However, even in the absence of an identifiable and curable cause, recovery is possible.

Resources

BOOKS

Isselbacher, Kurt, et al., ed. *Harrison's Principles of Internal Medicine.* New York: McGraw-Hill, 1998.

"Posttraumatic Stress Disorder." *Treatments of Psychiatric Disorders.* 3rd ed. Ed. Glen O. Garbbard. Washington, DC: American Psychiatric Press Inc., 2001.

PERIODICALS

Bourdette, Dennis N., et al. "Symptom Factor Analysis, Clinical Findings, and Functional Status in a Population-Based Control Study of Gulf War Unexplained Illness." *Journal of Occupational and Environmental Medicine* 43 (December 2001): 1026–1040.

Haley, R. W., et al. "Evaluation of Neurologic Function in Gulf War Veterans. A Blinded Case-Control Study." *Journal of the American Medical Association.* 277 (January 15, 1997): 223–230.

> ## KEY TERMS
>
> **Ataxia**—Lack of coordination.
>
> **Caloric testing**—Flushing warm and cold water into the ear stimulates the labyrinth and causes vertigo and nystagmus (involuntary movement of the eyes in a horizontal direction) if all the nerve pathways are intact.
>
> **Endemic**—Belonging or native to a particular locality or people.
>
> **Paresthesia**—An abnormal sensation often described as burning, numbness, tingling, or pin pricks.
>
> **Syndrome**—Common features of a disease or features that appear together often enough to suggest they may represent a single, as yet unknown, disease entity. When a syndrome is first identified, an attempt is made to define it as strictly as possible, even to the exclusion of some cases, in order to separate out a pure enough sample to study. This process is most likely to identify a cause, a positive method of diagnosis, and a treatment.

Knoke, James D., and Gregory C. Gray. "Hospitalizations for Unexplained Illnesses Among U.S. Veterans of the Persian Gulf War." *Emerging Infectious Diseases* 4 (April-June 1998): 211–219.

McDiarmid, Melissa, et al. "Surveillance of Depleted Uranium-Exposed Gulf War Veterans: Health Effects Observed in an Enlarged 'Friendly Fire' Cohort." *Journal of Occupational and Environmental Medicine* 43 (December 2001): 991–1000.

"Self-Reported Illness and Health Status Among Gulf War Veterans. A Population-Based Study. The Iowa Persian Gulf Study Group." *Journal of the American Medical Association* 277 (January 15, 1997): 238–245.

Spencer, Peter S., et al. "Self-Reported Exposures and Their Association With Unexplained Illness in a Population-Based Case-Control Study of Gulf War Veterans." *Journal of Occupational and Environmental Medicine* 43 (December 2001): 1041–1056.

Szegedy-Maszak, Marianne. "A Gulf War Legacy." *U.S. News & World Report* (December 24, 2001): 50.

ORGANIZATIONS

Office of the Special Assistant for Gulf War Illnesses. 5111 Leesburg Pike, Suite 901, Falls Church, Virginia, 22041. 703-578-8518. brostker@gwillness.osd.mil. <http://www.gulflink.osd.mil>.

The American Legion. Gulf War Veteran Issues. <http://www.legion.org/veterans/vt_gulfvet_info.htm>.

Veterans Administration. Persian Gulf Medical Information Helpline. 400 South 18th Street, St. Louis, Missouri 63103-2271. (800) 749-8387.

Veterans Administration. Persian Gulf Registry. 800-PGW-VETS (800-749-8387). <http://www.va.gov>.

Gulf War News. Office of the Special Assistant for Gulf War Illnesses, 5113 Leesburg Pike, Suite 901, Falls Church, Virginia 22041. (703) 578-8518. edipaolo@gwillness.osd.mil.

OTHER

Joseph, Stephen C., and the Comprehensive Clinical Evaluation Program (CCEP). "A Comprehensive Clinical Evaluation of 20,000 Persian Gulf War Vetrans." *Military Medicine* 162 (March 1997). [cited October 2002]. <http://www.defenselink.mil/pubs/foi/clinic.pdf>.

Paula Ford-Martin
Rebecca J. Frey, PhD

Gum disease

Definition

Gum disease is also called periodontal disease. It is defined as the inflammation of the structures that surround and support the teeth. If left untreated, gum disease may progress to the point where there is destruction of the jawbone. It is one of the most common causes of tooth loss. Periodontal disease is also a risk factor for coronary **heart disease** and preterm low birth weight.

Description

Gingivitis is the earliest stage of a gum infection. It may recur or even become chronic. If gingivitis is not treated properly, it may progress to periodontitis, an inflammation of the periodontal ligament that helps hold the teeth in the bone. Periodontitis is sometimes called pyorrhea, which means a pus discharge. Severe cases of periodontitis may affect the jawbone. A severe case of gum disease that comes on suddenly is a disease known as trench mouth. Trench mouth, or necrotizing ulcerative gingivitis, is also known as Vincent's infection. It is caused by an infection of both spirochetes and fusiform bacilli. It was once a major problem for soldiers during World War I. Currently, trench mouth is particularly common among teenagers and young adults under **stress**, often at examination time. Inflammation from trench mouth can also spread to nearby tissues of the face and neck.

Causes & symptoms

By far, the most common cause of gum disease is poor dental hygiene. Regular daily brushing and flossing of the teeth generally clears away food and bacteria

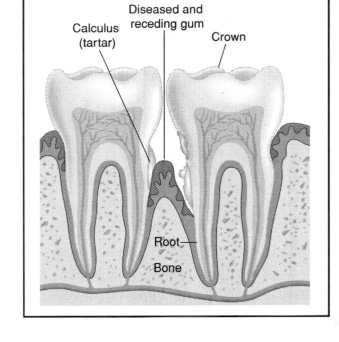

If not brushed away, plaque accumulates around teeth and hardens into calculus, or tartar. As tartar accumulates, the gum recedes. Gum disease can result in tooth loss. *(Illustration by Electronic Illustrators Group. The Gale Group.)*

buildup in the mouth. If the teeth are neglected, bacteria collect, and plaque forms on the teeth and gums. If the plaque is not removed, it mixes with saliva and hardens into tartar. Tartar irritates the gums and causes them to shrink away from the teeth, opening up spaces where more bacteria and plaque can collect. This cycle encourages increasingly severe inflammation and infection.

The mechanisms by which bacteria cause tissue destruction in advanced gum disease are not fully understood. Several bacterial products that diffuse through tissue are thought to play a role in gum disease. Toxins produced by some bacteria can kill cells. Studies show that the amount of endotoxin present correlates with the severity of periodontal disease. Other bacterial products include proteolytic enzymes, which are molecules that digest protein found in cells, thereby causing cell destruction. The human immune response has also been implicated in tissue destruction. As part of a normal immune response, white blood cells enter regions of inflammation to destroy bacteria. In the process of destroying bacteria, periodontal tissue is also destroyed.

Other factors can contribute to the development of gum disease. Smokers are more than two times as likely as nonsmokers to develop gum disease. Hormone levels contribute to the development of bacteria in the mouth. Thus **pregnancy**, puberty, **menopause**, and the use of

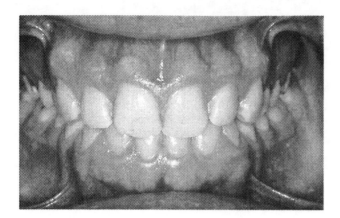

Gingivitis, an inflammation of the gums, is a common periodontal disease. *(Photograph by Edward H. Gill, Custom Medical Stock Photo. Reproduced by permission.)*

oral or injectable contraceptives may create a climate that favors the development of gum disease. Additional factors include **diabetes mellitus**, scurvy, pellagra, **allergies**, **leukemia**, **Crohn's disease**, **AIDS**, chemotherapy, nutritional deficiencies, hydrochloric acid deficiency, poorly fitted fillings, radiation treatments, and exposure to heavy metals (mercury, lead, arsenic, and nickel). Medications that may contribute to the development of gum disease include phenytoin for controlling seizures; cyclosporine, which is taken by people who have had organ transplants; and the **calcium** channel blockers used to control blood pressure and heartbeat.

The main symptoms of gingivitis are dark red swollen gums that are mushy and bleed easily. **Pain** is usually minimal. People with periodontitis have the same symptoms. In addition they may also have pain, loose teeth, and **bad breath**. Abscesses and pus may develop. The symptoms of trench mouth include sudden onset of illness accompanied by pain, bleeding gums, bad breath, and a grayish mucus that covers the gums.

Diagnosis

A dental examination and history will be taken. As the disease progresses, a dentist will be able to find hollowed pockets near the gums. X rays may be used to reveal the breakdown of bone. A smear of the gum area may be taken to determine the existence of any bacterial **infections**. The visualization of spirochetes can be used to confirm the diagnosis of trench mouth.

Treatment

Naturopathic treatment

Zinc, copper, folic acid, vitamin E, selenium, and **vitamin A** or beta-carotene are very helpful in slowing the progression of gum disease, especially if the patient has dietary deficiencies. Daily CoQ10 supplementation is also recommended. Mouthwashes that contain either a 0.1% folate solution or a 5% solution of zinc, or both, swished in the mouth and held there for at least a minute, can be taken twice daily.

Flavonoids help reduce inflammation and strengthen the gum tissue. A daily menu that includes foods rich in flavonoids is recommended. These foods include blueberries, **hawthorn** berries, onions, and grapes. Extracts of these foods may be used as well.

Homeopathy

The main homeopathic remedy for mild gum disease is *Mercurius solubilis hahnemanni* in a 6c potency. *Natrum muriaticum,* also in a 6c potency, is for more severe disease, especially if there is formation of pus. Homeopathic remedies can be taken four times daily for up to three days.

Ayurvedic medicine

Ayurvedic practitioners recommend a daily cup of water with the juice of a fresh lemon squeezed into it for bleeding gums. Five grams of amla powder in a cup of water daily is also recommended. The teeth can be brushed with catechu or **neem** powder or both.

Traditional Chinese medicine

According to **traditional Chinese medicine**, the gums are nourished by the liver's function. If the level of toxins in the body exceeds the liver's blood-cleansing limits, eventually the gums (and other parts of the body) become a breeding ground for disease. The Chinese also consider the liver as a reservoir of blood; it ensures that adequate blood and Qi (vital energy) are delivered to the muscles, gums, and joints.

Herbal therapies

The teeth can be brushed with a mixture of baking soda and hydrogen peroxide to clean them thoroughly and to fight infection. **Goldenseal** root powder, *Hydrastis canandensis,* can be used in the same way. **Myrrh**, *Commiphora molmol,* can be applied directly to the gums. *Aloe vera* may be applied directly to the gums to reduce pain and inflammation. In addition, a cup of water with a teaspoon of apple cider vinegar makes a good daily mouth rinse. An herbal mouth rinse can be prepared from 1 oz. hydrastis, 1 oz. myrrh, and 1 pint of water.

Allopathic treatment

Dentists may advise mouth rinses with warm salt water as well as such measures for symptom relief as over-the-counter anesthetic ointments. The dentist will scrape away the damaged gum tissue. The root surfaces may have to be scraped. If the gums are badly damaged, surgery is performed to remove and tighten the gum tissue. Bone loss may be addressed by a of variety techniques to encourage growth. If there is advanced disease, the teeth in the affected areas may have to be pulled. Any underlying medical conditions should be assessed and treated, as they may be contributing to the gum disease. Such dental problems as poorly aligned teeth or grinding of the teeth may need to be addressed. **Nutrition** should be improved. If a severe infection like trench mouth is present, antibiotics will be given. The antibiotics may be delivered directly to the infected gum and bone tissues to ensure that high concentrations of the antibiotic reach the infected area. Recently, physicians have discovered that the importance of treating serious gum infections with antibiotics spreads from the patient's mouth to his or her general health. By looking for markers of inflammation throughout the body after treating some patients with gum infections with antibiotics, and not treating others, they have found oral bacteria from gum infections in arterial plaque.

Infected abscesses, especially of bone, are difficult to treat and require long-term antibiotic treatment to prevent recurrence of infection. Patients with gum disease should be reevaluated after three months to assess progress and further treatment needs.

Expected results

With good dental habits, most simple cases of gum disease resolve. If the teeth and gums are not cared for or if the disease progresses for other reasons, there may be destruction of bone and a loss of teeth. Research indicates that the bacteria connected with plaque formation and chronic gum disease may enter the bloodstream and cause an infection that may bring on heart disease, **pneumonia**, or premature births.

Prevention

The teeth should be brushed and flossed daily, after meals. Fifteen minutes per day should be spent massaging the gums with **eucalyptus**, **witch hazel**, or vitamin E, rubbing a finger in a circular motion along the gum line. Toothbrushes should be changed monthly, since there may be a tendency for bacteria to accumulate on them. The toothbrush should also be soft to avoid any further injury to the gums. A dentist should regularly check the health of the gums and teeth of people who are prone to gum disease. A dental hygienist should clean the teeth regularly, especially if there is an increased tendency to form plaque.

A whole foods diet is highly recommended. It should include fresh fruit and vegetables, and plenty of

---

KEY TERMS

Flavonoids—Pigments found in plants that help protect human tissues against damage from free radicals and help to modify other physiological responses.

Gingivitis—Inflammation of the gums.

Pellagra—A deficiency disease caused by a lack of niacin in the diet. The symptoms of pellagra include the classic triad of diarrhea, dermatitis (patches of irritated skin), and dementia.

Plaque—A deposit of bacteria and other materials on the surface of teeth that contributes to tooth decay and the development of periodontal disease.

Tartar—A hard, yellowish-brown gritty deposit that collects on the teeth. It is also called dental calculus.

---

dietary fiber. Such processed foods as sugar and white bread and grains contribute to plaque formation and should be avoided. Foods high in **vitamin C** should be consumed daily. Vitamin C is important in maintaining healthy gums, and supplementation may also be needed. As **smoking** reduces vitamin C absorption, the use of tobacco products should be avoided. Calcium and **magnesium** supplementation is recommended to minimize the loss of bone in progressive gum disease.

Resources

BOOKS

Bunch, Bryan, ed. *The Family Encyclopedia of Diseases: A Complete and Concise Guide to Illnesses and Symptoms.* New York: Scientific Publishing, Inc., 1999.

The Burton Goldberg Group. *Alternative Medicine: The Definitive Guide.* Tiburon, CA: Future Medicine Publishing, 1995.

The Editors of Time-Life Books. *The Medical Advisor: The Complete Guide to Alternative and Conventional Treatments.* Alexandria, VA: Time-Life, Inc., 1997.

Lockie, Dr. Andrew, and Dr. Nicola Geddes. *The Complete Guide to Homeopathy: The Principles and Practice of Treatment with a Comprehensive Range of Self-Help Remedies for Common Ailments.* London: Dorling Kindersley, Ltd., 1995.

PERIODICALS

"Using Antibiotics for Gum Infection Helps Whole Body." *Health & Medicine Week* (April 8, 2002): 2.

Patience Paradox
Teresa G. Odle

Gymnema

Description

Gymnema (*Gymnema sylvestre*) is a climbing plant that grows in the tropical forests of central and southern India. The woody gymnema plant also grows in parts of Africa. Leaves of this long, slender plant have been used for more than 2,000 years in India to treat diabetes. Gymnema is also known as gurmar, gurmabooti, periploca of the woods, and meshasringi (ram's horn).

General use

In the past, powdered gymnema root was used to treat snake bites, **constipation**, stomach complaints, water retention, and liver disease. However, the Hindu word gurmar best describes the primary use of gymnema. Gurmar means sugar destroyer, and it has been used in **Ayurvedic medicine** for thousands of years to treat adult-onset diabetes, a condition once described as "honey urine."

Gymnema and diabetes

Diabetes is a consequence of abnormalities in the blood levels of insulin, the hormone that converts blood sugar into energy. Adult-onset diabetes is caused by the body's inability to adequately process insulin. Today it is known as Type II diabetes, non-insulin-dependent **diabetes mellitus** (NIDDM), and stable diabetes.

Type I diabetes, or juvenile diabetes, results from an insulin shortage. Type I diabetes is also called insulin-dependent diabetes mellitus (IDDM).

Thousands of years ago, Type II diabetes was treated with gymnema. The plant's sugar-destroying property was released when a person chewed on one or two leaves. Gymnema was said to paralyze a person's tongue to the taste of sugar and bitter tastes. That taste-blocking reaction lasted for several hours. During that time, leaves supposedly provided a slight block to the taste for salty foods, while the taste for acidic foods was not affected.

By blocking the taste buds from tasting sugar, gymnema blocked sugar in the digestive system, resulting in a decrease in blood sugar, also known as a hypoglycemic effect. This medicinal action has been studied since the late 1930s.

Gymnema has also been used in folk medicine as a remedy for **allergies**, urinary tract inflections, **anemia**, hyperactivity, digestion, **cholesterol**, and weight control. Most of those treatments did not prove to be effective. Gymnema lowers cholesterol slightly, but not enough to be regarded as a significant remedy.

Contemporary uses of gymnema

Currently, gymnema is known primarily for its sugar-blocking properties. It is used to treat high blood sugar in diabetics and has been promoted as a weight loss remedy. In India, gymnema has been used by both Type I and Type II diabetics, but is used mainly to treat Type II diabetics.

Some clinical trials in India indicated that gymnema could help with both types of diabetes. During the 1990s, Type II diabetics in India were studied, and gymnema proved successful for lowering blood sugar with continuous use for 18 to 24 months. In another study, people diagnosed as juvenile diabetics took gymnema along with insulin. In some cases, people were able to reduce their dosages of insulin.

In mid-2002, a U.S. clinical trial was reported to further support gymnema's use in managing Type I diabetes. Of those participating in the trial, about 16% were able to decrease usage of their prescription medication usage. The same research group also found gymnema beneficial for non-insulin dependent diabetics. While those results appeared promising, medical professionals caution that more research is still needed. That research would include double-blind studies and involve more people.

A weight-loss remedy?

Although gymnema won't make sugary foods taste bad, the sugar destroyer is said to curb the desire for sweets. Due to this sugar-blocking property, gymnema is marketed as a weight-loss remedy. People could take gymnema to help fight the desire for sweet treats. As a weight-loss remedy, gymnena has not been studied extensively, and some in the medical community were dubious about its effectiveness, an opinion held as of June 2000. Instead, the sugar destroyer is acknowledged as a potential treatment for diabetes.

Preparations

Gymnema is available commercially as a water-soluble extract that is standardized to contain 24% gymnemic acid. The usual dosage of is 400–600 mg of gymnema per day. However, the strengths of commercial products can vary. A person taking gymnema should follow the directions on the package.

When taken in capsule form, the dosage of gymnema is one 100-mg capsule taken three to four times daily.

Gymnema is also available in powdered form. The recommended dosage for powdered gymnema leaves is 0.5–1 tsp (2–4 g) per day. An herbal tea can be prepared by pouring 1 cup (240 ml) of boiling water over the powdered leaves. The mixture is covered and steeped for 10–15 minutes. The tea is strained before it is consumed.

Precautions

The United States Food and Drug Administration does not regulate gymnema and other herbal remedies. That means that the remedies have not proven to be effective and that ingredients are not standardized.

In addition, the safety of gymnema has not been established for use by children, pregnant women, nursing mothers, and people with severe kidney and liver diseases.

Before beginning any herbal treatment, people should consult a physician or health practitioner. Consulting a medical professional is particularly important before taking gymnema because the remedy could potentially lower blood sugar too much, resulting in a hypoglycemic reaction.

It is especially important for diabetics to consult with a doctor. Gymnema should not be regarded as a substitute for other medications. If people diagnosed with Type I or Type II diabetes are taking insulin to control their blood sugar, they cannot replace the insulin with gymnema.

In addition, diabetes can go undetected for some time. It may not be diagnosed until a person goes to a doctor after experiencing symptoms such as frequent urination, **dizziness**, and **fatigue**. Diabetes must be treated medically since complications from untreated diabetes can include kidney failure, **heart disease**, blindness, and loss of limbs.

Side effects

As of June 2000, gymnema was believed to be free of side effects when taken at the recommended dosages. However, more research could reveal side effects.

Interactions

Gymnema could interact with medications taken to reduce blood sugar levels. The herbal remedy could cause the drugs to work better, resulting in **hypoglycemia**.

Resources

BOOKS

Duke, James A. *The Green Pharmacy.* Emmaus, PA: Rodale Press, Inc., 1997.

> **KEY TERMS**
> . . . .
> **Ayurvedic medicine**—Ayurveda is the Sanskrit word for the science of life and longevity. The Ayurvedic treatment is based on the theory that health is a balance between the physical, emotional, and the spiritual.

Ritchason, Jack. *The Little Herb Encyclopedia.* Pleasant Grove, UT: Woodland Health Books, 1995.

Squier, Thomas Broken Bear with Lauren David Peden. *Herbal Folk Medicine.* New York: Henry Holt and Company, 1997.

PERIODICALS

Bone, Kerry. "Gymnema and Diabetes. (Phytotherapy Review & Commentary)." *Townsend Letter for Doctors and Patients* (June 2002):94.

ORGANIZATIONS

American Botanical Council. P.O. Box 201660, Austin TX, 78720. (512) 331-8868. http://www.herbs.org.

American Diabetes Association. P.O. Box 363, Mt. Morris, IL 61054-0363. http://www.diabetes.org.

Herb Research Foundation. 1007 Pearl St., Suite 200, Boulder, CO 80302. (303) 449-2265. http://www.herbs.org.

OTHER

"Diabetes: Herbal Remedies that may Help Control Blood Sugar." In *The Complete Natural Health Reference Guide.* Discovery Health. http://www.discoveryhealth.com (January 17, 2001).

Holistic Online. http://www.holisticonine.com (January 17, 2001).

Reitchenberg-Ullman, Judith. "Can You Just Say No to Sugar?" Healthworld Online. 1996. http://www.healthworldonline.com (January 17, 2001).

Liz Swain
Teresa G. Odle

Gypsywort *see* **Bugleweed**

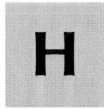

Hair loss

Definition

Hair loss, or *alopecia*, is total or partial baldness caused by hormonal changes or physical or mental **stress**.

Description

Hair loss occurs for many reasons. Some causes, such as hormonal changes, are considered natural, while others signal serious health problems. Some conditions are confined to the scalp, while others reflect disease processes throughout the body.

Causes & symptoms

Androgenetic alopecia occurs in both men and women, and is considered normal in adult males. Also known as male pattern baldness, it is easily recognized by the distribution of hair loss over the top and front of the head (leaving a horseshoe pattern of hair) and by the healthy condition of the scalp. Women with androgenetic alopecia experience hair thinning, particularly over the top of the scalp. The disorder is thought to be caused by a genetic predisposition that triggers the production of certain enzymes that convert testosterone into the hormone dihydrotestosterone (DHT). DHT is known to shrink hair follicles, and can cause partial or complete hair loss.

Alopecia areata and *alopecia circumscripta* refer to hair loss conditions that can be patchy or extend to complete baldness. The exact cause of alopecia areata is unknown, but it is thought to be triggered by an immune system disorder.

Oftentimes, conditions affecting the skin of the scalp will result in hair loss. The first clue to the specific cause is the pattern of hair loss, whether it be complete baldness (*alopecia capitis totalis*), patchy bald spots, thinning, or hair loss confined to certain areas. Also a factor is the condition of the hair and the scalp beneath it. Sometimes only the hair is affected; sometimes the skin is visibly diseased as well.

Fungal infections of the scalp usually cause patchy hair loss. The fungus, similar to the ones that cause **athlete's foot** and ringworm, often glows under ultraviolet light.

Complete hair loss is a common result of **cancer** chemotherapy, due to the toxicity of the drugs used. Placing a tourniquet around the skull just above the ears during the intravenous infusion of the drugs may reduce or eliminate hair loss by preventing the drugs from reaching the scalp. However, this technique may not be recommended in the treatment of certain types of cancer. An investigational topical gel that may prevent chemotherapy-related hair loss, known as GW 8510, was in clinical trials as of April 2000.

Systemic diseases often affect hair growth either selectively or by altering the skin of the scalp. One example is thyroid disorders. **Hyperthyroidism** (too much thyroid hormone) causes hair to become thin and fine. **Hypothyroidism** (too little thyroid hormone) thickens both hair and skin. Several autoimmune diseases also affect the skin and potentially the hair, notably lupus erythematosus.

Hair loss can also be caused by *trichotillomania*, a mental disorder or compulsion that causes a person to pull out his/her own hair. In some individuals severe mental or physical stress can cause hair loss, including major surgery or illness, significant life changes (i.e., divorce, death of a loved one), and drastic dietary changes. This type of hair loss is called *Telogen effluvium,* and is the second most common type of hair loss.

Diagnosis

Dermatologists are skilled in diagnosis by sight alone. For more obscure diseases, they may have to resort to a skin biopsy, removing a tiny bit of skin using a local anesthetic so that it can be examined under a microscope. Systemic diseases will require a complete

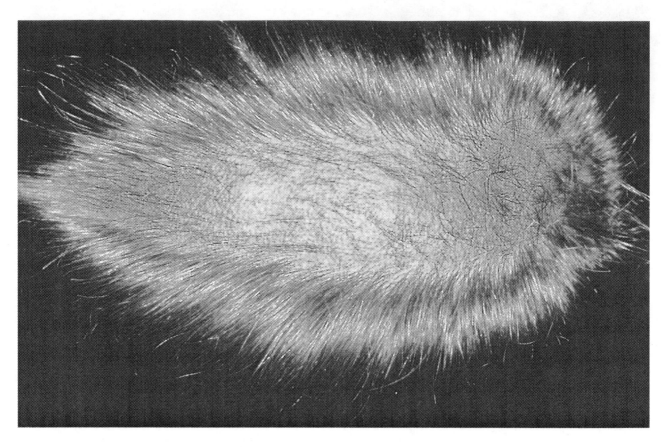

Balding on scalp. *(Custom Medical Stock Photo. Reproduced by permission.)*

evaluation by a physician, including specific tests to identify and characterize the problem.

Treatment

Traditional Chinese medicine (TCM) has a particular understanding of baldness that is different from the allopathic view. TCM recommends foods to eat and others to avoid, herbs to treat hair loss, and special hair massage. One Chinese approach is to first understand where there is weak energy in the body and to strengthen the qi (chi) of those organ systems. Treatment is not a one-shot approach but a well-rounded response.

Vitamins B_6 and **biotin** are thought to advocate healthy hair growth, as are the minerals **zinc**, **copper**, and **silica**. Fifty milligrams of silica a day is thought to encourage hair growth in young men with alopecia. The herb **horsetail** (*Equisetum arvense*) contains silica, and can be taken as an infusion, or tea. Copper and zinc have been shown to inhibit growth of the enzyme that causes DHT production. **Iron** supplements may be useful in individuals whose hair loss is caused by **anemia** or an inadequate intake of dietary iron.

The herbal remedies **saw palmetto** (*Serenoa repens*) and pygeum (*Pygeum africanum*) may be pre-scribed by an herbalist, naturopath, or holistic healthcare professional to stop or slow hair loss. Saw palmetto is thought to stop DHT production, and pygeum influences testosterone production. Both can be taken orally as a dietary supplement. The Chinese herb He Shou Wun (*Polygonum multiflorum*) can be taken orally or applied as a topical formula.

For hair loss caused by trichotillomania (hair pulling), **behavioral therapy** may be a useful treatment program. If the hair pulling or hair loss itself is triggered by stress, there are a number of stress reduction therapies that can promote **relaxation**, including **aromatherapy**, muscle relaxation exercises, **yoga**, **guided imagery**, and **biofeedback**.

Allopathic treatment

Successful treatment of underlying causes is most likely to restore hair growth, be it the completion of chemotherapy, effective cure of a scalp fungus, or control of a systemic disease. Drugs such as minoxidil (Rogaine) and finasteride (Propecia, Proscar) promote hair growth in a significant minority of patients, especially those with male pattern baldness and alopecia areata.

KEY TERMS

Athlete's foot—A fungal infection between the toes, officially known as tinea pedis.

Autoimmune disease—Certain diseases caused by the body's development of an immune reaction to its own tissues.

Chemotherapy—The treatment of diseases, usually cancer, with drugs (chemicals).

Hair follicles—Tiny organs in the skin, each one of which grows a single hair.

Lupus erythematosus—An autoimmune disease that can damage skin, joints, kidneys, and other organs.

Ringworm—A fungal infection of the skin, also known as tinea corporis.

Systemic—Affecting all or most parts of the body.

When used continuously for long periods of time, minoxidil produces satisfactory results in about one-quarter of patients with androgenic alopecia and as many as half the patients with alopecia areata. Both drugs have so far proved to be quite safe when used for this purpose. Side effects of Rogaine include some dryness and irritation of the scalp. Reported side effects of Propecia include infrequent cases of diminished sexual drive and **impotence**. Propecia is not approved for women because it can cause birth defects.

In 2001, a study was made of immunotherapy with diphencyprone to treat alopecia areata. A lag of three months from start of therapy to development of noticeable hair growth occurred. Researchers noted that the extent of the disease prior to therapy and age at time hair loss began affected treatment success. Patients who were older at onset of baldness had a better success rate than those who were younger. The study concluded that long-term therapy was required for effectiveness.

Over the past few decades there have appeared a multitude of hair replacement methods performed by both physicians and non-physicians. They range from simply weaving someone else's hair in with the remains of an individual's own hair to surgically transplanting thousands of hair follicles one at a time.

Expected results

The prognosis for individuals with hair loss varies with the cause. It is generally much easier to lose hair than to regrow it. Even when it returns, it is often thin and less attractive than the original crop.

Resources

BOOKS

American Society of Health-System Pharmacists Inc. *American Hospital Formulary Service Drug Information.* Bethesda, MD: American Society of Health-System Pharmacists Inc., 1998.

Bennett, J. Claude, and Fred Plum, eds. *Cecil Textbook of Medicine.* Philadelphia: W. B. Saunders, 1999.

PERIODICALS

Amichai, B., M. H. Grunwald, and R. Sobel. "5 Alpha-reductase Inhibitors—A New Hope in Dermatology?" *International Journal of Dermatology* (March 1997): 182–4.

Lewis, Eric J., et al. "Some Common—and Uncommon—Causes of Hair Loss." *Patient Care* (December 15, 1997): 50.

Watson, Fiona. "Dermatologists Must Sift Through Alternative Tx." *Dermatology Times* (November 1997): 5.

Wiseman, Marni C. "Protective Model for Immunotherapy of Alopecia Areata with Diphencyprone." *JAMA, The Journal of the American Medical Association* (November 21, 2001): 2384.

Paula Ford-Martin
Teresa G. Odle

Halitosis *see* **Bad breath**
Hangnail *see* **Ingrown nail**

Hangover

Definition

Hangover is the collection of physical and mental symptoms that occur after a person drinks excessive amounts of alcohol.

Description

Hangovers have probably been experienced since prehistoric time when alcohol was first discovered. A survey found that about 75% of the persons who drank enough to be intoxicated (drunk) sometimes experienced hangover. Although very prevalent, hangovers have not been extensively studied. It is known that ethanol is the primary chemical component of alcohol to produce the effects associated with drinking.

Whether hangover affects complex mental tasks and the performance of simple tasks is unclear. Studies on these areas have yielded conflicting results, presumably due to differences in methods. Clearly, alcohol consumption can affect sleep, and sleep deprivation is known to affect performance.

Causes & symptoms

The cause of hangover is believed to be multifactorial. Hangover is likely caused by a combination of direct effects of ethanol, effects of ethanol removal, effects of ethanol breakdown products, effects of other components of the alcoholic beverage, personal characteristics, and behaviors associated with alcohol use.

Direct effects of ethanol

Ethanol can directly affect the body by causing dehydration (loss of fluids), electrolyte (body chemicals) imbalance, stomach and intestinal irritation, low blood sugar, and sleep disruption. In addition, alcohol directly affects the circadian rhythm (internal 24-hour clock) causing a feeling similar to **jet lag**. Ethanol causes vasodilation (enlarged blood vessels) and affects bodily chemicals, like serotonin and histamine, which may contribute to the **headache** associated with hangover.

Effects of ethanol removal

Because hangover symptoms peak at around the same time that the blood alcohol concentration falls to zero, some researchers propose that hangover is actually a mild form of withdrawal. Excessive drinking causes changes in the chemical messenger system of the brain and, when the alcohol is removed, the system becomes unbalanced. Many of the symptoms of hangover are similar to those associated with mild withdrawal. Some differences exist, however, between hangover and withdrawal; specifically, hangover symptoms do not include the hallucinations, seizures, and the lengthy impairment of withdrawal.

Effects of ethanol breakdown products

In the body, ethanol is first broken down to acetaldehyde and then to acetate. Acetaldehyde is a reactive chemical that, at high concentrations, can cause sweating, rapid pulse, skin flushing, **nausea**, and **vomiting**. Some researchers believe that acetaldehyde causes hangover. Although there is no acetaldehyde in the blood when the blood alcohol concentration reaches zero, the toxic effects of acetaldehyde on the body may still persist.

Other factors

Most alcoholic beverages contain small amounts of other active compounds besides ethanol. These compounds add to the smell, taste, and appearance of the beverage. Gin or vodka, which contain almost pure ethanol, produce fewer hangover symptoms than alcoholic beverages that contain other alcohol compounds (such as red wine, brandy, or whiskey). For example, methanol is implicated in contributing to hangover. Red wine, whiskey, and brandy all contain high levels of methanol.

Some inherent personal traits place persons at risk of experiencing hangover. In some persons, high levels of acetaldehyde accumulate (because of a deficient enzyme) which causes them to experience more severe hangovers. Persons who are neurotic, angry, or defensive, feel guilty about drinking, experience negative life events, or have a family history of **alcoholism** have increased hangover symptoms.

Certain behaviors associated with drinking increase the chance of experiencing hangover. These include drug use, disruption of normal sleep patterns, restricted food intake, and cigarette use.

Hangover symptoms begin within several hours after a person has stopped drinking and may last up to 24 hours. The specific symptoms experienced may vary depending upon the individual, the occasion, and the type and amount of alcohol consumed. The physical symptoms of hangover include headache, **fatigue**, light and sound sensitivity, muscle aches, eye redness, thirst, nausea, vomiting, and stomach **pain**. Hangover can cause rapid heartbeat, tremor, increased blood pressure, and sweating. Mental symptoms associated with hangover are decreased sleep, changes in sleep stages, decreased attention, decreased concentration, **depression**, **dizziness**, **anxiety**, irritability, and a sense that the room is spinning (vertigo).

Treatment

Eating balanced meals, drinking extra water, and limiting total alcohol help to reduce or avoid hangover. There are also many alternative treatments to prevent or reduce hangover symptoms. Drinking additional alcohol to relieve hangover, although it reduces short-term symptoms, is not recommended. Some experts believe that drinking alcohol to relieve hangover is a sign of impending alcoholism. The primary measure to fight hangover is to drink plenty of water while drinking alcoholic beverages, before going to bed, and the day after. Sweating from exertion, **exercise**, sauna, or massage may also help.

Food therapy

Hangover symptoms may be reduced by taking in lots of extra water and fluids and by eating foods that are high in **vitamin C** and the B vitamins, which are believed to speed the removal of alcohol from the body. Oranges, guava, grapefruit, and strawberries are rich in vitamin C and beans, fish, and whole grains are rich in the B vitamins. A cocktail prepared from orange juice (1 cup), pineapple juice (1 cup), kiwi fruit (one), vitamin-B-enriched nutritional yeast (1 tablespoon), and honey (1 tablespoon) provides important nutrients which the body needs to recover from hangover. Juice therapists recommend drinking a mixture of carrot juice (8 oz), beet juice (1 oz), celery juice (4 oz), and **parsley** juice (1 oz) twice during hangover. The Chinese drink fresh tangerine juice and eat 10 strawberries to treat hangover.

Eating bland complex carbohydrates, such as crackers or toast, is easy on the stomach and helps to raise blood sugar levels. Drinking tea or coffee can relieve fatigue and possibly the headache. Throughout the world, traditional food remedies for hangover have certain things in common. These include eggs, tripe, hot spices, hearty soups, and fruit and vegetable juices. These foods all serve to replenish vitamins, minerals, and other nutrients lost by the body as it detoxifies alcohol.

Ayurveda

Ayurvedic practitioners believe that hangover reflects the symptoms of excess pitta. Immediate relief may be found after drinking water containing lime juice (1 teaspoon), sugar (one half teaspoon), salt (pinch), and baking soda (one half teaspoon). Orange juice containing cumin (pinch) and lime juice (1 teaspoon) helps hangover. Drinking cool lassi, water containing yogurt (1 tablespoon) and cumin powder (pinch), three or four times daily may relieve nausea, headache, and drowsiness.

Herbals

The following herbal remedies are useful in treating hangover symptoms:

- An Ayurvedic remedy is to take one half teaspoon of a mixture of *shatavari* (5 parts), *shanka bhasma* (one eighth part), *kama dudha* (one eighth part), and *jatamamsi* (3 parts) with water 2–3 times daily.

- An Ayurvedic antidote for alcohol toxicity is one half teaspoon of *tikta* (or **myrrh**, **aloe** vera, or *sudharshan*) with warm water three times during the day.

- Barberry (*Barberis vulgaris*) tea reduces hangover symptoms.

- Dandelion (*Taraxacum officinale*) and burdock (*Arctium lappa*) tea (with gentian extract, powdered **ginger**, and honey) can ease the nausea.

- Evening primrose (*Oenothera biennis*) oil helps to replenish lost gamma-linoleic acid.

- **Milk thistle** (*Silybum marinum*) reduces alcohol toxicity on the liver.

- *Nux vomica* (*Strychnos nux vomica*) is a homeopathic antidote for alcohol overconsumption.

- Siberian ginseng (*Eleutherococcus senticosus*) helps the body adjust to the **stress** of alcohol toxicity.

- Wintergreen (*Gaultheria procumbens*) tea with hot pepper (*Capsicum*) sauce relieves the headache.

Other hangover remedies

Various other remedies for hangover include:

- Acupressure. Point LI 4 (between the thumb and index finger) relieves headache and stomach ailments and the B2 points (upper edge of the eye socket) relieves headache accompanied by light sensitivity.

- Aromatherapy. The nausea of hangover may be relieved by drinking an aromatic cocktail of water, lemon juice, and a drop of **fennel** essential oil before breakfast.

- Imagery. The hangover sufferer may visualize being on a ship in a stormy ocean. The ocean gradually becomes calm until the ship is gently bobbing in the water.

- Probiotics. The bacteria *Bifidobacterium bifidus* is able to remove alcohol breakdown products. To fight hangover, naturopaths recommend taking *B. bifidus* before going to bed and again the following day.

- Supplements. Taking 50 mg of vitamin B_3 before going to bed may relieve hangover.

- Hydrotherapy. Drinking a glass of water containing **activated charcoal** powder before going to bed may absorb alcohol in the stomach and reduce hangover symptoms.

Allopathic treatment

Hangover symptoms may be relieved by taking antacids for nausea and stomach pain and aspirin or a nonsteroidal anti-inflammatory drugs (ibuprofen or naproxen) for headache and muscle pains. Acetaminophen (Tylenol) should be avoided while drinking or during hangover because alcohol enhances acetaminophen's toxic effects on the liver. **Caffeine**, usually taken as coffee, is historically used to treat hangover, although this has not been studied.

Expected results

There is no cure for hangover. Left untreated, hangover will resolve within several hours. Treatments may reduce the severity of certain symptoms.

Prevention

Hangover may be prevented by limiting the intake of alcohol, or drinking alcoholic beverages with a lesser incidence of causing hangover such as gin, vodka, or pure ethanol. Getting adequate sleep may reduce the fatigue associated with hangover. Drinking nonalcoholic beverages, both during and after drinking alcohol, may reduce dehydration and reduce hangover symptoms. Taking 120 mg of milk thistle before drinking can help the liver detoxify the alcohol.

KEY TERMS

Acetaldehyde—An intermediate product in the breakdown pathway of ethanol. Acetaldehyde is believed to cause hangover.

Dehydration—Loss of fluids from the body. Dehydration worsens some of the symptoms of alcohol.

Ethanol—The chemical which causes the effects and aftereffects of drinking alcoholic beverages.

Methanol—A liquid alcohol, used as a solvent or denaturant for ethanol.

Withdrawal—The physical and mental symptoms caused by removal of alcohol or other addictive substance from the body.

Resources

BOOKS

"Hangover." In *New Choices in Natural Healing: Over 1,800 of the Best Self-Help Remedies from the World of Alternative Medicine.* edited by Bill Gottlieb, et al. Rodale Press, Inc., 1995.

PERIODICALS

Cameron, Elizabeth. "Help for Hangovers." *Natural Health* 27 (November 1997): 58+.

Finnigan, Frances, Richard Hammersley, and Tracy Cooper. "An Examination of Next-Day Hangover Effects After a 100 mg/100 ml Dose of Alcohol in Heavy Social Drinkers." *Addiction* 93 (1998):1829-1838.

O'Neill, Molly. "Get Over It: Hangover Remedies for the Morning After." *New York Times Magazine* 149 (26 December 1999): 51+.

Maeder, Thomas. "After the Party." *Health* 13 (November/December 1999): 106+.

Swift, Robert and Dena Davidson. "Alcohol Hangover." *Alcohol Health & Research World* 22 (1998): 54+.

Belinda Rowland

Hardening of the arteries *see* **Atherosclerosis**

Hatha yoga

Definition

Hatha yoga is the most widely practiced form of yoga in America. It is the branch of yoga that concentrates on physical health and mental well-being. Hatha yoga uses bodily postures (*asanas*), breathing techniques (*pranayama*), and **meditation** (*dyana*) with the goal of bringing about a sound, healthy body and a clear, peaceful mind. There are nearly 200 hatha yoga postures, with hundreds of variations, which work to make the spine supple and to promote circulation in all the organs, glands, and tissues. Hatha yoga postures also stretch and align the body, promoting balance and flexibility.

Origins

Yoga was developed in ancient India as far back as 5,000 years ago; sculptures detailing yoga positions have been found in India which date back to 3000 B.C. Yoga is derived from a Sanskrit word which means "union." The goal of classical yoga to bring self-transcendence, or enlightenment, through physical, mental, and spiritual health. Many people in the West mistakenly believe yoga to be a religion, but its teachers point out that it is a system of living designed to promote health, peace of mind, and deeper awareness of ourselves. There are several branches of yoga, each of which is a different path and philosophy toward self-improvement. Some of these paths include service to others, pursuit of wisdom, non-violence, devotion to God, and observance of spiritual rituals. Hatha yoga is the path which has physical health and balance as a primary goal, for its practitioners believe that greater mental and spiritual awareness can be brought about with a healthy and pure body.

The origins of hatha yoga have been traced back to the eleventh century A.D. The Sanskrit word *ha* means "sun" and *tha* means "moon," and thus hatha, or literally sun-moon yoga, strives to balance opposing parts of the physical body, the front and back, left and right, top and bottom. Some yoga masters (*yogis*) claim that hatha yoga was originally developed by enlightened teachers to help people survive during the Age of Kali, or the spiritual dark ages, in which Hindus believe we are now living.

The original philosophers of yoga developed it as an eight-fold path to complete health. These eight steps include moral and ethical considerations (such as honesty, non-aggression, peacefulness, non-stealing, generosity, and sexual propriety), self-discipline (including purity, simplicity, devotion to God, and self-knowledge), posture, breath control, control of desires, concentration, meditation, and happiness. According to yogis, if these steps are followed diligently, a person can reach high levels of health and mental awareness.

As it has subsequently developed, hatha yoga has concentrated mainly on two of the eight paths, breathing and posture. Yogis believe breathing to be the most important metabolic function; we breathe roughly 23,000 times per day and use about 4,500 gallons of air, which

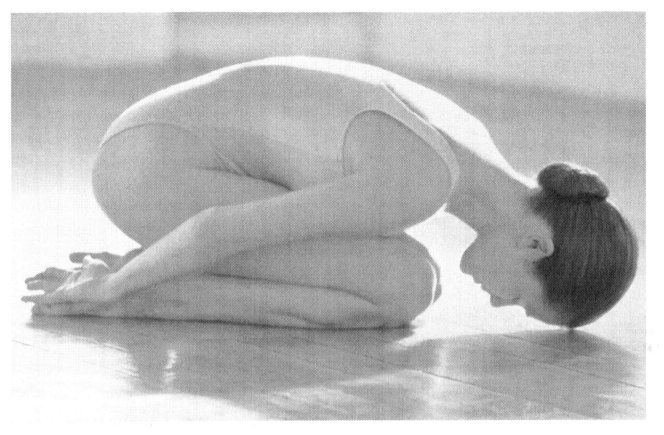

Woman in child's pose, a hatha yoga position. *(Photo Researchers, Inc. Reproduced by permission.)*

increases during **exercise**. Thus, breathing is extremely important to health, and *prana*, or life-force, is found most abundantly in the air and in the breath. If we are breathing incorrectly, we are hampering our potential for optimal health. *Pranayama*, literally the "science of breathing" or "control of life force," is the yogic practice of breathing correctly and deeply.

In addition to breathing, hatha yoga utilizes asanas, or physical postures, to bring about flexibility, balance and strength in the body. Each of these postures has a definite form and precise steps for achieving the desired position and for exiting it. These postures, yogis maintain, have been scientifically developed to increase circulation and health in all parts of the body, from the muscular tissues to the glands and internal organs. Yogis claim that although hatha yoga can make the body as strong and fit as any exercise program, its real benefits come about because it is a system of maintenance and balance for the whole body.

Yoga was brought to America in the late 1800s, when Swami Vivekananda, an Indian yogi, presented a lecture on yoga in Chicago. Hatha yoga captured the imagination of the Western mind, because accomplished yogis could demonstrate incredible levels of fitness, flexibility, and control over their bodies and metabolism.

Yoga has flourished in the West. Americans have brought to yoga their energy and zest for innovation, which troubles some Indian yogis and encourages others, as new variations and schools of yoga have developed. For instance, power yoga is a recent Americanized version of yoga which takes hatha yoga principles and speeds them up into an extremely rigorous aerobic workout, and many strict hatha yoga teachers oppose this sort of change to their philosophy. Other variations of hatha yoga in America now include Iyengar, Ashtanga, Kripalu, Integral, Viniyoga, Hidden Language, and Bikram yoga, to name a few. Sivananda yoga was practiced by Lilias Folen, who was responsible for introducing many Americans to yoga through public television.

Iyengar yoga was developed by B.K.S. Iyengar, who is widely accepted as one of the great living yogis. Iyengar uses classical hatha yoga asanas and breathing techniques, but emphasizes great precision and strict form in the poses, and uses many variations on a few postures. Iyengar allows the use of props such as belts, ropes, chairs, and blocks to enable students to get into postures they otherwise couldn't. In this respect, Iyengar yoga is good for physical therapy because it assists in the manipulation of inflexible or injured areas.

Ashtanga yoga, made popular by yogi K. Patabhi Jois, also uses hatha yoga asanas, but places an emphasis on the sequences in which these postures are performed. Ashtanga routines often unfold like long dances with many positions done quickly one after the other. Ashtanga is thus a rigorous form of hatha yoga, and sometimes can resemble a difficult aerobic workout. Ashtanga teachers claim that this form of yoga uses body heat, sweating, and deep breathing to purify the body.

Kripalu yoga uses hatha yoga positions but emphasizes the mental and emotional components of each asana. Its teachers believe that tension and long-held emotional problems can be released from the body by a deep and meditative approach to the yoga positions. Integral yoga seeks to combine all the paths of yoga, and is generally more meditative than physical, emphasizing spirituality and awareness in everyday life. Viniyoga tries to adapt hatha yoga techniques to each individual body and medical problem. Hidden Language yoga was developed by Swami Sivananda Radha, a Western man influenced by Jungian psychology. It emphasizes the symbolic and psychological parts of yoga postures and techniques. Its students are encouraged to write journals and participate in group discussions as part of their practice. Bikram yoga has become very popular in the late 1990s, as its popular teacher, Bikram Choudury, began teaching in Beverly Hills and has been endorsed by many famous celebrities. Bikram yoga uses the repetition of 26 specific poses and two breathing techniques to stretch and tone the whole body.

Benefits

In a celebrated 1990 study, *Dr. Dean Ornish's Program for Reversing Heart Disease* (Random House), a cardiologist showed that yoga and meditation combined with a low-fat diet and group support could significantly reduce the blockage of coronary arteries. Other studies have shown yoga's benefit in reducing stress-related problems such as high blood pressure and **cholesterol**. Meditation has been adopted by medical schools and clinics as an effective **stress** management technique. Hatha yoga is also used by physical therapists to improve many injuries and disabilities, as the gentleness and adaptability of yoga make it an excellent rehabilitation program.

Yoga has been touted for its ability to reduce problems with such varying conditions as **asthma**, backaches, diabetes, **constipation**, **menopause**, **multiple sclerosis**, **varicose veins**, and **carpal tunnel syndrome**. A vegetarian diet is the dietary goal of yoga, and this change of lifestyle has been shown to significantly increase longevity and reduce **heart disease**.

Yoga as a daily exercise program can improve fitness, strength, and flexibility. People who practice yoga correctly every day report that it can promote high levels of overall health and energy. The mental component of yoga can clarify and discipline the mind, and yoga practitioners say its benefits can permeate all facets of a person's life and attitude, raising self-esteem and self-understanding. Once individuals learn the basics of yoga, certain poses can be used to help with particular needs, such as improving memory and concentration or reducing bloating and **gas** after meals.

Description

A hatha yoga routine consists of a series of physical postures and breathing techniques. Routines can take anywhere from 20 minutes to two hours, depending on the needs and ability of the practitioner. Yoga should always be adapted to one's state of health; that is, a shorter and easier routine should be used when a person is fatigued. Yoga is ideally practiced at the same time every day, to encourage the discipline of the practice. It can be done at any time of day; some prefer it in the morning as a wake-up routine, while others like to wind down and de-stress with yoga at the end of the day.

Yoga asanas consist of three basic movements: backward bends, forward bends, and twisting movements. These postures are always balanced; a back bend should be followed with a forward bend, and a leftward movement should be followed by one to the right. Diaphragm breathing is important during the poses, where the breath begins at the bottom of the lungs. The stomach should move outward with the inhalation and relax inward during exhalation. The breath should be through the nose at all times during hatha asanas. Typically, one inhales during backward bends and exhales during forward bending movements.

The mental component in yoga is as important as the physical movements. Yoga is not a competitive sport, but a means to self-awareness and self-improvement. An attitude of attention, care, and non-criticism is important; limitations should be acknowledged and calmly improved. Patience is important, and yoga stretches should be slow and worked up to gradually. The body should be worked with, and never against, and a person should never overexert. A yoga stretch should be done only so far as proper form and alignment of the whole body can be maintained. Some yoga stretches can be uncomfortable for beginners, and part of yoga is learning to distinguish between sensations that are beneficial and those that can signal potential injury. A good rule is that positions should be stopped when there is sharp **pain** in the joints, muscles, or tendons.

Preparations

All that is needed to perform hatha yoga is a flat floor and adequate space for stretching out. A well-ventilated space is preferable, for facilitating proper breathing technique. Yoga mats are available that provide non-slip surfaces for standing poses. Loose, comfortable clothing should be worn. Yoga should be done on an empty stomach; a general rule is to wait three hours after a meal.

Yoga is an exercise that can be done anywhere and requires no special equipment. Yoga uses only gravity and the body itself as resistance, so it is a low-impact activity excellent for those who don't do well with other types of exercise. The mental component of yoga can appeal to those who get bored easily with exercise. By the same token, yoga can be a good stress management tool for those who prefer movement to sitting meditation.

Precautions

As with any exercise program, people should check with their doctors before starting yoga practice for the first time. Those with medical conditions, injuries, or spinal problems should find a yoga teacher familiar with their conditions before beginning yoga. Pregnant women, particularly after the third month of **pregnancy**, should only perform a few yoga positions with the supervision of an experienced teacher. Some yoga asanas can be very difficult, and potentially injurious, for beginners, so teachers should always be consulted as preparation for advanced yoga positions. Certain yoga positions should not be performed by those with fevers, or during **menstruation**.

Side effects

Those just beginning hatha yoga programs often report **fatigue** and soreness throughout the body, as yoga stretches and exercises muscles and tendons that are often long-neglected. Some yogic breathing and meditation techniques can be difficult for beginners and can cause **dizziness** or disorientation; these are best performed under the guidance of a teacher.

Training & certification

At this time, there are no generally accepted standards for yoga teacher certification in America, unlike in Europe and England, where yoga schools have been standardized. Some schools in America require teachers to study for many years, while some will grant beginning certificates in a much shorter time. When choosing teachers, students should search for qualities they may require, such as understanding, patience, knowledge of certain medical conditions, carefulness, and attention to individual details.

Yoga classes cost around 10 dollars per session. Many communities, schools, and health organizations offer discounted or free yoga classes as part of health awareness programs. Yoga can be reimbursed by insurance when it is part of physical therapy.

KEY TERMS

. . . .

Asana—Yoga posture or stance.

Diaphragm breathing—Method of deep breathing using the entire lungs.

Dyana—Yoga meditation.

Meditation—Technique of mental relaxation.

Prana—Yoga term for life-enhancing nutrient found in air, food and water.

Pranayama—Yoga method of breathing.

Resources

BOOKS

Bodian, Stephan, and Feuerstein, Georg. *Living Yoga* New York: Putnam, 1993.

Christensen, Alice. *20 Minute Yoga Workouts* New York: Fawcett, 1995.

Feuerstein, Georg. *Yoga for Dummies* New York: IDG Books, 1999.

Iyengar, B.K.S. *Light on Yoga.* New York: Schocken, 1975.

PERIODICALS

Schaeffer, Rachel. "Calm Digestive Upset with Yoga: If you Frequently Suffer from Bloating, Cramping, and Gas after Meals, these Poses can Help." *Natural Health* (July 2002):38–42.

Schaeffer, Rachel. "Sharpen Your Memory with Yoga: These Poses can Help you be Less Frazzled and Forgetful." *Natural Health* (August 2002):40–42.

Yoga Journal P.O. Box 469088, Escondido, CA 92046. http://www.yogajournal.com.

Yoga International Magazine R.R. 1 Box 407, Honesdale, PA 18431. http://www.yimag.com.

ORGANIZATIONS

International Association of Yoga Therapists (IAYT), 4150 Tivoli Ave., Los Angeles, CA 90066.

Douglas Dupler
Teresa G. Odle

Hawaiian massage *see* **Lomilomi**

Hawthorn

Description

Hawthorn is a dense, thorny shrub that grows 5–13 ft (1.5–4 m) high. It has white flowers that look like roses and is considered one of the most beautiful of all

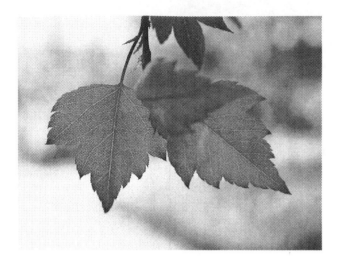

Hawthorn leaves. *(Photo by Kelly Quinn. Reproduced by permission.)*

the shrubs that flower in the spring. A member of the rose family, it has been planted along hedges to deter trespassers since the Middle Ages. Hawthorn grows throughout the world anywhere that is moist.

Hawthorn is the common name for *Crataegus oxyacantha* or other *Crataegus* species. There are more than 300 species throughout the world. Hawthorn's flowers, leaves, and fruit (berries) are used as medicine, although the flowers have an unpleasant smell and taste slightly bitter. The hawthorn fruit is sour.

Hawthorn is one of the oldest medicinal plants known in Europe, where it has been used since the Middle Ages for heart problems. The ancient Greeks and Native Americans also recognized hawthorn's heart-healthy properties.

Hawthorn also is called *Crataegus* extract, mayflower, maybush, and whitethorn. Common trade names for hawthorn include Cardiplant, Hawthorn Berry, Hawthorn Formula, Hawthorn Heart, Hawthorn Phytosome, and Hawthorn Power.

General use

Hawthorn most commonly is used to treat **heart disease** and to treat and prevent cardiovascular disorders. Herbalists consider hawthorn to be the world's best heart tonic. It increases blood flow to the heart by dilating the coronary arteries; lowers blood pressure and eases the heart's workload by dilating arteries in the arms and legs; and increases the force of the heart's contractions.

In Europe, scientific studies have shown that the hawthorn leaf expands the blood vessels and lets more oxygen-rich blood reach the heart muscles; increases the strength of the heartbeat and slightly increases its speed; and helps the heart by reducing resistance throughout the rest of the circulatory system. Hawthorn leaf is used for **angina** and weak heart. A 2001 report on a European study stated that patients using hawthorn extract reported improved **exercise** intolerance, **fatigue**, and shortness of breath.

Hawthorn also is a powerful antioxidant. There is strong evidence that **antioxidants** lower the risk of heart attacks, strokes, and deaths from heart diseases, but this has not been proven in studies. Antioxidants are believed to help the coronary arteries dilate and increase blood flow to the heart. They may prevent blockages from coming back after a surgical procedure called angioplasty.

Hawthorn is used, in conjunction with standard medical treatment, for heart failure classified as mild to moderate (stage II) by the New York Heart Association and to prevent angina. Mild to moderate heart failure includes patients with heart disease who do not have any limitations in their physical activities due to the heart disease. They are comfortable when resting and feel symptoms such as fatigue, palpitation, shortness of breath, or angina **pain** when performing ordinary physical activities.

Hawthorn has long been used in Europe to treat mild cases of heart failure. In Germany, the Federal Institute for Drugs and Medical Devices has approved the use of hawthorn leaf with flower extracts as a treatment for New York Heart Association functional stage II heart failure. The treatment also is listed in the German Pharmacopeia and approved in the German Commission E monographs. Several recent studies conducted outside the United States, primarily in Germany, have studied hawthorn's effects. In one study, patients who took hawthorn after having moderate heart attacks showed some improvement compared to patients who took a placebo; however, this study only lasted eight weeks. Other studies have shown that hawthorn can be used safely and effectively for congestive heart failure, that it can improve heart function in patients with chronic heart disease, and that it compared well with a heart drug called Captopril in treating stage II heart disease patients. Most of these studies only lasted eight weeks.

In 2003, a longer trial, consisting of 16 weeks of treatment of more than 200 patients, showed that use of hawthorn increased exercise capacity and decreased signs and symptoms on heart failure. Hawthorn was slightly more effective at a higher dose (1,800 mg per day).

Hawthorn also is taken in liquid form for **insomnia** and nervous conditions and is used as a gargle for sore throats. In folk medicine, hawthorn is used as a heart tonic and treatment, to regulate blood pressure, and as a sedative, but it hasn't been proven effective yet in clinical studies.

Preparations

Hawthorn is most commonly used in liquid or dry extracts or as capsules. It is collected and dried at room temperature. The dosage of hawthorn varies and the manufacturer's directions should always be followed. A typical dose of hawthorn might be 160 to 900 mg of extract given in two or three doses a day or 1 gram of crushed herb taken up to five times a day. Hawthorn should be taken for at least six weeks. It should be stored in a tightly sealed container and protected from the light.

Precautions

Hawthorn should only be used for diagnosed heart conditions. Women who are pregnant or breast feeding should take hawthorn only under the advice of a physician. Patients who are sensitive to other types of Rosaceae plants should not take hawthorn.

Hawthorn leaf only is useful for angina when it is used over a long period of time. It can sometimes prevent angina, but it cannot treat an angina attack.

Side effects

Hawthorn rarely has side effects. In high doses, hawthorn can cause a severe drop in blood pressure, arrhythmias, and sedation.

Interactions

Since hawthorn performs the same function as some nitrates, cardiac glycosides, central nervous system depressants, and medications for high blood pressure, lower doses of these medications might be needed. Consult a qualified practitioner for appropriate dosages.

Resources

BOOKS

Fetrow, Charles W. and Avila, Juan R. *Professional's Handbook of Complementary & Alternative Medicines.* Springhouse, 1999.

The PDR Family Guide to Natural Medicines & Healing Therapies. Three Rivers Press, 1999.

PDR for Herbal Medicines. Medical Economics Company, 1998.

PERIODICALS

Gaby, Alan R. "Hawthorn (Crateagus) Effective Against Heart Failure: Double-blind Study." *Townsend Letter for Doctors and Patients* , (May 2003): 32.

KEY TERMS

Angina—A type of pain in the chest caused by a temporary inadequate blood supply to the heart. Angina usually occurs after excitement or exertion.

Angioplasty—Surgery to dilate the narrowed or blocked part of a blood vessel.

Arrhythmia—An abnormal rate or rhythm of the heartbeat.

Cardiac glycosides—Drugs that block the enzyme that regulates the electrical activity of the heart

Cardiovascular—Related to the heart and lungs.

Dyspnea—Shortness of breath.

Palpitation—A feeling of irregular or rapid heartbeat.

"Heart Effects of Herbal Medicine." *Harvard Health Letter* (March 2000): 3.

"Herbs and Drugs for Your Heart: Sorting Out What's Safe." *Herbs for Health* (Nov/Dec 1999):28-29.

Walsh, Nancy. "Hawthorn Extract Limits CHF, Mild Heart Ailments." *Internal Medicine News* (October 1, 2001):9.

OTHER

onhealth. *"Hawthorn Leaf."* http://onhealth.com/alternative/resource/herbs/item,77150.asp

"Hawthorn for the Heart: A Cardiologist's Perspective." *Heart Watch*, from the publishers of *The New England Journal of Medicine*, http://www.allhealth.com/heartwatch/jul99/nejm/0,4802,7016_127324,00.html.

Lori De Milto
Teresa G. Odle

Hay fever

Definition

Hay fever, which is also called allergic **rhinitis**, is a common allergic condition. A main feature of the condition is an inflammation of the nasal passages, or rhinitis, caused by an allergic reaction to pollen. Hay fever usually occurs when airborne plant pollens are at their highest levels in the spring, summer, and early fall.

Description

Hay fever is one of the most common chronic diseases in the United States. It is estimated that about 35

SYMPTOMS OF HAY FEVER
Symptoms
Sneezing
Runny nose
Watery eyes
Postnasal drip
Sore throat and roof of mouth
Head congestion
Ear pressure
Sleep disturbances
Nasal discharge

million people in the United States are affected. Hay fever can develop at any age, but it shows up most often in childhood through the early 20s. The term "hay fever" is not quite accurate, since the pollen of hay grasses is only one of the many possible allergens involved, and there is no fever. Although an allergy to pollen does not appear to be inherited, the tendency to allergic sensitivity in general may run in families.

Causes & symptoms

Of all the causes of **allergies**, pollen is one of the most widespread. Trees, weeds, and grasses produce pollen in large amounts for seed production. These pollens are dispersed by the wind, and many never reach the intended targets. Instead, they are inhaled through the nose and throat. Different plants release their pollen at different times of the year, so the timing of hay fever symptoms varies from person to person, depending on which plants provoke a response.

For people with hay fever, inhaled pollen grains are identified by the body as foreign invaders. This is probably due to a dysfunction in the immune system. The mast cells of the immune system act as storage containers for highly reactive chemical granules, including histamine. Allergens trigger a release of these granules, and the mast cells spill their chemicals into neighboring blood vessels and nerve cells. Histamine dilates the blood vessels, causing fluids to escape into surrounding tissues. This results in swelling, pooling of fluid in the tissues, and redness of the nose and eyes. Histamine also stimulates **pain** receptors, and causes the itchiness and discomfort of the nose, eyes, and throat that are common hay fever symptoms.

Inflammation of the nose, or rhinitis, is the major symptom of hay fever. Inflammation causes **itching**,

sneezing, runny nose, redness, and tenderness. Swelling of the sinuses can constrict the eustachian tube that connects the inner ear to the throat, causing a feeling of congestion and popping in the ears. Mucus from the sinuses may run down the back of the throat, leading to throat irritation and redness. Seasonal **fatigue** and sinus headaches may also be indications of hay fever, as well as respiratory congestion and a decreased sense of smell. Severe allergies can lead to dark circles under the eyes, puffy eyelids, and creases under the eyes. Characteristically, children with hay fever may push their noses upward with the palm of their hand or twitch their noses to clear the congestion.

Virtually any type of tree or grass may cause hay fever, although plants with showy flowers usually produce a sticky pollen that is much less likely to become airborne. Among North American plants, weeds are the most prolific producers of allergenic pollen. Ragweed is the major culprit, but other plant pollens that routinely affect hay fever sufferers include sagebrush, lamb's-quarter, Russian thistle, and English **plantain**. Grasses include timothy grass, Kentucky bluegrass, Johnson grass, Bermuda grass, redtop grass, orchard grass, and sweet vernal grass. Trees that produce allergenic pollen include **oak**, ash, elm, hickory, pecan, box **elder**, and mountain cedar.

Diagnosis

The diagnosis of hay fever is usually simple. A thorough history of the illness is important in diagnosing allergies, including whether the symptoms vary according to time of day or the season, and possible exposures. When symptoms always appear during a particular season and disappear with the onset of cold weather, hay fever is almost certainly the culprit. For a more definitive diagnosis, a skin prick test is used, in which a diluted extract of the suspected allergen is injected superficially or scratched into the skin and the reaction is observed. Another test is a provocative challenge, which is performed by putting an extract of the suspected allergen onto the conjunctiva of the eye or in the nose or lungs. When such direct skin testing is not possible, various methods of testing the blood may be used. Other conditions causing rhinitis, such as infection, may have to be ruled out by a nasal smear, in which a sample of mucus is taken on a swab for examination.

Treatment

Alternative treatments for hay fever often focus on modulation of the body's immune response. They frequently center around diet and lifestyle adjustments. A healthy diet high in fiber and whole foods, including

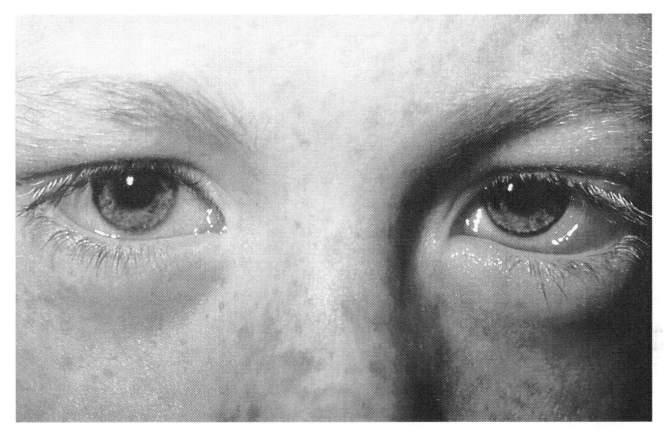

A child's red, watery, itchy eyes caused by hay fever. *(NMSB/ Custom Medical Stock Photo. Reproduced by permission.)*

generous amounts of vegetables, grains, nuts, and raw seeds should be maintained. Plenty of fluids should be consumed. Six to eight glasses of water daily are recommended, along with plenty of herbal teas. Raw vegetable juices are also beneficial, particularly carrot, celery, beet, cucumber, spinach, and **parsley**. Meat, dairy, and foods high in saturated fats may aggravate a hay fever condition, and should be limited in the diet. It is also best to avoid dairy products, wheat, eggs, citrus fruits, chocolate, peanuts, shellfish, food colorings, and preservatives, especially sulfites. These are all common food allergens that may worsen hay fever symptoms. **Caffeine**, alcohol, tobacco, and sugar should be avoided, as well.

Beneficial supplements for treating hay fever include vitamins A, E, and B complex. **Vitamin C**, especially the buffered type, is a natural antihistamine. In substantial amounts it can help stabilize the mucous membrane response to allergens. **Bioflavonoids** prevent the release of histamine, and can be taken in combination with vitamin C. **Essential fatty acids**, contained in **evening primrose oil**, **fish oil**, or **flaxseed** oil, are also recommended as a daily supplement. **Glutathione** peroxidase is an enzyme that blocks a key inflammatory reaction in the hay fever cycle. It can play a key role in

neutralizing the allergic reactions of hay fever. **Selenium** is a trace mineral that may help stop the inflammation due to allergens and reduce other allergy symptoms.

For symptom relief, nettles (*Urtica dioica*) have been reported to have the ability to clear the sinuses and to greatly reduce other symptoms. Tincture of **licorice** (*Glycerrhiza glabra*) is also recommended. A good tincture combination for hay fever is comprised of equal parts of **black cohosh** (*Cimicifuga racemosa*), Chinese **skullcap** (*Scutellaria baicalensis*), **pleurisy** root, orbutterflyweed (*Asclepias tuberosa*), **catnip** (*Nepeta cataria*), and **cayenne** pepper (*Capsicum frutescens*). Other western herbal remedies herbs found to be effective include **ginger** root (*Zingiber officinale*), **eyebright** (*Euphrasia officinalis*), **goldenseal** (*Hydrastis canadensis*), ephedra, horseradish (*Amoracia rusticana*), and **mullein** (*Verbascum thapsus*). **Bee pollen** may also be effective in alleviating or eliminating hay fever symptoms. Bee pollen should be taken a few months before the hay fever season starts. It desensitizes the body and can dramatically reduce hay fever symptoms.

Acute attacks of hay fever often respond to homeopathic remedies. Possible hay fever remedies include **Allium cepa**, **Arsenicum album**, euphrasia, **Ferrum**

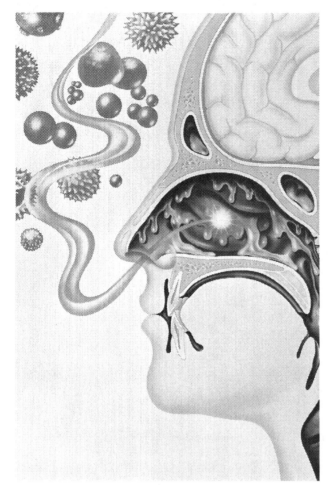

This illustration depicts excessive mucus production in the nose after inhalation of airborne pollen. *(Photo Researchers, Inc. Reproduced by permission.)*

phosphoricum, **gelsemium**, **Natrum muriaticum**, **Nux vomica**, sabadilla, and wyethia, depending on the associated symptoms. Since hay fever is often associated with deep-seated health problems, it is often best addressed with a constitutional remedy and the guidance of an experienced homeopathic practitioner.

Indoor allergens can cause increased sensitivity to outdoor allergens. Therefore allergy testing for allergens other than pollen should be done, and those allergens should be removed from the diet or the environment to the greatest extent possible.

Allopathic treatment

The goal of most medical approaches to hay fever treatment is reduction of symptoms. Avoidance of the allergens is best, but this is often not possible. When it is not possible, drug therapy is the major form of medical treatment used. Care should be taken, however, since a wide variety of antihistamines are available, and they all have potential side effects that impact function. These may include drowsiness, heart problems, and harmful interactions with other medications and medical conditions. The extended use of topical decongestants can cause rebound congestion that is worse than the original problem.

Antihistamines block the action of histamine. They are most effective when used preventively, before symptoms appear. Over-the-counter antihistamines are often sufficient to provide relief for hay fever symptoms. People with severe or frequent symptoms, however, may need stronger, prescription antihistamines. Azelastine, an antihistamine nasal spray, is effective and causes fewer side effects than oral antihistamines. When antihistamines do not relieve nasal symptoms, a nasal spray of cromolyn **sodium** is sometimes used. It works by preventing the release of histamine and similar chemicals.

Decongestants constrict blood vessels and counteract the effects of histamine. They may also be helpful in reducing symptoms such as nasal congestion. Nasal sprays are available that can be applied directly inside the nose. Oral decongestants are available as well. Phenylpropanolamine, phenylephrine, or pseudoephedrine are available in many preparations combined with antihistamines to increase the effectiveness of the drugs. Decongestants are stimulants and may cause increased heart rate and blood pressure, headaches, and agitation.

Corticosteroids may be prescribed to reduce severe symptoms. An intranasal corticosteroid spray can be quite useful in reducing inflammation of the mucous membranes. Severe symptoms that do not respond to other treatment may require a course of oral corticosteroids. Corticosteroids are best started before allergy season begins. They are especially effective because they work more slowly and last longer than most other types of medication.

Late in 2001, researchers reported the first of many new drugs that may change treatment of hay fever and **asthma**: omalizumab. A monoclonal antibody, omalizumab works by blocking immunoglobulin E (IgE), an antibody produced in excessive amounts in people suffering from hay fever.

Expected results

It is possible that hay fever can be outgrown if the immune system becomes less sensitive to the pollen. However, while hay fever may improve over time, it may also get worse or even lead to the development of new allergies. Hay fever treatment may sometimes cause uncomfortable and even dangerous side effects. However, most people can achieve acceptable hay fever relief with a combination of preventive strategies and treatment.

Prevention

There is no known way to prevent development of hay fever, but subsequent attacks may be reduced or prevented. Immunotherapy, also known as desensitization or allergy shots, involves injections of very small but gradually increasing amounts of an allergen over several weeks or months, with periodic boosters. This serves to acclimatize, or familiarize, the body to encountering the allergen without having a major allergic response. Individuals receiving allergy shots will be monitored closely following each shot because of the small risk of anaphylaxis. Full benefits of the shots may take up to several years to achieve, and even then about one person in five does not receive any benefit from the immunotherapy.

Reducing exposure to pollen may reduce symptoms of hay fever. Most trees produce pollen in the spring, while most grasses and flowers produce pollen during the summer, and ragweed and other late-blooming plants produce pollen during late summer and early autumn. People with hay fever should be aware of their particular "pollen season" and remain indoors whenever possible during that time. A pollen count can be used as a general guide for when it is most advisable to stay indoors to avoid contact with the pollen. Unfortunately, moving to a region with consistently low pollen counts is rarely effective, since new allergies often develop to the local flora.

Further strategies to prevent or reduce hay fever attacks include the following:

- Remain indoors with windows closed during the morning hours, when pollen levels are highest.

- Car windows should be kept rolled up while driving.

- A surgical facemask can be worn when outside.

- Forests and fields of grasses should be avoided, especially at the height of the pollen season.

- Clothes and hair should be washed after being outside.

- Air conditioners or air filters should be used in the home, and their filters should be changed regularly.

Resources

BOOKS

Adelman, Daniel C., et al., eds. *Manual of Allergy and Immunology.* 4th ed. Boston: Little, Brown & Co., 2002.

Weil, Andrew. *Natural Health, Natural Medicine: A Comprehensive Manual for Wellness and Self-Care.* New York: Houghton Mifflin Co., 1995.

PERIODICALS

Plaut, Marshall. "Immune-Based, Targeted Therapy for Allergic Diseases." *JAMA, The Journal of the American Medical Association.* (December 19, 2001): 3005.

KEY TERMS

. . . .

Allergen—A substance that provokes an allergic response.

Anaphylaxis—A possibly life-threatening allergic reaction causing increased sensitivity to an allergen. It can result in a sharp drop in blood pressure and difficulty breathing.

Antigen—A foreign protein to which the body reacts by making antibodies.

Granules—Small packets of reactive chemicals stored within cells.

Histamine—A chemical released by mast cells that activates pain receptors and causes cells to become leaky.

Mast cells—A type of immune system cell that is found in the lining of the nasal passages and eyelids, displays a type of antibody called immunoglobulin type E (IgE) on its cell surface, and participates in the allergic response by releasing histamine from intracellular granules.

Pollen count—The amount of pollen in the air; often broadcast on the daily news during allergy season. It tends to be lower after a heavy rain that washes the pollen out of the air and higher on warm, dry, windy days.

OTHER

drkoop.com Medical Encyclopedia. "Allergic rhinitis." [cited October 2002]. <http://www.drkoop.com>.

Merck & Co., Inc. "Disorders with Type I Hypersensitivity Reactions." [cited October 2002]. <http://www.merck.com/pubs/mmanual/section12/chapter148/148b.htm>.

Virtual Hospital of University of Iowa Health Care. [cited October 2002]. <http://www.vh.org>.

Patience Paradox
Teresa G. Odle

He shou wu *see* **Fo ti**

Head lice *see* **Lice infestation**

Headache

Definition

A headache is a **pain** in the head and neck region that may be either a disorder in its own right or a symp-

HEADACHE THERAPIES

	Description	Type
Acupressure	Press pointer fingers beneath cheekbones and parallel to pupils (Stomach 3) for one minute. Squeeze fleshy area between thumb and pointer finger (Large Intestine 4) for one minute.	Sinus
Aromatherapy	Massage mixture of lavender oil and sunflower oil in temples, sides of eyes, behind ears, and on the neck. Do same using eucalyptus.	Migraine, tension, and sinus
Chiropractic	Spinal or cervical manipulation to realign posture.	Tension
Diet and exercise	Avoid chocolate, cheeses, citrus, red wine, and foods containing sodium nitrates or MSG. Exercise regularly.	Migraine
Herbal remedies	Feverfew, hawthorn, skullcap, ginger, goldenseal, valerian, passionflower, and cayenne.	Migraine and tension
Homeopathy	Belladonna, bryonia, kali bichromicum, and nux vomica.	Sinus and tension
Home remedies	Simultaneous ice pack/warm foot soak; drink three cold glasses of water; inhale pure oxygen.	Migraine and cluster
Massage	Scalp massage	All
Mind/body	Meditation and relaxation and biofeedback.	Migraine
Osteopathy	Neuromuscular manipulation and massage of head, neck, and shoulders.	All

tom of an underlying medical condition or disease. The medical term for headache is cephalalgia.

Description

Headaches are divided into two large categories, primary and secondary, according to guidelines established by the International Headache Society (IHS) in 1988 and revised for republication in 2004. Primary headaches—accounting for more than 90% of all headaches— are not caused by an underlying medical condition. There are three major types of primary headaches: migraine, cluster, and tension. Secondary headaches are caused by another disease or medical condition, and account for fewer than 10% of headaches.

Rebound headaches, also known as analgesic abuse headaches, are a subtype of primary headache caused by overuse of headache drugs. They may be associated with medications taken for tension or migraine headaches.

Secondary headaches are classified as either traction or inflammatory headaches. Traction headaches result from the pulling, pushing, or stretching of pain-sensitive structures, such as a brain tumor pressing upon the outer layer of tissue that covers the brain. Inflammatory headaches are caused by infectious diseases of the ears, teeth, sinuses, or other parts of the head.

Headaches are very common in the North American adult population. The American Council for Headache Education (ACHE) estimates that 95% of women and 90% of men in the United States and Canada have had at least one headache in the past 12 months. Most of these are tension headaches. Migraine headaches are less common, affecting about 11% of the population in the United States and 15% in Canada. Several studies indicate that doctors tend to underdiagnose migraine headaches; thus the true number of patients with migraines may be considerably higher than the reported statistics. Cluster headaches are the least common type of primary headaches, affecting about 0.4% of adult males in the United States and 0.08% of adult females. Cluster headaches occur most commonly in adults between the ages of 20 and 40.

It is possible for patients to suffer from more than one type of headache. For example, patients with chronic tension headaches often have migraine headaches as well.

Causes & symptoms

Causes

A person feels headache pain when specialized nerve endings, known as nociceptors, are stimulated by pressure on or injury to any of the pain-sensitive structures of the head. Most nociceptors in humans are located in the skin or on the walls of blood vessels and internal organs. The bones of the skull and the brain itself do not contain these specialized pain receptors. The parts of the head that are sensitive to pain include the skin that covers the skull and upper spine; the 5th, 9th, and 10th cranial nerves, and the nerves that supply the upper part of the neck; and the large arteries located at the base of the brain, as well as those that supply the membranes covering the brain and spinal cord.

Tension headaches typically result from tightening of the face, neck, and scalp muscles as a result of emotional stress; physical postures that cause the head and neck muscles to tense (e.g., holding a phone against the ear with one's shoulder); emotional **depression** or **anxiety**; temporomandibular joint (TMJ) dysfunction; or arthritis of the neck. The tense muscles put pressure on the walls of the blood vessels that supply the neck and head, which stimulates the nociceptors in the tissues that line the blood vessels.

The causes of migraine headaches have been debated since the 1940s. Some researchers think that migraines are the end result of a **magnesium** deficiency in the brain, or of hypersensitivity to a neurotransmitter (brain chemical) known as dopamine. Another theory is that certain nerve cells in the brain become unusually excitable, setting off a chain reaction that leads to changes in the amount of blood flowing through the blood vessels and stimulation of their nociceptors. Specific genes associated with migraines were recently discovered. This finding suggests that genetic mutations may be responsible for the abnormal excitability of the nerve cells in the brains of patients with migraine headaches.

As of 2004, little is known about the causes of cluster headaches or changes in the central nervous system that produce them. Patients with cluster headaches are advised to quit **smoking** and minimize their use of alcohol because nicotine and alcohol appear to trigger these headaches. The precise connection between these chemicals and cluster attacks is not yet completely understood.

Symptoms

Tension headaches are less severe than other types of primary headache. They rarely last more than a few hours; 82% resolve in less than a day. Patients usually describe the pain of a tension headache as mild to moderate. The doctor will not find anything abnormal in the course of a general physical examination, although he or she may detect sore or tense areas (trigger points) in the muscles of the patient's forehead, neck, or upper shoulder area.

Migraine headaches are characterized by throbbing or pulsating pain of moderate or severe intensity lasting from four hours to as long as three days. The pain is typically felt on one side of the head; in fact, the English word "migraine" is a combination of two Greek words that mean "half" and "head." Migraine headaches wors-

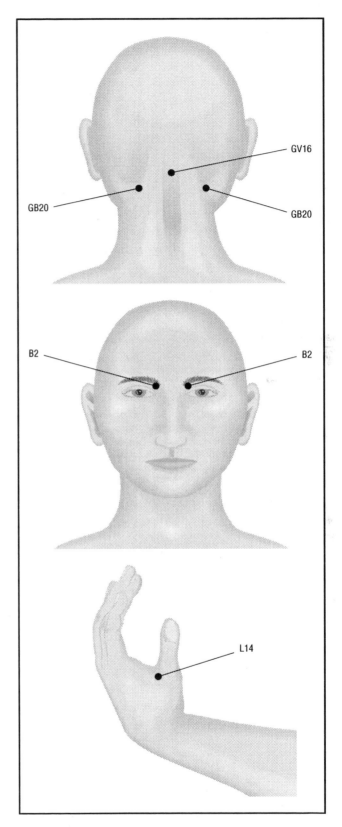

Acupressure points that help relieve headaches. (*Illustration by GGS Information Services, Inc. The Gale Group.*)

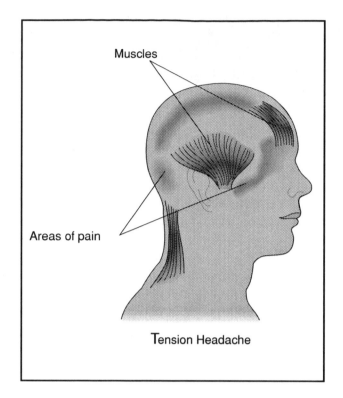

Muscles

Areas of pain

Tension Headache

Tension headache is the most common type of headache. It is caused by severe muscle contractions and triggered by stress or exertion. Tension headaches usually occur in the front of the head, although they also may appear at the top or the back of the skull, as shown in the illustration above. *(Illustration by Electronic Illustrators Group. The Gale Group.)*

en with physical activity, and are often accompanied by **nausea** and **vomiting**. Patients with migraine headaches are hypersensitive to lights, sounds, and odors.

Cluster headaches are recurrent brief attacks of sudden and severe pain on one side of the head. The pain is usually most intense in the area around the eye. Cluster headaches may last between five minutes and three hours, and may occur once every other day or as often as eight times per day. Some patients describe it as severe enough to make them consider suicide. Patients may pace the floor, weep, rock back and forth, or bang their heads against a wall in desperate attempts to stop the pain. In addition to severe pain, patients often have a runny or congested nose, watery or inflamed eyes, drooping eyelids, swelling in the area of the eyebrows, and heavy facial perspiration. Because of the nasal symptoms and the relative rarity of cluster headaches, they are sometimes misdiagnosed as sinusitis.

Diagnosis

Patient history

The differential diagnosis of headaches begins with a careful patient history that includes information about

head injuries or surgery on the head; eye problems or disorders; sinus **infections**; dental problems or extensive oral surgery; and medications that the patient takes regularly. Some primary care physicians give the patient a printed questionnaire that consists of 50–55 brief questions covering such matters as the timing and frequency of the headaches; family history of the same type of headache; signs of depression; correlation between headaches and weather changes; and so on. The doctor may also ask the patient to keep a headache diary to help identify foods, stress, lack of sleep, weather, and other factors that may trigger the pain.

Physical examination

A physical examination helps the doctor identify signs and symptoms that may be relevant to the diagnosis such as **fever**; difficulty breathing; nausea or vomiting; stiff neck; changes in vision or hearing; watering or inflammation of the nose and eyes; evidence of head trauma; skin **rashes** or other indications of an infectious disease; and abnormalities in the structure or alignment of the spinal column, teeth or jaw. In some cases, the doctor may refer the patient to a dentist or oral surgeon for a more detailed evaluation of the mouth and jaw.

Special tests and imaging studies

Laboratory tests are useful in identifying headaches caused by infections, **anemia**, or thyroid disease. These tests include a complete blood count (CBC); erythrocyte sedimentation rate (ESR); and blood serum chemistry profile. Patients who report visual disturbances and other neurologic symptoms may be given visual field tests and screened for **glaucoma** (a condition involving high fluid pressure inside the eye). Imaging studies may include x rays of the sinuses to check for infections; and CT or MRI scans, which can rule out brain tumors and cerebral aneurysms. Patients whose symptoms cannot be fully explained by the results of physical examinations and tests may be referred to a psychiatrist for evaluation of psychological factors related to their headaches.

Warning symptoms

There are warning signs associated with headache that indicate the need for prompt medical attention. Patients with any of the following symptoms should see a physician at once:

- Three or more headaches per week.
- Need for a headache pain reliever every day or almost every day.
- Need for greater than recommended doses of over-the-counter (OTC) headache medications.

- Headache accompanied by one-sided weakness, numbness, visual loss, speech difficulty, or other signs.

- Headache that becomes worse over a period of six months, especially if most prominent in the morning or if accompanied by neurological symptoms.

- Sudden onset of headache accompanied by fever and stiff neck.

- Change in the character of the headaches—for example, persistent severe headaches in a person who has previously had only mild headaches of brief duration.

- Recurrent headaches in a child.

- Recurrent severe headaches beginning after age 50.

Treatment

Alternative remedies can lessen the frequency and severity of headaches. Common treatments include:

- Acupressure. The stomach 3 and large intestine 4 points relieve sinus headaches.

- **Acupuncture**. A National Institutes of Health (NIH) panel concluded that acupuncture may be a useful treatment for headache.

- Aerobic exercise. Regular aerobic exercise reduces the frequency and intensity of headaches.

- Aromatherapy. Massage using the **essential oils** of lavender, **rosemary**, or **peppermint** relieves headache.

- Autogenic therapy. Headache may be relieved by learning to put oneself in a semi-hypnotic state.

- Chiropractic. Cervical manipulation may relieve tension headaches.

- Heat and/or cold. A hot shower or bath can ease tension headaches. Vascular headache may be relieved by placing an ice pack on the forehead, or the feet in hot water and a cold pack on the forehead (**hydrotherapy** treatment).

- Herbals. Feverfew (*Chrysanthemum parthenium*) can be used for migraine; goldenseal (*Hydrastis canadensis*) for sinus headache; valerian (*Valeriana officinalis*), skullcap (*Scutellaria lateriflora*), or passionflower (*Passiflora incarnata*) for tension headache; and cayenne (in nostrils) for cluster headache. A German remedy made from butterbur root (*Petasites hybridus*) is now available in the United States under the brand name Petadolex. The herb, Brahmi (*Bacopa monnieri*), is used in **Ayurvedic medicine** to treat headaches related to anxiety.

- Holistic medicine. Headaches may be caused by **constipation** and liver malfunction. Apple-spinach juice relieves constipation, and a blend of carrot, beet, celery, and **parsley** juices treats the liver.

- Homeopathy. Remedies are chosen for each patient and may include Belladonna (throbbing headache), Bryonia (splitting headache), Kali bichromicum (sinus headache), and Nux vomica (tension headache with nausea and vomiting).

- Massage. Firm massage of the forehead, neck, and scalp may relieve headache.

- Osteopathy. Headache is treated with neuromuscular manipulation and massage of the head, neck, and upper back.

- Pressure. A headband tied tightly around the head may relieve migraines in some patients.

- Reflexology. Headache is treated using the solar plexus, ear, eye, and head points.

- Relaxation techniques. Meditation, biofeedback, and **yoga** may relieve headache.

- Supplements. Vitamins B_2 and B_{12}, **niacin**, and magnesium (a mineral) may help treat or prevent headache.

- Transcutaneous electrical nerve stimulation (TENS). This effective headache treatment electrically stimulates nerves and blocks pain transmission.

- Visualization. This relaxation technique controls the images in the mind, replacing negative thoughts and images with positive ones that enhance relaxation.

Allopathic treatment

Medical

Tension headaches are usually relieved fairly rapidly by such over-the-counter analgesics as aspirin (300–600 mg every four hours), acetaminophen (650 mg every four hours), or other nonsteroidal anti-inflammatory drugs (NSAIDs) such as ibuprofen (brands include Advil or Motrin) or naproxen (brands such as Naprosyn or Aleve). For patients with chronic tension headaches, the doctor may prescribe a tricyclic antidepressant or benzodiazepine tranquilizer in addition to a pain reliever. A newer treatment for chronic tension headaches is botulinum toxin (Botox type A), which appears to work quite well for some patients.

Nonsteroidal anti-inflammatory drugs, including acetaminophen (e.g. Tylenol), ibuprofen, and naproxen are helpful for early or mild migraines. More severe attacks may be treated with dihydroergotamine; a group of drugs known as triptans; beta-blockers and **calcium** channelblockers; antiseizure drugs; antidepressants (SSRIs); meperidine (Demerol); or metoclopramide (Reglan). Some of these medications are also available as nasal sprays, intramuscular injections, or rectal suppositories for patients with severe vomiting.

Sumatriptan (known as the brand Imitrex) or indomethacin (Indameth or Indocin) may be prescribed to suppress a cluster headache.

Surgical

Headaches that are caused by brain tumors, head trauma, dental problems, or disorders affecting the spinal discs usually require surgical treatment. In addition, some plastic surgeons have reported success in treating chronic migraine patients by removing some muscle tissue near the eyebrows, cutting a branch of the trigeminal nerve, and repositioning the soft tissue around the temples (sides of the head).

Psychotherapy

Psychotherapy may be helpful to patients with chronic headaches by interrupting the "feedback loop" between emotional upset and the physical symptoms of headaches.

Expected results

The prognosis for primary headaches varies. Episodic tension headaches usually resolve completely in less than a day without affecting the patient's overall health. The long-term outlook for patients with migraines depends on whether they have one or more of the other disorders associated with migraine. These disorders include Tourette's syndrome, **epilepsy**, ischemic **stroke**, hereditary essential tremor, depression, anxiety, and others. For example, migraine with aura increases a person's risk of ischemic stroke by a factor of six.

The prognosis for secondary headaches depends on the seriousness and severity of the cause.

Prevention

Lifestyle modification is one measure that people can take to lower their risk of tension headaches. They should get enough sleep and eat nutritious meals at regular times. Skipping meals, using unbalanced fad **diets** to lose weight, and insufficient or poor-quality sleep can bring on tension headaches.

Some headaches may be prevented by avoiding substances and situations that trigger them, or by employing alternative therapies, such as yoga and regular exercise. Proper lighting may prevent headaches caused by eyestrain. Because food **allergies** are often linked with headaches, especially cluster strain headaches and migraines, identification and elimination of the allergy-causing food(s) from the diet can be an important preventive measure. Women with migraines often benefit by switching from oral contraceptives to another method of birth control, or by discontinuing estrogen replacement therapy. Prophylactic treatments for migraine include prednisone, calcium channel blockers, and methysergide.

Resources

BOOKS
American Psychiatric Association. *Diagnostic and Statistical Manual of Mental Disorders*, 4th ed., text revision. Washington, DC: American Psychiatric Association, 2000.
Pelletier, Kenneth R. *The Best Alternative Medicine*, Part II, "CAM Therapies for Specific Conditions: Headache." New York: Simon&Schuster, 2002.
Rapoport, Alan M., and Fred D. Sheftell. *Headache Disorders: A Management Guide for Practitioners*. Philadelphia: W.B. Saunders Company, 1996.
Somerville, Robert. *The Alternate Advisor: The Complete Guide to Natural Therapies and Alternative Treatments*. Alexandria, VA: Time-Life Books, 1997.
Ying, Zhou Zhong, and Jin Hui De. *Clinical Manual of Chinese Herbal Medicine and Acupuncture*. New York: Churchill Livingston, 1997.

PERIODICALS
Guyuron, B., T. Tucker, and J. Davis. "Surgical Treatment of Migraine Headaches." *Plastic and Reconstructive Surgery* 109 (June 2002): 2183-9.
Headache Classification Subcommittee of the International Headache Society. "The International Classification of Headache Disorders," 2nd ed. *Cephalalgia* 24 (2004) (Supplement 1): 1–150.
Mendizabai, Jorge, M.D. "Cluster Headache." *eMedicine*, 26 September 2003. <http://www.emedicine.com/neuro/topic70.htm>.
Sahai, Soma, M.D., Robert Cowan, M.D., and David Y. Ko, M.D. "Pathophysiology and Treatment of Migraine and Related Headache." *eMedicine*, 30 April 2002. <http://www.emedicine.com/neuro/topic517.htm>.
Singh, Manish K., M.D. "Muscle Contraction Tension Headache." *eMedicine*, 5 October 2001. <http://www.emedicine.com/neuro/topic231.htm>.
Vernon, H., C. S. McDermaid, and C. Hagino. "Systematic Review of Randomized Clinical Trials of Complementary/Alternative Therapies in the Treatment of Tension-Type and Cervicogenic Headache." *Complementary Therapies in Medicine*. (1999): 142–55.

ORGANIZATIONS
American Council for Headache Education (ACHE). 19 Mantua Road, Mt. Royal, NJ 08061. (609) 423-0043 or (800) 255-2243. <http://www.achenet.org/>.
National Headache Foundation. 428 West St. James Place, Chicago, IL 60614. (800) 843-2256. <http://www.headaches.org/>.

OTHER
National Institute of Neurological Disorders and Stroke (NINDS). "Headache—Hope Through Research." Bethesda, MD:

KEY TERMS

. . . .

Analgesics—A class of pain-relieving medicines, including aspirin and acetaminophen.

Biofeedback—A technique in which a person is taught to consciously control the body's response to a stimulus.

Cephalalgia—The medical term for headache.

Chronic—A condition that occurs frequently or continuously.

Neurotransmitter—Any of a group of chemicals that transmit nerve impulses across the gap (synapse) between two nerve cells.

Nociceptor—A specialized type of nerve cell that senses pain.

Primary headache—A headache that is not caused by another disease or medical condition.

Prophylactic—Treatment that prevents a disorder's symptoms from occurring.

Secondary headache—A headache that is caused by another disease or disorder.

Transcutaneous electrical nerve stimulation (TENS)—A treatment in which a mild electrical current is passed through electrodes on the skin to stimulate nerves and block pain signals.

NINDS, <http://www.ninds.nih.gov/health_and_medical/ pubs/headache_htr>.

NINDS. "Migraine Information Page." Bethesda, MD: NINDS, 2003. <http://www.ninds.nih.gov/health_and_medical/ pubs/migraineupdate.htm>.

Rebecca J. Frey, PhD

Hearing loss

Definition

Hearing loss is any degree of impairment of the ability to apprehend sound.

Description

Sound can be measured accurately. The term decibel (dB) is a measure of loudness and refers to a unit for expressing the relative intensity of sound on a scale from zero, for a nearly imperceptible sound, to 130, which is the level at which sound causes **pain** in the average person. A drop of more than 10 dB in the level of sound a person can hear is significant.

Sound travels as waves through a medium like air or water. These waves are collected by the external ear and cause the tympanic membrane (eardrum) to vibrate. The chain of ossicles (tiny bones) connected to the eardrum—the incus, malleus, and stapes—carries the vibration to the oval window (an opening to the inner ear), increasing its amplitude 20 times on the way. There, the energy causes a standing wave in the watery liquid (endolymph) inside the organ of Corti. (A standing wave is one that does not move.) The frequency of the sound determines the configuration of the standing wave. Many thousands of tiny nerve fibers detect the highs and lows of the standing wave and transmit their findings to the brain, which interprets the signals as sound.

To summarize, sound energy passes through the air of the external ear, the bones of the middle ear, and the liquid of the inner ear. It is then translated into nerve impulses, sent to the brain through nerves, and understood there as sound. It follows that there are five steps in the hearing process:

• air conduction through the external ear to the eardrum

• bone conduction through the middle ear to the inner ear

• water conduction to the organ of Corti

• nerve conduction into the brain

• interpretation by the brain

Hearing can be interrupted in a variety of ways at each of the five steps.

The external ear canal can be blocked with ear wax, foreign objects, infection, and tumors. Overgrowth of the bone can also narrow the passageway, making blockage and infection more likely. This condition can occur when the ear canal has been flushed with cold water repeatedly for years, as is the case with surfers, for whom the condition called "surfer's ear" is named.

The eardrum is so thin a physician can see through it into the middle ear. It can be ruptured by sharp objects, pressure from an infection in the middle ear, or even a firm cuffing or slapping of the ear. The eardrum is also susceptible to pressure changes during scuba diving.

Several conditions can diminish the mobility of the small bones (ossicles) in the middle ear. Otitis media, an infection in the middle ear, occurs when fluid cannot escape into the throat because the eustachian tube is blocked. The fluid (pus or mucus) that accumulates prevents the ossicles from moving as efficiently as they normally do, thus dampening the sound waves. In a disease called otosclerosis, spongy tissue grows around the bones

DECIBEL RATINGS AND HAZARDOUS LEVELS OF NOISE

Decibel Level	Example Of Sounds
30	Soft whisper
35	Noise may prevent the listener from falling asleep
40	Quiet office noise level
50	Quiet conversation
60	Average television volume, sewing machine, lively conversation
70	Busy traffic, noisy restaurant
80	Heavy city traffic, factory noise, alarm clock
90	Cocktail party, lawn mower
100	Pneumatic drill
120	Sandblasting, thunder
140	Jet airplane
180	Rocket launching pad

Above 110 decibels, hearing may become painful

Above 120 decibels is considered deafening

Above 135 decibels, hearing will become extremely painful and hearing loss may result if exposure is prolonged

Above 180 decibels, hearing loss is almost certain with any exposure

Source: FDA Consumer, Gale Encyclopedia of Psychology, 1996. *(Stanley Publishing. Reproduced by permission.)*

of the inner ear. This growth sometimes binds the stapes in the oval window, which interferes with its normal vibration and causes deafness. All the conditions mentioned so far—those that occur in the external and middle ear—are causes of what is known as *conductive* hearing loss.

The second category, sensory hearing loss, refers to damage to the organ of Corti and the acoustic nerve. Prolonged exposure to loud noise is the leading cause of sensory hearing loss. A million people have this condition, many identified during the military draft and rejected as being unfit for duty. The cause is often believed to be prolonged exposure to rock music. Occupational noise exposure is the other leading cause of noise-induced hearing loss (NIHL) and is ample reason for wearing ear protection on the job.

More unusual, but often undetected, is low-frequency hearing loss. Scientists discovered in 2001 that people with a particular gene mutation gradually lose their abilities to hear low-frequency sounds. Since those people with this type of hearing loss can still distinguish speech, they often remain unaware of the low-frequency changes in their hearing. The scientists believe that the same gene mutations might make some people more susceptible to high-frequency hearing loss, but further study is needed.

One-third of people older than 65 have presbycusis, which is sensory hearing loss due to **aging**. Both NIHL

and presbycusis are primarily loss of the ability to hear high-frequency sounds. In speech, consonants generally have a higher frequency than vowels. Yet in most languages, consonants provide us the clues needed for determining what a person is saying. So these people hear plenty of noise, they just cannot easily make out what it means. They have particular trouble differentiating speech from background noise.

Brain **infections** such as **meningitis**, drugs such as the aminoglycoside antibiotics (streptomycin, gentamycin, kanamycin, tobramycin), and Meniere's disease can also cause permanent sensory hearing loss. Meniere's disease combines attacks of hearing loss with attacks of vertigo. The symptoms may occur together or separately. High doses of salicylates such as aspirin and quinine can cause a temporary high-frequency loss, and prolonged high doses can lead to permanent deafness. There is also a hereditary form of sensory deafness and a congenital form most often caused by **rubella** (German **measles**).

Sudden hearing loss of at least 30 dB in less than three days is most commonly caused by cochleitis, a mysterious viral infection.

The final category of hearing loss is *neural* hearing loss. Permanent neural hearing loss most often results from damage to the acoustic nerve and the parts of the brain that control hearing. Strokes, **multiple sclerosis**, and acoustic neuromas are all possible causes of neural hearing loss.

Hearing can also be diminished by **tinnitus**, which is characterized by extra sounds generated by the ear. These sounds are referred to as tinnitus, and can be ringing, blowing, clicking, or anything else that no one but the patient hears. Tinnitus may be caused by loud noises, medication, **allergies**, or medical conditions—from the same kinds of disorders that can cause diminished hearing.

Diagnosis

Many common causes of hearing loss can be detected through an examination of the ears and nose combined with simple hearing tests performed in the physician's office. An audiogram (a test of hearing at a range of sound frequencies) often concludes the evaluation. These simple tests often produce a diagnosis. If the defect is in the brain or the acoustic nerve, further neurological testing and imaging will be required.

The audiogram has many uses in diagnosing hearing deficits. The pattern of hearing loss across the audible frequencies gives clues to the cause. Several alterations in the testing procedure can give additional information. For example, speech is perceived differently than pure tones. Adequate perception of sound combined with inability to recognize words points to a brain problem rather than a sensory or conductive deficit. Loudness perception is distorted by disease in certain areas but not in others. Acoustic neuromas often distort the perception of loudness.

Treatment

Conductive hearing loss can be treated with alternative therapies that are specific to the particular condition.

Nutritional therapy

The following dietary changes may help improve certain hearing impairment conditions:

- Alleviate accumulated wax in the ear by taking oral supplements with **essential fatty acids** such as flax oil and omega-3 oil.
- Identify and avoid potential allergenic foods. Children who are allergic to foods have an increased risk of getting chronic ear infections.
- Take nutritional supplements. B-complex vitamins and **iron** supplements may be helpful in preventing protein deficiency and **anemia**. These conditions depress immune function and increase the risk of chronic ear infections. Children suffering from frequent ear infections may need supplementation with strong **antioxidants** such as vitamins A and C, **zinc**, and **bioflavonoids**. High-potency multivitamin and mineral

supplements should contain most of these helpful nutrients as well as other essential vitamins and minerals.

Herbal therapy

There are several effective herbal treatments for hearing impairments. They include:

- Ginkgo biloba. Ginkgo may be effective in patients with hearing loss who often complain of ringing in the ears.
- Natural antibiotics such as **echinacea** and **goldenseal** can help prevent or treat ear infections.
- Certain Chinese herbal combinations can help alleviate tinnitus, ear infections, and chronic sinus infections that can lead to hearing loss.

Homeopathy

Homeopathic therapies may help patients who have sensory hearing loss. An experienced homeopathic physician will prescribe specific remedies based on knowledge of the underlying cause.

Acupuncture

Acupuncture may be able to improve hearing in some patients with sensory-neural deafness. It may be used to improve the circulation of fluids in the head that lead to chronic congestion and noises.

Other therapies

Other therapies that may help improve hearing in some patients include **Ayurvedic medicine**, **craniosacral therapy**, and **auditory integration training**.

Allopathic treatment

Conductive hearing loss can almost always be restored to some degree, if not completely.

- Matter in the ear canal can easily be removed, with a dramatic improvement in hearing.
- Surfer's ear gradually regresses if the patient avoids cold water or uses a special ear plug. In advanced cases, surgeons can grind away the excess bone.
- A middle-ear infection involving fluid is also simple to treat. If medications do not work, fluid may be surgically drained through the eardrum, which heals completely after treatment.
- Traumatically damaged eardrums can be repaired with a tiny skin graft.
- Otosclerosis may be surgically repaired through an operating microscope. In this intricate procedure, tiny artificial parts are substituted for the original ossicles.

Now available for complete conductive hearing loss are bone conduction hearing aids and even devices that can be surgically implanted in the cochlea.

Sensory and neural hearing loss, on the other hand, cannot readily be cured. Fortunately such hearing loss is rarely complete, and hearing aids can fill the deficit. In-the-ear hearing aids can boost the volume of sound by up to 70 dB. (Normal speech is about 60 dB.) Federal law now requires that aids be dispensed only by prescription.

Tinnitus can sometimes be relieved by adding white noise (such as the sound of wind or waves crashing on the shore) to the environment.

Decreased hearing is such a common problem that there are legions of organizations to provide assistance. Special language training, both in lip reading and signing, is available in most regions of the United States, as well as special schools and camps for children.

Prevention

Prompt treatment and attentive follow-up of middle-ear infections in children will prevent this cause of conductive hearing loss. Sensory hearing loss as a complication of epidemic disease has been greatly reduced by control of infectious childhood diseases, such as measles. Laws that require protection from loud noise in the workplace have substantially reduced incidences of noise-induced hearing loss. Surfers, cold-water fishermen, and other people who are regularly exposed to frigid water should use the right kind of ear plugs.

Resources

BOOKS

Alberti, R. W. "Occupational Hearing Loss." *Disorders of the Nose, Throat, Ear, Head, and Neck,* edited by John Jacob Ballenger. Philadelphia: Lea & Febiger, 1991.

Bennett, J. Claude, and Fred Plum, eds. *Cecil Textbook of Medicine*. Philadelphia: W. B. Saunders, 1996.

"Hearing and Ear Disorders." In *Alternative Medicine: The Definitive Guide,* compiled by The Burton Goldberg Group. Tiburon, Calif.: Future Medicine Publishing, 1999.

Tierney, Lawrence M., M.D., et al., eds. *Current Medical Diagnosis and Treatment*. Stamford, CT: Appleton & Lange, 1998.

PERIODICALS

Nadol, J. B. "Hearing Loss." *New England Journal of Medicine* 329 (1993): 1092–102.

"Scientist Identify Gene Linked to Low-Frequency Hearing Loss." *Genomics and Genetics Weekly* (December 14, 2001): 6.

Sodipo, Joseph O., and Phillip A. Okeowo. "Therapeutic Acupuncture for Sensory-Neural Deafness." *Am J Chin Med* 8, no. 4 (1980): 385–390.

KEY TERMS

Cochlea—A snail-shaped structure inside the inner ear, which contains the organ of Corti as well as fluid-filled compartments through which sound waves travel.

Decibel—A unit of the intensity of sound, a measure of loudness.

Meniere's disease—The combination of vertigo and decreased hearing caused by abnormalities in the inner ear.

Organ of Corti—A spiral structure inside the cochlea that converts vibration to signals that are passed to the brain.

Ossicles—A group of tiny bones in the middle ear that conduct sound through vibration. The bones are the malleus (or anvil), incus (or hammer), and stapes (or stirrup).

Otosclerosis—A disease that scars and limits the motion of the small conducting bones in the middle ear.

ORGANIZATIONS

Alexander Graham Bell Association for the Deaf. 3417 Volta Place NW, Washington, DC 20007-2778. (202) 337-5220. http:/www.agbell.org.

National Association of the Deaf. 814 Thayer Ave., Silver Spring, MD 20910-4500. (301) 587-1788. http://www.nad.org.

National Institute on Deafness and Other Communication Disorders, National Institutes of Health. 31 Center Dr., Bethesda, MD 20892. (301) 496-7243. Fax: (301) 402-0018. http://www.nih.gov/nidcd.

Self Help for Hard of Hearing People, Inc. 7910 Woodmont Avenue, Suite 1200, Bethesda, MD 20814. (301) 657-2248. http://www.shhh.org.

OTHER

DeafSource: An Internet Guide to Resources for Helping Professionals Working with Deaf and Hard of Hearing Individuals. http://home.earthlink.net/~drblood.

Mai Tran
Teresa G. Odle

Heart attack

Definition

A heart attack is the death of, or damage to, part of the heart muscle because its blood supply is severely reduced or stopped.

Description

Heart attack is the leading cause of death in the United States. Approximately every 29 seconds one American will have a heart attack, and once a minute one American will die from a heart attack. More than 1.5 million Americans suffer a heart attack every year, and almost half a million die, according to the American Heart Association. Most heart attacks are the end result of years of silent but progressive coronary artery disease, which can be prevented in many people. A heart attack is often the first symptom of coronary artery disease. According to the American Heart Association, 63% of women and 48% of men who died suddenly of coronary artery disease had no previous symptoms. Heart attacks are also called myocardial infarctions (MIs).

A heart attack occurs when one or more of the coronary arteries that supply blood to the heart are completely blocked and blood to the heart muscle is cut off. The blockage is usually caused by **atherosclerosis**, the build-up of plaque in the artery walls, and/or by a blood clot in a coronary artery. Sometimes, a healthy or atherosclerotic coronary artery has a spasm and the blood flow to part of the heart decreases or stops. Why this happens is unclear, but it can result in a heart attack.

About half of all heart attack victims wait at least two hours before seeking help. This increases their chance of sudden death or being disabled. The longer the artery remains blocked during a heart attack, the more damage will be done to the heart. That is why it is important to recognize the signs of a heart attack and seek prompt medical attention at the nearest hospital with 24-hour emergency cardiac care.

About one fifth of all heart attacks are silent, that is, the victim does not know one has occurred. Although the victim feels no **pain**, silent heart attacks can still damage the heart.

The outcome of a heart attack also depends on where the blockage is, whether the heart rhythm is disturbed, and whether another coronary artery supplies blood to that part of the heart. Blockages in the left coronary artery are usually more serious than in the right coronary artery. Blockages that cause an arrhythmia, an irregular heartbeat, can cause sudden death.

Causes & symptoms

Heart attacks are generally caused by severe coronary artery disease. Most heart attacks are caused by **blood clots** that form on atherosclerotic plaque. This blocks a coronary artery from supplying oxygen-rich blood to part of the heart. A number of factors increase the risk of developing coronary artery disease.

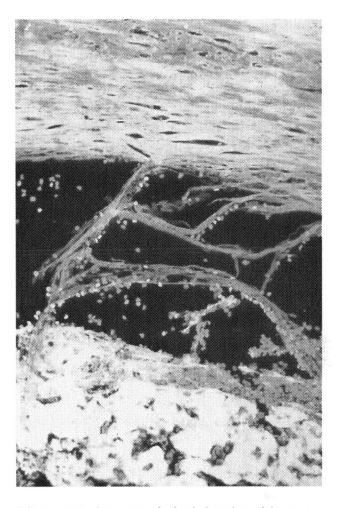

A fluorescent microscopy of a fresh thrombus of the coronary artery. *(Photograph by J.L. Carson, Custom Medical Stock Photo. Reproduced by permission.)*

Major risk factors significantly increase the risk of coronary artery disease. Those that cannot be changed are:

• Heredity. People whose parents have coronary artery disease are more likely to develop it as well. African Americans are also at increased risk, due to their higher rate of severe **hypertension** than whites.

• Gender. Men under the age of 60 years of age are more likely to have heart attacks than women of the same age.

• Age. Men over the age of 45 and women over the age of 55 are considered at risk. Older people (those over 65) are more likely to die of a heart attack. Older women are twice as likely to die within a few weeks of a heart attack than men. This may be because of other co-existing medical problems.

Major risk factors that can be changed are:

- **Smoking**. Smoking greatly increases both the chance of developing coronary artery disease and the change of dying from it. Smokers have two to four times the risk of non-smokers of sudden cardiac death and are more than twice as likely to have a heart attack. They are also more likely to die within an hour of a heart attack.

- High **cholesterol**. Cholesterol is a soft, waxy substance that is produced by the body, as well as obtained from eating foods such as meat, eggs, and other animal products. Cholesterol level is affected by age, sex, heredity, and diet. Risk of developing coronary artery disease increases as blood cholesterol levels increase. Total cholesterol of 240 mg/dL and over poses a high risk, and 200–239 mg/dL a borderline high risk. In LDL cholesterol, high risk starts at 130–159 mg/dL, depending on other risk factors. HDL (healthy cholesterol) can lower or raise the coronary risk also.

- High blood pressure. High blood pressure makes the heart work harder, and over time, weakens it. It increases the risk of heart attack, **stroke**, kidney failure, and congestive heart failure. A blood pressure of 140 over 90 or above is considered high. As the numbers increase, high blood pressure goes from Stage 1 (mild) to Stage 4 (very severe). When combined with **obesity**, smoking, high cholesterol, or diabetes, the risk of heart attack or stroke increases several times.

- Lack of physical activity. This increases the risk of coronary artery disease. Even modest physical activity is beneficial if done regularly.

- Use of certain drugs or supplements. Extreme caution is advised in the use of the herbal supplement **ephedra**. The supplement, which was marketed for weight loss and to improve athletic performance, was found to contribute to heart attack, seizure, stoke and death. In April 2003, the U.S. Food and Drug Administration (FDA) investigating controlling or banning the substance. While it was once believed that hormone replacement therapy (HRT) helped prevent **heart disease** in women, a large clinical trial called the Women's Health Initiative found the opposite to be true. In 2003, the FDA began requiring manufacturers of HRT to place warnings on the box listing adverse effects of estrogen, including increased risk of heart attack, stroke and blood clots. The labels also must mention that HRT should not be used as a preventive medicine for heart disease.

Contributing risk factors

Contributing risk factors have been linked to coronary artery disease, but their significance and prevalence are not known yet. Contributing risk factors are:

- Diabetes mellitus. The risk of developing coronary artery disease is seriously increased for diabetics. More than 80% of diabetics die of some type of heart or blood vessel disease.

- Obesity. Excess weight increases the strain on the heart, increases blood pressure and blood cholesterol, and increases the risk of developing coronary artery disease, even if no other risk factors are present. In fact, new research in 2002 shows that losing weight also reduces inflammation of the arteries in obese women, which is a risk factor equal to that of high cholesterol.

- **Stress** and anger. Some scientists believe that stress and anger can contribute to the development of coronary artery disease. Stress increases the heart rate and blood pressure, and can injure the lining of the arteries.

More than 60% of heart attack victims experience symptoms before the heart attack occurs. These sometimes occur days or weeks before the heart attack. Sometimes, people do not recognize the symptoms of a heart attack or are in denial that they are having one. Symptoms are:

- Uncomfortable pressure, fullness, squeezing, or pain in the center of the chest. This lasts more than a few minutes, or may go away and return.

- Pain that spreads to the shoulders, neck, or arms.

- Chest discomfort accompanied by lightheadedness, fainting, sweating, **nausea**, or shortness of breath.

All of these symptoms do not occur with every heart attack. Sometimes, symptoms disappear and then reappear. A person with any of these symptoms should immediately call an emergency rescue service or be driven to the nearest hospital emergency room.

Diagnosis

Experienced emergency care personnel can usually diagnose a heart attack simply by looking at the patient. To confirm this diagnosis, they talk with the patient, check heart rate and blood pressure, perform an electrocardiogram, and take a blood sample. The electrocardiogram shows which coronary artery is blocked. Electrodes covered with conductive jelly are placed on the patient's chest, arms, and legs. They send impulses of the heart's activity through an oscilloscope (a monitor) to a recorder, which traces them on paper. The blood test shows the leak of enzymes or other biochemical markers from damaged cells in the heart muscle. In 2003, the FDA cleared a new test for ruling out heart attacks in people who come to emergency rooms with severe chest pains. It is the first new blood test for evaluation of heart attacks since 1994 and is used along with an electrocardiogram.

Treatment

Heart attacks are treated with cardiopulmonary resuscitation (CPR) when necessary to start and keep the patient breathing and his heart beating. Upon arrival at the hospital, the patient is closely monitored. An electrical-shock device called a defibrillator may be used to restore a normal rhythm if the heartbeat is fluttering uncontrollably. Oxygen is often used to ease the heart's workload or to help a victim of a severe heart attack breathe easier. If oxygen is used within hours of the heart attack, it may help limit damage to the heart.

Alternative therapies aim at preventing the progression of heart disease that leads to a heart attack. Changes in lifestyle can also prevent second heart attacks.

Herbal medicine offers a variety of remedies that may have a beneficial effect on coronary artery disease. Oats (*Avena sativa*), **garlic** (*Allium sativum*), and guggul(*Commiphora mukul*) may help reduce cholesterol; linden (*Tilia europaea*) and **hawthorn** (*Crataegus* spp.) are sometimes recommended to control high blood pressure, a risk factor for heart disease. Tea (*Camellia sinensis*), especially **green tea**, is high in **antioxidants**, which studies have shown may have a preventative effect against atherosclerosis. A 2003 study found that black tea may reduce the risk of a heart attack by as much as 43% and that black tea's protective effects are even greater in women than in men.

Nutritional therapies have been shown to prevent coronary artery disease and stop, or even reverse, the progression of atherosclerosis. A low-fat, **high-fiber diet** is often recommended. It is essential to reduce the amount of meat and animal products consumed, as they are high in saturated fats. Whole grains, fresh fruits and vegetables, legumes, and nuts are recommended. Vitamin and mineral supplements that reduce, reverse, or protect against coronary artery disease include **chromium**; **calcium** and **magnesium**; B complex vitamins; the antioxidant vitamins B and E; L-carnitine; and **zinc**. These protective effects even work in the elderly, according to a 2003 report. A study revealed that those age 65 and older who ate the most cereal and bread fiber were 21% less likely to develop heart disease than those who ate the least. They also were less likely to have a heart attack or stroke.

Yoga and other bodywork, massage, **relaxation** therapies, **aromatherapy**, and **music therapy** may also help by reducing stress and promoting physical and mental wellbeing. A 1996 study in the United Kingdom found that participants who practiced **t'ai chi** had a resulting lowering in blood pressure. By evoking the body's relaxation response through **meditation** and deep breathing, blood pressure, metabolic rate, and hearth rate can all be reduced.

Allopathic treatment

Additional treatment after a heart attack can include close monitoring, electric shock, drug therapy, re-vascu-larization procedures, percutaneous transluminal coronary angioplasty and coronary artery bypass surgery.

Drugs to stabilize the patient and limit damage to the heart include thrombolytics, aspirin, anticoagulants, painkillers and tranquilizers, beta-blockers, ace-inhibitors, nitrates, rhythm-stabilizing drugs, and diuretics. Thrombolytic drugs that break up blood clots and enable oxygen-rich blood to flow through the blocked artery increase the patient's chance of survival if given as soon as possible after the heart attack. These include anisoylated plasminogen streptokinase activator complex (APSAC) or anistreplase (Eminase), recombinant tissue-type plasminogen activator (r-tPA, Retevase, or Activase), and streptokinase (Streptase, Kabikinase).

To prevent additional heart attacks, aspirin and an anticoagulant drug often follow the thrombolytic drug. These prevent new blood clots from forming and existing blood clots from growing. Anticoagulant drugs help prevent the blood from clotting. The most common anticoagulants are heparin and warfarin. Heparin is given intravenously while the patient is in the hospital; warfarin, taken orally, is often given later. Aspirin helps to prevent the dissolved blood clots from reforming.

To relieve pain, a nitroglycerine tablet taken under the tongue may be given. If the pain continues, morphine sulfate may be prescribed. Tranquilizers such as diazepam (Valium) and alprazolam (Ativan) may be prescribed to lessen the trauma of a heart attack.

Percutaneous transluminal coronary angioplasty and coronary artery bypass surgery are invasive revascularization procedures which open blocked coronary arteries and improve blood flow. They are usually performed only on patients for whom clot-dissolving drugs do not work, or who have poor **exercise** stress tests, poor left ventricular function, or **ischemia**. Generally, angioplasty is performed before coronary artery bypass surgery.

Percutaneous transluminal coronary angioplasty, usually called coronary angioplasty, is a non-surgical procedure in which a catheter (a tiny plastic tube) tipped with a balloon is threaded from a blood vessel in the thigh or arm into the blocked artery. The balloon is inflated and compresses the plaque to enlarge the blood vessel and open the blocked artery. The balloon is then deflated and the catheter is removed. Coronary angioplasty is successful about 90% of the time. For one third of patients, the artery narrows again within six months after the procedure. The procedure can be repeated. It is less invasive and less expensive than coronary artery bypass surgery.

In coronary artery bypass surgery, called bypass surgery, a detour is built around the coronary artery blockage with a healthy leg or chest wall artery or vein.

The healthy vein then supplies oxygen-rich blood to the heart. Bypass surgery is major surgery appropriate for patients with blockages in two or three major coronary arteries or severely narrowed left main coronary arteries, as well as those who have not responded to other treatments. About 70% of patients who have bypass surgery experience full relief from **angina**; about 20% experience partial relief. Long term, symptoms recur in only about three or four percent of patients per year. Five years after bypass surgery, survival expectancy is 90%, at 10 years it is about 80%, at 15 years it is about 55%, and at 20 years it is about 40%.

Expected results

The aftermath of a heart attack is often severe. Two-thirds of heart attack patients never recover fully. Within one year, 27% of men and 44% of women die. Within six years, 23% of men and 31% of women have another heart attack, 13% of men and 6% of women experience sudden death, and about 20% have heart failure. People who survive a heart attack have a chance of sudden death that is four to six times greater than others and a chance of illness and death that is two to nine times greater. Older women are more likely than men to die within a few weeks of a heart attack.

New statistics released in early 2002 revealed that about half of all deaths from heart disease happen before the patient can get to the hospital. Women were slightly more likely than men to die quickly after cardiac arrest and the risk of dying quickly from heart disease increased with age, to 61% of those over age 85. The study authors said that improved prevention and recognition of the warning symptoms of heart attack could lower the number of sudden deaths.

Prevention

Many heart attacks can be prevented through a healthy lifestyle, which can reduce the risk of developing coronary artery disease. For patients who have already had a heart attack, a healthy lifestyle and carefully following doctor's orders can prevent another heart attack. A heart healthy lifestyle includes eating right, regular exercise, maintaining a healthy weight, no smoking, moderate drinking, no illegal drugs, controlling hypertension, and managing stress.

A healthy diet includes a variety of foods that are low in fat (especially saturated fat), low in cholesterol, and high in fiber; plenty of fruits and vegetables; and limited **sodium**. Saturated fat raises cholesterol, and, in excessive amounts, it increases the amount of the proteins in blood that form blood clots. Polyunsaturated and monounsaturated fats are relatively good for the heart.

Fat should comprise no more than 30 percent of total daily calories. In 2002, new evidence suggested that a diet rich in **lutein**, the pigment found in dark green leafy vegetables, helps artery walls fight plaque and lessens risk of heart attack.

Cholesterol should be limited to about 300 mg per day. Many popular lipid-lowering drugs can reduce LDL-cholesterol by an average of 25–30% when combined with a low-fat, low-cholesterol diet. Soluble fiber can also help lower cholesterol. Fruits and vegetables are rich in fiber, vitamins, and minerals, and they are low calorie and nearly fat free. **Vitamin C** and beta-carotene, found in many fruits and vegetables, keep LDL-cholesterol from turning into a form that damages coronary arteries. Excess sodium can increase the risk of high blood pressure, and daily intake should be limited to 2,400 mg—about the amount in a teaspoon of salt.

Regular aerobic exercise can lower blood pressure, help control weight, and increase HDL ("good") cholesterol. Moderate intensity aerobic exercise lasting about 30 minutes four or more times per week is recommended for maximum heart health, according to the Centers for Disease Control and Prevention and the American College of Sports Medicine. Three 10-minute exercise periods are also beneficial. Aerobic exercise—activities such as walking, jogging, and cycling—uses the large muscle groups and forces the body to use oxygen more efficiently. It can also include everyday activities such as active gardening, climbing stairs, or brisk housework.

Maintaining a desirable body weight is also important. About one quarter of all Americans are overweight, and nearly one-tenth are obese, according to the Surgeon General's Report on Nutrition and Health. People who are 20% or more over their ideal body weight have an increased risk of developing coronary artery disease. Losing weight can help reduce total and LDL cholesterol, reduce triglycerides, and boost relative levels of HDL cholesterol.

Smoking has many adverse effects on the heart. It increases the heart rate, constricts major arteries, and can create irregular heartbeats. It also raises blood pressure, contributes to the development of plaque, increases the formation of blood clots, and causes blood platelets to cluster and impede blood flow. Heart damage caused by smoking can be repaired by quitting—even heavy smokers can return to heart health. Several studies have shown that ex-smokers face the same risk of heart disease as non-smokers within five to 10 years of quitting.

Drinking should be done in moderation. Modest consumption of alcohol can actually protect against coronary artery disease. This is believed to be because alcohol raises HDL ("good") cholesterol levels in some patients. The American Heart Association defines moderate consumption as one ounce of alcohol per day—roughly one cocktail, one 8-ounce glass of wine, or two 12-ounce glasses of beer. Excessive drinking is always bad for the heart. It usually raises blood pressure, and can poison the heart and cause abnormal heart rhythms or even heart failure. Illegal drugs, like cocaine, can seriously harm the heart and should never be used.

High blood pressure, one of the most common and serious risk factors for coronary artery disease, can be completely controlled through lifestyle changes and medication. People with moderate hypertension may be able to control it through lifestyle changes and medication.

Stress management means controlling mental and physical reactions to life's irritations and challenges. Techniques for controlling stress include thinking positively, getting enough sleep, exercising, and practicing relaxation techniques.

Daily aspirin therapy has been proven to help prevent blood clots associated with atherosclerosis. It can also prevent heart attacks from recurring, prevent heart attacks from being fatal, and lower the risk of strokes. Surprisingly, a 2002 study found that aspirin therapy is underused by people at risk for heart attacks. Patients should consult their doctors before taking aspirin regularly.

Resources

BOOKS

American Heart Association. *2000 Heart and Stroke Statistical Update*. Dallas, TX: American Heart Association, 1999.

DeBakey, Michael E., and Antonio M. Gotto Jr. *The New Living Heart*. Holbrook, MA: Adams Media Corporation, 1997.

Notelovitz, Morris, and Diana Tonnessen. *The Essential Heart Book for Women*. New York: St. Martin's Press, 1996.

PERIODICALS

"Aspirin Underused to Prevent Heart Attacks, Strokes." *Diabetes Week* (January 28, 2002): 15.

Cerrato, Paul L. "Tea Consumption May Benefit Heart and Bone." *Contemporary OB/GYN* (January 2003):101.

"Drugs or Angioplasty After a Heart Attack?" *Harvard Health Letter* 22, no. 10 (August 1997): 8.

Evans, Julie, et al. "Popeye's Favorite for Strong-to-the-Finish Arteries." *Prevention* (January 2002): 108.

"First New Blood Test to Evaluate Heart Attacks." *Biomedical Market Newsletter* (January-February 2003):42.

"How Weight Loss May Protect Your Heart" *Environmental Nutrition* (March 2002): 1.

Kirn, Timothy F. "FDA Probes Ephedra, Proposes Warning Label (Risk of Heart Attack, Seizure, Stroke)." *Clinical Psychiatry News* (April 2003):49.

Marble, Michelle. "FDA Urged to Expand Uses for Aspirin, Benefits for Women." *Women's Health Weekly* (February 10, 1997).

"More on Anger and Heart Disease." *Harvard Heart Letter.* (May 1997): 6-7.

KEY TERMS

Angina—Chest pain that happens when diseased blood vessels restrict the flow of blood to the heart. Angina is often the first symptom of coronary artery disease.

Atherosclerosis—A process in which the walls of the coronary arteries thicken due to the accumulation of plaque in the blood vessels. Atherosclerosis is the cause of coronary artery disease.

Coronary arteries—The two arteries that provide blood to the heart. The coronary arteries surround the heart like a crown, coming out of the aorta, arching down over the top of the heart, and dividing into two branches. These are the arteries where coronary artery disease occurs.

Myocardial infarction—The technical term for heart attack. Myocardial means heart muscle and infarction means death of tissue from lack of oxygen.

Plaque—A deposit of fatty and other substances that accumulate in the lining of the artery wall.

Mozaffarian, Dariush, et al. "Cereal, Fruit, and Vegetable Fiber Intake and the Risk of Cardiovascular Disease in Elderly Individuals." *JAMA* (April 2, 2003):1659.

Stephenson, Joan. "FDA Orders Estrogen Safety Warnings: Agency Offers Guidance for HRT Use." *JAMA* (February 5, 2003):537.

"Too Many Patients Never Make it to the Hospital Alive" *Medical Letter on the CDC & FDA* (March 31, 2002): 7.

ORGANIZATIONS

American Heart Association. National Center. 7272 Greenville Avenue, Dallas, TX 75231-4596. (800) AHA-USA1. http://www.americanheart.org

National Heart, Lung, and Blood Institute Information Center. P.O. Box 30105, Bethesda, MD 20824-0105. http://www.nhlbi.gov/nhlbi/nhbli.htm.

Texas Heart Institute Heart Information Service. P.O. Box 20345, Houston, TX 77225-0345. 1-800-292-2221. http://www.tmc.edu/thi/his.html.

Paula Ford-Martin
Teresa G. Odle

Heart disease

Definition

Heart disease is the narrowing or blockage of the arteries and vessels that provide oxygen and nutrient-rich

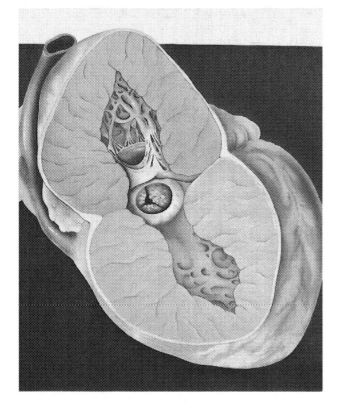

This illustration shows hypertrophic muscle in the heart. The lesions are due to an incompetent aortic valve. *(Illustration by Bryson Biomedical Illustrations, Custom Medical Stock Photo. Reproduced by permission.)*

blood to the heart. It is caused by **atherosclerosis**, an accumulation of fatty materials on the inner linings of arteries that restricts blood flow. When the blood flow to the heart is completely cut off, the result is a **heart attack** because the heart is starved of oxygen.

Description

Heart disease, also called coronary heart disease or coronary artery disease, is the leading cause of death for both men and women in the United States. According to the American Heart Association, deaths from coronary artery disease have declined somewhat since about 1990, but more than 40,000 people still died from the disease in 2000. About 13 million Americans have active symptoms of coronary artery disease.

Heart disease occurs when the coronary arteries become partially blocked or clogged. This blockage limits the flow of blood through the coronary arteries, the major arteries supplying oxygen-rich blood to the heart. The coronary arteries expand when the heart is working harder and needs more oxygen. If the arteries are unable to expand, the heart is deprived of oxygen (myocardial **ischemia**). When the blockage is limited, chest **pain** or

pressure called **angina** may occur. When the blockage cuts off the blood flow, the result is heart attack (myocardial infarction or heart muscle death).

Healthy coronary arteries are open, elastic, smooth, and slick. The artery walls are flexible and expand to let more blood through when the heart needs to work harder. The disease process is thought to begin with an injury to the linings and walls of the arteries. This injury makes them susceptible to atherosclerosis and production of **blood clots** (thrombosis).

Causes & symptoms

Heart disease is usually caused by atherosclerosis. **Cholesterol** and other fatty substances accumulate on the inner wall of the arteries. They attract fibrous tissue, blood components, and **calcium**. They then harden into artery-clogging plaques. Atherosclerotic plaques often form blood clots that can also block the coronary arteries (coronary thrombosis). Congenital defects and muscle spasms of arteries or heart muscles also block blood flow. Recent research indicates that infection from organisms such as **chlamydia** bacteria may be responsible for some cases of heart disease.

A number of major contributing risk factors increase the chance of developing heart disease. Some of these can be changed and some cannot. The greater the number of risk factors, the greater the chance of developing heart disease.

Major risk factors

Major risk factors significantly increase the chance of developing heart disease. These include:

- Heredity. People whose parents have heart disease are more likely to develop it. African-Americans are also at increased risk because they experience a high rate of severe **hypertension**.

- Gender. Men are more likely to have heart attacks than women and to have them at a younger age. Over the age of 60, however, women have heart disease at a rate equal to that of men.

- Age. Men who are 45 years of age and older and women who are 55 years of age and older are more likely to have heart disease. Occasionally, heart disease may strike men or women in their 30s. People over 65 are more likely to die from a heart attack. Older women are twice as likely as older men to die within a few weeks of a heart attack.

- **Smoking**. Smoking increases both the chance of developing heart disease and the chance of dying from it. Smokers are more than twice as likely as nonsmokers to have a heart attack and are two to four times more likely die from it.

- High cholesterol levels. Dietary sources of cholesterol are meat, dairy food, eggs, and other animal fat products. It is also produced by the body. Age, body fat, diet, **exercise**, heredity, and sex affect one's blood cholesterol. Total blood cholesterol is considered high at levels above 240 mg/dL and borderline at 200-239 mg/dL. High-risk levels of low-density lipoprotein (LDL cholesterol) begin at 130-159 mg/dL, depending on other risk factors. Risk of developing heart disease increases steadily as blood cholesterol levels increase above 160 mg/dL.

- High blood pressure. High blood pressure makes the heart work harder and weakens it over time. It increases the risk of heart attack, **stroke**, kidney failure, and congestive heart failure. A blood pressure of 140 over 90 or above is considered high. The risk of heart attack or stroke is raised several times for people with high blood pressure combined with **obesity**, smoking, high cholesterol levels, or diabetes.

- Lack of physical activity. Lack of exercise increases the risk of heart disease. Even modest physical activity, like walking, is beneficial if done regularly.

- Diabetes mellitus. The risk of developing heart disease is seriously increased for diabetics. More than 80% of diabetics die of some type of heart or blood vessel disease.

Contributing risk factors

Contributing risk factors have been linked to heart disease, but their significance is not known yet. Contributing risk factors are:

- Obesity. Excess weight increases the strain on the heart and increases the risk of developing heart disease even if no other risk factors are present. Obesity increases blood pressure and blood cholesterol and can lead to diabetes.

- Hormone replacement therapy (HRT). Even though physicians once believed that HRT could help prevent heart disease in women, the Women's Health Initiative (WHI) released information in 2002 and 2003 showing that use of combined hormones (estrogen and progestin) is harmful in women who already have coronary artery disease.

- **Stress** and anger. Some scientists believe that poorly managed stress and anger can contribute to the development of heart disease and increase the blood's tendency to form clots (thrombosis). Stress increases the heart rate and blood pressure and can injure the lining of the arteries.

- Chest pain (angina). Angina is the main symptom of coronary heart disease but it is not always present. Other symptoms include shortness of breath, chest heaviness, tightness, pain, a burning sensation, squeezing, or pressure either behind the breastbone or in the left arm, neck, or jaws. According to the American Heart Association, 63% of women and 48% of men who died suddenly of heart disease had no previous symptoms of the disease.

Diagnosis

Diagnosis begins with a visit to the physician, who will take a medical history, discuss symptoms, listen to the heart, and perform basic screening tests. These tests will measure blood lipid levels, blood pressure, **fasting** blood glucose levels, weight, and other indicators. Other diagnostic tests include resting and exercise electrocardiograms, echocardiography, radionuclide scans, and coronary angiography. The treadmill exercise (stress) test is an appropriate screening test for those with high risk factors even though they feel well.

An electrocardiogram (ECG) shows the heart's activity and may reveal a lack of oxygen (ischemia). Electrodes covered with conducting jelly are placed on the patient's chest, arms, and legs. They send impulses of the heart's activity through an oscilloscope (a monitor) to a recorder that traces them on paper. Another type of electrocardiogram, known as the exercise stress test, measures how the heart and blood vessels respond to exertion when the patient is exercising on a treadmill or a stationary bike. Both tests can be performed in a physician's office or outpatient facility.

Echocardiography, or cardiac ultrasound, uses sound waves to create an image of the heart's chambers and valves. A technician applies gel to a hand-held transducer, then presses it against the patient's chest. The heart's sound waves are converted into an image that can be displayed on a monitor. The test does not reveal the coronary arteries themselves but can detect abnormalities in the heart wall caused by heart disease. Typically performed in a doctor's office or outpatient facility, the test takes 30-60 minutes.

Radionuclide angiography enables physicians to see the blood flow of the coronary arteries. Nuclear scans are performed by injecting a small amount of a radiopharmaceutical, such as thallium, into the bloodstream. As the patient lies on a table, a camera that uses gamma rays to produce an image of the radioactive material passes over the patient and records pictures of the heart. Radionuclide angiography is usually performed in a hospital's nuclear medicine department. The radiation exposure is about the same as that in a chest x ray.

Coronary angiography is considered the most accurate method for making a diagnosis of heart disease but it is also the most invasive. During coronary angiography the patient is awake but sedated. The cardiologist inserts a catheter into a blood vessel and guides it into the heart. A contrast dye (a radiopaque substance that is visible on x ray) is injected into the catheter and x rays are taken. Coronary angiography is performed in a cardiac catheterization laboratory in either an outpatient or inpatient surgery unit.

Treatment

Herbal medicine has a variety of remedies that may have a beneficial effect on heart disease. **Garlic** (*Allium sativum*), **myrrh** (*Commiphora molmol*), oats (*Avena sativa*) may help reduce cholesterol and **hawthorn** (*Crataegus* spp.), linden (*Tilia europaea*), and **yarrow** (*Achillea millefolium*) are sometimes recommended to control high blood pressure, a risk factor for heart disease. Tea, especially **green tea** (*Camellia sinensis*), is high in **antioxidants**; studies have shown that it may have a preventative effect against atherosclerosis. Coenzyme Q10 has been shown to be beneficial for 70% of patients with congenitive heart failure. According to Dr. Elson Haas, taurine, an amino acid found in meat and fish proteins, is used to treat heart arrhythmia. Two grams three times a day for people with congestive heart failure showed improved cardiovascular functions.

Yoga and other bodywork, massage, **relaxation**, aromatherapy, and music therapies may also help prevent heart disease and stop, or even reverse, the progression of atherosclerosis. Vitamin and mineral supplements that reduce, reverse, or protect against heart disease include B-complex vitamins, calcium, **chromium**, **magnesium**, L-carnitine, **zinc**, and the antioxidant vitamins C and E. The effectiveness of vitamins C and E is still under debate, and physicians caution that they be used in moderation.

Traditional Chinese medicine (TCM) may recommend herbal remedies, massage, **acupuncture**, and dietary modification. A healthy diet (including cold **water** fish as a source of **essential fatty acids**) and exercise are important components of both alternative and conventional prevention and treatment strategies.

New reports on diet and heart disease have answered some questions, but others remain unclear. While one study concludes that four servings per day of fruit and vegetables are associated with a slight drop in risk of heart disease, eight or more servings per day can produce a significant drop in risk. Another study showed that consuming legumes at least four times per week lowered risk of heart disease from 11% to 22% compared with consuming legumes less than once a week. Research on antioxidants continues to send mixed messages, with some reports showing that vitamins E, C, and other antioxidants can help prevent heart disease, and other studies showing they have no effect. Many physicians and researchers therefore recommend that those wanting to follow healthy heart habits continue to eat a diet rich in antioxidants but recognize that there is probably no value in adding antioxidant supplements to a good diet.

Allopathic treatment

Heart disease can be treated in many ways. The choice of treatment depends on the patient and the severity of the disease. Treatments include lifestyle changes and drug therapy, coronary artery bypass surgery, and percutaneous transluminal coronary angioplasty, although these are not cures. Heart disease is a chronic disease requiring lifelong care.

Percutaneous transluminal coronary angioplasty, usually called coronary angioplasty, is a nonsurgical procedure. A catheter tipped with a balloon is threaded from a blood vessel in the thigh into the blocked artery. The balloon is inflated, compressing the plaque to enlarge the blood vessel and open the blocked artery. The balloon is then deflated and the catheter removed.

People with moderate heart disease may gain adequate control through lifestyle changes and drug therapy. Drugs such as nitrates, beta-blockers, and calcium-channel blockers relieve chest pain and complications of heart disease, but they cannot clear blocked arteries. Nitrates improve blood flow to the heart, and beta-blockers reduce the amount of oxygen required by the heart during stress. Calcium-channel blockers help keep the arteries open and reduce blood pressure.

Aspirin helps prevent blood clots from forming on plaque deposits, reducing the likelihood of a heart attack and stroke. Cholesterol-lowering medications are also indicated in most cases.

Coronary angioplasty is successful about 90% of the time, but for one-third of patients the artery narrows again within six months. The procedure can be repeated. It is less invasive and less expensive than coronary artery bypass surgery.

In coronary artery bypass surgery, a healthy vein from an arm, leg, or chest wall is used to build a detour around the coronary artery blockage. The healthy vessel then supplies oxygen-rich blood to the heart. Bypass surgery is major surgery. It is appropriate for those patients with blockages in two or three major coronary arteries, those with severely narrowed left main coronary arteries, and those who have not responded to other treatments. About 70% of patients who have bypass surgery experience full relief from angina; about 20% experience partial relief. Only about 3-4% of patients per year experience a return of symptoms.

Three other surgical procedures for unblocking coronary arteries are being studied and used on a limited basis. Atherectomy is a procedure in which the cardiologist shaves off and removes strips of plaque from the blocked artery. In laser angioplasty, a catheter with a laser tip is inserted into the affected artery to burn or break down the plaque. A metal coil called a stent can be implanted permanently to keep a blocked artery open. Stenting is becoming more common.

Expected results

Advances in medicine and the adoption of healthier lifestyles have caused a substantial decline in death rates from heart disease since the mid-1980s. New diagnostic techniques enable doctors to identify and treat heart disease in its earliest stages. New technologies and surgical procedures have extended the lives of many patients who would have otherwise died. Research on heart disease continues.

Prevention

A healthy lifestyle can help prevent heart disease and slow its progress. A heart-healthy lifestyle includes maintaining a healthy diet, regular exercise, weight maintenance, no smoking, moderate drinking, controlling hypertension, and managing stress. Cardiac rehabilitation programs are excellent to help prevent recurring coronary problems for people who are at risk and who have had coronary events and procedures.

Eating right

A healthy diet includes a variety of foods that are low in fat, especially saturated fat, low in cholesterol, and high in fiber. It includes plenty of fruits and vegetables and limited salt. Saturated fats should equal seven to 10% of calories, polyunsaturated fats should equal about 10%, monounsaturated fat should be 15%, and carbohydrates should total 55-60% of daily calories. Fat should comprise no more than 30% of total daily calories and should be taken preferably as **fish oil**, olive oil, seeds, and vegetable oil. New evidence shows that replacing saturated fat with unsaturated fat is more effective in lowering coronary heart disease risk than reducing total fat intake. Eating cold-water fish or taking comparable omega-3 polyunsaturated fatty acid supplements can help prevent cardiac death. In 2003, the American Heart Association began advocating daily servings of fatty fish or three fish oil capsules daily.

Cholesterol, a waxy substance containing fats, is found in foods such as meat, dairy, eggs, and other animal products. It is also produced in the liver. Soluble fiber can help lower cholesterol. Dietary cholesterol should be limited to about 300 milligrams per day. Many popular lipid-lowering drugs can reduce LDL cholesterol by an average of 25-30% when used with a low-fat, low-cholesterol diet.

Antioxidants are chemical compounds in plant foods. When people eat antioxidant-rich foods, they may improve the function of the arteries, prevent arterial plaque formation, and reduce their risk of **cancer**. Colorful vegetables and fruits are sources of antioxidants, and are rich in fiber, vitamins, and minerals. They are low-calorie and nearly fat-free. **Vitamin C** and beta-carotene, found in many fruits and vegetables, keep LDL-cholesterol from turning into a form that damages coronary arteries. Whole grains, especially whole oats and oat bran, reduce cholesterol.

Excess **sodium** can increase the risk of high blood pressure. Many processed foods contain large amounts of sodium. Daily intake should be limited to about 2,400 milligrams, about the amount in a teaspoon of salt.

The Food Guide Pyramid developed by the U.S. Departments of Agriculture and Health and Human Services provides easy-to-follow guidelines for daily heart-healthy eating.

Exercising regularly

Aerobic exercise can lower blood pressure, help control weight, and increase HDL (good) cholesterol. It also may keep the blood vessels more flexible. The Centers for Disease Control and Prevention and the American College of Sports Medicine recommend moderate to intense aerobic exercise lasting about 30 minutes four or more times per week for maximum heart health. People with heart disease or risk factors should consult a doctor before beginning an exercise program.

Maintaining a desirable body weight

People who are 20% or more over their ideal body weight have an increased risk of developing heart disease. Losing weight can help reduce total and LDL cholesterol, reduce triglycerides, and boost HDL cholesterol. It may also reduce blood pressure. Eating right and exercising are two key components of losing weight.

Quitting smoking

Smoking has many adverse effects on the heart. It increases the heart rate, constricts major arteries, and can create irregular heartbeats. It also raises blood pressure, contributes to the development of plaque, increases the formation of blood clots, and causes blood platelets to cluster and impede blood flow. When smokers quit the habit, heart damage can be repaired. Several studies have shown that ex-smokers face the same risk of heart disease as nonsmokers within five to 10 years after they quit.

Drinking in moderation

Modest consumption of alcohol may actually protect against heart disease because alcohol appears to raise levels of HDL cholesterol. The American Heart Association defines moderate consumption as one ounce of alcohol per day, roughly one cocktail, one 8-ounce glass of wine, or two 12-ounce glasses of beer. Excessive drinking is always bad for the heart. It usually raises blood pressure and can poison the heart and cause abnormal heart rhythms or even heart failure.

Seeking diagnosis and treatment for hypertension

High blood pressure, one of the most common and serious risk factors for heart disease, can be completely controlled through lifestyle changes and medication. Seeking out the diagnosis and treatment is critical because hypertension often exhibits no symptoms; many people do not know they have it. Moderate hypertension can be controlled by reducing dietary intake of sodium and fat, exercising regularly, managing stress, abstaining from smoking, and drinking alcohol in moderation.

Managing stress

Everyone experiences stress. Stress can sometimes be avoided and, when it is inevitable, it can be managed through relaxation techniques, exercise, and other methods.

Resources

BOOKS

American Heart Association. *2000 Heart and Stroke Statistical Update.* Dallas, TX.: American Heart Association, 1999.

DeBakey, Michael E., and Antonio M. Gotto, Jr. *Heart disease, and Surgical Treatment of Heart disease. In The New Living Heart.* Holbrook, MA: Adams Media Corporation, 1997.

Haas, Elson, M.D. *Staying Healthy with Nutrition: The Complete Guide to Diet and Natural Medicine.* Berkeley, CA: Celestial Arts, 1992.

Ody, Penelope. *The Complete Medicinal Herbal.* New York: DK Publishing. 1993.

PERIODICALS

Cerrato, Paul L. "Antioxidants, CAD, and Diabetes." *Contemporary OB/GYN* (January 2002): 111.

Dioreto, Stacy. "Legume Intake Lowers CHD Risk." *Patient Care* (January 30, 2002): 41.

"For Fighting Heart Disease, Vitamins C and E Fall Short." *Tufts University Health and Nutrition Newsletter* (January 2003): 2.

Mirzaei, H.A. "Role of Soy Protein in Lowering LDL Levels." *The Journal of Nutrition* (March 2002): 604S.

KEY TERMS

Atherosclerosis—A process in which the walls of the coronary arteries thicken due to the accumulation of plaque in the blood vessels. Atherosclerosis is the cause of heart disease.

Angina—Chest pain that occurs when diseased blood vessels restrict the flow of blood to the heart. Angina is often the first symptom of heart disease.

Beta-blocker—A drug that blocks some of the effects of fight-or-flight hormone adrenaline (epinephrine and norepinephrine), slowing the heart rate and lowering the blood pressure.

Calcium-channel blocker—A drug that blocks the entry of calcium into the muscle cells of small blood vessels (arterioles) and keeps them from narrowing.

Coronary arteries—The main arteries that provide blood to the heart. The coronary arteries surround the heart like a crown, coming out of the aorta, arching down over the top of the heart, and dividing into two branches. These are the arteries in which heart disease occurs.

HDL cholesterol—High-density lipoprotein cholesterol is a component of cholesterol that helps protect against heart disease. HDL is nicknamed good cholesterol.

LDL cholesterol—Low-density lipoprotein cholesterol is the primary cholesterol molecule. High levels of LDL increase the risk of coronary heart disease. LDL is nicknamed bad cholesterol.

Plaque—A deposit of fatty substances and calcium that accumulates in the lining of the artery wall.

Triglyceride—A fat that comes from food or is made from other energy sources in the body. Elevated triglyceride levels contribute to the development of atherosclerosis.

Sadovsky, Richard. "Omega-3 Fatty Acids and CHC Prevention." *American Family Prevention* (March 1, 2002): 952.

Wellbery, Caroline. "No HRT or Antioxidants in Women with Coronary Disease." *American Family Physician* (March 15, 2003): 1371.

Zoler, Michael L. "Heart Association Advocates Fish Oil Supplements." *Family Practice News* (January 15, 2003): 6.

ORGANIZATIONS

American Heart Association. National Center. 7272 Greenville Avenue, Dallas, Texas 75231. 1-800-AHA-USA1. <http://www.americanheart.org>.

OTHER

Lycos Health with Web MD. "Antioxidants." http://webmd. lycos.com/content/dmk/dmk_article_6463016.

Masley, Dr. Steven, M.D. The Vitality Center. http://www.dr-masley.com/index.htm.

Paula Ford-Martin
Teresa G. Odle

Heartburn

Definition

Heartburn is a burning sensation in the chest that can extend to the neck, throat, and face. It usually occurs after eating and is worsened by bending, lifting, or lying down.

Description

Heartburn, sometimes called acid **indigestion** or gastroesophageal reflux, is very common. More than one third of the population suffers from occasional heartburn, as do about one half of pregnant women. Some 50 million adult Americans complain of frequent heartburn. The occurrence of heartburn generally increases with age; however, it is common—and often overlooked—in infants and children.

Heartburn occurs when digestive juices from the stomach move back up into the esophagus, the tube connecting the throat to the stomach. The upper third of the esophagus consists of skeletal muscle that propels the food downward. The lower two-thirds of the esophagus is smooth muscle. The lower esophageal sphincter (LES) is a thick band of muscle that encircles the esophagus just above the uppermost part of the stomach. This sphincter is usually tightly closed—opening only when food passes from the esophagus into the stomach—and prevents the contents of the stomach from moving back into the delicate esophageal tissue. The stomach has a thick mucous coating that protects it from the strong hydrochloric acid it secretes to digest food. However the much-thinner esophageal mucous coating does not protect against stomach acid. Thus, if the LES opens inappropriately or fails to close completely, stomach acids can back up and burn the esophagus, causing heartburn.

Occasional heartburn is usually harmless. However, frequent or chronic heartburn (recurring more than twice per week) is called gastroesophageal reflux disease (GERD) and requires early management. Repeated episodes of GERD can lead to esophageal inflammation (esophagitis). If the esophagus is repeatedly subjected to

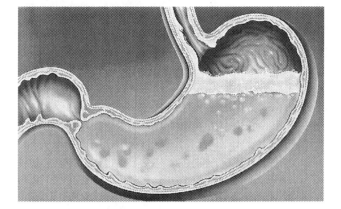

Illustration of foaming antacid on top of the contents of a human stomach. Heartburn is caused by a backflow of the stomach's acidic contents into the esophagus, causing inflammation and a sense of pain that can rise to the throat. *(Photograph by John Bavosi, Custom Medical Stock Photo. Reproduced by permission.)*

stomach acid and **digestive enzymes**, ulcerations, scarring, and thickening of the esophageal walls can result. This causes a narrowing of the interior of the esophagus that can affect swallowing and the peristaltic movements that send food downward. Repeated esophageal irritation also can result in Barrett's syndrome—changes in the types of cells lining the esophagus. Barrett's esophagus can develop into esophageal **cancer**.

Nighttime heartburn, affecting about 80% of heartburn sufferers, is more damaging to the esophagus than daytime heartburn. It often interferes with sleep and may trigger symptoms in **asthma** sufferers.

Gastroesophageal reflux may occur in children under age one, particularly pre-term babies or those with **cerebral palsy**. It also may be a cause of some migraine headaches. In addition, chronic heartburn can be a symptom of a gastric ulcer or coronary artery disease.

Causes & symptoms

Causes

Heartburn is caused by:

- a relaxed LES that does not close properly
- over-production of stomach acid
- increased stomach pressure
- a damaged esophagus with increased acid sensitivity

Many factors can contribute to LES malfunction:

- irregular eating, skipping meals
- **smoking**
- **caffeine**

- stress
- some medications, including diazepam (Valium), meperidine (Demerol), theophylline, morphine, prostaglandins, **calcium** channel blockers, nitrate heart medications, progesterone, and anticholinergic and adrenergic drugs (drugs that limit nerve reactions)
- paralysis and scleroderma (an autoimmune disease that hardens body organs)
- large meals that distend the stomach and prevent the LES from closing
- alcohol, which lowers the pressure on the LES, allowing it to relax and open. Alcohol also may irritate the esophageal lining
- weakening LES and loss of LES muscle tone with increasing age

Hiatal hernias are common among pregnant women, smokers, the obese, and those over age 50. The hiatus is an opening in the diaphragm (the large muscle that separates the chest cavity and the abdomen) through which the esophagus connects to the stomach. If the hiatus loses its tautness and shape, the stomach may protrude through, forming a pocket just below the LES where stomach acid can be trapped. These hiatal hernias can cause the LES to relax and open. Hiatal hernias may result in frequent and severe heartburn and GERD.

Various factors can increase stomach pressure, causing gastroesophageal reflux:

- obesity
- lying down within one or two hours of eating
- tight clothing
- **Pregnancy**, which causes the enlarged uterus to displace the stomach, delaying the removal of stomach contents

Eating too fast, chewing insufficiently, and smoking all increase stomach acid production. Smoking also dries up saliva that protects the esophagus from acid.

Many foods are known to contribute to heartburn:

- greasy, fried, or fatty foods
- spicy foods
- black pepper
- such acidic foods as tomatoes, pickles, and vinegar
- chocolate
- coffee with or without caffeine
- **Peppermint** or other mints

Symptoms

Heartburn itself is a symptom of gastroesophageal reflux and GERD. Heartburn sufferers may salivate excessively or regurgitate stomach contents into their mouths, leaving a sour or bitter taste.

Other symptoms of GERD include:

- difficult or painful swallowing
- sore throat
- hoarseness, **laryngitis**, **wheezing**, coughing
- **pneumonia**
- gingivitis, bad breath
- earache

Diagnosis

Heartburn usually is diagnosed by patient histories, symptoms, and clinical assessments. Additional procedures may be used to confirm the diagnosis, assess damage to the esophagus, and monitor the healing progress. The following diagnostic procedures are appropriate for anyone with frequent, chronic, or difficult-to-treat heartburn, or complicating GERD symptoms as listed above.

Esophageal manometry uses a thin flexible catheter placed down the esophagus. Small openings in the catheter sense pressure at various points on the esophagus while the muscle is at rest and during swallowing. The pressures are transmitted to a computer that analyzes the wave patterns.

An upper gastrointestinal (GI) series, or "barium swallow," can reveal esophageal narrowing, ulcerations, tumors, **hiatal hernia**, or reflux episodes as they occur. X rays are taken after a patient swallows a barium (a chemical element) suspension. This procedure takes about 15 minutes. However, it cannot detect structural changes associated with different degrees of esophagitis.

Upper GI endoscopy uses a thin flexible tube to view the inside of the esophagus directly. It is performed by a gastroenterologist, a physician specializing in diagnosis and treatment of disorders of the gastrointestinal tract, or by a gastrointestinal endoscopist. Upper GI endoscopy enables the physician to distinguish the degree of esophagitis and provides an accurate profile of esophageal damage. This procedure may include a biopsy—the removal of a small piece of tissue—to examine for Barrett's syndrome or malignancies. Patients with Barrett's esophagus may have frequent examinations of the esophageal lining for early detection of precancerous cells.

Other diagnostic tests include measurements of esophageal acidity (pH), usually over a 24-hour period, using an ambulatory acid probe. The patient is given a large capsule containing an acid-sensing probe, a battery, and a transmitter. Acid in the esophagus is measured by the probe, which then transmits the information to a recorder that the patient is wearing on his belt.

Note: A burning sensation in the chest is usually heartburn and is not associated with the heart itself. About 15 percent of the annual six million U. S. emergency room visits for chest pain are due to heartburn. However, **angina** (one type of temporary chest pain, pressure, or discomfort) sometimes is mistaken for severe heartburn. Chest pain that radiates into the arms and is not accompanied by regurgitation is a warning sign of a possible serious heart problem. Persistent chest pain should always be evaluated by a physician.

Treatment

Herbal remedies

These herbal remedies may be used to treat heartburn:

• **ginger** (*Zingiber officinalis*) as a tea or candied. (Ginger may cause heartburn in some people.)

• chamomile (*Matricaria chamomilla*) tea

• slippery elm (*Ulmus fulva*) tea

• cinnamon tea

• anise (*Pimpinella anisum*), caraway, dill, and/or **fennel** seed tea

• cardamom (*Elettaria cardamomum*) on buttered raisin toast

• turmeric (*Curcuma domestica*) added to warm water

• marsh mallow root (*Althaea officinalis*)

• licorice (*Glycyrrhiza glabra*), especially **deglycyrrhizinated licorice** (DGL) (The capsules or tablets may be dissolved in the mouth or in tea or two to four chewable 380-mg. wafers are taken about 20 minutes before eating. DGL should not be used more than three times per week, as repeated use can be toxic.)

• peppermint tea (Peppermint also can cause heartburn by relaxing the LES.)

• Ayurvedic (traditional East Indian) herbs

Homeopathic remedies

Homeopathic remedies for heartburn include:

• *Calcarea carbonica*

• *Nux vomica* after eating spicy foods

• *Carbo vegetalis* after eating rich foods

• *Arsenicum album* (for burning pain)

• *Natrum muriaticum* (for nervousness, tension, and pain)

• *Zinc metallicum* after eating too fast

Other remedies

A variety of other remedies and therapies may be used to treat heartburn:

• **Sodium** bicarbonate (baking soda) reduces esophageal acidity immediately. However, its effect is short-lived and it should not be used by people on sodium-restricted diets.

• Nutritional remedies include carrots, celery, **angelica**, fennel, and/or **parsley**. These can be combined in a juice taken before meals.

• Acupressure points Stomach 36, Spleen 6, Pericardium 6, and Conception Vessel 12. CV 12 should not be pressed just after eating or during pregnancy.

• In Chinese medicine, foods and herbs that balance and cool the qi (Chinese term for universal life energy), including radishes, radish seed, citrus fruit peels, and cardamom.

• Walking after a meal.

• Chewing gum after eating to help produce saliva for soothing the esophagus and washing acid back into the stomach.

• Relaxation therapy, visualization, and deep breathing.

Allopathic treatment

Drugs

Occasional heartburn is commonly treated with nonprescription antacids that neutralize the pH of stomach acid. The neutralized acid does not burn the esophagus. Antacids usually work within 15 minutes and their effects last one to two hours. Liquid or dissolving antacids usually act faster than tablets. However, antacids, if taken for too long, can cause side effects, including **diarrhea** or **constipation**.

Some antacids interfere with medications for kidney or **heart disease**. Heartburn sufferers with two or more episodes per week, or with an episode lasting more three weeks, should not rely on antacids as the sole treatment, since they may be at risk of kidney damage or other metabolic changes.

Common antacids include Maalox, Mylanta, Alka-Seltzer, Pepto-Bismol, Riopan, and Rolaids. The active ingredient in antacids such as Tums is calcium carbonate. Alginate (Gaviscon) is a foaming agent that coats the esophagus and the stomach to help prevent reflux. Other antacids are made from aluminum hydroxide, magaldrate, or **magnesium** hydroxide. Some antacids contain baking soda (sodium bicarbonate), which may interfere with vitamin and mineral absorption during pregnancy.

Histamine receptor (H2) blockers, such as famotidine (Pepcid), ranitidine (Zantac), nizatidine (Axid), and cimetidine (Tagamet), decrease stomach acid secretion. They relieve heartburn in about 75% of users. However, they take 30 to 45 minutes to act and usually are taken two to four times daily for several weeks. H2 blockers are both over-the-counter (OTC) and prescription medicines. They may have side effects or interactions with other medications.

Proton pump inhibitors (PPI) are for severe heartburn. They are the most effective drugs for inhibiting acid production and allowing the esophagus to heal in GERD. It may take up to five days for PPIs to take effect. They cannot be used by people with kidney or liver problems. Although it appears safe to take PPIs for at least 10 years, the lowest effective dosage reduces the risk of side effects that may include **headache**, diarrhea, stomach pain, and interactions with other medications. Common PPIs include lansoprazole (Prevacid), omeprazole (Prilosec), rabeprazole (Aciphex), pantoprazole (Protonix), and esomeprazole (Nexium). Prilosec OTC is available in 20-milligram doses to be taken once a day for 14 days to treat frequent heartburn.

Prokinetics are drugs that strengthen the LES (lower esophageal sphincter) and increase the rate of stomach emptying. These include metoclopramide (Reglan) and bethanechol (Urecholine). These drugs frequently have side effects.

Surgery

Laparoscopic Nissen fundoplication is a surgical procedure to increase pressure on the LES by stretching and wrapping the upper part of the stomach around it. It is performed under general anesthetic and takes one to two hours. The complete recovery period is less than two weeks.

GERD (gastroesophageal reflux disease) may be treated successfully by endoscopic suturing of the weakened LES to stop acid reflux. Studies have shown that symptoms usually improve with this procedure and the use of medications declines. Another procedure involves using electrodes to make tiny cuts in the LES tissues. The resulting scarring tightens the LES. These outpatient procedures take less than an hour. They are not used in cases of hiatal hernia or Barrett's esophagus.

If the esophagus has become narrowed and badly scarred from stomach acid, a procedure that stretches and widens the esophageal tissue may be used along with acid-suppressing medication. Enteryx is a liquid that can be injected into the LES where it forms a spongy muscle implant that strengthens the LES.

Prognosis

Occasional heartburn without esophageal damage has an excellent prognosis. Esophageal damage that is treated with a program that promotes healing also has an excellent prognosis. Infants usually outgrow gastroesophageal reflux by age one.

Untreated heartburn and GERD may lead to bleeding, esophageal ulcers, and **infections**. With treatment, the damaged tissue that forms ulcers can heal. About ten percent of patients with GERD experience esophageal narrowing from acid damage that leads to the formation of scar tissue in the lower esophagus. GERD also can cause laryngitis, **bronchitis**, and aspiration pneumonia. After five years of heartburn, the risk of developing Barrett's esophagus increases. About five percent of GERD patients have Barrett's syndrome. This condition is incurable and may lead to cancer. The prognosis for esophageal cancer is very poor. There is a strong likelihood of painful illness and a less than five percent chance of survival for more than five years.

Prevention

Due to the risk of GERD, Barrett's syndrome, and esophageal cancer, prevention of heartburn is very important. Heartburn usually is preventable with dietary and lifestyle changes.

Dietary adjustments to eliminate many causes of heartburn include:

- eating smaller, more frequent meals to reduce pressure on the LES
- eating slowly, chew thoroughly, and take deep breaths between bites
- avoiding caffeine, chocolate, onions, spicy foods, and mint, all of which tend to increase stomach acid and relax the LES
- avoiding fatty, fried, and greasy foods. Fatty foods relax the LES and slow stomach emptying, and fat consumption has been linked to GERD
- avoiding milk, **garlic**, peppers, and carbonated beverages
- avoiding nicotine
- avoiding citrus fruits and juices and tomato-based foods, which are acidic and can irritate an inflamed esophagus
- replacing meat at dinner with carbohydrates and easier-to-digest proteins such as rice, beans, and pastas
- avoiding alcohol
- adding the spice annato (*Bix orellana*) or bouquet garni to foods
- drinking tea made with crushed caraway seeds with meals
- controling body weight

KEY TERMS

Antacid—Common medication that neutralizes stomach acid for the short-term treatment of heartburn.

Barrett's esophagus or Barrett's syndrome—Changes in the type of cells lining the esophagus. Sometimes associated with the development of esophageal cancer.

Digestive enzymes—Proteins that catalyze the breakdown of large molecules (usually food) into smaller molecules.

Endoscopy—Procedure in which a thin flexible scope is placed down the esophagus to examine, biopsy, and/or suture the tissue.

Esophagitis—Inflammation of the esophagus.

Esophagus—Muscular tube, about 10 in (25 cm) long, connecting the throat to the stomach.

Fundoplication—Surgical procedure that increases pressure on the LES (lower esophageal sphincter), reducing reflux.

Gastroesophageal reflux—Upward flow of stomach contents into the esophagus, causing heartburn.

Gastroesophageal reflux disease (GERD)—Frequent (more than twice a week) gastroesophageal reflux.

Hiatal hernia—Protrusion of part of the stomach through the diaphragm to a position next to the esophagus.

Hiatus—Opening in the diaphragm through which the stomach connects to the esophagus.

Histamine receptor 2 (H2) blocker—Heartburn medication that reduces the production of stomach acid.

Lower esophageal sphincter (LES)—Muscle at the base of the esophagus that opens to allow food to enter the stomach and closes to prevent reflux back into the esophagus.

Manometry—Procedure that measures pressure. In esophageal manometry, a thin, flexible catheter is placed down the esophagus to measure pressure at various points.

Peristalsis—Sequence of muscle contractions that progressively squeezes the digestive tract to push food along.

Proton pump inhibitor (PPI)—Medication that inhibits stomach acid production in severe heartburn.

Ulceration—Wound or abrasion of surface tissue.

Lifestyle changes that can alleviate heartburn include:

- avoiding drugs known to contribute to heartburn, including aspirin or other nonsteroidal anti-inflammatories
- avoiding clothing that fits tightly around the abdomen
- not lying down until the stomach is empty—within about three hours of eating
- elevating the head of the bed six to nine inches to prevent nighttime heartburn
- avoiding strenuous **exercise** for two to three hours after a meal

Resources

BOOKS

Berkson, Lindsey. *Healthy Digestion the Natural Way: Preventing and Healing Heartburn, Constipation, Gas, Diarrhea, Inflammatory Bowel and Gallbladder Diseases, Ulcers, Irritable Bowel Syndrome, Food Allergies and More.* New York: Wiley, 2000.

Castleman, Michael. *Blended Medicine: The Best Choices in Healing.* Emmaus, PA: Rodale, 2000.

Cheskin, Lawrence J. and Brian E. Lacy. *Healing Heartburn.* Emmaus, PA: Rodale, 2000.

Goldmann, David R. and David A. Horowitz, editors. *American College of Physicians Complete Home Medical Guide.* 2nd ed. New York: DK, 2003.

Litin, Scott C., editor. *Mayo Clinic Family Health Book.* 3rd ed. New York: HarperResource, 2003.

Minocha, Anil, and Christine Adamec. *How to Stop Heartburn: Simple Ways to Heal Heartburn and Acid Reflux.* New York: Wiley, 2001.

Shimberg, Elaine Fantle. *Coping with Chronic Heartburn: What You Need to Know About Acid Reflux and GERD.* New York: St. Martin's Press, 2001.

Sklar, Jill, and Annabel Cohen. *Eating for Acid Reflux: A Handbook and Cookbook for Those with Heartburn.* Emeryville, CA: Marlowe & Company, 2003.

PERIODICALS

"Gastrointestinal Reflux: New Guidelines Set Standard on Test to Diagnose Acid Reflux, Heartburn." *Health & Medicine Week* (December 22, 2003): 284–285.

"New Bard Endoscopic Suturing System Treats Chronic Heartburn." *Journal of Clinical Engineering* 28 (April-June 2003): 88–90.

Sadovsky, Richard. "Management of Refractory Heartburn: A Review." *American Family Physician* 69 (February 1, 2004): 698.

Savarino, Vincenzo and Pietro Dulbecco. "Optimizing Symptom Relief and Preventing Complications in Adults with Gastro-Oesophageal Reflux Disease." *Digestion* 69, Supplement 1 (2004): 9–16.

Urbach, David R., et al. "Whither Surgery in the Treatment of Gastroesophageal Relux Disease (GERD)?" *Canadian Medical Association Journal* 170 (January 20, 2004): 219–221.

ORGANIZATIONS

American Gastroenterological Association (AGA). 4930 Del Ray Avenue, Bethesda, MD 20814. (310 654-2055. <http://www.gastro.org/>.

National Digestive Diseases Information Clearinghouse. 2 Information Way, Bethesda, MD 20892–3570. (800) 891-5389. (301) 654-3810. nddic@info.niddk.nih.gov. <http://digestive.niddk.nih.gov/.>.

The National Heartburn Alliance. 303 East Wacker Drive, Suite 440, Chicago, IL 60601. (877) 471-2081. nhbainformation @heartburnalliance.org. <http://www.heartburnalliance.org/>.

Margaret Alic, PhD

Heavy metal poisoning

Definition

Heavy metal poisoning is the toxic accumulation of heavy metals in the soft tissues of the body.

Description

Heavy metals are chemical elements that have a specific gravity (a measure of density) at least five times that of water. The heavy metals most often implicated in human poisoning are lead, mercury, arsenic, and cadmium. Some heavy metals, such as **zinc, copper, chromium, iron**, and **manganese**, are required by the body in small amounts, but can be toxic in larger quantities. Heavy metals may enter the body through food, water, or air, or by absorption through the skin. Once in the body, they compete with and displace essential minerals such as zinc, copper, **magnesium**, and **calcium**, and interfere with organ system function. People may come in contact with heavy metals in industrial work, pharmaceutical manufacturing, and agriculture. Children may be poisoned as a result of playing in contaminated soil.

Sources of exposure for some heavy metals

- lead: old paint, leaded gasoline, old pipes
- mercury: contaminated fish, industrial and agricultural wastes
- cadmium: industrial waste, insecticides, old galvanized pipes
- arsenic: insecticides and industrial processes, some drinking water

Causes & symptoms

Symptoms will vary, depending on the nature and quantity of the heavy metal, and whether it was ingested or inhaled. Patients who ingest a heavy metal may complain of cramps, **nausea, vomiting, diarrhea**, stomach **pain, headache**, sweating, and a metallic taste in the mouth. Mercury can cause skin **burns** if it has touched the skin, and inhaled mercury vapor can cause severe inflammation of the lungs. If lead is inhaled in the form of lead dust, **insomnia**, headache, mania, and convulsions may occur. In severe cases of heavy metal poisoning, patients exhibit obvious impairment of cognitive, motor, and language skills. The expression "mad as a hatter" comes from the mercury poisoning prevalent in seventeenth-century France among hatmakers who soaked animal hides in a solution of mercuric nitrate to soften the hair.

Diagnosis

Heavy metal poisoning may be detected using blood, urine, and stool tests, hair and tissue analysis, or x rays. In children, blood lead levels above 80 mcg/dl generally indicate **lead poisoning**; however, significantly lower levels (>.30 mcg/dL) can cause mental retardation and other cognitive and behavioral problems in chronically exposed children. The Centers for Disease Control and Prevention considers a blood lead level of 10 mcg/dl or higher in children a cause for concern. In adults, symptoms of lead poisoning are usually seen when blood lead levels exceed 80 mcg/dl for a number of weeks. Blood levels of mercury should not exceed 3.6 mcg/dl, while urine levels should not exceed 15 mcg/dl. Symptoms of mercury poisoning may appear when mercury levels exceed 20 mcg/dl in blood and 60 mcg/dl in urine. Mercury levels in hair may be used to gauge the severity of chronic mercury exposure, but a 2002 report says that these tests have questionable validity.

Since arsenic is rapidly cleared from the blood, blood arsenic levels may not be very useful in diagnosis. Arsenic in the urine (measured in a 24-hour collection following 48 hours without eating seafood) may exceed 50 mcg/dl in people with arsenic poisoning. If acute arsenic poisoning is suspected, an x ray may reveal ingested arsenic in the abdomen (since arsenic is opaque to x rays). Arsenic may also be detected in the hair and nails for months following exposure. Cadmium toxicity is generally indicated when urine levels exceed 10 mcg/dl of creatinine and blood levels exceed 5 mcg/dl.

Treatment

Emergency treatment of acute poisoning, especially in children, can be handled by calling a poison control line (800-222-1222) or by dialing 911. Alternative practitioners often rely on the same chelating agents used by standard doctors to treat heavy metal poisoning, but also use natural supplements and additional techniques to assist the body's own **detoxification** processes. One highly contested issue between alternative medicine and mainstream dentistry surrounds mercury poisoning. Alternative practitioners believe that there is a large body of evidence suggesting that silver amalgam tooth fillings, which contain mercury, are a major factor in mercury poisoning. For those with high mercury levels in their bodies, they recommend that all mercury-containing tooth fillings be removed by a holistic dentist. The National Institutes of Health hope to put some of the debate over amalgam fillings to rest with two clinical trials on fillings currently underway. However, the results are not expected until 2005.

Dietary changes are used to support the treatment of heavy metal poisoning. Detoxification **diets** are predominantly vegetarian, and reduce or avoid foods that may **stress** the immune system, such as processed foods, fried foods, sugar, fat, alcohol, **caffeine**, meat, and dairy products. Organic foods are recommended to avoid exposure to pesticides and chemicals. Detoxification diets include plenty of high-fiber foods, including oat bran and **psyllium** seeds, to help cleanse the digestive tract. Apples, pears, and legumes are high in pectins, which are believed to have chelating effects on heavy metals. Foods high in **antioxidants** are recommended, such as fruits, vegetables, and fresh juices. Sulfur-containing foods such as **garlic**, onions, and eggs (organically produced) are utilized, as are dark-green leafy vegetables that contain high amounts of chlorophyll. Foods that may contain heavy metals are avoided, including many fish and shellfish. Factory-farmed chicken and eggs are avoided as well, because chickens are often fed fish meal. A 2002 study reported that eating tofu may reduce lead levels in the blood. Tofu is rich in calcium, which may help reduce the blood's ability to absorb and retain lead.

Nutritional supplements include antioxidant vitamins A, C, and E, and multimineral supplements that contain calcium, iron, magnesium, copper, chromium, **selenium**, and zinc. Cysteine, **methionine**, L-gluthione, and DMSA (dimethyl succinate) are other supplements. Herbal support includes herbs that have detoxification effects, such as **milk thistle**, burdock, and numerous others. **Spirulina** and **chlorella** sea algae are used as well, and **acidophilus** helps rebuild the digestive tract.

Homeopathic remedies, which prompt the body's detoxification mechanisms, have shown success with heavy metal poisoning. Detoxification therapies are also highly recommended, including **fasting**, sweating, colonics, and therapeutic vomiting. **Ayurvedic medicine** has an intensive detoxification and healing program called **panchakarma**.

Allopathic treatment

In an emergency, patients should call 911 or a poison control hotline (800) 222-1222. The treatment for most heavy metal poisoning is **chelation therapy**. A chelating agent specific to the metal involved is given orally, intramuscularly, or intravenously. The three most common chelating agents are edetate calcium disodium, dimercaprol (BAL), and penicillamine. Succimer (DMSA) is used for children suffering from lead poisoning. The chelating agent encircles and binds the metal in the body's tissues, forming a complex that is then released from the tissue and travels in the bloodstream. The complex is filtered out of the blood by the kidneys and excreted in the urine. This process may be lengthy and painful, and typically requires hospitalization. Chelation therapy is effective in treating lead, mercury, and arsenic poisoning, but is not useful in treating **cadmium poisoning**. To date, no treatment has been proven effective for cadmium poisoning. In cases of acute mercury or arsenic ingestion, vomiting may be induced. Washing out the stomach (gastric lavage) may also be useful. The patient may also require treatment such as intravenous fluids for complications of poisoning such as shock, **anemia**, and kidney failure.

Expected results

The chelation process can only halt further effects of the poisoning; it cannot reverse neurological damage already sustained.

Prevention

Because exposure to heavy metals is often an occupational hazard, protective clothing and respirators should be provided and worn on the job. Protective clothing should then be left at the work site and not worn home, where it could carry toxic dust to family members. Industries are urged to reduce or replace the heavy metals in their processes wherever possible. Exposure to environmental sources of lead, including lead-based paints, plumbing fixtures, vehicle exhaust, and contaminated soil, should be reduced or eliminated.

Resources

BOOKS

Goldberg, Burton. *Chronic Fatigue, Fibromyalgia and Environmental Illness.* Tiburon, CA: Future Medicine, 1998.

Lappe, Marc. *Chemical Deception: The Toxic Threat to Health and the Environment.* San Francisco: Sierra Club, 1991.

Lawson, Lynn. *Staying Well in a Toxic World.* Chicago: Noble, 1993.

PERIODICALS

Kales, Stefanos N., and Rose H. Goldman. "Mercury Exposure: Current Concepts, Controversies, and a Clinic's Experience." *Journal of Occupational and Environmental Health* (February 2002): 143–146.

"Should Amalgam Fillings be Banned? Evidence on the Risks of Mercury Fillings is Mixed. Should They be Outlawed Anyway?." *Natural Health* (March 2002): 26.

"Tofu May Lower Lead Levels in Blood." *Townsend Letter for Doctors and Patients* (February–March 2002): 23.

ORGANIZATIONS

American Association of Poison Control Centers. 3201 New Mexico Avenue, Suite 310. Washington, DC 20016. (800) 222-1222. <http://www.aapcc.org>.

American Holistic Medical Association. 12101 Menaul Blvd. NE, Suite C., Albuquerque, NM 87112. (505) 292-7788. info@holisticmedicine.org. <http://www.holisticmedicine.org>.

Center for Occupational and Environmental Medicine. 7510 Northforest Drive, North Charleston, SC 29420. (843) 572-1600. allanl@coem.com. <http://www.coem.com>.

OTHER

A Citizen's Toxic Waste Manual. Greenpeace USA, 1436 U St. NW, Washington, DC 20009. (202) 462-1177.

Douglas Dupler
Teresa G. Odle

Heel spurs

Definition

A heel spur is a bony projection on the sole (bottom) of the heel bone. This condition may accompany or re-sult from severe cases of inflammation to the structure called *plantar fascia*. The plantar fascia is a fibrous band of connective tissue on the sole of the foot, extending from the heel to the toes.

Description

Heel spurs are a common foot problem resulting from excess bone growth on the heel bone. The bone growth is usually located on the underside of the heel bone, and may extend forward toward the toes. A painful tear in the plantar fascia between the toes and heel can produce a heel spur and/or inflammation of the plantar fascia. Because this condition is often correlated to a decrease in the arch of the foot, it is more prevalent after the ages of six to eight years, when the arch is fully developed.

Causes & symptoms

One frequent cause of injury to the plantar fascia is *pronation*. Pronation is defined as the inward and downward action of the foot that occurs while walking, so that the foot's arch flattens toward the ground (fallen arch). A condition known as excessive pronation creates a mechanical problem in the foot, and the portion of the plantar fascia attached to the heel bone can stretch and pull away from the bone. This damage can occur especially while walking and during athletic activities.

Some symptoms at the beginning of this condition include **pain** and swelling, and discomfort when pushing off with the toes during walking. This movement of the foot stretches the fascia that is already irritated and inflamed. If this condition is not treated, pain will be noticed in the heel when a heel spur develops in response to the stress. This is a common condition among athletes and others who run and jump a significant amount.

An individual with the lower legs turning inward, a condition called *genu valgus* or "knock knees," can have a tendency toward excessive pronation. This can lead to a fallen arch and problems with the plantar fascia and heel spurs. Women tend to suffer from this condition more than men. Heel spurs can also result from an abnormally high arch.

Other factors leading to heel spurs include a sudden increase in daily activities, an increase in weight, or a thinner cushion on the bottom of the heel due to old age. A significant increase in training intensity or duration may cause inflammation of the plantar fascia. High-heeled shoes, improperly fitted shoes, and shoes that are too flexible in the middle of the arch or bend before the toe joints will cause problems with the plantar fascia and possibly lead to heel spurs.

Bone spurs may cause sudden, severe pain when putting weight on the affected foot. Individuals may try to walk on their toes or ball of the foot to avoid painful pressure on the heel spur. This compensation during walking or running can cause additional problems in the ankle, knee, hip, or back.

Diagnosis

A thorough history and physical exam is always necessary for the proper diagnosis of heel spurs and other foot conditions. X rays of the heel area are helpful, as excess bone production will be visible.

Treatment

Acupuncture and **acupressure** can used to address the pain of heel spurs, in addition to using friction massage to help break up scar tissue and delay the onset of bony formations. Physical therapy may help relieve pain and improve movement. The **Feldenkrais** method could be especially helpful for retraining some of the compensation movements caused by the pain from the spur. **Guided imagery** or a light massage on the foot may help to relieve some of the pain. Other treatments include low-gear cycling, and pool running. Some chiropractors approve of moderate use of aspirin or ibuprofen, or other appropriate anti-inflammatory drugs. **Chiropractic** manipulation is not recommended, although chiropractors may offer custom-fitted shoe orthotics and other allopathic-type treatments outlined below.

Allopathic treatment

Heel spurs and plantar fascitis (inflammation of the plantar fascia) are usually controlled with conservative treatment. Early intervention includes stretching the calf muscles while avoiding reinjury to the plantar fascia. Decreasing or changing activities, losing excess weight, and improving the fit of shoes are all important measures to decrease foot pain. Modification of footwear includes well-padded shoes with a raised heel and better arch support. Shoe inserts recommended by a healthcare professional are often very helpful when used with exercises to increase the strength of the foot muscles and arch. The inserts prevent excessive pronation and continued tearing of the plantar fascia.

To aid in the reduction of inflammation, applying ice for 10–15 minutes after activities and the use of anti-inflammatory medications, such as aspirin or ibuprofen, can be helpful. Corticosteroid injections may also be used to reduce pain and inflammation. Physical therapy can be beneficial with the use of heat modalities, such as ultrasound, that create a deep heat and reduce inflammation. If the pain caused by inflammation is constant, keeping the foot raised above the heart and/or compressed by wrapping with a bandage will help. Taping can help speed the healing process by protecting the fascia from reinjury, especially during stretching and walking.

In 2000, a number of U.S. podiatrists were experimenting with a new technology known as Extracorporeal Pressure Wave Treatment (EPWT). This technology is similar to lithotripsy, which uses sound waves to break up **kidney stones**. Cost of EPWT was roughly comparable to that of surgery. Initial reports from practitioners using the treatment were positive.

Heel surgery

When chronic heel pain fails to respond to conservative treatment, surgical treatment may be necessary. Heel surgery can provide pain relief and restore mobility. The type of procedure used is based on examination and usually consists of releasing the excessive tightness of the plantar fascia, called a plantar fascia release. The procedure may also include removal of heel spurs.

Expected results

Usually, heel spurs are curable with conservative treatment. If not, heel spurs are curable with surgery, although there is the possibility of them growing back. About 10% of those who continue to see a physician for plantar fascitis have it for more than a year. If there is limited success after approximately one year of conservative treatment, patients are often advised to have surgery.

Prevention

To prevent this condition, wearing properly fitted shoes with good arch support is very important. If a person is overweight, weight loss can help diminish stress on the feet and help prevent foot problems. For those who **exercise** frequently and intensely, proper stretching is always necessary, especially when there is an increase in activities or a change in running technique. It is not recommended to attempt to work through the pain, as this can change a mild case of heel spurs and plantar fascitis into a long-lasting and painful episode of the condition.

In 2002, researchers attempted to compare the effects of various running techniques on pronation and resulting injuries like stress **fractures** and heel spurs. They suggested that it is possible to teach runners to stride in such a way as to minimize impact forces. One way is to lower running speed. Another is to take longer rest periods following a run.

Resources

BOOKS
Perkins, Kenneth E. "Lower Extremity Orthotics in Geriatric Rehabilitation." In *Geriatric Physical Therapy,* edited by

Andrew Guccione. St. Louis, MO.: Mosby Year Book Inc., 1993.

PERIODICALS

Feeny, Tracy. "If The Shoe Fits." *Advance Magazine for Physical Therapists.* (July 1997): 7.

Hreljac, Alan. "Technique Impacts Overuse Injuries in Runners — Research Suggests Impact Forces and Rate of Pronation Influence Risk of Injury." *Biomechanics.* (September 1, 2002): 51.

ORGANIZATIONS

American Orthopedic Foot and Ankle Society. 222 South Prospect, Park Ridge, IL 60068.

American Podiatry Medical Association. 9312 Old Georgetown Road, Bethesda, MD 20814.

OTHER

Roberts. *Plantar Fascitis.* http:\\www.heelspurs.com (1998).

David Helwig

Heliotrope *see* **Valerian**

Hellerwork

Definition

Hellerwork is a system of bodywork that combines deep tissue massage, body movement education, and verbal dialogue. It is designed to realign the body's structure for overall health, improvement of posture, and reduction of physical and mental **stress**.

Origins

Joseph Heller (1940–) developed Hellerwork, a system of structural integration patterned after **Rolfing**.

Although Heller received a degree in engineering and worked for NASA's Jet Propulsion Laboratory in Pasadena, CA, he became interested in humanistic psychology in the 1970s. He spent two years studying bioenergetics and Gestalt therapy as well as studying under the architect and futurist Buckminster Fuller (1895–1983), the flotation tank therapy developer John Lilly, the family therapist Virginia Satir, and the body movement pioneer **Judith Aston**.

During this period, he trained for six years with Dr. Ida P. Rolf (1896-1979), the founder of Rolfing, and became a certified Rolfer in 1972. After Heller developed his own system of bodywork, he founded Hellerwork in 1979 and established a training facility in Mt. Shasta, California, where he continues his work.

Benefits

Hellerwork improves posture and brings the body's natural structure into proper balance and alignment. This realignment can bring relief from general aches and pains; improve breathing; and relieve physical and mental stress. Hellerwork has also been used to treat such specific physical problems as chronic back, neck, shoulder, and joint **pain** as well as repetitive stress injuries, including **carpal tunnel syndrome**. Hellerwork is also used to treat and prevent athletic injuries.

Description

Hellerwork is based largely on the principles of Rolfing, in which the body's connective tissue is manipulated or massaged to realign and balance the body's structure. Because Heller believes that physical realignment is insufficient, however, he expanded his system to include movement education and verbal dialogue as well as deep tissue massage.

Connective tissue massage

The **massage therapy** aspect of Hellerwork is designed to release the tension that exists in the deep connective tissue, called fascia, and return it to a normal alignment. The fascia is plastic and highly adaptable; it can tighten and harden in response to the general effects of gravity on the body, other ongoing physical stresses, negative attitudes and emotions, and periodic physical traumas. One example of ongoing physical stress is carrying a briefcase, which pulls down the shoulder on one side of the body. Over time, the connective tissue becomes hard and stiff; the body becomes adapted to that position even when the person is not carrying a briefcase. In trying to adjust to the uneven weight distribution, the rest of the body becomes unbalanced and pulled out of proper alignment.

JOSEPH HELLER 1940–

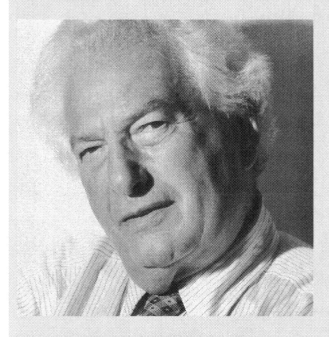

(AP/Wide World Photos. Reproduced by permission.)

Born in Poland, Joseph Heller attended school in Europe until age 16, when he immigrated to the United States. Living in Los Angeles, he attended the California Institute of Technology in Pasadena and graduated in 1962 with a degree in engineering. He worked for 10 years at the National Aeronautics and Space Administration's Jet Propulsion Laboratory (JPL) in Pasadena as an aerospace engineer. During his service at JPL, Heller became interested in humanistic psychology. After leaving JPL in 1972, he became director of Kairos, a center for human development in Los Angeles. He spent two years studying bioenergetics and gestalt. He also trained under Buckminster Fuller, flotation tank therapy developer John Lilly, self-esteem trainer Virginia Satir, and body movement pioneer Judith Aston.

He became a certified Rolfer in 1972 and spent the next six years studying structural integration under **Rolfing** founder Ida P. Rolf. He became the first president of the Rolf Institute in 1975. During his training with Rolf, Heller began developing his own system of bodywork. He left the institute in 1978 and moved to Northern California, where he founded Hellerwork. He conducts classes and continues his work today at his headquarters, 406 Berry St., Mt. Shasta, CA 96067.

Ken R. Wells

Heller believes that as people age, more of these stress and trauma patterns become ingrained in the connective tissue, further throwing the body out of alignment. As stress accumulates, the body shortens and stiffens, a process commonly attributed to **aging**. Hellerwork seeks to recondition the body and make the connective tissue less rigid.

Movement education

The second component of Hellerwork, movement education, trains patients in the proper physical movements needed to keep the body balanced and correctly aligned. Movement education focuses on such common actions as sitting, standing, and walking. Hellerwork practitioners also teach better patterns of movement for activities that are specific to each individual, such as their job and favorite sports or social activities.

Verbal dialogue

Verbal dialogue is the third aspect of Hellerwork. It is designed to teach awareness of the relationships among emotions, life attitudes, and the body. Hellerwork practition-

ers believe that as patients become responsible for their attitudes, their body movements and patterns of self-expression improve. Dialogue focuses on the theme of each session and the area of the body that is worked on during that session.

Hellerwork consists of eleven 90-minute sessions costing about $90–100 each. The first three sessions focus on the surface layers of the fascia and on developmental issues of infancy and childhood. The next four sessions are the core sessions and work on the deep layers of tissue and on adolescent developmental issues. The final four treatments are the integrative sessions, and build upon all the previous ones, while also looking at questions of maturity.

Preparations

No advance preparations are required to begin Hellerwork treatment. The treatment is usually done on a massage table with the patient wearing only undergarments.

Precautions

Since Hellerwork involves vigorous deep tissue massage, it is often described as uncomfortable and

KEY TERMS

· ·

Bioenergetics—A system of therapy that combines breathing and body exercises, psychological therapy, and the free expression of emotions to release blocked physical and psychic energy.

Bodywork—A term that covers a variety of therapies that include massage, realignment of the body, and similar techniques to treat deeply ingrained stresses and traumas carried in the tissues of the body.

Chronic—Referring to a disease or condition that progresses slowly but persists or reoccurs over time.

Fascia—The sheet of connective tissue that covers the body under the skin and envelops the muscles and various organs.

Gestalt therapy—A form of therapy that focuses on helping patients reconnect with their bodies and their feelings directly, as contrasted with verbal intellectual analysis.

Kinesiology—The study of the anatomy and physiology of body movement, particularly in relation to therapy.

Rolfing—A deep-tissue therapy that involves manipulating the body's fascia to realign and balance

sometimes painful, especially during the first several sessions. As it requires the use of hands, it may be a problem for people who do not like or are afraid of being touched. It is not recommended as a treatment for any disease or a chronic inflammatory condition such as arthritis, and can worsen such a condition. Anyone with a serious medical condition, including **heart disease**, diabetes, or respiratory problems, should consult a medical practitioner before undergoing Hellerwork.

Side effects

There are no reported serious side effects associated with Hellerwork when delivered by a certified practitioner to adults and juveniles.

Research & general acceptance

As most alternative or holistic treatments, there is little mainstream scientific research documenting the effectiveness of Hellerwork therapy. Since the deep tissue massage aspect of Hellerwork is similar to Rolfing, however, several scientific studies of Rolfing may be useful

in evaluating Hellerwork. A 1988 study published in the *Journal of the American Physical Therapy Association* indicated that Rolfing stimulates the parasympathetic nervous system, which can help speed the recovery of damaged tissue. A 1997 article in *The Journal of Orthopaedic and Sports Physical Therapy* reported that Rolfing can provide effective and sustained pain relief from lower back problems.

Training & certification

Hellerwork practitioners are certified by Hellerwork and must complete 1,250 hours of training, including courses in anatomy, psychology, massage, and kinesiology.

Resources

BOOKS

Bradford, Nikki, ed. *Alternative Healthcare.* San Diego, CA: Thunder Bay Press, 1997.

Claire, Thomas. *Bodywork: What Type of Massage to Get and How to Make the Most of It.* New York: William Morrow and Co., 1995.

Golten, Roger. *The Owner's Guide to the Body.* London: Thorsons, 1999.

Heller, Joseph. *Bodywise.* Berkeley, CA: Wingbow Press, 1991.

Levine, Andrew S., and Valerie J. Levine. *The Bodywork and Massage Sourcebook.* Lincolnwood, IL: Lowell House, 1999.

Nash, Barbara. *From Acupressure to Zen: An Encyclopedia of Natural Therapies.* Alameda, CA: Hunter House, Inc., 1996.

ORGANIZATIONS

Hellerwork. 406 Berry St., Mt. Shasta, CA 96067. (530) 926-2500. http://www.hellerwork.com.

Ken R. Wells

Hemorrhoids

Definition

Hemorrhoids, which are also called piles, is a condition of weakened and swollen veins in the anus or lower rectum. They often go unnoticed and usually clear up after a few days, but can also cause long-lasting discomfort of the rectum such as **pain**, **itching**, and bleeding. Hemorrhoids can be divided into two types: Internal hemorrhoids lie inside the anus or lower rectum; external hemorrhoids lie outside the anal opening. Both can be present at the same time. Sometimes a blood clot forms in an external hemorrhoid and inflammation and a painful lump develops. This condition is called a thrombosed hemorrhoid.

Description

Hemorrhoids are a very common medical complaint. More than 75% of Americans have hemorrhoids at some point in their lives, typically after age 30. Men are more likely than women to suffer from hemorrhoids that are serious enough to require professional treatment.

During a bowel movement, veins in the anus are protected from damage by expanding to drain blood away from the area. The veins are normally somewhat elastic, and they snap back to their regular size after defecation is finished. However, repeated straining due to constipation or hardened stools causes the veins to be swollen and stretched out of shape. The swelling also triggers nerves in the area, causing itchiness and a sensation of fulless in the bowel. In addition, straining may cause the rupture of blood vessels and bleeding at the anus.

Causes & symptoms

Aging, **obesity**, pregnancy, chronic constipation or chronic **diarrhea**, excessive use of enemas or laxatives, straining during bowel movements, and spending too much time on the toilet are all factors that can contribute to the development of hemorrhoids. In some people there is also a genetic tendency to have fragile veins that are prone to developing hemorrhoids and **varicose veins**.

The most common symptom of internal hemorrhoids is bright red blood in the toilet bowl or on one's feces or toilet paper. When hemorrhoids remain inside the anus they are almost never painful, but they can protrude outside the anus and become irritated and sore. Such hemorrhoids are called prolapsed hemorrhoids. These sometimes move back into the anal canal on their own or can be pushed back inside; however, they may remain permanently outside the anus until treated by a doctor. Small external hemorrhoids usually do not produce symptoms. Larger ones, however, can be painful and interfere with sitting, walking, defecating, and cleaning the anal area after a bowel movement.

Diagnosis

Diagnosis of hemorrhoids begins with a visual examination of the anus, followed by an internal manual examination. The doctor may also insert an anoscope, a small tube with a light that can be used to view the anal canal. More serious problems may be ruled out using a sigmoidoscope or colonoscope to inspect the colon.

Treatment

An herbal sitz bath using **witch hazel**, *Hamamelis virginiana,* may shrink hemorrhoids and ease discomfort. A strong infusion should be prepared by adding a

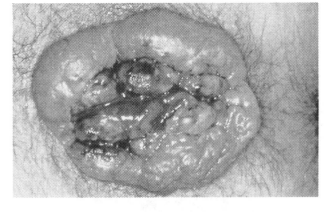

Clinical photo of a thrombosed external hemorrhoid. *(Custom Medical Stock Photo. Reproduced by permission.)*

gallon of boiling **water** to eight ounces of the dry herb, and then letting this mixture steep overnight. The infusion can be used several times as a 15-minute soak. Witch hazel can also be wiped directly over external hemorrhoids. In addition, an ointment formulated of **plantain**, *Plantago* spp. and **yarrow**, *Achillea millefolium,* will reportedly reduce pain and swelling.

Chinese herbal medicine may be formulated to treat Spleen Qi deficiency or heat in the lower burner. Hemp seeds are recommended for constipation. Daily helpings of foods that soften the stools and make them easier to pass are recommended by **traditional Chinese medicine** (TCM); examples of these include carrots, broccoli, dried persimmons and unripe figs. **Acupuncture** and **acupressure** are also recommended.

Homeopathy offers a gentle treatment solution for hemorrhoids. It is, therefore, especially appropriate for use during pregnancy. Suggested remedies include *Aeschulus hippocastanum* 30c, *Hamamelis virginiana* 6c, and *Calcarea fluorica* 6c. Homeopathic and herbal rectal suppositories are available.

Allopathic treatment

Hemorrhoids can often be dealt with effectively by dietary and lifestyle changes. Avoiding constipation is important; therefore adding fiber to the diet is recommended. Bulk laxatives and fiber supplements such as Metamucil or Citrucel may be suggested. After each bowel movement, wiping with a moistened tissue or pad sold for that purpose helps lessen irritation. A warm sitz bath for about 10 or 15 minutes two to four times a day can ease hemorrhoid pain. A cool compress or ice pack to reduce swelling is also recommended. Many people find temporary relief using over-the-counter hemorrhoid creams and foams. These products, however, are not receommended during pregnancy.

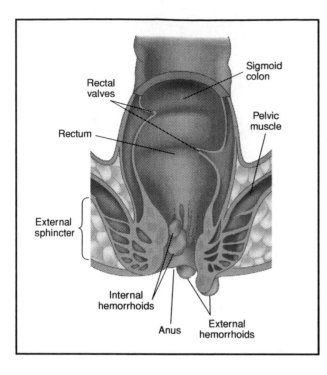

Sigmoid colon

Rectal valves

Pelvic muscle

Rectum

External sphincter

Internal hemorrhoids

Anus

External hemorrhoids

Sitting for long periods, pregnancy, constipation, and straining to defecate all contribute to hemorrhoids, which are caused by congestion in the veins of the lower rectum or anus. *(Illustration by Electronic Illustrators Group. The Gale Group.)*

When painful hemorrhoids do not respond to home-based remedies, professional medical treatment is necessary. Rubber band ligation is probably the most widely used of the many treatments for internal hemorrhoids. It is also the least costly for the patient. This procedure is performed on an outpatient basis. An applicator is used to place one or two small rubber bands around the base of the hemorrhoid, cutting off the blood supply. After 3 to 10 days in the bands, the hemorrhoid falls off, leaving a sore that heals in a week or two. Because internal hemorrhoids are located in a part of the anus that is not sensitive to pain, anesthesia is unnecessary and the procedure is painless in most cases. The procedure may need to be repeated a few weeks later. After five years, 15–20% of patients experience a recurrence of internal hemorrhoids, but in most cases all that is needed is another banding.

External hemorrhoids, and some prolapsed internal hemorrhoids, are removed by conventional surgery in a hospital. Depending on the circumstances, this procedure may require anesthesia. Full healing takes two to four weeks, but most people are able to resume normal activities at the end of a week. Hemorrhoids seldom return after surgery.

Expected results

Hemorrhoids are rarely life-threatening. Most clear up after a few days without medical treatment. However,

KEY TERMS

Anus—The opening at the lower end of the rectum. The anus and rectum are both part of the large intestine.

Constipation—A condition marked by difficulty passing stools, infrequent stools, or insufficient stools.

Defecate—Pass feces through the anus for elimination.

Heat—In traditional Chinese medicine (TCM), a disease condition characterized by intolerance for cold, deficient fluids, and irritability, as well as other traits.

Ligation—Tying off a blood vessel or other tube with wire or suture, usually during surgery.

Lower burner—A TCM term for the kidneys.

Prolapsed—Referring to an organ fallen down from its normal body position.

Qi—In TCM, the vital energy that is the foundation for all physical and mental activity.

Rectum—The lower section of the large intestine. After food has passed through the stomach and intestines and been digested, the leftover material, enters the rectum, in the form of feces, where it stays until defecation.

Sitz bath—A warm water bath, sometimes including medications or herbs, that is taken in the sitting position, with water covering only the hips and buttocks.

Spleen—In TCM, all the organs considered necessary for extracting and using nutrients.

Varicose veins—Swollen veins that can no longer maintain proper blood pressure.

because **colorectal cancer** and other digestive system diseases can cause anal bleeding and other hemorrhoid symptoms, people should always consult a healthcare practitioner when hemorrhoid symptoms occur.

Prevention

A **high-fiber diet**, daily **exercise**, and losing excess weight are recommended to maintain healthy digestion and elimination. To prevent hemorrhoids by strengthening the veins of the anus, rectum, and colon and increasing circulation, blackberries, blueberries, cherries and **vitamin C** are recommended. Tinctures of **butcher's broom** (*Ruscus aculeatus*, and **horse chestnut** (*Aesculus hippocastanum*), plant pigments (called flavonoids) found in fruit and fruit products, tea, and soy also are recommended. It should be noted that horse chestnut, along with commercial hemorrhoid preparations, is contraindicated during pregnancy.

Drinking water with a high-fiber meal or supplement will cause the stools to be softer and easier to pass, reducing straining. Constipation should be avoided, and good toilet habits should be cultivated. Promptly responding to the urge to defecate will help encourage regular bowel movements. Defecation should be done without rushing or straining. A squatting position over the toilet or having the feet raised on a small bench or footstool will also improve elimination. Reading, working or watching television are discouraged, because they entail prolonged sitting on the toilet, which increases the strain placed on the anal and rectal veins. Perfumed soaps or toilet waters may irritate the anal area and should be avoided, as should excessive cleansing, rubbing, or wiping.

Resources

BOOKS

The Burton Goldberg Group, eds. *Alternative Medicine: The Definitive Guide*. Fife, WA: Future Medicine Publishing, 1999.

Lininger, D.C., Skye, editor-in-chief, et al. *The Natural Pharmacy*. Rocklin, CA: Prima Health, 1998.

Simons, Anne M.D., Bobbie Hasselbring, and Michael Castleman. *Before You Call the Doctor: Safe, Effective Self-Care for Over 300 Common Medical Problems*. New York: Fawcett Columbine, 1992.

PERIODICALS

Pfenninger, John L. "Modern Treatments for Internal Haemorrhoids." *British Medical Journal*, 1997.

Surrell, James. "Nonsurgical Treatment Options for Internal Hemorrhoids." *American Family Physician* (September 1995).

ORGANIZATIONS

National Digestive Diseases Information Clearinghouse. 2 Information Way, Bethesda, MD 20892-3570. http://www.niddk.nih.gov/health/digest/nddic.htm

Patience Paradox

Hepar sulphuris

Description

Hepar sulphuris is a homeopathic remedy that was created by Samuel Hahnemann, the father of **homeopathy**. Hahnemann combined the inner layer of oyster shells (*Calcium carbonica*) with flowers of **sulfur** and burned them to create *Hepar sulphuris calcareum,* or *Hepar sulph.* as it is commonly called. It is also known as

calcium sulfide or Hahnemann's calcium sulfide. *Hepar* is the Latin word for liver, and as certain compounds of sulfur had the color of liver, the remedy was so named.

Calcium sulfide was once used as a treatment for mercury poisoning, **gout**, **itching**, rheumatism, goiter, and swellings from **tuberculosis**. Now it is used in veterinary medicine, and in the manufacture of medicine, luminous paint, and hair removal products.

Although *Hepar sulph.* has the chemical properties of two other remedies, *Calcium carbonica* and sulfur, the actions of the remedies are different.

General use

Homeopaths prescribe *Hepar sulph.* for colds, coughs, sore throats, **croup**, abscesses, earaches, inflamed cuts and **wounds**, **asthma**, arthritis, **emphysema**, herpes, **constipation**, conjunctivitis, *Candida albicans* **infections**, **syphilis**, sinusitis, and skin infections.

The main indications for *Hepar sulph.* are as follows. The patient is overly sensitive to **pain**, touch, and cold. Pains are sharp, as if a splinter or piece of glass were being poked into the skin. A **sore throat** may feel like a fish bone is stuck in it and the pain increases upon swallowing. The slightest pressure causes much pain and the patient may faint from the pain. The patient cannot tolerate the cold and any exposure to cold air causes **chills**. If a hand or foot slips outside the bedcovers the patient will become chilled. Any slight exertion will cause the patient to perspire. The patient's sweat is cold and profuse and smells sour and offensive, like rotten cheese. Bodily discharges are yellow and thick and also smell offensive. If a **cough** is present, it is a dry, hacking cough with rattling of mucus in the chest.

The typical *Hepar sulph.* patients are delicate, oversensitive persons who tend to be scrawny in build and have enlarged glands. They are slow persons with flabby muscles, and often have light hair. They catch cold easily, dislike the cold, crave sour foods such as pickles and vinegar, and may dislike fats.

Mentally they are irritable, impulsive, angry, obstinate, anxious, fearful, impatient, sad, and depressed. They are very hard to get along with. Nothing pleases them and they dislike company. Often the desire to commit violence is present. They have poor memories. The *Hepar sulph.* patient is usually in a hurry—he drinks and eats fast and talks rapidly.

Hepar sulph. ailments generally arise from exposure to cold dry wind, suppression of perspiration and skin eruptions. Typical patients suffer from a lack of internal warmth, so all symptoms are made worse from exposure to cold conditions: cold air, cold weather, and cold wind.

Fresh air, lying on the painful side, any pressure or touch, or being uncovered also aggravate the symptoms. Symptoms are worse in the morning and at night. Bed warmth and heat tend to make the symptoms better. The patient craves warmth and can often be found wrapped up in the bedcovers or wearing several layers of clothing.

Specific indications

The action of *Hepar sulph.* prevents the formation of pus and hastens healing of abscesses. In fact, *Hepar sulph.* is one of the best remedies for abscesses, but is useful only before the **abscess** is open. The *Hepar sulph.* abscess is swollen and painful, with needle-like pains.

Hepar sulph. colds are frequently brought on by exposure to cold, dry weather. A cold wind causes **sneezing** and a runny nose. At first the mucus is watery, then it becomes thick, yellow, and offensive smelling. The nose is swollen, red, and tender and the sense of smell may be lost. A hoarse voice, sore throat, and cough may develop. The patient may also be constipated.

The *Hepar sulph.* cough is of a dry, barking nature with thick, sticky, yellow mucus. The chest becomes sore from coughing. The cough is worse in the evening, and the patient may cough straight through to midnight or sometimes all night long. The patient may gag or choke while coughing. *Hepar sulph.* may be used in the treatment of croup when the symptoms for cough are exhibited. Croup coughs are generally worse in the morning, and the patient may have difficulty bringing up mucus.

The sore throat is accompanied by a splinter-like pain and swollen tonsils. The patient may feel as if there were a fish bone caught in the throat. The throat becomes worse from coughing or swallowing cold drinks.

Fevers are hot and often are accompanied by chills. A cold, sour sweat may be present, although it doesn't give any relief to the patient. If **diarrhea** is present, it is accompanied by a rumbling sensation in the abdomen.

Earaches with sharp, tearing pains may occur suddenly and be accompanied by abscesses in the ears. If the eardrum ruptures there may be a bloody, offensive discharge.

Eye irritations may indicate this remedy. The eyes are red and inflamed, and may discharge a fluid. Toothaches are accompanied by bleeding gums and mouth abscesses.

Slow-to-heal cuts and wounds may be cured by *Hepar sulph.* The tissues surrounding the wound are inflamed and the pain is splinter-like.

Pains in the finger, hip, and shoulder joints are caused by exposure to the cold and are of a sore, bruised nature.

Hepar sulph. has a positive effect on such skin problems as **eczema, boils,** and herpes. The eczema is crusty, scabby, and oozing and generally appears in the bends of joints. Other eruptions may be moist, dry, itchy, and filled with pus. The boils are red, inflamed, and sore.

This remedy is often indicated in liver problems. Symptoms include stitching pains in the right side, a soreness that is aggravated by pressing on the area, sensitive **hemorrhoids**, and constipation.

A burning in the bladder or frequent urge to urinate may be present. The urine flows in a slow stream or in drops.

Preparations

Finely powdered oyster shell is mixed with flowers of sulfur and heated in an airtight container. The resulting white powder is dissolved in hot hydrochloric acid, mixed with milk sugar and diluted.

Hepar sulph. is available at health food and drug stores in various potencies in the form of tinctures, tablets, and pellets.

Precautions

If symptoms do not improve after the recommended time period, the patient should consult homeopath or health-care practitioner. Do not exceed the recommended dose.

Side effects

There are no side effects, but individual aggravations may occur.

Interactions

When taking any homeopathic remedy, the patient should not use **peppermint** products, coffee, or alcohol. These products are known as antidotes in homeopathy. They counteract the homeopathic remedies.

Resources

BOOKS

Cummings, Stephen M.D., and Dana Ullman, M.P.H. *Everybody's Guide to Homeopathic Medicines.* New York, NY: Jeremy P. Tarcher/Putnam, 1997.

Kent, James Tyler. *Lectures on Materia Medica.* Delhi, India: B. Jain Publishers, 1996.

Jennifer Wurges

Hepatitis

Definition

Hepatitis is inflammation of the liver. Infectious or viral hepatitis is caused by a viral infection. The three most common forms of viral hepatitis recognized to cause liver disease are hepatitis A, hepatitis B, and hepatitis C (previously called hepatitis non-A, non-B). Other recognized types of hepatitis are hepatitis D, hepatitis E, and hepatitis G.

Description

Hepatitis A

Hepatitis A is an inflammation of the liver caused by the hepatitis A virus (HAV). It is usually not very severe, generally starting within two to six weeks after contact with the virus, and lasting no longer than two months.

Hepatitis A is commonly known as infectious hepatitis because it spreads relatively easily from those infected to their close contacts. Once the infection ends, there is no lasting, chronic phase of illness. However, it is not uncommon to have a second episode of symptoms about a month after the first (a relapse).

Epidemics of HAV infection can infect dozens and even hundreds of persons. Major outbreaks of hepatitis A have been linked to infected food handlers contaminating prepared foods. Many types of food also can be infected by sewage containing HAV, and shellfish are a common culprit.

Certain groups have an increased risk of contracting hepatitis A. These include:

• children and employees at daycare centers

• individuals living in crowded and/or unsanitary conditions

• sexually active individuals

• tourists visiting an area where hepatitis A is common

Hepatitis B

More than 300 million people throughout the world are infected by the hepatitis B virus (HBV). Hepatitis B occurs in both rapidly developing (acute) and long-lasting (chronic) forms, and is one of the most frequent chronic infectious diseases worldwide. Commonly called "serum hepatitis," hepatitis B ranges from mild to very severe. Some people who are infected by HBV develop no symptoms, but they may carry HBV in their blood and pass the infection on to others. In its chronic form, HBV infection may destroy the liver through a scarring process called **cirrhosis.**

When a person is infected by HBV, the virus enters the bloodstream and body fluids, and is able to pass through tiny breaks in the skin, mouth, or the genital area. This infection can occur during birth, when a mother with hepatitis B may pass HBV on to her infant. The virus also may be transmitted through contaminated needles and through unprotected sex with an HBV infected individual. Casual contact cannot transmit hepatitis B.

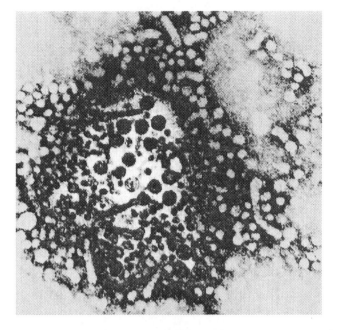

Hepatitis A virus, magnified 225,000 times. *(Custom Medical Stock Photo. Reproduced by permission.)*

Hepatitis C

Hepatitis C, or HCV, causes a rapidly developing and often long-lasting disease. Spread mainly by contact with infected blood, HCV is the major cause of "transfusion hepatitis," which can develop in patients who are given blood, although, donated blood is regularly tested for hepatitis C as of the early 2000s. The existence of a third hepatitis virus (in addition to the A and B viruses) became clear in 1974, although HCV was first identified in 1989.

Hepatitis C is generally mild in its early, acute stage, but it is much more likely to produce chronic liver disease than hepatitis B. About two of every three persons who are infected by HCV may continue to have the virus in their blood and become carriers who can transmit the infection to others.

The most common way of transmitting hepatitis C is when blood containing the virus enters another person's bloodstream through a break in the skin or the mucosa (inner lining) of the mouth or genitals. HCV may be passed from an infected mother to the infant she is carrying (however, the risk of infection from breast milk is very low). It also can be spread through sexual intercourse, especially if one partner is acutely infected at the time.

Hepatitis D

Hepatitis D (or delta), occurs only in patients who also are infected by the hepatitis B virus. Infection by the hepatitis delta virus (HDV) either occurs at the same time as hepatitis B, or develops later when infection by HBV has entered the chronic stage.

Delta hepatitis can be quite severe, but is seen only in patients already infected with HBV. In the late 1970s Italian physicians discovered that some patients with hepatitis B had another type of infectious agent in their liver cells. Later the new virus, HDV, was confirmed by experimentally infecting chimpanzees. When both viruses are present, acute infection tends to be more serious. Furthermore, patients with both **infections** are more likely to develop chronic liver disease than those with HBV alone, and, when it occurs, it is more severe.

Hepatitis E

Hepatitis E also is known as epidemic non-A, non-B hepatitis. Like hepatitis A, it is an acute and short-lived illness that sometimes can cause liver failure. HEV, discovered in 1987, is spread by the fecal-oral route. It is present in countries in which human waste has contaminated the drinking **water** supply. Large outbreaks (epidemics) have occurred in Asian and South American countries where there is poor sanitation. In the United States and Canada no outbreaks have been reported, but persons traveling to a region where it is present may return with HEV.

Hepatitis G

HGV, also called hepatitis GB virus, was first described in early 1996. Little is known about the frequency of HGV infection, the nature of the illness, or how to prevent it. What is known is that transfused blood containing HGV has caused some cases of hepatitis. For this reason, patients with hemophilia and other bleeding conditions who require large amounts of blood or blood products are at risk of constructing hepatitis G. HGV has been identified in 1–2% of blood donors in the United States. Also at risk are patients with kidney disease who undergo hemodialysis treatments, and those who inject intravenous drugs. It is possible that an infected mother can pass on the virus to her newborn infant, or that sexual transmission can occur.

Often patients with hepatitis G are infected at the same time by the hepatitis B or C virus, or both. In about three of every thousand patients with acute viral hepatitis, HGV is the only virus present. There is some indication that patients with hepatitis G may continue to carry the virus in their blood for many years, and so might be a source of infection for others.

Causes & symptoms

Hepatitis A

The time between exposure to HAV and the onset of symptoms ranges from two to seven weeks and averages about one month. The virus is passed in the feces, especially late in the incubation period, before symptoms first appear. The virus can live for several hours on the skin surface, and during this time may be transmitted to others. Infected persons are most contagious starting about a week before symptoms develop, and remain contagious until the time **jaundice** (yellowing of the skin and/or eyes) is noted.

Often the first symptoms to appear are **fatigue**, muscle and joint aches, **nausea**, and a loss of appetite. Low-grade **fever** is common, and the liver often enlarges, causing **pain** or tenderness in the upper right part of the abdomen. Jaundice then develops, typically lasting seven to ten days.

Hepatitis B

In the United States, a majority of acute HBV infections occur in teenagers and young adults. Half of these youth never develop symptoms, and only about 20% of infected patients develop severe symptoms and jaundice. The remaining 30% of patients have only flu-like symptoms and will probably not even be diagnosed as having hepatitis unless certain tests are done. Acute hepatitis B is characterized by loss of appetite, nausea, and pain or tenderness in the right upper part of the abdomen. Compared to patients with hepatitis A or C, those with HBV infection require more bed rest.

An HBV infection lasting longer than six months is said to be chronic. After this time it is much less likely for the infection to disappear. Not all carriers of the virus develop chronic liver disease; in fact, most have no symptoms. However, about one in every four HBV carriers develop cirrhosis. Patients are also likely to have an enlarged liver and spleen. The most serious complication of chronic HBV infection is liver **cancer**.

Hepatitis C

More than half of all patients who develop hepatitis C have no symptoms or signs of liver disease. Some, however, may have a minor illness with flu-like symptoms. About one in four patients with hepatitis C will develop jaundice, and some patients lose their appetite and frequently feel tired. Patients also may experience nausea.

In most patients, HCV can still be found in the blood six months after the start of acute infection, and these patients are considered carriers. If the virus persists for one year, it is unlikely to disappear completely. About 20% of chronic carriers develop cirrhosis (scarring) of the liver when the virus damages or destroys large numbers of liver cells, which are then replaced by scar tissue. Cirrhosis may develop only after a long period of time—as long as 20 years—has passed. Many patients will not develop cirrhosis and instead have a mild, chronic form of infection called chronic persistent hepatitis.

Hepatitis D

The delta virus is a small and incomplete viral particle. Perhaps this small size is why it cannot cause infection on its own. Its companion virus, HBV, actually forms a covering over the HDV particle. In chronically ill patients (those whose virus persists longer than six months), cirrhosis typically occurs.

When HBV and HDV infections develop at the same time—a condition called coinfection—recovery is the rule. Only 2–5% of patients become chronic carriers (the virus remains in their blood more than six months after infection). It may be that HDV actually keeps HBV from reproducing as rapidly as it would if it were alone, making chronic infection less likely.

When HBV infection occurs first and is followed by HDV infection, the condition is called superinfection. Between one-half and two-thirds of patients with superinfection develop severe acute hepatitis. Once the liver cells contain large numbers of HBV viruses, HDV tends to reproduce more actively. Massive infection and liver failure are more common in superinfection. The risk of liver cancer, however, is no greater than from hepatitis B alone.

As with other forms of hepatitis, the earliest symptoms are nausea, loss of appetite, joint pains, and fatigue. There may be fever and an enlarged liver may cause discomfort or pain in the right upper part of the abdomen. Jaundice may develop later.

Hepatitis E

There are at least two strains of HEV, one found in Asia and another in Mexico. The virus may start dividing in the gastrointestinal tract, but it grows mostly in the liver. After an incubation period of two to eight weeks, infected persons develop jaundice, fever, nausea, a loss of appetite, and discomfort or pain in the right upper part of the abdomen. Most often the illness is mild and disappears within a few weeks with no lasting effects.

Hepatitis E never becomes a chronic illness, but on rare occasions the acute illness damages and destroys so many liver cells that the liver can no longer function. This is called fulminant liver failure, and may end in death. The great majority of patients who recover from acute infection do not continue to carry HEV and cannot pass the infection on to others.

Hepatitis G

Some researchers believe that there may be a group of GB viruses, rather than just one. Others remain doubtful that HGV actually causes illness. If it does, the type of acute or chronic illness that results is not clear. When diagnosed, acute HGV infection has usually been mild and brief. There is no evidence of serious complications, but it is possible that, like other hepatitis viruses, HGV can cause severe liver damage resulting in liver failure. The virus has been identified in as many as 20% of patients with longlasting viral hepatitis, some of whom also have hepatitis C.

Diagnosis

A health care professional will conduct a thorough medical history and physical examination of the patient when hepatitis is suspected. Blood tests for specific antigens and antibodies that are present in the different subtypes of hepatitis will confirm the diagnosis, although these tests cannot detect all types of hepatitis. Liver function tests that measure enzyme levels may also be performed.

Treatment

Once symptoms appear, no antibiotics or other medicines will shorten the course of infectious hepatitis. Patients should rest in bed as needed, follow a healthy diet, and avoid drinking alcohol or taking any medications that could further damage the liver. Any medication that can cause liver damage should be avoided, and non-critical surgery should be postponed.

An herbalist or naturopathic health care professional may recommend a preparation of **milk thistle** (*Silybum marianum*) for the treatment of hepatitis. Milk thistle is thought to promote the growth of new liver cells, and to prevent toxins from penetrating through healthy liver cells by binding itself to the cell membranes. It is frequently prescribed by herbalists for the treatment of cirrhosis, hepatitis, and other liver disorders. A large controlled trial sponsored by the National Center for Complementary and Alternative Medicine (NCCAM) and the National Institutes of health (NIH) on milk thistle's medicinal value in the treatment of hepatitis and liver injury was scheduled to begin in the year 2000. **Licorice** (*Glycyrriza glabra*) may also be used for hepatitis. Its properties include protecting the liver and enhancing the immune system. Extended use of licorice should not be undertaken without medical consultation, since **potassium** deficiency may result.

Vitamin C may be taken as a nutritional supplement. It has been shown to help diminish acute hepatitis and help prevent hepatitis in hospitalized patients. Liver extracts are effective in liver regeneration, and have been used for over a century. Thymus extracts enhance the immune system, which may help the body fight a hepatitis virus.

A practitioner of Chinese herbal medicine may recommend *Fructus Schisandrae Chinensis,* which improves liver function; *Fructus Citrulli Vulgaris,* which helps to expel jaundice; or other herbs for hepatitis symptoms.

Allopathic treatment

A natural body protein, interferon alpha, now can be made in large amounts by genetic engineering, and improves the outlook for many patients who have chronic hepatitis C. The protein can lessen the symptoms of infection and improve liver function. In 2003, a synthetic analogue was added to improve the treatment's effectiveness. Fever and flu-like symptoms are frequent side effects of this treatment. Approximately one-half of patients respond positively to the treatment, although only about 20% receive lasting effects. Several new treatment drugs have been tested and found beneficial in suppressing hepatitis B since early 2003. One of these drugs also helps those patients infected with both hepatitis B and HIV.

When hepatitis destroys most or all of the liver, the only hope may be a liver transplant. However, even when the procedure is successful, disease often recurs and cirrhosis may actually develop more rapidly than before.

Expected results

Hepatitis A

Most patients with acute hepatitis A, even when severe, begin feeling better in two to three weeks, and recover completely in four to eight weeks. After recovering from hepatitis A, a person no longer carries the virus and remains immune for life. In the United States, serious complications are infrequent and deaths are rare. In the United States, as many as 75% of adults over the age of 50 will have blood test evidence of previous hepatitis A.

Hepatitis B

Each year an estimated 150,000 persons in the United States get hepatitis B. More than 10,000 will require hospital care, and as many as 5,000 will die from complications of the infection. About 90% of those infected will have only acute disease. A large majority of these patients will recover within three months. It is the remaining 10% with chronic infection who account for most serious complications and deaths from HBV infection. In the United States, perhaps only 2% of all infected will become chronically ill. People infected with both HIV and hepatitis B are most likely to die than from either disease alone. Even when no symptoms of liver disease develop, chronic carriers remain a threat to others by serving as a source of infection.

Hepatitis C

In roughly one-fifth of patients who develop hepatitis C, the acute infection will subside, and they will recover completely within four to eight weeks and have no later problems. Other patients face two risks: they themselves may develop chronic liver infection and possibly serious complications such as liver cancer, and they will continue carrying the virus and may pass it on to others. The overall risk of developing cirrhosis is about 15% for all patients infected by HCV. Liver failure is less frequent in patients with chronic hepatitis C than it is for those with other forms of hepatitis. In those people who also have **AIDS**, hepatitis C infection increases the chance for liver cancer.

Hepatitis D

A large majority of patients with coinfection of HBV and HDV recover from an episode of acute hepatitis. However, about two-thirds of patients chronically infected by HDV go on to develop cirrhosis of the liver. If severe liver failure develops, the chance of a patient surviving is no better than 50%. A liver transplant may improve this figure to 70%.

Hepatitis E

In the United States hepatitis E is not a fatal illness, but elsewhere 1–2% of those infected die of advanced liver failure. In pregnant women the death rate is as high as 20%. It is not clear whether having hepatitis E once guarantees against future HEV infection.

Hepatitis G

What little is known about the course of hepatitis G suggests that illness is mild and does not last long. When more patients have been followed up after the acute phase, it will become clear whether HGV can cause severe liver damage.

Prevention

The best way to prevent any form of viral hepatitis is to avoid contact with blood and other body fluids of infected individuals. The use of condoms during sex also is advisable. Travelers should avoid water and ice if unsure of their purity, or they can boil water before drinking it. All foods eaten should be packaged, well cooked, or, in the case of fresh fruit, peeled. Caution should be exercised when getting tattoos or body piercing, since a 2003 report said that only about one-half of tattoo and piercing shops follow the government's guidelines concerning infection control. These practices can pass hepatitis and HIV infection.

There are vaccines available for both hepatitis A and hepatitis B. Individuals in a high-risk group and travelers should be vaccinated for hepatitis A, and much of the general population can be vaccinated for hepatitis B.

Resources

BOOKS

Fauci, Anthony S. et al., eds. *Harrison's Principles of Internal Medicine.* 14th edition. New York: McGraw Hill, 1998.

PERIODICALS

"Antiviral Effective Against Hepatitis B Virus in HIV-Coinfected." *Virus Weekly* (January 28, 2003): 16.

Bauer, Jeff. "Co-infection with Hepatitis B and HIV Increases Men's Risks of Death from Liver Disease." *RN* (March 2003): 97.

Eckler, Jody A. Lambright. "Preventing Hepatitis." *Nursing* 29, no. 8 (August 1999): 66.

Elliott, William T. "Warfarin Effectively Prevents Venous Thromboembolism (Pharmacology Watch)." *Critical Care Alert* (April 2003).

"Hepatitis C Drug Launched." *Chemist and Druggist* (January 25, 2003):24.

"Hepatitis C Virus Presents Risk for Liver Cancer in Adults with AIDS." *Cancer Weekly* (January 7, 2003):35.

"Some Tattoo, Piercing Shops Still Unsafe." *AIDS Weekly* (March 24, 2003):23.

ORGANIZATIONS

Hepatitis Foundation International. 30 Sunrise Terrace, Cedar Grove, NJ 07009-1423. (800)891-0707. Fax: (973)857-5044. http://www.hepfi.org/.

OTHER

Centers for Disease Control. *Hepatitis.* http://www.cdc.gov/ncidod/diseases/hepatitis/.

Hep Net: The Hepatitis Information Network. http://www.hep-net.com/.

Paula Ford-Martin
Teresa G. Odle

Herbalism, traditional Chinese

Definition

Chinese herbalism is one of the major components of **traditional Chinese medicine** (TCM), or Oriental medicine (OM). In TCM, herbs are often used in conjunction with such other techniques as **acupuncture** or massage. Chinese herbalism is a holistic medical system, meaning that it looks at treating a patient as a whole person, looking at the mental and spiritual health as well as the physical health, of the individual. Illness is seen as a disharmony or imbalance among these aspects of the individual. Chinese herbalism has been practiced for over 4,000 years.

One of the earliest and certainly the most important Chinese herbal text is the *Huang Ti Nei Ching*, or *Yellow Emperor's Classic of Internal Medicine*. It is believed to have been authored by Huang Ti during his reign over China, which started about 2697 B.C. Since that time, herbal practices have been more extensively documented and refined. In modern China, traditional Chinese herbalism is taught alongside conventional Western pharmacology. Chinese herbal remedies have been used in the West only relatively recently, over the past two decades. These remedies are more gentle and natural than conventional medicines. In addition, they have fewer unpleasant side effects. Individuals with chronic disorders in particular are increasingly drawn to the holistic aspect of Chinese herbalism and TCM in general.

Origins

Historical background

Traditional Chinese medicine originated in the region of eastern Asia that today includes China, Tibet, Vietnam, Korea, and Japan. Tribal shamans and holy men who lived as hermits in the mountains of China as early as 3500 B.C. practiced what was called the "Way of Long Life." This regimen included a diet based on herbs and other plants; kung-fu exercises; and special breathing techniques that were thought to improve vitality and life expectancy.

After the Han dynasty, the next great age of Chinese medicine was under the Tang emperors, who ruled from A.D. 608–906. The first Tang emperor established China's first medical school in A.D. 629. Under the Song (A.D.) 960–1279 and Ming (A.D. 1368–1644) dynasties, new medical schools were established, their curricula and qualifying examinations were standardized, and the traditional herbal prescriptions were written down and collected into encyclopedias. One important difference

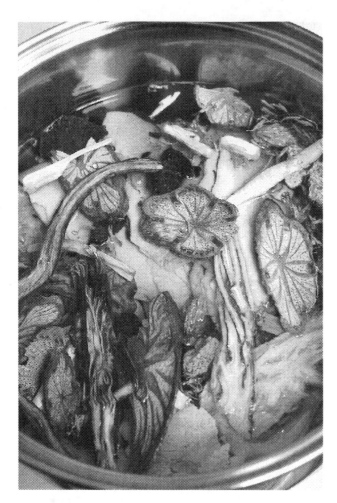

Chinese herbs being boiled to make traditional Chinese medicines. *(Photo Researchers, Inc. Reproduced by permission.)*

between the development of medicine in China and in the West is the greater interest in the West in surgical procedures and techniques.

Philosophical background: the cosmic and natural order

In Taoist thought, the Tao, or universal first principle, generated a duality of opposing principles that underlie all the patterns of nature. These principles, yin and yang, are mutually dependent as well as polar opposites. They are basic concepts in traditional Chinese medicine. Yin represents everything that is cold, moist, dim, passive, slow, heavy, and moving downward or inward; while yang represents heat, dryness, brightness, activity, rapidity, lightness, and upward or outward motion. Both forces are equally necessary in nature and in human well-being, and neither force can exist without the other. The dynamic interaction of these two principles is reflected in the cycles of the seasons, the human life cycle, and other natural phenomena. One objective of traditional Chinese medicine is to keep yin and yang in harmonious balance within a person.

In addition to yin and yang, Taoist teachers also believed that the Tao produced a third force, primordial energy or qi (also spelled chi or ki). The interplay between yin, yang, and qi gave rise to the Five Elements of water, metal, earth, wood, and fire. These entities are all reflected in the structure and functioning of the human body.

The human being

Traditional Chinese physicians did not learn about the structures of the human body from dissection because they thought that cutting open a body insulted the person's ancestors. Instead they built up an understanding of the location and functions of the major organs over centuries of observation, and then correlated them with the principles of yin, yang, qi, and the Five Elements. Thus wood is related to the liver (yin) and the gall bladder (yang); fire to the heart (yin) and the small intestine (yang); earth to the spleen (yin) and the stomach (yang); metal to the lungs (yin) and the large intestine (yang); and water to the kidneys (yin) and the bladder (yang). The Chinese also believed that the body contains Five Essential Substances, which include blood, spirit, vital essence (a principle of growth and development produced by the body from qi and blood), fluids (all body fluids other than blood, such as saliva, spinal fluid, sweat, etc.), and qi.

Benefits

Because it is a safe and inexpensive solution to health problems of all kinds, Chinese herbalism is very popular in China. In recent years, herbalism has been modernized with the introduction of quality control. For example, herbs are subjected to absorption spectrometry to determine levels of heavy metals found in some. Because they are standardized, Chinese herbs are safer for self-treatment. This approach puts the individual, not the physician, in charge of the individual's health; that is a basic goal of Chinese herbalism.

Chinese herbalism offers unique advice regarding what foods can help and what can hinder, and a herbalist can help an individual discover what he is allergic to. In addition, Chinese herbs stimulate the immune system and provide beneficial nutrients, aside from their role in curing illness.

At M.D. Anderson Hospital in Texas, medical research has confirmed that patients undergoing chemotherapy were shown to have an improved degree of immune function when they took the tonic herb astragalus (*huang qi*). (It is well known that chemotherapy suppresses the immune system.) Research also showed that T-cell and macrophage activity and interferon production were increased in patients using the Chinese herbs **ganoderma**, lentinus, and polyporus, helping the body fight **cancer** cells. Agents also found in ganoderma were found to inhibit platelet aggregation and thrombocyte formation, which would be helpful to counter circulation and heart problems.

An ingredient of ginseng was found to promote adrenal function, which would give the herb properties of enhancing many hormone functions in the body.

Description

Chinese herbal treatment differs from **Western herbalism** in several respects. In Chinese practice, several different herbs may be used, according to each plant's effect on the individual's Qi and the Five Elements. There are many formulas used within traditional Chinese medicine to treat certain common imbalance patterns. These formulas can be modified to fit specific individuals more closely.

A traditional Chinese herbal formula typically contains four classes of ingredients, arranged in a hierarchical order: a chief (the principal ingredient, chosen for the patient's specific illness); a deputy (to reinforce the chief's action or treat a coexisting condition); an assistant (to counteract side effects of the first two ingredients); and an envoy (to harmonize all the other ingredients and convey them to the parts of the body that they are to treat).

Methods of diagnosis

A Chinese herbalist will not prescribe a particular herb on the strength of symptoms only, but will take into consideration the physical condition, emotional health, and mental state of the patient. He or she may look at the condition of the patient's hair, skin, and tongue, as well as the appearance of the eyes, lips, and general complexion. The practitioner then listens to the sounds the body makes when breathing. He or she may smell the breath, **body odor**, or sputum in diagnosis.

TCM practitioners take an extensive medical history of a patient. He or she may ask about dietary habits, lifestyle, and sleep patterns. The patient will be questioned about chief medical complaints, as well as on his or her particular emotional state and sexual practices.

Chinese herbalists employ touch as a diagnostic tool. They may palpate the body or use light massage to assess the patient's physical health. Another chief component of Chinese medical diagnosis is **pulse diagnosis**, or sphygmology. This is a very refined art that takes practitioners years to master. Some practitioners can detect 12 different pulse points that correspond to the 12 major organs in Chinese medicine. There are over 30 pulse qualities that practitioners are able to detect on each point. The strength, speed, quality, and rhythm of the pulse, to name a few, will be determined before a diagnosis is given.

Herbs

Chinese herbs may be used alone or in combination. Relatively few are used alone for medicinal purposes. Practitioners believe that illness can be effectively treated by combining herbs based on their various characteristics and the patient's overall health. Every herb has four basic healing properties: nature, taste, affinity, and effect.

An herb's nature is described according to its yin or yang characteristics. Yang, or warming, herbs treat cold deficiencies. They are frequently used in the treatment of the upper respiratory tract, skin, or extremities. Yin, or cooling, herbs, treat conditions of excessive heat. They are most often used to treat internal conditions and problems with organs. Herbs can also be neutral in nature.

An herb's taste does not refer to its flavor, but to its effect on qi, blood, fluids, and phlegm. Sour herbs have a concentrating action. They are prescribed to treat bodily excess conditions, such as **diarrhea**, and concentrate qi. Bitter herbs have an eliminating or moving downward action. They are used to treat coughs, **constipation**, and heart problems. Sweet or bland herbs have a harmonizing action. They are used as restorative herbs and to treat **pain**. Spicy herbs have a stimulating action. They are prescribed to improve blood and qi circulation. Salty herbs have a softening action. They are used to treat constipation and other digestion problems.

An herb's affinity describes its action on a specific bodily organ. (Note that Chinese medicine does not have the anatomical correlation for organ names. They correspond more closely to the organ's function.) Sour herbs have an affinity for the Liver and Gallbladder. Bitter herbs act on the Heart and Small Intestine. Sweet and bland herbs affect the Stomach and Spleen. Spicy herbs have an affinity for the Lungs and Large Intestine, whereas salty herbs act on the Kidneys and Bladder.

Chinese herbs are lastly classified according to their specific actions, which are divided into four effects. Herbs that dispel are used to treat an accumulation, sluggishness, or spasm by relaxing or redistributing. Herbs with an astringent action are used to consolidate or restrain a condition characterized by discharge or excessive elimination. Herbs that purge treat an obstruction or "poison" by encouraging elimination and **detoxification**. Tonifying herbs nourish, support, and calm where there is a deficiency.

Treatment of diabetes

The incidence of diabetes has increased quite dramatically in recent years, especially in the United States, where in general people take less **exercise**, and food is taken in greater quantity with a general reduction in quality. This increase has led to a scramble to find new solutions to the problem, and many researchers have focused their interest on Chinese herbal remedies. In the search for more effective and more convenient treatments, the alkaloid berberine has come under close scrutiny for its many uses, among them the treatment of diabetes. In trials, rats given a mixture of berberine and alloxan showed less likelihood of incurring a rise in blood sugar. Patients suffering from type II diabetes who were given between 300 and 600 mg of berberine daily for between one and three months showed a reduction in blood sugar levels, when the drug was taken in conjunction with a controlled diet.

Treatment of AIDS and cancer

Independent researchers are investigating indications that Chinese herbalism can reduce the toxicity of chemotherapy and other medications, in addition to stimulating immune responses.

Treatment of diarrhea associated with cholera

A team of researchers in Japan has found that some traditional Chinese herbal formulations inhibit the toxin produced by *Vibrio cholerae*, the microorganism that causes cholera. These preparations appear to be helpful when given in addition to oral rehydration treatment for diarrhea associated with cholera.

Treatment of atopic dermatitis

Some physicians have found Chinese herbal remedies useful in relieving the symptoms of atopic **dermatitis**, a chronic disorder of the skin that is difficult to treat. Herbal remedies have the advantage of relieving the **itching** and inflammation associated with atopic dermatitis without the long-term toxic side effects of conventional medications.

Preparations

Those who are unfamiliar with Chinese herbs and their uses should consult a practitioner before starting any treatment. Once a remedy is prescribed, it may be purchased at Oriental markets or health food stores. Most Chinese remedies prepared for Western markets are standardized and sold in ready-to-use formulations, with instructions for dosage. A Chinese herbalist may prescribe herbs to be made into tea or taken as capsules.

Precautions

It is best to avoid Chinese herbs that are not sold in a standardized form. Herbs can vary considerably in potency, depending on the time and place of their harvesting. In addition, cases have been reported in Europe as well as the United States of dried Chinese herbs contaminated by sewage or other forms of pollution.

When treating a patient, the herbalist will aim to gently "nudge" the system into shape, rather than producing any immediate reaction. A return to health, therefore, may take time, and it is important that the patient realize the principles underlying the treatment. Some practitioners estimate that treatment will take a month for every year that a chronic condition has existed. The advantage of the slow pace is that if there is a bad reaction to any herb, which is rare, it will be mild because the treatment itself is gentle.

As with most naturopathic therapies, Chinese herbal remedies work best when taken in conjunction with a healthy lifestyle and program of exercise.

Side effects

Some Chinese herbs are incompatible with certain prescription drugs or foods. Others should not be taken during **pregnancy**. Because of possible interactions, persons who are interested in taking traditional Chinese herbal remedies should not try to diagnose or treat themselves with these preparations.

Recent studies indicate that some herbs used in Chinese medicines may cause liver damage. Women appear to be more susceptible to such reactions than men. Damage to the liver may range from minor problems involving higher levels of certain enzymes called transaminases, to chronic **hepatitis**, **cirrhosis**, and acute liver failure requiring transplantation. Because of these risks, persons considering Chinese herbal treatments should consult a medical doctor before going to the herbalist. *It is essential for patients to inform their doctors about all medications or preparations they are taking, including alternative and over-the-counter remedies as well as prescription drugs.*

Research & general acceptance

At present, there is renewed interest in the West in traditional Chinese medicine and Chinese herbalism. Of the 700 herbal remedies used by traditional Chinese practitioners, over 100 have been tested and found effective by the standards of Western science. Several United States agencies, including the National Institutes of Health, the Office of Alternative Medicine, and the Food and Drug Administration are currently investigating Chinese herbal medicine as well as acupuncture and *Tui na* massage. In general, however, Western studies of Chinese medicine focus on the effects of traditional treatments and the reasons for those effects, thus attempting to fit traditional

KEY TERMS

Absorption spectrometry—A scientific procedure to determine the chemical composition of an unknown substance.

Interferon—A substance proved to be necessary in the body to help fight cancer cells.

Immune function—The body's defense system against bacteria, viruses and fungi, and any malfunction of the organism.

Pharmacodynamics—The study of the relationships and interactions of drugs.

Platelet aggregation—The clumping together of blood cells, possibly forming a clot.

Qi—The Chinese term for life force or vital energy.

Thrombocyte—Another name for platelet.

Chinese medicine within the Western framework of precise physical measurements and scientific hypotheses.

Training & certification

Practitioners of Oriental medicine can obtain certification in Chinese herbalism through the National Commission for the Certification of Acupuncture and Oriental Medicine, (NCCAOM). Some states have adopted the NCCAOM examination as all or part of their criteria for licensing. In California, the standards are higher, and these qualifications are not accepted. The licensing titles given by states vary, but herbalists are required to be a doctor of Oriental medicine (OMD or DOMO). In 1990, the U.S. Secretary of Education recognized the National Accreditation Commission for Schools and Colleges of Acupuncture and Oriental Medicine as an accrediting agency.

Resources

BOOKS

Molony, David. *The American Association of Oriental Medicine's Complete Guide to Chinese Herbal Medicine.* New York: Berkeley Publishing Group, 1998.

PERIODICALS

Oi, H., D. Matsuura, M. Miyake, et al. "Identification in Traditional Herbal Medications and Confirmation by Synthesis of Factors That Inhibit Cholera Toxin-Induced Fluid Accumulation." *Proceedings of the National Academy of Sciences of the USA* 99 (March 5, 2002): 3042-3046.

Stedman, C. "Herbal Hepatotoxicity." *Seminars in Liver Disease* 22 (2002):195-206.

Vender, R. B. "Alternative Treatments for Atopic Dermatitis: A Selected Review." *Skin Therapy Letter* 7 (February 2002): 1-5.

ORGANIZATIONS

National Center for Complementary and Alternative Medicine <http://nccam.nih.gov/nccam/>.

The California Association of Acupuncture and Oriental Medicine <http://www.CAAOM.ORG/medicine/overview.htm>

For help with herbs and a list of practitioners http://www.crane-herb.com/.

Institute of Chinese Materia Medica, China Academy of Traditional Chinese Medicine. *Beijing, 100700.*

Patricia Skinner
Rebecca J. Frey, PhD

Herbalism, Western

Definition

Western herbalism is a form of the healing arts that draws from herbal traditions of Europe and the Americas, and that emphasizes the study and use of European and Native American herbs in the treatment and prevention of illness. Western herbalism is based on physicians' and herbalists' clinical experience and traditional knowledge of medicinal plant remedies preserved by oral tradition and in written records over thousands of years. Western herbalism, like the much older system of **traditional Chinese medicine**, relies on the synergistic and curative properties of the plant to treat symptoms and disease and maintain health.

Western herbalism is based upon pharmocognosy, the study of natural products. Pharmocognosy includes the identification, extraction methods, and applications of specific plant constituents responsible for specific therapeutic actions, such as the use of digoxin from digitalis leaf for heart failure. These constituents are extracted, purified and studied in clinical research. They may be concentrated to deliver standardized, set doses. Sometimes, the natural constituent can be synthesized in the laboratory, or changed and patented. Practitioners may choose to use fresh medicinal plants, simple extracts, or standardized extracts.

In standardized extracts, a specific quantity of a constituent is called a marker compound, and it may or may not be the active constituent(s) in the plant medicine. The products should be produced under good manufacturing processes and according to the traditional *National Formulary, the U. S. Dispensatory,* or the *U. S. Pharmacopeia.*

Origins

Over 2,500 years ago Hippocrates wrote, "In medicine one must pay attention not to plausible theorizing

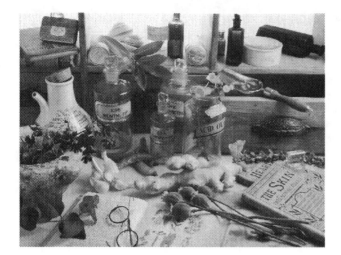

A selection of Western herbal medical equipment and traditional herbs, including foxglove (upper right), ginger (center right), and periwinkle (lower left). *(Photo Researchers, Inc. Reproduced by permission.)*

but to experience and reason together." This Greek physician and herbalist from the fourth century B.C. is considered the father of Western medicine. He stressed the importance of diet, water quality, climate, and social environment in the development of disease. Hippocrates believed in treating the whole person rather than merely isolating and treating symptoms. He recognized the innate capacity of the body to heal itself, and emphasized the importance of keen observation in the medical practice. He recommended simple herbal remedies to assist the body in restoring health.

Ancient Greek medicine around the fifth century B.C. was a fertile ground for contrasting philosophies and religions. Greek physicians were influenced by the accumulated medical knowledge from Egypt, Persia, and Babylon. Medical advances flourished and practitioners and scholars were free to study and practice without religious and secular constraints. In the fourth century B.C., Theophrastus wrote the *Historia Plantarum*, considered to be the founding text in the science of botany.

During the first century A.D. Dioscorides, a Greek physician who traveled with the Roman legions, produced five medical texts. His herbal text, known as the *De Materia Medica,* is considered to be among the most influential of all western herbal texts. It became a standard reference for practitioners for the next 1,500 years. This influential book also included information on medicinal herbs and treatments that had been used for centuries in Indian **Ayurvedic medicine**. Galen of Pergamum, who also lived in the first century A.D., was a Roman physician and student of anatomy and physiology. He authored a recipe book containing 130 antidotes

and medicinal preparations. These elaborate mixtures, known as galenicals, sometimes included up to 100 herbs and other substances. This complex approach to herbal medicine was a dramatic change from the simple remedies recommended by Hippocrates and employed by traditional folk healers. Galen developed a rigid system of medicine in which the physician, with his specialized knowledge of complex medical formulas, was considered the ultimate authority in matters of health care. The Galenic system, relying on theory and scholarship rather than observation, persisted throughout the Middle Ages. The galenical compounds, along with bloodletting, and purging, were among the drastic techniques practiced by the medical professionals during those times; however, traditional herbal healers persisted outside the mainstream medical system.

During the eighth century a medical school was established in Salerno, Italy, where the herbal knowledge accumulated by Arab physicians was preserved. The Arabian Muslims conducted extensive research on medicinal herbs found in Europe, Persia, India, and the Far East. Arab businessmen opened the first herbal pharmacies early in the ninth century. The *Leech Book of Bald*, the work of a Christian monk, was compiled in the tenth century. It preserved important medical writings that had survived from the work of physicians in ancient Greece and Rome.

The Middle Ages in Europe were a time of widespread death by plagues and pestilence. The Black Plague of 1348, particularly, and other health catastrophes in later years, claimed so many lives that survivors began to lose faith in the dominant Galenic medical system. Fortunately, the knowledge of traditional herbal medicine had not been lost. Medieval monks who cultivated extensive medicinal gardens on the monastery grounds also patiently copied the ancient herbal and medical texts. Folk medicine as practiced in Europe by traditional healers persisted, even though many women herbalists were persecuted as witches and enemies of the Catholic Church and their herbal arts were suppressed.

The growing spice trade and explorations to the New World introduced exotic plants, and a whole new realm of botanical medicines became available to Europeans. Following the invention of the printing press in the fifteenth century, a large number of herbal texts, also simply called herbals, became available for popular use. Among them were the beautifully illustrated works of the German botanists Otto Brunfels and Leonhard Fuchs published in 1530, and the Dutch herbal of Belgian physician Rembert Dodoens, a popular work that was later reproduced in English. In 1597, the physician and gardener John Gerard published one of the most famous of the English herbals, still in print today. Gerard's herbal, known as *The Herball or General Historie of Plantes* was not an original work. Much of the content was taken from the translated text of his Belgian predecessor Dodoens. Gerard did, however, include descriptions of some of the more than one thousand species of rare and exotic plants and English flora from his own garden.

The correspondence of astrology with herbs was taught by Arab physicians who regarded astrology as a science helpful in the selection of medicines and in the treatment of diseases. This approach to Western herbalism was particularly evident in the herbal texts published in the sixteenth and seventeenth centuries. One of the most popular and controversial English herbals is *The English Physician Enlarged* published in 1653. The author, Nicholas Culpeper, was an apothecary by trade. He also published a translation of the Latin language *London Pharmacopoeia* into English. Culpeper was a nonconformist in loyalist England, and was determined to make medical knowledge more accessible to the apothecaries, the tradesmen who prescribed most of the herbal remedies. Culpeper's herbal was criticized by the medical establishment for its mix of magic and astrology with **botanical medicine**, but it became one of the most popular compendia of botanical medicine of its day. Culpeper also accepted the so-called "Doctrine of Signatures," practiced by medieval monks in their medicinal gardens. This theory teaches that the appearance of plants is the clue to their curative powers. Plants were chosen for treatment of particular medical conditions based on their associations with the four natural elements and with a planet or sign. The place where the plant grows, its dominant physical feature, and the smell and taste of an herb determined the plant's signature. Culpeper's herbal is still in print in facsimile copies, and some pharmocognosists and herbalists in the twenty-first century voice the same criticisms that Culpeper's early critics did.

European colonists brought their herbal knowledge and plant specimens to settlements in North America, where they learned from the indigenous Americans how to make use of numerous nutritive and medicinal plants native to the New World. Many European medicinal plants escaped cultivation from the early settlements and have become naturalized throughout North America. The first record of Native American herbalism is found in the manuscript of the native Mexican Indian physician, Juan Badianus, published in 1552. The American folk tradition of herbalism developed as a blend of traditional European medicine and Native American herbalism. The pioneer necessity for self-reliance contributed to the perseverance of folk medicine well into the twentieth century.

In Europe in the seventeenth century, the alchemist Paracelsus changed the direction of Western medicine with the introduction of chemical and mineral medicines.

He was the son of a Swiss chemist and physician. Paracelsus began to apply chemicals, such as arsenic, mercury, **sulfur**, **iron**, and **copper** sulfate to treat disease. His chemical approach to the treatment of disease was a forerunner to the reliance in the twentieth century on chemical medicine as the orthodox regimen treatment prescribed in mainstream medical practice.

The nineteenth and twentieth centuries brought a renewed interest in the practice of western herbalism and the development of natural therapies and health care systems that ran counter to the mainstream methods of combating disease symptoms with synthetic pharmaceuticals.

In the late eighteenth century, the German physician **Samuel Hahnemann** developed a system of medicine known as **homeopathy**. This approach to healing embraces the philosophy of "like cures like." Homeopathy uses extremely diluted solutions of herbs, animal products, and chemicals that are believed to hold a "trace memory" or energetic imprint of the substance used. Homeopathic remedies are used to amplify the patient's symptoms with remedies that would act to produce the same symptom in a healthy person. Homeopathy holds that the symptoms of illness are evidence of the body's natural process of healing and eliminating the cause of the disease.

In 1895, the European medical system known as naturopathy was introduced to North America. Like homeopathy, this medical approach is based on the Hippocratic idea of eliminating disease by assisting the body's natural healing abilities. The naturopath uses nontoxic methods to assist the body's natural healing processes, including nutritional supplements, herbal remedies, proper diet, and **exercise** to restore health.

Western herbalism is regaining popularity at a time when the world faces the stress of overpopulation and development that threatens the natural biodiversity necessary for these valuable medicinal plants to survive. The American herb market is growing rapidly and increasing numbers of individuals are choosing alternative therapies over mainstream allopathic Western medicine. It is projected that by the year 2002 consumers will spend more than seven billion dollars a year on herbal products.

Though research into the efficacy and safety of traditional herbal remedies is increasing, it has been limited by the high costs of clinical studies and laboratory research, and by the fact that whole plants and their constituents are not generally patentable (therefore, there is no drug profit after market introduction). Outside the United States, herbalism has successfully combined with conventional medicine, and in some countries is fully integrated into the nations' health care systems. At the beginning of the twenty-first century, 80% of the world's population continues to rely on herbal treatments. The World Health Organization promotes traditional herbal medicine for treatment of many local health problems, particularly in the Third World, where it is affordable and already well integrated into the cultural fabric.

In the United States, the re-emergence in interest in holistic approaches to health care is evident. Citizens are demanding access to effective, safe, low-cost, natural medicine. Legislative and societal change is needed, however, before natural therapies can be fully integrated into the allopathic health care system and provide citizens with a wide range of choices for treatment. If the current trend continues, U. S. citizens will benefit from a choice among a variety of safe and effective medical treatments.

Benefits

The benefits of botanical medicine may be subtle or dramatic, depending on the remedy used and the symptom or problem being addressed. Herbal remedies usually have a much slower effect than pharmaceutical drugs. Some herbal remedies have a cumulative effect and work slowly over time to restore balance, and others are indicated for short-term treatment of acute symptoms. When compared to pharmaceutical drugs, herbal remedies prepared from the whole plant have relatively few side effects. This characteristic is due to the complex chemistry and synergistic action of the full range of phytochemicals present in the whole plant, and the relatively lower concentrations. They are generally safe when used in properly designated therapeutic dosages, and less costly than the isolated chemicals or synthetic prescription drugs available from western pharmaceutical corporations.

Description

Herbs are generally defined as any plant or plant part that may be used for medicinal, nutritional, culinary, or other beneficial purposes. The active constituents of plants (if known) may be found in varying amounts in the root, stem, leaf, flower, and fruit, etc. of the plant. Herbs may be classified into many different categories. Some Western herbalists categorize herbal remedies according to their strength, action, and characteristics. Categories may include sedatives, stimulants, laxatives, febrifuges (to reduce **fever**), and many others. One system of classification is based on a principle in traditional Chinese medicine that categorizes herbs into four classes: tonics, specifics, heroics, or cleansers and protectors. Within these broad classifications are the numerous medicinal actions of the whole herb, which may be due to a specific chemical or combination of chemicals in the plant.

• Tonics. Herbs in this classification are also known as alteratives in western herbalism. They are generally mild in their action and act slowly in the body, providing gentle stimulation and **nutrition** to specific organs and systems. Tonic herbs act over time to strengthen and nourish the whole body. These herbs are generally safe and may be used regularly, even in large quantities. These tonic herbs are known as "superior" remedies in traditional Chinese medicine. The therapeutic dose of tonic remedies is far removed from the possible toxic dose. **American ginseng** is an example of a tonic herb.

• Specifics. Herbs in this classification are strong and specific in their therapeutic action. They are generally used for short periods of time in smaller dosages to treat acute conditions. Herbs classified as specifics are not used beyond the therapeutic treatment period. **Echinacea** is a specific herb.

• Heroic. These herbs offer high potency but are potentially toxic, and should not be used in self-treatment. Because the therapeutic dosage may be close to the lethal dosage, these herbs are presented cautiously and closely monitored or avoided by trained clinicians. They should not be used continuously or without expert supervision. Poke (*Phytolacca americana*) is an example of a heroic remedy.

• Cleansers and protectors. These herbs, plants, and plant tissues remove wastes and pollutants, while minimally affecting regular body processes. An example of a cleanser is pectin. Pectins are the water-soluble substances that bind cell walls in plant tissues, and some researchers believe that they help remove heavy metals and environmental toxins from the body.

Preparations

Herbal preparations are commercially available in a variety of forms, including tablets or capsules, tinctures, teas, fluid extracts, douches, washes, suppositories, dried herbs, and many other forms. The medicinal properties of herbs are extracted from the fresh or dried plant parts by the use of solvents appropriate to the particular herb. Alcohol, oil, water, vinegar, glycerin, and propylene glycol are some of the solvents used to extract and concentrate the medicinal properties. Steam distillation and cold-pressing techniques are used to extract the **essential oils**. The quality of any herbal remedy and the potency of the phytochemicals found in the herb depend greatly on the conditions of weather and soil where the herb was grown, the timing and care in harvesting, and the manner of preparation and storage.

Precautions

Herbal remedies prepared by infusion, decoction, or alcohol tincture from the appropriate plant part, such as the leaf, root, or flower, are generally safe when ingested in properly designated therapeutic dosages. However, many herbs have specific contraindications for use when certain medical conditions are present. Not all herbal remedies may be safely administered to infants or small children. Many herbs are not safe for use by pregnant or lactating women. Some herbs are toxic, even deadly, in large amounts, and there is little research on the chronic toxicity that may result from prolonged use. Herbal remedies are sold in the United States as dietary supplements and are not regulated for content or efficacy. Self-diagnosis and treatment with botanical medicinals may be risky. A consultation with a clinical herbalist, naturopathic physician, or certified clinical herbalist is prudent before undertaking a course of treatment.

Essential oils are highly concentrated and should not be ingested as a general rule. They should also be diluted in water or in a non-toxic carrier oil before application to the skin to prevent **contact dermatitis** or photo-sensitization. The toxicity of the concentrated essential oil varies depending on the chemical constituents of the herb.

An American professor of pharmacognosy, Varro E. Tyler, believes that "herbal chaos" prevails in the United States with regard to herbs and phytomedicinals. In part he blames the herb producers and marketers of crude herbs and remedies for what he terms unproven hyperbole, poor quality control, deceptive labeling, resistance to standardization of dosage forms, and continued sale of herbs determined to be harmful.

A new warning about Western herbalism has been made necessary by technology. The Internet has a number of sites available with unregulated and often unhealthy advice about use of herbal remedies. Many herbalists and allopathic physicians urge patients to use caution when seeking Internet information on herbal treatments. One cancer-related study found that only 36% of the web sites found in a search offered information that complied with regulatory guidelines about unsubstantiated claims about treatment or cure of disease.

Side effects

Herbs contain a variety of complex phytochemicals that act on the body as a whole or on specific organs and systems. Some of these chemical constituents are mild and safe, even in large doses. Other herbs contain chemicals that act more strongly and may be toxic in large doses or when taken continuously. Drug interactions are possible with certain herbs when combined with certain pharmaceutical drugs. Some herbs are tonic in a small amount and toxic in larger dosages.

In 2002, a report to the American Academy of Pediatrics cautioned members to watch for signs of adverse effects to the cardiovascular system of children from certain herbal remedies that are often not revealed by their families. For example, **ephedra** causes increases in heart rate and blood pressure. Other examples of child and adolescent patients with heart complications from herbs given to them that their parents assumed would be harmless were given by the presenter. Another report said that even adult patients fail to inform their physicians about herbal products they are using, and that patients do not think of them as medicines. Yet many herbal products can interact with allopathic medicines and either cancel their effects or cause adverse effects. For example, **garlic**, ginseng, ginkgo, **feverfew**, **licorice**, and other common remedies have anticoagulant properties that can put patients as risk of bleeding during surgery.

Research & general acceptance

Western herbalism is experiencing a revival of popular and professional interest. The number of training schools and qualified herbal practitioners is growing to meet the demand. Western herbalism is incorporated into the medical practice of licensed naturopathic doctors, who receive special training in clinical herbalism. Folk herbalists, heir to the continuing oral traditions passed from generation to generation in many rural areas, as well as amateur self-taught herbalists, keep the practice of botanical medicine alive at the grassroots level. Traditional Western herbalism relies on traditional use and materia medica, folk wisdom, and recent clinical research and advances in the extraction processes. These advances provide increased quality control on the concentration and potency of the active ingredients. Western physicians, educated in allopathic medicine, typically receive no training in the use of herbs. These doctors rely on pharmaceutical drugs for their patients, and some cite the following reasons for continuing to do so: lack of standardized dosages, lack of quality control in the preparation of herbal medicinals, and the dearth of clinical research verifying the safety and effectiveness of many traditional herbal remedies.

Herbalism is widely practiced throughout Europe, particularly in England, France, Italy, and Germany, where phytomedicinals are available in prescription form and as over-the-counter remedies. In Germany, plant medicines are regulated by a special government body known as the Commission E. In the United States, however, despite increasing popularity, traditional herbalism is not integrated into the allopathic medical system. Phytomedicinals are sold as dietary supplements rather than being adequately researched and recognized as safe and effective drugs. The Dietary Supplement Health and Education Act of 1994 circumvented a U. S. Food and Drug Administration (FDA) effort to effectively remove botanicals from the marketplace and implement regulations restricting sale. Massive popular outcry against the proposed regulations on the sale of herbs and phytomedicinals resulted in this Congressional action. In 2000, U.S. President Bill Clinton, by executive order, created the White House Commission on Alternative Medicine in an effort to hold alternative medicine therapies "to the same standard of scientific rigor as more traditional health care interventions." That commission is charged with recommending federal guidelines and legislation regarding the use of alternative medical therapies in the twenty-first century.

Training & certification

In the United States, courses of study in Western herbalism are available in almost all 50 states. The study of traditional herbalism is part of the course curriculum in Naturopathic medical colleges that offer four-year degree programs leading to licensure as a Doctor of Naturopathy. The oldest of these institutions is the National College of **Naturopathic Medicine**, established in 1956. Western clinical herbalism is taught through a growing number of institutions and organizations offering training and certification through residential and apprenticeship programs, and by correspondence. Some programs are comprehensive, with curricula in physiology, clinical diagnosis and treatment, ethnobotany, pharmacognosy, phytotherapy, plant identification, ethical wildcrafting and cultivation, and preparation and application of herbal remedies. Other programs are brief, geared more to the amateur herbalist and gardener. The Southwest School of Botanical Medicine in Bisbee, Arizona, is one of the oldest herbal schools, established in 1978. No licensing body yet exists in the United States to regulate the practice of herbal medicine.

In the United States herbal remedies are sold as dietary supplements. They are not regulated as to content and efficacy, and few are prepared in standardized dosages. Many of the supplements commercially available base claims for efficacy on traditional use and anecdotal evidence that has not been duplicated by clinical studies. In Germany, Commission E evaluates the safety and efficacy of the 300 herbs and herb combinations sold in that country. No equivalent regulatory commission exists in the United States. Permits are required in some states for the wildcrafting of rare and endangered herbs, such as **goldenseal** and American ginseng, two commercially valuable herbs in high demand in the growing medical botanicals industry.

Resources

BOOKS

The Burton Goldberg Group. *Alternative Medicine, The Definitive Guide.* Fife, WA: Future Medicine Publishing, Inc., 1993.

> ## KEY TERMS
>
> **Phyto-, as in phytochemical, phytomedicinal, and phytotherapy**—Pertaining to a plant or plants.
>
> **Wildcrafting**—Gathering of herbs or other natural materials.

Kowalchik, Claire, and William H. Hylton, *Rodale's Illustrated Encyclopedia of Herbs.* Emmaus, PA: Rodale Press, 1987.
Lust, John. *The Herb Book.* New York: Bantam Books, 1974.
McIntyre, Anne. *The Medicinal Garden.* New York: Henry Holt and Company, Inc., 1997.
Murray, Michael T. *The Healing Power of Herbs,* 2nd ed. Rocklin, CA: Prima Publications, Inc., 1995.
Weiss, Gaea and Shandor Weiss. *Growing & Using The Healing Herbs.* New York: Wings Books, 1992.

PERIODICALS

Deneen, Sally, with Tracey, Rembert, "Uprooted, The Worldwide Plant Crisis Is Accelerating." *E Magazine* (July/August 1999) : 36-40.
Liebmann, Richard, N.D. "United Plant Savers—Planting the Future." *PanGaia* 22 (Winter 1999-2000) : 23- 26.
McNamara, Damian. "Alternative Therapies Can Cause Serious Problems (Cardiovascular Effects, Drug Interactions)." *Pediatric News* (February 2002) : 38.
McNamara, Damian. "Warn Patients About Bad Herbal Advice on Web." *Family Practice News* (January 1, 2002) : 8.
Torpy, Janet M. "Integrating Complementary Therapy Into Care." *JAMA, The Journal of the American Medical Association* (January 16, 2002) : 306.

ORGANIZATIONS

National Center for the Preservation of Medicinal Herbs. 3350 Beech Grove Road, Rutland, Ohio 45775. (740)742- 4401.
United Plant Savers. P.O. Box 98, East Barre, Vermont 05649. (802)479-9825. http://www.plantsavers.org.

OTHER

Hobbs, Christopher. "Specific and Tonic Immune Herbs: Exploring a Practical System of Western Herbalism." Health World. <http://www.healthy.net/asp/templates/article.asp?PageType=Article&ID=960>.
Oracle Tree New Age Mall. "Western Medical Astrology: A Brief History." <http://ww.oracletree.com/avalonphysics/wesmedas.html>.
Tyler, Varro E., Ph.D. *Herbs and Health Care in the Twenty-First Century.* <http://www.richters.com/newdisplay.cgi?page=OttoRichter/1995.html>.
Wicke, Roger, Ph.D. "A World History of Herbology and Herbalism: Oppressed Arts." Rocky Mountain Herbal Institute. <http://www.rmhiherbalorg/a/f.ahrl.hist.html>.

Clare Hanrahan
Teresa G. Odle

Herniated disk

Definition

Disk herniation is a breakdown of a fibrous cartilage material (annulus fibrosus) that makes up the intervertebral disk. The annulus fibrosus surrounds a soft gel-like substance in the center of the disk called the nucleus pulposus. Pressure from the vertebrae above and below may cause the nucleus pulposus to be forced against the sides of the annulus. The constant pressure of the nucleus against the sides of the annulus will cause the fibers of the annulus to break down. As the fibers of the annulus break down, the nucleus will push toward the outside of the annulus and cause the disk to bulge in the direction of the pressure. This condition most frequently occurs in the lumbar region and is also commonly called a herniated nucleus pulposus, prolapsed disk, ruptured disk, or a slipped disk.

Description

The spinal column is made up of 24 vertebrae that are joined together and permit forward and backward bending, side bending, and rotation of the spine. There are seven cervical (neck), twelve thoracic (chest region), and five lumbar (low back) vertebra. There are intervertebral disks between each of the 24 vertebrae as well as a disk between the lowest lumbar vertebrae and the large bone at the base of the spine called the sacrum.

Disk herniation most commonly affects the lumbar region. However, disk herniation can also occur in the cervical spine. The incidence of cervical disk herniation is most common between the fifth and sixth cervical vertebrae. The second most common area for cervical disk herniation occurs between the sixth and seventh cervical vertebrae. Disk herniation is uncommon in the thoracic region.

The peak age for occurrence of disk herniation is between 20 and 45 years of age. Studies have shown that males are more commonly affected than females in lumbar disk herniation by a 3:2 ratio. Long periods of sitting or a bent-forward work posture may lead to an increased incidence of disk herniation.

There are four classifications of disk pathology:

- A protrusion occurs when a disk bulges without rupturing the annulus fibrosus.

- A prolapse occurs when the nucleus pulposus pushes to the outermost fibers of the annulus fibrosus but does not break through them.

- An extrusion occurs when the outermost layer of the annulus fibrosus is torn and the material of the nucleus moves into the epidural space.

- A sequestration occurs when fragments from the annulus fibrosus or the nucleus pulposus have broken free and lie outside the confines of the disk.

Causes & symptoms

Any direct or, forceful in a vertical direction pressure on the disks can cause the disk to push its nucleus into the fibers of the annulus or into the intervertebral canal. A herniated disk may occur suddenly from lifting, twisting, or direct injury, but more often it will occur from constant compressive loads over time. There may be a single incident that causes symptoms to be felt, but very often the disk was already damaged and bulging prior to any one particular incident.

Depending on the location of the herniation, the herniated material can also press directly on nerve roots or on the spinal cord. Pressure on the nerve roots or spinal cord may cause a shock-like pain sensation down the arms if the herniation is in the cervical vertebrae or down the legs if the herniation is in the lumbar region.

In the lumbar region a herniation that presses on the nerve roots or the spinal cord may also cause weakness, numbness, or problems with bowels, bladder, or sexual function. It is unclear if a herniated disk causes pain by itself without pressing on neurological structures. It is likely that irritation of the disk or the adjacent nerve roots may cause muscle spasm and pain in the region of the disk pathology.

Diagnosis

Several radiographic tests are useful for confirming a diagnosis of disk herniation and locating the source of pain. X rays show structural changes of the lumbar spine. Myelography is a special x ray of the spine in which a dye or air is injected into the patient's spinal canal. The patient lies strapped to a table as the table tilts in various directions and spot x rays are taken. X rays showing a narrowed dye column in the intervertebral disk area indicate possible disk herniation.

Computed tomography scan (CT scans) exhibit the details of pathology necessary to obtain consistently good treatment results. Magnetic resonance imaging (MRI) analysis of the disks can accurately detect the early stages of disk **aging** and degeneration. Electromyograms (EMGs) measure the electrical activity of the muscle contractions and possibly show evidence of nerve damage.

A number of physical examination procedures may be used to determine if a herniated disk is pressing on a nerve root. While these tests may not identify the definitive presence of a herniated disk, they are very useful for

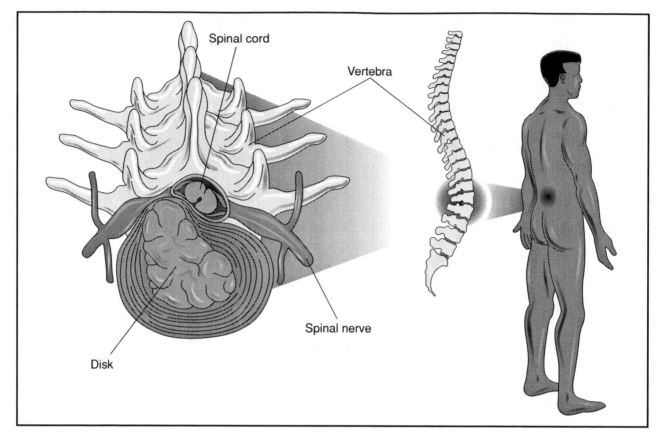

A herniated disk refers to the rupture of a ring of fibrocartilagenous material called the annulus fibrosus, which surrounds the intervertebral disk. When rupture occurs, pressure from the vertebrae above and below may force the disk's center portion, a gel-like substance, outward, placing additional pressure on the adjacent spinal nerve and causing pain and damage to the nerve. *(Illustration by Electronic Illustrators Group. The Gale Group.)*

indicating if there is pressure on a nerve root from some structure such as a herniated disk. The straight leg raise test may be used to identify pressure on nerve roots in the lumbar region while the Spurling's test (involving neck motion) may be used to identify compression of nerve roots in the cervical region. Compression of nerve roots in the cervical, thoracic, or lumbar regions may be apparent with the slump test.

Treatment

It is unclear if herniated disks cause pain themselves, or if they must press on a nerve root to cause pain. Pain may also occur with herniated disks as a result of mechanical or neurological irritation of surrounding structures such as muscles, tendons, ligaments, or joint capsules. Therefore, many treatment strategies will be primarily focused on managing symptoms that occur in conjunction with a herniated disk. Unless a serious neurological problem exists, most symptoms of a herniated disk will resolve on their own. Yet, the interventions listed below may greatly speed the time required to resolve symptoms associated with a herniated disk.

Chiropractic manipulations are often used to treat herniated disks. There is often significant joint restriction that accompanies a herniated disk and the manipulative therapy is effective at helping to mobilize movement restrictions in the spine. Mobilizing the spine will help the patient get back to moderate activity levels sooner. The earlier an individual can return to moderate activity levels, the quicker they can expect a resolution of their symptoms. Chiropractic manipulations are generally done with a greater frequency when a condition is in an acute stage. The frequency of treatments will be reduced as the condition improves.

Osteopathic therapy, considered by some to be an alternative treatment, may use manipulations or manual therapy techniques very similar to those of chiropractors. However, osteopathic physicians often employ more manual therapy techniques that focus on the role of the muscles and other soft tissues in producing pain sensations with herniated disks. Osteopathic physicians may also recommend use of the same medications prescribed by allopathic physicians. Some osteopaths also perform surgery for herniated disks.

Acupuncture involves the use of fine needles inserted along the pathway of the pain to move energy through the body and relieve the pain. Neurological irritation is considered to be a frequent source of pain with a herniated disk. Many believe acupuncture is particularly effective for pain management and addressing this neurological irritation. Acupuncture can also help break the cycle of pain and muscle spasm that often accompanies a herniated disk.

Massage therapists focus on muscular reactions to the herniated disk. Neurological irritation that comes with a herniated disk will often cause excessive muscle spasms in the lower back muscles. These spasms will perpetuate dysfunctional movements in the joints of the spine and may exaggerate compressive forces on the intervertebral disk. By relaxing the muscles, massage therapists will attempt to manage the symptoms of disk herniation until proper movement can be restored. Proper movement and avoidance of aggravating postures, like sitting for long periods, will often be a great help in completely resolving the symptoms.

Allopathic treatment

Unless serious neurologic symptoms occur, herniated disks can initially be treated with pain medication. Pain medications, including anti-inflammatories, muscle relaxants, or in severe cases, narcotics, may be used if needed. Bed rest is sometimes prescribed. However, bed rest is frequently discouraged as a treatment for herniated disks unless movement is severely painful. It has become apparent that prolonged periods of bed rest may aggravate symptoms, slow down the healing time, and cause other complications.

Epidural steroid injections have been used to decrease pain by injecting an anti-inflammatory drug, usually a corticosteroid, around the nerve root to reduce inflammation and **edema** (swelling). This treatment partly relieves the pressure on the nerve root as well as resolves the inflammation.

Physical therapists are skilled in treating acute back pain caused by disk herniation. The physical therapist can provide noninvasive therapies, such as ultrasound or **diathermy,** to project heat deep into the tissues of the back or administer manual therapy, if mobility of the spine is impaired. They may help improve posture and develop an **exercise** program for recovery and long-term protection. Traction can be used to decrease pressure on the disk. A lumbar support can be helpful for a herniated disk at this level as a temporary measure to reduce pain and improve posture.

Surgery may be used for conditions that do not improve with conservative treatment. There are several surgical approaches to treating a herniated disk. A number of surgical procedures may be used to remove a portion of the intervertebral disk that may be pressing on a nerve root. When a portion of the disk is removed through a surgical procedure it is called a discectomy. Sometimes a spinal fusion will be performed after disk material has been removed. In this process a portion of bone is taken from the pelvis and placed between the bodies of the vertebrae. A spinal fusion will limit motion at that vertebral segment, but may be helpful in the event that significant disk material has been removed.

Chemonucleolysis is an alternative to surgical removal of the disk. Chymopapain, a purified enzyme derived from the papaya plant, is injected into the disk space to reduce the size of the herniated disks. The reduction in size of the disk relieves pressure on the nerve root. In 2002, Tokyo doctors produced evidence that a growth factor called vascular endothelial growth factor (VEGF) may speed up the process of injured disk resorption.

In September 2002, a noted orthopedic and spine authority named John Engelhardt became the first American to receive an artificial disk replacement (using the Bristol disk) in an operation in Switzerland. The artificial disk technology was still in clinical trials in the United States and was not expected to be approved until about 2005 or later.

Expected results

Only a small percentage of patients with unrelenting neurological involvement, leading to chronic pain of the spine, need to have a surgical procedure performed. This fact strongly suggests that many patients with herniated disks respond well to conservative treatment. Alternative therapies can play a significant role in managing the pain and discomfort for the majority of patients with a herniated disk. In fact, magnetic resonance imaging (MRI) studies of the lumbar spine have indicated that many people without any back pain at all have herniated disks. This finding means it is unclear what role the herniated disk plays in many back pain cases. For many of these patients, proper symptom management of pain and improvement in joint motion and mobility through manual therapies will be enough to fully resolve their symptoms. For those patients who do require surgery, options are available for newer and less invasive procedures that will allow a quicker healing time.

Prevention

Proper exercises to strengthen the lower back and abdominal muscles are key in preventing excess **stress** and compressive forces on lumbar disks. Good posture will help prevent problems on cervical, thoracic, and lumbar disks. A good flexibility program is critical for

Jensen, M., et al. "Magnetic Resonance Imaging of the Lumbar Spine in People Without Back Pain." *New England Journal of Medicine* 331 (July 14, 1994): 69.

Whitney Lowe
Teresa G. Odle

Herpes genitalis *see* **Genital herpes**

Herpes simplex *see* **Canker sores; Cold sores**

Herpes zoster *see* **Shingles**

KEY TERMS

Annulus fibrosus—The outer portion of the intervertebral disk made primarily of fibrocartilage rings.

Epidural space—The space immediately surrounding the outer most membrane of the spinal cord.

Excision—The process of cutting out, removing, or amputating.

Fibrocartilage—Cartilage that consists of dense fibers.

Nucleus pulposus—The center portion of the intervertebral disk that is made up of a gelatinous substance.

prevention of muscle spasm that can cause an increase in compressive forces on disks at any level. Proper lifting of heavy objects is important for all muscles and levels of the individual disks. Good posture in sitting, standing, and lying down is helpful for the spine. Losing weight, if needed, can prevent weakness and unnecessary stress on the disks caused by **obesity**.

Such alternative treatments as chiropractic, **massage therapy**, or acupuncture may play a very important role in prevention of herniated disk problems. Regular use of these approaches may help maintain proper muscular tone and reduce the cumulative effects of postural strain that may lead to the development of disk problems.

Resources

BOOKS

Hammer, W. *Functional Soft Tissue Examination and Treatment by Manual Methods*, 2nd ed. Gaithersburg, MD: Aspen, 1999.

Kessler, R.M. *Management of Common Musculoskeletal Disorders: Physical Therapy Principles and Methods*. Philadelphia: J.B. Lippincott Co., 1990.

Liebenson, C. *Rehabilitation of the Spine*. Baltimore: Williams & Wilkins., 1996.

Maciocia, G. *Foundations of Chinese Medicine*. London: Churchill Livingstone, 1989.

Magee, D.J. *Orthopedic Physical Assessment*. Philadelphia: W.B. Saunders,1992.

Waddell, G. *The Back Pain Revolution*. London: Churchill Livingstone, 1998.

PERIODICALS

"Factor Could Speed Absorption of Herniated Disks." *Pain & Central Nervous System Week* (July 29, 2002): 2.

"Industry Authority Becomes First American to Receive Artificial Cervical Disk." *Medical Devices & Surgical Technology Week* (September 22, 2002): 3.

Hiatal hernia

Definition

A hiatal hernia is an abnormal protrusion of the stomach up through the diaphragm and into the chest cavity.

Description

A hiatal or diaphragmatic hernia is different from abdominal hernias in that it is not visible on the outside of the body. With a hiatal hernia, the stomach bulges upward through the esophageal hiatus (the hole through which the esophagus passes) of the diaphragm. This type of hernia occurs more often in women than in men, and it is treated differently from other types of hernias.

Causes & symptoms

A hiatal hernia may be caused by **obesity**, **pregnancy**, **aging**, or previous surgery. About 50% of all people with hiatal hernias do not have any symptoms. For those who do have symptoms, they include **heartburn**, usually 30–60 minutes after a meal, or mid-chest **pain** due to gastric acid from the stomach being pushed up into the esophagus. The pain and heartburn are usually worse when lying down. Frequent belching and feelings of abdominal fullness may also occur.

Diagnosis

The diagnosis for a hiatal hernia is based on a person's reported symptoms. The doctor may then order tests to confirm the diagnosis. If a barium swallow is ordered, the person drinks a chalky white barium solution, which will help any protrusion through the diaphragm to show up on the x ray that follows. Currently, a diagnosis of hiatal hernia is more frequently made by endoscopy. This procedure is done by a gastroenterologist (a specialist in

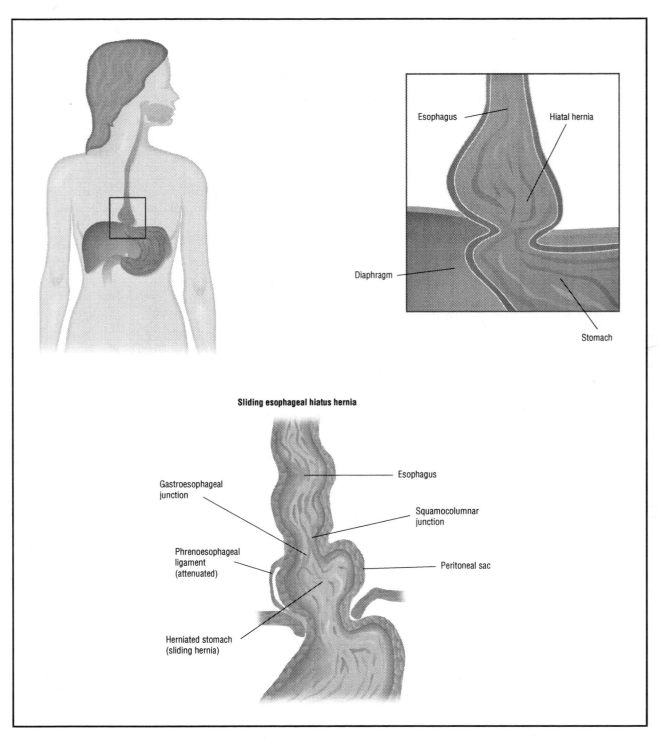

Esophagus

Hiatal hernia

Diaphragm

Stomach

Sliding esophageal hiatus hernia

Esophagus

Gastroesophageal
junction

Squamocolumnar
junction

Phrenoesophageal
ligament
(attenuated)

Peritoneal sac

Herniated stomach
(sliding hernia)

(Illustration by GGS Information Services, Inc. The Gale Group.)

digestive diseases). During an endoscopy the person is given an intravenous sedative and a narrow tube is inserted through the mouth and esophagus, into the stomach where the doctor can visualize the hernia. The procedure takes about 30 minutes and may cause some discomfort, but usually no pain. It is done on an outpatient basis.

Treatment

Dietary and lifestyle adjustments to control a hiatal hernia include:

• Avoiding reclining after meals.

• Avoiding spicy foods, acidic foods, alcohol, and tobacco.

- Eating small frequent bland meals to keep pressure on the esophageal sphincter.

- Eating a high-fiber diet.

- Raising the head of the bed several inches with blocks to help both the quality and quantity of sleep.

Visceral manipulation done by a trained therapist can help return the stomach to its proper positioning. **Deglycyrrhizinated licorice** (DGL), helps balance stomach acid by improving the protective substances that line the stomach and intestines and by improving blood supply to these tissues. DGL does not interrupt the normal function of stomach acid.

Allopathic treatment

There are several types of medications that help to manage the symptoms of a hiatal hernia. Antacids are used to neutralize gastric acid and decrease heartburn. Drugs that reduce the amount of acid produced in the stomach (H2 blockers) are also used. This class of drugs includes famotidine (sold under the name Pepcid), cimetidine (Tagamet), and ranitidine (Zantac). Omeprazole (Prilosec) is not an H2 blocker, but is another drug that suppresses gastric acid secretion and is used for hiatal hernias. Another option may be metoclopramide (Reglan), a drug that increases the tone of the muscle around the esophagus and causes the stomach to empty more quickly.

Expected results

Hiatal hernias are treated successfully with medication and diet modifications 85% of the time. The prognosis remains excellent even if surgery is required in adults who are otherwise in good health.

Prevention

Some hernias can be prevented by maintaining a reasonable weight, avoiding heavy lifting and **constipation**, and following a moderate **exercise** program to maintain good abdominal muscle tone.

Resources

BOOKS

Bare, Brenda G. and Suzanne C. Smeltzer. *Brunner and Suddarth's Textbook of Medical-Surgical Nursing.* 8th edition. Philadelphia: Lippincott-Raven Publishers, 1996.

Polaske, Arlene L. and Suzanne E. Tatro. *Luckmann's Core Principles and Practice of Medical Surgical Nursing.* Philadelphia: W.B. Saunders Company, 1996.

PERIODICALS

Kingsley, A.N., I.L. Lichtenstein, and W.K. Sieber. "Common Hernias In Primary Care." *Patient Care.* (April 1990): 98-119.

Paula Ford-Martin

KEY TERMS

Endoscopy—A diagnostic procedure in which a tube is inserted through the mouth into the esophagus and stomach. It is used to visualize various digestive disorders, including hiatal hernias.

Herniorrhaphy—Surgical repair of a hernia.

Incarcerated hernia—A hernia that cannot be reduced, or pushed back into place, inside the intestinal wall.

Reducible hernia—A hernia that can be gently pushed back into place or that disappears when the person lies down.

Strangulated hernia—A hernia that is so tightly incarcerated outside the abdominal wall that the intestine is blocked and the blood supply to that part of the intestine is cut off.

Hibiscus

Description

Hibiscus is the name given to more than 250 species of herbs, shrubs, and trees of the mallow or Malvaceae family. The most commonly used species of hibiscus for medicinal purposes are *Hibiscus sabdariffa*, commonly known as the roselle; *Hibiscus rosa-sinensis*, also called China rose and common hibiscus; and *Hibiscus syriacus*, known as the Rose of Sharon. These three shrubs are native to tropical climates, but are now grown around the world. Hibiscus is renowned for its beauty as well as its medicinal uses, and gardeners cultivate the plant for its showy flowers.

General use

Hibiscus is used for a variety of ailments partly because there are so many species. Roselle lowers fevers and high blood pressure, increases urination, relieves coughs, and has been found to have antibacterial properties. All parts of the plant are used, from the seeds to the roots. Common hibiscus is used mainly for respiratory problems, but is also widely used for skin disorders or to treat fevers. Rose of Sharon is used externally as an emollient, but is also taken internally for gastrointestinal disorders.

Fever

As a natural febrifuge, roselle contains citric acid, which is a natural coolant. In Pakistan and Nepal, it is the flowers that are used as a treatment for **fever**. Common hibiscus has been found to be particularly useful for children's fevers.

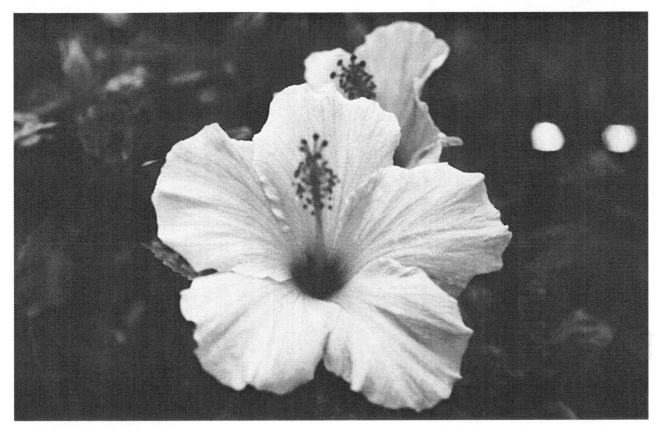

Hibiscus flower. *(Photo by Kelly Quinn. Reproduced by permission.)*

Respiratory disorders

Common hibiscus is used to treat coughs by placing extracts from the plant in the patient's bath or in **water** used for steam inhalations. Hibiscus is often combined with other herbs to make a **cough** syrup. Hibiscus is used widely in Cuba, where the tropical climate contributes to respiratory illnesses, and where hibiscus is readily found.

Hypertensive conditions

Roselle and rose of Sharon contain hypotensive compounds that lower the blood pressure. Roselle's ability to lower blood pressure may be due to its diuretic and laxative effects. The plant contains ascorbic and glycolic acids, which increase urination.

Skin conditions

Hibiscus is a natural emollient, used for softening or healing the skin. The leaves and flowers of the roselle are used all around the world for their emollient qualities. When the leaves are heated, they can be placed on cracked feet or on **boils** and ulcers to promote healing. Since the herb is a cooling herb, when applied externally it cools the surface of the skin by increasing blood flow to the epidermis and dilating the pores of the skin. A lotion made from a decoction of hibiscus leaves can be used to soothe **hemorrhoids**, **sunburn**, open sores, and **wounds**.

Other conditions

Hibiscus has been credited with a wide range of healing properties. In Colombia, the plant is used to treat **hair loss** and scurvy; in Samoa, it is commonly given to women who are suffering from menstrual cramps or who are in **childbirth**, as the leaves ease labor pains. In the Cook Islands and the Philippines, the flowers are used to induce abortions. In a 1962 study, hibiscus was confirmed to be hypotensive, as well as antispasmodic, anthelminthic, and antibacterial. In subsequent studies, the plant was found to effectively work against such diseases as ascariasis and **tuberculosis**. Studies in France, Malaysia, and Egypt have found that the plant has anticarcinogenic effects.

Preparations

A decoction of hibiscus can be made by pouring 1 cup of boiling water over 2 tsp of dried blossoms or 1 tsp of crumbled blossom. Steep for 10 minutes. In addition, many commercial herbal teas contain hibiscus.

KEY TERMS

Abortifacient—A substance that induces abortions.

Anthelminthic—A medication that destroys or expels parasitic worms from the digestive tract.

Antispasmodic—A medication that prevents or relieves involuntary muscular cramps.

Emollient—A substance that softens and smoothes the skin.

Febrifuge—A substance or medication that lowers or dispels fevers.

Precautions

Since there are over 250 species of hibiscus, it is essential to identify the species of the herb before taking it. Since some species of hibiscus are used as abortifacients, the plant should not be used by women who are pregnant or nursing.

Side effects

Some drinks made from roselle can have alcoholic effects. The plant can also be mildly hallucinogenic.

Interactions

There are no known interactions between hibiscus and standard pharmaceutical preparations. Because it is a tart plant, however, it may not mix harmoniously with other tannic herbs. Mint leaves or rose hips are good to blend with hibiscus.

Resources

BOOKS

Chevallier, Andrew. *Encyclopedia of Medicinal Plants*. London: Dorling Kindersley Publishers, 1996.

Keys, John D. *Chinese Herbs*. New York: Charles E. Tuttle Co., 1976.

Katherine Y. Kim

Hiccups

Definition

Hiccups are the result of an involuntary, spasmodic contraction of the diaphragm followed by the closing of the throat.

Description

Virtually everyone experiences hiccups, but they rarely last long or require a doctor's care. Occasionally, a bout of hiccups will last longer than two days, earning it the name "persistent hiccups." Very few people will experience intractable hiccups, in which hiccups last longer than one month.

A hiccup involves the coordinated action of the diaphragm and the muscles that close off the windpipe (trachea). The diaphragm is a dome-shaped muscle separating the chest and abdomen. It is normally responsible for expanding the chest cavity for inhalation. Sensation from the diaphragm travels to the spinal cord through the phrenic nerve and the vagus nerve, which pass through the chest cavity and the neck. Within the spinal cord, nerve fibers from the brain monitor sensory information and adjust the outgoing messages that control contraction. These messages travel along the phrenic nerve.

Irritation of any of the nerves involved in this loop can cause the diaphragm to undergo an involuntary contraction, or spasm, pulling air into the lungs. When this spasm occurs, it triggers a reflex in the throat muscles. Less than a tenth of a second afterward, the trachea is closed off, making the characteristic "hic" sound.

Causes & symptoms

Hiccups can be caused by disorders of the central nervous system, by injury or irritation to the phrenic and vagus nerves, and by toxic or metabolic disorders affecting the central or peripheral nervous systems. They may be of unknown cause or may be a symptom of psychological **stress**. Hiccups often occur after drinking carbonated beverages or alcohol. They may also follow overeating or rapid temperature changes. Persistent or intractable hiccups may be caused by any condition that irritates or damages the relevant nerves, including:

- overstretching of the neck
- laryngitis
- heartburn (gastroesophageal reflux)
- irritation of the eardrum (which is innervated by the vagus nerve)
- general anesthesia
- surgery
- bloating
- tumor
- infection
- diabetes

Diagnosis

Hiccups are diagnosed by observation and by hearing the characteristic sound. Diagnosing the cause of intractable hiccups may require imaging studies, blood tests, pH monitoring in the esophagus, and other tests.

Treatment

Most cases of hiccups will disappear on their own. Home remedies, which interrupt or override the spasmodic nerve circuitry, are often effective. Such remedies include:

• Holding one's breath for as long as possible.

• Breathing into a paper bag.

• Swallowing a spoonful of sugar or peanut butter.

• Bending forward from the waist and drinking water from the wrong side of a glass.

Acupressure techniques can also be helpful in eliminating hiccups. Acupressure is a Chinese medicine treatment that involves placing pressure on different points of the body, called acupoints. It is based on the premise that good health is based on a harmony of energy flow, or *qi*, throughout the body. By placing pressure on acupoints, qi is balanced and harmony—and health—is restored to the patient.

To treat hiccups through acupressure, rest the heels of the palms on both cheekbones while placing hands over the eyes. Massage the temples by pulling the thumbs in towards the palm. After massaging, remove the hands from the eyes and lightly press the tip of the nose with a fingertip.

Allopathic treatment

Treating any underlying disorder will usually cure the associated hiccups. Chlorpromazine (Thorazine) relieves intractable hiccups in 80% of cases. Metoclopramide (Reglan), carbamazepam, valproic acid (Depakene), and phenobarbital are also used. As a last resort, surgery to block the phrenic nerve may be performed, although it may lead to significant impairment of respiration.

Expected results

Most cases of hiccups last no longer than several hours, with or without treatment.

Prevention

Some cases of hiccups can be avoided by drinking in moderation, avoiding very hot or very cold food, and avoiding cold showers. When carbonated beverages are

drunk through a straw, more **gas** is delivered to the stomach than when they are sipped from a container; therefore, avoid using straws.

Resources

BOOK

Hurst, J. Willis, ed. *Medicine for the Practicing Physician.* 4th ed. Stamford, Conn.: Appleton & Lange, 1996.

Paula Ford-Martin

High blood pressure *see* **Hypertension**
High cholesterol *see* **Cholesterol**

High-fiber diet

Definition

Fiber is the material that gives plants texture and support. Dietary fiber is found in many plant foods, including fruits, vegetables, beans, nuts, and whole grains. Although fiber is primarily made up of carbohydrates, it does not have a lot of calories and usually is not broken down by the body for energy. Fiber is sometimes called roughage.

There are two types of fiber: soluble and insoluble. Insoluble fiber, as the name implies, does not dissolve in **water** because it contains high amounts of cellulose. Insoluble fiber is found in grain brans, fruit pulp, and vegetable peels or skins. Soluble fiber is the type of fiber that dissolves in water. It can be found in a variety of such fruits, grains, and vegetables as apples, oatmeal and oat bran, rye flour and dried beans.

Although the two types of fiber share some common characteristics such as being partially digested in the stomach and intestines and being low in calories, each type has its own specific health benefits. Insoluble fiber speeds up the movement of foods through the digestive system and adds bulk to the stools; it helps to treat **constipation** or **diarrhea** and prevents colon **cancer**. On the other hand, only soluble fiber can lower blood **cholesterol** levels. This type of fiber works by attaching itself to the cholesterol so that it can be eliminated from the body. This process prevents cholesterol from recirculating and being reabsorbed into the bloodstream.

Origins

High-fiber diet therapy is actually a return to nature and the plant-based **diets** used by our ancestors since the beginning of time. In fact, our ancestors consumed large quantities of fiber-containing foods such as fruits, vegetables and whole grain products every day. As technology advanced, however, people began to turn away from these unprocessed healthful foods and began eating more highly processed and fat-laden foods. As a result, the incidence of coronary **heart disease**, diabetes, and cancers has steadily risen. Naturopathic physicians, who practice natural healing methods, have long advocated high-fiber diets as a major preventive and therapeutic treatment for these and other diseases. Extensive medical research has now confirmed that a high-fiber diet prevents or treats a wide variety of diseases ranging from constipation to heart disease and cancer.

Benefits

A high-fiber diet helps prevent or treat the following health conditions:

• High blood cholesterol levels. Fiber effectively lowers blood cholesterol levels. It appears that soluble fiber binds to the cholesterol molecule and moves it through the digestive tract so that it can be excreted from the body. This mechanism prevents cholesterol from being reabsorbed into the bloodstream. In 2003, research confirmed the long-term effects of high-fiber diets on lowering bad cholesterol in people with Type II diabetes.

• Constipation. A high-fiber diet is a useful non-drug treatment for constipation. Fiber in the diet adds more bulk to the stools, making them softer. Fiber also shortens the length of time that foods remain in the digestive tract. It is important, however, for people increasing their fiber intake to drink more water as well, in order to get the benefit of using dietary fiber to relieve constipation.

• **Hemorrhoids**. Fiber in the diet adds more bulk and softens the stool, thus reducing the **pain** and bleeding associated with hemorrhoids.

• Diabetes. A common problem for diabetics is the rapid rise of insulin levels following meals. Soluble fiber in the diet delays the emptying of the stomach contents into the intestines. This delay helps to slow the rise of blood sugar levels following a meal and thus gives diabetics greater control over their condition.

• Obesity. Dietary fiber makes a person feel full more rapidly. It can thus help a person lose weight by making the appetite easier to control.

• Colon and **colorectal cancer**. Insoluble fiber in the diet speeds up the movement of the stools through the gastrointestinal tract. The faster that food and its byproducts travel through the digestive tract, the less time there is for potential cancer-causing substances to work on the food. Diets that are high in insoluble fiber help to prevent the accumulation of toxic substances that cause cancer of the colon.

• **Breast cancer**. A high dietary consumption of fats is associated with an increased risk of breast cancer. Because fiber reduces fat absorption in the digestive tract, it may prevent breast cancer. In 2003, a study confirmed these findings and showed that women who consumed more fiber and **vitamin E** also had a lower risk of developing benign breast disease, a condition that can lead to breast cancer.

• **Prostate cancer**. Though research is still relatively new, Dr. **Dean Ornish** presented new data in April 2002 in a study that showed how a high-fiber vegan diet could slow or even stop prostate cancer for men in early stages of the disease. Men who submitted to an extremely low-fat vegan diet consisting of fruits, vegetables, whole grains, beans and soy products instead of dairy, and who gave up alcohol and agreed to **exercise** three hours a week, relax and meditate one hour a day showed improvements in markers for prostate cancer indicators. Patients should not try this regimen unless they first discuss it with their doctors. In addition, it should complement other physician–ordered treatments.

Description

The American Dietetic Association recommends eating 25–35 g of fiber daily. A person can meet this fiber requirement by consuming two to three servings of fruits and three to five servings of vegetables every day. To increase fiber intake, a person should eat more of the following high-fiber foods: whole grains, beans, fruits (preferably with skins on), roots and leafy vegetables, broccoli or carrots. As an added bonus, he or she will also receive other health benefits provided by the vitamins, minerals, **antioxidants** and cancer-fighting phytochemicals in these foods.

Preparations

For the greatest benefit to health, people should have both soluble and insoluble fiber in their diet, preferably in a 50:50 ratio. The following foods are good sources of insoluble fiber:

- wheat bran
- whole wheat products
- cereals made from bran or shredded wheat
- crunchy vegetables
- barley
- grains
- whole-wheat pasta
- rye flour

Good sources of soluble fiber include:

- oats
- oat bran
- oatmeal
- apples
- citrus fruits
- strawberries
- dried beans
- barley
- rye flour
- potatoes
- raw cabbage
- pasta

Precautions

High-fiber therapy must be part of a balanced diet that includes adequate water intake and also provides the proper amounts of essential vitamins and minerals, including **calcium**, **iron** and **zinc**.

Side effects

Some side effects such as loose bowel movements, excessive **gas**, or occasional stomach pain have been reported from high-fiber diets. However, a 2002 report told of a study that followed more than 1,000 women on varying amounts of fiber intake. Those with higher dietary fiber consumption did not report expected symptoms of bloating, gas and stomach upset, so most people can enjoy the benefits of fiber with minimal side effects.

Research & general acceptance

As a result of the large volume of scientific evidence supporting the use of fiber in disease prevention and

> ### KEY TERMS
>
> **Cellulose**—The primary substance composing the cell walls or fibers of all plant tissues.
>
> **Hemorrhoid**—A varicose vein in the area around the anus. Hemorrhoids sometimes cause pain and bleeding.
>
> **Naturopathy**—A school of alternative medicine that focuses on natural healing. Therapies provided by practitioners of naturopathy often include diet, exercise, supplement and hydrotherapy and may also include osteopathic and chiropractic treatments.
>
> **Roughage**—Another name for dietary fiber.

treatment, high-fiber diet treatments have been accepted and advocated by practitioners of alternative and conventional medicine alike. High-fiber diets have been endorsed by the American Heart Association, the American Dietetic Association, the National Cancer Institute, the National Research Council, and the United States Department of Health and Human Services.

Resources

BOOKS

Murray, Michael, and Joseph Pizzorno. *Encyclopedia of Natural Medicine,* revised 2nd edition. Rocklin, CA: Prima Health, 1998.

Winick, Myron. *The Fiber Prescription.* New York: Fawcett Columbine, 1992.

PERIODICALS

"Fight Prostate Cancer with High Fiber Vegan Diet." *Natural Life* (July-August 2002): 8.

"High-fiber Diet Increases Triglycerides in Type 2 Diabetics." *Diabetes Week* (March 24, 2003): 17.

Mangels, Reed. "High Fiber Diet without the Worry of Discomfort." *Vegetarian Journal* (July-August 2002): 20–21.

Sullivan, Michele G. "More Fiber, Less Fat may Reduce Breast Cancer Risk." *Family Practice News* (January 15, 2003): 30.

ORGANIZATIONS

American Association of Naturopathic Physicians. P.O. Box 20386. Seattle, WA 98102. (206) 323-7610.

Mai Tran
Teresa G. Odle

High-protein diet *see* **Atkins diet**

High sensitivity C-reactive protein test

Definition

The high sensitivity C-reactive protein (hsCRP) test is a blood assay used to estimate an individual's risk for **heart disease** and **stroke**. The test also measures the presence of inflammation or infection.

Origins

In the late twentieth century, the primary methods of measuring a person's risk of heart disease included traditional factors such as age, family history of heart disease or stroke, past heart disease, **smoking**, **obesity**, and tests that measured lipids in the bloodstream, including low-density lipoprotein (LDL). Low-density lipoproteins ("bad" **cholesterol**) were previously considered the gold standard in risk factor prediction.

In the 1990s and early twenty-first century, several new tests came into widespread use. These tests are considered better predictors of heart disease risk. They include blood tests to measure the levels of homocysteine, lipoprotein(a), fibrinogen, and highly sensitive C-reactive protein. They are called emerging or nontraditional risk factors.

Benefits

Knowing one's highly sensitive C-reactive protein levels can help a person manage and lower his or her risk for heart disease. Factors that lower highly sensitive CRP levels include weight loss, regular **exercise**, a healthy diet, and smoking cessation. Medicines may also be needed. Medications include a class of drugs called statins, with brand names such as Lipitor, Zocor, Crestor, and Pravachol. Other interventions may include Zetia, a cholesterol absorption inhibitor, and a class of drugs called thiazoladinediones, such as the diabetes brand-name medications Avandia and Actos.

According to the American Heart Association, the three risk levels associated with high sensitivity CRP levels are:

• Low risk: under 1 milligram per liter of blood.

• Average risk: 1 to 3 milligrams per liter of blood.

• High risk: More than 3 milligrams per liter of blood.

Description

C-reactive protein is produced by the liver and is not normally found in the blood in high amounts. It is rapidly produced following an injury, bacterial or fungal infection, or inflammation. It disappears quickly once the injury, illness, or inflammation heals or resolves. High CRP levels following surgery or an injury are a good indication that an infection is present. Until early in this century, the blood test used to detect CRP levels could only measure them down to 3 milligrams per liter of blood or higher. Improvements in technology have permitted more precise measurements of CRP levels ranging from less than 0.3 milligrams to 3 milligrams per liter of blood. The more precise measurement is called the high sensitivity C-reactive protein (hsCRP) test.

While levels under 3 milligrams per liter of blood do not necessarily indicate the presence of infection, they do indicate the presence of an inflammatory reaction. Researchers found that these lower amounts of CRP in the body are extremely useful in predicting coronary heart disease (CHD). However, since CRP levels vary on different days, at least two separate measurements are needed to adequately determine a person's CHD risk level.

To take the high sensitivity CRP test, a healthcare worker draws blood from a vein, into a tube. In the laboratory, the tube of blood spins at high speed within a machine called a centrifuge. The blood cells sink to the bottom and the liquid stays on the top. This straw-colored liquid on the top is the plasma. To measure the high sensitivity CRP, a person's plasma is combined with other substances. From the resulting reaction, the amount of CRP in the plasma is determined.

A study released in 2003 by the College of American Pathologists found varying outcomes when it compared results from five different methods in identifying hsCRP. A 2001 study by several university medical departments found that six out of nine hsCRP testing methods did not produce results as accurate as the manufacturers claimed. In 2003 the Centers for Disease Control and Prevention announced that it would attempt to address these issues.

Preparations

Unlike some blood tests that require **fasting**, the high sensitivity C-reactive protein test can be done either before or after eating. No other preparations are needed.

Each high sensitivity CRP test requires a 5-milliliter blood sample. A healthcare worker usually ties a tight band (tourniquet) on the person's upper arm. The blood is drawn from a vein in the arm, usually at the inside of the elbow or on the back of the hand. The needle insertion site is cleaned with antiseptic. A small needle is inserted through the skin and into the vein, allowing the blood sample to flow into a collection tube or syringe. Once the blood is collected, the needle is removed from the puncture site. Collecting the blood sample takes several minutes or less.

Precautions

The primary risk to the patient is a mild stinging or burning sensation during the drawing of blood, with minor swelling or bruising afterward. Some patients may feel faint or lightheaded when blood is drawn.

Side effects

There are generally no side effects associated with the test. Any weakness, fainting, sweating, or other unusual reaction should be immediately reported.

Research & general acceptance

Several large-scale scientific studies have shown that high sensitivity C-reactive protein levels are a strong predictor of future heart attacks and strokes among apparently healthy men and women. Research has also shown that hsCRP test will play an important role in preventing heart disease, according to an article in the March 2001 issue of *Circulation*. The Centers for Disease Control and Prevention, and the American Heart Association, recommend limited use of hsCRP testing for assessing heart disease risk. The two groups recommend the test only when a physician is undecided about a course of treatment for a patient who is considered at intermediate risk for CHD. According to an article in the February 2003 issue of the *Harvard Health Letter*, a growing number of physicians believe everyone should be tested, and this test may eventually supplant cholesterol testing as a predictor of CHD.

Training & certification

Nurses are usually the health care professionals that administer high sensitivity CRP tests. Nurses can also help educate patients regarding the role that a proper diet and regular exercise can play in reducing the risk of CHD. However, only a physician can recommend specific treatment and prescribe needed medication.

Resources

BOOKS

Deron, Scott J. *C-Reactive Protein: Everything You Need to Know About it and Why It's More Important Than Cholesterol to Your Health*. New York, NY: McGraw-Hill, 2003.

Hirsch, Anita. *Good Cholesterol, Bad Chloresterol: An Indispensable Guide to the Facts About Cholesterol* New York, NY: Marlowe and Co., 2002.

Myers, Robert. *Heart Disease: Everything You Need to Know (Your Personal Health)*. Richmond Hill, ON: 2004.

KEY TERMS

Anticoagulant—Medication that prevents blood clotting.

C-reactive protein—A protein produced in the liver that is not normally found in the blood in high amounts. It is elevated when infection or inflammation are present. A test that measures this substance in the bloodstream serves as a predictor of heart disease or stroke.

Centrifuge—A machine that rotates rapidly and uses centrifugal force to separate substances of different densities.

Cholesterol—A compound found in animal tissue and blood, of which high levels in the blood are linked to clogged arteries, heart disease, and gallstones.

Cholesterol absorption inhibitor—A substance that decreases the absorption of cholesterol in the intestines.

Diabetes—A group of metabolic disorders in which the body produces insufficient insulin or is resistant to the insulin it does produce, causing glucose levels to rise in the blood.

Fasting—Avoiding food for a period of time.

Fibrinogen—A protein that is important in blood clotting.

Homocysteine—An amino acid derived from protein in food that can build up in the blood and contribute to the development of heart disease.

Lipids—Organic compounds that are greasy, insoluble in water, but soluble in alcohol. Fats, waxes, and oils are examples of lipids.

Lipoprotein(a)—A type of bad cholesterol that increases the risk of heart attack or stroke.

Low-density lipoprotein—LDL, the so-called bad cholesterol.

Plasma—A clear yellowish fluid that is a component of blood.

Statins—A class of drugs used primarily, but not exclusively, to treat high cholesterol.

Thiazoladinediones—A class of drugs typically used to treat diabetes and insulin resistance.

Rosenfeld, Isadore. *Dr. Isadore Rosenfeld's Breakthrough Health 2004: 167 Up-to-the-Minute Medical Discoveries, Treatments, and Cures that Can Save Your Life, From America's Most Trusted Doctor!* Emmaus, PA: Rodale, 2004.

PERIODICALS

Futterman, Laurie G., and Louis Lemberg. "High-Sensitivity C&-Reactive Protein is the Most Effective Prognostic Measurement of Acute Coronary Events." *American Journal of Critical Care* (September 2002): 482–6.

Rifai, Nader, and Paul M. Ridker. "High-Sensitivity C-Reactive Protein: A Novel and Promising Marker of Coronary Heart Disease." *Clinical Chemistry* (March 2001): 403-11.

Roberts, William L., et al. "Evaluation of Nine Automated High-Sensitivity C-Reactive Protein Methods: Implications for Clinical and Epidemiological Applications. Part 2." *Clinical Chemistry* (March 2001): 418–25.

Sandovsky, Richard. "Inflammatory Markers in Coronary Artery Disease." *American Family Physician* (March 1, 2004): 1245.

Seppa, N. "Early Warning? Inflammatory Protein is Tied to Colon Cancer Risk." *Science News* (Feb. 7, 2004): 84–5.

(No author.) "AHA/CDC Panel Issues Recommendations on CRP testing." *Medical Laboratory Observer* (March 2003): 6.

(No author.) "Why Do We Need Another Test?" *Harvard Health Letter* (February 2003).

ORGANIZATIONS

American Heart Association National Center. 7272 Greenville Avenue, Dallas, TX 75231-4596. 800-242-8721. <http://www.americanheart.org>.

Ken R. Wells

HIV infection *see* **AIDS**

Hives

Definition

Hives are an allergic skin reaction causing localized redness, swelling, and **itching**.

Description

Hives are a reaction of the body's immune system that causes areas of the skin to swell, itch, and become reddened. (The affected areas are called wheals.) When the reaction is limited to small areas of the skin, it is called urticaria. Involvement of larger areas, such as whole sections of a limb, is called angioedema.

Causes & symptoms

Causes

Hives are an allergic reaction. The body's immune system is normally responsible for protection from foreign invaders. When it becomes sensitized to normally harmless substances, the resulting reaction is called an allergy. An attack of hives is set off when such a substance, called an allergen, is ingested, inhaled, or otherwise contacted. It interacts with immune cells called mast cells, which reside in the skin, airways, and digestive system. When mast cells encounter an allergen, they release histamine and other chemicals, both locally and into the bloodstream. These chemicals cause blood vessels to become more porous, allowing fluid to accumulate in tissue and leading to the swollen and reddish appearance of hives. Some of the chemicals released sensitize **pain-related** nerve endings, causing the affected area to become itchy and sensitive.

A wide variety of substances may cause hives in sensitive people. Common culprits include:

• prescription and nonprescription drugs (Aspirin and penicillin are the two most commonly known causes of allergic reactions in adults.)

• nuts, especially peanuts, walnuts, and Brazil nuts

• fish, mollusks, and shellfish

• eggs

• wheat

• milk

• strawberries

• food additives and preservatives

• influenza vaccines

• tetanus toxoid vaccine

• gamma globulin

• bee, wasp, and hornet stings

• bites of mosquitoes, fleas, and scabies.

In addition, hives may also result from the body's response to certain physical conditions, such as emotional **stress**, rubbing, cold wind, heat contact (**prickly heat** rash), wearing tight clothing, or **exercise** after a heavy meal.

Symptoms

Urticaria is characterized by redness, swelling, and itching of small areas of the skin. These patches usually grow and recede in less than a day, but may be replaced by others in other locations. Angioedema is characterized by more diffuse swelling. Swelling of the airways may cause **wheezing** and respiratory distress. In severe cases, airway obstruction may occur.

Diagnosis

Hives are easily diagnosed by visual inspection. The cause of hives is usually apparent, but may require a careful medical history in some cases.

Treatment

Home remedies

To deal with the symptoms of hives, an oatmeal bath may help to relieve itching. **Chickweed** (*Stellaria media*), applied as a poultice (crushed or chopped herbs applied directly to the skin) or added to bath water, may also help relieve itching.

Nutritional therapy

Naturopaths or nutritionists will try to determine what allergic substance is causing the reaction and help the patient eliminate or minimize its effects. They may also recommend **vitamin C**, **vitamin B$_{12}$**, and quercetin (a flavonoid) supplements to help control acute or chronic hives.

Homeopathic therapy

The following homeopathic remedies have been used to relieve itching, redness or swelling associated with hives:

• *Urtica urens*

• **Apis** *(Apis mellifica)*

• *Sulfur*

Allopathic treatment

Mild cases of hives are treated with antihistamines, such as diphenhydramine (Benadryl). More severe cases may require such oral corticosteroids prednisone. Topical corticosteroids are not effective. In 2002, the Food and Drug Administration (FDA) approved the allergy drug Claritin for over-the-counter use for patients with urticaria. The drug comes in tablet and syrup form and carries little risk. Its release for over-the-counter use was delayed until the company that manufactures the drug could add instructions for patients about self-diagnosis of hives. They cautioned it should be used only for recurrent hives that had already been diagnosed by a physician, not for acute or severe urticaria. Airway swelling may require emergency injection of epinephrine (adrenaline).

Expected results

Most cases of hives clear up within one to seven days without treatment, provided the cause (allergen) is found and avoided.

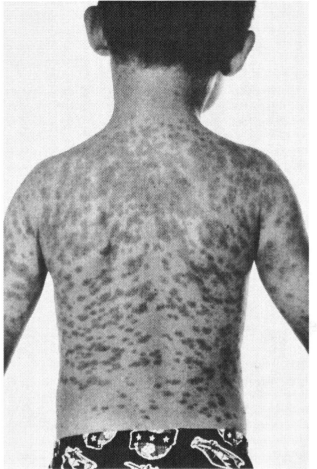

An unidentified rash on young boy's back. *(Custom Medical Stock Photo. Reproduced by permission.)*

Prevention

Preventing hives depends on avoiding the allergen causing them. Analysis of new items in the diet or new drugs taken may reveal the likely source of the reaction. Chronic hives may be aggravated by stress, **caffeine**, alcohol, or tobacco; avoiding these may reduce the frequency of reactions.

Resources

BOOKS

Jonas, Wayne B., and Jennifer Jacobs., "Skin Rashes." *Healing with Homeopathy: The Doctor's Guide.* New York, NY: Warner Books, 1996.

Lawlor, G. J., Jr., T.J. Fischer, and D.C. Adelman. *Manual of Allergy and Immunology.* Boston, MA: Little, Brown and Co., 1995.

Murray, Michael T. and Joseph E. Pizzorno. "Hives." *Encyclopedia of Natural Medicine.* Revised 2nd ed. Rocklin, CA: Prima Publishing, 1998.

Novick, N. L. *You Can Do Something About Your Allergies.* NY: Macmillan, 1994.

PERIODICALS

Franklin, Deanna. "FDA Panel Recommends OTC Approval of Claritin (Urticaria Indication Debated)." *Family Practice News* (June 15, 2002):26–31.

Mai Tran
Teresa G. Odle

Hodgkin's disease

Definition

Hodgkin's disease, also called Hodgkin's lymphoma, is a type of **cancer** involving tissues of the lymphatic system, or lymph nodes. Its cause is unknown, although some interaction between individual genetic makeup, family history, environmental exposures, and infectious agents is suspected.

Description

Hodgkin's lymphoma can occur at any age, although the majority of these lymphomas occur in people aged 15–34, and over the age of 60. Lymphoma is a cancer of the lymphatic system. Depending on the specific type, a lymphoma can have any or all of the characteristics of cancer: rapid multiplication of cells, abnormal cell types, loss of normal arrangement of cells with respect to one another, and invasive ability.

Causes & symptoms

Hodgkin's lymphoma usually begins in a lymph node. The node enlarges and—similar to enlarged lymph nodes due to infectious causes—may or may not cause any **pain**. Hodgkin's lymphoma progresses in a fairly predictable way, traveling from one group of lymph nodes to another unless it is treated. More advanced cases of Hodgkin's involve the spleen, liver, and bone marrow.

The features and prognosis of patients with Hodgkin's disease and non-Hodgkin's lymphoma (NHL)

differ significantly. However, research in 2001 found that among patients with human immunodeficiency virus (HIV), Hodgkin's disease appears very similar to HIV-related non-Hodgkin's lymphoma. NHL occurs much more often in patients with HIV, but in recent years, a small but significant increase in Hodgkin's disease has been seen in HIV-infected patients.

Constitutional symptoms—symptoms that affect the whole body—are common. They include **fever**, weight loss, heavy sweating at night, and **itching**. Some patients note pain after drinking alcoholic beverages.

As the lymph nodes swell, they may push against nearby structures, resulting in other local symptoms. These symptoms include pain from pressure on nerve roots as well as loss of function of specific muscle groups served by the compressed nerves. Kidney failure may result from compression of the ureters, the tubes which carry urine from the kidneys to the bladder. The face, neck, or arms may swell due to pressure slowing the flow in veins that should drain blood from those regions (superior vena cava syndrome). Pressure on the spinal cord can result in leg paralysis. Compression of the trachea and/or bronchi (airways) can cause **wheezing** and shortness of breath. Masses in the liver can cause the accumulation of certain chemicals in the blood, resulting in jaundice—a yellowish discoloration of the skin and the whites of the eyes.

As Hodgkin's lymphoma progresses, a patient's immune system becomes less and less effective at fighting infection. Thus, patients with Hodgkin's lymphoma become increasingly more susceptible to both common **infections** caused by bacteria and unusual (opportunistic) infections caused by viruses, fungi, and protozoa.

Diagnosis

Diagnosis of Hodgkin's lymphoma requires the removal of a sample of a suspicious lymph node (biopsy) and careful examination of the tissue under a microscope. In Hodgkin's lymphoma, certain characteristic cells—Reed-Sternberg cells—must be present in order to confirm the diagnosis. These cells usually contain two or more nuclei—oval centrally-located structures within cells that house their genetic material. In addition to the identification of these Reed-Sternberg cells, other cells in the affected tissue sample are examined. The characteristics of these other cells help to classify the specific subtype of Hodgkin's lymphoma.

Once Hodgkin's disease has been diagnosed, staging is the next important step. Staging involves computed tomography (CT) scans of the abdomen, chest, and pelvis, to identify areas of lymph node involvement. In rare cases, a patient must undergo abdominal surgery so that lymph nodes in the abdominal area can be biopsied (staging laparotomy). Some patients have their spleens removed during this surgery, both to help with staging and to remove a focus of the disease. Bone marrow biopsy is also required unless there is obvious evidence of vital organ involvement. Some physicians also order a lymphangiogram—a radiograph of the lymphatic vessels.

Staging is important because it helps to determine what kind of treatment a patient should receive. On one hand, it is important to understand the stage of the disease so that the treatment chosen is sufficiently strong to provide the patient with a cure. On the other hand, all the available treatments have serious side effects, so staging allows the patient to have the type of treatment necessary to achieve a cure, and to minimize the severity of short and long-term side effects from which the patient may suffer.

Treatment

Hodgkin's disease is a life-threatening disease. A correct diagnosis and appropriate treatment with surgery, chemotherapy, and/or radiation therapy are critical to controlling the illness.

Acupuncture, **hypnotherapy**, and **guided imagery** may be useful tools in treating pain symptoms associated with Hodgkin's. Acupuncture involves the placement of a series of thin needles into the skin at targeted locations on the body known as acupoints in order to harmonize the energy flow within the human body.

In guided imagery, the patient creates pleasant and comfortable mental images that promote **relaxation** and improve a patient's ability to cope with discomfort and pain symptoms. Other guided imagery techniques involve creating a visual mental image of the pain. Once the pain can be visualized, the patient can adjust the image to make it more pleasing and thus more manageable.

A number of herbal remedies are also available to lessen pain symptoms and promote relaxation and healing. However, individuals should consult with their healthcare professionals before taking them. Depending on the preparation and the type of herb, these remedies may interact with or enhance the effects of other prescribed medications.

Allopathic treatment

Treatment of Hodgkin's lymphoma has become increasingly effective over the years. The type of treatment used for Hodgkin's depends on the information obtained by staging, and may include chemotherapy (treatment with a combination of drugs), and/or radiotherapy (treatment with radiation to kill cancer cells).

Both chemotherapy and radiation therapy have unfortunate side effects. Chemotherapy can result in **nausea, vom-**

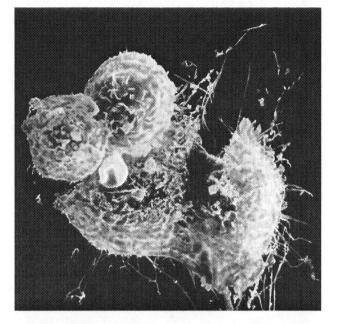

A scanning electron micrograph (SEM) of dividing Hodgkin's cells from the pleural effusions (abnormal accumulations of fluid in the lungs) of a 55-year-old male patient. *(Photograph by Dr. Andrejs Liepins, Photo Researchers, Inc. Reproduced by permission.)*

iting, hair loss, and increased susceptibility to infection. Radiation therapy can cause **sore throat,** difficulty in swallowing, **diarrhea,** and growth abnormalities in children. Both forms of treatment, especially in combination, can result in sterility (the permanent inability to have offspring), as well as heart and lung damage. A 2003 study showed a link between radiation therapy for Hodgkin's disease and increased risk for later **breast cancer.** However, adding chemotherapy to the regimen decreased the chance for breast cancer, perhaps by inducing premature **menopause.**

Expected results

Hodgkin's is one of the most curable forms of cancer. Current treatments are quite effective, especially with early diagnosis. Children have a particularly high rate of cure from the disease, with about 75% still living cancer-free 20 years after their original diagnosis. Adults with the most severe form of the disease have about a 50% cure rate. In 2003, new research noted that even after complete remission, some patients showed signs of thyroid dysfunction, most likely from the immune problems caused by Hodgkin's disease. The researchers recommended thyroid examinations every year during follow-up of the disease.

Prevention

While Hodgkin's disease cannot be prevented, researchers continue to study risk factors for the disease.

In 2003, a study showed a possible link between exposure to the **measles** virus around the time of **pregnancy** or birth. As research continues, these and other discoveries may help people control certain risk factors for Hodgkin's disease and other cancers.

Resources

BOOKS

Dollinger, Malin, et al. *Everyone's Guide to Cancer Therapy.* Kansas City, MO: Andrews McMeel Publishing, 1997.

Freedman, Arnold S. and Lee M. Nadler. "Hodgkin's Disease." In *Harrison's Principles of Internal Medicine,* edited by Anthony S. Fauci, et al. New York: McGraw-Hill, 1998.

PERIODICALS

"Chemotherapy May Suppress Breast Cancer Risk in Hodgkin Disease Survivors." *Women's Health Weekly* (July 31, 2003): 52.

"HIV-Positive Hodgkin Patients' Disease Looks Like NHL." *Cancer Weekly* (December 18, 2001):22.

"The Risk of Hodgkin Disease May be Association with Exposure to Infections." *Blood Weekly* (June 12, 2003):10.

"Thyroid Should be Examined Once a Year During Follow-up for Hodgkin Disease." *Clinical Trials Week* (March 24, 2003): 70.

ORGANIZATIONS

The Lymphoma Research Foundation of America, Inc. 8800 Venice Boulevard, Suite 207, Los Angeles, CA 90034. (310) 204-7040. http://www.lymphoma.org.

Paula Ford-Martin
Teresa G. Odle

Holistic dentistry

Definition

Holistic dentistry, also referred to as biologic dentistry, is an alternative approach that focuses on the use of non-toxic restorative materials for dental work, and emphasizes the unrecognized impact that dental toxins and dental **infections** may have on a person's overall health. While traditional dentistry focuses only on the areas above the neck, holistic dentistry looks at the patient as a whole system and how the mouth relates to the rest of the body.

Origins

Applying a biological concept to the practice of dentistry began in the late 1800s, when the National Dental Association recognized the harmful effects of mercury (amalgam) fillings, and mandated that members of the association not use these on their patients. As of 1997, this warning has been recognized and acted upon by several foreign countries that have either banned the use of mercury in fillings or are in the process of doing so. Supporters of holistic dentistry state that mercury in amalgam fillings causes ill effects when placed as an implant in the body.

Further beginnings of holistic dentistry are linked to a 1925 article by the dentist Weston A. Price (1870–1948). A former director of research for the American Dental Association, Price claimed in an article for the *Journal of the American Medical Association* that such degenerative diseases as heart troubles, kidney and bladder disorders, arthritis, rheumatism, mental illness, lung problems, and several kinds of bacterial infections arise from root canal therapy, or endodontics. To come to this conclusion, Price conducted research that involved implanting teeth from the root canals of individuals with symptoms of severe heart problems and kidney disease under the skin of healthy rabbits. These same conditions arose in the rabbits, and within three days they died. Price then implanted the same tooth in another rabbit and found a similar response, but he also found that implanting a normal extracted tooth did not affect the rabbits.

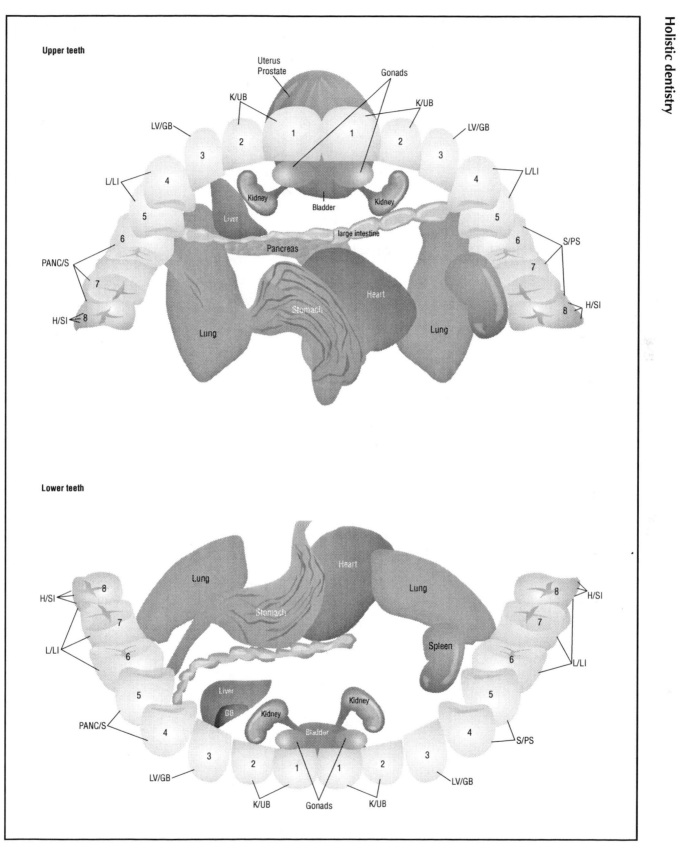

Upper teeth

Lower teeth

Teeth acupuncture points that correspond to major organs. *(Illustration by GGS Information Services, Inc. The Gale Group.)*

Price's root canal research became known as the "focal infection" theory, and because of its popularity, led to the extraction of millions of endodontically treated teeth. Further research conducted during the 1930s ridiculed Price's theory by calling it invalid, ending the once-recommended extractions.

Price also maintained that sugar causes not only tooth decay, but is responsible for physical, mental, moral, and social decay. This judgment came about as he and anthropologist Francis Pottenger observed primitive areas throughout the world whose natives did not have cavities. Although concluding that the lack of sugar in their **diets** led to good oral health, critics have since pointed out that Price overlooked the fact that malnourished people do not typically get many dental cavities.

Support of Price's theories continued, especially from a dentist named Melvin Page. Page coined the phrase "balancing body chemistry" and considered tooth decay an "outstanding example of systemic chemical imbalances." In an attempt to aid these problems, Page marketed a mineral supplement with claims that widespread mineral deficiencies were an underlying cause of several health conditions, including goiter, heart trouble, **tuberculosis**, and diabetes. He also claimed that drinking cow's milk was unnatural and the underlying cause of colds, sinus infections, colitis, and **cancer**. There is no research supporting Price's statements, and his mineral supplement was never supported by the Federal Trade Commission (FTC).

The origins of holistic dentistry remain with Price's manuscripts and photographs at the Price-Pottenger **Nutrition** Foundation in La Mesa, California. Founded in 1965, the Foundation promotes nutrition, megavitamin therapy, **homeopathy**, and **chelation therapy**.

Since the late 1800s, supporters of holistic dentistry continue to state their concerns regarding several procedures and recommendations of conventional dentistry including the use of fluoride in drinking water and in teeth cleansers.

Benefits

Holistic dentistry is said to be an emerging new field of probiotic dental medicine—a type of medicine that supports the life process. Those who practice this form of biologic dentistry claim that it is aesthetic, relatively nontoxic, and individually biocompatible, or life supporting. A holistic dentist uses physiologic and electronic methods to locate areas of chronic disease that are difficult to locate by current standard methods.

The benefits of holistic dentistry are said to be the result of its incorporation of hypnosis, homeopathy, **aromatherapy**, nutrition, and herbology.

Hypnosis

When hypnosis is used, patients are able to relax their bodies and minds by concentrating on suggestions of **relaxation**. The patient is fully aware of what is happening during their treatment and no drugs are used. Many holistic dentists employ specialist hypnotherapists to provide treatment that is highly effective and cannot cause any harm or produce any side effects.

Homeopathy

Homeopathy is used by holistic dentists as a natural approach to their practice. The therapy is a safe and natural alternative that is nonaddictive and effective with both adults and children. Homeopathic remedies are used to improve the psychological or emotional condition of patients without the drugging effects of conventional tranquilizers. The three main remedies considered by holistic dentists include: *aconite* (**foxglove**); *gelsemium* (yellow jasmine); and *argentum nitricum* (silver nitrate).

Aromatherapy

Aromatherapy uses the pure oil essences from plants and flowers that act as hormone-like stimulants to improve a patient's health balance. Used because they are natural and gentle, oils like **lavender**, bergamot, sandalwood, and basil are beneficial in their power to soothe, relax, and calm. Some holistic dentists use these oils to make their offices more inviting to the patient.

Nutrition

Holistic dentists believe that **stress** and tension are often linked to diet. Dietary excesses or deficiencies increase the body's needs for essential vitamins and minerals, and the stress and tension accelerate any fears or **phobias** of the patient.

Botanical medicine & herbal medicine

Holistic dentistry may use herbs to promote relaxation. The sedative properties of **chamomile**, limeflower, vervain, **rosemary**, and **valerian** are relied upon in place of conventional drugs.

Holistic dentists may incorporate **acupuncture** and physical therapy into their use of clinical dentistry. The more modern sciences of **neural therapy**, hematology, immunology, and electroacupuncture may also be incorporated into a holistic dental practice.

Description

Biological dentistry's main concern is the toxicity of metals and their release from fillings and replacement appliances (such as metal partials and crowns that have nickel) used in dentistry. According to supporters of holistic dentistry, the metal ions separate from their original structures to diffuse, migrate to, and become absorbed in the tissues of the body, affecting the overall integrity of the immune system. An additional biological concern is "oral galvanism," or the direct electrical currents generated by separated metals throughout fluids and tissues in the body. Hidden or residual infection, or the abnormal changes in the soft connective tissue containing dental material that cannot be processed, is believed to cause local and general defenses that put the body in a continuous state of active conflict, often leading to chronic disease.

According to those who practice holistic dentistry, there may be several major types of dental problems that can cause illness or dysfunction in the body, including:

- silver (amalgam) fillings that typically contain 50% mercury silver

- root canals

- cavitations, or neuralgia-inducing cavitational osteonecrosis (NICO), a term coined by the oral pathologist J.E. Bouguot in the 1980s

- electro-oral galvanism from dissimilar metals

- temporomandibular joint syndrome (TMJ), a painful condition of the jaw and its supporting muscles

The main goals of a holistic dentist include identifying areas that need treatment and providing treatment to patients that will not create stress. Holistic dentists work in conjunction with other health care providers to investigate whether a hidden infection of dental origin exists, and whether it may be the source of or contributing factor to overall health problems. A biological approach to dentistry ensures the use of treatment and therapies that cause the least disturbance to the immune system. In order to determine the appropriate method of treatment, a holistic dentist must thoroughly review the patient's medical and dental background.

Preparations

While the method of biological dentistry varies for each holistic dentist, the keys to preparing their patients remain education and communication. Treatment is individualized.

A typical initial visit consists of an interview process, examination and x rays. Pictures of the patient's mouth are often collected with state-of-the-art equipment that uses film providing 50% less radiation than standard systems. The second meeting is typically called a "Review of Findings" appointment that educates the patient about the mouth and proactive treatment choices.

Precautions

Although proponents of holistic dentistry continue to increase, so do critics of their alternative methods. Believers in biologic dentistry claim that root canal-treated teeth cause NICO and other chronic systemic diseases and require removal of all these teeth and the healthy teeth surrounding them. Critics state that these extreme measures are bizarre and dangerous. According to a 1994 article in *Milwaukee Magazine*, a group of local patients filed suit against several holistic practitioners who had removed several of their perfectly healthy teeth after guaranteeing improvement of their diseases. These patients experienced no relief from their ongoing health problems after the extractions.

Side effects

Certain side effects have been reported as a result of treatments used by holistic dentists. Patients who were treated with **auriculotherapy**, or acupuncture of the ear, have experienced complications from unsterile needles.

When correcting a "bad bite," holistic dentists often place a plastic appliance called a mandibular orthopedic repositioning appliance (MORA) between the teeth. The long-term use of MORAs has been reported to cause the patient's teeth to move out of proper alignment, leading to the need for orthodontics or facial reconstructive surgery to correct the deformity.

With amalgam fillings being one of the main concerns of holistic dentists, many have turned to using nontoxic composite materials, but these too have come under scrutiny. The plastics used in the composites have been linked to leaching compounds that may be dangerous to health.

Research & general acceptance

While dentistry has been reportedly undergoing a quiet revolution with the emergence of holistic dentists, their complementary methods remain under criticism. The nutritional supplements they prescribe to "balance the body chemistry" and the methods holistic dentists use to reach their recommended treatment continually attract negative comments. Hair analysis, computerized dietary analysis, or blood chemistry screening tests are used by some practitioners as a basis for recommending supplements. Critics state that hair analysis is not a reliable tool for measuring the body's nutritional state, and computer analysis, while useful for determining the composition of a person's diet, is being used by dentists who may not be qualified to perform dietary counseling. Blood chemistry screenings are processed in laboratories, but while the results may indicate a "normal" reading, holistic dentists use a narrower range to read the results, indicating to patients that their bodies are out of balance and need treatment.

Amalgam (mercury) fillings have been an issue of research for both the traditional and holistic dentist. While holistic supporters ban the use of amalgram, scientific testing has shown that the amount of mercury absorbed from fillings is only a small fraction of the average daily intake from food. The U.S. Public Health Service concluded in 1992 that it was inappropriate to recommend restricting the use of dental amalgam. In 2002, a report said that a U.S. representative in California introduced a bill in Congress that would prevent dentists from using amalgam fillings nationwide by the year 2006 because of their mercury content. The American Dental Association opposes banning amalgam and says that it does not add to mercury levels in the brain. Results from two trials being conducted by the National Institutes of Health on amalgams will not be released until about 2005.

Although supportive research is limited regarding the alternative methods used by holistic dentists, advocates of the complementary treatment continue to grow. With the formation of the Holistic Dental Association in 1978, a shift to treating the entire patient's health needs is emerging from dentists, dental hygienists, and health care practitioners from all fields who endorse these ideas.

Many of the medical services provided by holistic dentists are paid for by health care insurance in the United States (excluding HMOs and Medicare). Insurance typically pays for "usual and customary" treatments, such as laboratory tests, doctor visits, medical treatment, and x rays, but it will not cover "experimental drugs."

Training & certification

Holistic dentists are those who have been trained as an authorized practitioner of dentistry through a school of medicine acquiring a degree as a Doctor of Dental Surgery (D.D.S.). Their focus is one that combines conventional teachings with new, complementary methods to treat their patients' health needs.

Resources

PERIODICALS

Gleeson, Carolyn. "Holistic Dentistry." *Shared Vision Magazine* (February 2000).

Harder, Patty A. "Dentistry the Holistic Way!" *Holistic Health News* (September 30, 1995).

Kramien, Liz. "It's All In Your Head." *To Your Health, The Magazine of Healing and Hope* (February 28,1998).

Mihaychuk, Nina. "The Role of Root Canal Therapy (Endodontics) in Holistic Dentistry." *Lilipoh* (July 31, 1998).

"Should Amalgam Fillings be Banned? Evidence on the Risks of Mercury Fillings is Mixed. Should They be Outlawed Anyway?." *Natural Health* (March 2002): 26.

KEY TERMS
· ·

Homeopathy—The principal of "like cures like," the use of minute quantities of remedies that if used in large doses would produce the effects of the disease being treated.

Mercury—A metallic element that is a silvery liquid at ordinary temperatures.

Probiotic—Favoring the support of life; related to promoting life and life conditions.

Toxins—Poisonous substances of animal or plant origin having a protein structure.

Smith, Gerald H. "Biological Dentistry." *Health & Happiness: A Newsletter for Better Living* (1997).

Varley, Peter. "Fear of the Dentist." *Homeopathy* (April 30, 1996).

ORGANIZATIONS

Holistic Dental Association. P.O. Box 5007, Durango, Colorado 81301. <http://www.holisticdental.org>.

OTHER

Barrett, Stephen and William T. Jarvis. "Holistic Dentistry: A Brief Overview." <http://www.quackwatch.com>.

"Biological Holistic Dentistry." <http://www.dancris.com>.

"Cavitational Osteopathosis and Biological Dentistry." <http:// www.quackwatch.com>.

Beth Kapes
Teresa G. Odle

Holistic medicine

Definition

Holistic medicine is a term used to describe therapies that attempt to treat the patient as a whole person. That is, instead of treating an illness, as in orthodox allopathy, holistic medicine looks at an individual's overall physical, mental, spiritual, and emotional well-being before recommending treatment. A practitioner with a holistic approach treats the symptoms of illness as well as looking for the underlying cause of the illness. Holistic medicine also attempts to prevent illness by placing a greater emphasis on optimizing health. The body's systems are seen as interdependent parts of the person's whole being. The body's natural state is one of health, and an illness or disease is an imbalance in the body's systems. Holistic therapies tend to emphasize proper **nutrition** and avoidance of substances—such as chemicals—that pollute the body. Their techniques are noninvasive.

Some of the world's health systems that are holistic in nature include **naturopathic medicine**, **homeopathy**, and **traditional Chinese medicine**. Many alternative or natural therapies have a holistic approach, although that is not always the case. The term complementary medicine is used to refer to the use of both allopathic and holistic treatments. It is more often used in Great Britain but is gaining acceptance in the United States.

There are no limits to the range of diseases and disorders that can be treated in a holistic way, as the principle of holistic healing is to balance the body, mind, spirit, and emotions so that the person's whole being functions smoothly. When an individual seeks holistic treatment for a particular illness or condition, other health problems improve without direct treatment due to improvement in the performance of the immune system, which is one of the goals of holistic medicine.

Origins

The concept of holistic medicine is not new. In the 4th century BC, Socrates warned that treating only one part of the body would not have good results. Hippocrates considered that many factors contribute to the health or otherwise of a human being, including weather, nutrition, emotional factors. In our time, a host of different sources of pollution can interfere with health. And of course, holistic medicine existed even before older Greece in some ancient healing traditions, such as those from India and China, which date back over 5,000 years. However, the term "holistic" only became part of everyday language in the 1970s, when Westerners began seeking an alternative to allopathic medicine.

Interestingly, it was only at the beginning of the twentieth century that the principles of holistic medicine fell out of favor in Western societies, with the advent of major advances in what we now call allopathic medicine. Paradoxically, many discoveries of the twentieth century have only served to confirm many natural medicine theories. In many cases, researchers have set out to debunk holistic medicine, only to find that their research confirms it, as has been the case, for example, with many herbal remedies.

Benefits

Many people are now turning to holistic medicine, often when suffering from chronic ailments that have not been successfully treated by allopathic means. Although many wonderful advances and discoveries have been made in modern medicine, surgery and drugs alone have a very poor record for producing optimal health because they are designed to attack illness. Holistic medicine is particularly helpful in treating chronic illnesses and maintaining health through proper nutrition and **stress** management.

Description

There are a number of therapies that come under the umbrella of holistic medicine. They all use basically the same principles, promoting not only physical health, but also mental, emotional, and spiritual health. Most emphasize quality nutrition. Refined foods typically eaten in modern America contain chemical additives and preservatives, are high in fat, **cholesterol**, and sugars, and promote disease. Alternative nutritionists counter refined foods by recommending whole foods whenever possible and minimizing the amount of meat—especially red meat—that is consumed. Many alternative therapies promote **vegetarianism** as a method of **detoxification**.

The aim of holistic medicine is to bring all areas of an individual's life, and most particularly the energy flowing through the body, back into harmony. Ultimately, of course, only the patient can be responsible for this, for no practitioner can make the necessary adjustments to diet and lifestyle to achieve health. The practice of holistic medicine does not rule out the practice of allopathic medicine; the two can complement each other.

A properly balanced holistic health regimen, which takes into consideration all aspects of human health and includes noninvasive and nonpharmaceutical healing methods, can often completely eradicate even acute health conditions safely. If a patient is being treated with allopathic medicine, holistic therapies may at least support the body during treatment and alleviate the symptoms that often come with drug treatments and surgery. In addition, holistic therapies focus on the underlying source of the illness, to prevent recurrence.

Here are some of the major holistic therapies:

- herbal medicine
- homeopathy
- naturopathic medicine
- traditional Chinese medicine
- Ayurvedic medicine
- nutritional therapies
- **chiropractic**
- stress reduction
- psychotherapy
- massage.

Because holistic medicine aims to treat the whole person, holistic practitioners sometimes may advise treatment from more than one type of practitioner. This precaution ensures that all aspects of health are addressed. Some practitioners also specialize in more than one therapy and so may be able to offer more comprehensive assistance.

Preparations

To choose a holistic practitioner, a person should conscious the following questions:

- How did you hear of this therapist? A personal referral can sometimes be more reliable than a professional one. What do other professionals say about this therapist? What qualifications, board certification, or affiliations does this practitioner have?

- How do you feel personally about this practitioner? Do you feel comfortable in his/her office and with his/her staff? Is your sense of well-being increased? Are you kept waiting for appointments?

- Do you have confidence in this practitioner, and does he/she respect you as a person? Does he/she show an interest in your family, lifestyle, and diet? Are various treatment options explained to you?

- Is your personal dignity respected?

- Do you feel that this practitioner is sensitive to your feelings and fears regarding treatment?

- Is this practitioner a good advertisement for his/her profession? Signs of stress or ill health may mean that you would be better off choosing another practitioner.

- Do you feel that you are rushed into decisions, or do you feel that you are allowed time to make an informed choice regarding treatment?

- Are future health goals outlined for you? And do you feel that the practitioner is taking your progress seriously?

- Do you feel unconditionally accepted by this practitioner?

- Would you send your loved ones to this practitioner?

If you answered yes to all the above, then you have found a suitable practitioner. The cost of treatment by a holistic therapist varies widely depending on the level of qualification and the discipline, so it is best to discuss how much treatment can be expected to cost with a practitioner before beginning a course of therapy. Some forms of holistic treatment may be covered by health insurance.

Precautions

Many people who try holistic therapies focus on one area of their health only, often detoxification and nutrition. However, practitioners stress that it is only when all areas of a person's potential well-being are tackled that total health and happiness can be achieved. They stress that the spiritual and emotional health contribute just as much as physical and mental health to a person's overall state of well-being.

When seeking treatment from a holistic practitioner, it is important to ensure that they are properly qualified. Credentials and reputation should always be checked. In addition, it is important that allopathic physicians and alternative physicians communicate with me another about a patient's care.

Side effects

One of the main advantages of holistic therapies is that they have few side effects when used correctly. If a reputable practitioner is chosen and guidelines are adhered to, the worst that typically happens is that when lifestyle is changed, and fresh nutrients are provided, the body begins to eliminate toxins that may have accumulated in the cells over a lifetime.

Often holistic therapy results in what is known in alternative medicine circles as a "healing crisis." This comes about when the cells eliminate poisons into the blood stream all at the same time, throwing the system into a state of toxic overload until it can clear the "backlog." Symptoms such as **nausea**, headaches, or sensitivities to noise and other stimulations may be experienced.

The answer to most patients who are otherwise healthy patients is often just to lie quietly in a darkened room and take herbal teas. However, in the case of someone who has a serious illness, such as arthritis, colitis, diabetes, or **cancer**, it is strongly advised that they seek the help of a qualified practitioner. Therapists can help patients achieve detoxification in a way that causes the least stress to their bodies.

Research & general acceptance

Traditionally, holistic medicine, in all its different forms, has been regarded with mistrust and skepticism on the part of the allopathic medical profession. This situation is gradually changing. As of the year 2004, many insurance companies will provide for some form of alternative, or complementary treatment.

In addition, many allopathic physicians, recognizing the role alternative medicine can play in overall health and well being, are actually referring patients to reputable practitioners, particularly chiropractors and **relaxation** therapists, for help with a varied range of complaints.

Training & certification

Holistic or alternative medicine practitioners are usually affiliated with an organization in their field. Training varies widely with the category, and ranges from no qualifications at all—experience only—to holding a Ph.D. from an accredited university. Again, credentials and memberships should be checked by prospective patients.

An excellent source for qualified practitioners is the American Board of Holistic Medicine (AHBM), which was incorporated in 1996. Also, the American Holistic Medicine Association has a comprehensive list of practitioners in all types of therapies across the United States, which they call "the holistic doctor finder." However, these groups stress that it is the responsibility of the patient to check each practitioner's credentials prior to treatment.

The ABHM has established the core curriculum upon which board certification for holistic medicine will be based. It includes the following twelve categories:

Body

Physical and environmental health

- nutritional medicine
- exercise medicine
- environmental medicine

Mind

Mental and emotional health

- behavioral medicine

Spirit

Spiritual health

- spiritual attunement
- social health

The six specialized areas:

- biomolecular diagnosis and therapy
- botanical medicine
- energy medicine
- ethnomedicine—including traditional Chinese medicine, Ayurveda, and Native American medicine
- homeopathy
- manual medicine

Founded in 1978 for the purpose of uniting practitioners of holistic medicine, membership of the AHMA is open to licensed medical doctors (MDs) and doctors of osteopathic medicine (DOs) from every specialty, and to medical students studying for those degrees. Associate membership is open to health care practitioners who are certified, registered or licensed in the state in which they practice. The mission of the AHMA is to support practitioners in their personal and professional development as healers, and to educate mainstream physicians about holistic medicine.

KEY TERMS

. . . .

Detoxification—Treating the body in such a way that it eliminates poisons accumulated in the cells.

Healing crisis—An uncomforatable when the body begins to eliminates toxins at an accelerated rate.

Resources

BOOKS

Goldberg, Burton. *Alternative Medicine: The Definitive Guide.* Fife, WA: Future Medicine Publishing, 1993.

Jensen, Dr. Bernard. *Foods That Heal.* Garden City, NY: Avery Publishing Group Inc., 1993.

Murray, Michael, and Joseph Pizzorno. *Encyclopedia of Natural Medicine, 2nd edition* Rocklin, CA: Prima Health, 1998.

ORGANIZATIONS

American Holistic Medicine Association http://www.holistic medicine.org/index.html.

Holistic medicine Website http://www.holisticmed.com/whatis. html.

American Holistic Health Association Dept. R P.O. Box 17400 Anaheim, CA 92817-7400 USA Phone: (714) 779-6152 E-mail: ahha@healthy.net http://www.healthy.net/pan/chg/ ahha/rosen.html.

Patricia Skinner

Holy thistle *see* **Blessed thistle**

Homeopathy

Definition

Homeopathy, or homeopathic medicine, is a holistic system of treatment that originated in the late eighteenth century. The name homeopathy is derived from two Greek words that mean "like disease." The system is based on the idea that substances that produce symptoms of sickness in healthy people will have a curative effect when given in very dilute quantities to sick people who exhibit those same symptoms. Homeopathic remedies are believed to stimulate the body's own healing processes. Homeopaths use the term "allopathy," or "different

HOMEOPATHIC REMEDIES

Name	Description
Aconite	Commonly known as monkshood, aconite is highly toxic. A nontoxic, diluted extract of aconite is used in homeopathy to treat symptoms similar to that of poison.
Allium cepa	Commonly known as red onion, homeopathic physicians use a dilute extract of red onion to treat symptoms similar to that of red onion—watery eyes, burning, etc.
Apis	Commonly known as the honeybee, apis as a homeopathic remedy is made from the body of the bee. It is used to treat symptoms similar to that of a bee sting—redness, swelling, etc.
Arnica	Commonly known as the mountain daisy, arnica is used by homeopathic physicians to treat bruises, sprains, and strains.
Arsenicum album	Also known as ars alb, arsenicum album is a diluted form of arsenic, a metallic poison. It is used by homeopathic physicians to treat symptoms similar to the effects of arsenic poisoning—dehydration, burning pain, etc.
Belladonna	Commonly known as deadly nightshade, belladonna is used in homeopathy to treat symptoms of dry mouth, nausea, delirium, etc.
Bryonia	Commonly known as wild hops, bryonia is used in homeopathy to treat vomiting, diarrhea, inflammation, etc.
Calcarea carbonica	Also known as calcium carbonate or calc carb, it is used in homeopathy to treat symptoms of exhaustion, depression, and anxiety.
Cantharis	Commonly known as Spanish fly, cantharis is used in homeopathy to treat conditions with symptoms of abdominal cramps, vomiting, diarrhea, convulsions, etc.
Chamomilla	Derived from German chamomile, it is used in homeopathy to treat irritability, impatience, etc. It is most often prescribed to children.
Ferrum phosphoricum	Also known as ferrum phos or iron phosphate, it is used to treat symptoms of low energy and anemia.
Gelsemium	Also known as yellow jasmine, it is used to treat conditions that affect vision, balance, thought, and locomotion.
Hepar sulphuris	Derived from the inner layer of oyster shells, hepar sulphuris is used to treat infection.

disease," to describe the use of drugs used in conventional medicine to oppose or counteract the symptom being treated.

Origins

Homeopathy was founded by the German physician **Samuel Hahnemann** (1755-1843), who was much disturbed by the medical system of his time, believing that its cures were crude and some of its strong drugs and treatments did more harm than good to patients. Hahnemann performed experiments on himself using Peruvian bark, which contains quinine, a **malaria** remedy. He concluded that in a healthy person, quinine creates the same symptoms as malaria, including fevers and **chills**, which is the reason why it is effective as a remedy. He then began to analyze the remedies available in nature by

what he called provings. Provings of homeopathic remedies are still compiled by dosing healthy adults with various substances and documenting the results, in terms of the dose needed to produce the symptoms and the length of the dose's effectiveness. The provings are collected in large homeopathic references called *materia medica* or materials of medicine.

Hahnemann formulated these principles of homeopathy:

• Law of Similars (like cures like)

• Law of the Infinitesimal Dose (The more diluted a remedy is, the more potent it is.)

• Illness is specific to the individual.

Hahnemann's Law of Similars was based on thinking that dated back to Hippocrates in the fourth century

HOMEOPATHIC REMEDIES (CONTD.)

Name	Description
Hypericum	Commonly known as St. John's wort, hypericum is used to treat nerve damage.
Ignatia	Derived from seeds of a plant, this homeopathic remedy is prescribed to treat conditions with symptoms such as headache, cramping, and tremors.
Ipecac	Ipecac induces vomiting and causes gastrointestinal distress. Homeopaths prescribe it to treat similar symptoms.
Kali bichromicum	Commonly known as potassium bichromate, kali bichromicum is a poison used also in textile dyes, wood stain, etc. Homeopaths use it to treat localized pain.
Lachesis	Derived from the venom of the bushmaster snake, this homeopathic remedy is used to treat conditions that cause the same symptoms as the venom itself.
Ledum	Also known as marsh tea, ledum is used to treat infections, most often from animal bites, stings, cuts, etc.
Lycopodium	Commonly known as club moss, lycopodium is used to treat diarrhea, digestive upset, etc.
Mercurius vivus	Also known as quicksilver, it is used to treat symptoms of sweats, shaking, nausea, etc.
Natrum muriaticum	Commonly known as salt, it is used to treat conditions that cause excessive thirst and salt cravings.
Nux vomica	It is used to treat symptoms caused by overeating and too much caffeine or alcohol.
Phosphorus	It is used to treat symptoms of excessive thirst, fatigue, and nervousness.
Pulsatilla	It is used to treat conditions that are accompanied by discharge, such as bedwetting, sinusitis, etc.
Rhus toxicodendron	Commonly known as poison ivy, homeopaths use it to treat conditions with symptoms of fever, swollen glands, and restlessness.
Ruta	It is used to treat conditions with bruising, such as tennis elbow, sciatica, etc.
Sepia	Sepia is the discharge used by the cuttlefish to disappear from a predator. Homeopaths use sepia to treat symptoms of apathy and weakness.
Silica	Also called flint, silica is used by homeopaths to treat conditions that cause weakness, sweating, and sensitivity to cold.
Sulphur	It is used to treat conditions with symptoms of itching, burning pains, and odor.

B.C. It is the same thinking that provided the basis for the vaccines discovered by Edward Jenner and Louis Pasteur. These vaccines provoke a reaction in the individual that protects against the actual disease. Allergy treatments work the same way. By exposing a person to minute quantities of the allergen, the person's tolerance levels are elevated.

The Law of the Infinitesimal Dose has always caused controversy among those outside the field of homeopathy. Hahnemann contended that as he diluted his remedies with **water** and alcohol and succussed, or shook, them, the remedies actually worked more effectively. In fact, diluted homeopathic remedies may have no chemical trace of the original substance. Practitioners believe that the electromagnetic energy of the original substance is retained in the dilution, but the toxic side effects of the remedy are not. It is this electrochemical "message" that stimulates the body to heal itself.

Homeopathic practitioners believe that illness is specific to an individual. In other words, two people with severe headaches may not receive the same remedies. The practitioner will ask the patient questions about lifestyle, dietary habits, and personality traits, as well as specific questions about the nature of the headache and when it occurs. This information gathering is called profiling or case-taking.

In the early 1900s, homeopathy was popular in America, with over 15 percent of all doctors being homeopaths. There were 22 major homeopathic medical schools, including Boston University and the University of Michigan. However, with the formation of the American Medical Association, which restricted and closed

SAMUEL HAHNEMANN 1755–1843

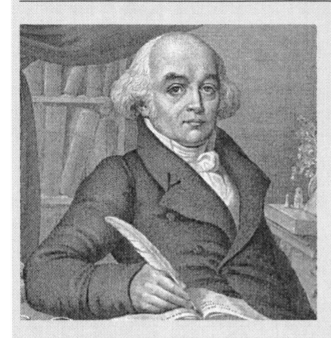

(Corbis Corporation. Reproduced by permission.)

Samuel Christian Hahnemann created and developed the system called homeopathy. It is also known as *similia similibus curentor* or "let like be cured by like.". Although his new methods initially met with ridicule and criticism, by the time of his death they were accepted the world over as a result of the great success he had with his new cure.

Hahnemann was born in Meissen, Saxony (now part of Germany) into a financially challenged middle class family. His parents initially educated him at home, where his father taught him never to accept anything he learned without first questioning it. He graduated as a physician from the University of Erlangen in 1779 after studying at Leipzig and Vienna. He was also fluent in English, German, Italian, French, Greek, Arabic, Latin and Hebrew.

At age 27 he married his first wife, Johanna Henriette Kuchler, the daughter of an apothecary, with whom he had 11 children.

Living in poverty, Hahnemann began practicing medicine in 1781 and translating scientific texts to supplement his income. However, disillusioned with medicine, he eventually gave it up entirely.

He discovered the concept of homeopathy when he considered the effect of quinine on **malaria**, and went on to cure soldiers and then sufferers of a typhus epidemic with astounding success. He documented his discoveries in the Organon, a treatise on his work. Homeopathy also proved its worth in 1831 when there was an outbreak of cholera. Hahnemann used homeopathic treatment with a 96% success rate, compared to the 41% of allopathic medicine. He also wrote his *Materia Medica Pura*.

In 1834, Hahnemann met his second wife, Marie Melanie d'Hervilly. Despite a great difference in age, they were happily married until his death in Paris on July 2, 1843, at the age of 88.

Patricia Skinner

down alternative practices, homeopathy declined for half a century. When the 1960s revived back-to-nature trends and distrust of artificial drugs and treatments, homeopathy began to grow again dramatically through the next decades. In 1993, *The New England Journal of Medicine* reported that 2.5 million Americans used homeopathic remedies and 800,000 patients visited homeopaths in 1990, and homeopathy has continued to grow. Homeopathy is much more popular in Europe than in the United States. French pharmacies are required to make homeopathic remedies available along with conventional medications. Homeopathic hospitals and clinics are part of the national health system in Britain. Homeopathy is also practiced in India and Israel, among other countries.

Benefits

Homeopathic physicians seek to cure their patients on the physical, mental and emotional levels, and each treatment is tailored to a patient's individual needs. Homeopathy is generally a safe treatment, as it uses medicines in extremely diluted quantities, and there are usually minimal side effects. Its nontoxicity makes some consider it a good choice for the treatment of children. Another benefit of homeopathy is the cost of treatments; homeopathic remedies are inexpensive, often a fraction of the cost of conventional drugs.

Homeopathic treatment has been shown to be effective in treating many conditions. Colds and flu may be effectively treated with aconite and bryonia. **Influenza** sufferers in a double-blind study found that they were twice as likely to recover in 48 hours when they took homeopathic remedies. Studies have been published in British medical journals confirming the efficacy of homeopathic treatment for **rheumatoid arthritis**. Homeopathic remedies are considered effective in treating infections, circulatory problems, respiratory problems, **heart disease, de-**

pression and nervous disorders, migraine headaches, **allergies**, arthritis, and diabetes. Homeopathy is a treatment to explore for acute and chronic illnesses, particularly if these are found in the early stages and where there is not severe damage. Homeopathy can be used to assist the healing process after surgery or chemotherapy.

Description

A visit to a homeopath is usually a different experience from a visit to a regular physician. Surveys have shown that homeopathic doctors spend much more time during initial consultations than conventional doctors spend. This is because a homeopath does a thorough case-taking to get a complete picture of a person's general health and lifestyle, as well as particular symptoms, on the physical, mental and emotional levels. Some symptoms can be so subtle that the patient is not always completely aware of them, and the doctor must spend time getting to know the patient.

The initial visit often includes a long questionnaire about a patient's medical and family history, and then a long interview with the doctor, who prompts the patient with many questions. Sometimes a homeopathic doctor will use lab tests to establish a patient's general level of health. The initial interview usually lasts between one and two hours.

The purpose of homeopathy is the restoration of the body to homeostasis, or healthy balance, which is its natural state. The symptoms of a disease are regarded as the body's own defensive attempts to correct its imbalance, rather than as enemies to be defeated. Because a homeopath regards symptoms as positive evidence of the body's inner intelligence, he or she will prescribe a remedy designed to stimulate this internal curative process, rather than suppress the symptoms.

In homeopathy, the curative process extends beyond the relief of immediate symptoms of illness. Healing may come in many stages, as the practitioner treats layers of symptoms that are remnants of traumas or chronic disease in the patient's past. The stages are related to Hering's Laws of Cure, named for Constantine Hering, the father of homeopathy in America. Hering believed that healing starts from the deepest parts of the body to the extremities, and from the upper parts of the body to the lower parts. Hering's Laws also state that homeopaths should treat disease symptoms in reverse chronological order, from the most recent to the oldest, restoring health in stages. Sometimes, the patient may feel worse before feeling better. This temporary worsening is called a healing crisis.

When prescribing a remedy, homeopaths will match a patient's symptoms with the proper remedy in a repertory or *materia medica* that has been compiled through-

out the history of homeopathy. Classical homeopaths prescribe only one remedy at a time. However, it is becoming more common, especially in Europe, to use combination formulas of several remedies for the treatment of some combinations of symptoms.

The cost of homeopathic care can vary. The cost of visits will be comparable to conventional medicine, with initial visits ranging from $50 to $300. Non-M.D. homeopaths can charge from $50 to $250. Follow-up visits are less, at about $35 to $100. Homeopathic medicine is significantly cheaper than pharmaceuticals, and most remedies cost between $2 and $10. Some doctors provide remedies without charge. Homeopaths rarely use lab tests, which reduces the cost of treatment further. In general, homeopathy is much more economical than conventional medicine. In 1991, the French government did a study on the cost of homeopathic medicine, and found that it costs half as much to treat patients, considering all treatment costs involved.

When homeopaths are licensed professionals, most insurance companies will pay for their fees. Consumers should consult their insurance policies to determine individual regulations. Insurance usually will not cover homeopathic medicine, because it is sold over the counter.

Precautions

Although homeopathic remedies sometimes use substances that are toxic, they are diluted and prescribed in non toxic doses. Remedies should be prescribed by a homeopathic practitioner. Those preparing to take homeopathic remedies should also avoid taking *antidotes*, which are substances that homeopathic doctors believe cancel the effects of their remedies. These substances include alcohol, coffee, prescription drugs, **peppermint** (in toothpaste and mouthwash), camphor (in salves and lotions), and very spicy foods. Homeopathic medicine should also be handled with care, and should not be touched with the hands or fingers, which may contaminate it.

Side effects

A homeopathic aggravation sometimes occurs during initial treatment with homeopathic remedies. This means that symptoms can temporarily worsen during the process of healing. Although this is usually mild, the aggravation can sometimes be severe. Homeopaths see aggravation as a positive sign that the remedy is a good match for the patient's symptoms. The healing crisis, which happens when the patient is undergoing treatment for layers of symptoms, may also cause the patient to feel worse before feeling better. Some patients can experience emotional disturbances like weeping or depression, if suppressed emotional problems led to the illness in the first place.

Research & general acceptance

Since the early 1900s, when the American Medical Association and pharmacists waged a battle against it, homeopathy has been neglected and sometimes ridiculed by mainstream medicine. Aside from politics, part of the reason for this hostility is that there are some aspects of homeopathy that have not been completely explained scientifically. For instance, homeopaths have found that the more they dilute and succuss a remedy, the greater effect it seems to have on the body. Some homeopathic remedies are so diluted that not even a single molecule of the active agent remains in a solution, yet it still works; studies have demonstrated this paradox, yet can't explain it. Also, homeopathy puts an emphasis on analyzing symptoms and then applying remedies to these symptoms, rather than working by classifying diseases. Thus, some people with the same disease may require different homeopathic medicines and treatments. Furthermore, conventional medicine strives to find out how medicines work in the body before they use them; homeopathy is less concerned with the intricate biochemistry involved than with whether a remedy ultimately works and heals holistically. For all these reasons, conventional medicine claims that homeopathy is not scientific, but homeopaths are quick to reply that homeopathy has been scientifically developed and studied for centuries, with much documentation and success.

There continue to be many studies that affirm the effectiveness of homeopathic treatments. Among the most celebrated, the *British Medical Journal* in 1991 published a large analysis of homeopathic treatments that were given over the course of 25 years. This project involved more than 100 studies of patients with problems ranging from vascular diseases, respiratory problems, infections, stomach problems, allergies, recovery from surgeries, arthritis, trauma, psychological problems, diabetes, and others. The study found improvement with homeopathic treatment in most categories of problems, and concluded that the evidence was "sufficient for establishing homeopathy as a regular treatment for certain indications."

For example, a study in early 2002 was reported on in a pediatric journal that showed symptom improvement for children with uncomplicated acute otitis media (**ear infection**) who received individualized homeopathic remedies. Although the authors concluded that more research was needed, results were positive enough to justify a larger study.

Training & certification

The Council on Homeopathic Education is the only organization that accredits training programs in classical homeopathy. To date, it has accredited five institutions: Bastyr University of Natural Health Sciences in Seattle; Ontario College of **Naturopathic Medicine** in Toronto; Hahnemann Medical Clinic in Albany, California; the National College of Naturopathic Medicine in Portland, and the International Foundation for Homeopathy, also in Seattle. Other well-known training programs include the Pacific Academy of Homeopathic Medicine in Berkeley, California, and the New England School of Homeopathy in Amherst, Massachusetts.

There are several organizations that certify homeopathic practitioners:

• The National Center for Homeopathy is the largest homeopathic organization, with more than 7,000 members. It also runs the Council on Homeopathic Education, and provides a listing of all its members and their credentials. Address: 801 N. Fairfax St., #306, Alexandria, VA 22314, phone (703) 548-7790.

• The American Institute of Homeopathy is the oldest national medical body. It provides a list of D.Ht.s (Diplomates in Homeopathy) certified by the American Board of Homeotherapeutics. Address: 1585 Glencoe, Denver, CO 80220, phone (303) 898-5477.

• The Council for Homeopathic Certification was created in 1992 to establish a certification exam and a code of ethics. It confers upon qualified practitioners a C.C.H. (Certification in Classical Homeopathy). Address: P.O. Box 157, Corte Madera, CA 94976.

• The Homeopathic Academy of Naturopathic Physicians offers a certification based on a competency exam, the "Diplomate in the Homeopathic Academy of Naturopathic Physicians" (D.H.A.N.P.).

• The North American Society of Homeopaths certifies non-physician homeopaths. Address: 10700 Old County Rd. 15, #350, Minneapolis, MN 55441, phone (612) 593-9458.

Resources

BOOKS

Castro, Miranda. *The Complete Homeopathy Handbook.* New York: St. Martin's, 1990.

Jonas, Wayne B., M.D., and Jennifer Jacobs, M.D. *Healing With Homeopathy.* New York: Warner, 1996.

Ullman, Dana, M.P.H. *The Consumer's Guide to Homeopathy.* New York: Putnam, 1996.

Weiner, Dr. Michael. *The Complete Book of Homeopathy.* New York: Avery, 1996.

PERIODICALS

Homeopathy Today. 801 N. Fairfax St. #306, Alexandria, VA 22314, phone (703) 548-7790.

Simillimum. P.O. Box 69565, Portland, OR 97201, phone (503) 795-0579.

Walsh, Nancy. "Homeopathy Shows Some Promise in AOM (Obstacles to Study this Therapy Remain)." *Pediatric News* (January 2002): 16.

OTHER

Ayurvedic Institute. <http://www.ayurveda.com/>.

National Center for Homeopathy. <http://www.healthy.net/nch/>.

North American Society for Homeopaths. <http://www.homeopathy.org/>.

Homeopathy, acute prescribing

Definition

Acute homeopathic prescribing is that part of **homeopathy** that treats illness of abrupt onset requiring immediate attention. In homeopathic medicine, acute refers primarily to the speed of onset and self-limiting character of the disorder rather than its seriousness. Colds, **influenza**, sore throats, insect stings, cuts, **bruises**, **vomiting**, **diarrhea**, **fever**, muscle aches, and short-term **insomnia** are all examples of conditions that are treated by acute prescribing. The remedies given in acute homeopathic prescribing are intended to stimulate the body's internal ability to heal itself; they do not kill germs or suppress symptoms. Acute prescribing can be done—within limits—by patients at home, as well as by homeopathic practitioners. Study courses, self-treatment guides, and homeopathic home medicine kits are now available by mail order from homeopathic pharmacies and educational services.

Origins

Homeopathy is a gentle, painless, holistic system of healing developed during the 1790s by Samuel Hahnemann, a German physician. Experimenting on himself with the anti-malarial drug quinine, Hahnemann noticed that large doses of the medicine actually caused malaria-like symptoms, while smaller doses cured the symptoms. From this, he advanced his concept of *Similia similibus curentur*, or "let like be cured with like." Hahnemann then developed an extensive system of medicine based on this concept. He named it homeopathy, from the Greek words *homoios* (the same) and *pathos* (suffering).

Homeopathic remedies are almost always made from natural materials—plant, animal, or mineral substances—that have been treated to form mother tinctures or nonsoluble powders. Liquid extracts are then potentized, or increased in power, by a series of dilutions and succussions, or shakings. It is thought that succussion is necessary to transfer the energy of the natural substance to the solution. In addition, the potency of the remedy is regarded as increasing with each dilution. After the tincture has been diluted to the prescribed potency, the resulting solution is added to a bottle of sucrose/lactose tablets, which are stored in a cool, dark place. If the remedy is not soluble in water, it is ground to a fine powder and triturated with powdered lactose to achieve the desired potency.

Proponents of homeopathy over the years have included Louisa May Alcott, Charles Dickens, Benjamin Disraeli, Johann Wolfgang Goethe, Nathaniel Hawthorne, William James, Henry Wadsworth Longfellow, Pope Pius X, John D. Rockefeller, Harriet Beecher Stowe, William Thackeray, Daniel Webster, and W. B. Yeats. England's royal family has employed homeopathic practitioners since the 1830s.

Benefits

Homeopathic physicians seek to cure their patients on physical, mental, and emotional levels, and each treatment is tailored to a patient's individual needs. Homeopathy is generally a safe treatment, as it uses medicines in extremely diluted quantities, and there are usually minimal side effects. Its nontoxicity makes it a good choice for the treatment of children. Another benefit of homeopathy is the cost of treatments; homeopathic remedies are inexpensive, often a fraction of the cost of conventional drugs.

Acute homeopathic prescribing is thought to benefit a wide range of ailments. These include altitude sickness, Bell's palsy, the **common cold**, **allergies**, coughing, dengue fever, dysentery, earaches, migraine headaches, fever, **food poisoning**, grief, influenza, **motion sickness**, shock, **sore throat**, surgical complications, and reactions to vaccinations and drug therapy. Acute remedies may also be prescribed for treat insect stings, animal bites, and problems related to poison **oak** and poison ivy. Homeopathy may be further employed in treating injuries including black eyes, **burns**, bruises, concussions, cuts, damaged tendons and ligaments, dislocations, **fractures**, herniated discs, **nosebleeds**, puncture **wounds**, sprains, and strains.

Description

Homeopathic prescribing differs in general from allopathic medicine in its tailoring of remedies to the patient's overall personality type and totality of symptoms, rather than to the disease. Whereas a conventional physician would prescribe the same medication or treatment regimen to all patients with the common cold, for example, a homeopathic practitioner would ask detailed questions about each patient's symptoms and the modalities, or factors, that make them better or worse. As a result, the homeopath might prescribe six different remedies for six different patients with the same illness. In acute prescribing homeopathy, consultations are more brief compared to constitutional homeopathic prescribing. A typical patient might spend just 10–15 minutes with the practitioner, compared to more than an hour for constitutional prescribing.

Homeopathic classification of symptoms

Homeopathic practitioners use the word symptom in a more inclusive fashion than traditional medicine. In homeopathy, symptoms include any change that the patient experiences during the illness, including changes in emotional or mental patterns.

Homeopaths classify symptoms according to a hierarchy of four categories for purposes of acute prescribing:

• Peculiar symptoms. These are symptoms unique to the individual that do not occur in most persons with the acute disease. Homeopaths make note of peculiar symptoms because they often help to determine the remedy.

• Mental and emotional symptoms. These are important general symptoms that inform the homeopath about the patient's total experience of the disorder.

• Other general symptoms. These are physical symptoms felt throughout the patient's body, such as tiredness, changes in appetite, or restlessness.

• Particular symptoms. Particular symptoms are localized in the body; they include such symptoms as **nausea**, skin **rashes**, **headache**, etc.

During homeopathic case-taking, the practitioner will evaluate the intensity of the patient's symptoms, assess their depth within the patient's body, note any peculiar symptoms, evaluate the modalities of each symptom, and make a list of key symptoms to guide the selection of the proper medicine.

Homeopathic remedies

There are several hundred homeopathic remedies. Homeopathic medicines are usually formulated from diluted or triturated natural substances, including plants, minerals, or even venom from snakes or stinging insects. Some remedies may be given in a spray, ointment, or cream, but the most common forms of administration are liquid dilutions and two sizes of pellets, or cylindrical tablets (for triturated remedies). A dose consists of one drop of liquid; 10–20 small pellets; or 1–3 large pellets. Since the remedies are so dilute, the exact size of the dose is not of primary importance. The frequency of dosing is considered critical, however; patients are advised not to take further doses until the first has completed its effect.

Homeopathic remedies can be kept indefinitely with proper handling. Proper handling includes storing the remedies in the original bottles and discarding them if they become contaminated by sunlight or other intense light; temperatures over 100°F (37.8°C); vapors from camphor, mothballs, or perfume; or from other homeopathic remedies being opened in the same room at the same time.

Preparations

Case-taking

The first step in acute prescribing is a lengthy interview with the patient, known as case-taking. In addition to noting the character, location, and severity of the patient's symptoms, the homeopath will ask about their modalities. The modalities are the circumstances or factors (e.g., weather, time of day, body position, behavior or activity, etc.) that make the symptoms either better or worse. Case-taking can be done by the patient or a family member as well as by a homeopath.

Selection and administration of a remedy

The choice of a specific remedy is guided by the patient's total symptom profile rather than by the illness. Homeopathic remedies are prescribed according to the law of similars, which holds that a substance that produces specific symptoms in healthy people cures those symptoms in sick people when given in highly diluted forms. For example, a patient with influenza who is irritable, headachy, and suffering from joint or muscle pains is likely to be given *bryonia* (wild **hops**), because this plant extract would cause this symptom cluster in a healthy individual.

Patients are instructed to avoid touching homeopathic medicines with their fingers. The dose can be poured onto a piece of white paper or the bottle's cap and tipped directly into the mouth. Homeopathic remedies are not taken with water; patients should not eat or drink anything for 15–20 minutes before or after taking the dose.

Precautions

Homeopathic acute prescribing is not recommended for the treatment of chronic conditions requiring constitutional prescribing, for severe **infections** requiring antibiotic treatment, or for conditions requiring major surgery. It is also not recommended for the treatment of mental health problems.

Persons who are treating themselves with homeopathic remedies should follow professional guidelines regarding the limitations of home treatment. Most homeopathic home treatment guides include necessary information regarding symptoms and disorders that require professional attention.

Homeopathic remedies may lose their potency if used at the same time as other products. Some homeopathic practitioners recommend the avoidance of mint and mentholated products (toothpastes, candies, chewing gum, mouth rinses), as well as camphor and camphorated products (including **eucalyptus** and Tiger Balm), patchouli and other **essential oils**, moth balls, strong perfumes, aftershaves, scented soaps, **stress**, x rays, coffee, nicotine, recreational drugs (**marijuana**) and certain therapeutic drugs (most notably cortisone and prednisone) during treatment. Patients are also advised to avoid electric blankets and dental work, as these are thought to adversely affect homeopathic therapy. Homeopathic remedies should never be placed near magnets.

Practitioners caution that high-potency preparations should be used only under the supervision of a homeopathic practitioner.

Side effects

Homeopathic medicines are so diluted that sometimes no trace of the original substance can be detected. These medicines are therefore considered non-toxic and generally free of harmful side effects. There may, however, be individual reactions to homeopathic medicine.

An intensified healing response may occur as treatment begins, which causes symptoms to worsen, but the phenomenon is temporary. In some patients, old symptoms may re-appear from past conditions from which recovery was not complete. Such phenomena are taken as positive indications that the healing process has commenced.

Research & general acceptance

As Samuel Hahnemann's healing system grew in popularity during the 1800s, it quickly attracted vehement opposition from the medical and apothecary professions. Since the early 1900s, when the American Medical Association and pharmacists waged a battle against it, homeopathy has been neglected and sometimes ridiculed by mainstream medicine. Aside from politics, part of the reason for this hostility is that there are some aspects of homeopathy which have not been completely explained scientifically. For instance, homeopaths have found that the more they dilute and succuss a remedy, the greater effect it seems to have on the body. Some homeopathic remedies are so diluted that not even a single molecule of the active agent remains in a solution, yet homeopaths maintain it still works. Also, homeopathy puts an emphasis on analyzing symptoms and then applying remedies to these symptoms, rather than working by classifying diseases. Thus, some people with the same disease may require different homeopathic medicines and treatments. Furthermore, conventional medicine strive to find out how physicians work in the body before they use them; homeopathy is less concerned with the intricate biochemistry involved than with whether a remedy ultimately works and heals holistically. For all these reasons, conventional medicine claims that homeopathy is not scientific, while homeopaths are quick to reply that homeopathy has been scientifically developed and studied for centuries with much documentation and success.

There continue to be many studies on the effectiveness of homeopathic treatments. Among the most celebrated, the *British Medical Journal* in 1991 published a large analysis of homeopathic treatments that were given over the course of 25 years. This project involved more than 100 studies of patients with problems ranging from vascular diseases, respiratory problems, infections, stomach problems, allergies, recovery from surgeries, arthritis, trauma, psychological problems, diabetes, and others. The study found improvement with homeopathic treatment in most categories of problems, and concluded that the evidence was "sufficient for establishing homeopathy as a regular treatment for certain indications."

A 2002 pediatric journal article reported on a study that showed some individualized homeopathic remedies eased the symptoms of uncomplicated acute otitis media (ear infections) in children. While the authors admitted more research was needed, they said the positive results justified further study on homeopathic remedies for childhood ear infections.

In the United Kingdom and other countries where homeopathy is especially popular, some medical doctors incorporate aspects of acute prescribing homeopathy into their practices. Countries in which homeopathy is popular include France, India, Pakistan, Sri Lanka, Brazil, and Argentina. Large homeopathic hospitals exist in London and Glasgow, and homeopathic medical centers can be found in India and South America.

Training & certification

It takes three to four years of training to become a qualified homeopath. Naturopathic physicians study homeopathy during their four-year medical school programs, and other practitioners may study homeopathy in post-graduate courses. The Council on Homeopathic Education is the only organization that accredits training programs in classical homeopathy. To date, it has accredited five institutions: Bastyr University of Natural Health Sciences in Seattle, Washington; Ontario College of **Naturopathic Medicine** in Toronto; Hahnemann Medical Clinic in Albany, California; the National College of Naturopathic Medicine in Portland, Oregon; and the International Foundation for Homeopathy, also in Seattle. Other well-known training programs include the Pacific Academy of Homeopathic Medicine in Berkeley, California, and the New England School of Homeopathy in Amherst, Massachusetts.

There are several organizations that certify homeopathic practitioners:

• The National Center for Homeopathy is the largest homeopathic organization, with over 7,000 members. It also runs the Council on Homeopathic Education, and provides a listing of all its members and their credentials.

• The American Institute of Homeopathy is the oldest national medical body. It provides a list of D.Ht.s (Diplomates in Homeopathy) certified by the American Board of Homeotherapeutics.

• The Council for Homeopathic Certification was created in 1992 to establish a certification exam and a code of ethics. It confers upon qualified practitioners a C.C.H. (Certification in Classical Homeopathy).

• The Homeopathic Academy of Naturopathic Physicians offers a certification based on a competency exam, the "Diplomate in the Homeopathic Academy of Naturopathic Physicians" (D.H.A.N.P.).

• The North American Society of Homeopaths certifies non-physician homeopaths.

Resources

BOOKS

Cummings, Stephen, and Dana Ullman. *Everybody's Guide to Homeopathic Medicines.* Los Angeles: Jeremy P. Tarcher, Inc., 1991.

KEY TERMS

Acute prescribing—Homeopathic treatment for self-limiting illnesses with abrupt onset.

Allopathy—Conventional medical treatment of disease symptoms that uses substances or techniques to oppose or suppress the symptoms.

Law of similars—The basic principle of homeopathic medicine that governs the selection of a specific remedy. It holds that a substance of natural origin that produces certain symptoms in a healthy person will cure those same symptoms in a sick person.

Modalities—The factors and circumstances that cause a patient's symptoms to improve or worsen.

Mother tincture—The first stage in the preparation of a homeopathic remedy, made by soaking a plant, animal, or mineral product in a solution of alcohol.

Potentization—The process of increasing the power of homeopathic preparations by successive dilutions and successions of a mother tincture.

Succussion—The act of shaking diluted homeopathic remedies as part of the process of potentization.

Trituration—The process of diluting a nonsoluble substance for homeopathic use by grinding it to a fine powder and mixing it with lactose powder.

MacEoin, Beth. *Homeopathy.* New York: HarperCollins Publishers, 1994.

Strohecker, James. *Alternative Medicine: The Definitive Guide.* Tiburon, Calif.: Future Medicine Publishing, Inc., 1999.

Ullman, Dana. *Discovering Homeopathy: Your Introduction to the Science and Art of Homeopathic Medicine.* Berkeley, Calif.: North Atlantic Books, 1991.

Vithoulkas, George. *Homeopathy: Medicine of the New Man.* New York: Fireside Books (Simon & Schuster), 1992.

PERIODICALS

Walsh, Nancy. "Homeopathy Shows Some Promise in AOM (Obstacles to Study this Therapy Remain)." *Pediatric News* (January 2002): 16.

ORGANIZATIONS

The American Institute of Homeopathy. 1585 Glencoe, Denver, CO 80220. (303) 898-5477.

The Council for Homeopathic Certification. P.O. Box 157, Corte Madera, CA 94976.

The International Foundation for Homeopathy. 2366 Eastlake Avenue East, #301, Seattle, WA 98102. (425)776-4147.

The National Center for Homeopathy. 801 North Fairfax Street, Suite 306, Alexandria, VA 22134. (703) 548-7790.

The North American Society of Homeopaths. 10700 Old County Rd. 15, #350, Minneapolis, MN 55441. (612) 593-9458.

Patricia Skinner

Homeopathy, constitutional prescribing

Definition

Constitutional homeopathic prescribing, also called classical prescribing, is a holistic system of medicine that has been practiced for more than 200 years. Unlike acute homeopathic prescribing, constitutional prescribing refers to the selection and administration of homeopathic preparations over a period of time for treatment related to what practitioners call miasmic disorders, those caused by an inherited predisposition to a disease. The term miasm comes from a Greek word meaning stain or pollution. As in acute prescribing, constitutional prescribing is holistic in that it is intended to treat the patient on the emotional and spiritual levels of his or her being as well as the physical. Constitutional prescribing is also aimed at eventual cure of the patient, not just suppression or relief of immediate symptoms.

Origins

Homeopathy was developed during the 1790s by **Samuel Hahnemann**, a German physician. Experimenting on himself with the anti-malarial drug quinine, Hahnemann noticed that large doses of the medicine actually caused malaria-like symptoms, while smaller doses cured the symptoms. From this, he advanced his concept of *Similia similibus curentur*, or "let like be cured with like." Hahnemann then developed an extensive system of medicine based on this concept. He named it homeopathy, from the Greek words *homoios* (the same) and *pathos* (suffering).

There are several hundred homeopathic remedies. They are almost always made from natural materials—plant, animal, or mineral substances—that have been treated to form mother tinctures or nonsoluble powders. Liquid extracts are then potentized, or increased in power, by a series of dilutions and successions, or shakings. It is thought that succussion is necessary to transfer the energy of the natural substance to the solution. In addition, the potency of the remedy is regarded as increasing with each dilution. After the tincture has been diluted to the prescribed potency, the resulting solution is added to a bottle of sucrose/lactose tablets, which are stored in a cool, dark place. If the remedy is not soluble in water, it is ground to a fine powder and triturated with powdered lactose to achieve the desired potency.

Proponents of homeopathy over the years have included Louisa May Alcott, Charles Dickens, Benjamin Disraeli, Johann Wolfgang von Goethe, Nathaniel Hawthorne, William James, Henry Wadsworth Longfellow, Pope Pius X, John D. Rockefeller, Harriet Beecher Stowe, William Thackeray, Daniel Webster, and W. B. Yeats. England's royal family has employed homeopathic practitioners since the 1830s.

Benefits

Homeopathic physicians seek to cure their patients on physical, mental, and emotional levels, and each treatment is tailored to a patient's individual needs. Homeopathy is generally a safe treatment, as it uses medicines in extremely diluted quantities, and there are usually minimal side effects. Its nontoxicity makes some consider it a good choice for the treatment of children. Another benefit of homeopathy is the cost of treatments; homeopathic remedies are inexpensive, often a fraction of the cost of conventional drugs.

Classical homeopathy has been used to treat a wide range of diseases and conditions, most of which tend to be long-term. These include: **alcoholism**, **allergies**, **anxiety**, arthritis, **asthma**, bladder conditions, **chronic fatigue syndrome**, **depression**, drug dependencies, gastrointestinal problems, Gulf War sickness, **headache**, hearing problems, herpes, hypersensitivity, immune disorders, **insomnia**, joint problems, kidney conditions, liver problems, **Lyme disease**, lower back problems, **malaria**, **menopause**, menstrual problems, migraine, **multiple sclerosis**, paralysis, **phobias**, **shingles**, sinus problems, skin disorders, repetitive **stress** injury, rheumatism, vertigo, vision problems, and yeast **infections**.

Description

Constitutional prescribing is based on the patient's symptom profile and specific aspects of homeopathic theory.

Homeopathic classification of symptoms

Homeopathic practitioners use the word symptom in a more inclusive fashion than traditional medicine. In homeopathy, symptoms include any change that the patient experiences during the illness, including changes in emotional or mental patterns.

Homeopaths classify symptoms according to a hierarchy of four categories:

• Peculiar symptoms. These are symptoms unique to the individual that do not occur in most persons. Homeopaths make note of peculiar symptoms because they often help to determine the remedy.

• Mental and emotional symptoms. These are important general symptoms that inform the homeopath about the patient's total experience of the disorder.

• Other general symptoms. These are physical symptoms felt throughout the patient's body, such as tiredness, changes in appetite, or restlessness.

• Particular symptoms. Particular symptoms are localized in the body; they include such symptoms as **nausea**, skin **rashes**, or headaches.

Miasms

Homeopaths regard the patient's symptom profile as a systemic manifestation of an underlying chronic disorder called a miasm. Miasms are serious disturbances of what homeopaths call the patient's vital force that are inherited from parents at the time of conception. Hahnemann believed that the parents' basic lifestyle, their emotional condition and habitual diet, and even the atmospheric conditions at the time of conception would affect the number and severity of miasms passed on to the child. Hahnemann himself distinguished three miasms: the psoric, which he considered the most universal source of chronic disease in humans; the syphilitic; and the sycotic, which he attributed to **gonorrhea**. Later homeopaths identified two additional miasms, the cancernic and the tuberculinic. The remaining major source of miasms is allopathic medicine. It is thought that specific allopathic treatments—particularly smallpox vaccinations, cortisone preparations, major tranquilizers, and antibiotics—can produce additional layers of miasms in the patient's constitution. Constitutional prescribing evaluates the person's current state or miasmic picture, and selects a remedy intended to correct or balance that state. The homeopath may prescribe a different remedy for each miasmic layer over time, but gives only one remedy at a time directed at the person's current state. The basic principle governing the prescription of each successive remedy is the law of similars, or "like cures like."

Hering's laws of cure

The homeopathic laws of cure were outlined by Constantine Hering, a student of Hahnemann who came to the United States in the 1830s. Hering enunciated three laws or principles of the patterns of healing that are used by homeopaths to evaluate the effectiveness of specific remedies and the overall progress of constitutional prescribing:

• Healing progresses from the deepest parts of the organism to the external parts. Homeopaths consider the person's mental and emotional dimensions, together with the brain, heart, and other vital organs, as a person's deepest parts. The skin, hands, and feet are considered the external parts.

• Symptoms appear or disappear in the reverse of their chronological order of appearance. In terms of constitutional treatment, this law means that miasms acquired later in life will resolve before earlier ones.

• Healing proceeds from the upper to the lower parts of the body.

Healing crises

Homeopaths use Hering's laws to explain the appearance of so-called healing crises, or aggravations, in the course of homeopathic treatment. It is not unusual for patients to experience temporary worsening of certain symptoms after taking their first doses of homeopathic treatment. For example, a person might notice that arthritic pains in the shoulders are better but that the hands feel worse. Hering's third law would indicate that the remedy is working because the symptoms are moving downward in the body. In constitutional prescribing, a remedy that removes one of the patient's miasmic layers will then allow the symptoms of an older miasm to emerge. Thus the patient may find that a physical disease is followed by a different set of physical problems or by emotional symptoms.

Preparations

The most important aspects of preparation for constitutional prescribing are the taking of a complete patient history and careful patient education.

Case-taking

Homeopathic case-taking for constitutional prescribing is similar to that for acute prescribing, but more in-depth. The initial interview generally takes one to two hours. The practitioner is concerned with recording the totality of the patient's symptoms and the modalities that influence their severity. Also included are general characteristics about the patient and his or her lifestyle choices. For example, a practitioner might ask the patient if he or she likes being outside or is generally hot or cold. There is also an emphasis on the patient's lifetime medical history, particularly records of allopathic treatments.

Patient education

Homeopaths regard patients as equal partners in the process of recovery. They will take the time to explain the theories underlying constitutional prescribing to the patient as well as taking the history. Patient education is especially important in constitutional prescribing in order to emphasize the need for patience with the slowness of results and length of treatment, and to minimize the possibility of self-treatment with allopathic drugs if the patient has a healing crisis.

Homeopathic remedies

In constitutional prescribing, one dose of the selected remedy is given. Patients then wait two to six weeks before following up with the homeopath, while the body begins the healing process. At the follow-up visit, the remedy may be repeated, or a different remedy prescribed. The preparation, selection, administration, and storage of remedies for constitutional prescribing are the same as for acute prescribing. These procedures are described more fully in the article on acute prescribing.

Precautions

Constitutional homeopathic prescribing is not appropriate for diseases or health crises requiring emergency treatment, whether medical, surgical, or psychiatric. In addition, constitutional prescribing should not be self-administered. Although home treatment kits of homeopathic remedies are available for acute self-limited disorders, the knowledge of homeopathic theory and practice required for constitutional evaluation is beyond the scope of most patients.

Patients are instructed to avoid touching homeopathic medicines with their fingers. The dose can be poured onto a piece of white paper or the bottle's cap and tipped directly into the mouth. Homeopathic remedies are not taken with water; patients should not eat or drink anything for 15–20 minutes before or after taking the dose.

Homeopathic remedies may lose their potency if used at the same time as other products. Some homeopathic practitioners recommend the avoidance of mint and mentholated products (toothpastes, candies, chewing gum, mouth rinses), as well as camphor and camphorated products (including **eucalyptus** and Tiger Balm), patchouli and other **essential oils**, moth balls, strong perfumes, aftershaves, scented soaps, stress, x rays, coffee, nicotine, recreational drugs (**marijuana**) and certain therapeutic drugs (most notably cortisone and prednisone) during treatment. Patients are also advised to avoid electric blankets and dental work, as these are thought to adversely affect homeopathic therapy. Homeopathic remedies should never be placed near magnets.

Side effects

Homeopathic medicines are so diluted that sometimes no trace of the original substance can be detected. These medicines are therefore considered non-toxic and generally free of harmful side effects. The primary risks to the patient from constitutional homeopathic treatment are the symptoms of the healing crisis and individual reactions to homeopathic medicine. The complexity of constitutional prescribing requires homeopaths to have detailed knowledge of the *materia medica* and the repertories, and to take careful and extensive case notes.

An intensified healing response may occur as treatment begins, which causes symptoms to worsen, but the phenomenon is temporary. In some patients, old symptoms may re-appear from past conditions from which recovery was not complete. Such phenomena are taken as positive indications that the healing process has commenced.

Research & general acceptance

As Samuel Hahnemann's healing system grew in popularity during the 1800s, it quickly attracted vehement opposition from the medical and apothecary professions. Since the early 1900s, when the American Medical Association and pharmacists waged a battle against it, homeopathy has been neglected and sometimes ridiculed by mainstream medicine. Aside from politics, part of the reason for this opposition is that there are some aspects of homeopathy which have not been completely explained scientifically. For instance, homeopaths have found that the more they dilute and succuss a remedy, the greater effect it seems to have on the body. Some homeopathic remedies are so diluted that not even a single molecule of the active agent remains in a solution, yet homeopaths maintain that it still works. Also, homeopathy puts an emphasis on analyzing symptoms and then applying remedies to these symptoms, rather than working by classifying diseases. Thus some people with the same disease may require different homeopathic medicines and treatments. Furthermore, conventional medicine strives to find out how medicines work in the body before they use them; homeopathy is less concerned with the intricate biochemistry involved than with whether a remedy ultimately works and heals holistically. For all these reasons, conventional medicine claims that homeopathy is not scientific, while homeopaths are quick to reply that homeopathy has been scientifically developed and studied for centuries, with much documentation and success.

There continue to be many studies on the effectiveness of homeopathic treatments. Among the most celebrated, the *British Medical Journal* in 1991 published a large analysis of homeopathic treatments that were given over the course of 25 years. This project involved more than 100 studies of patients with problems ranging from vascular diseases, respiratory problems, infections, stomach problems, allergies, recovery from surgeries, arthritis, trauma, psychological problems, diabetes, and others. The study found improvement with homeopathic treatment in most categories of problems, and concluded that the evidence was "sufficient for establishing homeopathy as a regular treatment for certain indications."

In early 2002, a study in England sought to prove homeopathy's effect on treating chronic **fatigue** syndrome. Homeopathic consultations with patients took place monthly and the homeopaths in the study were allowed to choose any remedies they deemed appropriate and changed them as needed. Patients who received homeopathic treatments reported feeling more rested, less tired, and fitter than those in the placebo control group. Overall, nearly two-thirds of chronic fatigue patients reported some improvement.

In the United Kingdom and other countries where homeopathy is especially popular, some medical doctors incorporate aspects of **acute prescribing homeopathy** into their practices. Countries in which homeopathy is popular include France, India, Pakistan, Sri Lanka, Brazil, and Argentina. Large homeopathic hospitals exist in London and Glasgow, and homeopathic medical centers can be found in India and South America.

Training & certification

It takes three to four years of training to become a qualified homeopath. Naturopathic physicians study homeopathy during their four-year medical school programs, and other practitioners may study homeopathy in post-graduate courses. The Council on Homeopathic Education is the only organization that accredits training programs in classical homeopathy. As of 2004, it has accredited five institutions: Bastyr University of Natural Health Sciences in Seattle, Washington; Ontario College of **Naturopathic Medicine** in Toronto; Hahnemann Medical Clinic in Albany, California; the National College of Naturopathic Medicine in Portland, Oregon; and the International Foundation for Homeopathy, also in Seattle. Other well-known training programs include the Pacific Academy of Homeopathic Medicine in Berkeley, California, and the New England School of Homeopathy in Amherst, Massachusetts.

There are several organizations that certify homeopathic practitioners:

• The National Center for Homeopathy is the largest homeopathic organization, with over 7,000 members. It also runs the Council on Homeopathic Education, and provides a listing of all its members and their credentials.

• The American Institute of Homeopathy is the oldest national medical body. It provides a list of D.Ht.s (Diplo-

---

KEY TERMS

. . . .

Aggravation—Another term used by homeopaths for the healing crisis.

Allopathy—Conventional medical treatment of disease symptoms that uses substances or techniques to oppose or suppress the symptoms.

Constitutional prescribing—Homeopathic treatment for long-term or chronic disorders related to inherited predispositions to certain types of illnesses.

Healing crisis—A temporary worsening of the patient's symptoms during successive stages of homeopathic treatment.

Law of similars—The basic principle of homeopathic medicine that governs the selection of a specific remedy. It holds that a substance of natural origin that produces certain symptoms in a healthy person will cure those same symptoms in a sick person.

Laws of cure—A set of three rules used by homeopaths to assess the progress of a patient's recovery.

Materia medica—In homeopathy, reference books compiled from provings of the various natural remedies.

Miasm—In homeopathic theory, a general weakness or predisposition to chronic disease that is transmitted down the generational chain.

Modalities—The factors and circumstances that cause a patient's symptoms to improve or worsen, including weather, time of day, effects of food, and similar factors.

Repertories—Homeopathic reference books consisting of descriptions of symptoms. The process of selecting a homeopathic remedy from the patient's symptom profile is called repertorizing.

---

mates in Homeopathy) certified by the American Board of Homeotherapeutics.

• The Council for Homeopathic Certification was created in 1992 to establish a certification exam and a code of ethics. It confers upon qualified practitioners a C.C.H. (Certification in Classical Homeopathy).

• The Homeopathic Academy of Naturopathic Physicians offers a certification based on a competency exam, the "Diplomate in the Homeopathic Academy of Naturopathic Physicians" (D.H.A.N.P.).

• The North American Society of Homeopaths certifies non-physician homeopaths.

Resources

BOOKS

Cummings, Stephen, and Dana Ullman. *Everybody's Guide to Homeopathic Medicines.* Los Angeles: Jeremy P. Tarcher, Inc., 1991.

MacEoin, Beth. *Homeopathy.* New York: HarperCollins Publishers, 1994.

Strohecker, James. *Alternative Medicine: The Definitive Guide.* Tiburon, Calif.: Future Medicine Publishing, Inc., 1999.

Ullman, Dana. *Discovering Homeopathy: Your Introduction to the Science and Art of Homeopathic Medicine.* Berkeley, Calif.: North Atlantic Books, 1991.

Vithoulkas, George. *Homeopathy: Medicine of the New Man.* New York: Fireside Books (Simon & Schuster), 1992.

PERIODICALS

Walsh, Nancy. "Homeopathy May Help Patients with Chronic Fatigue Syndrome." *Clinical Psychiatry News* (March 2002): 27.

ORGANIZATIONS

The American Institute of Homeopathy. 1585 Glencoe, Denver, CO 80220. (303) 898-5477.

The Council for Homeopathic Certification. P.O. Box 157, Corte Madera, CA 94976.

The International Foundation for Homeopathy. 2366 Eastlake Avenue East, #301, Seattle, WA 98102. (425)776-4147.

The National Center for Homeopathy. 801 North Fairfax Street, Suite 306, Alexandria, VA 22134. (703) 548-7790.

The North American Society of Homeopaths. 10700 Old County Rd. 15, #350, Minneapolis, MN 55441. (612) 593-9458.

Patricia Skinner

Honeysuckle

Description

Honeysuckle is a large, volubilate shrub of the genus *Lonicera*. There are over 300 species of honeysuckle in the Caprifoliaceae family, found from Asia to North America. The shrub reaches heights of 20–30 ft (6–9 m), with thin, hairy branches. It has ovoid leaves that range 1.2–3.2 in (3–8 cm) long by 0.6–1.6 in (1.5–4.0 cm) wide. The plant flowers in late spring or early summer, depending on the species. Japanese honeysuckle (*Lonicera japonica*) blooms in the spring from April to May, with fragrant white flowers touched with a shade of purple that fade to yellow as they mature. The species of honeysuckle that is found in North America, the United Kingdom, and western Asia, *Lonicera caprifolium*, flowers in June. Generally, honeysuckle flowers are 1.2–1.6 in (3–4) cm long, with an inner tube of approximately the same length. All varieties of honeysuckle are famous for this tube, which is extracted and sucked for its sweet nectar. The shrub also produces a black berry. Despite the sweetness of its fragrance and nectar, the medicinal parts of the plant are bitter, due to the saponin in its stem, the 8% tannin in the leaves and the 1% insitol in its flowers.

General use

Japanese honeysuckle (*L. japonica*, also called Japanese *jin yin hua,* which means gold and silver flower) and common honeysuckle (*L. caprifolium*, also called Italian honeysuckle, Dutch honeysuckle, and woodbine) are both widely used for their medicinal qualities. Although the Chinese most commonly use the bud of the flower in their medical practice, in other countries it is mostly the flowers and leaves that are used for their healing properties. Japanese honeysuckle works well as a detoxifier, and is best used for acute **infections** and inflammations. As an alterative, which cleanses and purifies the blood, and an antipyretic, which reduces fever with its cooling properties, Japanese honeysuckle is best used for such ailments as sore throats, swollen eyes, headaches, etc.

Acute infections and inflammations

Japanese honeysuckle is most useful in treating acute illnesses, infections and inflammations. At the onset of a cold, honeysuckle should be taken in combination with chrysanthemum flowers. Several popular Chinese formulas, such as *yin chaio* and *ganmaoling,* contain this herbal combination. Because it is a natural antibiotic, honeysuckle can also be used to treat infections caused by staphylococcal or streptococcal bacteria. Honeysuckle should be used for acute conditions, and is not meant to be used in the treatment of chronic illnesses.

Skin infections

Honeysuckle works well against internal infections, and it can also be used externally for skin irritation and infections. Honeysuckle has been found useful in alleviating **rashes** ranging from skin diseases to poison **oak**. For these types of skin ailments, honeysuckle is best used as a poultice. For cuts and abrasions that may become infected, a honeysuckle infusion can be applied externally. It is in treating skin infections that the stems of honeysuckle are used.

Circulatory system

John Gerard, a master herbalist of the sixteenth century, said that honeysuckle's "floures, be steeped in oile,

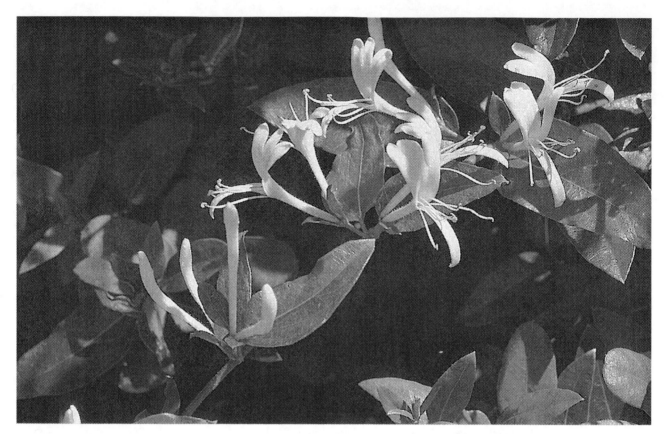

Honeysuckle. (*© PlantaPhile, Germany. Reproduced by permission.*)

and set in the Sun, are good to annoint the body that is bennumed, and growne very cold." Indeed, *L. caprifolium* as a fixed oil is good for the circulatory system. When it is heated and smoothed onto the skin, it has been shown to have a vasodilatory effect, causing the blood to flow into the dermis, which is the thick layer of skin beneath the epidermis.

Asthma and coughs

L. caprifolium can be used for **asthma** on account of its antispasmodic properties. An herbal infusion of the leaves is the best method for treating asthma. A decoction of honeysuckle flowers can be used for coughs.

Other uses

The seeds of *L. caprifolium* can be used as a diuretic. *L. villosa*, also known as American honeysuckle, has been used as a kidney stimulant. *L. japonica* has been used to treat dysentery, and **diarrhea**.

Preparations

Three teaspoons of the leaf infusion can be taken three times a day. For skin irritation, honeysuckle should be made into an infusion or poultice and applied externally to the skin. When honeysuckle is compounded in capsule form, 10–17 g can be taken daily.

Precautions

Although honeysuckle poultices are used for skin irritations, there have been cases of contact dermititis reported from pulling up Japanese honeysuckle. A patient that had come into contact with *L. japonica* reported developing a line of itchy **blisters**. People often taste honeysuckle tubes for their nectar; however, several cases of plant poisoning have been reported in children. The symptoms include gastrointestinal discomfort and muscle cramps.

Side effects

There are no known side effects from using honeysuckle.

Interactions

No known adverse drug interactions have been reported with honeysuckle.

KEY TERMS

Alterative—A substance that cleanses and purifies the blood.

Antipyretic—A substance or medication that combats fever with cooling properties.

Antispasmodic—A substance or medication that prevents spasms or cramps.

Vasodilatory—Having the effect of relaxing or widening the blood vessels.

Resources

BOOKS

Hallowell, Michael. *Herbal Healing*. Vonore, TN: Avery Publishing Group, 1994.

Mabey, Richard. *The New Age Herbalist*. London: Gaia Books, 1988.

Ritchason, Jack. *The Little Herb Encyclopedia*. Pleasant Grove, UT: Woodland Health Books, 1995.

Katherine Y. Kim

Hops

Description

Hops come from the large perennial vine *Humulus lupulus*. This plant is native to North America and Europe, but is cultivated in many other places. The vine grows to a height of 25 ft (8 m). It has heart-shaped dark green leaves and yellowish green flowers. Each plant produces either male or female flowers. Only the female flowers, called strobiles, are used medicinally. Strobiles are picked in autumn and either used fresh or dried.

General use

Hops have been cultivated to be used in the brewing of beer since at least A. D. 1000, but they also have a mixed history of use in healing. Ancient Hebrews used hops to help ward off plague. In North America, several Native American tribes independently discovered the healing properties of hops and used them as a sedative and sleep aid, to relieve **toothache**, and to improve digestion. By the end of the 1800s, hops were being routinely used in mainstream medicine in the United States as a sedative and digestive tonic. Although hops were sometimes used as a sleep aid in Europe, until relatively recently their major use in Europe was in the brewing of beer, to which they add a bitter flavor and act as a preservative.

Today European herbalists are much more enthusiastic about the healing properties of hops. They are used in three ways: as a sedative, to aid digestion, and as an antibiotic.

Hops' best known medicinal function is as a mild sedative and sleep aid. For centuries pillows filled with hops have been prescribed for people who have difficulty falling asleep. Hops extracts taken orally are also said to promote sleep. Hops are chemically complex and contain many different compounds. Scientists have separated out several components that are sedative in nature, although it is not clear whether hops contain enough of these compounds to actually make a person sleepy. Studies are ongoing, but the German Federal Health Agency's Commission E, established in 1978 to independently review and evaluate scientific literature and case studies pertaining to herb and plant medications, has approved hops for sleep problems, restlessness, and **anxiety**. Hops belongs to the same family of herbs as **marijuana**, and some people claim it produces a mild, relaxed, euphoric feeling when smoked. There is no scientific evidence for this claim.

The second major use of hops is as an aid to digestion. It has been used for centuries in both **traditional Chinese medicine** and Native American healing to stimulate the appetite, ease digestion, and aid in relieving **colic**. It is believed that hops stimulates the secretions of the stomach.

The German E Commission has also concluded that hops may act as a digestive aid. Scientists have isolated another extract from the plant that in the laboratory inhibits spasms in the digestive tract and other smooth muscle. Follow-up studies in people have not yet been done.

Chinese healers use hops to treat **tuberculosis** and as an antibiotic. Test-tube studies show that the bitter acids in hops inhibit the growth of certain bacteria and fungi, including the common bacteria *Staphylococcis aureus* (responsible for staph **infections**) and *Bacillus subtilis*; but do not inhibit *Escherichia coli*, a bacterium that causes digestive upsets. This antibacterial action may account for the preservative effect of hops in brewed beer. A 1999 study also showed that some compounds isolated from hops were effective in test-tube studies in reducing the proliferation of certain types of human breast and **ovarian cancer** cells. As of 2002, hops extract is being studied as a possible **cancer** chemopreventive.

There has been much debate in the healing community about whether hops contain a compound related to or easily converted into estrogen, the main female hormone. Some herbalists believe that the presence of an estrogenic compound accounts for the dampening of male sexual arousal and the control of sexual nervous tension

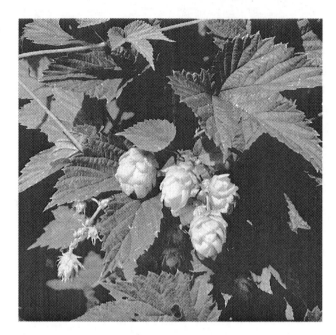

Hops plants. *(Photograph by Bill Howes. Frank Lane Picture Agency/Corbis- Bettmann. Reproduced by permission.)*

ascribed to fresh hops. Other herbalists disagree, maintaining that those effects are related only to the relaxing or sedative properties of hops. In 2002, however, a team of British researchers reported on the activity of a phytoestrogen that was recently discovered in the female flowers of hops plants. The compound, known as 8-prenylnaringenin, appears to be stronger than previously identified phytoestrogens.

In addition to their uses in healing, hops are used as an ingredient in perfume and occasionally as a tobacco or food flavoring. Their main food use and commercial value is in beer.

Preparations

Fresh and dried hops have different properties and are used to treat different symptoms. Fresh or newly dried hops, usually dampened with glycerin to reduce the rustling noise, are used in sleep pillows to help ease a restless or anxious person into sleep. As the hops age, they change in chemical composition. For this reason, the hops in pillows should be changed every few months. Fresh hops can also be made into a tea that is taken to combat **insomnia**. The tea is made by steeping about two teaspoons of fresh hops in one cup (250 ml) of boiling **water** for five minutes.

Dried hops change in composition when exposed to light, heat, or moisture. They should be stored in a container that excludes moisture and light, and should be kept at room temperature. Dried hops are used to treat di-

gestive and other complaints. They can be prepared in a myriad of different ways. As a tincture, about 1/2 tsp (2 ml) can be taken three times a day. Capsules are available commercially to take before meals to aid digestion. Dry extract or powder can be added to boiling water to make a tea. Compresses are made by soaking a pad in the infusion or diluted tincture. An essential oil is produced by steam distillation. Hops are also used in combination with other herbs in commercially available remedies.

Precautions

Hops are not recommended for people suffering from **depression**. Their sedative action may accentuate depressive symptoms in these people. Some herbalists recommend that pregnant women and those with estrogen sensitive **breast cancer** avoid hops because of the possibility that they contain an estrogenic compound. Hops are included on the United States Food and Drug Administration's list of foods "Generally Recognized As Safe" (GRAS).

Side effects

There are no known side effects if hops are used in the recommended dosages. Some people who pick fresh hops may develop a skin rash (**contact dermatitis**).

Interactions

There has been little scientific study of the interaction of hops and pharmaceuticals. As noted above, however, people who are depressed or who are taking medications for depression should consult a doctor before using hops.

Resources

BOOKS

Chevallier, Andrew. *Encyclopedia of Medicinal Plants.* Boston, MA: DK Publishers, 1996.

Lawless, Julia. *The Illustrated Encyclopedia of Essential Oils.* Rockport, MA: Element.

PDR for Herbal Medicines. Montvale, NJ: Medical Economics Company, 1998.

Peirce, Andrea. *The American Pharmaceutical Association Practical Guide to Natural Medicines.* New York: William Morrow and Company, 1999.

Weiner, Michael A., and Janet Weiner. *Herbs That Heal.* Mill Valley, CA: Quantum Books, 1999.

PERIODICALS

Kapadia, G. J., M. A. Azuine, H. Tokuda, et al. "Inhibitory Effect of Herbal Remedies on 12-o-Tetradecanoylphorbol-13-Acetate-Promoted Epstein-Barr Virus Early Antigen Activation." *Pharmacological Research* 45 (March 2002): 213–222.

KEY TERMS

Phytoestrogen—Any of several compounds found in plants that possess estrogen-like activity.

Tincture—An alcohol-based extract prepared by soaking plant parts.

Milligan, S., J. Kalita, V. Pocock, et al. "Oestrogenic Activity of the Hop Phyto-Oestrogen, 8-Prenylnaringenin." *Reproduction* 123 (February 2002): 235–242.

Tish Davidson
Rebecca J. Frey, PhD

Horehound

Description

Horehound (*Marrubium vulgare L.*), commonly known as white horehound, is a European native of the Lamiaciae or mint family. Other names for this ancient remedy include houndsbane, marrubium, eye of the star, seed of Horus, marvel, bulls' blood, and houndsbane. Horehound is a hardy perennial that has naturalized throughout North America; it may be found in sunny, wayside places, thriving even in poor, dry soil. The common name horehound comes from the Old English words *har* and *hune*, meaning downy plant. This descriptive name refers to the white hairs that give this herb its distinctive hoary appearance. Another suggested derivation is from the name of the Egyptian god of sky and light, Horus. Horehound is one of the oldest known **cough** remedies. It was one of the herbs in the medicine chests of the Egyptian pharaohs. In Roman times, Caesar's antidote for poison included horehound. The generic name is believed to be derived from the Hebrew word *marrob*, meaning bitter juice. Horehound is one of the bitter herbs used in the Jewish Passover rites. Throughout its long history, white horehound has been valued not only as a folk remedy for coughs and congested lungs, but also as a magic herb for protection against the spells attributed to witches.

Black horehound (*Ballota nigra*), also known as black stinking horehound, is the smelly relative of white horehound. It belongs to the same family of plants as white horehound and is credited with some of the same medicinal applications. Both black and white horehound have been used to treat the bites of snakes and mad dogs, to rid the system of intestinal **worms**, and as antidotes to vegetable poisons. Black horehound is considered to be especially useful in quelling the **nausea** associated with **motion sickness**, or to stop the **vomiting** brought on by nervous tension. It also acts as an emmenagogue, restoring a healthy balance to the menstrual cycle.

White horehound is a bushy plant that grows nearly 2 ft (61 cm) tall from a short, stout, and woody root. The small oval leaves are bitter to the taste, with a musky aroma. They are wrinkled and dark green on top, and pale with downy white hairs on the underside. The leaves are opposite and deeply veined, growing on hairy, square, branching stems also covered with downy white hairs. The lower leaves of white horehound have long stalks, while the upper leaves are smaller and stalkless. The small white flowers form dense whorls at the leaf axils, blooming in the second year of growth from June to August. Flowers are tubular with two lips. Four small shiny dark brown seeds are carried in each nutlet after flowering. Horehound seeds have tiny barbs to attach to animal fur and clothing, while horehound blossoms attract bees to the garden.

General use

White horehound is best known as a time-honored cough remedy, found in syrup, candy and tea preparations. The aerial parts of the plant are used medicinally. The active ingredients include sesquiterpene **bitters**, marrubin, volatile oil, tannins, flavonoids, and mucilage. White horehound is antiseptic. An infusion used as a wash, or a preparation of horehound salve is useful to disinfect **wounds**. A cold infusion of white horehound acts as a bitter digestive tonic and will stimulate the flow of bile from the gall bladder. It is diuretic and may also relieve flatulence and stimulate appetite. White horehound stimulates discharge of bronchial mucus, loosening and expelling phlegm. It is beneficial in the treatment of **croup, bronchitis**, and **whooping cough**, and has been in the past in the treatment of **tuberculosis**, once known as consumption. White horehound is also said to normalize cardiac arrhythmias. A warm infusion is diaphoretic, meaning that it will promote sweating. It has been used to break fevers and to treat **jaundice** and typhoid **fever**. The finely chopped leaves, mixed with honey and chewed slowly, will ease a **sore throat** and relieve hoarseness. The herb was also used following **childbirth** to promote expulsion of the placenta. White horehound combines well with other herbs in medicinal infusions, including elecampane (*Inula helenium L.*) and **licorice** (*Glycyrrhiza glabra*).

Many of the time-tested traditional uses for this safe herbal remedy have not been clinically proven. White

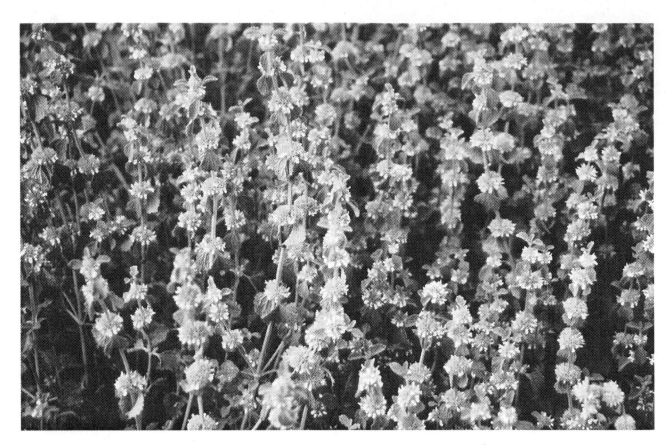

Horehound plant (*Marrubium vulgare*). *(Photo by Henriette Kress. Reproduced by permission.)*

horehound has been approved for treatment of bronchial problems and as an appetite stimulant by the German E Commission—an advisory group on herbal medicines in that country. The U.S. Food and Drug Administration (FDA), however, has declared horehound ineffective for its traditional medicinal use as a sore throat remedy, while approving it as a safe food additive.

It is possible, however, that horehound may prove to be useful in herbal treatments for inflammation. In 2002, French researchers reported isolating new glycoside compounds in horehound, one of which has anti-inflammatory activity. In addition, a group of American researchers studying traditional Mexican herbal remedies for **headache**, **asthma**, arthritis, fever, and menstrual cramps found that horehound has a high antioxidant content that may explain its inclusion in folk remedies for these conditions.

Preparations

Tincture: Combine 4 oz of finely-cut fresh horehound leaf (or 2 oz of dry powdered herb) with 1 pt of brandy, gin, or vodka in a glass container. There should be enough alcohol to cover the plant parts and have a 50/50 ratio of alcohol to **water**. Cover and store the mixture away from light for about two weeks, shaking sever-

al times each day. Strain and store in a tightly-capped dark glass bottle. A standard dose is 10–15 drops of the tincture in water, up to three times a day.

Infusion: Place 2 oz of fresh horehound leaves in a warmed glass container. Bring 2.5 cups of fresh, nonchlorinated water to the boiling point and add it to the herbs. Cover. Infuse the tea for about ten minutes. Strain and sweeten to taste. Drink warm or cold, depending on the intended results. The prepared tea will store for about two days in the refrigerator. Drink three cups a day.

Syrup: Using fresh leaves, prepare a strong infusion of horehound using twice the amount of fresh herb. Combine the infusion with a 50/50 mixture of honey and brown sugar. Use 24 oz of sweetener for each 2.5 cups of the herbal infusion. Heat the mixture in a glass or enamel pot and stir frequently as the mixture thickens. Cool and pour into clearly-labeled glass bottles. Refrigerate for storage. One teaspoonful of syrup may be taken three times a day, or every two hours if needed in acute illness.

Precautions

Pregnant women should not self-medicate with horehound herbal preparations. Lactating women should also consult with a qualified herbalist before using the herb internally. Infants and children under two years of age should not be given horehound. Do not use horehound medicinally if there is chronic disease of the gastrointestinal tract, such as ulcers, esophageal reflux, colitis, or diverticulosis. Large doses of horehound may have a purgative action. Very large doses may cause irregular heartbeat.

Side effects

When horehound is taken internally, it may interfere with the absorption of **iron** and other minerals.

Interactions

No interactions have been reported as of 2002 between horehound and standard pharmaceutical preparations. However, some anesthesiologists recommend that patients scheduled for any surgery requiring total anesthesia should discontinue all herbal preparations for 1–2 weeks before the operation. The reason for this precaution is that some herbal preparations appear to interfere with the action of inhaled anesthetics.

Resources

BOOKS

Bremnes, Lesley. *The Complete Book of Herbs.* New York: Henry Holt, 1995.

Duke, James A., Ph.D. *The Green Pharmacy.* Emmaus, PA: Rodale Press, 1997.

Hoffmann, David. *The New Holistic Herbal,* 2nd ed. Boston: Element, 1986.

Hutchens, Alma R. *A Handbook of Native American Herbs.* Boston: Shambhala Publications, Inc., 1992.

PDR for Herbal Medicines. Montvale, NJ: Medical Economics Company, 1998.

Prevention's 200 Herbal Remedies. Emmaus, PA: Rodale Press, Inc., 1997.

Tyler, Varro E., Ph.D. *The Honest Herbal.* New York: Pharmaceutical Products Press, 1993.

Weiss, Gaea, and Shandor Weiss. *Growing & Using the Healing Herbs.* New York: Wings Books, 1992.

PERIODICALS

Sahpaz, S., et al. "Isolation and Pharmacological Activity of Phenylpropanoid Esters from *Marrubium vulgare.*" *Journal of Ethnopharmacology* 79 (March 2002): 389-392.

Sahpaz, S., T. Hennebelle, and F. Bailleul. "Marruboside, a New Phenylethanoid Glycoside from *Marrubium vulgare L.*" *Natural Product Letters* 16 (June 2002): 195-199.

Vanderjagt, T. J., R. Ghattas, D. J. Vanderjagt, et al. "Comparison of the Total Antioxidant Content of 30 Widely Used Medicinal Plants of New Mexico." *Life Sciences* 70 (January 18, 2002): 1035-1040.

KEY TERMS

Antioxidant—An enzyme or other organic substance that is able to counteract the damaging effects of oxidation in living tissue.

Diaphoretic—A medication given to induce sweating.

Emmenagogue—A substance or medication given to bring on a woman's menstrual period.

Infusion—The most potent form of extraction of an herb into water. Infusions are steeped for a longer period of time than teas.

Mucilage—A gummy or gelatinous substance found in some plants, including horehound.

Tincture—The extraction of an herb into an alcohol solution for either internal or external use.

ORGANIZATIONS

Herb Research Foundation. 1007 Pearl St., Suite 200, Boulder, CO 80302. (303) 449-2265. <www.herbs.org>.

New York Botanical Garden. Bronx River Parkway at Fordham Road, Bronx, NY 10458. (718) 817-8700. <www.nybg.org>.

OTHER

Grieve, M. "A Modern Herbal." http://www.botanical.com.

Clare Hanrahan
Rebecca J. Frey, PhD

Horse chestnut

Description

The European horse chestnut, *Aesculus hippocastanum*, is the horse chestnut most frequently used in herbal medicine. It is a member of the Hippocastanaceae family. Horse chestnuts are in an entirely different botanical family from the well-known sweet chestnut tree, *Castanea vesca*. Horse chestnuts exist in nature as both a tree and a shrub, and are found in all temperate regions of Europe, Asia, and North America.

There are 15 recognized species of horse chestnut. The European horse chestnut is believed to have originated in the Balkan region of eastern Europe but is now grown in every country in the Northern Hemisphere.

The name *Aesculus* is actually a misnomer, coming originally from the word *esca*, meaning food. It was applied by ancient peoples to a certain species of oak; somehow the name was transferred over the years to the horse chestnut. The name *hippocastanum* is thought to refer to the horse chestnut's ability to heal horses and cattle of respiratory illnesses. Another possibility may be that it is named for the small horseshoe-like markings that are present on the branches of the horse chestnut tree.

Horse chestnut trees grow in nearly any soil but seem to prefer a sandy loam. They grow very rapidly into tall straight trees that can reach heights of over 100 ft (approximately 30 m) tall, with widely spreading branches. The bark is grayish-green or grayish-brown in color, and the tree limbs are thick and have corky, elongated, wart-like eruptions that appear from a distance like ribbing. The interior of horse chestnut bark is pinkish-brown, with fine lines running its length. It is odorless and its taste is very bitter and astringent.

The characteristic horseshoe markings found on the branches are actually the scars from where leaves previously grew. Horse chestnut wood is seldom if ever used for lumber due to its soft and spongy character. Large leaf and flower buds are clearly visible even during winter months but are encased in a scaly, resinous protective covering that prevents damage from frost or damp. This thick sticky coating melts with the beginning of warm weather in spring, and flowers and leaves appear with remarkable rapidity, usually within three to four weeks.

The leaves are dark green, rough in texture, and large, with minutely serrated edges. Horse chestnut leaves can be nearly 1 ft (0.3 m) in length. They somewhat resemble a hand with five to nine leaf sections emerging from a palm-like base to form the finger-like projections. European horse chestnuts produce clusters of white flowers with a pale scarlet tinge at the throat or yellow mottling. American horse chestnut flowers can be white, pale pink, or yellow, depending upon the species. All types of horse chestnut trees, with their graceful wide limbs and showy flowers, are grown for their ornamental beauty.

The fruit of the horse chestnut is a dark brown smooth-surfaced nut approximately 2 in (5 cm) in diameter. It has a polished appearance except for the rounded dull tan-colored scar on the side that was attached to the seed vessel. Horse chestnuts are encased in a light green spine-covered coating that divides into three parts and drops away prior to the nut dropping from the tree. Horse chestnut nuts contain mostly carbohydrates which are generally indigestible until boiled. They also contain saponins, tannin, flavones, two glycosides, aesculin and fraxin, some crude protein, a fatty oil, ash and water.

Horse chestnuts native to North America are called buckeyes because of their large seeds which resembling the eye of a buck, or male deer.

American horse chestnuts are divided into four types:

- Ohio buckeye, or *Aesculus glabra*, is a medium-sized tree which grows from the southern United States to the prairies of western Canada. It is the state tree of Ohio, hence the state's nickname of the Buckeye State.

- Yellow buckeye, *Aesculus octandra*, or *Aesculus flava*, is a tree which grows to heights of 40 ft (12 m) or more. It is fairly common across the central portion of the United States. Its leaves are somewhat smoother than those of other horse chestnuts.

- Red buckeye, or *Aesculus pavia*, is a shrub or small tree that generally is found in the southern United States. In early summer it develops brilliantly scarlet flowers in large clusters, and has dense foliage. The tree species of red buckeye grows to heights of between 15–20 ft (5–7 m) tall.

- California buckeye, or *Aesculus californica*, is a horse chestnut tree found all along the Pacific coast.

General use

Horse chestnuts have been used as fodder for feeding farm animals, and some Native American peoples have included them in their diet. However, the outer covering of the horse chestnut nut is toxic, and the nut itself has to be boiled prior to being eaten safely. Its wood, which is too soft for furniture-making or construction, is used in building crates and other packing cases.

Both the bark and the fruit from horse chestnut trees are used medicinally to strengthen and tone the circulatory system, especially the venous system. It is used both internally and externally to treat varicose veins, **phlebitis**, and hemorrhoids. Horse chestnut preparations are particularly effective in treating varicose ulcers. Due to its ability to improve circulation, it is also helpful for the relief of leg cramps. Its bark also has narcotic and fever-reducing properties. A compound known as aescin, which is present in the horse chestnut fruit, is now often added to external creams and preparations used for the treatment of **varicose veins**, varicose ulcers, bruises, and sports injuries.

Horse chestnut preparations using the seed, bark, twigs, and leaves are all utilized in traditional Chinese medicine. Chinese herbalists consider horse chestnut to be a part of treatment not only for circulatory problems, but use it as an astringent, as a diuretic, for reduction of **edema** or swelling, to reduce inflammation, as an expectorant in respiratory problems, and to fight viruses.

Preparations

Horse chestnut bark is removed in the spring in strips 4 or 5 in (10–13 cm) long, about 1 in (2.5 cm) thick and broad. The fruit of the horse chestnut is gathered in the autumn, when they fall from the tree. Both the bark and the fruit are dried in sunlight or with artificial heat, and are either kept whole or ground to a powder for storage. A decoction made of 1 or 2 tsp of the dried, pulverized bark or fruit left to simmer for 15 minutes in 1 cup of **water** can be either taken internally three times a day or used externally as a lotion. Horse chestnut preparations are also available as tinctures, extracts, capsules, and external ointments and lotions.

Precautions

The outer husks of the horse chestnut fruit are poisonous. There are also reported cases of poisoning from eating raw horse chestnuts.

Side effects

There have been reported cases of gastrointestinal irritation, **nausea**, and **vomiting** from taking large doses of horse chestnut. There are also rare reports of rash and **itching**, and even rarer cases of kidney problems.

Interactions

Horse chestnut's ability to reduce blood coagulation, or clotting, indicates that it should not be given to those with bleeding disorders or who are taking anticoagulant drugs. It is known to add to the action of such blood thinning drugs as warfarin or aspirin.

Resources

BOOKS

Grieve, M., and C.F. Leyel. *A Modern Herbal: The Medical, Culinary, Cosmetic and Economic Properties, Cultivation and Folklore of Herbs, Grasses, Fungi, Shrubs and Trees With All of Their Modern Scientific Uses.* NY: Barnes and Noble Publishing, 1992.

Hoffman, David, and Linda Quayle. *The Complete Illustrated Herbal: A Safe and Practical Guide to Making and Using Herbal Remedies.* NY: Barnes and Noble Publishing, 1999.

Taber, Clarence Wilbur. *Taber's Cyclopedic Medical Dictionary.* Philadelphia: F.A.Davis Co., 1997.

OTHER

Hobbs, Christopher. "Herbal Advisor." http://www2.allherb.com/.

Healing People. http//www.healingpeople.com. Support@healing people.com.

Joan Schonbeck

Horsetail

Description

Horsetail is a perennial plant that is found in or near watery areas such as marshes, streams, or rivers. Horsetail grows in temperate northern hemisphere areas of Asia, Europe, North America, and North Africa. It flourishes where it can root in **water** or clay soil.

Horsetail is a derivative of larger plants that grew 270 million years ago during the carboniferous period. It belongs to the Equisetaceae family and is a relative of the fern.

There are over 20 species of horsetail. The species most commonly used medicinally is field horsetail (*Equisetum arvense*). *E. arvense* grows up to 1.5 ft (0.5 m) in corn fields and wet meadows. Wood horsetail (*E. sylvaticum*) grows in copses and on hedgebanks, usually to a height of 1-2 ft (0.3-0.6 m). This species is used as food for horses in parts of Sweden. River horsetail (*E. maximum*) is the largest of the European species of horsetail. Found in bogs, ditches, and on banks of rivers and ponds, *E. maximum* grows to a height of 3-6 ft (1-2 m).

Horsetail has no leaves or flowers and grows in two stages. The first stage occurs during the early spring. At this time, a fertile hollow stem appears that resembles asparagus. After these stems have withered and died, the second stage begins. During this stage, which occurs during the summer months, thin green barren stems branch out from the plant. It is during this stage that horsetail is gathered for medicinal use.

Horsetail was named for its bristly appearance. The genus name *Equisetum* is derived from the Latin words *equus*, meaning horse, and *seta*, meaning bristle. Other names for horsetail include shave-grass, bottle-brush, and paddock-pipes.

Horsetail contains silicon, **potassium**, aluminum, **manganese**, saponins, phytosterols, phenolic acids, cafeic acids, alkaloids, and tannins. Fifteen types of **bioflavonoids** are also present. These bioflavonoids are believed to be responsible for horsetail's strong diuretic action. The high silicon content of the herb strengthens connective tissue, ligaments, bones, hair, and fingernails.

Origins

The medicinal use of horsetail dates back to ancient Roman and Greek times. The Greeks used horsetail as a wound healer, a diuretic, and an agent to stop bleeding. Nicholas Culpeper, a popular seventeenth-century herbalist, wrote of horsetail's beneficial properties in stopping bleeding, and treating ulcers, **kidney stones**, **wounds**, and skin inflammation. In the nineteenth centu-

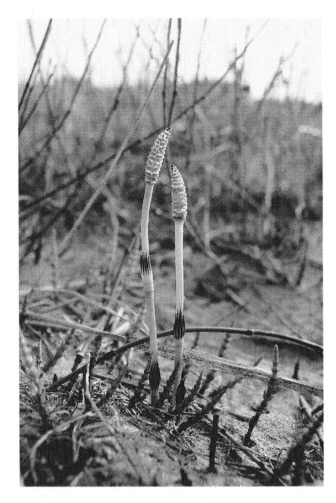

Horsetail plants. *(Photograph by Robert J. Huffman. Field Mark Publications. Reproduced by permission.)*

ry, horsetail was also used to treat **gonorrhea**, prostatitis, and **urinary incontinence**.

The North American native peoples used horsetail to treat a number of kidney and bladder ailments. The Cherokee used horsetail to aid the kidneys. Chippewa natives made a decoction out of horsetail stems and used it to treat painful or difficult urination. The Okanagan-Colville and Potowatami peoples made a horsetail infusion as a diuretic to aid kidney function.

Horsetail's reedy exterior and **silica** content have made it a popular metal polisher and natural abrasive cleanser. One species is so rich in silica that it was imported from Holland for the purpose of polishing metal, hence the nickname Dutch rushes. Another nickname is pewterwort, so named because it was used to scour pewter. Dairy maids of England used horsetail to scour their milk pails, while early Americans used it to scrub their metal pots and pans.

Horsetail has been used internally and externally as a folk medicine to treat rheumatism and **gout**, coughs and **asthma**, **acne**, brittle hair and fingernails, and as a blood purifier. Shoots of a larger species of horsetail were sometimes eaten by the poorer classes, although the food lacked taste and wasn't very nutritious.

General use

Herbalists still use horsetail to treat a variety of kidney and bladder problems. Horsetail has properties that help bladder and kidney tissue. Its tonifyng effects help to reduce inflammation in such conditions as kidney stones, bladder and **kidney infections**, weak bladder, weak kidney, and urinary incontinence.

The German Commission E has approved horsetail as an effective treatment for kidney and bladder inflammations, **edema**, urinary tract **infections**, and bacterial infections. It is also used as a component in diuretic drugs.

Silica and horsetail

Horsetail is rich in minerals, particularly silica deposited in its stems. Silica helps to promote the body's absorption of **calcium**, an important component in tissue repair and bone and cartilage formation. Horsetail's silica and silicic acid content ranges from 5-8%, making it a good source for strengthening weak connective tissues, and healing bones, **fractures**, and torn ligaments. Horsetail is also used to treat arthritis and **osteoporosis**, as the silicon in horsetail may replace lost silicon in the affected bones.

Horsetail may be a possible remedy for senility. Senility often occurs when there is more aluminum in the blood than silicon. One theory suggests that when the silicon and aluminum levels are balanced, the symptoms of senility will disappear.

Wound healer

Horsetail's ability to stop blood flow has made it useful in treating **nosebleeds**, internal bleeding, heavy menstrual bleeding, bleeding **hemorrhoids**, and bleeding wounds. Often a compress made from fresh horsetail juice is placed on the wound to stop the flow of blood. The healing effect may be strongest when horsetail is taken both internally and externally.

Other uses

Horsetail is also used to remedy brittle nails, bleeding wounds, **hair loss**, cystic ulcers, **rheumatoid arthritis**, gout, gonorrhea, digestive disturbances, **bronchitis**, lung disorders, **tuberculosis**, poor teeth and gums, **varicose veins**, and fallen arches. Skin ailments such as **sties**, **rashes**, itchy **eczema**, or eye inflammation may be treated with an external compress made from horsetail tea.

Preparations

Horsetail is gathered in the spring and early summer, after the fertile stems have died and the barren shoots have grown. The plant is cut above the root and the stems are used dried or fresh. Horsetail is available in dried bulk, powder, capsules, tablets, or tincture forms.

It is recommended that commercial preparations of horsetail contain no more than 3% blackish rhizome fragments and no more than 5% stems or branches from other horsetail species. Standard preparations generally contain 10% silicic acid and 7% silica.

Taken as a dietary supplement, horsetail is a good source of calcium and silica. Horsetail can be made into a tea (infusion or decoction) and consumed internally. Horsetail may also be used in full body baths, sitz baths, foot baths, compresses, hair rinses, and poultices.

For the capsule form, two capsules can be taken with water up to two times daily.

To make a tea, 1 cup of boiling water can be poured over 2 tsp of dried horsetail and steeped for 15 minutes. Up to 4 cups of the cold tea can be drunk daily for bladder or kidney ailments. The tea may be used externally as a hair rinse for **dandruff** or an oily scalp.

About 10-60 drops of the tincture can be used daily.

Precautions

Pregnant or nursing women and people with severe kidney or liver disease should consult their health practitioner before using horsetail. People with high blood pressure or heart problems should not take horsetail. Horsetail contains low levels of nicotine and may not be safe for young children. Horsetail shouldn't be taken internally for more than three days, and people should not take more than the normal dosage. Long-term use or high doses of horsetail have caused irreversible kidney damage due to too much silica. It is best to follow dosage guidelines and use properly harvested horsetail since the older shoots are higher in silica.

Commercial preparations that are processed at high temperatures are recommended since the heat destroys a potentially harmful enzyme, thiaminase, found in crude horsetail.

When horsetail is gathered for medicinal use, plants with brown spots aren't collected. Brown spots may indicate the presence of a toxic fungus. Horsetail that grows near an industrial or waste site or in heavily fertilized areas should not be harvested since it can pick up nitrates and **selenium** from the soil. The correct species of horsetail should be collected. Marsh horsetail (*E. palustre*) is poisonous.

KEY TERMS

Decoction—An herbal tea created by boiling herbs in water. Roots, bark, and seeds are used in decoctions; boiling the herbs brings out their medicinal properties.

Diuretic—A substance that promotes urination.

Edema—A condition that occurs when fluid accumulates in the tissues of the body.

Incontinence—The inability to control urination.

Infusion—An herbal tea created by steeping herbs in hot water. Generally, leaves and flowers are used in infusions.

Perennial—A plant that lives for many years and comes back yearly without replanting.

Sitz bath—A bath in which only the hips and buttocks are soaked.

Side effects

Mild side effects include **diarrhea**, upset stomach, and increased urination.

Severe side effects that may require medical attention are kidney **pain**, lower back pain, pain while urinating, **nausea**, or **vomiting**. These symptoms may signal kidney damage. Heart palpitations can occur if horsetail is overused. If this happens, immediate medical attention is required.

Interactions

People taking digitalis-type drugs should consult their health practitioner before taking horsetail.

Resources

BOOKS

American Herb Association. *Complete Book of Herbs*. Illinois: Publications International, Ltd., 1997.

Fischer-Rizzi, Susanne. *Medicine of the Earth*. Cambridge, MA: Rudra Press, 1996.

Jennifer Wurges

Hot flashes

Definition

Hot flashes, experienced by large numbers of women and some men as a result of surgical, chemical, or age-induced changes in estrogen levels, are characterized by a rapid rise and discharge of heat with perspiration, discomfort, and possible redness. Ranging from mild to severe in intensity, they may be preceded by an "aura-like" experience, and may be followed by a subsequent feeling of chill. With natural age-related **menopause**, hot flashes may begin as early as two years prior to the cessation of menses and continue as long as five or more years afterward. Statistically, the average experience is approximately four years of hot flashes of varying intensities.

Description

Approximately 20% of women without **breast cancer** and 50–75% of women taking tamoxifen subsequent to breast **cancer** will reportedly seek a doctor's advice for the management of hot flashes. For women without breast cancer, this seems to be a conservative estimate, given that another source notes that as many as 75% of Caucasian women experience perimenopausally related hot flashes, beginning an average of two years prior to the cessation of **menstruation**. On average, 85% of these women experience hot flashes for more than one year. Statistics are mixed with regard to overall duration. One study reported that only 20% of women reported still having hot flashes after four years, while another reported 25–50% of women continuing to have them as long as five years. Hot flashes appear to be more common amongst African American women than among Caucasian, Japanese, Hispanic, or Chinese women, while Mayan Indian women report no symptoms associated with menopause at all.

Hot flashes may be preceded by a prodromal experience, or set of signs, of rapid heart rate, **anxiety**, and **dizziness** or weakness. There is considerable variation in the experience of hot flashes. As the flash comes on, there is a feeling of sudden heat that may produce as little as a beading of perspiration on the upper lip, or a sudden and uncontrollable drenching. The sudden feeling of heat may be followed by a cold, clammy sensation as evaporation of perspiration occurs. The episode may last from 30 seconds to five minutes; an average of four minutes is reported. One clinical source reported that patients most commonly describe the onset of hot flashes as coming between two and four in morning, disrupting sleep, often resulting in a need to change nightclothes or even bed linens; but another source noted that the most common time of onset was between six and eight in the morning and six and ten at night.

A stressful incident may precede the hot flash, and keeping a journal of these events as a means of identifying triggers may be helpful. Depending on the intensity, severity, and timing, embarrassment may also accompany the hot flash when others witness the sudden, unmistakable signs of the experience. Breast cancer, premature onset of menopause, faster onset of menopause, tamoxifen therapy in women and antiandrogenic therapies in women and men, may contribute to more severe and longer-lasting hot flashes. One source noted that each person individually may themselves experience a wide variation of symptoms, dependent on their unique biochemical, environmental, and psychosocial factors.

Causes & symptoms

The exact cause and mechanism of hot flashes is not well understood. What is recognized is that as estrogen levels are depleted, whether due to surgical, chemical, or natural age-related changes, the area in the brain that regulates several functions including body temperature—the hypothalamus—becomes "confused." The core body temperature set point is lowered, and the threshold between acceptable and nonacceptable body heat levels is more easily crossed. When that occurs, signals are sent to the rest of the body of a sudden need to discharge heat, accomplished through the sudden release of perspiration from the sweat glands. Studies reveal measurable rises in skin temperature. Other hypothalamic signals cause awakenings from sleep, changes in blood pressure and heart rate, and anxiety states (alertness), as if the body is in "fight or flight" mode.

A summary of common accompanying symptoms include:

- sleep disruptions
- **fatigue**
- night sweats
- heart palpitations
- irritability
- short-term memory loss
- attention span changes
- **depression** and weepiness
- uncharacteristic rage or impatience
- dryness of eyes and vagina
- reduced libido and interest in sex
- accelerated bone loss

Diagnosis

In most cases, diagnosis of hot flashes is not difficult. What may be difficult is assessing existing levels of hormones, anticipating the duration of menopause and menopausal symptoms, and finding safe, effective treatment options. Family history, personal medical history, including history of pregnancies and births, a physical examination, such diagnostic assessments as blood workups for thyroid and adrenal (**stress** coping) function, and hormonal assays (blood or saliva) may be recommended. Bone density testing, and depending on history, more regular mammograms and Pap tests, though not diagnostic of hot flashes, may become advisable.

Treatment

Several alternative treatments are effective.

Phyto- (plant-derived) hormones

The most widely proclaimed remedies in this category include **black cohosh** (*Cimicifuga racemosa*), wild yam (*Dioscorea villosa*), **dong quai** (*Angelica sinensis*), **red clover** (*Trifollium pratense*), and **licorice** (*Glycyrrhiza glabra*). Also in this category are soy and two soy isoflavones—genistein and daidzein. Of all of these, black cohosh, wild yam, and soy have shown the greatest efficacy. The have also incited controversy.

Black cohosh may be the most well-studied of all the phytoestrogens. In North America, Native American women have traditionally used it. The German Commission E, whose stamp of approval makes prescriptive use of black cohosh reimbursable, recommends, according to one source, use for no longer than six months at doses of 20–40 mg daily [of the concentrate]. Apart from safety issues, use of black cohosh by women also taking tamoxifen is not as effective because of competition for estrogen receptor sites. For women not taking tamoxifen simultaneously, the reported improvement over placebo in the use of black cohosh was 25–30%. Given that the **placebo effect** generates a 30–50% improvement, these statistics may mean as high as a 75–80% reduction with black cohosh. Other combination formulas may include black cohosh in an unconcentrated and unstandardized product, and may be safer for longer periods of time.

A study examining the reduction of hot flashes from use of soy flour showed a 40% reduction, 15% greater than placebo. However, considerable controversy about an estrogen-additive effect in women at risk or with a history of breast or **uterine cancer**, and in men at risk of **prostate cancer**, warrants caution. One study noted that the soy isoflavones stimulated tumor growth and opposed any beneficial effects tamoxifen might have.

Dong quai was reported to be equivalent to placebo with regard to hot flashes, with an advisory caution. Dong quai belongs to a family of herbs that contain warfarin (Coumadin)-like substances, and is therefore contraindicated for use in persons on Coumadin (warfarin) or other blood-thinning therapies.

Wild yam and licorice have both been used and recommended for their progesterone-like qualities. Many of the progesterone creams available without prescription have wild yam as a basic source ingredient. Many of these creams also contain pharmaceutical-grade (concentrated and standardized) amounts of progesterone. Without monitoring use by saliva sampling, a worsening of hot flashes may be provoked by progesterone's estrogen suppressive capacity. Licorice has been historically included in many combination herbals in **traditional Chinese medicine** as a synergistic (exponentially additive) element; however, caution is advised for persons with high blood pressure.

A study of red clover using of 252 women divided into three groups, two each using a separate red clover supplement for 12 weeks and one control group, reported a 40% improvement and no significant side effects. An average of eight hot flash episodes was reduced to an average of five in the two trial groups. When compared with estrogen's 90% improvement statistic, these results were considered disappointing.

Traditional Chinese medicine (TCM)

TCM divides menopause into "hot" and "cold" menopause on the basis of a thorough history taking and examination of the tongue and pulses (six different pulses). Both **acupuncture** and Chinese herbology may be employed to reduce stress, facilitate the movement of Chi (or Qi, the body's internal energy flow), and balance body systems. While some critics claim TCM is no more effective than placebo in controlling hot flashes or the symptoms of menopause, with "few documented benefits," others point to the survival of this tradition in medicine for thousands of years and believe that something more than a placebo effect is evidenced.

Vitamins and vitamin E therapy

Vitamin E therapy is perhaps one of the most historically recommended therapies in North America for hot flashes, in a dosing range from 400–1,000 International Units (IU) daily. Since the 1940s, vitamin E has been believed to be useful in reducing hot flashes and another common symptoms of estrogen deficiency—vaginal dryness. One vitamin company at least, has built a reputation on the clinical benefits of vitamin E therapy. Nevertheless, one source reports on the basis of a "well designed trial" that the success of vitamin E therapy (40%) for the reduction of hot flashes is comparable to placebo (30%). Other studies regarding the antioxidant properties of vitamin E suggest that when the vitamin is combined simultaneously with **vitamin C** supplementation, a beneficial synergistic antioxidant effect is obtained. A tamoxifen-related trial by the National Cancer Institute recommends use of vitamin E, with C and 200–250 mg of vitamin B_6.

The entire **vitamin B complex** might also be recommended for its support of the nervous system and stress reduction.

Dietary changes

Weight and fitness have been demonstrated to be factors in the management of hot flashes. Weight is recommended to be height-proportionate. Women with less body fat may have as difficult a time as women with too much body fat. Fitness is especially important, and **exercise** has been demonstrated to improve stamina and attitude, which contribute to tolerance.

Nuts, whole grains, apples, celery, **alfalfa**, and beans have all been recommended as useful dietary adjuncts. One source reports that a general dietary "housecleaning back to basics," eliminating highly refined and processed foods, including "fast foods" and "junk food," reducing or eliminating sugar and sugar-substitute products like aspartame, eating more vegetables than fruit, and including in the diet **essential fatty acids** like flax or fish oils, may go a long way toward stabilizing the nervous system and supporting more normal activity in the hypothalamus.

Natural hormone replacement therapy

Yes, there really is such a thing. Licensed practitioners and others in the healthcare community have recognized for some time that there is a relationship between high estrogen (estradiol or E2) levels and **fibrocystic breast disease**, **uterine fibroids**, **endometriosis** and fertility dysfunction. Saliva sampling was developed as an alternate means of effectively monitoring not just the levels of circulating hormone, but the amount of biologically active circulating hormone. The pioneer laboratory, DiagnosTechs, Inc. of Kent, Washington, developed a female hormone profile that tracks the interplay of estrogen and progesterone across the span of a menstruating woman's cycle. They also developed a post menopausal panel to assess the more static balances of women after menstruation ceases, and a testosterone panel for men. Information from these kinds of tests are valuable **aids** in assessing an individual's existing hormone values, especially when compared to statistical data of physiologically effective ranges. This information allows for safer, more precise and individual—not one size fits all—use of hormone replacement therapy.

A special class of pharmacist, known as a compounding pharmacist, is able to formulate a hormone replacement of "molecularly identical" phytohormones (usually soy and wild yam), standardized to a calculated milligram strength, for use by prescription. These natural estrogen replacements make broadest use of the weakest, most gentle fraction of estrogen, estriol (E3).

The other fractions are estradiol (E2)—the most potent—and estrone (E1). Although natural hormones are available in capsules, the most commonly recommended forms are sublingual (under the tongue) drops, or a topical cream or gel, in order to avoid adding further burden to the liver. The liver is responsible for metabolizing the chemistry of the body, and by the time hormone replacement therapy is usually needed, the liver has been hard at work for many years. Drops and creams also allow for individual tailoring. **Natural hormone replacement therapy**, however, must be used with the same caution as pharmaceutical synthetics, even though its compounds may be safer and reduce the health risks that have become associated with synthetic hormone replacement therapy or no treatment at all. Without clinical trials, statistical proof and good data remain unavailable. The International Academy of Compounding Pharmacists (IACP) maintains a website to help locate compounding pharmacists: http://www.iacprx.org/about_iacp/ The American Association of Naturopathic Physicians maintains a website of licensed members at: http://www.naturopathic.org

Liver support and detoxification

Because the liver is the primary organ for metabolizing hormones, therapies that include a liver support or **detoxification** may assist in the smooth transitioning through menopause. This might be especially important in persons whose hot flashes are surgically or chemically induced, as the need for both of these kinds of interventions was likely preceded by hormone related illness. Colon cleansing and increased intake of dietary and soluble fibers may also be recommended. Sources of dietary and soluble fiber include whole grains and grain brans, most vegetables, many fruits and fruit pectin, psyllium, and guar gum.

Allopathic treatment

Premarin and Prempro

For many years, the standard remedy for relief of hot flashes was Premarin, a product derived from the urine of pregnant mares. During **pregnancy**, levels of the most potent fraction of estrogen, estradiol (E2), are downgraded to a less potent fraction, estrone (E1). (Estrone is more potent than estriol, or E3.) Mares were kept pregnant, catheterized for urine collection, and dehydrated for more concentrated urine. That fact alone was enough to dissuade some women from using it. However, no other single remedy had been shown to have the efficacy (96%)of reducing or eliminating hot flashes like estrogen (as Premarin) hormone replacement therapy.

Mares have similar but unidentical estrogens compared to humans. One of the substances specific to mares estrogen is genetically toxic to humans. Furthermore, in the normal female's physiology, estrogen is opposed by progesterone, another female reproductive hormone. Supplementing estrogen by using Premarin, unopposed by progesterone, resulted frequently in a condition known as hyperestrogenism and increased risks and rates of breast and uterine cancer. Ignoring a possible genetic toxicity of premarin, subsequent prescriptions for hormone replacement therapy concentrated on opposing premarin's estrogen in a combination patented hormone drug called Prempro. In the summer of 2002, results of the Women's Health Initiative study were released, statistically demonstrating the increased health risks (breast cancer, **stroke** and **heart attack**) of these modalities. Along with results of other studies suggesting that estrogen replacement therapy was also not as protective against **osteoporosis** as had once been believed, serious reconsideration of hot flashes management was prompted. The current trend in synthetic hot flashes management and hormone replacement therapy is a multi-faceted approach which may include the short-term use of estrogen. Several the other synthetic options are discussed below.

The progestins

Depomedroxyprogesterone acetate (MPA) has been reviewed and found, at doses of 150 mg every one to two months [as an injection], for women with endometrial cancer to be 85% effective in reducing hot flashes when compared with estrogen. Oral doses of 10 mg/day were 87% effective. Reported side effects included: irregular vaginal bleeding, weight gain and bloating, breast tenderness and mood swings.

Blood pressure medications (antihypertensives)

Blood pressure medications—alpha-adrenergic agonist antihypertensives—that inhibit the stress trigger pathways involved in hot flashes, reduce hot flashes 20% to 65%. Drugs and dosages used include: clonidine, at 0.05–0.2 mg/day; lefoxidine, at 0.1 mg/day; and methyldopa, at 250 mg three times daily. Side effects of dizziness and **dry mouth** were reported.

Bellergal

The twice daily use of 40 mg of bellergal—a potent hypnotic-sedative combination of ergotamine tartrate, belladona alkaloids, and phenobarbitol— reduces hot flashes by 60% when compared to the placebo rate of 22%. This drug is one of the older synthetic remedies prescribed for hot flashes, due to its effects on the nervous system. It has the very undesirable effect of being addictive, and avoidance of alcohol is strongly advised.

Megestrol acetate

One of the newer drugs for relief of hot flashes, studied under rigorous clinical trial according to one source, a 20 mg twice daily oral dose, megestrol acetate is considered to show high promise for use in both men and women. It is considered as a treatment for breast cancer in high continuous doses. Initial dosing is reported to start at 40 mg daily, and then be tapered up or down after a month, to a maximum of 80 mg daily. Side effects noted were fluid retention and bloating.

Selective serotonin reuptake inhibitors (SSRIs)

New attention is being paid to this class of drugs, especially to Prozac (fluoxetine), Paxil (paroxetine), and Effexor (venlafaxine). Venlafaxine is sometimes also notated as an 'NSRI' or a norepinephrine serotonin reuptake inhibitor. Norepinephrine is an adrenal hormone related to feelings of ambition and depression. By relieving deficits that may affect mood and hot flashes, these reuptake inhibitors are showing a 50% to 75% efficacy in decreasing hot flashes in 60% of women, making them better than trial placebo (22% to 30%) by about half. Eighty per cent of the benefit was achieved in the first week. The noted dose on Paxil is 10 mg. daily for the first week, followed by 20 mg daily thereafter. Dosing for Effexor was noted at 75 mg twice daily of a time released formula. The study using 75 mg followed studies using considerably less, 12.5 mg twice daily. Side effects include **sexual dysfunction**, and, according to one source, possible weight gain from increased carbohydrate craving.

Prognosis

Though some hot flashes for some women may be severe, occur over several years, be embarrassing, disruptive, mood-altering, fatigue-inducing, and correlated with other age-related deficiencies sufficient to make a grown person cry, they are not life-threatening. The statistics, according to one source, that "in virtually all reported studies, hot flashes respond to placebo in 30% to 50% of women," may mean that an average 40% reduction in hot flashes may be obtained by visiting a health care professional, allopathic or alternative, talking about concerns, and instituting lifestyle changes representing a kind of pampering or self-care. In other words, hot flash sufferers may feel statistically justified in adopting new ways of living they might have been contemplating previously but have not yet adopted.

Prevention

Hot flashes may represent an invitation or opportunity to experiment with new modalities. Prevention, in the strictest sense, is not a likely option unless one is a Mayan Indian woman or healthy male. However, many suggestions offer significant improvements in quality of life that may be helpful, including:

- Saliva sampling: Consider working with a healthcare professional who can offer advice and hormone testing of the bio-available levels through saliva sampling, and who may also be able to quantitatively advise and monitor natural hormone replacement therapy. A post-menopausal saliva panel costs between $85 and $100, and may be covered by insurance. Sampling intervals may vary according to need.

- Obtaining and maintaining optimum body weight: Adipose (fat) tissue stores estrogen, which may complicate safe hormone replacement therapy, while making heat distribution more difficult. A deficiency of adipose tissue may add to stress and lower immunity.

- Exercising regularly: Exercise not only tones the muscles and improves distribution of all hormones, it also reduces stress, builds endorphins (hormones related to feeling well), and quiets the nervous system.

- Avoiding dietary triggers: Sugar, spicy foods, **caffeine** and alcohol may all adversely affect the ability of the hypothalamus to regulates body temperature.

- Avoiding life style triggers: Diet pills, saunas, hot tubs, hot showers, and **smoking** are all to be avoided.

- Wearing layered cotton clothing and using cotton bed linens: Breathable natural fibers or sport fibers that wick away perspiration may help transfer heat; layering more easily allows quicker responses to heating and chilling.

- Meditating and breathing deeply: Also included in this category are **yoga**, hypnosis, massage, **biofeedback** techniques, visualization, and **relaxation** exercises. These techniques reduce stress and oppose or quiet the nerve pathways involved in increased triggering of hot flashes.

- Air conditioning: One source suggested liberal use of the air conditioner and even the freezer (at home and supermarket) when a hot flash happens; turning down the thermostat of the furnace in winter as low as possible was also suggested.

Resources

BOOKS

Rosensweet, David. M.D., *Menopause and Natural Hormones.* Naples, FL: Life Medicine & Healing, 2002.

PERIODICALS

Fitzpatrick, Lorraine A., M.D., and Richard J. Santen, M.D. "Hot Flashes: The Old and the New, What is Really True?" *Mayo Clinic Proceedings* (November 2002): 1155–1158.

KEY TERMS

Bellergal—A potent combination of ergotamine tartrate (a blood vessel-constricting substance often used for migraines), belladona alkaloids (a potentially poisonous substance with sedative and antispasmodic effects), and phenobarbitol (an hypnotic, long acting sedative and anti-convulsant). Bellergal is one of the early synthetic patented formulations prescribed for relief of hot flashes due to its actions on the central nervous system, but now avoided due to its addictive capacity.

Estrogen—One of the primary reproductive hormones in women and present in men. Three fractions of estrogen have been identified: E1 or estrone is moderately active; E2 or estradiol is the most potent; and, E3 or estriol is the least potent and most often recommended for use in natural hormone replacement therapy, often in an 80% to 10% to10% combination of E3 to E1 and E2.

Hormone replacement therapy (HRT)—A term used for the supplementation of hormones in the treatment of hormone deficiency related symptoms and illnesses. HRT often uses synthetic patented hormonal drugs. Natural soy or wild yam based hormone replacement therapy is also available using hormones molecularly identical to human hormones and therefore unpatentable.

Progesterone—Another of the primary reproductive hormones in women that has an estrogen-suppressing and pregnancy term-supporting role. Natural progesterone levels often decline long before declining estrogen levels may produce hot flashes. Prior to estrogen replacement therapy, progesterone therapy may be recommended to balance estrogen and reduce the risk of estrogen-related health risks like fibroids of breast and uterus, and breast or endometrial cancer.

Standardization—A process by which active ingredients in compounds are quantified to insure a desired level of potency.

Synergy—A condition in which the action of a sum of parts is greater than the individual actions of those parts added together, something like "one plus one is greater than two."

OTHER

"All About Hot Flashes." breastcancer.org, PO Box 222, Narberth, PA 19072-0222. [cited, June 3, 2004]. <http://www.breastcancer.org/bey_cope_meno_hot-Flash_pf.html>.

Caruso, David B. "Managing Menopause." CBS Broadcasting, Inc. November 18, 2002 [cited June 3, 2004]. <http://www.nci.nih.gov/cancer_information/doc.aspx>.

Hopson, Krista. "U-M Study Works to Take the Heat Off Menopause." University of Michigan Health Minute. February 3, 2003 [Cited June 3, 2004]. &<http://www.med.umich.edu/opm/newspage/2003/hot-flashes.htm>.

"Remedies For Hot Flashes." CBSNews.com. August 13, 2003. [cited June 3, 2004]. <http://www.cbsnews.com/stories/2003/08/12/earlyshow/contributors/emilysenay/main 567971.shtml>.

Tanner, Lindsey. "Menopause Remedy Makers Get Tough." The Associated Press. November 26, 2002 [cited, June 3, 2004]. <http://www.cbsnews.com/stories/2002/11/26/health/main530881.shtml>.

Tanner, Lindsey. "Red Clover No Help For Menopause." The Associated Press. July 9, 2003 [cited June 3, 2004]. <http://www.cbsnews.com/stories/2003/07/09/health/main562392.shtml>.

"What Are Hot Flashes and What Can I Do About Them?" FamiliesFirst.com. Last updated, January 21, 2003. [cited June 3, 2004]. <http://www.families_first.com/hotflashes/faq/faq08.htm>.

Katherine E. Nelson, N.D.

Hou xiang see **Agastache**

Houndsbane see **Horehound**

Huang qi see **Astragalus**

Huckleberry see **Bilberry**

Humor therapy

Definition

Humor therapy is the art of using humor and laughter to help heal people with physical or mental illness.

Origins

The benefits of humor therapy were acknowledged as far back as the book of Proverbs in the Old Testament, which contains verses like Prov. 17:22: "A cheerful heart is a good medicine, but a downcast spirit dries up the bones." The earliest historical reference to humor therapy is from the fourteenth century, when French surgeon Henri de Mondeville wrote, "Let the surgeon take care to regulate the whole regimen of the patient's life for joy and happiness, allowing his relatives and special friends to cheer him, and by having someone tell him jokes." In the sixteenth century, Martin Luther used a form of humor therapy as part of his pastoral counseling of depressed people. He advised them not to isolate themselves but to surround themselves with friends who could joke and make them laugh. Many of Luther's own letters to other people include playful or humorous remarks.

Modern humor therapy dates from the 1930s, when clowns were brought into hospitals to cheer up children hospitalized with polio. In his 1979 book, *Anatomy of an Illness*, author Norman Cousins brought the subject of humor therapy to the attention of the medical community. Cousins, himself a physician, details how he used laughter to help ease his **pain** while undergoing treatment for rheumatoid arthritis of the spine (ankylosing spondylitis). The benefits of laughter in treating the sick captured the public's attention in the 1998 movie *Patch Adams*, starring Robin Williams as the real-life doctor Hunter "Patch" Adams. The movie is based on Adams' experiences treating the poor in rural West Virginia, as related in his 1983 book *Gesundheit!*.

Benefits

It may seem difficult to measure the benefits of laughter in medicine, but a number of clinical studies have helped verify the adage that laughter is the best medicine. In general, laughter improves the physical, mental, emotional, and spiritual health of individuals. Laughter appears to release tension in the diaphragm and relieve pressure on the liver and other internal organs. It stimulates the immune system, reduces stress, and helps balance the body's natural energy fields or auras. People who have developed a strong sense of humor generally have a better sense of well-being and control in their lives.

A strong advocate of humor therapy is Dr. Michael R. Wasserman, president and chief medical officer of GeriMed of America, Inc., a primary care physician management company for seniors. "A few years ago I came down with **pneumonia**, pulled out videotapes of *I Love Lucy* reruns and laughed myself back to good health," he said. "Clearly, humor and laughter have a positive effect on one's attitude and health overall. While we don't know all of the specifics, our immune system appears to benefit from these emotions."

Description

Humor therapy is used in both mainstream and alternative medicine. It can take many forms, but generally it is simply the recognition by physicians, nurses, and other health care practitioners of the value of mixing humor and laughter with medication and treatment. It is especially important with children and the elderly. Patients can also help themselves to heal by adding more humor and laughter to their lives.

Hospitals, hospices, nursing homes, and other medical care facilities can also turn to professionals for help in bringing humor to their patients. One example is the Big Apple Circus Clown Care Unit, which has programs in hospitals throughout the New York metropolitan area and major children's hospitals throughout the United States, including Children's Hospital in Boston. Professional clowns perform three days a week at the bedsides of hospitalized children to help ease the **stress** of serious illnesses. The clowns use juggling, mime, magic tricks, music, and gags to promote the healing power of humor. Instead of stethoscopes, thermometers, and hypodermics, the "doctors of delight" make their "clown rounds" with Groucho Marx disguises, funny hats, and rubber chickens.

Preparations

No advance preparation is required, except possibly a good repertoire of jokes and gags for the therapist.

Precautions

Not everyone will appreciate humor therapy. Some people may consider humor for the sick or injured as inappropriate or harmful. Therefore, it is important to know or sense when humor will be therapeutic and when it will be inappropriate. It should be used cautiously at first in situations in which the sensitivity of the person to whom it is directed is uncertain or unknown.

Side effects

The only adverse side effect of humor therapy is that it can cause mental hurt, sadness, and alienation in persons who are not receptive to it, or if it is used insensitively.

Research & general acceptance

Humor therapy is widely accepted in the alternative health community and is finding growing acceptance with mainstream health practitioners, especially registered nurses. Numerous scientific studies done in a clinical setting support the benefits of humor therapy. Two 1989 studies done at the Loma Linda (CA) University School of Medicine showed that laughter stimulates the immune system, counteracting the immunosuppressive effects of stress. These findings have been supported by other studies at the UCLA Medical School Department of Behavioral Medicine, the Ohio State University School of Medicine, and the VA Medical Center in San Diego.

While several studies have demonstrated that humor therapy raises the level of salivary immunoglobin A, they have also been challenged. Other research focuses on the

---

KEY TERMS

Aura—An energy field surrounding the human body, discernible by its various colors.

Gesundheit—A German expression wishing good health, usually used when a person sneezes.

Immunosuppressive—Anything that acts to suppress or weaken the body's immune system, thus making it more susceptible to disease.

---

effects of humor therapy on natural killer (NK) cell assays, which are considered to give clearer and more replicable results. The general conclusion is that laughter has the potential to reduce stress and stress hormone levels, consequently reducing their effects on the immune system. Humor therapy may well be a useful complementary therapy for oncology patients.

Training & certification

Although no official training or certification is required, there are a few institutions that teach humor therapy. Further information is available from the American Association for Therapeutic Humor listed below.

Resources

BOOKS

Adams, Patch, and Maureen Mylander. *Gesundheit!: Bringing Good Health to You, the Medical System, and Society Through Physician Service, Complementary Therapies, Humor, and Joy.* Rochester, VT: Inner Traditions International Ltd., 1998 (Revised).

Klein, Allen. *The Courage to Laugh: Humor, Hope, and Healing in the Face of Death and Dying.* Boston: J.P. Tarcher, 1998.

Wooten, Patty. *Compassionate Laughter: Jest for Your Health!* Salt Lake City, UT: Commune-A-Key, 1996.

ORGANIZATIONS

American Association for Therapeutic Humor. 222 S. Meramec, Suite 303. St. Louis, MO 63105. (314) 863-6232. <http://www.aath.org>.

International Center for Health & Humor. 2930 Hidden Valley Road, Edmond, OK 73013. (405) 341-8115. http://www.humorandhealth.com.

OTHER

Humor and Health Journal. Bimonthly newsletter. P.O. Box 16814. Jackson, MS 39236. (601) 957-0075.

Jest for the Health of It Services. Consultant, Patty Wooten. P.O. Box 8484. Santa Cruz, CA 95061. (831) 460-1600. http://www.jesthealth.com.

Ken R. Wells

Huna

Definition

Huna is an esoteric Polynesian psychology that claims to use the powers of the mind to accomplish healing and spiritual development. Max Freedom Long, who rediscovered Huna in the 1920s, defined it as a system of religious psychiatry because it contains elements of religion, psychology, and psychic science.

Origins

Huna practitioners believe their teachings are ancient and sacred, although at least one writer has claimed they actually have modern origins. In the Hawaiian language, the word *huna* means "secret" or "that which is hidden," referring to a tradition of hiding these teachings. The word is also said to be taken from *kahuna*, a priest or teacher who was the "keeper of the secret." Huna has traditionally been passed on through oral communication and in chants rather than in writing.

Huna was outlawed in the nineteenth century by Christian missionaries to the Hawaiian Islands. Max Freedom Long, who founded the Huna Fellowship in 1945, spent years decoding the language of Huna knowledge. He published eight books on Huna between the 1920s and his death in 1971. Serge Kahili King, a non-Polynesian kahuna, founded One Order of Huna International in 1973.

Benefits

Huna claims to offer the following benefits to its adherents:

- becoming a complete person psychologically

- solving personal problems, including financial or social issues

- having a higher level of physical, emotional, and spiritual energy

- handling the demands and stresses of daily life more effectively

- acquiring the ability to heal oneself and others

- learning how to accumulate mana (vital force) in order to attain personal goals

- growing spiritually

- changing one's future

Description

The specific teachings and customs associated with Huna vary somewhat from island to island. All agree, however, on the concept of three spirits or minds in the human being. According to Huna, the complete being consists of a physical body inhabited by two of the three minds: the "low self" which is below the level of consciousness, and the "middle self" which is the conscious mind. The middle self is what others perceive as one's personality. The third spirit or mind, the High Self, is outside the body. Each person has a transparent shadow body that completely duplicates the physical body. This shadow body is called the *aka*. The aka is like a pattern or blueprint that connects the three selves. It has a sticky and stretchy quality that allows it to form connections between an individual and another person or object. When someone touches, looks at, or even thinks of something, a thread or cord from the aka attaches to it, forming an energy channel between the person and another person or object. Illness develops when there is a conflict between the conscious mind and the patterns of the aka.

The third mind or self, the High Self, is not God but a person's divine connection with God. Ideally all three selves or minds in a person should be in continual contact with one another. The low self is the communication link between the middle self and the High Self. It obtains information directly from the senses and is the seat of the emotions. It has a limited ability to reason and reacts to events only on the basis of previous programming even if this programming has been incorrect or negative. Blockages in the low self caused by fear, anger, or negative programming interrupt communication with the High Self. The function of the kahuna is to remove these blocks. Kahunas use a wide range of techniques including telepathy, rituals, massage, body stroking, herbs, dream work to clear the mind of limiting beliefs and fears, meditative movements known as *kalana hula,* and a variety of other self-development techniques to establish harmony among people, objects, locations, and circumstances. An example of the latter is *Ho' oponopono*, which refers to counseling and mediation to balance relationships.

The three minds or selves use a form of subtle energy called *mana,* which is stored in the aka. The low self takes energy from food and turns it into mana, or basic life energy. The kahunas, who serve as conduits for the healing qualities of mana, use breathing techniques to increase a person's mana. The basic breathing technique involves drawing a deep breath, holding it, and willing the mana into a body part that needs healing, into the hands, or into an object like a crystal or talisman. A person's mana is also increased by living correctly. Huna emphasizes the importance of living and speaking positively, and of doing no harm to others.

Practitioners of Huna also emphasize that their way of life is accessible to everyone and can be practiced by everyone; that is, it does not depend on having unusual psychic gifts or on joining a small group of "chosen" ini-

Hydrotherapy

KEY TERMS
. . . .

Aka—In Huna, the shadow body of the low self. The aka forms threads or cords between the low self and other persons, objects, or the High Self. These aka threads serve as energy channels.

High Self—The Huna term for the level of the personality that functions as a guardian spirit and forms the person's connection with God.

Kahuna—A native Hawaiian priest or healer.

Low self—The Huna term for the subconscious mind. The word "low" does not mean inferior in value, but refers only to what is below the level of consciousness.

Mana—The Hawaiian word for life energy. According to Huna, mana can be transferred from the conscious mind into parts of the body needing healing or into talismans or crystals to charge them with energy.

Middle self—The Huna term for the conscious mind, including the ability to reason. The middle self is what others recognize as an individual's personality.

tiates. All humans have the basic capacity to practice and benefit from Huna.

Precautions

As of 2000, Huna is considered an unproved therapy for major physical disorders and should not be used to the exclusion of proven medical treatments. Huna is said to promote general wellness, and should therefore be used only in conjunction with other healing methods in cases of potentially serious illness.

Side effects

There are no known physical side effects to Huna healing. The system's emphasis on speaking only positive things, being of service to others, and not hurting others might well have beneficial side effects in a person's life. In addition, the Huna Fellowship maintains that Huna does not require anyone to give up other religious affiliations or belief systems. This understanding minimizes the possibility of emotional **stress** caused by conflicting loyalties.

Research & general acceptance

The healing methods of Huna are unproved by medical research, although medical practitioners acknowledge that benefits may be achieved through a **placebo effect**.

Training & certification

Training consists of brief courses (usually less than one week) offered in Hawaii and elsewhere. The methods can also be self-taught, using books, videos, and other teaching materials that can be obtained from Huna Research. Huna healers and teachers can be found in many countries of the world.

Resources

ORGANIZATIONS

Aloha International. P.O. Box 665. Kilauea, HI 96754. (808) 828-0302. http://www.huna.org/.

Huna Research, Inc. 1760 Anna Street. Cape Girardeau, MO 63701-4504. (573) 334-3478.

David Helwig

Hydrotherapy

Definition

Hydrotherapy, or **water** therapy, is the use of water (hot, cold, steam, or ice) to relieve discomfort and promote physical well-being.

Origins

The therapeutic use of water has a long history. Ruins of an ancient bath were unearthed in Pakistan and date as far back as 4500 B.C. Bathhouses were an essential part of ancient Roman culture. The use of steam, baths, and aromatic massage to promote well being is documented since the first century. Roman physicians Galen and Celsus wrote of treating patients with warm and cold baths in order to prevent disease.

By the seventeenth and eighteenth centuries, bathhouses were extremely popular with the public throughout Europe. Public bathhouses made their first American appearance in the mid 1700s.

In the early nineteenth century, Sebastien Kneipp, a Bavarian priest and proponent of water healing, began treating his parishioners with cold water applications after he himself was cured of **tuberculosis** through the same methods. Kneipp wrote extensively on the subject, and opened a series of hydrotherapy clinics known as the Kneipp clinics, which are still in operation today. Around the same time in Austria, Vincenz Priessnitz was treating patients with baths, packs, and showers of cold spring water. Priessnitz also opened a spa that treated over 1,500 patients in its first year of operation, and be-

VINZENZ PRIESSNITZ 1799–1851

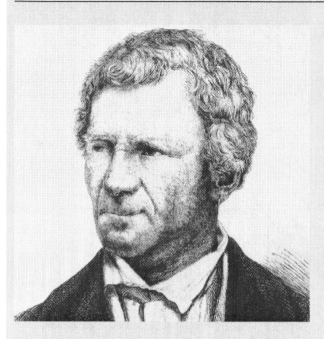

(Betmann/CORBIS. Reproduced by permission.)

Hydrotherapy inventor Vinzenz Priessnitz was the son of a Silesian farmer from a remote Austrian territory in the Jeseniky Mountains. From the age of 12, Priessnitz dutifully provided for his blind father, his elderly mother, and his sister. His formal education was sporadic at best. However, Priessnitz possessed a level head and a high degree of intelligence along with a keen and active mind. As he matured he became extremely aware of his surroundings in nature.

At age 16, Priessnitz fell from a horse and was seriously hoofed by the animal. He received the morbid prognosis that he might be crippled at best, or might die at worst. He set to treating his own chest wound with cold packs, in emulation of a doe that he had once observed bathing a wound in a cool mountain stream. The hydrotherapy regimen proved highly effective and drew considerable attention to his small hometown of Gräfenberg. In 1822 he rebuilt the family home, renovating its wooden frame into a solid brick spa structure. The spa, known as the castle, housed as many as 1,500 guests each year by 1839. Among the guests were medical professionals who were intent upon exposing the therapy as a sham.

Detractors notwithstanding, word of the simple and effective treatment spread to Vienna, where Priessnitz traveled on occasion to provide counsel at the emperor's court. Priessnitz, for his remarkable discovery, received the Austrian Gold Civil Merit Medal First Class, the highest civilian honor of the Austrian government.

Priessnitz died on November 28, 1851. He was survived by a wife, Zofie Priessnitz, and a young son, Vinzenz Pavel. Joseph Schindler took over the operation of the spa at Gräfenberg following the death of its founder.

Gloria Cooksey

came a model for physicians and other specialists to learn the techniques of hydrotherapy.

Benefits

Hydrotherapy can soothe sore or inflamed muscles and joints, rehabilitate injured limbs, lower fevers, soothe headaches, promote **relaxation**, treat **burns** and frostbite, ease labor pains, and clear up skin problems. The temperature of water used affects the therapeutic properties of the treatment. Hot water is chosen for its relaxing properties. It is also thought to stimulate the immune system. Tepid water can also be used for **stress** reduction, and may be particularly relaxing in hot weather. Cold water is selected to reduce inflammation. Alternating hot and cold water can stimulate the circulatory system and improve the immune system. Adding herbs and **essential oils** to water can enhance its therapeutic value. Steam is frequently used as a carrier for essential oils that are inhaled to treat respiratory problems.

Since the late 1990s, hydrotherapy has been used in critical care units to treat a variety of serious conditions, including such disorders of the nervous system as Guillain-Barré syndrome.

Description

Water can be used therapeutically in a number of ways. Common forms of hydrotherapy include:

- Whirlpools, Jacuzzis, and hot tubs. These soaking tubs use jet streams to massage the body. They are frequently used by physical therapists to help injured patients regain muscle strength and to soothe joint and muscle **pain**. Some midwives and obstetricians also approve of the use of hot tubs to soothe the pain of labor.

- Pools and Hubbard tanks. Physical therapists and rehabilitation specialists may prescribe underwater pool exercises as a low-impact method of rebuilding muscle strength in injured patients. The buoyancy experienced

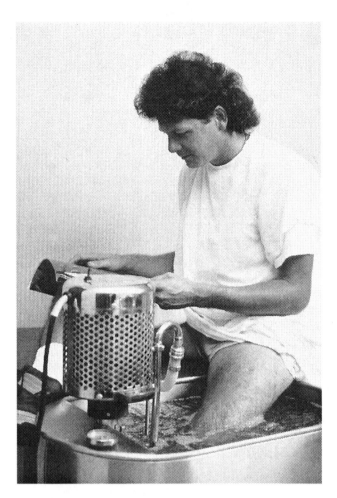

This patient is treating his injured left leg with a whirlpool bath. *(Custom Medical Stock Photo. Reproduced by permission.)*

during pool immersion also helps ease pain in such conditions as arthritis. The Arthritis Foundation has put together a set of Aquatic Program exercises that have been shown to improve isometric strength and range of motion in **osteoarthritis** patients.

• Baths. Tepid baths are prescribed to reduce a **fever**. Baths are also one of the oldest forms of relaxation therapy. Aromatherapists often recommend adding essential oils of **lavender** (*Lavandula angustifolia*) to a warm to hot bath to promote relaxation and stress reduction. Adding Epsom salts (**magnesium** sulfate) or Dead Sea salts to a bath can also promote relaxation and soothe rheumatism and arthritis.

• Showers. Showers are often prescribed to stimulate the circulation. Water jets from a shower head are also used to massage sore muscles. In addition, showering hydrotherapy has been shown to be preferable to immersion hydrotherapy for treating burn patients.

• Moist compresses. Cold, moist compresses can reduce swelling and inflammation of an injury. They can also

be used to cool a fever and treat a **headache**. Hot or warm compresses are useful for soothing muscle aches and treating abscesses.

• Steam treatments and saunas. Steam rooms and saunas are recommended to open the skin pores and cleanse the body of toxins. Steam inhalation is prescribed to treat respiratory **infections**. Adding botanicals to the steam bath can increase its therapeutic value.

• Internal hydrotherapy. **Colonic irrigation** is an enema that is designed to cleanse the entire bowel. Proponents of the therapy say it can cure a number of digestive problems. Douching, another form of internal hydrotherapy, directs a stream of water into the vagina for cleansing purposes. The water may or may not contain medications or other substances. Douches can be self-administered with kits available at most drug stores.

Preparations

Because of the expense of the equipment and the expertise required to administer effective treatment, hydrotherapy with pools, whirlpools, Hubbard tanks, and saunas is best taken in a professional healthcare facility, and/or under the supervision of a healthcare professional. However, baths, steam inhalation treatments, and compresses can be easily administered at home.

Bath preparations

Warm to hot bath water should be used for relaxation purposes, and a tepid bath is recommended for reducing fevers. Herbs can greatly enhance the therapeutic value of the bath for a variety of illnesses and minor discomforts.

Herbs for the bath can be added to the bath in two ways—as essential oils or whole herbs and flowers. Whole herbs and flowers can be placed in a muslin or cheesecloth bag that is tied at the top to make an herbal bath bag. The herbal bath bag is then soaked in the warm tub, and can remain there throughout the bath. When using essential oils, add five to 10 drops of oil to a full tub. Oils can be combined to enhance their therapeutic value. Marjoram (*Origanum marjorana*) is good for relieving sore muscles; **juniper** (*Juniperus communis*) is recommended as a detoxifying agent for the treatment of arthritis; lavender, ylang ylang (*Conanga odorata*), and **chamomile** (*Chamaemelum nobilis*) are recommended for stress relief; cypress (*Cupressus sempervirens*), **yarrow** (*Achillea millefolium*), geranium (*Pelargonium graveolens*), clary **sage** (*Salvia sclaria*), and myrtle (*Myrtus communis*) can promote healing of **hemorrhoids**; and spike lavender and juniper (*Juniperus communis*) are recommended for rheumatism.

To prepare salts for the bath, add one or two handfuls of Epsom salts or Dead Sea salts to boiling water until they are dissolved, and then add them to the tub.

A sitz bath, or hip bath, can also be taken at home to treat hemorrhoids and promote healing of an episiotomy. There is an special apparatus available for taking a seated sitz bath, but it can also be taken in a regular tub partially filled with warm water.

Steam inhalation

Steam inhalation treatments can be easily administered with a bowl of steaming water and a large towel. For colds and other conditions with nasal congestion, aromatherapists recommend adding five drops of an essential oil that has decongestant properties, such as **peppermint** (*Mentha piperita*) and **eucalyptus** blue gum (*Eucalyptus globulus*). Oils that act as expectorants, such as myrtle (*Myrtus communis*) or **rosemary** (*Rosmarinus officinalis*), can also be used. After the oil is added, the individual should lean over the bowl of water and place the towel over the head to trap the steam. After approximately three minutes of inhaling the steam with eyes closed, the towel can be removed.

Other herbs and essential oils that can be beneficial in steam inhalation include:

- Tea tree oil (*Melaleuca alternifolia*) for **bronchitis** and sinus infections.

- Sandalwood (*Santalum album*), virginian cedarwood (*Juniperus virginiana*), and frankincense (*Boswellia carteri*) for sore throat.

- Lavender (*Lavandula angustifolia*) and **thyme** (*Thymus vulgaris*) for cough.

Compresses

A cold compress is prepared by soaking a cloth or cotton pad in cold water and then applying it to the area of injury or distress. When the cloth reaches room temperature, it should be resoaked and reapplied. Applying gentle pressure to the compress with the hand may be useful. Cold compresses are generally used to reduce swelling, minimize bruising, and to treat headaches and sprains.

Warm or hot compresses are used to treat abscesses and muscle aches. A warm compress is prepared in the same manner as a cold compress, except steaming water is used to wet the cloth instead of cold water. Warm compresses should be refreshed and reapplied after they cool to room temperature.

Essential oils may be added to moist compresses to increase the therapeutic value of the treatment. Peppermint, a cooling oil, is especially effective when added to cold compresses. To add oils to compresses, place five drops of the oil into the bowl of water the compress is to be soaked in. Never apply essential oils directly to a cloth, as they may irritate the skin in undiluted form.

Precautions

Individuals with paralysis, frostbite, or other conditions that impair the nerve endings and cause reduced sensation should take hydrotherapy treatments only under the guidance of a trained hydrotherapist, physical therapist, or other appropriate healthcare professional. Because these individuals cannot accurately sense temperature changes in the water, they run the risk of being seriously burned without proper supervision. Diabetics and people with **hypertension** should also consult their healthcare professional before using hot tubs or other heat hydrotherapies.

Hot tubs, Jacuzzis, and pools can become breeding grounds for bacteria and other infectious organisms if they are not cleaned regularly, maintained properly, kept at the appropriate temperatures, and treated with the proper chemicals. Individuals should check with their healthcare provider to ensure that the hydrotherapy equipment they are using is sanitary. Those who are using hot tubs and other hydrotherapy equipment in their homes should follow the directions for use and maintenance provided by the original equipment manufacturer.

Certain essential oils should not be used by pregnant or nursing women or by people with specific illnesses or physical conditions. Individuals suffering from any chronic or acute health condition should inform their healthcare provider before starting treatment with any essential oil.

Such essential oils as cinnamon leaf, juniper, lemon, eucalyptus blue gum, peppermint, and thyme can be extremely irritating to the skin if applied in full concentration. Oils used in hydrotherapy should always be diluted in water before they are applied to the skin. Individuals should never apply essential oils directly to the skin unless directed to do so by a trained healthcare professional and/or aromatherapist.

Colonic irrigation should be performed only by a healthcare professional. Pregnant women should never douche, as the practice can introduce bacteria into the vagina and uterus. They should also avoid using hot tubs without the consent of their healthcare provider.

The vagina is self-cleansing, and douches have been known to upset the balance of vaginal pH and flora, promoting **vaginitis** and other infections. Some studies have linked excessive vaginal douching to increased incidence of **pelvic inflammatory disease** (PID).

Side effects

Most forms of hydrotherapy are well tolerated. There is a risk of allergic reaction (also known as **contact dermatitis**) for some patients using essential oils and herbs in their bath water. These individuals may want to test for allergic sensitization to herbs by performing a skin patch test (i.e., rubbing a small amount of diluted herb on the inside of their elbow and observing the spot for redness and irritation). People who experience an allergic reaction to an essential oil should discontinue its use and contact their healthcare professional for further guidance.

The most serious possible side effect of hydrotherapy is overheating, which may occur when an individual spends too much time in a hot tub or Jacuzzi. However, when properly supervised, this is a minimal risk.

Research & general acceptance

Hydrotherapy treatments are used by both allopathic and complementary medicine to treat a wide variety of discomforts and disorders. Not as well accepted are invasive hydrotherapy techniques, such as colonic irrigation, enemas, and douching. These internal cleansing techniques can actually harm an individual by upsetting the natural balance of the digestive tract and the vagina. Most conventional medical professionals agree that vaginal douches are not necessary to promote hygiene in most women, and can actually do more harm than good.

Training & certification

Hydrotherapy is practiced by a number of physical therapists, medical doctors (especially those specializing in rehabilitation), nurses, and naturopathic physicians. Medical doctors, physical therapists, and nurses are licensed throughout the United States. Naturopaths are licensed in a number of states. Aromatherapists, who frequently recommend water-based treatments with herbs and essential oils, are not licensed, although there are certification programs available for practitioners.

Resources

BOOKS

Chaitow, Leon. *Hydrotherapy: Water Therapy for Health and Beauty.* Boston: Element Books, 1999.

Lawless, Julia. *The Complete Illustrated Guide to Aromatherapy.* Boston: Element Books, 1997.

Pelletier, Dr. Kenneth R. *The Best Alternative Medicine, Part I: Naturopathic Medicine.* New York: Simon and Schuster, 2002.

PERIODICALS

Baird, Carol L. "First-Line Treatment for Osteoarthritis: Part 2: Nonpharmacologic Interventions and Evaluation." *Orthopaedic Nursing* 20 (November-December 2001): 13–20.

KEY TERMS

Contact dermatitis—Skin irritation as a result of contact with a foreign substance.

Episiotomy—An incision made in the perineum during labor to assist in delivery and to avoid abnormal tearing of the perineum.

Essential oil—A volatile oil extracted from the leaves, fruit, flowers, roots, or other components of a plant and used in aromatherapy, perfumes, foods, and beverages.

Hubbard tank—A large water tank or tub used for underwater exercises.

Jacuzzi—A trademark name for a whirlpool bath.

Sitz bath—A bathtub shaped like a chair, which allows a person to bathe in a sitting position so that only the hips and buttocks are immersed. The name comes from the German word for "sit."

Barker, K. L., H. Dawes, P. Hansford, and D. Shamley. "Perceived and Measured Levels of Exertion of Patients with Chronic Back Pain Exercising in a Hydrotherapy Pool." *Archives of Physical Medicine and Rehabilitation* 84 (September 2003): 1319–1323.

Cider, A., M. Schaufelberger, K. S. Sunnerhagen, and B. Andersson. "Hydrotherapy—A New Approach to Improve Function in the Older Patient with Chronic Heart Failure." *European Journal of Heart Failure* 5 (August 2003): 527–535.

Johnson, Kate. "Hydrotherapy Greatly Eases Delivery Stress, Pain." *OB GYN News* 34 (November 1999): 27.

Keegan, L. "Therapies to Reduce Stress and Anxiety." *Critical Care Nursing Clinics of North America* 15 (September 2003): 321–327.

Mayhall, C. G. "The Epidemiology of Burn Wound Infections: Then and Now." *Clinical Infectious Diseases* 37 (August 15, 2003): 543–550.

Molter, N. C. "Creating a Healing Environment for Critical Care." *Critical Care Nursing Clinics of North America* 15 (September 2003): 295–304.

Taylor, S. "The Ventilated Patient Undergoing Hydrotherapy: A Case Study." *Australian Critical Care* 16 (August 2003): 111–115.

ORGANIZATIONS

American Association of Naturopathic Physicians. 8201 Greensboro Drive, Suite 300, McLean, Virginia 22102. (206) 298-0126. <http://naturopathic.org>.

Canadian Naturopathic Association/Association canadienne de naturopathie. 1255 Sheppard Avenue East at Leslie, North York, ON M2K 1E2. (800) 551-4381 or (416) 496-8633. <http://www.naturopathicassoc.ca>.

Paula Ford-Martin
Rebecca J. Frey, PhD

Hyperactivity *see* **Attention-deficit hyperactivity disorder**

Hypercortisolemia

Definition

Cortisol is an essential glucocorticoid hormone, a subgroup of steroid hormones, the major hormone secreted by the adrenal glands. Hormones are messenger substances, substances produced in one gland or area of the body that move through the blood and stimulate activity in other glands or areas. Glucocorticoid hormones affect carbohydrate and protein metabolism. Steroid hormones are hormones related to **cholesterol**. Hypercortisolemia refers to high amounts of circulating cortisol and may be a pathological or non-pathological condition.

Description

Pathological hypercortisolemia, or Cushing's syndrome, named after the United States surgeon, Harvey Cushing (1869–1939), may result from a **lung cancer**, tumor of the pituitary or adrenal glands, or from kidney failure. Nonpathological hypercortisolemia is a normal response of **pregnancy**, and to such traumas, as accidents or surgery (including circumcision, studies show), some forms of **depression** and **stress**. Over time, continued exposure to trauma and stress may produce chronic hypercortisolemia and result in serious long-term debilitating illness.

Causes & symptoms

The natural regulation of cortisol is governed by a circular feedback response system. Output is initiated when pituitary gland secretions of adrenocorticotropin hormone (ACTH) travel to and stimulate the adrenal glands located atop the kidneys near the middle of the upper back. From the adrenals, cortisol travels to its target tissues, initiating a series of reactions known as the "flight-or-fight" response. Information from these target tissues is monitored by the brain. If the messages received tell the brain that more help is needed, the pituitary gland is stimulated to secrete more ACTH, which stimulates increased secretion of cortisol. The most significant feedback factor is stress. When stress levels are reported to the brain as high, high levels of cortisol are released in response. When stress remains high indefinitely, cortisol levels may also remain high indefinitely, producing a series of biochemical, physiological and even anatomical reactions.

Normally, cortisol output has a diurnal and circadian rhythm, rising in the morning, falling at night, and changing with the seasons. Changes related to work-sleep cycles affect this rhythm, and changes in the rhythm affect night time sleep patterns. Changes in the length of daylight hours, blindness, and loss of consciousness also affects the rhythm.

Cortisol target tissues include:

• liver

• bone

• blood vessels

• kidney

• muscle

• brain

• immune system

Long-term exposure to cortisol, whether natural or synthetic—from such steroid drugs as prednisone, dexamethasone (Decadron), and Methylprednisone (Medrol)—may eventually result in such changes as **osteoporosis**, muscle weakening and wasting, high blood pressure, increased abdominal fat deposition, immune dysfunction, steroid-induced diabetes, and cardiovascular disease. Another serious consequence may be the eventual **fatigue** and failure of the adrenal glands. Cushing's syndrome classic symptoms include, in addition to "normal" long-term symptoms, a "moon face" (rounded), thinning of the skin accompanied by purple or pink stretch marks and easy bruising, **acne**, increased facial and body hair and decreased scalp hair in women, and fatigue.

Diagnosis

Initial diagnosis may be made through the office of a family practice physician or internist on the basis of signs and symptoms, physical examination, and lab work including testing levels of circulating cortisol. Three types of testing are available to check cortisol levels: 24-hour urine collection; blood testing; and, saliva sampling. The 24-hour urine collection test is done at home beginning after the first urination of the morning and finishing after the first urination of the following day. This test can be done on infants. No special preparation is necessary. The test is described as not uncomfortable. Special considerations were reported to include emotional or physical stress and medications: lithium, diuretics, estrogen, tricyclic antidepressants, ketoconazole, and glucocorticoids. Blood testing requires a visit to a lab, where blood is drawn and then analyzed. This test can be performed on infants, children and adults. Preparation for the test may include discontinuation of medications similar to those medications listed above, as advised by one's healthcare provider. Some people experience **pain** or trauma with blood drawing, which may affect test results. Results may also be affected by the timing of the blood draw, since cortisol normally varies rhythmically. Risks of a blood test include bruising, pain, excessive bleeding, infection, fainting or the need for multiple punctures. Saliva sampling is done at home by collecting four samples at specific times of day. Unlike the urine collection method that produces a daily average, or the blood test that produces a single-spot sampling, saliva sampling produces a time-wave pattern for a more amplified diagnosis. Preparation includes discontinuation of medications listed with the other two methods, as well as a short list of foods and drinks, antacids, tooth brushing, and **smoking** prior to sampling. Cost comparisons were not reported. Test results may suggest followup care with an endocrinologist, who is a specialist in glandular and hormonally related disease, for further testing and diagnosis.

Treatment

Preventive alternative care may focus on stress reduction primarily. Since stress may be induced by emotional demands, dietary and nutritional imbalances, subclinical illness (illness which may not have fully shown itself), and physical inactivity, an alternative-minded medical doctor, a licensed naturopathic physician, or other professional alternative healthcare provider may first work to reestablish balance through lifestyle changes specific to individual need. Treatment may include counseling; dietary and nutritional therapies; energy therapies, such as **Reiki**, tai-chi, qi gong, **chakra balancing** or Healing Touch; **Traditional chinese medicine**, including chinese herbals and **acupuncture**; **chiropractic**; **Ayurvedic medicine**; environmental medicine; **homeopathy**; **relaxation** therapy; **biofeedback**; craniosacral work; massage; **exercise** therapies; **shamanism**; and faith-based therapies, including prayer, **meditation**, **yoga** and other spiritual exercises. Dietary supplement products to block cortisol or correct underlying dietary and nutritional insufficiencies are also being advertised. Assistance from a professional healthcare provider is recommended.

Allopathic treatment

Initial allopathic care may focus on antidepressants, hypoglycemics (drugs that lower blood sugar), sedatives, or anti-hypertensives (drugs that lower blood pressure), medications to correct underlying or related imbalances. Discontinuance of such steroidal medications as prednisone, dexamethasone (Decadron), and methylprednisone (Medrol) may be warranted or advised. Treatment may also include higher protein recommendations to combat muscle wasting, or therapies which support kidney function.

Prognosis

In hypercortisolemia that has not progressed to serious disease, prognosis may be very good when commit-

KEY TERMS

Circadian—Events that occur on a 24 hour rhythmic cycle; a biological clock.

Diurnal—Events that happen in the daytime, daily; associated with circadian rhythms.

Feedback response—A response to information carried back to the brain, or to other areas or glands from target tissues that generates a follow up response.

Ketoconazole—An antifungal medication.

Osteoporosis—A condition referring to bone that is thinned and weakened; loss of bone mass. It results from the process of osteopenia, or bone loss.

Pathological or nonpathological—Terms indicating whether a condition is considered a disease state.

Prognosis—Referring to the expected outcome of a disease and its treatment.

Target tissues—Tissues specifically receptive to a given hormone.

Tricyclics—A type of antidepressant; Elavil, for example.

ted changes in lifestyle are made. The prognosis may be further improved when medications are avoided which either intensify the imbalance, or overlook or disguise an underlying cause, thereby adding further stress. In Cushing's syndrome, or where hypercortisolemia has progressed to chronic disease, prognosis may be complicated by a need for difficult surgery, chemotherapy, or radiation. Follow up supplemental administration of cortisol may be required. Where surgery or other direct control of adrenal output is not an option, administration of cortisol output suppressing medications may be necessary.

Prevention

Given that stress is the single most influential feedback signal to the brain, a reasonable conclusion is that stress reduction is the single most influential prevention. Lifestyle changes, strategies, and therapies that reduce or eliminate stress, directly by reducing burden, or indirectly by improving underlying health, are key. One theory in medicine is that if preventive intervention can be made before an organ or gland is exhausted, especially if supportive, strengthening or tonifying remedies and therapies are also employed, good health can be restored, and a higher quality of life preserved.

Resources

BOOKS

Berne, Robert M., and Matthew N. Levy, Bruce M. Koeppen, Bruce A. Stanton. *Physiology,* 4th ed. St. Louis, MO: Mosby, Inc., 1998.

Ferri, Fred. *Ferri's Clinical Advisor, Instant Diagnosis and Treatment.* St. Louis, MO:Mosby, Inc., 2003.

Ganong, William F. *Review of Medical Physiology,* 18th ed. Stromford, CT: Appleton & Lange. 2003.

OTHER

Ball, David. "Hypercortisolemia Cited in Link Between Depression and Cardiovascular Disorders." *Psychosomatic Medicine* April 9, 2002. [Cited May 5, 2004]. <http://www.docguide.com/news/content.nsf/NewsPrint>.

"Glucocorticoid Hormones." *UCSF Division of Endocrinology and Metabolism.* March 24, 2000 [Cited May 5, 2004]. <http://mountzion.ucsfmedicalcenter.org/endocrinology/adrenal/gluco.html>.

Gunnar, Megan R. et al. "The Effects of Circumcision on Serum Cortisol and Behavior." *Psychoneuroendocrinology.* February 23, 1981. [Cited May 5, 2004]. <http://www.cirp.org/library/pain/gunnar>.

Gur, Ali. "Cortisol and Hypothalamic-pituitary-gonadal Axis Hormones in Follicular-phase Women with Fibromyalgia and Chronic Fatigue Syndrome and Effect of Depressive Symptoms on these Hormones." *Arthritis Research Therapy* 2004. [Cited May 5, 2004] <http://arthritis-research.com/content/6/3/R232>.

Katy Nelson, ND

Hypericum *see* **St. John's wort**

Hyperopia

Definition

Hyperopia (farsightedness) is an eye condition in which incoming rays of light reach the retina before they converge into a focused image.

Description

When light passes through the lens and cornea of the eye, its velocity decreases. The surfaces of the lens and cornea are not perpendicular to the incoming light, so the direction of the light changes. The greater the curvature of the lens system, the greater the change in the direction of the light.

When parallel light rays pass through the lens system of the eye, they are bent so they converge at a point some distance behind the lens. With perfect vision, this point of convergence where the light rays are focused lies on the retina. Hyperopia is the condition in which the point of

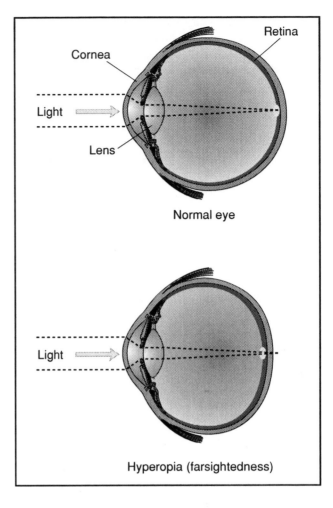

Normal eye

Hyperopia (farsightedness)

Hyperopia, or farsightedness, is a condition of the eye where incoming rays of light impinge on the retina before converging into a focused image, resulting in difficulty seeing nearby objects clearly. *(Illustration by Electronic Illustrators Group. The Gale Group.)*

focus of parallel light rays from an object lies behind the retina. This condition exists when the eyeball depth is too short for the curvature of its lens system.

There is a connection between the focusing of the lens of the eye (accommodation) and convergence of the eyes (the two eyes turning in to look at a close object). A good example is during reading, when the lens accommodates to make the close-up material clear and the eyes turn in to look at the print and keep it from doubling. Because of this connection between accommodation and convergence, if the lens needs to accommodate and focus for distance (to bring the image back onto the retina), the eyes may appear to turn in.

Causes & symptoms

Babies are generally born slightly hyperopic, but this symptom tends to decrease with age. There is normal variation in eyeball length and curvature of the lens and cornea, and some combinations of these variables give rise to eyes in which the cornea is too flat for the distance between the cornea and the retina. If the hyperopia is not too severe, the lens may be able to accommodate and bring the image back onto the retina. This accomodation results in clear distance vision, but the constant focusing could cause headaches or eyestrain. If the lens cannot accommodate for the full extent of the hyperopia, the distant image is blurry. If the eyes are focused for distance and the person is looking at a nearby object, the lens needs to accommodate further. This need may result in blurry nearby objects or headaches during close work.

Symptoms depend on the degree of hyperopia. Some individuals may have no symptoms, while others have blurry near vision and clear distance vision, and those with the most severe cases have blurry near and distance vision. Headaches and eyestrain may also occur, particularly when doing close work. An eye turned in (esotropia) may be a result of hyperopia, particularly in children. A turned eye could also signal a more serious problem, so a physician should be consulted.

Diagnosis

Because it is possible to have good visual acuity with some degree of hyperopia it, is important to relax accommodation before an eye exam. This is done with the use of eye drops and is called a cycloplegic exam, or cycloplegic refraction. The patient's visual status can be determined with a hand-held instrument called a retinoscope and/or by having the patient read from an eye chart while placing different lenses in front of the patient's eyes. The patient should be driven home after such an exam because the drops cause blurred vision for several hours.

Treatment

Herbals

Bilberry (*Vaccinium myrtillus*) increases the flow of blood through the vessels of the eye. Eye drops of **eyebright** (*Euphrasia officinalis*) tea can relieve eyestrain and, taken orally with rosemary (*Rosemarinus officinalis*) in white wine, can improve vision. **Schisandra** (*Schisandra chinensis*) improves visual clarity.

Homeopathy

Rue (*Ruta graveolens*) can be prescribed for eyestrain. A homeopathic practitioner should be consulted for a proper recommendation.

Supplements

Vitamins A and C, **magnesium**, zinc, and **selenium** can help strengthen the retina and improve vision.

Flavonoids—present in bilberry and eyebright—improve visual clarity.

Deconditioning

Persons whose vision changes according to their emotional state may have vision problems because of negative conditioning. Exploration and deconditioning may improve their vision.

Ayurveda

Head massage and nasya (placing drops in the nose) using warm Jivantal taila oil (which contains *Asparagus racemosus*, *Glycyrrhiza glabra*, *Leptadenia reticulata*, *Sida cordifolia*, *Sida retusa*, and **sesame oil**) may improve vision in persons who are hyperopic.

Chinese medicine

Performing qigong eye exercises significantly reduced hyperopia in children. In another study, children with hyperopia were cured following treatment with plum-blossom needle tapping plus external application of Huoxue Zengshi Ye (Infusion for Promoting Blood Circulation and Improving Eyesight) and Huoxue Zengshi Dan (Pellets for Promoting Blood Circulation and Improving Eyesight).

Bates method

The **Bates method** involves the use of therapeutic eye exercises to help strengthen and train the eye muscles. Some patients have found the eye exercises to help, although the method has not been tested in a clinical setting.

Other

Other movement exercises or disciplines can be useful including massage, **Feldenkrais movement therapy**, **yoga** and t'ai chi. A practitioner should be consulted to determine what would be most helpful for particular individuals.

Allopathic treatment

The usual treatment for hyperopia is corrective lenses (spectacles or contact lenses). Special contact lenses (vision orthotics) that are worn overnight temporarily reshape the cornea for ideal vision on the following day.

There are now several different surgical methods used to correct hyperopia. One approach is to implant corrective contact lenses behind the patient's iris. Another approach, called laser in situ keratomileusis (LASIK), is to surgically increase the curvature of the eye's existing cornea or lens using a laser. Many surgeries are successful, but complications, including worsening of vision, may occur.

In mid-2002, the Food and Drug Administration (FDA) approved a new surgical technique to correct hyperopia. Called conductive keratoplasty, it involves no cutting or removal of tissue. An ophthalmologist uses a small probe about the size of a human hair to pass radiofrequency waves that produce heat into the corneal tissue. The waves shrink the tissue and reshape the cornea.

Expected results

The prognosis for fully corrected vision is excellent for patients with low to moderate degrees of hyperopia. Patients with very high hyperopia may not achieve full correction.

Hyperopia increases the chances of chronic glaucoma, but vision loss from **glaucoma** is preventable.

Prevention

Hyperopia is usually present at birth and cannot be prevented. Eyestrain may be prevented by resting the eyes when they become overworked, blinking often, and periodically changing the eyes' focus while driving or doing close work for extended periods of time.

Resources

BOOKS
Newell, Frank W. *Ophthalmology: Principles and Concepts.* 8th edition. St. Louis: Mosby, 1996.

PERIODICALS
"Eye Zapper for Hyperopia." *Chemistry and Industry* (May 6, 2002):7.

"Eyes Wide Open About LASIK." *Harvard Health Letter* 24 (October 1999): 1+.

Hongfeng, Cheng and Ma Yuying. "Treatment of Juvenile Ametropia by Auricular-Plaster Therapy Combined with Plum-Blossom Needle Tapping: A Report of 200 Cases." *Journal of Traditional Chinese Medicine* 18 (1998): 47–48.

Lieberath, Frederik. "High Tech Eyes." *Harper's Bazaar* (September 1999): 529+.

Preboth, Monica. "FDA Approves Surgical Device to Treat Farsightedness." *American Family Physician* (June 1, 2002): 2389.

ORGANIZATIONS
American Academy of Ophthalmology. PO Box 7424, San Francisco, CA 94120-7424. (415) 561-8500. http://www.eyenet.org/.

American Optometric Association. 243 North Lindbergh Boulevard, St. Louis, MO 63141. (800) 365-2219. http://www.aoanet.org/.

KEY TERMS

Close work—Tasks that cause the eyes to focus on something close at hand, such as reading, writing, computer work, and sewing.

Cornea—The clear, dome-shaped outer covering of the front of the eye.

Iris—The colored ring of muscle that controls the amount of light allowed to reach the retina.

Pupil—The black hole in the center of the iris through which light enters on the way to the lens and retina.

Refraction—Method of determining the optical status of the eyes. Lenses are placed before the patient's eyes while the patient reads from an eye chart.

Retina—The inner, light-sensitive layer of the eye that transforms images into electrical messages which are sent to the brain.

OTHER
Edmiston, D. "Hyperopia." http://eyeinfo.com/hyperopia.html/.

"Treating Vision Disorders." AlternativeMedicine.com. http://www.alternativemedicine.com

Belinda Rowland
Teresa G. Odle

Hyperparathyroidism

Definition

Hyperparathyroidism is the overproduction by the parathyroid glands of a hormone called parathyroid hormone (parathormone). Parathyroid glands are four pea-sized glands located just behind the thyroid gland in the front of the neck. Parathyroid hormone (parathormone) helps regulate the levels of **calcium** and phosphorus in the body.

Description

Thyroid glands and parathyroid glands, despite their similar names and proximity, are entirely separate, and each produces hormones with different functions.

Hyperparathyroidism may be primary or secondary. It most often occurs in patients over age 30, and most commonly in patients 50 to 60 years old. It rarely occurs in children or the elderly. Women are affected by the dis-

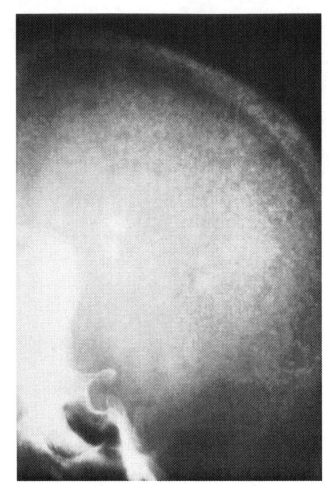

X ray of skull showing lighter areas of bone demineralization. *(Custom Medical Stock Photo. Reproduced by permission.)*

ease up to three times more often than men. It is estimated that 28 of every 100,000 people in the United States will develop hyperparathyroidism each year.

Normally, parathyroid glands produce the parathormone as calcium levels drop and lower to meet the demands of a growing skeleton, pregnancy, or lactation. However, when one or more parathyroid glands malfunction, it can lead to overproduction of the hormone and elevated calcium level in the blood. Therefore, a common result of hyperparathyroidism is hypercalcemia, or an abnormally high level of calcium in the blood.

Primary hyperparathyroidism occurs as a malfunction of one of the glands, usually as a result of a benign tumor called an adenoma. Secondary hyperparathyroidism occurs as the result of an abnormality outside the parathyroid glands related to the body's metabolism, or chemical changes in living cells that help provide the body's energy. These changes cause a resistance to the function of the parathyroid hormones. Primary hyper-

parathyroidism is one of the most common endocrine disorders, led only by diabetes and **hyperthyroidism**.

Causes & symptoms

Often, there are no obvious symptoms to give rise to suspicion of hyperparathyroidism, and it is first diagnosed when a patient is discovered to be hypercalcemic during a routine blood chemistry profile. Patients may believe they have been feeling fine, but realize improvements in sleep, irritability, and memory following treatment. When symptoms are present, they may include development of gastric ulcers or **pancreatitis** because high calcium levels can cause inflammation and **pain** in the linings of the stomach and pancreas.

Most of the symptoms of hyperparathyroidism are those present as a result of hypercalcemia, such as **kidney stones**, **osteoporosis**, or bone degradation resulting from the bones giving up calcium. Muscle weakness, central nervous system disturbances such as **depression**, psychomotor and personality disturbances, and even coma can occur. Patients also may experience heartburn, **nausea**, constipation, or abdominal pain. In secondary hyperparathyroidism, patients may show such signs of calcium imbalance as deformities of the long bones. Symptoms of the underlying disease also may be present.

Most commonly, hyperparathyroidism occurs as the result of a single adenoma, or benign tumor, in one of the parathyroid glands. About 90 percent of all cases of hyperparathyroidism are caused by an adenoma. The tumors seldom are cancerous. They will grow to a much larger size than the parathyroid glands, often to the size of a walnut. Genetic disorders or multiple endocrine tumors also can cause a parathyroid gland to enlarge and oversecrete hormone. In 10 percent or fewer of patients with primary hyperparathyroidism, there is enlargement of all four parathyroid glands. This condition is called parathyroid hyperplasia.

Diagnosis

Diagnosis of hyperparathyroidism most often is made when a blood test (radioimmunoassay) reveals high levels of parathyroid hormone and calcium. A blood test that specifically measures the amount of parathyroid hormone has made diagnosis simpler. Hypercalcemia is mild or intermittent in some patients, but persistent hypercalcemia is an excellent indicator of primary hyperparathyroidism. Dual energy x-ray absorptiometry (DEXA or DXA), a tool used to diagnose and measure osteoporosis, may be used once the diagnosis is made to show reduction in bone mass for primary hyperparathyroidism patients. Once a diagnosis of hyperparathyroidism is reached, the physician will probably order further tests to evaluate complications. For example, abdominal radiographs might reveal kidney stones.

For secondary hyperparathyroidism, normal or slightly decreased calcium levels in the blood and variable phosphorous levels may be visible. A patient history of familial kidney disease or convulsive disorders may suggest a diagnosis of secondary hyperparathyroidism. Other tests may reveal a disease or disorder that is causing the secondary hyperparathyroidism.

Treatment

Nutritional therapy

Limiting intake of soft drinks can help to prevent hyperparathyroidism. Soda drinks contain high levels of phosphorus. High **phosphorus** intake can cause hypocalcemia that leads to secondary hyperparathyroidism. In patients with hyperparathyroidism, forcing fluids and reducing intake of calcium-rich foods can help decrease calcium levels prior to surgery or if surgery is not necessary. These patients should not take any supplements that contain calcium without a doctor's approval.

Allopathic treatment

Hyperparathyroidism cases will usually be referred to an endocrinologist, who is a physician specializing in hormonal problems, or a nephrologist, who specializes in kidney and mineral disorders.

Patients with mild cases of hyperparathyroidism may not need immediate treatment if they have only slight elevations in blood calcium level and normal kidneys and bones. These patients should be regularly checked, probably as often as every six months, by physical examination and measurement of kidney function and calcium levels. A bone densitometry—a test to diagnose and monitor osteoporosis or thinning of bones—measurement should be performed every one or two years. After several years with no worsened symptoms, the length of time between tests may be increased.

Patients with more advanced hyperparathyroidism usually will have all or half of the affected parathyroid gland or glands surgically removed. This surgery is relatively safe and effective. The primary risks are those associated with general anesthesia. There are some instances in which the surgery can be performed with the patient under regional, or cervical (neck) block, anesthesia. Often such studies as ultrasonography—a test with high-frequency sound waves (ultrasound) that are bounced off tissues and echoes are converted to pictures called sonograms— prior to surgery help pinpoint the affected areas.

Treatment of secondary hyperparathyroidism involves removing or treating the underlying cause. In 2004, a new drug therapy was shown to lower parathyroid levels and improve calcium and phosphorus function in patients receiving dialysis (a blood-purifying treatment often performed on people with kidney diseases) who had uncontrolled secondary hyperparathyroidism. The drug, called cinacalcet, was approved by the U.S. Food and Drug Administration for people who have chronic kidney disease with secondary hyperparathyroidism.

Expected results

Removal of the enlarged parathyroid gland or glands (parathyroidectomy) cures the disease 95 percent of the time. Relief of bone pain may occur in as few as three days. In 2004, a study showed that parathyroidectomy improved depression in patients with hyperparathyroidism. As many as 54 percent of patients who had the procedure no longer needed antidepressant medications after having the surgery. In up to five percent of patients undergoing surgery, chronically low calcium levels may result, and these patients will require calcium supplements or **vitamin D** treatment.

Damage to the kidneys as a result of hyperparathyroidism is often irreversible. Prognosis is generally good; however, complications of hyperparathyroidism such as osteoporosis, bone **fractures**, kidney stones, peptic ulcers, pancreatitis, and nervous system difficulties may worsen prognosis.

Prevention

Secondary hyperparathyroidism may be prevented by early treatment of the disease causing it. Early recognition and treatment of hyperparathyroidism may prevent hypercalcemia. Since the cause of primary hyperparathyroidism, the adenoma which causes parathyroid enlargement, is largely unknown, there are no prescribed prevention methods.

Resources

BOOKS

Murray, Michael T. "Calcium." In *Encyclopedia of Nutritional Supplements: The Essential Guide for Improving Your Health Naturally.* Rocklin, CA: Prima Publishing, 1996.

Trattler, Ross. *Better Health Through Natural Healing.* New York, NY: McGraw-Hill Book Company, 985.

PERIODICALS

Allerheiligen, David A., Joe Schoeber, Robert E. Houston, Virginia K. Mohl, and Karen M. Wildman. "Hyperparathyroidism." *American Family Physician* 58 (April 15, 1998): 1795–1803.

"Parathyroidectomy Improves Depression in Patients with Hyperparathyroidism." *Drug Week* (April 23, 2003): 161.

KEY TERMS

Demineralization—A loss or decrease of minerals in the bones.

Endocrine—A system of organs and glands that secrete hormones directly into the blood lymph.

Phosphorous—An essential element in the diet, important in building bones.

"Positive New Data for Amgen's Sensipar for Secondary Hyperparathyroidism." *Pharma Marketletter* (April 12, 2004).

Taniegra, Edna D. "Hyperparathyroidism." *American Family Physician* (January 15, 2004): 333.

ORGANIZATIONS

Osteoporosis and Related Bone Diseases-National Resource-Center. 1150 17th S. NW, Ste. 500, Washington, DC 20036. (800) 624-BONE.

The Paget Foundation. 200 Varick Street, Suite 1004, New York, NY 10014-4810. (800) 23-PAGET.

OTHER

"Endocrine disorder and endocrine surgery." Endocrine Web. <http://www.endocrineweb.com>.

Mai Tran
Teresa G. Odle

Hypertension

Definition

Hypertension is the medical term for high blood pressure. Blood pressure is the force of blood pushing against the walls of arteries as it flows through them. Arteries are the blood vessels that carry oxygenated blood from the heart to the body's tissues.

Description

As blood flows through arteries, it pushes against the inside of the artery walls. The more pressure the blood exerts on the artery walls, the higher the blood pressure. The size of small arteries also affects the blood pressure. When the muscular walls of arteries are relaxed, or dilated, the pressure of the blood flowing through them is lower than when the artery walls are narrow, or constricted.

Blood pressure is highest when the heart beats to pump blood out into the arteries. When the heart relaxes to fill with blood again, the pressure is at its lowest point. Blood pressure when the heart beats is called systolic pressure. Blood pressure when the heart is at rest is called diastolic pressure. When blood pressure is measured, the systolic pressure is stated first and the diastolic pressure second. Blood pressure is measured in millimeters of mercury (mm Hg). For example, if a person's systolic pressure is 120 and diastolic pressure is 80, it is written as 120/80 mm Hg. The American Heart Association considers blood pressure above 140 over 90 high for adults.

Hypertension is a major health problem, especially because it has no symptoms. Many people have hypertension without knowing it. In the United States, about 50 million people age sixty and older have high blood pressure. Hypertension is more common in men than women and in people over the age of 65 than in younger persons. More than half of all Americans over the age of 65 have hypertension. It is also more common in African-Americans than in white Americans.

Hypertension is serious because people with the condition have a higher risk for **heart disease** and other medical problems than people with normal blood pressure. Serious complications can be avoided by getting regular blood pressure checks and treating hypertension as soon as it is diagnosed.

If left untreated, hypertension can lead to the following medical conditions:

- arteriosclerosis, also called **atherosclerosis**
- blindness
- **heart attack**
- **stroke**
- enlarged heart
- kidney damage

Arteriosclerosis is hardening of the arteries. The walls of arteries have a layer of muscle and elastic tissue that makes them flexible and able to dilate and constrict as blood flows through them. High blood pressure can make the artery walls thicken and harden. When artery walls thicken, the inside of the blood vessel narrows. **Cholesterol** and fats are more likely to build up on the walls of damaged arteries, making them even narrower. **Blood clots** can also get trapped in narrowed arteries, blocking the flow of blood.

Arteries narrowed by arteriosclerosis may not deliver enough blood to organs and other tissues. Reduced or blocked blood flow to the heart can cause a heart attack. If an artery to the brain is blocked, a stroke can result.

Hypertension makes the heart work harder to pump blood through the body. The extra workload can make the heart muscle thicken and stretch. When the heart becomes too enlarged it cannot pump enough blood. If the hypertension is not treated, the heart may fail.

The kidneys remove the body's wastes from the blood. If hypertension thickens the arteries to the kidneys, less waste can be filtered from the blood. As the condition worsens, the kidneys fail and wastes build up in the blood. Dialysis or a kidney transplant are needed when the kidneys fail. About 25% of people who receive kidney dialysis have kidney failure caused by hypertension.

Causes & symptoms

Many different actions or situations can normally raise blood pressure. Physical activity can temporarily raise blood pressure. Stressful situations can make blood pressure go up. When the **stress** goes away, blood pressure usually returns to normal. These temporary increases in blood pressure are not considered hypertension. A diagnosis of hypertension is made only when a person has multiple high blood pressure readings over a period of time.

The cause of hypertension is not known in 90–95% of the people who have it. Hypertension without a known cause is called primary or essential hypertension. When a person has hypertension caused by another medical condition, it is called secondary hypertension. Secondary hypertension can be caused by a number of different illnesses. Many people with kidney disorders have secondary hypertension. The kidneys regulate the balance of salt and **water** in the body. If the kidneys cannot rid the body of excess salt and water, blood pressure goes up. **Kidney infections**, a narrowing of the arteries that carry blood to the kidneys, called renal artery stenosis, and other kidney disorders can disturb the salt and water balance.

Cushing's syndrome and tumors of the pituitary and adrenal glands often increase levels of the adrenal gland hormones cortisol, adrenalin, and aldosterone, which can cause hypertension. Other conditions that can cause hypertension are blood vessel diseases, thyroid gland disorders, some prescribed drugs, **alcoholism**, and **pregnancy**.

Even though the cause of most hypertension is not known, some people have risk factors that give them a greater chance of getting hypertension. Many of these risk factors can be changed to lower the chance of developing hypertension or as part of a treatment program to lower blood pressure.

Risk factors for hypertension include:

- age over 60
- male sex
- race (The African-American community has a higher incidence of hypertension.)
- heredity

The effects of hypertension on the heart and kidney. Hypertension has caused renal atrophy and scarring, and left ventricular hypertrophy in the sectioned heart (at right). *(Photograph by Dr. E. Walker, Photo Researchers, Inc. Reproduced by permission.)*

- salt sensitivity
- obesity
- inactive lifestyle
- heavy alcohol consumption
- use of oral contraceptives

Some risk factors for hypertension can be changed, while others cannot. Age, male sex, and race are risk factors that a person cannot deter. Some people inherit a tendency to get hypertension. People with family members who have hypertension are more likely to develop it than those whose relatives are not hypertensive. People with these risk factors can avoid or eliminate the other risk factors to lower their chance of developing hypertension.

Diagnosis

Because hypertension does not cause symptoms, it is important to have blood pressure checked regularly. Blood pressure is measured with an instrument called a sphygmomanometer. A cloth-covered rubber cuff is wrapped around the upper arm and inflated. When the cuff is inflated, an artery in the arm is squeezed to momentarily stop the flow of blood. Then, the air is let out of the cuff while a stethoscope placed over the artery is used to detect the sound of the blood spurting back through the artery. This first sound is the systolic pressure, the pressure when the heart beats. The last sound heard as the rest of the air is released is the diastolic pressure, the pressure between heartbeats. Both sounds are recorded on the mercury gauge on the sphygmomanometer.

A number of such factors as **pain**, stress, or **anxiety** can cause a temporary increase in blood pressure. For this reason, hypertension is not diagnosed on the basis of only one high blood pressure reading. If a blood pressure reading is 140/90 or higher for the first time, the physician will have the person return for another blood pressure check. Diagnosis of hypertension usually is made based on two or more readings after the first visit. Sometimes, patients have high blood pressure only while in the doctor's office. This phenomenon, called "white-coat hypertension" has usually been dismissed as mere anxiety over visiting the doctor. In late 2001, an Italian study questioned dismissal of these patients as not being hypertensive and encouraged further study.

Systolic hypertension of the elderly is common and is diagnosed when the diastolic pressure is normal or low, but the systolic is elevated, e.g.170/70 mm Hg. This condition usually coexists with hardening of the arteries (atherosclerosis).

Blood pressure measurements are classified in stages according to severity:

• normal blood pressure: lower than 130/85 mm Hg

• high normal: 130–139/85–89 mm Hg

• mild hypertension: 140–159/90–99 mm Hg

• moderate hypertension: 160–179/100–109 mm Hg

• severe hypertension: 180–209/110–119

• very severe hypertension: 210/120 or higher

A typical physical examination to evaluate hypertension includes:

• medical and family history

• physical examination

• ophthalmoscopy: examination of the blood vessels in the eye

• chest x ray

• electrocardiograph (ECG)

• blood and urine tests

The medical and family history help the physician determine if the patient has any conditions or disorders that might contribute to or cause the hypertension. A family history of hypertension might suggest a genetic predisposition to the disorder.

The physical exam may include several blood pressure readings at different times and in different positions. The physician uses a stethoscope to listen to sounds made by the heart and blood flowing through the arteries. The pulse, reflexes, height, and weight are checked and recorded. Internal organs are palpated, or felt, to determine if they are enlarged.

Because hypertension can cause damage to the blood vessels in the eyes, the eyes may be checked with an instrument called an ophthalmoscope. The physician will look for thickening, narrowing, or hemorrhages in the blood vessels.

A chest x ray can detect an enlarged heart, other heart abnormalities, or lung disease.

An electrocardiogram (ECG) measures the electrical activity of the heart. It can detect if the heart muscle is enlarged and if there is damage to the heart muscle from blocked arteries.

Urine and blood tests may be done to further evaluate health and to detect the presence of disorders that might cause hypertension.

Treatment

There is no cure for primary hypertension, but blood pressure can almost always be lowered with the correct treatment. The goal of treatment is to lower blood pressure to levels that will prevent heart disease and other complications of hypertension. In secondary hypertension, the disease that is responsible for the hypertension is treated in addition to the hypertension itself. Successful treatment of the underlying disorder may cure the secondary hypertension.

Treatment to lower blood pressure usually includes changes in diet and getting regular **exercise**. Patients with mild or moderate hypertension who do not have damage to the heart or kidneys may first be treated primarily with lifestyle changes.

Lifestyle changes that may reduce blood pressure by about 5–10 mm Hg include:

• reducing salt intake

• reducing fat intake

• losing weight

• getting regular exercise

• quitting **smoking**

• reducing alcohol consumption

• managing stress

Natural remedies approved by a physician may also lower or even prevent hypertension. **Aromatherapy** as a treatment option uses **essential oils** either inhaled from a bottle in times of anxiety or massaged daily into the skin at bedtime in the area beneath the collarbone. Blue **chamomile** and **lavender** are known for their stress relief and **relaxation** effects.

Food therapy has also been shown to affect blood pressure. Muscles that regulate blood pressure have been noted to dilate with the intake of celery; celery juice has also been found to have a mild diuretic effect. Eating fresh fruits and vegetables, which are high in **potassium** and **magnesium**, lowers systemic **sodium** and fluid levels in the circulatory system. A 2001 study showed that reducing intake of sodium decreases blood pressure in participants with or without hypertension. **Garlic** intake has also been linked with lowering blood pressures. Taken either via enteric-coated capsules or fresh garlic cloves, allicin is thought to be the ingredient that brings down the blood pressure.

Relaxation and **meditation** can help lower blood pressure. Focusing on relaxing music can also slow the heart rate and lower blood pressure, as can imagery (envisioning coolness seeping into the pores and throughout the body, sensing that blood pressure is within normal range). **Yoga** experts cite two specific poses, the corpse pose and the knee squeeze, when used in combination with breathing exercises, as being particularly helpful in relieving tension and improving blood flow.

Allopathic treatment

Patients whose blood pressure remains higher than 139/90 will most likely be advised to take antihypertensive medication. Numerous drugs have been developed to treat hypertension. The choice of medication will depend on the stage of hypertension, side effects, other medical conditions the patient may have, and other medicines the patient is taking.

Patients with mild or moderate hypertension are initially treated with monotherapy, a single antihypertensive medicine. If treatment with a single medicine fails to lower blood pressure sufficiently, a different medicine may be tried or another medicine may be added to the first. Patients with more severe hypertension may initially be given a combination of medicines to control their hypertension. Combining antihypertensive medicines with different types of action often controls blood pressure with smaller doses of each drug than would be needed for monotherapy.

Antihypertensive medicines fall into several classes:

• diuretics

• beta-blockers

• **calcium** channel blockers

• angiotensin-converting enzyme inhibitors (ACE inhibitors)

• alpha-blockers

• alpha-beta blockers

• vasodilators

• peripheral-acting adrenergic antagonists

• centrally-acting agonists

Diuretics help the kidneys eliminate excess salt and water from the body's tissues and the blood. This helps reduce the swelling caused by fluid buildup in the tissues. The reduction of fluid dilates the walls of arteries and lowers blood pressure.

Beta-blockers lower blood pressure by acting on the nervous system to slow the heart rate and reduce the force of the heart's contraction. They are used with caution in patients with heart failure, **asthma**, diabetes, or circulation problems in the hands and feet.

Calcium channel blockers block the entry of calcium into muscle cells in artery walls. Muscle cells need calcium to constrict, so reducing their calcium keeps them more relaxed and lowers blood pressure.

ACE inhibitors block the production of substances that constrict blood vessels. They also help reduce the buildup of water and salt in the tissues. They are often given to patients with heart failure, kidney disease, or diabetes. ACE inhibitors may be used together with diuretics.

Alpha-blockers act on the nervous system to dilate arteries and reduce the force of the heart's contractions.

Alpha-beta blockers combine the actions of alpha and beta blockers.

Vasodilators act directly on arteries to relax their walls so blood can move more easily through them. They lower blood pressure rapidly and are injected in hypertensive emergencies when patients have dangerously high blood pressure.

Peripheral-acting adrenergic antagonists act on the nervous system to relax arteries and reduce the force of the heart's contractions. They usually are prescribed together with a diuretic. Peripheral acting adrenergic antagonists can cause slowed mental function and lethargy.

Centrally-acting agonists also act on the nervous system to relax arteries and slow the heart rate. They are usually used with other antihypertensive medicines.

In 2001, a medical device company announced findings about the effectiveness of a breathing device to work along with antihypertensive medications. By helping patients alter breathing patterns to lengthen the phase in which they exhale, they could slow breathing and see beneficial effects on blood pressure accumulate. The device is available through prescription only, but is pending over-the-counter-clearance from the Food and Drug Administration (FDA.)

Expected results

There is no cure for hypertension. However, it can be well controlled with the proper treatment. The key to avoiding serious complications of hypertension is to detect

KEY TERMS

. . . .

Arteries—Blood vessels that carry blood to organs and other tissues of the body.

Arteriosclerosis—Hardening and thickening of artery walls.

Cushing's syndrome —A disorder in which too much of the adrenal hormone, cortisol, is produced; it may be caused by a pituitary or adrenal gland tumor.

Diastolic blood pressure—Blood pressure when the heart is resting between beats.

Hypertension—High blood pressure.

Renal artery stenosis —Disorder in which the arteries that supply blood to the kidneys constrict.

Sphygmomanometer—An instrument used to measure blood pressure.

Systolic blood pressure—Blood pressure when the heart contracts (beats).

Vasodilator—Any drug that relaxes blood vessel walls.

Ventricle —One of the two lower chambers of the heart.

and treat it before damage occurs. Because antihypertensive medicines control blood pressure, but do not cure it, patients must continue taking the medications to maintain reduced blood pressure levels and avoid complications.

Prevention

Prevention of hypertension centers on avoiding or eliminating known risk factors. Even persons at risk because of age, race, or sex or those who have an inherited risk can lower their chance of developing hypertension.

The risk of developing hypertension can be reduced by making the same lifestyle changes recommended for treating hypertension.

Resources

BOOK

Bellenir, Karen, and Peter D. Dresser, eds. *Cardiovascular Diseases and Disorders Sourcebook.* Detroit: Omnigraphics, 1995.

Texas Heart Institute. *Heart Owner's Handbook.* New York: John Wiley and Sons, 1996.

PERIODICALS

Boschart, Sherry. "Guided Breathing Exercise May Help Cut Hypertension (Preliminary Trial Results)." *Internal Medicine News* 34, no. 21 (November 1, 2001): 30–31.

"Study Suggests White-Coat Hypertension is Not Harmless." *Medical Devices and Surgical Technology Week* (December 23, 2001): 26.

Vollmer, William M., et al. "Effects of Diet and Sodium Intake on Blood Pressure: Subgroup Analysis of the DASH-Sodium Trail." *Annals of Internal Medicine* 135, no. 12 (December 18, 2001): 1019–1020.

ORGANIZATION

American Heart Association. 7272 Greenview Avenue, Dallas, TX 75231-4596. (800) AHS-USA1. <http://www.amhrt.org>.

National Heart, Lung, and Blood Institute. Information Center. PO Box 30105, Bethesda, MD 20824-0105. (301) 251-1222.

Texas Heart Institute. Heart Information Service, PO Box 20345, Houston, TX 77225-0345. (800) 292-2221.

Kathleen Wright
Teresa G. Odle

Hyperthermia

Definition

Hyperthermia involves raising the body's core temperature as a means of eradicating tumors. The treatment simulates **fever**. Some therapies actually bring on fever through the introduction of fever-causing organisms, while others raise body temperature by directly heating the blood.

Origins

Hyperthermia dates back to investigations begun in 1883 by William B. Coley, M.D., a general surgeon at New York City's Memorial Hospital. Coley was intrigued by a paper published in 1868 by an American family physician named Busch. Busch's paper described a patient with an untreatable sarcoma of the face. Though Busch had been unable to help the patient overcome her **cancer**, the patient went into remission spontaneously after suffering a bout of the skin infection known as erysipelas. The erysipelas resulted in a high fever ranging from 104°F to 105.8°F (40°C to 41°C). Over the next 20 years, Coley performed a series of experiments to study the effects of elevated temperature on various forms of cancer. After experimenting on animals, Coley moved to treating human cancer patients, injecting them with bacteria to induce high fevers. The bacteria he used are known as Coley's toxins. He reported much success with his method, especially against soft-tissue sarcomas and sarcomas of the bone. Yet his treatment also had serious side effects due to the **infections** he was introducing.

In spite of its drawbacks, Coley's work intrigued a few other researchers. A study published in *Cancer Research* in 1957 showed that in a review of 450 cases of supposed spontaneous remissions of cancer, 150 of the patients had suffered acute infections that raised their body temperatures. In the 1960s, a Cleveland surgeon and **breast cancer** specialist, George Crile Jr., published several studies of his experiments in eliminating tumors in mice using heat. Another doctor, Harry Leveen of South Carolina, began building machines that used radio frequencies to heat either the whole body or affected parts. But Leveen's machines were not approved by the Food and Drug Administration (FDA) and Leveen took his inventory to the University of Bangor in Wales. Hyperthermia did not receive much attention in the United States after this point, but practitioners in other countries, particularly Germany, Italy, and Mexico, have reported good results with it. An international congress on hyperthermia has been held each year since 1977.

Benefits

Hyperthermia has been shown in several studies to reduce malignant tumors either alone or in combination with chemotherapy. A 1998 study of patients with breast and **ovarian cancer** found that hyperthermia therapy increased the effectiveness of chemotherapy. This study suggested that patients undergoing hyperthermia might be successfully treated with lower doses of chemotherapy. A 2003 study demonstrated that women with breast cancer were less likely to experience spread of the cancer to distant lymph nodes or the lungs if they received a combination of whole-body hyperthermia and chemotherapy. A form of localized hyperthermia used to treat benign enlarged prostate glands can be performed in a doctor's office in as little as an hour, and this method does not have the side effects, such as **impotence** and incontinence, that often accompany traditional prostate surgery.

Newer methods of hyperthermia involving noninvasive (no penetration of skin) microwave technology have been introduced in other countries and were making their way to the United States in early 2002. This technology offered excellent results for some cancer patients in improving five-year survival rates for some aggressive forms of cancer when combined with other cancer therapy procedures.

Description

Hyperthermia therapy involves raising the body's internal temperature, and this can be brought about by several methods. Hyperthermia can involve the whole body, or just an affected local region. For reducing an enlarged prostate, doctors use a device approved by the FDA in 1996 that delivers microwaves to the prostate, while **water** cools the surrounding tissue to prevent **burns**. For whole-body hyperthermia, a method used in Europe employs a tent-like device that delivers infrared light to the body. The patient is injected with toxins to provoke a mild fever and then monitored under lights. The lights produce a slow rise in temperature, optimally to 107.6°F (42°C). A prominent practitioner of hyperthermia in Mexico directly heats the patient's blood. Under sedation, the doctor inserts a catheter into each leg near the groin. The two catheter tubes are connected to a heat exchanger. The heat exchanger heats the patient's blood, bringing up the entire body temperature. The patient is monitored by thermometers in the esophagus and rectum. Body temperature is raised to 107.6°F (42°C) for about one hour.

Side effects

The side effects of hyperthermia depend on how it is delivered. Cardiac problems are possible. The patient should be closely monitored during the procedure and after. For treatment of the prostate, localized hyperthermia seems to be without the side effects of traditional prostate surgery.

Research & general acceptance

Though research into hyperthermia as a cancer treatment began in the United States, most active practitioners are in Europe or Mexico as of 2004. However, the heat therapy for **prostate enlargement** was approved in the United States in 1996. Localized hyperthermia was being studied in the late 1990s for treatment of other conditions, including menorrhagia (heavy menstrual periods) and malignant tumors of the liver and rectum. Whole body hyperthermia continues to be studied and tested for its impact on cancers, and a test underway in 1999 in Texas examined this therapy for patients with **AIDS**. Several studies in 2003 showed hyperthermia's positive effects on cellular immune response in cancer patients, especially when used along with chemotherapy. One study suggested that the effectiveness of certain chemotherapy drugs used for **leukemia** patients could be enhanced by adding hyperthermia to the treatment.

Training & certification

Practitioners performing hyperthermia are certified medical doctors and such trained assistants as nurses and anesthesiologists.

Resources

PERIODICALS

"BSD Medical Licenses Right to NIH Non-invasive Deep Hyperthermia Cancer Therapy." *BIOTECH Patent News* (February 2002).

"Cancer (therapy)." *Women's Health Weekly* (August 10, 1998): 17.

"Hyperthermia and Ifosfamide Induced Cytotoxicity is Subadditive." *Proteomics Weekly* (March 24, 2003):10.

"Hyperthermia Improves Immune Response to Human Hepatocellular Carcinoma." *Vaccine Weekly* (July 30, 2003):10.

Jack, David. "Waxing Hot and Cold in the Surgical Arena." *The Lancet* (April 11, 1998): 1110.

Key, Sandra, and Michelle Marble. "Hyperthermia Treatment Evaluated" *Cancer Weekly Plus* (February 8, 1999): 14.

Walker, Morton. "Medical Journalist Report of Innovative Biologics: Whole Body Hyperthermia Effect on Cancer." *Townsend Letter for Doctors & Patients* (June 30, 1998): 60–66.

"Whole-body Hyperthermia and Metronomic Chemotherapy Prevent Cancer Metastasis." *Angiogenesis Weekly* (April 11, 2003):4.

Wu, Corrina, Shannon Brownlee, and Anna Mulrine. "Zapping a Problem Prostate." *U.S. News & World Report* (May 20, 1996): 71.

Angela Woodward
Teresa G. Odle

Hyperthyroidism

Definition

Hyperthyroidism is the overproduction of thyroid hormones by an overactive thyroid gland.

Description

Located in the front of the neck, the thyroid gland produces the hormones thyroxine (T_4) and triiodothyronine (T_3) that regulate the body's metabolic rate by helping to form protein ribonucleic acid (RNA) and increasing oxygen absorption in every cell. In turn, the production of these hormones is controlled by a thyroid-stimulating hormone (TSH) that is produced by the pituitary gland. When production of the thyroid hormones increases despite the level of TSH being produced, hyperthyroidism occurs. The excessive amount of thyroid hormones in the blood increases the body's metabolism, creating both mental and physical symptoms.

The term hyperthyroidism covers any disease that results in an overabundance of thyroid hormone. Other names for hyperthyroidism, or specific diseases within the category, include Graves' disease, diffuse toxic goiter, Basedow's disease, Parry's disease, and thyrotoxicosis. Hyperthyroidism affects 2.5 million people in the United States, but could affect up to 4.5 million people because more than half of the people with thyroid disease don't know they have it. Although it occurs at all ages, hyperthyroidism is most likely to occur after the age of 15. There is a form of hyperthyroidism called neonatal Graves' disease, which occurs in infants born of mothers with Graves' disease. Occult hyperthyroidism may occur in patients over age 65 and is characterized by a distinct lack of typical symptoms. Diffuse toxic goiter occurs in as many as 80% of patients with hyperthyroidism.

Causes & symptoms

Hyperthyroidism is often associated with the body's production of auto-antibodies in the blood that cause the thyroid to grow and secrete excess thyroid hormone. This condition, as well as other forms of hyperthyroidism, may be inherited. Regardless of the cause, hyperthyroidism produces the same symptoms, including weight loss with increased appetite, shortness of breath and fatigue, intolerance to heat, heart palpitations (strong, very fast heartbeats), increased frequency of bowel movements, weak muscles, **tremors, anxiety**, and difficulty sleeping. Women also may notice decreased menstrual flow and irregular menstrual cycles.

Patients with Graves' disease often have a goiter (visible enlargement of the thyroid gland), although as many as ten percent do not. These patients also may have bulging eyes. Thyroid storm, a serious form of hyperthyroidism, may show up as sudden and acute symptoms, some of which mimic typical hyperthyroidism but with the addition of **fever**, substantial weakness, extreme restlessness, confusion, emotional swings or psychosis, and perhaps even coma.

Diagnosis

Physicians will look for physical signs and symptoms indicated by patient history. On inspection, the physician may note symptoms such as a goiter or eye-bulging. Other symptoms or family history may be clues to a diagnosis of hyperthyroidism. An elevated basal (lowest range of normal) body temperature above 98.6 degrees Fahrenheit (37 degrees centigrade) may be an indication of a heightened basal metabolic rate (which measures the energy used to maintain vitality) and hyperthyroidism. A simple blood test can be performed to determine the amount of thyroid hormone in the patient's blood. The diagnosis usually is straightforward with this combination of clinical history, physical examination, and routine blood hormone tests.

Radioimmunoassay, or a test to show concentrations of thyroid hormones with the use of a radioisotope (a chemical element capable of radioactive or atomic transformations) mixed with fluid samples, helps confirm the diagnosis. A thyroid scan is a nuclear medicine procedure involving injection of a radioisotope dye that will tag the thyroid and help produce a clear image of inflammation or involvement of the entire thyroid.

Other tests can determine thyroid function and thyroid-stimulating hormone levels. Ultrasonography (a test whereby high-frequency sound waves (ultrasound) are bounced off tissues and echoes are converted to pictures (sonograms), computed tomography or (CT) scan (an x-ray computer procedure that produces a detailed picture of a cross-section of the body), and magnetic resonance imaging (MRI) (an x-ray technique that produces a detailed image of the inner body using a powerful magnet, radio waves, and a computer) may provide visual confirmation of a diagnosis or help to determine the extent of involvement.

Treatment

Alternative treatments for hyperthyroidism include nutritional therapy, herbal therapy, and **homeopathy**, the use of tiny doses of diluted and harmless remedies to catalyze healing.

Nutritional therapy

Consumption of such foods as broccoli, Brussels sprouts, cabbage, cauliflower, kale, rutabagas, spinach, turnips, peaches, and pears can help naturally suppress thyroid hormone production. Dairy products and any stimulants such as tea, coffee, soda, and other caffeinated drinks should be avoided. Under the supervision of a trained physician, high dosages of certain vitamin/mineral combinations can help alleviate hyperthyroidism.

Homeopathy

An experienced homeopath may give patients specific remedies tailored to their overall personality profile as well as their specific symptoms. Symptomatic treatments may include Iodium or *Natrum muriaticum.*

Other therapies

Other alternative treatments that may help relieve hyperthyroidism symptoms include **traditional Chinese medicine** and Western herbal medicine. **Stress** reduction techniques such as **meditation** also may prove beneficial. Patients should contact experienced herbalists for specific preparations and treatment.

Allopathic treatment

Allopathy is the theory or system of medical practice that combats disease by use of remedies that produce

SYMPTOMS OF HYPERTHYROIDISM
Symptoms
Goiter
Weight loss with increased appetite
Trembling hands
Heightened blood pressure
Excessive nervousness
Increased bowel movements
Accelerated heart rate

effects different from those produced by the disease. Treatment will depend on the specific disease and individual circumstances such as age, severity of disease, and other conditions affecting a patient's health.

Antithyroid drugs

Antithyroid drugs often are administered to help the patient's body cease overproduction of thyroid hormones. In 2004, some drugs used to interfere with the thyroid gland's uptake of **iodine** were propylthiouracil (PTU) and methimazole (Tapazole®). Medication may work for young adults, pregnant women, and others. Women who are pregnant should be treated with the lowest dose required to maintain thyroid function in order to minimize the risk of **hypothyroidism** (underactive thyroid gland function) in the infant.

Radioactive iodine

Radioactive iodine often is prescribed to damage cells that make thyroid hormone. The cells need iodine to make the hormone, so they will absorb any iodine found in the body. The patient may take an iodine capsule daily for several weeks, resulting in the eventual shrinkage of the thyroid, reduced hormone production, and a return to normal blood levels. A single large oral dose of radioactive iodine simplifies treatment but should only be given to patients who are not of reproductive age or are not planning to have children, since a large amount can concentrate in the reproductive organs (gonads).

Surgery

Patients treated with thyroidectomy, or surgery involving of partial or total removal of the thyroid, most often suffer from large goiter and have suffered relapses, even after repeated attempts to address the disease through drug therapy with iodine. Following thyroidectomy or iodine therapy, patients must be carefully monitored for years to watch for signs of hypothyroidism, or insufficient produc-

KEY TERMS

Goiter—Chronic enlargement of the thyroid gland.

Gonads—Organs that produce sex cells—the ovaries and testes.

Metabolic—Pertaining to metabolism, or the chemical processes that take place in the body, which result in growth, energy, elimination of waste, and other body functions.

Palpitation—A subjective feeling of a rapid and forceful heartbeat.

Radioisotope—A chemical tagged with radioactive compounds that is injected during a nuclear medicine procedure to highlight organs or tissue.

Thyroidectomy—Removal of the thyroid gland.

tion of thyroid hormones. Hypothyroidism can occur as a complication of thyroid production suppression.

Expected results

Hyperthyroidism generally is treatable and carries a good prognosis. Most patients lead normal lives with proper treatment. The majority of patients who receive radioactive iodine report feeling better within about three to six weeks of treatment. Thyroid storm, however, can be life-threatening and can lead to heart, liver, or kidney failure. Some patients who undergo radioactive iodine treatment or surgery become hypothyroid.

Prevention

There are no known prevention methods for hyperthyroidism, since its causes are either inherited or not completely understood. The best prevention tactic is knowledge of family history and close attention to symptoms and signs of the disease. Careful attention to prescribed therapy can prevent complications of the disease.

Resources

BOOKS

The Burton Goldberg Group. *Alternative Medicine.* Puyallup, WA: Future Medicine Publishing Inc., 1994.

Zand, Janet, Allan N. Spreen, and James B. LaValle. "Hyperthyroidism." *Smart Medicine for Healthier Living.* Garden City Park, NY: Avery Publishing Group, 1999.

PERIODICALS

Lazarus, John H. "Hyperthyroidism." *The Lancet* 340 (February 1, 1997): 339–342.

"Thyroid Disorders; Facts to Know." *NWHRC Health Center—Thyroid Disorders* (March 2, 2004).

"Thyroid Disorders; Treatment." *NWHRC Health Center—Thyroid Disorders* (March 2, 2004).

ORGANIZATIONS

The Thyroid Foundation of America. 350 Ruth Sleeper Hall RSL 350, Parkman Street, Boston, MA 02114. (800) 832–8321. <http://www.clark.net/pub/tfa>.

OTHER

"Endocrine disorder and endocrine surgery." Endocrine Web. <http://www.endocrineweb.com>.

Mai Tran
Teresa G. Odle

Hypnotherapy

Definition

Hypnotherapy is the treatment of a variety of health conditions by hypnotism or by inducing prolonged sleep.

Origins

Hypnotherapy is thought to date back to the healing practices of ancient Greece and Egypt. Many religions such as Judaism, Christianity, Islam, and others have attributed trance-like behavior to spiritual or divine possession.

An Austrian physician, Franz Mesmer (1734–1815), is credited with being the first person to scientifically investigate the idea of hypnotherapy in 1779 to treat a variety of health conditions. Mesmer studied medicine at the University of Vienna and received his medical degree in 1766. Mesmer is believed to have been the first doctor to understand the relationship of psychological trauma to illness. He induced a trance-like state, which became known as mesmerization, in his patients to successfully treat nervous disorders. These techniques became the foundation for modern-day hypnotherapy.

Mesmer's original interest was in the effect of celestial bodies on human lives. He later became interested in the effects of magnetism and found that magnets could have tremendous healing effects on the human body. Mesmer believed that the human body contained a magnetic fluid that promoted health and well being. It was thought that any blockage to the normal flow of this magnetic fluid would result in illness, and that the use of the Mesmerism technique could restore the normal flow.

Mesmer performed his technique by passing his hands up and down the patient's body. The technique

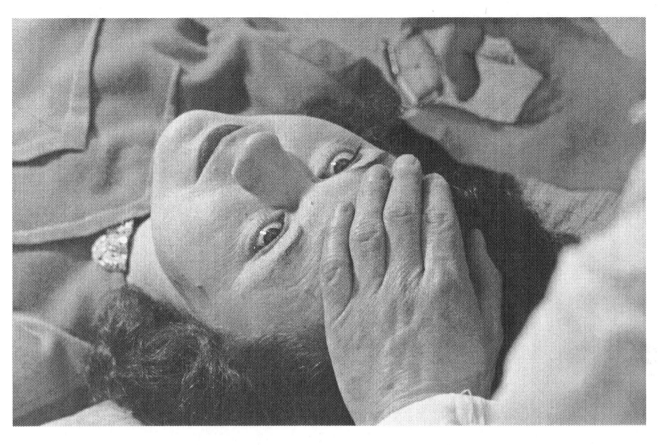

A psychiatrist hypnotises a volunteer in a London Clinic. (© *Hulton-Deutsch Collection/Corbis. Reproduced by permission.*)

was supposed to transmit magnetic fluid from his hands to the bodies of his patients. During this time period, there was no clear delineation between health conditions that were physical or psychological in nature. Although Mesmer did not realize it at that time, his treatments were most effective for those conditions that are now known to be primarily psychosomatic.

Mesmer's technique appeared to be quite successful in the treatment of his patients, but he was the subject of scorn and ridicule from the medical profession. Because of all the controversy surrounding mesmerism, and because Mesmer's personality was quite eccentric, a commission was convened to investigate his techniques and procedures. The very distinguished panel of investigators included Benjamin Franklin, the French chemist Antoine-Laurent Lavoisier, and the physician Jacques Guillotin. The commission acknowledged that patients did seem to obtain noticeable relief from their conditions, but the whole idea was dismissed as being medical quackery.

Other pioneers in this field, such as James Braid and James Esdaile, discovered that hypnosis could be used to successfully anesthetize patients for surgeries. James Braid accidentally discovered that one of his patients began to enter a hypnotic state while staring at a fixed light as he waited for his eye examination to begin. Since mesmerism had fallen out of favor, Braid coined the term hypnotism, which is derived from the Greek word for sleep. Braid also used the techniques of monotony, rhythm, and imitation to assist in inducing a hypnotic state. These techniques are generally still in use.

Around 1900, there were very few preoperative anesthetic drugs available. Patients were naturally apprehensive when facing surgery. One out of 400 patients would die, not from the surgical procedure, but from the anesthesia. Dr. Henry Munro was one of the first physicians to use hypnotherapy to alleviate patient fears about having surgery. He would get his patients into a hypnotic state and discuss their fears with them, telling them they would feel a lot better following surgery. Ether was the most common anesthetic at that time, and Dr. Munro found that he was able to perform surgery using only about 10% of the usual amount of ether.

It took more than 200 years for hypnotherapy to become incorporated into mainstream medical treatment. In 1955, the British Medical Association approved the use of hypnotherapy as a valid medical treatment, with the American Medical Association (AMA) giving its approval in 1958.

DR. FRANZ MESMER 1734–1815

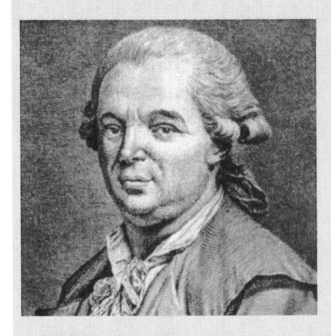

Corbis-Bettmann. Reproduced by permission.

Franz Mesmer was born on May 23, 1734, in the village of Itznang, Switzerland. At age 15 he entered the Jesuit College at Dillingen in Bavaria, and from there he went in 1752 to the University of Ingolstadt, where he studied philosophy, theology, music, and mathematics. Eventually he decided on a medical career. In 1759 he entered the University of Vienna, receiving a medical degree in 1766.

Mesmer settled in Vienna and began to develop his concept of an invisible fluid in the body that affected health. At first he used magnets to manipulate this fluid but gradually came to believe these were unnecessary; that, in fact, anything he touched became magnetized and that a health-giving fluid emanated from his own body. Mesmer believed a rapport with his patients was essential for cure and achieved it with diverse trappings. His treatment rooms were heavily draped, music was played, and Mesmer appeared in long violet robes.

Mesmer's methods were frowned upon by the medical establishment in Vienna, so in 1778 he moved to Paris, hoping for a better reception for his ideas. In France he achieved overwhelming popularity except among the physicians. On the basis of medical opinion, repeated efforts were made by the French government to discredit Mesmer. Mesmer retired to Switzerland at the beginning of the French Revolution in 1789, where he spent the remaining years of his life.

Critics focused attention of Mesmer's methods and insisted that cures existed only in the patient's mind. The nineteenth-century studies of Mesmer's work by James Braid and others in England demonstrated that the important aspect of Mesmer's treatment was the patient's reaction. Braid introduced the term "hypnotism" and insisted that hypnotic phenomena were essentially physiological and not associated with a fluid. Still later studies in France by A. A. Liebeault and Hippolyte Bernheim attributed hypnotic phenomena to psychological forces, particularly suggestion. While undergoing this scientific transformation in the nineteenth century, mesmerism in other quarters became more closely associated with occultism, spiritualism, and faith healing, providing in the last instance the basis for Christian Science.

Benefits

Hypnotherapy is used in a number of fields including **psychotherapy**, surgery, dentistry, research, and medicine. Hypnotherapy is commonly used as an alternative treatment for a wide range of health conditions, including weight control, **pain** management, and **smoking** cessation. It is also used to control pain in a variety of such conditions as **headache**, facial **neuralgia**, arthritis, **burns**, musculoskeletal disorders, **childbirth**, and many more. Hypnotherapy is being used in place of anesthesia, particularly in patients who prove to be allergic to anesthetic drugs, for such surgeries as hysterectomies, cesarean sections, certain cardiovascular procedures, thyroidectomy, and others. Dentists use hypnotherapy with success on patients who are allergic to all types of dental anesthetics. Hypnotherapy is also useful in helping patients overcome **phobias.**

Hypnotherapy is used for nonmedical patients as well as those who wish to overcome bad habits. Hypnotherapy has been shown to help those who suffer from performance **anxiety** in such activities as sports and speaking in public. In academic applications, it has also been shown to help with learning, participating in the classroom, concentrating, studying, extending attention span, improving memory, and helping remove mental blocks about particular subjects.

In more general areas, hypnotherapy has been found to be beneficial for such problems as motivation, procrastination, decision-making, personal achievement and development, job performance, buried or repressed memories, **relaxation**, and **stress** management.

Description

Hypnotherapy involves achieving a psychological state of awareness that is different from the ordinary state of consciousness. While in a hypnotic state, a variety of phenomena can occur. These phenomena include alterations in memory, heightened susceptibility to suggestion, paralysis, sweating, and blushing. All of these changes can be produced or removed in the hypnotic state. Many studies have shown that roughly 90% of the population is capable of being hypnotized.

This state of awareness can be achieved by relaxing the body, focusing on one's breathing, and shifting attention away from the external environment. In this state, the patient has a heightened receptivity to suggestion. The usual procedure for inducing a hypnotic trance in another person is by a direct command repeated in a soothing, monotonous tone of voice.

Preparations

Ideally, the following conditions should be present to successfully achieve a state of hypnosis:

- willingness to be hypnotized
- rapport between the patient or client and the hypnotherapist
- a comfortable environment conducive to relaxation

Precautions

Hypnotherapy can have negative outcomes. When used as entertainment, people have been hypnotized to say or do things that would normally embarrass them. There have been instances where people already dangerously close to psychological breakdown have been pushed into an emotional crisis during what was supposed to be a harmless demonstration of hypnosis. A statement from the World Hypnosis Organization (WHO) warns against performing hypnosis on patients suffering from psychosis, organic psychiatric conditions, or antisocial personality disorders. Because there are no standard licensing requirements, there is a risk that the hypnotist will have difficulty in controlling or ending a hypnotic state that has been induced in the patient.

There is a commonly held belief that a person cannot be coerced into doing things that he or she would not normally do while under hypnosis. The hynotherapist should take care, however, not to give suggestions during hypnosis that are contrary to the patient's moral code.

Many religions do not condone the practice of hypnotherapy. Leaders of the Jehovah's Witnesses and Christian Science religions oppose the use of hypnotherapy and advise their members to avoid it completely, whether for entertainment or therapy. The Church of Jesus Christ of Latter-Day Saints approves it for medical purposes, but cautions members against allowing themselves to be hypnotized for entertainment or demonstration purposes.

In 1985, the AMA convened a commission that warned against using hypnotherapy to aid in recollection of events. The commission cited studies that showed the possibility of hypnotic recall resulting in confabulation or an artificial sense of certainty about the course of events. As a result, many states limit or prohibit testimony of hypnotized witnesses or victims.

Side effects

Experiments have been conducted to determine any side effects of hypnotherapy. Some subjects have reported side effects such as headache, stiff neck, drowsiness, cognitive distortion or confusion, **dizziness**, and anxiety. However, most of these effects cleared up within several hours of the hypnotherapy session.

Research & general acceptance

Research on the effectiveness of hypnotherapy on a variety of medical conditions is extensive. In one study, the use of hypnotherapy did not seem to alter the core symptoms in the treatment of **attention-deficit hyperactivity disorder** (ADHD); however, it did seem useful in managing the associated symptoms, including sleep disturbances and tics.

Hypnotherapy is being studied in children who have common chronic problems and to aid in relieving pain. Children are particularly good candidates for hypnotherapy because their lack of worldly experience enables them to move easily between the rational world and their imagination. Studies with children have shown responses to hypnotherapy ranging from diminished pain and anxiety during a number of medical procedures; a 50% range in reduction of symptoms or a complete resolution of a medical condition; and a reduction in use of antinausea medication and **vomiting** during chemotherapy for childhood cancers.

In 2002, a report compiled several study results on hypnosis. One recent study evaluated how self-hypnosis relieved pain and anxiety in patients undergoing angioplasty with local anesthesia. Those patients needed less sedation and less procedure time. Another study found that pregnant adolescents counseled in hypnosis needed less anesthesia during delivery and less pain medication afterward. They also left the hospital sooner.

The use of hypnotherapy with **cancer** patients is another area being investigated. A meta-analysis of 116 studies showed positive results of using hypnotherapy with cancer patients. Ninety-two percent showed a positive effect on **depression**; 93% showed a positive effect on physical well-being; 81% showed a positive effect on vomiting; and 92% showed a positive effect on pain. In 2002, the National Hospice and Palliative Care Association reported that it recognizes hypnosis therapy as one effective tool to help terminally ill patients deal with their fears, feelings, and emotions; and to promote relaxation.

Training & certification

In the early twenty-first century, anyone could be a hypnotherapist. It is very easy to learn how to hypnotize someone, and the fact that hypnotism dates back to ancient times proves the ease with which a trance can be induced. There are no licensing procedures in place that limit the practice of hypnotherapy to medical professionals. Hypnotherapists are not regulated in any way; there are no uniform education or certification requirements to perform hypnotherapy.

The National Board for Hypnotherapy and Hypnotic Anaesthesiology (NBHA) has specific membership requirements and also offers varying levels of professional recognition. Certification as a Clinical Hypnotherapist (C.Ht.) requires a minimum of 200 hours of classroom instruction and, independent study and life learning experience in the medical, dental, psychological, or peer counseling professions. Certification as a Medical Hypnotherapist (C.M.H.) requires meeting the standards for the Clinical Hypnotherapist level plus attending a residential training course or home study training course that requires a clinical practicum/internship approved by the NBHA. Certification as a Hypno-Anesthesia Therapist (Ct.H.A.) requires the successful completion of an NBHA-approved course in Visualization and **Guided Imagery** for Pain Management, and a passing score on the examination. Certification as a Registered Hypnotic Anaesthesiologist (R.H.A.) requires two years of continuous membership in the NBHA at the Ct.H.A. level, and completion of advanced training seminars. The highest level of certification that can be obtained in this organization is Fellow (F.B.H.A.). Requirements for achieving this level of certification include membership at the R.H.A. level and a graduate degree from an accredited university, plus submitting a comprehensive thesis.

There is an ongoing debate regarding the issue of clinically trained versus lay hypnotists. The position of the American Society of Clinical Hypnotists (ASCH) is that the training of lay hypnotists is unethical. This organization supports only the training of those persons who are pursuing an advanced degree in the health sciences. ASCH further believes that hypnotherapy is a treatment modality to be used in conjunction with other forms of treatment, not a treatment that stands alone. Medical professionals believe that lay hypnotists keep the view of hypnotherapy in low esteem by the general public. They also believe that their practices are impacted economically by the lay hypnotists.

ASCH and the Society for Clinical and Experimental Hypnosis (SCEH) are two organizations that are trying to set up formal screening, training, and accrediting standards. Both of these organizations offer formal training to medical professionals at their annual meetings.

Resources

BOOKS

Elman, Dave. *Hypnotherapy*. Glendale, CA: Westwood Publishing Co., 1964.

Kappas, John G. *Professional Hypnotism Manual: Introducing Physical and Emotional Suggestibility and Sexuality*. Tarzana, CA: Panorama Publishing Company, 1987.

Murphy, Michael. *The Future of the Body: Explorations Into the Further Evolution of Human Nature*. Los Angeles, CA:: Jeremy P. Tarcher, Inc., 1992.

Shrader, Wesley. *The Amazing Power of Hypnosis: What It Can Do for You*. New York: Doubleday & Company, Inc., 1976.

Targ, Russell and Jane Katra. *Miracles of Mind: Exploring Nonlocal Consciousness and Spiritual Healing*. Novato, CA: New World Library, 1998.

PERIODICALS

Baumgaertel, Anna. "Attention-Deficit/Hyperactivity Disorder: Alternative and Controversial Treatments for Attention-Deficit/Hyperactivity Disorder." *Pediatric Clinics of North America* (October 1999).

Devine, E.C., and S.K. Westlake. "The Effects of Psychoeducational Care Provided to Adults with Cancer: Meta-Analysis of 116 Studies." *Oncology Nursing Forum* (1995).

"Hypnosis: Theory and Application Part II." *Harvard Mental Health Letter* (June 2002).

"Hypnotherapy is no Longer Just a Party Trick: Hospices Can Use It to Relieve Pain and Grief." *Hospice Management Advisor* (April 2002): 42–44.

Margolis, Clorinda G. "Hypnotic Trance: The Old and the New." *Primary Care Clinics in Office Practice*.

Newell, Sallie and Rob W. Sanson-Fisher. "Australian Oncologists' Self-Reported Knowledge and Attitudes about Nontraditional Therapies used by Cancer Patients." *Medical Journal of Australia* (February 7, 2000).

ORGANIZATIONS

American Board of Hypnotherapy. 16842 Von Karman Avenue, Suite 476, Irvine, CA 92714. http://www.hypnosis.com/.

American Psychotherapy & Medical Hypnosis Association. 210 S. Sierra, Reno, NV 89501. http://members.xoom.com/Hypnosis/.

American Society of Clinical Hypnosis. 200 E. Devon Avenue, Des Plaines, IL 60018.

International Council for Medical and Clinical Therapists. 7361 McWhorter Place, Suite 300, Annandale, VA 22003-5469. http://www.ultradepth.com/ICMCT.htm.

International Medical and Dental Hypnotherapy Association. 4110 Edgeland, Suite 800, Royal Oak, MI 48073-2285. http://www.infinityinst.com.

The National Board for Hypnotherapy and Hypnotic Anaesthesiology. 7841 West Ludlow Drive, Suite A, Peoria, AZ 85381. http://www.nbha-medicine.com/index.html.

National Guild of Hypnotists. PO Box 308, Merrimack, NH. http://www.ngh.net

Society for Clinical and Experimental Hypnosis. 6728 Old McLean Village Drive, McLean, VA 22101.

World Hypnosis Organization, Inc. 2521 W. Montrose Avenue, Chicago, IL 60618. http://www.worldhypnosis.org/about.html.

Kim Sharp
Teresa G. Odle

Hypoglycemia

Definition

The condition called hypoglycemia is literally translated as low blood sugar. Hypoglycemia occurs when blood sugar (or blood glucose) concentrations fall below a level necessary to properly support the body's need for energy and stability throughout its cells.

Description

Carbohydrates are the main dietary source of the glucose that is manufactured in the liver and absorbed into the bloodstream to fuel the body's cells and organs. Glucose concentration is controlled by hormones, primarily insulin and glucagon. Glucose concentration is also controlled by epinephrine (adrenalin) and norepinephrine, as well as growth hormone. If these regulators are not working properly, levels of blood sugar can become either excessive (as in hyperglycemia) or inadequate (as in hypoglycemia). If a person has a blood sugar level of 50 mg/dl or less, he or she is considered hypoglycemic, although glucose levels vary widely from one person to another.

Hypoglycemia can occur in several ways.

Drug-induced hypoglycemia

Drug-induced hypoglycemia, a complication of diabetes, is the most commonly seen and most dangerous form of hypoglycemia.

Hypoglycemia occurs most often in diabetics who must inject insulin periodically to lower their blood sugar. While other diabetics are also vulnerable to low

blood sugar episodes, they have a lower risk of a serious outcome than do insulin-dependent diabetics. Unless recognized and treated immediately, severe hypoglycemia in the insulin-dependent diabetic can lead to generalized convulsions followed by amnesia and unconsciousness. Death, though rare, is a possible outcome.

In insulin-dependent diabetics, hypoglycemia known as an insulin reaction or insulin shock can be caused by several factors. These include overmedicating with manufactured insulin, missing or delaying a meal, eating too little food for the amount of insulin taken, exercising too strenuously, drinking too much alcohol, or any combination of these factors.

Idiopathic or reactive hypoglycemia

Idiopathic or reactive hypoglycemia (also called postprandial hypoglycemia) occurs when some people eat. A number of reasons for this reaction have been proposed, but no single cause has been identified.

In some cases, this form of hypoglycemia appears to be associated with malfunctions or diseases of the liver, pituitary, adrenals, liver, or pancreas. These conditions are unrelated to diabetes. Children intolerant of a natural sugar (fructose) or who have inherited defects that affect digestion may also experience hypoglycemic attacks. Some children with a negative reaction to aspirin also experience reactive hypoglycemia. It sometimes occurs among people with an intolerance to the sugar found in milk (galactose), and it also often begins before the onset of diabetes.

Fasting hypoglycemia

Fasting hypoglycemia sometimes occurs after long periods without food, but it also happens occasionally following strenuous **exercise**, such as running in a marathon.

Other factors sometimes associated with hypoglycemia include:

• pregnancy
• a weakened immune system
• a poor diet high in simple carbohydrates
• prolonged use of drugs, including antibiotics
• chronic physical or mental **stress**
• heartbeat irregularities (arrhythmias)
• **allergies**
• breast cancer
• high blood pressure treated with beta-blocker medications (after strenuous exercise)
• upper gastrointestinal tract surgery

Causes & symptoms

When carbohydrates are eaten, they are converted to glucose that goes into the bloodstream and is distributed throughout the body. Simultaneously, a combination of chemicals that regulate how the body's cells absorb that sugar is released from the liver, pancreas, and adrenal glands. These chemical regulators include insulin, glucagon, epinephrine (adrenaline), and norepinephrine. The mixture of these regulators released following digestion of carbohydrates is never the same, since the amount of carbohydrates that are eaten is never the same.

Interactions among the regulators are complicated. Any abnormalities in the effectiveness of any one of the regulators can reduce or increase the body's absorption of glucose. Gastrointestinal enzymes such as amylase and lactase that break down carbohydrates may not be functioning properly. These abnormalities may produce hyperglycemia or hypoglycemia, and can be detected when the level of glucose in the blood is measured.

Cell sensitivity to these regulators can be changed in many ways. Over time, a person's stress level, exercise patterns, advancing age, and dietary habits influence cellular sensitivity. For example, a diet consistently overly rich in carbohydrates increases insulin requirements over time. Eventually, cells can become less receptive to the effects of the regulating chemicals, which can lead to glucose intolerance.

Diet is both a major factor in producing hypoglycemia as well as the primary method for controlling it. **Diets** typical of Western cultures contain excess refined carbohydrates, especially in the form of simple carbohydrates such as sweeteners, which are more easily converted to sugar. In poorer parts of the world, the typical diet contains even higher levels of carbohydrates. Fewer dairy products and meat are eaten, and grains, vegetables, and fruits are consumed. This dietary trend is balanced, however, since people in these cultures eat more complex carbohydrates, eat smaller meals, and usually use carbohydrates more efficiently through physical labor.

Early symptoms of severe hypoglycemia, particularly in the drug-induced type of hypoglycemia, resemble an extreme shock reaction. Symptoms include:

- cold and pale skin
- numbness around the mouth
- apprehension
- heart palpitations
- emotional outbursts
- hand tremors
- mental cloudiness
- dilated pupils
- sweating
- fainting

Mild attacks, however, are more common in reactive hypoglycemia and are characterized by extreme tiredness. Patients first lose their alertness, then their muscle strength and coordination. Thinking grows fuzzy, and finally the patient becomes so tired that he or she becomes "zombie-like," awake but not functioning. Sometimes the patient will actually fall asleep. Unplanned naps are typical of the chronic hypoglycemic patient, particularly following meals.

Additional symptoms of reactive hypoglycemia include headaches, double vision, staggering or an inability to walk, a craving for salt and/or sweets, abdominal distress, premenstrual tension, chronic colitis, allergies, ringing in the ears, unusual patterns in the frequency of urination, skin eruptions and inflammations, **pain** in the neck and shoulder muscles, memory problems, and sudden and excessive sweating.

Unfortunately, a number of these symptoms mimic those of other conditions. For example, the **depression**, **insomnia**, irritability, lack of concentration, crying spells, **phobias**, forgetfulness, confusion, unsocial behavior, and suicidal tendencies commonly seen in nervous system and psychiatric disorders may also be hypoglycemic symptoms. It is very important that anyone with symptoms that may suggest reactive hypoglycemia see a doctor.

Because all of its possible symptoms are not likely to be seen in any one person at a specific time, diagnosing hypoglycemia can be difficult. One or more of its many symptoms may be due to another illness. Symptoms may persist in a variety of forms for long periods of time. Symptoms can also change over time within the same person. Some of the factors that can influence symptoms include physical or mental activities, physical or mental state, the amount of time passed since the last meal, the amount and quality of sleep, and exercise patterns.

Diagnosis

Drug-induced hypoglycemia

Once diabetes is diagnosed, the patient then monitors his or her blood sugar level with a portable machine called a glucometer. The diabetic places a small blood sample on a test strip that the machine can read. If the test reveals that the blood sugar level is too low, the diabetic can make a correction by eating or drinking an additional carbohydrate.

Reactive hypoglycemia

Reactive hypoglycemia can be diagnosed only by a doctor. Symptoms usually improve after the patient has gone on an appropriate diet. Reactive hypoglycemia was diagnosed more frequently 10–20 years ago than today. Studies have shown that most people suffering from its symptoms test normal for blood sugar, leading many doctors to suggest that actual cases of reactive hypoglycemia are quite rare. Some doctors think that people with hypoglycemic symptoms may be particularly sensitive to the body's normal postmeal release of the hormone epinephrine, or are actually suffering from some other physical or mental problem. Other doctors believe reactive hypoglycemia is actually the early onset of diabetes that occurs after a number of years. There continues to be disagreement about the cause of reactive hypoglycemia.

A common test to diagnose hypoglycemia is the extended oral glucose tolerance test. Following an overnight fast, a concentrated solution of glucose is drunk and blood samples are taken hourly for five to six hours. Though this test remains helpful in early identification of diabetes, its use in diagnosing chronic reactive hypoglycemia has lost favor because it can trigger hypoglycemic symptoms in people with otherwise normal glucose readings. Some doctors now recommend that blood sugar be tested at the actual time a person experiences hypoglycemic symptoms.

Treatment

Treatment of the immediate symptoms of hypoglycemia can include eating sugar. For example, a patient can eat a piece of candy, drink milk, or drink fruit juice. Glucose tablets can be used by patients, especially those who are diabetic. Effective treatment of hypoglycemia over time requires the patient to follow a modified diet. Patients are usually encouraged to eat small but frequent meals throughout the day and, avoid excess simple sugars (including alcohol), fats, and fruit drinks.

One of the herbal remedies commonly suggested for hypoglycemia is a decoction (an extract made by boiling) of gentian (*Gentiana lutea*). It should be drunk warm 15–30 minutes before a meal. Gentian is believed to help stimulate the endocrine (hormone-producing) glands.

In addition to the dietary modifications recommended above, people with hypoglycemia may benefit from supplementing their diet with **chromium**, which is believed to help improve blood sugar levels. Chromium is found in whole-grain breads and cereals, cheese, molasses, lean meats, and **brewer's yeast**. Eating oats can help stabilize blood sugar levels. Daily supplements of **vitamin E** are also recommended. People with hypoglycemia should avoid alcohol, **caffeine**, and cigarette smoke, since these substances can cause significant swings in blood sugar levels.

Allopathic treatment

Those patients with severe hypoglycemia may require fast-acting glucagon injections that can stabilize their blood sugar within approximately 15 minutes.

Prevention

Drug-induced hypoglycemia

Preventing hypoglycemic insulin reactions in diabetics requires taking glucose readings through frequent blood sampling. Insulin can then be regulated based on those readings. Maintaining proper diet is also a factor. Programmable insulin pumps implanted under the skin have proven useful in reducing the incidence of hypoglycemic episodes for insulin-dependent diabetics. In early 2002, scientists announced that a new therapy involving a synthetic insulin called insulin glargine in combination with one of several other short-acting insulins could provide a new alternative for diabetics at risk for hypoglycemia. The synthetic insulin combination acted safely in all patients, including children, and did not cause hypoglycemia like rapid-acting insulins.

Reactive hypoglycemia

The onset of reactive hypoglycemia can be avoided or at least delayed by following the same kind of diet used to control it. While not as restrictive as the diet diabetics must follow to keep tight control over their disease, it is quite similar.

There are a variety of diet recommendations for the reactive hypoglycemic. Patients should:

• Avoid overeating.

• Never skip breakfast.

• Include protein in all meals and snacks, preferably from sources low in fat, such as the white meat of chicken or turkey, most fish, soy products, or skim milk.

• Restrict intake of fats (particularly saturated fats, such as animal fats), and avoid refined sugars and processed foods.

• Keep a "food diary." Until the diet is stabilized, a patient should note what and how much he/she eats and drinks at every meal. If symptoms appear following a meal or snack, patients should note them and look for patterns.

• Eat fresh fruits, but restrict the amount eaten at one time. Patients should remember to eat a source of pro-

KEY TERMS

. . . .

Adrenal glands—Two organs that sit atop the kidneys; these glands make and release such hormones as epinephrine.

Epinephrine—Also called adrenaline, a secretion of the adrenal glands (along with norepinephrine) that helps the liver release glucose and limits the release of insulin. Norepinephrine is both a hormone and a neurotransmitter, a substance that transmits nerve signals.

Fructose—A type of natural sugar found in many fruits, vegetables, and in honey.

Glucagon—A hormone produced in the pancreas that raises the level of glucose in the blood. An injectable form of glucagon, which can be bought in a drug store, is sometimes used to treat insulin shock.

Postprandial—After eating or after a meal.

tein whenever they eat high sources of carbohydrate like fruit. Apples make particularly good snacks because, of all fruits, the carbohydrate in apples is digested most slowly.

• Follow a diet that is high in fiber. Fruit is a good source of fiber, as are oatmeal and oat bran, which slow the buildup of sugar in the blood during digestion.

A doctor can recommend a proper diet, and there are many cookbooks available for diabetics. Recipes found in such books are equally effective in helping to control hypoglycemia.

Expected results

Like diabetes, there is no cure for reactive hypoglycemia, only ways to control it. While some chronic cases will continue through life (rarely is there complete remission of the condition), others will develop into type II (adult-onset) diabetes. Hypoglycemia appears to have a higher-than-average incidence in families where there has been a history of hypoglycemia or diabetes among their members, but whether hypoglycemia is a controllable warning of oncoming diabetes has not yet been determined by clinical research.

Resources

BOOKS

Ruggiero, Roberta. *The Do's and Don'ts of Low Blood Sugar.* Hollywood, FL: Frederick Fell Publishers.

PERIODICALS

Hartnett, Terry. "Early Results Show Promise for Synthetic Insulin." *Diabetes Week* (March 18, 2002): 4.

ORGANIZATIONS

Hypoglycemia Association, Inc. 18008 New Hampshire Ave., PO Box 165, Ashton, MD 20861-0165.

National Hypoglycemia Association, Inc. PO Box 120, Ridgewood, NJ 07451. (201) 670-1189.

Paula Ford-Martin
Teresa G. Odle

Hypothyroidism

Definition

Hypothyroidism, or a condition of insufficient thyroid hormone in the body, develops when the thyroid gland fails to produce or secrete as much thyroxine (T_4) and triiodothyronine (T_3) as the body needs. Because T_4 regulates such essential functions as heart rate, digestion, physical growth, and mental development, an insufficiency of this hormone can slow life-sustaining processes, damage organs and tissues in every part of the body, and lead to life-threatening complications.

Description

Hypothyroidism is one of the most common chronic diseases in the United States. Symptoms may not appear until years after the thyroid has stopped functioning, and they are often mistaken for signs of other illnesses, **menopause**, or **aging**. Although this condition is believed to affect as many as 11 million adults and children, as many as two of every three people with hypothyroidism may not know they have the disease.

The thyroid gland influences almost every organ, tissue, and cell in the body. It is shaped like a butterfly and located just below the Adam's apple. The thyroid stores **iodine** the body gets from food and uses this mineral to create T_4 and T_3. Low T_4 levels can alter weight, appetite, sleep patterns, body temperature, sex drive, and a variety of other physical, mental, and emotional characteristics.

There are three types of hypothyroidism. The most common is primary hypothyroidism, in which the thyroid doesn't produce an adequate amount of T_4. Secondary hypothyroidism develops when the pituitary gland does not release enough of the thyroid-stimulating hormone (TSH) that prompts the thyroid to manufacture T_4. Tertiary hypothyroidism results from a malfunction of the hypothalamus, the part of the brain that controls the endocrine system. Drug-induced hypothyroidism, an adverse reaction to medication, occurs in two of every 10,000 people, but rarely causes severe hypothyroidism.

Hypothyroidism is at least twice as common in women as it is in men. Although hypothyroidism is most common in women who are middle-aged or older, the disease can occur at any age. Newborn infants are tested for congenital (acquired in utero (Latin)) thyroid deficiency (cretinism) using a test that measures the levels of thyroxine and TSH in the infant's blood. Treatment within the first few months of life can prevent mental retardation and physical abnormalities. Older children who develop hypothyroidism suddenly stop growing.

Factors that increase a person's risk of developing hypothyroidism include age, weight, and medical history. Women are more likely to develop the disease after age 50; men, after age 60. **Obesity** (excessively fat condition) also increases the risk. A family history of thyroid problems or a personal history of high **cholesterol** levels or such autoimmune diseases as lupus, **rheumatoid arthritis**, or diabetes can make an individual more susceptible to hypothyroidism.

Causes & symptoms

Hypothyroidism is most often the result of Hashimoto's disease, also known as chronic thyroiditis (inflammation of the thyroid gland). In this disease, the immune system fails to recognize that the thyroid gland is part of the body's own tissue and attacks it as if it were a foreign body. The attack by the immune system impairs thyroid function and sometimes destroys the gland. Other causes of hypothyroidism include:

- Radiation (the process whereby an element like radium emits rays). Radioactive (the quality some atoms have of producing energy) iodine used to treat **hyperthyroidism** (overactive thyroid) or radiation treatments for head or neck cancers can destroy the thyroid gland.

- Surgery. Removal of the thyroid gland because of **cancer** or other thyroid disorders can result in hypothyroidism.

- Viruses (very small organisms that cause disease)and bacteria (very small one-cell organisms that divide and can cause disease). **Infections** that depress thyroid hormone production usually cause permanent hypothyroidism.

- Human immunodeficiency virus (HIV). Among viruses, HIV, the virus that causes acquired immunodeficiency syndrome, or **AIDS**, may cause overt hypothyroidism. A 2004 report said that hypothyroidism occurs more often in HIV-infected patients taking highly active antiretroviral therapy (HAART).

SYMPTOMS OF HYPOTHYROIDISM
Symptoms
Goiter
Weight gain
Tingling or numbness in the hands
Heightened sensitivity to cold
Lethargy
Decreased heart rate

- Medications. Nitroprusside, lithium, or iodides can induce hypothyroidism. Because patients who use these medications are closely monitored by their doctors, this side effect is very rare.

- Pituitary gland malfunction. This is a rare condition in which the pituitary gland fails to produce enough TSH to activate the thyroid's production of T_4.

- Congenital defect. One of every 4,000 babies is born without a properly functioning thyroid gland.

- Diet. Because the thyroid makes T_4 from iodine drawn from food, an iodine-deficient diet can cause hypothyroidism. Adding iodine to table salt and other common foods has eliminated iodine deficiency in the United States. Certain foods (cabbage, rutabagas, peanuts, peaches, soybeans, spinach) can interfere with thyroid hormone production.

- Environmental contaminants. Certain industrial chemicals, such as PCBs, found in the local environment at high levels may also cause hypothyroidism.

Hypothyroidism sometimes is referred to as a "silent" disease because early symptoms may be so mild that no one realizes anything is wrong. Untreated symptoms become more noticeable and severe, and can lead to confusion and mental disorders, breathing difficulties, heart problems, fluctuations in body temperature, and death.

Someone who has hypothyroidism will probably have more than one of the following symptoms:

- **Fatigue**
- decreased heart rate
- progressive hearing loss
- weight gain
- problems with memory and concentration
- depression
- goiter (enlarged thyroid gland)
- muscle **pain** or weakness

- loss of interest in sex; decreased libido
- numb, tingling hands
- dry skin
- swollen eyelids
- dryness, loss, or premature graying of hair
- extreme sensitivity to cold
- **constipation**
- irregular menstrual periods
- hoarse voice

Hypothyroidism usually develops gradually. When the disease results from surgery or other treatment for hyperthyroidism, symptoms may appear suddenly and include severe muscle cramps in the arms, legs, neck, shoulders, and back. It's important to see a doctor if any of these symptoms appear unexpectedly. When hypothyroidism remains undiagnosed and untreated, a person may eventually develop myxedema. Symptoms of this rare but potentially deadly complication include enlarged tongue, swollen facial features, hoarseness, and physical and mental sluggishness.

Myxedema coma is characterized by unresponsiveness, irregular and shallow breathing, and a drop in blood pressure and body temperature. The onset of this medical emergency can be sudden in people who are elderly or have been ill, injured, or exposed to very cold temperatures; who have recently had surgery; or who use sedatives or antidepressants. Without immediate medical attention, myxedema coma can be fatal.

Diagnosis

The diagnosis of hypothyroidism is based on the patient's observations, medical history, physical examination, and thyroid function tests. Doctors who specialize in treating thyroid disorders (endocrinologists) are most apt to recognize subtle symptoms and physical indications of hypothyroidism. A blood test known as a thyroid-stimulating hormone (TSH) assay, tests of T_4 and T_3 levels, a thyroid nuclear medicine scan, and thyroid ultrasound are used to confirm the diagnosis. A woman being tested for hypothyroidism should let her doctor know if she is pregnant or breastfeeding. All patients should be sure their doctors are aware of any recent procedures involving radioactive materials or contrast media.

The TSH assay is extremely accurate, but some doctors doubt the test's ability to detect mild hypothyroidism. They advise patients to monitor their basal (resting) body temperature for below-normal readings that could indicate the presence of hypothyroidism. These readings should be taken for five consecutive days, starting on the second day of the menstrual cycle for female patients. The normal temperature reading is 97.5°F (36.4°C).

Treatment

Alternative treatments are aimed primarily at strengthening the thyroid gland and will not eliminate the need for thyroid hormone medications. They include nutritional therapy, herbal therapy, and **exercise**.

Nutritional therapy

If a person is experiencing symptoms resembling those of hypothyroidism, it is best to talk to a family physician immediately for appropriate diagnosis and treatments. Nutritional therapy should only be complementary and not used to replace conventional treatment for this disorder. In 2004, a study found that feeding soy formula to infants with congenital hypothyroidism led to prolonged increases in TSH levels. The study authors recommended close follow-up and frequent TSH measures if infants are put on soy-based formulas.

A naturopath or a nutritionist may recommend the following dietary changes to improve mild hypothyroidism:

- Avoiding eating the following raw foods: cabbage, mustard, spinach, cassava roots, peanuts, soybeans, and peaches. They may interfere with thyroid hormone production if not cooked.
- Eating foods with high iodine content such as fish, shellfish, and seaweed.
- Taking multivitamin and mineral supplements daily. Vitamins A, B_2, B_3, B_6, E, and **zinc** are needed for normal thyroid hormone production.
- Strengthening thyroid function with thyroid preparations sold at local food stores. They are used to treat mild hypothyroidism only. Available products include thyroid extracts, iodine, zinc, or tyrosine. Most Americans may not need iodine supplements, as the daily requirement can easily be met by eating iodine-rich foods or using iodized salt. Consuming more than 600 mcg of iodine per day may result in toxicity.

Herbal therapies

Herbal remedies to improve thyroid function and relieve thyroid symptoms include **Siberian ginseng** (for treatment of fatigue), *Panax ginseng,* and bladder wrack (*Fucus vesiculosus,*) which can be taken in capsule form or as a tea.

Homeopathic remedies

Homeopathic treatments (tiny doses of diluted, safe remedies to promote healing) may gradually reduce the need for supplemental thyroid hormone in some patients. Homeopathic remedies for hypothyroidism include homeopathic thyroid as well as others based on the patient's individualized symptoms.

Exercise

Exercise improves thyroid function by stimulating production of thyroid hormone and making body tissues more responsive to the effects of thyroid hormone. It also increases the metabolic (chemical changes in cells providing energy to the body) rate and helps hypothyroid patients lose weight.

Allopathic treatment

In allopathic treatment—medical practice that combats disease with remedies that produce effects different from those produced by the disease—natural or synthetic thyroid hormones are used to restore normal (euthyroid) thyroid hormone levels. Synthroid, or synthetic T_4, is easy to take and works for about 80% of patients. In addition, some patients need additional T_3. However, physicians have not agreed for many years on adding this therapy. In 2004, a study showed there were no benefits to adding T_3 to traditional T_4 therapy. Synthetic hormones are more effective than natural substances, but it may take several months to determine the correct dosage. Patients start to feel better within 48 hours, but symptoms will return if they stop taking the medication.

Most doctors prescribe levothyroxine **sodium** tablets, and most people with hypothyroidism will take the medication for the rest of their lives. Aging, other medications, and changes in weight and general health can affect how much replacement hormone a patient needs, and regular TSH tests are used to monitor hormone levels. Patients should not switch from one brand of thyroid hormone to another without a doctor's permission.

Possible side effects of too much T_4 or T_3 include **osteoporosis** (after long-term use), occasional **anxiety**, heart palpitations (very fast, strong heartbeat), **insomnia**, and occasional episodes of mania (acting crazed).

Regular exercise and a **high-fiber diet** can help maintain thyroid function and prevent constipation.

Expected results

Thyroid hormone replacement therapy generally maintains normal thyroid hormone levels unless treatment is interrupted or discontinued. In 2004, a study showed that treating hypothyroidism reduces risk of cardiac disease, particularly from **atherosclerosis**, or hardened arteries from plaque buildup.

KEY TERMS

Cretinism—Severe hypothyroidism that is present at birth.

Endocrine system—The network of glands that produces hormones and releases them into the bloodstream. The thyroid gland is part of the endocrine system.

Hypothalamus—The part of the brain that controls the endocrine system.

Myxedema—A condition that can result from a thyroid gland that produces too little of its hormone. In addition to a decreased metabolic rate, symptoms may include anemia, slow speech, an enlarged tongue, puffiness of the face and hands, loss of hair, coarse and thickened skin, and sensitivity to cold.

Pituitary gland—A small oval endocrine gland attached to the hypothalamus. The pituitary gland releases TSH, the hormone that activates the thyroid gland.

Thyroid-stimulating hormone (TSH)—A hormone secreted by the pituitary gland that controls the release of T_4 by the thyroid gland.

Thyroxine (T_4)—A thyroid hormone that regulates many essential body processes.

Triiodothyronine (T_3)—A thyroid hormone similar to thyroxine but more powerful. Preparations of triiodothyronine are used in treating hypothyroidism.

Prevention

Primary hypothyroidism can't be prevented, but routine screening of adults can detect the disease in its early stages and prevent complications.

Resources

BOOKS

The Editors of Time-Life Books. *The Medical Advisor: The Complete Guide to Alternative and Conventional Treatments.* Alexandria, VA: Time-Life Books, 1996.

Langer, Stephen and James F. Scheer. *Hypothyroidism: The Unsuspected Illness.* New Canaan, CT:Keats Publishing, 1995.

Murray, Michael, and Joseph Pizzorno. *Encyclopedia of Natural Medicine.* Rocklin, CA: Prima Health, 1998.

Walker, Lynne Paige and Ellen Hodgson Brown. *The Alternative Pharmacy.* Paramus, NJ: Prentice Hall Press, 1998.

Wood, Lawrence C., David S. Cooper, and E. Chester Ridgway. *Your Thyroid: A Home Reference.* New York: Ballantine Books, 1996.

PERIODICALS

Conrad, S.C., H. Chiu, and B. L. Silverman. "Soy Formula Complicates Management of Congenital Hypothyroidism." *Archives of Disease in Childhood* (January 2004):37–41.

Elliott, William T. "T$_4$ Alone is OK for Hyperthyroidism Therapy." *Critical Care Alert* (February 2004):S2–S3.

Sadovsky, Richard. "Treating Hypothyroidism Reduces Atherosclerosis Risk." *American Family Physician* (February 1, 2004):656.

Zepf, Bill. "Hypothyroidism Common in Patients Infected With HIV." *American Family Physician* (March 15, 2004):1508.

ORGANIZATIONS

American Thyroid Association. Montefiore Medical Center. 111 E. 210th St., Bronx, NY 10467.

Endocrine Society. 4350 East West Highway, Suite 500, Bethesda, MD 20814-4410. (301) 941-0200.

Thyroid Foundation of America, Inc. Ruth Sleeper Hall, RSL 350, Boston, MA 02114-2968. (800) 832-8321 or (617) 726-8500.

Thyroid Society for Education and Research. 7515 S. Main St., Suite 545. Houston, TX 77030. (800) THYROID or (713) 799-9909.

Mai Tran
Teresa G. Odle

Hyssop

Description

Hyssop (*Hyssopus officinalis*) is a member of the Lamiaceae or mint family. This aromatic evergreen, classified by botanists as a sub-shrub, should not be confused with several distinct species of plants also called hyssop, including giant hyssop, hedge hyssop, prairie hyssop, or wild hyssop. Hyssop is native to southern Europe and Asia. The London surgeon and apothecary John Gerard, author of the *Herball or Generall Historie of Plantes,* brought hyssop to England in 1597. The attractive herb soon became a component in many ornamental knot gardens. The sun-loving hyssop has naturalized throughout North America, and grows wild in chalky soil and on dry and rocky slopes in the Mediterranean.

Hyssop has a short and fibrous rhizome. The stalk emerges from a woody base and divides into numerous erect, square, and branching stems that may reach a height of 2 ft (61 cm). The small leaves are opposite, without stems, and lance-shaped, with fine hairs and smooth margins. They have a somewhat bitter taste. Flowers have a tubular, two-lipped corolla, and four sta-

mens. They bloom in successive whorls in the leaf axils at the top of the stems, only growing along one side. The blooms may be in shades of rose, purple, mauve, blue, and sometimes white, depending on the variety. Hyssop comes into flower from June through October, and the blossoms are well loved by bees. The perennial hyssop is a sweet and warming aromatic with a camphor-like scent. This garden favorite is especially useful in companion planting. Hyssop attracts the white butterfly, a pest to cabbage and broccoli, thus sparing the food crops from the infestation. The herb also has been used to increase the yield of grapevines and the flavor of the fruit when it is planted nearby.

The Hebrew people called this herb *azob*, meaning "holy herb." Hyssop was used in ancient times as a cleansing herb for temples and other sacred places. It was also used to repel insects. The Romans used hyssop to bring protection from the plague and prepared an herbal wine containing hyssop. In ancient Greece, the physicians Galen and Hippocrates valued hyssop for inflammations of the throat and chest, pleurisy, and other bronchial complaints. In the early seventeenth and eighteenth centuries, hyssop tea and tincture were used to treat **jaundice** and dropsy.

General use

The flowers and leaves of hyssop are considered medicinally valuable by some herbalists; however, the German Commission E has not approved hyssop for any medicinal purposes. The herb has some antimicrobial and antiviral properties. It is especially useful in helping the immune system to combat respiratory infections and colds. Hyssop taken in a warm infusion acts as an expectorant and will help to expel phlegm and break up congestion in the lungs. It is frequently recommended for the treatment of congested sinuses and catarrh. It is also a beneficial herb for treatment of the **cold sore** virus, *Herpes simplex*. An infusion has also been used to relieve the distress of **asthma**. Hyssop is a diaphoretic which means that it acts to promote perspiration. It will help to reduce fever and eliminate toxins through the skin. Hyssop also acts as a carminative and digestive aid, relieving flatulence and relaxing the digestive system. This versatile herb is also a nervine, which means that it calms anxiety. It is useful in children's digestive and respiratory herbal formulas, as well.

Used externally as a skin wash, a decoction of the flowering tops can help the healing of **burns** and relieve skin inflammations. The fresh crushed leaves promote healing of bruises, and relieve the discomfort of insect bites and stings. When applied as a hair rinse, hyssop may help eliminate head lice. Hyssop preparations have also been used to relieve muscular pain and rheumatism

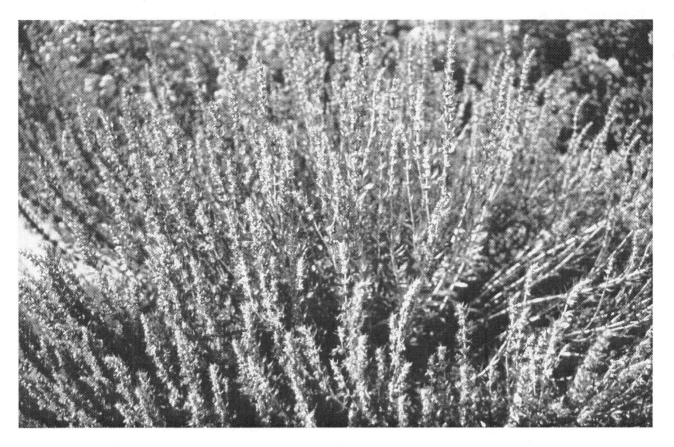

Hyssop (*Hyssopus officinalis*). *(Photo by Henriette Kress. Reproduced by permission.)*

when taken as a tea or a bath additive. The hot vapors of a steaming decoction of hyssop may bring relief of **earache** and inflammation.

A research study published in 2002 confirmed the results of studies done in the early 1990s, which found that hyssop leaf extract demonstrates strong anti-HIV activity. The specific compounds responsible for this antiviral action, however, were not identified in these studies. Moreover, none of these studies tested the efficacy of hyssop in human subjects. The volatile oil of hyssop contains camphene, pinenes, terpinene, the glycoside hyssopin, flavonoids (including diosmin and hesperidin), tannins, acids, resin, gum, and the bitter substance known as marrubiin. Marrubiin is also found in white horehound (*Marrubium vulgare*).

More recently, researchers have discovered that essential oil of hyssop is an effective muscle relaxant. The component that has been identified as most likely responsible for this effect is isopinocamphone.

Preparations

One should harvest hyssop when the herb reaches a height of about 1.5 ft (46 cm). Frequent cuttings from the tops of mature plants will keep the foliage tender for use in salads, soups, or teas. Used sparingly in culinary preparations, hyssop's tender shoots are a digestive aid, especially with greasy meats. When harvesting the herb for medicinal uses, one should use the flowering tops. Gather the herb on a sunny August day after the dew has dried. Hang the branches to dry in a warm, airy room out of direct sunlight. Remove leaves and flowers from the stems and store in clearly labeled, tightly sealed, dark-glass containers.

Infusion: Place 3 tbsp dried, or twice as much fresh, hyssop leaf and blossom in a warm glass container. Bring 2.5 cups of fresh, nonchlorinated water to the boiling point, and add it to the herbs. Cover and infuse the tea for 10–15 minutes. Strain and drink warm. The prepared tea will store for about two days if kept in a sealed container in the refrigerator. Hyssop tea may be enjoyed by the cupful up to three times a day. Hyssop may be combined with white **horehound** for additional expectorant action to relieve coughs. For sore throats, a warm infusion of hyssop combined with sage (*Salvia officinalis*) is a home remedy recommended by some herbalists.

Tincture: Combine four ounces of finely-cut fresh or powdered dry herb with one pint of brandy, gin, or vodka, in a glass container. The alcohol should be sufficient to cover the plant parts. Place the mixture away from light for about two weeks, shaking several times each day. Strain and store in a tightly-capped, dark glass bottle. A standard dose is 1–2 ml of the tincture three times a day.

Essential oil: The commercially available essential oil of hyssop is obtained by steam distillation of the flowering tops. The oil is highly aromatic and is used in perfumes, **aromatherapy**, and to flavor liqueurs, especially Chartreuse and Benedictine. The oil has a warm and pungent aroma with a slight camphor-like smell. It may be used in dilute form as an external nonirritating application on **bruises**, cuts, eczema, and **dermatitis**, as a chest rub for bronchitis and the congestion of colds, and as an additive to bath water to relieve nervous exhaustion and melancholy.

Precautions

Only moderate amounts of hyssop essential oil should be used. Do not use the herb continuously in any form for long periods of time. Pregnant women, children, and persons with **epilepsy** should avoid any use of this potent essential oil. High doses (10–30 drops for adults) may cause convulsions due to the ketone known as pinocamphone. Pregnant or lactating women should not use any form of hyssop.

Side effects

Hyssop can cause **nausea**, upset stomach, and **diarrhea** in susceptible persons. Symptoms of overdose include **dizziness**, tightness in the chest, and disturbances of the central nervous system.

Interactions

No interactions between hyssop and standard pharmaceuticals have been reported as of early 2003.

Resources

BOOKS
Lawless, Julia. *The Complete Illustrated Guide to Aromatherapy.* Rockport, MA: Element Books Inc., 1997.
McIntyre, Anne. *The Medicinal Garden.* New York: Henry Holt and Company, Inc., 1997.
PDR for Herbal Medicines. Montvale, NJ: Medical Economics Company, 1998.
Prevention's 200 Herbal Remedies. Emmaus, PA: Rodale Press, Inc., 1997.
Tyler, Varro E. *The Honest Herbal.* New York: Pharmaceutical Products Press, 1993.

PERIODICALS
Bedoya, L. M., S. S. Palomino, M. J. Abad, et al. "Screening of Selected Plant Extracts for In Vitro Inhibitory Activity on Human Immunodeficiency Virus." *Phytotherapy Research* 16 (September 2002): 550-554.
Lu, M., L. Battinelli, C. Daniele, et al. "Muscle Relaxing Activity of *Hyssopus officinalis* Essential Oil on Isolated Intestinal Preparations." *Planta Medica* 68 (March 2002): 213-216.

ORGANIZATIONS
American Herbalists Guild. 1931 Gaddis Road, Canton, GA 30115. (770) 751-6021. <www.americanherbalistsguild.com>.
Herb Research Foundation. 1007 Pearl Street, Boulder, CO 80302.(303) 449-2265.

OTHER
Hoffmann, David L. "Hyssop." Herbal Materia Medica. http://www.healthy.net/asp/templates/book.asp?PageType=Book&ID=603.

Clare Hanrahan
Rebecca J. Frey, PhD

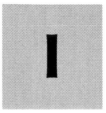

IBD *see* **Inflammatory bowel disease**

IBS *see* **Irritable bowel syndrome**

Iceland moss

Description

Iceland moss (*Cetraria islandica*) is a lichen (a moss-like plant) that grows on the ground in mountains, forests, and arctic areas. In addition to Iceland, the lichen is found in Scandinavia, Great Britain, North America, Russia, and other areas in the Northern Hemisphere. Iceland moss also grows in Antarctica.

The plant's thallus (shoot) curls from 1–4 in (2.5–10 cm) tall. The dried thallus is used as an herbal remedy. Iceland moss is also known as Iceland lichen, cetraria, fucus, muscus, and eryrngo-leaved (spiny-leaf) liverwort.

General use

Iceland moss is rich in **calcium**, **iodine**, **potassium**, phosphorous, and vitamins. The lichen is a bitter-tasting plant that is said to smell like seaweed when it is wet. Despite these unappetizing characteristics, Iceland moss has long been used in Scandinavia and Europe as a food source and a remedy for numerous conditions.

Historic uses of Iceland moss

People in countries including Iceland, Sweden, Norway, Finland, and Russia have used Iceland moss for food and medicine. When used for nourishment, the Iceland moss was ground into flour, which was used to bake bread. Boiling the plant was said to remove the bitter taste, so the plant was boiled and made into a jelly. The lichen became part of a gelled dessert with ingredients that could include chocolate, almonds, or lemon.

In addition, Iceland moss was boiled in milk, a beverage served as a remedy for such conditions as malnutrition. The milk-and-lichen beverage was served to sick people, frail children, and the aged. It was also used for serious conditions when the person was vomiting.

Iceland moss also had numerous folk medicine uses. The lichen was a folk remedy for **tuberculosis**, lung disease, chest ailments, and problems with the kidney and bladder. Iceland moss was also used to treat **wounds** that did not heal, **diarrhea**, problems with lactation, fevers, and **gastritis**.

Furthermore, people in Norway ate Iceland moss during a seven-year famine that started in 1807. The Russians found another use for the lichen during World War II, when they prepared a version of molasses with Iceland moss.

Contemporary uses of Iceland moss

The acids in Iceland moss have an antibiotic effect. It is a mild antimicrobial and a demulcent—a remedy that soothes irritated or inflamed mucous membranes. The lichen is used to treat inflammation of the mouth and pharynx, and for treatment of the **common cold**, fever, dry **cough**, and bronchitis. It is also used for people who have a tendency toward infection. Furthermore, the bitter herb is a remedy for digestive complaints, loss of appetite, and **gastroenteritis**. Iceland moss boiled in milk is still used as a tonic beverage for people recovering from illnesses. In addition, the lichen has been used to treat diabetes.

Preparations

In Europe, Iceland moss cough drops are sold in pharmacies. The lichen is also sold in other forms for a range of conditions. In the United States, Iceland moss is generally found in powdered form and is usually consumed as a tea. It can also be used as a gargle to soothe a sore throat .

Iceland moss tea is made by pouring 1 cup of boiling **water** over 1–2 tsp of powdered Iceland moss. The mixture is covered and steeped for 10–15 minutes.

Sweetener can be added to the tea, or the herb can be mixed with cocoa or chocolate. The average daily dosage of Iceland moss is 1–3 tsp.

An Iceland moss decoction can be made by putting 2 tsp of shredded lichen in 2 cups of cold water. The mixture is simmered for 10 minutes. It is then strained to squeeze out the juice. One cup of the decoction is consumed in the morning and another at night. Iceland moss can also be taken as a tincture.

In addition, Iceland moss can be used topically for skin rashes and fungus.

Precautions

Iceland moss is safe when taken in proper dosages. However, Iceland moss is not regulated by the FDA. Before beginning herbal treatment, people should consult a physician, health practitioner, or herbalist to discuss potential cautions.

Powdered Iceland moss must be soaked in lye for 24 hours or filtered through ash in order to properly extract the lichen acids. One study found that poorly prepared Iceland moss may contain toxic levels of lead. A person should talk to an experienced herbalist or other health practitioner to determine a proper source for Iceland moss, and should not attempt to prepare it themselves.

In rare cases, external use of Iceland moss has caused sensitivity reactions.

Side effects

Side effects include the rare sensitivity reaction, and the risk of **lead poisoning** in poorly prepared Iceland moss. In excessive doses or with prolonged use, Iceland moss may cause gastric irritation and liver problems.

Interactions

There are no known interactions with standard pharmaceuticals associated with use of Iceland moss.

Resources

BOOKS

Duke, James A. *The Green Pharmacy*. Emmaus, Penn.: Rodale Press, Inc., 1997.

Medical Economics Company. *PDR for Herbal Medicines*. Montvale, N.J.: Medical Economics Company, 1998.

Ritchason, Jack. *The Little Herb Encyclopedia*. Pleasant Grove, Utah: Woodland Health Books, 1995.

Squier, Thomas Broken Bear, with Lauren David Peden. *Herbal Folk Medicine*. New York: Henry Holt and Company, 1997.

ORGANIZATIONS

American Botanical Council. P.O. Box 201660, Austin, TX 78720. (512) 331-8868. http://www.herbs.org.

Herb Research Foundation. 1007 Pearl St., Suite 200, Boulder, CO 80302. (303) 449-2265. http://www.herbs.org.

OTHER

Holistic OnLine. http://www.holisticonine.com.

Moore, Michael. Southwest School of Botanical Medicine. http://chili.rt66.com/hrbmoore.

MotherNature.com Health Encyclopedia. http://www.mother-nature.com/ency.

OnHealth Network Company. "Iceland Moss." http://www.on-health.com/alternative/resource/herbs/item,77157.asp (August 8, 2000).

Liz Swain

Ignatia

Description

Ignatia is a homeopathic remedy that is derived from the bean of a small tree that is native to the Philippine Islands and China. The tree belongs to the Loganiaceae family, and has long, twining, smooth branches. On the branches grows a fruit that is the size and shape of a pear. Inside the fruit are almond-shaped seeds, or beans, that have a fine, downy covering and are blackish gray or clear brown in color.

The Latin name is *Ignatius amara*, amara being the Latin work for bitter. The bean was named after St. Ignatius Loyola, a Spanish Jesuit who was responsible for bringing the beans to Europe from the Philippines in the seventeenth century. As a result, the beans are often called St. Ignatius beans. The missionaries were introduced to the beans by the locals, who wore the beans as amulets to prevent disease. The bean was then used as a treatment for **gout, epilepsy**, cholera, and **asthma**.

The beans contain a substantial amount of strychnine, a bitter substance that is often used in rat poison. Strychnine is fatal to humans if taken in large doses. Small doses cause headaches, loss of appetite, cramps, muscle twitching, trembling, frightening dreams, cold sweat, nervous laughter, and giddiness.

General use

Ignatia is one of the best remedies for conditions brought about by emotional upset such as grief, shock, jealousy, fear, anger, **depression**, embarrassment, fright, or ridicule. Homeopaths frequently recommend ignatia when the patient is suffering from romantic disappointment or the loss of a spouse, relative, friend, or pet. The remedy helps the patient bear the grief and suffering common to emotional upsets.

Suppression of the emotions is the general cause of ignatia complaints. Men and women of all ages may benefit from Ignatia when they are grieving, but Ignatia is particularly well suited for sensitive, delicate women and children. It is recommended for children who develop ailments after being punished, teenagers who are suffering from a lost love, women who have had a miscarriage, and elderly folk who grieve silently. Ignatia is a good remedy for children who suffer from extreme trembling after a fright. Ignatia is frequently prescribed in cases of physical or sexual abuse. Women who suffer from nervousness, confusion, or forgetfulness during their menstrual cycles may also benefit from Ignatia.

Persons who require the interaction of Ignatia are idealistic, introspective, moody, quarrelsome, sensitive to **pain**, timid, easily startled, weepy, and depressed. As a result of their grief they become fearful, apprehensive, and antisocial. They dislike consolation and desire to be alone. When in the company of others they are secretive and try to hold in their emotions, although they sigh frequently and loudly. When alone, they are prone to frequent bouts of sobbing alternating with nervous laughter. They are conscientious about performing tasks correctly.

Ignatia is a remedy of contradictions. It is used to treat symptoms that are often paradoxical and erratic. For example, symptoms of **nausea** are relieved by eating, a **sore throat** is better from swallowing solids, and simple foods are harder to digest than heavier foods. Symptoms may be relieved after passing a hard stool. Lying on the painful side may make the symptoms better. Eating causes the patient to have more hunger. She may crave sour or hard to digest foods. She may also want to remain uncovered when cold. The patient dislikes fresh air and is sensitive to coffee and tobacco.

General symptoms are aggravated by cold air, emotional excitement, mental exertion, sweets, and consolation.

They are worse in the morning, evening, night, and before and during **menstruation**. Symptoms may appear at regular intervals, such as headaches that occur every seven days. Symptoms are improved by warmth and eating.

Ignatia is also used as a remedy for headaches, sore throat, trembling, nervousness, **insomnia**, heart palpitations, **gas**, **indigestion**, weakness, and weeping. Other conditions include **irritable bowel syndrome**, painful **hemorrhoids**, or a dry, tickling **cough**.

The cough is a dry, irritating cough that is often accompanied by a stitching pain in the chest. Suppression of the cough is helpful. The patient is made worse by coughing or lying in bed, and the cough is worse in the evening. Ignatia is often used in the treatment of **whooping cough** or **croup**.

The **fever** is often accompanied by extreme thirst and **chills**. The patient feels better when uncovered, and is worse in the afternoon.

Headaches typical of Ignatia start gradually and stop suddenly. The pain is gathered in the forehead. The patient may complain of a sensation as if a nail were being driven through her head. Headaches are often caused by emotional upset and are worse in a smoky room.

A sore throat accompanied by stitching pains and a sensation as if there were a lump in the throat is often present as a result of suppressed emotions. The throat is worse in the evening and is better from swallowing.

When indigestion is present, the patient may feel as though her stomach were empty. She may suffer from sour-tasting belches that ameliorate her symptoms.

Preparations

Ignatia is prepared by grinding the bean into a powder and steeping the powder in alcohol. The mixture is strained and diluted until it becomes a non-toxic substance. It is then succussed to create the final preparation.

During an emotional crisis, take a single dose of 30X or 30C. If the symptoms are unchanged after eight hours, try another remedy. If the dose helps, repeat the dose only when the symptoms worsen. Do not take more than two times a day for three days.

Precautions

If symptoms do not improve after the recommended time period, consult your homeopath or health-care practitioner.

Do not exceed the recommended dose.

Ignatia may cause insomnia and should be taken in the morning.

Side effects

The only side effects are individual aggravations that may occur.

Interactions

When taking any homeopathic remedy, do not use **peppermint** products, coffee, or alcohol. These products may cause the remedy to be ineffective.

Resources

BOOKS

Cummings, Stephen M.D., and Dana Ullman, M.P.H. *Everybody's Guide to Homeopathic Medicines.* New York, NY: Jeremy P. Tarcher/Putnam, 1997.

Kent, James Tyler. *Lectures on Materia Medica.* Delhi, India: B. Jain Publishers, 1996.

Jennifer Wurges

Imagery *see* **Guided imagery**

Immuno-augmentation therapy

Definition

Immuno-augmentation therapy (IAT), also called immuno-augmentative or immuno-augmentive therapy, is a **cancer** treatment aimed at restoring the immune system with injections of a mixture of blood factors.

Origins

The theory behind IAT was formulated in the 1950s by Dr. Lawrence Burton. After earning his doctorate in experimental zoology in 1955 from New York University, Burton moved to the California Institute of Technology (Caltech) as a postdoctoral fellow in the laboratory of H. K. Mitchell. There, he and his coworkers discovered a tumor-inducing factor (TIF) in fruit flies. A few years later, Burton and his colleague, Dr. Frank Friedman, joined the cancer research staff of Dr. Antonio Rottino at St. Vincent's Hospital in New York City. Rottino was one of the first scientists to conclude that there was a connection between the body's immune system and cancer.

Burton and the development of IAT

After Burton and his colleagues reported finding an inhibitor of fruit-fly TIF in mice and human tissue, Mitchell published a retraction of the papers he had coauthored with Burton. Mitchell claimed that Burton's assay for TIF—on which Burton was basing his recent work—could not be repeated independently. Undeterred, Burton continued using fruit flies and mice to develop a mixture of blood proteins to slow or stop the proliferation of cancer cells.

By the mid-1960s, Burton was making sensational presentations. In 1966, at an American Cancer Society (ACS) seminar for science writers, Burton injected mice with his "unblocking factor." Their tumors shrunk in less than an hour. Although newspaper headlines read "15-Minute Cancer Cure," the medical community was unconvinced. Professional journals refused to publish Burton's papers and he eventually lost his research funding. The American Cancer Society (ACS) placed Burton's IAT on its list of unproven methods.

In 1973, Burton and Friedman left St. Vincent's and, with independent funding, founded the Immunology Researching Foundation in Great Neck, New York. They began treating cancer patients with IAT. The following year they submitted an investigational new drug application to the United States Food and Drug Administration (FDA) in order to begin clinical trials of IAT. However, when FDA officials asked Burton for his experimental evidence, he withdrew his application.

Burton and Friedman eventually patented four substances that they claimed to have isolated from human blood:

• deblocking protein

• tumor antibody 1

• tumor antibody 2

• tumor complement

Burton claimed that when used in the correct combination, these substances restored normal immune function in cancer patients.

During the 1970s and early 1980s, the National Cancer Institute (NCI) tried to evaluate IAT. Burton refused to disclose his methods for isolating his blood substances, and an agreement regarding evaluation methods could not be reached.

The Bahamian clinic

Hostility from the medical establishment drove Burton to close his New York clinic in 1977. With private funding, he founded the Immunology Researching Centre (IRC), Ltd. in Freeport on Grand Bahama Island. This not-for-profit organization was licensed to treat people who had been diagnosed with cancer. In 1978, representatives from the Bahamian Ministry of Health and the Pan American Health Organization found violations in admissions, treatment, and evaluation of the clinic's patients. They could not determine the blood components used in IAT, and found no records of patient survival rates. They concluded that there was no evidence that IAT was effective, and recommended that the facility be closed.

However, the Bahamian health authority did not close the clinic until 1985. At that time it was announced that blood supplies across the United States were contaminated with the human immunodeficiency virus (HIV). Burton's clinic was no exception. Indeed the clinic had treated **Kaposi's sarcoma** in patients with acquired immune deficiency syndrome (**AIDS**). Although no HIV **infections** were ever traced to the clinic, and some scientists questioned the HIV screening used by the authorities, the sera used in IAT were found to carry **hepatitis** virus and infectious bacteria. At least two cases of hepatitis were traced to the sera. The Bahamian government, at the apparent insistence of the FDA and the NCI, closed the clinic for seven months, until screening and sterilization methods for serum production were improved. IAT had been legalized in Florida and Oklahoma in the early 1980s; however, Florida rescinded its law when the clinic closed. In 1986, the FDA banned the import of IAT drugs.

The closing of Burton's clinic and the ban on sera import enraged many patients and their families. They formed the Immuno-Augmentative Therapy Patient Association (IATPA), later renamed People Against Cancer, and began lobbying the United States Congress. In 1986, the Office of Technology Assessment (OTA), then a research branch of Congress, was told to investigate alternative cancer therapies. OTA worked with Burton to develop procedures for an IAT clinical trial on colon cancer patients. However the arrangement broke down, and the OTA concluded that there was no reliable data with which to evaluate IAT.

During the 1990s, the IRC opened additional clinics in Germany and Mexico. Burton died in 1993 and his long-time associate, Dr. R. John Clement, took over IRC operations. In 2003, Clement founded the ITL Cancer Clinic, a new operating company for the IRC. This new, expanded clinic offered additional mainstream and alternative treatments combined with IAT.

Benefits

As of 2004, no one claims that IAT cures cancer. Proponents claim that the therapy can stop the spread of many cancers and may send the cancer into remission. They claim that by treating deficiencies or imbalances in the immune system, the body is able treat itself, resulting in an extended lifespan and enhanced quality of life. Sometimes the disease has spread too far within the body to respond to IAT. Furthermore, if chemotherapy or radiation treatment has over-suppressed the immune system, response to IAT may be slow.

IAT is claimed to have about a 19% effectiveness rate. Various cancers respond differently to IAT:

• Bladder cancer responds favorably.

• Brain cancer: astrocytomas (noncapsulated brain tumors arising in brain cells called astrocytes), grades I and II, respond favorably; grade III does not respond well; glioblastoma multiforme (the fastest-growing type of brain tumor) is not a candidate for IAT.

• Breast cancer: all types respond, although inflammatory cancers respond poorly.

• Cervical cancer: responds in early stages; mixed results in late stages.

• Colorectal cancer: good response in most stages; metastasis to the liver disqualifies it for IAT.

• Head and neck cancers respond favorably.

• Leukemias: adult chronic types respond to IAT.

• Lung cancers: adeno- and squamous-cell (large-cell) cancers and mesotheliomas respond well to IAT; small-cell, oat-cell, and undifferentiated cancers are not candidates for IAT.

• Lymphoma: responses vary.

• Melanomas: extremely variable responses.

• Myeloma responds well, even at late stages.

• Pancreatic cancer: good response in some cases, although IAT may be inappropriate because of disease complications.

• Prostate cancer responds at all stages.

• Skin metastases do not respond to IAT.

Description

Both conventional cancer immunotherapy and IAT are based on enhancement of the immune system. Sometimes called immune enhancement or immune modulation, conventional immunotherapy is used at many U. S. clinics. Clinical trials have found it useful for treating various cancers, including melanoma, lymphoma, kidney, and bladder cancers.

IAT components and treatment

Three serum factors are used in IAT:

• Tumor antibody factor (TAF), more commonly called tumor necrosis factor (TNF), may induce antibodies that destroy tumors.

• Tumor complement factor (TCF) is said to induce antibody formation.

• Deblocking protein factor (DPF) is claimed to remove an endogenous blocking protein that prevents the immune system from detecting the cancer.

TAF and DPF are isolated from the blood of healthy donors. TCF is isolated from the clotted blood of cancer patients.

IAT patients are screened for imbalances in immune system components. During the initial treatment, blood factors are measured once or twice per day, five days per week. In addition to measuring the serum factors used in treatment, the blood is analyzed for blocking protein factor (BPF). High levels of BPF and low levels of DPF and TCF are claimed to cause immunosuppression or immunodeficiency, enabling the cancer to grow and spread. Based on this data, a computer calculates the amount of each serum to be injected into the patient.

Treatment varies from one to 12 daily injections. Treatment is on an outpatient basis for an average of 10–12 weeks. Following outpatient treatment, patients are given supplies of sera and a computerized prescription for home injections. Home treatment may last weeks, months, or the rest of one's life. Patients typically return to the clinic for about two weeks, every four to six months. They undergo measurements of tumor activity and IAT responses, in conjunction with conventional methods for determining tumor regression, and symptom and disease remission.

Approximate costs

IAT is expensive:

• Four weeks of initial and intensive therapy—$7,500.

• Each week thereafter—$700.

• Costs for megadoses of oral supplements. **Metabolic therapies**, including vitamins, minerals, animal or plant extracts, or other nutrients, are prescribed on an individual basis and administered orally or intravenously. Intravenous infusions cost about $150 each.

• Home maintenance supplies—$50 per week.

These fees do not include:

• Special medications or nutrients not used in routine IAT.

• Laboratory or other tests performed outside of the clinic.

• Outside physician or hospital services.

• Medical aids or equipment not prescribed or supplied by the clinic.

• Transportation, lodging, and living expenses during outpatient treatment.

IAT usually is not covered by insurance.

Preparations

Under Bahamian law, IAT patients must have been previously diagnosed with cancer. Patients are screened to determine if IAT is appropriate for their type of cancer. Typically, patients travel to an IAT clinic, where they are given a physical exam, and blood and urine tests, to determine the status of their immune system. IAT appears to be more effective on patients who have not had chemotherapy.

IAT patients are asked to abstain from tobacco and to limit alcohol consumption during treatment. **Lung cancer** patients must have stopped **smoking** prior to treatment at the IRC. In addition, patients should:

• avoid dietary animal fats

• avoid excess vitamin C

• take antioxidant supplements that are recommended

Precautions

Proponents of IAT claim that it is nontoxic, safe, and effective. However, there have been no controlled clinical studies of IAT, and scientists have not been able to replicate Burton's original results with mice. In addition:

• IAT sera have not been tested for safety by accepted medical standards.

• Some medical practitioners caution that the unregulated IAT sera may contain infectious agents transmitted in human blood.

• Relying on IAT in place of conventional cancer treatments may have serious health consequences.

Side effects

Anecdotal reports from patients indicate that the side effects of IAT are minor and include:

KEY TERMS

Adenocarcinoma—A cancerous tumor derived from epithelial (surface) cells or a gland-like tumor.

Antibody—A protein that recognizes and destroys a specific foreign antigen, such as a cancer cell.

Best-case series—A preliminary study that relies on assumptions about patient outcomes without a specific treatment, compared with similar patients receiving the best available conventional treatments. There are no control cases.

Blocking protein factor (BPF)—A serum component that may prevent the immune system from recognizing cancer cells.

Complement—A large group of serum proteins that are involved in the immune response.

Deblocking protein factor (DPF)—A serum component used in IAT that is claimed to inactivate or remove BPF.

Immune system—The body system that fights infection and disease.

Mesothelioma—A tumor consisting of spindle cells or fibrous tissue, usually in the lining of the lung.

Metastasis, pl. metastases—A secondary tumor; the process by which cancerous cells form secondary tumors in distant parts of the body.

Serum, pl. sera—The clear liquid that remains after cellular components are removed from blood by clotting; a blood derivative containing an antitoxin for diagnostic or therapeutic use.

Tumor—An overgrowth of body tissue.

Tumor antibody factor (TAF)—A component of IAT sera, possibly tumor necrosis factor (TNF), that may induce antibodies that destroy tumors.

Tumor complement factor (TCF)—A component of IAT sera that stimulates antibody production.

Tumor-inducing factor (TIF).—A blood component that can initiate tumor growth.

• fatigue

• pain at the injection site

• flu-like symptoms

• pain and **edema** (fluid accumulation) during IAT given to bone cancer patients

Research & general acceptance

There is no scientific evidence that IAT is an effective cancer treatment. Nor is there scientific evidence that IAT sera contain specific components. In 1980, Met-Path, a biomedical firm, terminated a contract with Burton after they could not identify or measure a substance that Burton claimed was present in IAT serum. Most anecdotal claims and testimonials for IAT's effectiveness against cancer are without supporting evidence.

In 1984, researchers at the University of Pennsylvania Cancer Center collected data from 79 patients who had received IAT at Burton's clinic. They concluded that reliable comparisons with those receiving conventional cancer treatment were not possible; however, their survey did find extended survival times among the IAT patients. They suggested that a well-controlled prospective study be performed.

In April 2003, the United States Agency for Healthcare Research and Quality (AHRQ) issued a report on IAT. Using criteria developed by the NCI, they conducted a "best-case series" to examine nine cancer patients treated with IAT. Their cancers included:

• hodgkin's lymphoma

• non-small cell carcinoma of the lung

• poorly-differentiated nodular lymphoma

• peritoneal mesothelioma (two cases)

• ovarian adenocarcinoma

• squamous cell carcinoma of the vocal cords (two cases)

• adenocarcinoma of the colon

The report concluded that IAT warranted further study. It recommended either a random controlled clinical trial or a prospective case series with treatment protocol and documentation established prior to treatment.

Training & certification

IAT practitioners are usually medical doctors.

Resources

BOOKS

Cassileth, B. *The Alternative Medicine Handbook.* New York: W. W. Norton & Co., 1998.

Pelton, Ross, and Lee Overholser. *Alternatives in Cancer Therapy: The Complete Guide to Non-traditional Treatments.* New York: Fireside, 1994.

Sackman, Ruth. *Rethinking Cancer: Non-Traditional Approaches to the Theories, Treatments and Prevention of Cancer.* Garden City Park, NY: Square One Publishers, 2003.

PERIODICALS

Green, Saul. "Immunoaugmentative Therapy." *Journal of the American Medical Association (JAMA)* 270, no. 14 (October 13, 1993): 1719-24.

ORGANIZATIONS

ITL Cancer Clinic (Bahamas) Ltd. P.O. Box F-42689, Freeport, Grand Bahama, Bahamas. (877) 785-7460. 242-352-7455. info@immunemedicine.com. burtonh101@aol.com. <http://www.iatclinic.com>. <http://www.immunemedicine.com>.

People Against Cancer. 604 East Street, P.O. Box 10, Otho, IA 50569. (515) 972-4444. info@PeopleAgainstCancer.net. <http://www.peopleagainstcancer.net>.

OTHER

"Best-Case Series for the Use of Immuno-Augmentation Therapy and Naltrexone for the Treatment of Cancer. Summary." *Evidence Report/Technology Assessment: No. 7. AHRQ Publication No. 03-E029.* April 2003 [cited April 29, 2004]. <http://www.ahrq.gov/clinic/epcsums/immaugsum.htm>.

&"Immuno-Augmentative Therapy." *Cancer Facts.* National Cancer Institute. October 27, 1999 [cited April 29, 2004]. <http://cis.nci.nih.gov/fact/9_15.htm>.

"Immuno-Augmentive Therapy." *Making Treatment Decisions.* American Cancer Society. 2000 [cited April 29, 2004]. <http://www.cancer.org/docroot/ETO/content/ETO_5_3X _Immuno-Augmentive_Therapy.asp?sitearea=ETO>.

Margaret Alic

Impetigo

Definition

Impetigo is a contagious bacterial infection of the skin. It primarily afflicts children and the elderly. Ecthyma is a more severe form of impetigo with sores affecting a deeper layer of the skin. It often leaves scarring and discoloration of the skin.

Description

The first sign of impetigo is a clear, fluid-filled bump, called a vesicle, which appears on the skin. The vesicle soon dries out and develops a scab-like, honey-colored crust, which breaks open and leaks fluid. These vesicles usually appear grouped closely together, and they may spread out and cover a large area of the skin. Impetigo often affects the area around the nose and mouth; however, it can spread to anywhere on the skin, but especially the arms and legs, as well as the diaper areas of infants. The condition called ecthyma is a form of impetigo in which the sores that develop are larger, filled with pus, and covered with brownish-black scabs that may lead to scarring. Impetigo **infections** most commonly occur during warmer weather.

Causes & symptoms

Impetigo is most frequently caused by the bacteria *Staphylococcus aureus,* also known as "staph," and less frequently, by group A beta-hemolytic streptococci, also known as "strep." These bacteria are highly contagious. Impetigo can quickly spread from one part of the body to another through scratching. It can also be spread to other people if they touch the infected sores or if they have contact with the soiled clothing, diapers, bed sheets, or toys of an infected person. Such factors as heat, humidity, crowded conditions, and poor hygiene increase the chance that impetigo will spread rapidly among large groups.

Impetigo tends to develop in areas of the skin that have already been damaged through some other means such as injury, insect bite, sunburn, **diaper rash**, chicken pox, or herpes, especially oral herpes. The sores tend to be very itchy, and scratching may lead to the spread of the disease. Keeping the hands washed with antibacterial soap and fingernails well trimmed are good precautions for limiting further infection.

Diagnosis

Observation of the appearance, location and pattern of sores is the usual method of diagnosis. Fluid from the vesicles can be cultured and examined to identify the causative bacteria.

Treatment

Echinacea tincture can be applied directly to the skin. The homeopathic remedy *Antimonium tartaricum* can be used when impetigo affects the face.

Bag Balm, an anti-bacterial salve, can be applied to sores to relieve **pain** and heal the skin.

A tincture of the pansy flower, *Viola tricolor,* can be taken internally twice daily for a week to speed healing.

Burdock root oil can be directly applied to the skin to help it heal.

Topical washes with **goldenseal**, **grapefruit seed extract** (which may sting), or tea tree oil are also recommended.

Allopathic treatment

Uncomplicated impetigo is usually treated with a topical antibiotic cream such as mupirocin (Bactroban). Oral antibiotics are also commonly prescribed. Patients are advised to wash the affected areas with an antibacterial soap and **water** several times per day, and to otherwise keep the skin dry. Scratching is discouraged, and the suggestion is that nails be cut or that mittens be worn—especiallly with young children. Ecthyma is treated in the same manner, but at times may require surgical debridement, or removal of the affected area.

Expected results

The vast majority of those with impetigo recover quickly, completely, and uneventfully. However, there is a chance of developing a serious disease, or sequela, especially if the infection is left untreated. Local spread of the infection can cause osteomyelitis, septic arthritis, cellulitis, or lymphangitis. If large quantities of the bacteria begin to circulate in the bloodstream, there is also a danger of developing a systemic infection such as glomerulonephritis or **pneumonia**.

Prevention

Prevention of impetigo involves good hygiene. In order to avoid spreading the infection from one person to another, those with impetigo should be isolated until all sores are healed, and their used linen, clothing, and toys should be kept out of contact with others.

Resources

BOOKS

Foley, Denise, et al. *The Doctors Book of Home Remedies for Children: From Allergies and Animal Bites to Toothache and TV Addiction, Hundreds of Doctor-Proven Techniques and Tips to Care for Your Kid.* Emmaus, PA: Rodale Press, 1999.

Shaw, Michael, ed., et al. *Everything You Need to Know About Diseases.* Springhouse, PA: Springhouse Corporation, 1996.

Weed, Susun. *Healing Wise.* New York: Ash Tree Publishing, 1989

OTHER

The Nemours Foundation. http://kidshealth.org/parent/general/infections/impetigo.html.

Patience Paradox

Impotence

Definition

Impotence, also known as erectile dysfunction, is the inability to achieve or maintain an erection long enough to engage in sexual intercourse.

Description

Under normal circumstances, when a man is sexually stimulated, his brain sends a message down the spinal cord and into the nerves of the penis. The nerve endings in the penis release chemical messengers, called neurotransmitters, that signal the arteries that supply blood to the corpora cavernosa (the two spongy rods of tissue that span the length of the penis) to relax and fill with blood. As they expand, the corpora cavernosa close off other veins that would normally drain blood from the penis. As the penis becomes engorged with blood, it enlarges and stiffens, causing an erection. Problems with blood vessels, nerves, or tissues of the penis can interfere with an erection.

Causes & symptoms

It is estimated that as many as 20 million American men frequently suffer from impotence and that it strikes up to half of all men between the ages of 40 and 70. Doctors used to think that most cases of impotence were psychological in origin, but they now recognize that, at least in older men, physical causes may play a primary role in 60% or more of all cases. In men over the age of 60, the leading cause is **atherosclerosis**, or narrowing of the arteries, which can restrict the flow of blood to the penis. Injury or disease of the connective tissue, such as Peyronie's disease, may prevent the corpora cavernosa from completely expanding. Damage to the nerves of the penis from certain types of surgery or neurological conditions, such as Parkinson's disease or **multiple sclerosis**, may also cause impotence. Men with diabetes are especially at risk for impotence because of their high risk of both atherosclerosis and a nerve disease called diabetic neuropathy.

Some drugs, including certain types of blood pressure medications, antihistamines, tranquilizers (especially when taken before intercourse), and antidepressants known as selective serotonin reuptake inhibitors (SSRIs, including Prozac and Paxil) can interfere with erections. **Smoking**, excessive alcohol consumption, and illicit drug use may also contribute. In some cases, low levels of the male hormone testosterone may contribute to erectile failure. Finally, such psychological factors as **stress**, guilt, or **anxiety**, may also play a role, even when the impotence is primarily due to organic causes.

Diagnosis

When diagnosing the underlying cause of impotence, the doctor begins by asking the man a number of questions about when the problem began, whether it only happens with specific sex partners, and whether he ever wakes up with an erection. (Men whose dysfunction occurs only with certain partners or who wake up with erections are more likely to have a psychological cause for their impotence.) Sometimes, the man's sex partner is also interviewed. In some cases, domestic discord may be a factor.

The doctor also obtains a thorough medical history to find out about past pelvic surgery, diabetes, cardiovascular disease, kidney disease, and any medications the man may be taking. The physical examination should include a genital examination, hormone tests, and a glucose test for diabetes. Sometimes a measurement of blood flow through the penis may be taken.

Alternative health practitioners often forgo such extensive testing and rely on information obtained from the patient. Usually the fact that the man cannot get or maintain an erection is reason enough to begin alternative or holistic therapy.

Treatment

A number of herbs have been promoted for treating impotence. The most widely touted is **yohimbe** (*Corynanthe yohimbe*), derived from the bark of the yohimbe tree native to West Africa. It has been used in Europe for about 75 years to treat erectile dysfunction. The FDA approved yohimbe as a treatment for impotence in the late 1980s. It is sold as an over-the-counter dietary supplement and as a prescription drug under brand names such as Yocon, Aphrodyne, Erex, Yohimex, Testomar, Yohimbe, and Yovital.

There is no clear medical research that indicates exactly how or why yohimbe works in treating impotence. It is generally believed that yohimbe dilates blood vessels and stimulates blood flow to the penis, causing an erection. It also prevents blood from flowing out of the penis during an erection. It may also act on the central nervous system, specifically the lower spinal cord area where sexual signals are transmitted. Studies show it is effective in 30–40% of men with impotence. It is primarily effective in men with impotence caused by vascular, psychogenic (originating in the mind), or diabetic problems. It usually does not work in men whose impotence is caused by organic nerve damage. In healthy men without impotence, yohimbe in some cases appears to increase sexual stamina and prolong erections.

The usual dosage of yohimbine (yohimbe extract) to treat erectile dysfunction is 5.4 mg three times a day. It may take three to six weeks for it to take effect. Most commercially available supplements don't contain enough yohimbe to be effective. Doctors recommend obtaining a prescription for yohimbe to get enough active ingredient for success.

Ginkgo (*Ginkgo biloba*) is also used to treat impotence, although it has not been shown to help the condition in controlled studies and probably has more of a psychological effect. In addition, ginkgo carries some risk of abnormal blood clotting and should be avoided by men taking such blood thinners, as coumadin. Other herbs promoted for treating impotence include true unicorn root (*Aletrius farinosa*), **saw palmetto** (*Serenoa repens*), ginseng (*Panax ginseng*), and **Siberian ginseng** (*Eleuthrococcus senticosus*). **Nux vomica** (*Strychnos nux-vomica*) has been recommended, especially when impotence is caused by excessive alcohol, cigarettes, or dietary indiscretions. Nux vomica can be very toxic if taken improperly, so it should be used only under the strict supervision of a physician trained in its use.

There are quite a few Chinese herbal remedies for impotence, usually combinations of herbs and sometimes such animal parts as deer antler and sea horse.

Allopathic treatment

Years ago, the standard treatment for impotence was a penile implant or long-term **psychotherapy**. Although physical causes are now more readily diagnosed and treated, individual or marital counseling is still an effective treatment for impotence when emotional factors play a role. Fortunately, other approaches are now available to treat the physical causes of impotence.

The most common treatment today is with the prescription drug sildenafil citrate, sold under the brand name Viagra. An estimated 20 million prescriptions for the pill have been filled since it was approved by the FDA in March 1998. It is also the most effective treatment, with a success rate of more than 60%. The drug boosts levels of a substance called cyclic GMP, which is responsible for widening the blood vessels of the penis. In clinical studies, Viagra produced headaches in 16% of men who took it, and other side effects included flushing, **indigestion**, and stuffy nose.

The primary drawback to Viagra, which works about an hour after it is taken, is that the FDA cautions men with **heart disease** or low blood pressure to be thoroughly examined by a physician before obtaining a prescription. At least 130 men have died while taking Viagra. Shortly after use of the drug skyrocketed, concerns were expressed over cardiovascular effects from Viagra. However, studies reported in 2002 that sildenafil had no effect on cardiac symptoms in older men who used it. Instead, cardiac events reported with use of Viagra are more likely the result of the physical demands of sexual activity in patients using the drug who were already at higher risk for cardiovascular disease.

In the summer of 2002, two investigational drugs were announced to become available in the near future to also treat erectile dysfunction. Vardenafil and tadalafil both helped men who also had such conditions as diabetes, high blood pressure and benign prostatic hypertrophy. The drugs are awaiting final FDA approval.

Vardenafil and tadalafil belong to the same group of chemical compounds as sildenafil, namely phosphodiesterase type 5 (PDE-5) inhibitors. Some men cannot benefit from sildenafil or the two newer PDE-5 inhibitors because they have low levels of nitric oxide. British investigators reported in late 2002 that three different types of compounds are being studied as possible medications for men with low levels of nitric oxide. They are Rho-kinase inhibitors, soluble guanylate cyclase activators, and nitric oxide-releasing PDE-5 inhibitors.

Other medications under investigation as treatments for impotence are topical agents. Topical means that they are applied externally to the skin rather than being injected or taken by mouth. If approved, these drugs would provide a noninvasive alternative for men who cannot take sildenafil or other oral medications for impotence.

Other traditional therapies for impotence include vacuum pump therapy, injection therapy involving injecting a substance into the penis to enhance blood flow, and a penile implantation device. In rare cases, if narrowed or diseased veins are responsible for impotence, surgeons may reroute the blood flow into the corpus cavernosa or remove leaking vessels.

A newer approach to the treatment of erectile dysfunction is gene therapy. As of late 2002, several preclinical studies have shown promise, but none of the gene-based strategies so far have yet been tested for safety.

Expected results

With proper diagnosis, impotence can nearly always be treated or coped with successfully. Unfortunately, fewer than 10% of impotent men seek treatment.

Prevention

There is no specific treatment to prevent impotence. Perhaps the most important measure is to maintain general good health and avoid atherosclerosis by exercising regularly, controlling weight, controlling **hypertension** and high **cholesterol** levels, and not smoking. Avoiding excessive alcohol intake may also help.

Resources

BOOKS

"Erectile Dysfunction." Section 17, Chapter 220 in *The Merck Manual of Diagnosis and Therapy*, edited by Mark H. Beers, MD, and Robert Berkow, MD. Whitehouse Station, NJ: Merck Research Laboratories, 1999.

Miller, Lucinda G., and Wallace J. Murray, eds. *Herbal Medicinals: A Clinician's Guide*. Binghamton, N.Y.: Haworth Press, 1999.

Pelletier, Kenneth R., MD. *The Best Alternative Medicine*, Part II, "CAM Therapies for Specific Conditions: Impotence." New York: Simon & Schuster, 2002.

Robbers, James E., and Varro E. Tyler. *Tyler's Herbs of Choice: The Therapeutic Use of Phytomedicinals*. Binghamton, N.Y.: Haworth Press, 1998.

Ryan, George. *Reclaiming Male Sexuality: A Guide to Potency, Vitality, and Prowess*. New York: M. Evans and Co., 1997.

PERIODICALS

Campbell, Adam. "Soft Science: The Exclusive World on Which Sex Supplements May Help and Which Won't." *Men's Health* (May 2002): 100.

Cellek, S., R. W. Rees, and J. Kalsi. "A Rho-Kinase Inhibitor, Soluble Guanylate Cyclase Activator and Nitric Oxide-Releasing PDE5 Inhibitor: Novel Approaches to Erectile Dysfunction." *Expert Opinion on Investigational Drugs* 11 (November 2002): 1563–1573.

Christ, G. J. "Gene Therapy for Erectile Dysfunction: Where Is It Going?" *Current Opinion in Urology* 12 (November 2002): 497–501.

Cowley, Geoffrey. "Looking Beyond Viagra." *Newsweek* (April 24, 2000): 77.

Gresser, U., and C. H. Gleiter. "Erectile Dysfunction: Comparison of Efficacy and Side Effects of the PDE-5 Inhibitors Sildenafil, Vardenafil and Tadalafil—Review of the Literature." *European Journal of Medical Research* 7 (October 29, 2002): 435–446.

"Is Viagra Safe?" *Internal Medicine Alert* (June 29, 2002): 90.

Norton, Patrice G.W. "Investigational Drugs in Erectile Dysfunction. (Vardenafil, Tadalafil)." *Internal Medicine News* (June 1, 2002): 50.

Yap, R. L., and K. T. McVary. "Topical Agents and Erectile Dysfunction: Is There a Place?" *Current Urology Reports* 3 (December 2002): 471–476.

"Yohimbe Tree Bark: Herbal Viagra Better Gotten by Rx." *Environmental Nutrition* (February 1999): 8.

ORGANIZATIONS

American Foundation for Urologic Disease. 1128 North Charles Street, Baltimore, MD 21201. (800) 242-2383. <http://www.afud.org>.

American Urological Association (AUA). 1120 North Charles Street, Baltimore, MD 21201. (410) 727-1100. <www.auanet.org>.

Center for Biologics Evaluation and Research (CBER), U. S. Food and Drug Administration (FDA). 1401 Rockville Pike, Rockville, MD 20852-1448. (800) 835-4709 or (301) 827-1800. <www.fda.gov/cber>.

Impotence Institute of America, Impotents Anonymous. 10400 Little Patuxent Parkway, Suite 485, Columbia, MD 21044-3502. (800) 669-1603.

National Kidney and Urologic Diseases Information Clearinghouse. 3 Information Way, Bethesda, MD 20892-3580. 800-891-5390. http://www.niddk.nih.gov/health/kidney/nkudic.htm.

OTHER

"Yohimbine." Drkoop.com. http://www.drkoop.com/hcr/drugstory/ pharmacy/leaflets/english/d01386a1.asp.

Ken R. Wells
Rebecca J. Frey, PhD

Indian medicine *see* **Ayurvedic medicine**
Indian paint *see* **Bloodroot; Goldenseal**
Indian plantago *see* **Psyllium**
Indian tobacco *see* **Lobelia**

Indigestion

Definition

Indigestion, which is sometimes called dyspepsia, is a general term covering a group of nonspecific symptoms in the digestive tract. It is often described as a feeling of fullness, bloating, **nausea**, **heartburn**, or gassy discomfort in the chest or abdomen. The symptoms develop during meals or shortly afterward. In most cases, indigestion is a minor problem that often clears up without professional treatment.

Description

Indigestion or dyspepsia is a widespread condition, estimated to occur in 25% of the adult population of the United States. Most people with indigestion do not feel sick enough to see a doctor; nonetheless, it is a common reason for office visits. About 3% of visits to primary care doctors are for indigestion.

Causes & symptoms

Physical causes

The symptoms associated with indigestion have a variety of possible physical causes, ranging from commonplace food items to serious systemic disorders:

• Diet. Milk, milk products, alcoholic beverages, tea, and coffee cause indigestion in some people because they stimulate the stomach's production of acid.

EFFECTIVE THERAPIES FOR INDIGESTION	
Therapy	**Description**
Acupressure	Massage the soft flesh between the thumb and point finger (Large Intestine 4) and press two fingers width away from the navel on both sides of the stomach (Stomach 25)
Aromatherapy	Ingest one drop of tarragon, marjoram, or rosemary accompanied by honey or other edible oil (safflower, almond, etc.)
Herbal medicine	Lavender, chamomile, peppermint, goldenseal, or lemon balm tea
Hydrotherapy	Hot water bottle or hot compress on abdomen
Massage	Abdominal massage
Traditional Chinese medicine (TCM)	Chinese herbal formulas such as Po Chai and Pill Curing

- Medications. Certain prescription drugs as well as over-the-counter medications can irritate the stomach lining. These medications include nonsteroidal anti-inflammatory drugs (NSAIDs, or over-the-counter **pain killers** like aspirin), some antibiotics, digoxin, theophylline, corticosteroids, **iron** (ferrous sulfate), oral contraceptives, and tricyclic antidepressants.

- Disorders of the pancreas and gallbladder. These include inflammation of the gallbladder or pancreas, **cancer** of the pancreas, and gallstones.

- Intestinal parasites. **Parasitic infections** that cause indigestion include amebiasis, fluke and tapeworm **infections**, giardiasis, and strongyloidiasis.

- Systemic disorders, including diabetes, thyroid disease, and collagen vascular disease.

- Cancers of the digestive tract.

- Conditions associated with women's reproductive organs. These conditions include menstrual cramps, **pregnancy**, and pelvic inflammatory disease.

Psychologic & emotional causes

Indigestion often accompanies an emotional upset, because the part of the nervous system involved in the so-called "fight-or-flight" response also affects the digestive tract. People diagnosed with **anxiety** or somatoform disorders frequently have problems with indigestion. Many people in the general population, however, will also experience heartburn, "butterflies in the stomach," or stomach cramps when they are in upsetting situations—such as school examinations, arguments with family members, crises in their workplace, and so on. Some people's digestive systems appear to react more intensely to emotional **stress** due to hypersensitive nerve endings in their intestinal tract.

Specific gastrointestinal disorders

In some cases, the patient's description of the symptoms suggests a specific digestive disorder as the cause of the indigestion. Some doctors classify these cases into three groups:

ESOPHAGITIS TYPE. Esophagitis is an inflammation of the tube that carries food from the throat to the stomach (the esophagus). The tissues of the esophagus can become irritated by the flow (reflux) of stomach acid backward into the lower part of the esophagus. If the patient describes the indigestion in terms of frequent or intense heartburn, the doctor will consider gastroesophageal reflux disease (GERD) as a possible cause. GERD is a common disorder in the general population, affecting about 30% of adults. In 2001, a study showed that **obesity** impairs the antireflux action. Those that are overweight have more severe reflux than most patients. Nighttime GERD affects 79% of adults with heartburn and is potentially more destructive to the esophagus than daytime indigestion. Another study found that acid reflux leads to **cough** and **wheezing** problems, particularly in people with **asthma**.

GERD also affects some infants and children, and is a common cause of babies spitting up formula. In most cases, the condition resolves itself, but children older than one year with regularly occurring pain in the lower chest or upper abdomen should cause concern. If a child is bothered by these symptoms during sleep or activities, a physician should be consulted.

PEPTIC ULCER TYPE. Patients who smoke and are over 45 are more likely to have indigestion of the peptic ulcer type. This group also includes people who find that their indigestion is relieved by taking antacids or eating a small amount of food. Patients in this category are often found to have *Helicobacter pylori* infections. *H. pylori* is a rod-shaped bacterium that lives in the tissues of the stomach and causes irritation of the mucous lining of the stomach walls. Most people with *H. pylori* infections do not develop chronic indigestion, but the organism appears to cause peptic ulcer disease (PUD) in a vulnerable segment of the population.

NONULCER TYPE. Most cases of chronic indigestion—as many as 65%—fall into this third category. Nonulcer dyspepsia is sometimes called functional dyspepsia because it appears to be related to abnormalities in the way that the stomach empties its contents into the intestine. In some people, the stomach empties either too slowly or too rapidly. In others, the stomach's muscular contractions are irregular and uncoordinated. These disorders of stomach movement (motility) may be caused by hypersensitive nerve endings in the stomach tissues. Patients in this group are likely to be younger than 45 and have a history of taking medications for anxiety or **depression**.

Diagnosis

Patient history

Because indigestion is a nonspecific set of symptoms, patients who feel sick enough to seek medical attention are likely to go to their primary care doctor. The history does not always point to an obvious diagnosis. The doctor can, however, use the process of history-taking to evaluate the patient's mood or emotional state in order to assess the possibility of a psychiatric disturbance. In addition, asking about the location, intensity, timing, and recurrence of the indigestion can help the doctor weigh the different diagnostic possibilities.

An important part of the history-taking is asking about symptoms that may indicate a serious illness. These warning symptoms include:

• weight loss

• persistent vomiting

• difficulty or pain in swallowing

• vomiting blood or passing blood in the stools

• anemia

Imaging studies

If the doctor thinks that the indigestion should be investigated further, he or she will order an endoscopic examination of the stomach. An endoscope is a slender tube-shaped instrument that allows the doctor to look at the lining of the patient's stomach. If the patient has indigestion of the esophagitis type or nonulcer type, the stomach lining will appear normal. If the patient has PUD, the doctor will be able to see breaks or ulcerated areas in the tissue. He or she may also order ultrasound

imaging of the abdomen, or a radionuclide scan to evaluate the motility of the stomach.

Laboratory tests

BLOOD TESTS. If the patient is over 45, the doctor will have the patient's blood analyzed for a complete blood cell count, measurements of liver enzyme levels, electrolyte and serum **calcium** levels, and thyroid function.

TESTS FOR *HELICOBACTER PYLORI*. Doctors can now test patients for the presence of *H. pylori* without having to take a tissue sample from the stomach. One of these noninvasive tests is a blood test and the other is a breath test.

Treatment

Nutritional supplements

Nutritionists or naturopaths may recommend the following to improve digestion:

• Stay away from foods that may cause an upset stomach. These include spicy, fried, cured, or junk foods, cucumbers, onions, peppers, tomatoes, beans, soda pop, or beverages containing **caffeine**.

• Eat lighter but more frequent meals.

• Avoid smoking.

• Adopt a **high-fiber diet** to improve regularity and treat such digestive problems as **constipation**, **hemorrhoids**, irritable bowel disease, and colon cancer. A high-fiber diet provides such additional health benefits as boosting the immune system function and preventing **heart disease**, cancer, and other diseases.

• Increase water intake. Proper hydration helps the digestive system work better.

• Improve poor digestive enzyme function with hydrochloric acid and pancreatic enzyme supplements such as lipase, amylase, and protease.

• Thickening a baby's food can help with reflux (add one tablespoon of dry rice cereal to each ounce of formula or breast milk). Hold babies upright after feedings rather than putting them down right away.

Herbal medicine

Practitioners of Chinese traditional herbal medicine might recommend medicines derived from peony (*Paeonia lactiflora*), **hibiscus** (*Hibiscus sabdariffa*), or hare's ear (*Bupleurum chinense*) to treat indigestion. Western herbalists are likely to prescribe **fennel** (*Foeniculum vulgare*), lemon balm (*Melissa officinalis*), or peppermint (*Mentha piperita*) to relieve stomach cramps and heartburn.

Homeopathy

Homeopaths tailor their remedies to the patient's overall personality profile as well as the specific symptoms. Depending on the patient's reaction to the indigestion and some of its likely causes, the homeopath might choose *Lycopodium*, *Carbo vegetalis*, *Nux vomica*, or *Pulsatilla*.

Diet and stress management

Many patients benefit from the doctor's reassurance that they do not have a serious or fatal disorder. Cutting out alcoholic beverages and drinks containing caffeine often helps. The patient may also be asked to keep a record of food intake, daily schedule, and symptom severity. Food diaries sometimes reveal psychological or dietary factors that influence indigestion.

Other treatments

Some alternative treatments are aimed at lowering the patient's stress level or changing attitudes and beliefs that contribute to indigestion. These therapies and practices include **Reiki, reflexology**, hydrotherapy, therapeutic massage, **yoga**, and **meditation**.

Allopathic treatment

Since most cases of indigestion are not caused by serious disorders, many doctors prefer to try medications and other treatment measures before ordering an endoscopy. Many patients with acid reflux treat themselves with over-the-counter remedies. For nighttime GERD, a 2001 study recommends a dose of a proton pump inhibitor before breakfast and another dose before dinner. Some medicines are also approved for use in infants and children with indigestion that doesn't resolve itself.

Medications

Patients with the esophagitis type of indigestion are often treated with H_2 antagonists. H_2 antagonists are drugs that block the secretion of stomach acid. They include ranitidine (Zantac) and famotidine (Pepcid).

Patients with motility disorders may be given prokinetic drugs. Prokinetic medications such as metoclopramide (Reglan) and cisapride (Propulsid) speed up the emptying of the stomach and increase intestinal motility.

Removal of H. pylori

Antibiotic therapy may be given to wipe out *H. pylori* bacteria from the gastrointestinal tract.

Expected results

Most cases of mild indigestion do not need medical treatment. For patients who consult a doctor and are given an endoscopic examination, 5–15% are diagnosed with GERD and 15–25% with PUD. About 1% of patients who are endoscoped have stomach cancer. Most patients with functional dyspepsia do well on either H_2 antagonists or prokinetic drugs, depending on the cause of their indigestion.

Prevention

Indigestion can often be prevented by attention to one's diet, general stress level, and ways of managing stress. Specific preventive measures include:

• stopping smoking

- cutting down on or eliminating alcohol, tea, or coffee

- avoiding foods that are highly spiced or loaded with fat

- eating slowly and keeping mealtimes relaxed

- practicing yoga or meditation

- not taking aspirin or other medications on an empty stomach

- keeping one's weight within normal limits

Resources

BOOKS

Cummings, Stephen, MD, and Dana Ullman, MPH. *Everybody's Guide to Homeopathic Medicines.* New York: G. P. Putnam's Sons, 1991.

Gach, Michael Reed, and Carolyn Marco. *Acu-Yoga: Self-Help Techniques to Relieve Tension.* Tokyo and New York: Japan Publications, Inc., 1998.

Murray, Michael, and Joseph Pizzorno. *Encyclopedia of Natural Medicine.* Rocklin, CA: Prima Health, 1998.

PERIODICALS

Avidan, B., et al. "Temporal Associations Between Coughing or Wheezing and Acid Reflux in Asthmatics." *Gut* 49, no. 6 (December 2001): 767.

"Fast Lives Bring on the Burn." *Chemist and Druggist* (November 10, 2001): 37.

Wajed, Shahjehan A. "Elevated Body Mass Disrupts the Barrier to Gastroesophageal Reflux." *JAMA—The Journal of the American Medical Association* (December 5, 2001): 2650.

"What You Should Know about Gastroesophageal Reflux (GER) in Infants and Children." *American Family Physician* (December 1, 2001).

Zoler, Mitchell L. "Nighttime GERD Affects 79% of Adults with Heartburn." *Internal Medicine News* (October 15, 2001).

Mai Tran
Teresa Norris

Infant massage

Definition

Infant massage refers to massage therapy as specifically applied to infants. In most cases, oil or lotion is used as it would be on an adult subject by a trained and licensed massage therapist. Medical professionals caring for infants might also use massage techniques on infants born prematurely, on those with motor or gastrointestinal problems, or on those who have been exposed to cocaine in utero.

Origins

The practice of massaging infants dates back to ancient times, particularly in Asian and Pacific Island cultures; that is, massage was a component of the baby's regular bath routine among the Maoris and Hawaiians. Touch in these cultures is considered healthful both physically and spiritually. In the West, however, infant massage has received more attention in recent years in conjunction with the popularity of natural **childbirth** and midwife-assisted births. Dr. Frédéric Leboyer, a French physician who was one of the leaders of the natural childbirth movement, helped to popularize infant massage through his photojournalistic book on the Indian art of baby massage.

Infant massage was introduced formally into the United States in 1978, when Vimala Schneider McClure, a **yoga** practitioner who served in an orphanage in Northern India, developed a training program for instructors at the request of childbirth educators. An early research study by R. Rice in 1976 had showed that premature babies who were massaged surged ahead in weight gain and neurological development over those who were not massaged. From McClure's training in India, her knowledge of **Swedish massage** and reflexology, along with her knowledge of yoga postures that she had already adapted for babies, she became the foremost authority on infant massage. In 1986 she founded the International Association of Infant Massage (IAIM), which has 27 chapters worldwide as of 2000.

Benefits

Research from experiments conducted at the Touch Research Institutes at the University of Miami School of Medicine and Nova Southeastern University has been cited for the clinical benefits massage has on infants and children. Tiffany Field, Ph. D., director, noted that the research ".. suggests that touch is as important to infants and children as eating and sleeping. Touch therapy triggers many physiological changes that help infants and children grow and develop. For example, massage can stimulate nerves in the brain which facilitate food absorption, resulting in faster weight gain. It also lowers level of **stress** hormones, resulting in improved immune function."

The benefits of infant massage include:

- relaxation

- relief from stress

- interaction with adults

- stimulation of the nervous system

The results of several studies showed that infant massage alleviates the stress that newborns experience as a result of the enormous change that birth brings about in their

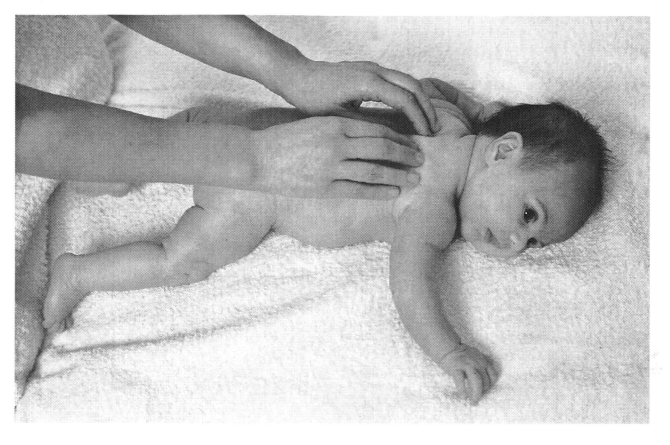

Infant massage. *(Photo Researchers, Inc. Reproduced by permission.)*

lives after the 6–9 months they have spent in the womb. Both premature infants and full-term babies need the relaxation that comes from massaging and moving their limbs and muscles. In infants with **colic**, massage provides the relief necessary to disperse **gas**, ease muscle spasms, tone the digestive system and help it work efficiently. Some techniques even help bring relief from teething and emotional stress. The stimulation an infant receives from massage can aid circulation, strengthen muscles, help digestion, and relieve **constipation**. The bonding that occurs with massage between a parent and child enhances the entire process of bonding that comes with contact through all of the senses, including touch, voice, and sight. It affords a physical experience of quality time between the parents and the child as well as with any significant others in a baby's life.

Description

Various techniques are used in infant massage, with the different strokes specific to a particular therapy. Special handling is used for treating a baby with gas and colic. Some of the strokes are known as "Indian milking," which is a gentle stroking of the child's legs; and the "twist and squeeze" **stroke**, a gentle squeeze of the muscles in the thigh and calf. The light "feather" strokes

often employed in regular Swedish massage are applied at the end of a massage. The procedure is not unlike certain forms of adult massage, but with extra care taken for the fragility of the infant.

There are also specific Chinese techniques of pediatric massage, including massage of children with special needs. In China, these forms of massage can be given by medical professionals, but parents are often taught how to do the simpler forms for home treatment of their children.

Preparations

If lotions or oils are used, care is taken to ensure their safety on a baby's delicate skin. The most important consideration is to use vegetable oils rather than mineral oils, which can clog the pores in the skin. The oil that is used should be warmed in the caregiver's hands before applying it to the baby's skin. The environment in which the massage is given to an infant should be comfortably warm, and as calm and nonthreatening as possible.

Precautions

Extreme caution is necessary when performing infant massage. Strokes are made with the greatest delicacy in order not to harm the infant in any way. Proper techniques are taught by licensed massage therapists ensuring that the infant is treated with appropriate physical touch. Anyone who is unfamiliar with handling a baby should receive appropriate instruction before beginning infant massage.

Side effects

No adverse side effects have been reported when infant massage is done properly after careful instruction, or by a licensed massage therapist who specializes in infant care.

Research & general acceptance

In addition to the study already noted regarding touch therapy, a website devoted to infant massage lists research published as early as 1969, and cites hundreds of individual projects that have been conducted throughout the world focusing on infant massage. Many of the studies are related to the benefits of massage and touch for premature infants and others born with such risk factors as drug dependence. Conclusions regarding the benefits are overwhelmingly positive. The proliferation of therapists licensed in infant massage across the United States and worldwide indicates that infant massage is increasingly recognized as a legitimate health care treatment.

Training & certification

The International Association of Infant Massage (IAIM) has developed a basic course for licensing infant massage therapists. The pioneer in the field, Vimala McClure, began to prepare a course of instruction in the 1970s. The course is introduced in four-day sessions around the United States. Licensing is obtained by those who complete the course, pass a take-home examination, and complete a teaching practicum with five families over a three-month period. IAIM listed its course in 2000 as costing $550.00 if paid in full two weeks prior to training, and $595 after that. It includes a $100 nonrefundable deposit due one month before training. The cities where the basic course was offered in 2000 included Augusta, GA; Gaithersburg, MD; Chicago, IL; Boston, MA; Washington, DC; Charlottesville, VA; Minneapolis, MN; and Albuquerque, NM. In 2000, the International Institute of Infant Massage in Albuquerque also offered an Infant Massage Instructor Certification Course specifically geared to men, entitled "Men Teaching Fathers," and scheduled to last four days.

The licensing of massage therapists varies from state to state, as infant massage qualifies for consideration as medical treatment. Infant massage is becoming an increasingly popular discipline within the field. Numerous websites provide listings for infant massage specialists throughout the United States. The IAIM course is recognized as the official course for infant massage.

Resources

BOOKS

Auckett, Amelia. *Baby Massage: Parent-Child Bonding through Touching.* New York: Newmarket Press, 1982.

Cline, Kyle. *Chinese Massage for Infants and Children: Traditional Techniques for Alleviating Colic, Teething Pain, Earache, and Other Common Childhood Conditions.* Rochester, VT: Inner Traditions International, Limited, 1999.

Fan, Ya-Li. *Chinese Pediatric Massage Therapy: Traditional Techniques for Alleviating Colic, Colds, Earaches, and Other Common Childhood Conditions,* ed. Bob Flaws. Boulder, CO: Blue Poppy Enterprises, 1999.

Gordon, Jay, and Brenda Adderly. *Brighter Baby: Boosting Your Child's Intelligence, Health and Happiness through Infant Therapeutic Massage.* New York: Regnery Publishing, Inc. 1999.

Heinl, Tina. *The Baby Massage Book: Shared Growth through the Hands.* Boston, MA: Sigo Press, 1991.

Leboyer, Frédéric. *Loving Hands: The Traditional Indian Art of Baby Massage.* New York: Knopf, 1976.

McClure, Vimala Schneider. *Infant Massage: A Handbook for Loving Parents.* New York: Bantam Books, 1989.

Walker, Peter. *Baby Massage: A Practical Guide to Massage and Movement for Babies and Infants.* New York: St. Martin's Press, 1996.

ORGANIZATIONS

International Association of Infant Massage. P.O. Box 1045. Oak View, CA 93022.

International Institute of Infant Massage. 605 Bledsoe Rd. NW. Albuquerque, NM 87107. (505) 341-9381. Fax: (505) 341-9386. http://www.infantmassage.com.

OTHER

Gentle Touch Infant Massage Video. Gentle Touch, Inc. 1996.

Jane Spehar

Infections

Definition

An infection is a condition in which viruses, bacteria, fungi, or parasites enter the body and cause a state of disease. Such invaders are called pathogens. They damage cells of the body by adhering to and damaging the cell walls, releasing toxic substances or causing allergic reactions. The body has a set series of responses to infection, which mostly involve body chemicals, body tissues, and the immune system. It was recently reported that infection is the fourth leading cause of death in the United States and kills more people than **cancer** and **heart disease** combined.

Description

Pathogens are everywhere in a person's daily environment: They may enter the body through breathing, ingested food or **water**, sexual contact, open **wounds**, or contact with contaminated objects. Having entered the body, pathogens begin to reproduce. Most pathogens are kept in check before they have a chance to multiply. If, however, the body is unable to keep the pathogens in balance, serious disease and even death may occur. Chronic infections may develop if the body has only limited control over a given pathogen. In that case, the infection will have a tendency to flare up in response to **stress** and weakness. Sepsis is a serious condition in which pathogens spread and circulate throughout the body via the bloodstream. This type of infection affects the entire body.

The body has many natural barriers to infection. For example, the harmless bacteria normally found on the skin, known as commensals, inhibit the growth of many pathogens. Sweat and oil gland secretions also protect the skin; and the skin itself offers a significant physical barrier that no bacteria are able to penetrate. Damage to the skin from **burns**, insect bites, surgery, or injuries may leave the skin open to infection. In addition to the physical barrier of the skin, many of the body's secretions such as tears, sweat, urine, and saliva contain chemicals that destroy pathogens.

The mucous membranes that line the passageways of the body secrete mucus, which contains enzymes and chemicals that kill or disable pathogens. The pathogens are then trapped in the mucus and filtered out or swallowed. Commensal bacteria also live on the mucous membranes; there they inhibit the spread and multiplication of pathogens just as they do on the skin. The digestive tract contains stomach acid, pancreatic enzymes, and other secretions that protect against infection. Peristalsis and the shedding of the lining of the intestinal tract also help to remove pathogens. The acid pH of the stomach and vagina is protective, as well as the length of the urethra in males. The flushing action of urine and feces as they are excreted also protect against infection.

A **fever** is defined as the elevation of the body temperature to at least 100°F (37.8°C). Fevers are a helpful part of the body's response to an infection, since most pathogens do not thrive at higher temperatures while the immune system's white blood cells (WBCs) work best in a warm environment. If the fever reaches levels of 102°F (38.9°C) or higher, it may have to be brought down to avoid seizures, dehydration, and tissue damage.

The second level of the body's defenses is the immune system. The white blood cells are a major part of this system. In response to the invasion of pathogens, WBCs are released from the bone marrow into the bloodstream. The main function of these WBCs, depending on their type, is to engulf pathogens and render them harmless, detoxify poisons, produce and release antibodies and chemicals, and clean up wastes left by other WBCs. The spleen, thymus, lymph system, and liver all have roles in the immune response. Successful removal of pathogens from the body often gives immunity against infection by that pathogen in the future.

Pathogens can be persistent. They may secrete enzymes, destroying tissues in the body to spread the infection more quickly and effectively. They may secrete chemicals that counteract the actions of the WBCs. Some pathogens release toxins that kill the surrounding cells. Many also have methods to evade being engulfed and destroyed. In addition, the body's own commensal bacteria may become pathogenic if something upsets their balanced state in the body. This loss of balance may often result from chronic illness, low stomach acid, recurrent use of antibiotics, cross-contamination through medical or sexual exploration, or a compromised immune system.

Causes & symptoms

Infections are caused by pathogens invading the tissues of the body and beginning to multiply. Headaches, muscle aches, fever, **chills**, and **fatigue** are common symptoms of infections. Many of these symptoms are due to inflammation and the response of the immune system to the pathogens. For example, during an infection, the blood supply is increased to the affected areas; as the blood rushes to the site of infection, it causes the skin to redden. The blood vessels also become more readily able to release WBCs into the tissues; when the WBCs die and decay they form a thick fluid known as pus. Enzymes released by the WBCs may also be responsible for **pain** and swelling.

More specific symptoms of infection vary according to the site and type of the infection. Some of these symptoms include:

• Gastrointestinal system: **Diarrhea, vomiting, nausea, stomachaches,** cramps, **gas** pains, and dehydration.

• Respiratory system: Coughing, **sneezing, sore throat,** congestion, fever, **bronchitis,** and runny nose.

• Urinary system: Increased frequency and urgency of urination; pain on urination; blood, pus, or other discharge in the urine; bad-smelling urine or discharge; and vaginal **itching**.

• Skin: **Rashes,** sores, itching, and **blisters**; redness, swelling, tenderness, and pain.

• Joints: Local pain, stiffness, redness, and swelling.

Risk factors for infections include chronic disease; severe emotional stress; broken skin; changes in the pH of various body fluids; malnutrition; surgery; rupture of amniotic membranes; invasive medical or dental procedures; tissue injuries or destruction; decreased flow of body fluids; changes in peristalsis; decreased output of stomach acid; recurrent use of antibiotics; and suppressed immune function. Many infections have a high probability of being passed from person to person. This is especially true of respiratory diseases, which can be transmitted through contact with the sputum and droplets produced by coughing or sneezing. Contact with infected waste products, open sores, skin eruptions, infected clothing and bedclothes, and sexual contact are circumstances which often lead to the further spread of infections.

New concerns about infections continue to baffle researchers and clinicians into the twenty-first century. First, the world faces the threat of infection from bioterrorism, and Americans faced a scare from deliberate distribution of anthrax spores through the United States postal system following the September 11, 2001, terrorist attack. The year 1999 saw the first reports of the West Nile virus in the United States, and reported cases of the disease began spreading after that date. Further, clinicians worry about widespread antibiotic resistance, as individuals and the public at large become exposed to more antibiotics for longer periods of time.

Diagnosis

Many infections are minor and self-limiting. Some infections, however, are serious; some can even lead to permanent impairment or death. If an infection does not clear up within a few days, or if it gets worse, a healthcare provider should be consulted. Infections are initially diagnosed by the patient's presentation and by a history of the illness or injury and the symptoms.

A complete blood count (CBC) is a simple clinical test that can be used to diagnose an infection. Increases in the total WBC count usually indicate a bacterial infection; decreases tend to indicate a viral infection or a very severe infection, both of which may cause the destruction of WBCs faster than they can be produced. Increases in specific types of white blood cells known as neutrophils, lymphocytes, and monocytes also point to an infection. An increase in eosinophils may be due to a parasitic infection. A blood chemistry panel may be taken to determine whether there are chemical changes that may have been brought on by an infection.

A serious illness may require further evaluation and diagnostic tests. Additional laboratory tests can be performed using blood, feces, or samples of the infected tissue. Ultrasound, computed tomography (CT) scans, and magnetic resonance imaging (MRI) may also be used. In some cases, a tissue sample (biopsy) is taken from the affected site for microbial culture tests and microscopic examination.

Treatment

Herbal therapy

Echinacea spp. enhances the action of the immune system. It can be taken for up to six weeks to prevent or heal infections. **Goldenseal** (*Hydrastis canadensis*) has strong antibiotic qualities. **Garlic** (*Allium sativum*) is also antibiotic. **Licorice** (*Glycyrrhiza glabra*) has significant antiviral activity. It reduces the bad effects of stress on the health, and has been used to treat herpes, staphylococcal and streptococcal infections, typhus, cholera, **pneumonia**, and infections caused by *Candida albicans*. *Astragalus membranaceus* is a Chinese herb that may be used to enhance the immune system as well as to prevent the recurrence of chronic infections. **Pau d'arco** (*Tabebuia impetiginosa*) is recommended for internal **fungal infections**, while the topical use of **tea tree oil** (*Melaleuca alternfolia*) is recommended for some external infections.

Dietary modifications

A healthful balanced diet and lifestyle are important supports of the immune function. Reishi (*Ganoderma lucidum*), shiitake (*Lentinus edodes*), and **maitake** (*Grifola frondosa*) mushrooms are renowned for their ability to strengthen the immune system and their antimicrobial properties. Regular supplementation with **vitamin C, vitamin A** or beta-carotene, **zinc**, and **bioflavonoids** is also recommended to boost the immune response.

Sugary foods, including honey, may depress the immune system. Very high levels of fat in the diet may also interfere. Alcohol decreases the functioning of the immune system. All of these substances should be avoided during the course of an infection. Food **allergies** should be considered, especially in the case of chronic colds, throat infections, and ear infections. Once allergens have been identified, they should be avoided. Patients should increase their intake of fluids, including soups, teas, diluted fruit and vegetable juices, and pure water.

Aromatherapy

Aromatherapy may be a useful supportive measure in infectious conditions. An essential oil of cedarwood (*Cedrus atlantica*) is recommended in fungal infections; **essential oils** of tea tree (*Melaleuca alternifolia*) and patchouli are also recommended. It should be remembered, however, that essential oils are very concentrated, toxic to the liver and kidneys, and should be used only in very small doses (drops).

Acupuncture

Acupuncture is helpful in stimulating the immune system. It reduces the effects of stress, improves circulation, and increases the production of RBCs and WBCs. It has been used for thousands of years to treat infectious diseases.

Hydrotherapy

Constitutional **hydrotherapy** is the use of applications of hot water alternated with cold. It is effective in respiratory infections and in stimulating the immune system. For proper administration of hydrotherapy, a naturopath or other healthcare provider familiar with its techniques should be consulted.

Allopathic treatment

Minor infections are often relieved by over-the-counter medications. A high fever or joint pain may be a sign of an infection spreading throughout the body. A physician should be contacted. Infections from bites and puncture wounds should also receive medical attention and possibly a **tetanus** injection.

Serious infections may be treated with antibiotics. Antibiotics are effective against many parasitic and fungal infections as well as bacteria. Antibiotics may also be given during a viral infection even though they have no effect on viruses. This measure is taken to prevent bacterial infections, which may occur due to the weakened state brought on by the virus. In the case of viral infections, antiviral drugs are used to reduce symptoms. Their usefulness, however, is limited because viruses quickly mutate and develop resistance to them.

Antifungal drugs are often applied directly to fungal infections. They may be taken orally, applied topically, or injected. Fungal infections often require several weeks of treatment and repeated courses of the drug. Both antifungal and antiviral drugs tend to be somewhat toxic to people as well as to the pathogens.

Expected results

Most minor infections resolve within a week. Chronic infections may last for years. Serious infections need to be attended by a physician, as tissue damage and death may be an imminent outcome. **Anemia** may result from severe infections, since RBCs or their production may be affected.

KEY TERMS

Allergen—Any substance, usually a protein, that induces an allergic reaction in a particular individual.

Antibiotic—An agent able to kill or interfere with the development of bacteria and other microorganisms.

Commensal bacteria—Bacteria that live in or on the human body and are in an often beneficial relationship with the human host. For example, some bacteria in the digestive tract produce needed B vitamins.

Pathogens—Microorganisms capable of causing disease.

Peristalsis—The smooth muscle contractions that move food, bile, and urine through their respective passageways.

pH—A comparative measure of the acidity or alkalinity of a solution.

Vaccine—Any preparation introduced into the body to prevent a disease by stimulating antibodies against it.

Prevention

Various vaccines are available to prevent major infections. These vaccines are made from deactivated parts of viruses or bacteria that confer future immunity to infection by those pathogens. Vaccinations for **mumps**, **measles**, chicken pox, tetanus, **hepatitis**, diphtheria, **whooping cough**, and pneumonia are widely available in the United States. They are routinely given to infants and children to provide lifetime immunity from these diseases. An anthrax vaccine is available but as of early 2002, reports say that a new, improved vaccine is needed in the United States, since the vaccine requires six doses over 18 months for full protection, with a booster every 12 months.

Good hygienic practices should be maintained. They include keeping the body clean as well as keeping food, utensils, and areas of preparation clean and free of contamination. Meat, seafood, and dairy products should be properly refrigerated. Breaks in the skin should be cleaned and disinfected to avoid further infection. Direct contact with people known or suspected to have infections should be limited, depending on the nature of the disease.

The health of the immune system should be maintained. A positive mental outlook is important, together with appropriate amounts of sleep, **relaxation**, and stress

---

reduction. A healthful diet should be followed, with decreased sugar, salt, saturated fats, and chemical additives. Good lifestyle habits, such as giving up **smoking** and taking regular physical **exercise**, should be cultivated.

Resources

BOOKS

Burton Goldberg Group. *Alternative Medicine: The Definitive Guide*. Fife, WA: Future Medicine Publishing, 1995.

Editors of Time-Life Books. *The Medical Advisor: The Complete Guide to Alternative and Conventional Treatments*. Alexandria, VA: Time-Life, Inc., 1997.

Lininger, Skye, et al. *The Natural Pharmacy*. Rocklin, CA: Prima Health, 1998.

Murray, Michael, and Joseph Pizzorno. *Encyclopedia of Natural Medicine*. Rocklin, CA: Prima Publishing, 1991.

PERIODICALS

Ford-Jones, E. Lee. "Human Surveillance for West Nile Virus Infection in Ontario in 2000." *JAMA, The Journal of the American Medical Association* 287, no. 12 (March 27, 2002): 1508.

Marwick, Charles. "Improved Anthrax Vaccine is Needed, Claims Report." *British Medical Journal* (March 16, 2002): 630.

Torpy, Janet M. "New Threats and Old Enemies: Challenges for Critical Care Medicine." *JAMA, The Journal of the American Medical Association* (March 27, 2002): 1513.

Patience Paradox
Teresa G. Odle

Infectious mononucleosis *see*
Mononucleosis

Infertility

Definition

Infertility is the failure of a couple to conceive a **pregnancy** after trying to do so for at least one full year. In primary infertility, pregnancy has never occurred. In secondary infertility, one or both members of the couple have previously conceived, but are unable to conceive again after a full year of trying.

Description

Approximately 20% of couples struggle with infertility at any given time. Infertility has increased as a problem over the last 30 years. Some studies blame this increase on social phenomena, including the tendency for marriage and starting a family to occur at a later age. For women, fertility decreases with increasing age:

- Infertility in married women ages 16–20 = 4.5%.
- Infertility in married women ages 35–40 = 31.8%.
- Infertility in married women over the age of 40 = 70%.

Presently, individuals often have several sexual partners before they marry and try to have children. This increase in numbers of sexual partners has led to an increase in sexually transmitted diseases. Scarring from these **infections**, especially from **pelvic inflammatory disease** (infection of the female reproductive organs) seems to be in part responsible for the rise in infertility. Furthermore, use of some forms of the contraceptive called the intrauterine device (IUD) has contributed to an increased rate of pelvic inflammatory disease, with subsequent scarring. A study in 2001 found that **copper** IUDs have probably been wrongfully blamed for tubal infertility, while infection from the sexually transmitted disease **chlamydia** was likely the cause.

To understand the causes of infertility, it is first necessary to understand the basics of human reproduction. Fertilization occurs when a sperm from the male merges with an egg (ovum) from the female, creating a zygote that contains genetic material (DNA) from both the father and the mother. If pregnancy is then established, the zygote will develop into an embryo, then a fetus, and ultimately, if all goes well, a baby will be born.

Sperm are small cells that carry the father's genetic material. The sperm are mixed into a fluid called semen, which is discharged from the penis during sexual intercourse. The whiplike tail of the sperm allows the sperm to swim up the female reproductive tract, in search of an egg.

The ovum is the cell that carries the mother's genetic material. Once a month, a single mature ovum is produced, and leaves the ovary in a process called ovulation. This ovum enters a tube leading to the uterus (the fallopian tube) where fertilization occurs.

When fertilization occurs, the resulting cell (which now contains genetic material from both the mother and the father) is called the zygote. This single cell will divide into multiple cells and the resulting cluster of cells (called a blastocyst) moves into the womb (uterus). The uterine lining (endometrium) has been preparing itself to receive a pregnancy by growing thicker. If the blastocyst successfully attaches itself to the wall of the uterus, then pregnancy has been achieved.

Causes & symptoms

Unlike most medical problems, infertility is an issue requiring the careful evaluation of two separate individuals, as well as an evaluation of their interactions with each other. In about 3–4% of couples, no cause for their infertility will be discovered. About 40% of the time, infertility is due to a problem with the male; about 40% of the time, infertility is due to the female; and about 20% of the time, there are fertility problems with both the male and the female.

The main factors involved in causing infertility include:

• male problems: 35%

• ovulation problems: 20%

• tubal problems: 20%

• **endometriosis**: 10%

• cervical factors: 5%

Male factors

Male infertility can be caused by a number of different characteristics of the sperm. To check for these characteristics, a sample of semen is obtained and examined under the microscope (semen analysis). Four basic characteristics are usually evaluated:

• Sperm count refers to the number of sperm present in a semen sample. The normal number of sperm present in just 1 ml of semen is over 20 million. A man with only 5–20 million sperm is considered subfertile and a man with fewer than 5 million sperm is considered infertile.

• Sperm are also examined to see how well they swim (sperm motility) and to be sure that most have normal structure.

• Not all sperm within a specimen of semen will be perfectly normal. Some may be immature, and some may have abnormalities of the head or tail. A normal semen sample will contain no more than 25% abnormal forms of sperm.

• Volume of the semen sample is important. An abnormal amount of semen could affect the ability of the sperm to successfully fertilize an ovum.

Any number of conditions result in abnormal findings in the semen analysis. Men can be born with testicles that have not descended properly from the abdominal cavity (where testicles develop originally) into the scrotal sac, or may be born with only one instead of the normal two testicles. Testicle size can be smaller than normal. Past infection (including **mumps**) can affect testicular function, as can a past injury. The presence of abnormally large veins (varicocele) in the testicles can increase testicular temperature, which decreases sperm count. History of having been exposed to various toxins, drug use, excess alcohol use, use of anabolic steroids, certain medications, diabetes, thyroid problems, or other endocrine disturbances can have direct effects on the formation of sperm (spermatogenesis). A study published in late 2001 linked certain organic solvents that men en-

counter in the workplace as possible causes of low sperm count. The types of solvents are most likely encountered in such occupations as those of professional printers, painters, and decorators. Theories suggest solvents like glycol ethers, which are know to affect animals' reproductive systems, are the most harmful.

Problems with the male anatomy can cause sperm to be ejaculated not out of the penis, but into the bladder; and scarring from past infections can interfere with ejaculation.

Studies continue to uncover reasons for male infertility. In 2001, researchers reported that a certain protein lacking in the sperm could prevent formation of the structure on the head of the sperm that contains enzymes that help penetrate the egg, allowing conception. The finding should lead to further study of the molecular basis of male fertility.

Ovulatory problems

The first step in diagnosing ovulatory problems is to make sure that an ovum is being produced each month. A woman's morning body temperature is slightly higher around the time of ovulation. A woman can measure and record her temperatures daily and a chart can be drawn to show whether or not ovulation has occurred. Luteinizing hormone (LH) is released just before ovulation. A simple urine test can be done to check if LH has been released around the time that ovulation is expected.

Pelvic adhesions & endometriosis

Pelvic adhesions cause infertility by blocking the fallopian tubes and preventing the sperm from reaching the egg. Pelvic adhesions are fibrous scars. These scars can be the result of past infections, such as pelvic inflammatory disease, or infections following abortions or prior births. Previous abdominal surgeries can also leave behind scarring.

Endometriosis is the abnormal location of uterine tissue outside of the uterus. When uterine tissue is planted elsewhere in the pelvis, it still bleeds on a monthly basis with the start of the normal menstrual period. This leads to irritation within the pelvis around the site of this abnormal tissue and bleeding, and may cause scarring. Endometriosis may lead to pelvic adhesions.

A hysterosalpingogram (HSG) can show if the fallopian tubes are blocked. This is an x-ray exam that tests whether dye material can travel through the patient's fallopian tubes. Scarring also can be diagnosed by examining the pelvic area through the use of a laparoscope that is inserted into the abdomen through a tiny incision made near the navel.

Cervical factors

The cervix is the opening from the vagina into the uterus through which the sperm must pass. Mucus produced by the cervix helps to transport the sperm into the uterus. Injury to the cervix or scarring of the cervix after surgery or infection can result in a smaller than normal cervical opening, making it difficult for the sperm to enter. Injury or infection can also decrease the number of glands in the cervix, leading to a smaller amount of cervical mucus. In other situations, the mucus produced is the wrong consistency (perhaps too thick) to allow sperm to travel through. In addition, some women produce antibodies (immune cells) that are specifically directed to identify sperm as foreign invaders and to kill them.

Cervical mucus can be examined under a microscope to diagnose whether cervical factors are contributing to infertility. The interaction of a live sperm sample from the male partner and a sample of cervical mucus from the female partner can also be examined. This procedure is called a post-coital test.

Treatment

Conventional treatment for infertility usually involves invasive and, expensive procedures. There are many alternative treatments available that can increase the chance of conception. Some have been proven effective in clinical studies.

General measures to increase fertility include monitoring ovulation and timing intercourse (optimal chance for conception is within six days prior to and including the day of ovulation); and quitting **smoking**, excessive drinking, and drug use. To improve sperm quality, men can wear boxer shorts instead of briefs.

Both men and women can increase fertility by eating a well-balanced diet. Good food choices include legumes (especially soy), dark-colored vegetables, fruits, seeds, nuts, and sufficient good quality protein including meat, fish, and eggs. Some people think that refined sugar, processed cheeses, foods made with white flour, and chemical preservatives should be avoided. Adequate sleep is also important.

Supplements

Dietary supplements that can enhance fertility include:

- Multivitamins can help treat infertility in women.
- Vitamin E has antioxidant activity that prevents reproductive damage in men and women. It can increase sperm count and motility in men and balance hormones in women.

- **Vitamin C** has antioxidant activity that prevents reproductive damage in men and women. Also, a study found that vitamin C supplementation led to improved sperm count and decreased sperm clumping in infertile men.
- Folic acid (with a multivitamin) improved fertility in a study of infertile women.
- **Zinc** deficiency is often associated with low sperm count. Studies have found that zinc supplementation can improve male fertility.
- Arginine supplementation led to major increases in sperm count and motility in a study of infertile men.
- **Selenium** has antioxidant activity. Selenium supplementation led to increased sperm count and motility and decreased number of abnormal sperm in a study of infertile men.
- Beta-carotene supplementation can increase sperm count and motility.
- B vitamins (B_2, B_6, and B_{12}) are important for optimal fertility.

Herbal and Chinese medicine

The following may be taken by women to treat infertility:

- Dong quai (*Angelica sinensis*) has been used to regulate menstrual cycles and for infertility.
- Licorice helps to balance levels of estrogen and testosterone and is used for infertility.
- Red clover (*Trifolium pratense*) has a beneficial effect on the uterus, can calm the nervous system, and can balance hormone levels.
- Nettle (*Urtica dioica*) supports the uterus and hormonal system.
- Raspberry leaf strengthens the mucous lining of the uterus.
- Chasteberry (*Vitex agnus-castus*) balances hormone production.
- Ladies mantle (*Alchemilla vulgaris*) balances hormone production.
- Shatavari (*Asparagus racemosus*) is an Ayurvedic remedy for infertility and works by balancing hormones.
- *Rehmannia* is an Ayurvedic remedy for infertility.
- Myrrh (*Commiphora myrrha*) is an Ayurvedic remedy for infertility.
- False unicorn (*Chamaelirium luteum*) balances hormone levels.
- Pomegranate essence balances the reproductive system.

The following may be taken by men to treat infertility:

• Ginseng may increase the formation of sperm, testosterone levels, and sexual activity.

• Pygeum may help infertile men who have a reduced secretion of semen.

• Pine bark extract improves sperm shape.

• Chasteberry (*Vitex agnus-castus*) balances hormone production.

• Shatavari (*Asparagus racemosus*) is an Ayurvedic remedy for infertility and works by balancing hormones. May increase sperm production.

• Saw palmetto (*Serenoa serrulata*) increases the production of testosterone and strengthens the reproductive system.

• Ashwaganda (*Withania omnifera*) is an Ayurvedic remedy that improves the quality of semen and sperm count.

• Chinese herbals must be specifically designed and used to treat infertility in males.

Other treatments

A variety of other alternative treatments may be used for infertility:

• stress reduction

• cognitive behavior therapy

• visualization

• homeopathy

• reflexology

• essential oils

• acupuncture

Allopathic treatment

The first step in the treatment of infertility is to perform thorough physical exams and testing of both partners in the hope of finding the source of infertility. For the woman this involves blood testing and ultrasound examinations at specific days during the menstrual cycle. This may include an endometrial biopsy in which a sample of the lining of the uterus is taken and examined. Hysteroscopy, in which a special camera examines the inside of the uterus, may be performed.

Pelvic adhesions can be treated during laparoscopy. The adhesions are cut using special instruments. Endometriosis can be treated with certain medications, but may also require surgery to repair any obstruction caused by adhesions.

Treatment of cervical factors includes antibiotics in the case of an infection, steroids to decrease production of anti-sperm antibodies, and artificial insemination techniques to completely bypass the cervical mucus.

Treatment of ovulatory problems depends on the cause. If a thyroid or pituitary problem is responsible, simply treating that problem can restore fertility. Medications that stimulate ovulation are clomiphene citrate (Clomid) that is taken by mouth and follicle stimulating hormone (Pergonal, Fertinex, and Follistim) that is given by injection. These drugs increase the risk of multiple births (twins, triplets, etc.) and may cause side effects.

Treatment of male infertility includes addressing known reversible factors first; for example, discontinuing any medication known to have an effect on spermatogenesis or ejaculation, as well as decreasing alcohol intake, and treating thyroid or other endocrine disease. Varicoceles can be treated surgically. Testosterone in low doses can improve sperm motility.

Other treatments of male infertility include collecting semen samples from multiple ejaculations, pooling them, and depositing them into the female's uterus during ovulation. When the male partner's sperm is proven to be absolutely unable to produce pregnancy, donor sperm may be used. Depositing the male partner's sperm or donor sperm by mechanical means into the female is called artificial insemination.

Assisted reproductive techniques include in vitro fertilization (IVF), gamete intrafallopian transfer (GIFT), and zygote intrafallopian tube transfer (ZIFT). These are usually used after other techniques to treat infertility (surgery, medications, and/or insemination) have failed.

IVF involves the use of drugs to induce the simultaneous production of many eggs from the ovaries, which are retrieved surgically or via ultrasound-guided needle aspiration through the vaginal wall. The ova and sperm are combined in a laboratory, where several of the ova may be fertilized. Cell division is allowed to take place up to the pre-embryo stage. While this takes place, the female may be given progesterone to ensure that her uterus is ready for implantation. Two or more pre-embryos are transferred to the female's uterus.

Success rates of IVF are still rather low. The national average success rate of IVF is approximately 27% but some centers have higher pregnancy rates. Because most IVF procedures put more than one embryo into the uterus, the chance for a multiple birth (twins or more) is greatly increased.

GIFT involves retrieval of both multiple ova and semen, and the mechanical placement of both within the female's fallopian tubes, where fertilization may occur.

KEY TERMS

Blastocyst—A cluster of cells representing multiple cell divisions that have occurred in the fallopian tube after successful fertilization of an ovum by a sperm. This is the developmental form that must enter the uterus and implant to achieve pregnancy.

Cervix—The opening from the vagina leading into the uterus.

Embryo—The stage of development of a baby between the second and eighth weeks after conception.

Endometrium—The lining of the uterus.

Fallopian tube—The tube leading from the ovary into the uterus.

Ovary—The female organ in which eggs (ova) are stored and mature.

Ovum—The reproductive cell of the female that contains genetic information and participates in the act of fertilization. Also popularly called the egg.

Semen—The fluid that contains sperm, which is ejaculated by the male.

Sperm—The reproductive cell of the male that contains genetic information and participates in the act of fertilization of an ovum.

Spermatogenesis—The process by which sperm develop to become mature sperm, capable of fertilizing an ovum.

Zygote—The result of the sperm successfully fertilizing the ovum. The zygote is a single cell that contains the genetic material of both the mother and the father.

ZIFT involves the same retrieval of ova and semen, and fertilization and growth in the laboratory up to the zygote stage, at which point the zygotes are placed in the fallopian tubes. Both GIFT and ZIFT have higher success rates than IVF.

Expected results

In general, it is believed that about half of the couples who undergo a complete evaluation of infertility followed by treatment will ultimately have a successful pregnancy. About 5% of those couples who choose to not undergo evaluation or treatment will go on to conceive after a year or more.

Resources

BOOKS

Hornstein, Mark D., and Daniel Schust. "Infertility." In *Novak's Gynecology,* edited by Jonathan S. Berek. Baltimore: Williams and Wilkins, 1996.

Maleskey, Gale. "Infertility." *Nature's Medicines: from Asthma to Weight Gain, from Colds to High Cholesterol—the Most Powerful All-Natural Cures.* Emmaus, PA: Rodale Press, 1999.

Martin, Mary C. "Infertility" In *Current Obstetric and Gynecologic Diagnosis and Treatment,* edited by Alan H. Cecherney and Martin L. Pernoll. Norwalk, CT: Appleton & Lange, 1994.

Ying, Zhou Zhong, and Jin Hui De. "Common Diseases of Gynecology." In *Clinical Manual of Chinese Herbal Medicine and Acupuncture.* New York: Churchill Livingston, 1997.

PERIODICALS

Alfieri, Rosemarie Gionta. "Natural Options for Fertility." *Let's Live,* 67 (May 1999): 37+.

"Copper IUD Not the Cause of Tubal Occlusion." *Contemporary OB/GYN* 46, no. 12 (December 2001): 111.

"Low Sperm Count Linked to Organic Solvents." *Health and Medicine Week* (October 1, 2001).

"New Study Provides Insight into Male Infertility." *Gene Therapy Weekly* (December 13, 2001).

Rosenbaum, Joshua. "Beat the Clock: Treatments for Infertility." *American Health* (December 1995): 70+.

Trantham, Patricia. "The Infertile Couple." *American Family Physician* (September 1, 1996): 1001+.

Veal, Lowana. "Complementary Therapy and Infertility: an Icelandic Perspective." *Complementary Therapies in Nursing & Midwifery* 4 (1998): 3–6.

ORGANIZATIONS

American Society for Reproductive Medicine. 1209 Montgomery Highway, Birmingham, AL 35216-2809. (205) 978-5000. <http://www.asrm.com>.

International Center for Infertility Information Dissemination. <http://www.inciid.org>.

RESOLVE. 1310 Broadway, Somerville, MA 02144-1779. (617) 623-1156. <http://www. resolve.org>.

Belinda Rowland
Teresa Norris

Inflammatory bowel disease

Definition

Inflammatory bowel disease (IBD) is the general name for ulcerative colitis and Crohn's disease. The disease is characterized by swelling, ulcerations, and loss of function of the intestines.

Description

The primary problem in IBD is inflammation, as the name suggests. Inflammation is a process that often occurs to fight off foreign invaders in the body, including viruses, bacteria, and fungi. In response to such organisms, the body's immune system begins to produce a variety of cells and chemicals intended to stop the invasion. These immune cells and chemicals, however, also have direct effects on the body's tissues, resulting in heat, redness, swelling, and loss of function. No one knows what starts the cycle of inflammation in IBD, but the result is a swollen, boggy intestine.

In ulcerative colitis, the inflammation affects the lining of the rectum and large intestine. It is thought that the inflammation typically begins in the last segment of large intestine, which empties into the rectum (sigmoid colon). This inflammation may spread through the entire large intestine, but only rarely affects the very last section of the small intestine (ileum). The rest of the small intestine remains normal.

Crohn's disease is a form of IBD that affects both the small and large intestines. The inflammation of ulcerative colitis occurs only in the lining of the intestine (unlike Crohn's disease which affects all of the layers of the intestinal wall). As the inflammation continues, the tissue of the intestine begins to slough off, leaving pits (ulcerations) that often become infected.

IBD can occur in all age groups, with the most common age of diagnosis being 15–35 years of age. Men and women are affected equally. Whites are more frequently affected than other racial groups, and people of Jewish origin have three to six times greater likelihood of suffering from IBD. IBD is familial; an IBD patient has a 20% chance of having other relatives who are fellow sufferers.

Causes & symptoms

No specific cause of IBD has been identified. Although no organism (virus, bacteria, or fungi) has been found to set off the cycle of inflammation, some researchers continue to suspect that an organism is responsible. Other researchers are concentrating on identifying some change in the cells of the colon that would make the body's immune system accidentally begin treating those cells as foreign. Additional evidence for a disorder of the immune system includes the high number of other immune disorders that frequently accompany IBD. The condition has also been linked to physical, mental, and emotional **stress**.

The first symptoms of IBD are abdominal cramping and **pain**, a sensation of urgent need to have a bowel movement (defecate), and blood and pus in the stools.

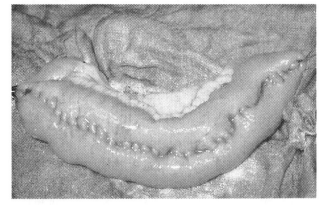

A specimen of a colon indicating ulcerative colitis. *(Photo Researchers, Inc. Reproduced by permission.)*

Some patients experience **diarrhea**, **fever**, and weight loss. If the diarrhea continues, signs of severe fluid loss (dehydration) begin to appear, including low blood pressure, fast heart rate, and **dizziness**.

Severe complications of IBD include perforation of the intestine, toxic dilation (enlargement) of the colon, and the development of colon **cancer**. Intestinal perforation occurs when long-standing inflammation and ulceration of the intestine weaken the wall to such an extent that a hole occurs. This is a life-threatening complication, because the contents of the intestine (which contain a large number of bacteria) spill into the abdomen. The presence of bacteria in the abdomen can result in a massive infection called peritonitis.

Toxic dilation of the colon is thought to occur because the intestinal inflammation interferes with the normal function of the muscles of the intestine. This allows the intestine to become lax, and its diameter begins to increase. The enlarged diameter thins the walls further, increasing the risk of perforation and peritonitis. When the diameter of the intestine is quite large and infection is present, the condition is referred to as "toxic megacolon."

Patients with IBD have a significant risk of developing colon cancer. This risk seems to begin around 10 years after diagnosis. The overall risk of developing cancer seems to be greatest for those patients with the largest extent of intestine involved. The risk becomes statistically greater every year:

• At 10 years, the risk of cancer is about 0.5–1%.

• At 15 years, the risk of cancer is about 12%.

• At 20 years, the risk of cancer is about 23%.

• At 24 years, the risk of cancer is about 42%.

Patients with IBD also have a high chance of experiencing other disorders, including inflammation of the joints (arthritis), inflammation of the vertebrae (spondylitis), ulcers in the mouth and on the skin, the development of painful, red bumps on the skin, inflammation of several areas of the eye, and various disorders of the liver and gallbladder.

Diagnosis

IBD is first suspected based on the symptoms that a patient is experiencing. Examination of the stool will usually reveal the presence of blood and pus (white blood cells). Blood tests may show an increase in the number of white blood cells, which is an indication of inflammation occurring somewhere in the body. The blood test may also reveal **anemia**, particularly when a great deal of blood has been lost in the stool.

The most important allopathic method of diagnosis is endoscopy, during which a doctor passes a flexible tube with a tiny fiberoptic camera device through the rectum and into the colon. The doctor can then examine the lining of the intestine for signs of inflammation and ulceration. A tiny sample (biopsy) of the intestine will be removed through the endoscope, which will be examined under a microscope for evidence of IBD. X-ray examination is helpful to determine the amount of affected intestine. However, x-ray examinations requiring the use of barium should be delayed until treatment has begun. Barium is a chalky solution that the patient drinks or is given through the rectum and into the intestine (enema). The presence of barium in the intestine allows more detail to be seen on x ray films.

Treatment

Treatment for IBD targets the underlying inflammation, as well as the problems occurring due to continued diarrhea and blood loss. The use of alternative medicines in the treatment of IBD is common. IBD sufferers have used a variety of treatments; however, few controlled studies of their effectiveness have been performed.

Chamomile tea is used to treat IBD. Chamomile is known to have anti-inflammatory, antispasmodic, and antibacterial properties. The patient should steep dried flowers for 10 to 15 minutes and drink three to four cups daily. Chamomile can cause allergic reactions in those who are allergic to other daisies. Other antispasmodics include **valerian**, wild yam, and **cramp bark**.

There is some preliminary evidence that alteration of the kinds of bacteria in the intestine prevents or controls colitis. Intestinal bacteria can be manipulated through use of **probiotics** or prebiotics. Probiotics refers to treatment with beneficial microbes either by ingestion or through a suppository. Prebiotics refers to dietary changes that favor the overgrowth of beneficial microbes. Preliminary animal and human studies have shown that *Lactobacilli* and related bacteria can control colitis and prolong remission. Ingestion of the nondigestable carbohydrates inulin or lactulose as prebiotics stimulates growth of these beneficial bacteria.

In a related treatment, preliminary evidence suggests that ingestion of parasitic worm eggs eases the symptoms of IBD. Within two to three weeks, five out of the six IBD patients who ingested the eggs went into complete remission which lasted one month. The tiny, harmless worms cannot reproduce in humans and are passed out within a few months.

Ingestion of enteric coated **fish oil** capsules may reduce the IBD relapse rate. A small study found that patients taking fish oil supplements had a lower relapse rate (59%) than those on placebo (90%).

Seventy-two percent of ulcerative colitis patients taking a Kui Jie Qing enema (alum, Halloysite, Calamine, *Indigo naturalis*, and plum-blossom tongue-pointing pills) daily were considered cured, as compared with 5% of those who were taking anti-inflammatory drugs. Fifty-three percent of ulcerative colitis patients taking Jian Pi Ling tablet and root of *Sophorae flavescentis* plus the flower of *sophora* enema were considered cured, as compared with 28% of those taking sulfasalazine and dexamethasone and 19% of those taking a placebo tablet and the enema. There are many other Chinese herbs that are useful in treating diarrhea and mucus in the bowel. Sometimes these are effective when drugs are not.

Forty-five percent of ulcerative colitis patients on an enzyme-potentiated hyposensitization protocol (B-glucuronidase enzyme and 1,3-cyclohexanediol with egg, milk, wheat, potato, and yeast) were improved, as compared with 6% of those on placebo.

Nutritionists often recommend changes in the diet for patients with inflammatory bowel disease. Food **allergies** and certain kinds of food are linked with the increased incidence of the disease. Eliminating diary and wheat products, common allergens, often alleviates symptoms. The incidence of Crohn's disease is increasing in areas where people consume a diet high in refined sugars and carbohydrates and saturated fats and low in dietary fiber. Elimination **diets** or those restricted in refined foods have sometimes proved successful in the alleviation of inflammatory bowel disease.

Dietary supplements are generally beneficial in the treatment of digestive disorders. Some typical recommendations include:

- vitamin C: 4000 mg daily
- vitamin B$_6$: 250 mg daily

- magnesium (aspartate): 400 mg daily
- vitamin E: 800 IU daily
- glutamine: 3000 mg daily, taken between meals
- garlic, deodorized: 2000 mg daily
- deglycyrrhizinated **licorice**: chew as needed.

Other treatments for IBD include **acupuncture**, macrobiotics, **cat's claw** (*Uncaria tomentosa*), **slippery elm**, **acupressure**, **biofeedback**, **relaxation** techniques, and **hypnotherapy**.

Allopathic treatment

Inflammation is often treated with an immune-suppressive drug called sulfasalazine. Because of poor absorption, sulfasalazine stays primarily within the intestine, where it is broken down into its two components: an antibiotic and an anti-inflammatory. It is believed to be primarily the anti-inflammatory component, salicylic acid, that is active in treating IBD. For patients who do not respond to sulfasalazine, steroid medications (such as prednisone) are the next choice.

Depending on the degree of blood loss, a patient with IBD may require blood transfusions and fluid replacement through a needle in the vein (intravenous or IV). Medications that can slow diarrhea must be used with great care, because they may actually cause the development of toxic megacolon.

A patient with toxic megacolon requires close monitoring and care in the hospital. He or she will usually be given steroid medications through an IV, and may be put on antibiotics. If these measures do not improve the situation, the patient will have to undergo surgery to remove the colon. This is done because the risk of death after perforation of toxic megacolon is greater than 50%.

A patient with proven cancer of the colon, or even a patient who shows certain precancerous signs, will need a colectomy (colon removal). When a colectomy is performed, a piece of the small intestine (ileum) is pulled through an opening in the abdomen and fashioned surgically to allow attachment of a special bag to catch the body's waste (feces). This opening, which will remain for the duration of the patient's life, is called an ileostomy.

Expected results

Remission refers to a disease becoming inactive for a period of time. The rate of remission of IBD (after a first attack) is nearly 90%. Those individuals whose colitis is confined primarily to the left side of the large intestine have the best prognosis. Those individuals with extensive colitis, involving most or all of the large intes-

---

KEY TERMS

Endoscopy—A medical examination in which an instrument called an endoscope is passed into an area of the body (the bladder or intestine, for example). The endoscope usually has a fiber-optic camera, which allows a greatly magnified image to be projected onto a video screen, to be viewed by the operator.

Immune system—The system of the body that is responsible for producing various cells and chemicals that fight off infection by viruses, bacteria, fungi, and other foreign bodies. In autoimmune disease, these cells and chemicals are turned against the body itself.

Inflammation—The result of the body's attempts to fight off and wall off an area that is infected. Inflammation results in the classic signs of redness, heat, swelling, and loss of function.

---

tine, have a much poorer prognosis. Recent studies show that about 10% of these patients have died within 10 years after diagnosis. About 20–25% of all IBD patients will require colectomy. Unlike the case for patients with Crohn's disease, however, such radical surgery results in a cure of the disease.

Resources

BOOKS

Glickman, Robert. "Inflammatory Bowel Disease: Ulcerative Colitis and Crohn's Disease." In *Harrison's Principles of Internal Medicine,* edited by Anthony S. Fauci, et al. New York: McGraw-Hill, 1998.

Long, James W. *The Essential Guide to Chronic Illness.* New York: HarperPerennial, 1997.

Saibil, Fred. *Crohn's Disease and Ulcerative Colitis.* Buffalo, NY: Firefly Books, 1997.

PERIODICALS

"Alternative Therapies Commonly Used by Patients with Inflammatory Bowel Disease." *Nutrition Research Newsletter* 18 (June 1999):13+.

Campieri, Massimo and Paolo Gionchetti. "Probiotics in Inflammatory Bowel Disease: New Insight to Pathogenesis or a Possible Therapeutic Alternative?" *Gastroenterology* 116 (1999):1246-1249.

Coghlan, Andy. "Wonderful Worms." *New Scientist* 163 (August 7, 1999):4.

Hilsden, Robert J. and Marja J. Verhoef. "Complementary and Alternative Medicine: Evaluating its Effectiveness in Inflammatory Bowel Disease." *Inflammatory Bowel Diseases* 4 (1998):318-323.

Martin, Frances L. "Ulcerative Colitis." *American Journal of Nursing* 97 (August 1997): 38+.

Peppercorn, Mark A., and Susannah K. Gordon. "Making Sense of a Mystery Ailment: Inflammatory Bowel Disease." *Harvard Health Letter* 22 (December 1996): 4+.

"Ulcerative Colitis: Manageable, With a Brighter Outlook." *Mayo Clinic Health Letter* 13 (December 1995): 1+.

ORGANIZATIONS

Crohn's and Colitis Foundation of America, Inc. 386 Park Avenue South, 17th Floor, New York, NY 10016-8804. (800) 932-2423.

Belinda Rowland

Influenza

Definition

Usually referred to as the flu or grippe, influenza is a highly infectious respiratory disease. Its name comes from the Italian word for "influence," because people in eighteenth-century Europe thought that the disease was caused by the influence of bad weather. We now know that flu is caused by a virus. When the influenza virus is inhaled, it attacks cells in the upper respiratory tract, causing such typical flu symptoms as **fatigue**, **fever** and **chills**, a hacking **cough**, and body aches. Although the stomach or intestinal "flu" is commonly blamed for stomach upsets and **diarrhea**, the influenza virus affects humans less often than is commonly believed.

Description

Influenza is considerably more debilitating than the **common cold**. Influenza outbreaks occur suddenly, and infection spreads rapidly. The annual death toll attributable to influenza and its complications averages 20,000 in the United States alone. In the 1918-1919 Spanish flu pandemic, the death toll reached a staggering 20–40 million worldwide. Approximately 500,000 of these fatalities occurred in North America.

Influenza outbreaks occur on a regular basis. The most serious outbreaks are pandemics, which affect millions of people worldwide and last for several months. The 1918-19 influenza outbreak serves as the primary example of an influenza pandemic. Pandemics also occurred in 1957 and 1968 with the Asian flu and Hong Kong flu, respectively.

Epidemics are widespread regional outbreaks that occur every two to three years and affect 5–10% of the population. A regional epidemic is shorter lived than a pandemic, lasting only several weeks. Finally, there are smaller outbreaks each winter that are confined to specific locales.

There are three types of influenza viruses, identified as A, B, and C. Influenza A can infect a range of animal species, including humans, pigs, horses, and birds, but only humans are infected by types B and C. Influenza A is responsible for most flu cases, while infection with types B and C virus are less common and cause a milder illness.

In the United States, 90% of all deaths from influenza occur among persons older than 65. Flu-related deaths have increased substantially in the United States since the 1970s, largely because of the **aging** of the American population. In addition, elderly persons are vulnerable because they are often reluctant to be vaccinated against flu.

A new concern regarding influenza is the possibility that hostile groups or governments could use the virus as an agent of bioterrorism. A report published in early 2003 noted that Type A influenza virus has a high potential for use as such an agent because of the virulence of the Type A strain that broke out in Hong Kong in 1997 and the development of laboratory methods for generating large quantities of the virus. The report recommended the stockpiling of present antiviral drugs and speeding up the development of new ones.

Causes & symptoms

Approximately one to four days after infection with the influenza virus, the victim develops an array of symptoms. Symptoms are usually sudden, although the sequence can be quite variable. They include the onset of **headache**, **sore throat**, dry cough, and chills, nasal congestion, fatigue, malaise, overall achiness and a fever that may run as high as 104°F (40°C). Flu victims feel extremely tired and weak, and may not return to their normal energy levels for several days or weeks.

Influenza complications usually arise from bacterial **infections** of the lower respiratory tract. Signs of a secondary respiratory infection often appear just as the patient seems to be recovering. These signs include high fever, intense chills, chest pains associated with breathing, and a productive cough or sinus discharge with thick yellowish-green sputum. If these symptoms appear, medical treatment is often necessary. Other secondary infections, such as sinus or ear infections, may also require medical intervention. Heart and lung problems and other chronic diseases, can be aggravated by influenza, which is a particular concern with elderly patients.

With children and teenagers, it is advisable to be alert for symptoms of Reye's syndrome, a rare but serious complication that occurs when children are given aspirin. Symptoms of Reye's syndrome are **nausea** and **vomiting**,

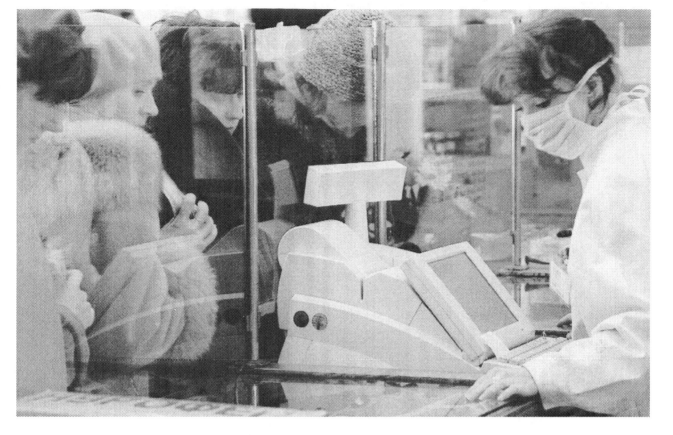

A pharmacy worker in Russia wears a mask to protect herself from a flu epidemic in 1999. *(A/P Wide World Photos. Reproduced by permission.)*

and more seriously, such neurological problems as confusion or delirium. The syndrome is primarily associated with the use of aspirin to relieve flu symptoms in children.

Diagnosis

Although there are specific laboratory tests to identify the flu virus strain from respiratory samples, doctors typically rely on a set of symptoms and the presence of influenza in the community for diagnosis. Specific tests are useful to determine the type of flu in the community, but they do little for individual treatment. Doctors may administer such tests as throat or sinus cultures or blood tests to identify secondary infections.

Since 1999, however, seven rapid diagnostic tests for flu have become commercially available. These tests appear to be especially useful in diagnosing flu in children, allowing doctors to make more accurate treatment decisions in less time.

Treatment

The patient should drink plenty of fluids and eat nutritious foods. Chicken soup with **ginger**, scallions, and rice noodles is nutritious and has healing powers. Rest, to allow the body to fight infection, is very important. Gargling with salt **water** (half teaspoon salt in one cup of water) helps to soothe a sore throat. A vaporizer with **eucalyptus** or Vicks VapoRub will make the patient feel more comfortable by easing breathing and aiding sleep. Applying Vicks ointment over chest and back will assist and speed recovery. Returning to normal activities too quickly invites a possible relapse or complications.

Herbals

Herbal teas and other preparations can be taken to stimulate the immune system, for antiviral activity, and to relieve symptoms. The following herbs are used to treat influenza:

- Ginger (*Zingiber officinalis*) reduces fever and **pain**, has a sedative effect, settles the stomach, and suppresses cough.

- Forsythia (*Forsythia suspensa*) fruit can be taken as a tea for its anti-inflammatory, fever-reducing, and antimicrobial properties.

- **Honeysuckle** (*Lonicera japonica*) flower can be taken as a tea for its anti-inflammatory, fever-reducing, and antimicrobial properties.

- Anise seed (*Pimpinella anisum*) can be added to tea to expel phlegm, induce sweating, ease nausea, and ease stomach gas.

- Slippery elm (*Ulmus rubra*) can be taken as a tea or slurry to soothe sore throat and ease cough.

- Echinacea (*Echinacea purpurea* or *angustifolia*), in clinical studies, reduced flu symptoms including sore throat, chills, sweating, fatigue, weakness, body aches, and headaches. The usual dosage is 500 mg thrice on the first day, then 250 mg four times daily thereafter.

- **Goldenseal** (*Hydrastis canadensis*) has fever reducing, antibacterial, anti-inflammatory, and antitussive properties. The usual dose is 125 mg three to four times daily. Goldenseal shouldn't be taken for more than one week.

- Astragalus (*Astragalus membranaceus*) boosts the immune system and improves the body's response to **stress**. The common dose is 250 mg of extract four times daily.

- Cordyceps (*Cordyceps sinensis*) modulates and boosts the immune system and improves respiration. The usual dose is 500 mg two to three times daily.

- Elder (*Sambucus nigra*) has antiviral activity, increases sweating, decreases inflammation, and decreases nasal discharge. In a study, elderberry extract reduced flu symptoms within two days whereas placebo took six days. The usual dose is 500 mg of extract thrice daily. Also use 2 tsp of dried flowers in 1 cup of water as a tea.

- Schisandra (*Schisandra chinensis*) helps the body fight disease and increases endurance.

- Grape (*Vitis vinifera*) seed extract has antihistamine and anti-inflammatory properties. The usual dose is 50 mg three times daily.

- Eucalyptus (*Eucalyptus globulus*) or **peppermint** (*Mentha piperita*) **essential oils** added to a steam vaporizer may help clear chest and nasal congestion.

- Boneset infusion (*Eupatorium perfoliatum*) relieves aches and fever.

- **Yarrow** (*Achillea millefolium*) relieves chills.

Other remedies

Acupuncture and **acupressure** are said to stimulate natural resistance, relieve nasal congestion and headaches, fight fever, and calm coughs, depending on the points used.

A homeopathic remedy called *Oscillococcinum* may be taken at the first sign of flu symptoms and repeated for a day or two. This remedy is said to shorten the duration of flu by one or two days. Although oscillococcinum is a popular flu remedy in Europe, however, a research study published in 2003 found it to be ineffective.

Other homeopathic remedies recommended vary according to the specific flu symptoms present. *Gelsemium* (*Gelsemium sempervirens*) is recommended to combat weakness accompanied by chills, a headache, and nasal congestion. *Bryonia* (*Bryonia alba*) may be used to treat muscle aches, headaches, and a dry cough. For restlessness, chills, hoarseness, and achy joints, poison ivy (*Rhus toxicodendron*) is recommended. Finally, for achiness and a dry cough or chills, *Eupatorium perfoliatum* is suggested.

Hydrotherapy can be utilized. A bath to induce a fever will speed recovery from the flu. While supervised, the patient should take a bath as hot as he/she can tolerate and remain in the bath for 20–30 minutes. While in the bath, the patient drinks a cup of yarrow or elderflower tea to induce sweating. During the bath, a cold cloth is held on the forehead or at the nape of the neck to keep the temperature down. The patient is assisted when getting out of the bath (he/she may feel weak or dizzy) and then gets into bed and covers up with layers of blankets to induce more sweating.

Supplemental vitamins are recommended for treating influenza, and include 500–2000 mg **vitamin C**, 400 IU to 500 IU of **vitamin E**, 200 micrograms to 300 micrograms **selenium**, and 25,000 IU beta-carotene. **Zinc** lozenges are helpful, as is supplemental zinc at 25 mg per day for two weeks or more.

Traditional Chinese medicine (TCM) uses mixtures of herbs to prevent flu as well as to relieve symptoms once a person has fallen ill. There are several different recipes for these remedies, but most contain ginger and Japanese honeysuckle in addition to other ingredients.

Allopathic treatment

Because influenza is a viral infection, antibiotics are useless in treating it. However, antibiotics are frequently used to treat secondary infections.

Over-the-counter medications are used to treat flu symptoms. Any medication that is designed to relieve such symptoms as pain and coughing will provide some relief. The best medicine for symptoms is an analgesic, such as aspirin, acetaminophen, or naproxen. Without a doctor's approval, aspirin is generally not recommended for people under 18 owing to its association with Reye's syndrome, a rare aspirin-associated complication seen in children recovering from viral infections. Children should receive acetaminophen or ibuprofen to treat their symptoms.

There are four antiviral drugs marketed for treating influenza as of 2003. To be effective, treatment should begin no later than two days after symptoms appear. Antivirals may be useful in treating patients who have weakened immune systems or who are at risk for developing serious complications. They include amantadine (Symmetrel, Symadine) and rimantadine (Flumandine), which work against Type A influenza; and zanamavir (Relenza) and oseltamavir phosphate (Tamiflu), which work against both Types A and B influenza. Amantadine and rimantadine can cause such side effects as nervousness, **anxiety**, lightheadedness, and nausea. Severe side effects include seizures, delirium, and hallucination, but are rare and are nearly always limited to people who have kidney problems, seizure disorders, or psychiatric disorders. The new drugs zanamavir and oseltamavir phosphate have few side effects but can cause **dizziness**, jitters, and **insomnia**.

Expected results

Following proper treatment guidelines, healthy people under the age of 65 usually suffer no long-term consequences associated with flu infection. The elderly and the chronically ill are at greater risk for secondary infection and other complications, but they can also enjoy a complete recovery.

Most people recover fully from an influenza infection, but it should not be viewed complacently. Influenza is a serious disease, and approximately 1 in 1,000 cases proves fatal.

Prevention

The Centers for Disease Control and Prevention recommend that people get an influenza vaccine injection each year before flu season starts. In the United States, flu season typically runs from late December to early March. Vaccines should be received two to six weeks prior to the onset of flu season to allow the body enough time to establish immunity.

Each season's flu vaccine contains three virus strains that are the most likely to be encountered in the coming flu season. The virus strains used to make the vaccine are inactivated and will not cause illness. When there is a good match between the anticipated flu strains and the strains used in the vaccine, the vaccine is 70-90% effective in people under 65. Because immune response diminishes somewhat with age, people over 65 may not receive the same level of protection from the vaccine, but even if they do contract the flu, the vaccine diminishes the severity and helps prevent complications.

It should be noted that certain people should not receive an influenza vaccine. Infants six months and younger have immature immune systems and will not benefit from the vaccine. Because the vaccines are prepared using hen eggs, people who have severe **allergies** to eggs or other vaccine components should not receive the influenza vaccine. Some persons may receive a course of amantadine or rimantadine, which are 70-90% effective in preventing influenza.

Certain groups are strongly advised to be vaccinated because they are at greater risk for influenza-related complications:

• All people 65 years and older.

• Residents of nursing homes and chronic-care facilities.

• Adults and children who have chronic heart or lung problems.

• Adults and children who have chronic metabolic diseases, such as diabetes and renal dysfunction, as well as severe **anemia** or inherited hemoglobin disorders.

• Children and teenagers who are on long-term aspirin therapy.

• Anyone who is immunocompromised, including HIV-infected persons, **cancer** patients, organ transplant recipients, and patients receiving steroids, chemotherapy, or radiation therapy.

• Anyone in contact with the above groups, such as teachers, care givers, health-care personnel, and family members.

• Travelers to foreign countries.

As of early 2003, researchers are working on developing an intranasal flu vaccine in aerosol form. An aerosol vaccine using a weakened form of Type A influenza virus has been tested in pilot studies and awaits further clinical trials.

The following dietary supplements may be taken to help prevent influenza:

• Elderberry prevents influenza virus from infecting cells.

• Astragalus: 250–500 mg daily.

• Multivitamins with zinc.

• Vitamin C; 500 mg.

• Echinacea; at the first sign of malaise or infection, take 3–5 ml of tincture or 2 tablets three or four times daily for three to 10 days.

Resources

BOOKS

Pelletier, Kenneth R., MD. *The Best Alternative Medicine*, Part II, "CAM Therapies for Specific Conditions: Colds/Flu." New York: Simon & Schuster, 2002.

"Respiratory Viral Diseases: Influenza." Section 13, Chapter 162 in *The Merck Manual of Diagnosis and Therapy*, edited by Mark H. Beers, MD, and Robert Berkow, MD. Whitehouse Station, NJ: Merck Research Laboratories, 1999.

PERIODICALS

Elkins, Rita. "Combat Colds and Flu." *Let's Live.* 68 (January 2000): 81+.

Jonas, W. B., T. J. Kaptchuk, and K. Linde. "A Critical Overview of Homeopathy." *Annals of Internal Medicine* 138 (March 4, 2003): 393–399.

Krug, R. M. "The Potential Use of Influenza Virus as an Agent for Bioterrorism." *Antiviral Research* 57 (January 2003): 147–150.

La Valle, James B., and Ernie Hawkins. "Colds and Flu: A Natural Approach." *Drug Store News.* 20 (12/14/98): CP17+.

Oxford, J. S., S. Bossuyt, S. Balasingam, et al. "Treatment of Epidemic and Pandemic Influenza with Neuraminidase and M2 Proton Channel Inhibitors." *Clinical Microbiology and Infection* 9 (January 2003): 1–14.

Roth, Y., J. S. Chapnik, and P. Cole. "Feasibility of Aerosol Vaccination in Humans." *Annals of Otology, Rhinology, and Laryngology* 112 (March 2003): 264–270.

Shortridge, K. F., J. S. Peiris, and Y. Guan. "The Next Influenza Pandemic: Lessons from Hong Kong." *Journal of Applied Microbiology* 94 (2003 Supplement): 70S–79S.

Storch, G. A. "Rapid Diagnostic Tests for Influenza." *Current Opinion in Pediatrics* 15 (February 2003): 77–84.

Thompson, W. W., D. K. Shay, E. Weintraub, et al. "Mortality Associated with Influenza and Respiratory Syncytial Virus in the United States." *Journal of the American Medical Association* 289 (January 8, 2003): 179–186.

ORGANIZATIONS

Centers for Disease Control and Prevention. 1600 Clifton Road, NE, Atlanta, Georgia 30333. (888) CDC-FACTS (888-232-3228). <http://www.cdc.gov/>.

National Institute of Allergy and Infectious Diseases (NIAID). 31 Center Drive, MSC 2520, Bethesda, MD 20892-2520. <http://www.niaid.nih.gov>.

OTHER

NIAID Fact Sheet: Flu. Bethesda, MD: NIAID, January 2003. <http://www.niaid.nih.gov/factsheets/flu.htm>.

Belinda Rowland
Rebecca J. Frey, PhD

Ingrown nail

Definition

Ingrown nail refers to the condition in which the edge of a nail cuts into the adjacent skin fold, causing **pain**, redness, and swelling.

Description

Ingrown nail (onychocryptosis) occurs when the nail plate (the horny covering) grows into and cuts the skin alongside the nail (lateral nail fold). Ingrown toenails make up 3–5% of all foot problems. Most cases of ingrown nail occur in men between the ages of 10–30 years. In this age group, males are affected twice as often as females. In older adults, the incidence is equal. There are three major types of ingrown nail: subcutaneous ingrown nail, in which the nail grows under the skin; overcurvature of the nail plate; and hypertrophy (overgrowth) of the lateral nail fold.

Ingrown nails occur most often on the big toe. Penetration of the nail into the skin causes inflammation (swelling and redness). Infection by bacteria or fungi may follow. Severe infection may lead to **abscess** formation, characterized by an oozing pus-filled blister. Small translucent red bumps called granulation tissue may develop along the lateral nail fold.

Causes & symptoms

Ingrown nails are most commonly caused by incorrect cutting of the nails and wearing poorly-fitting shoes. Other causes of ingrown nail include:

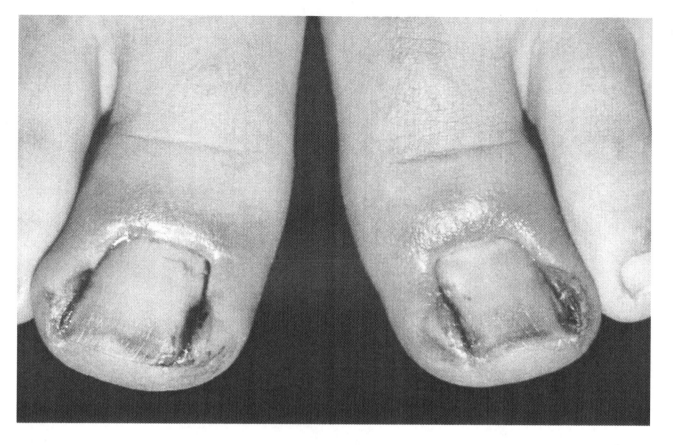

Ingrown toenails. *(Custom Medical Stock Photo. Reproduced by permission.)*

- abnormally long toes

- overcurvature of the nail

- excessive sweating

- shoes that put pressure on the toes (pointed-toe, high-heeled)

- poor foot hygiene

- high lateral nail folds

- discrepancy between the widths of the nail and nail bed

- improper alignment of the large toenail

- repeated trauma to the large toe

Persons who are at increased risk of developing ingrown nails include people with arthritis, immune system deficiencies, neoplasms (tumors), **obesity**, and circulatory disorders.

The symptoms of ingrown nail include swelling, redness, and pain in the lateral nail fold. Increased swelling, pus drainage, and ulceration (tissue destruction) can occur as the condition progresses. Advanced onychocryptosis is characterized by long-term swelling, the formation of granulation tissue, and lateral fold overgrowth.

Diagnosis

Ingrown nail is easily diagnosed in a physical examination done by a family physician, a podiatrist (foot specialist), or a dermatologist (skin specialist).

Treatment

Because of the possibility of serious complications, a physician should be consulted for treatment of severe and/or infected ingrown nails. Alternative treatments for treating ingrown nail include:

- Ayurveda. Ayurvedic principles state that persons whose constitutions are dominated by vata and kapha have stronger nails and are prone to ingrown nails. Ingrown nails are treated with warm water soaks followed by application of a solution of equal parts tea tree and **neem** oils under the nails.

- Herbal therapy. When an ingrown nail is forming, the toe should be soaked for 15–30 minutes in five drops each of hypericum and **calendula** tinctures diluted in 1/2 pint of warm water. Afterward, the toe should be wrapped in linen, placing it between the fold and the nail.

- Homeopathy. Preparations of *Hepar sulph.* or *Silica* in 6c potency may be taken every 12 hours for two weeks, to reduce the inflammation around the nail.

- Hydrotherapy. To treat ingrown nail, the patient should soak the foot in hot, soapy water for 20 minutes, trim the nail square, wrap the toe in a hot compress, and cover it with a dry cloth overnight. In the morning, the patient should trim the nail into a U shape and place a bit of cotton between the nail and the fold. The cotton should be kept in place until the nail grows out.

- Massage. If an ingrown nail is developing, the patient should gently push the skin away from the nail. Repeated massage of the overgrown lateral nail folds can reduce pain and separate the fold away from the nail.

Allopathic treatment

Nonsurgical

Nonsurgical methods of treating ingrown nails focus on eliminating infection with medications and separating the ingrown nail from the lateral nail fold. Whenever possible, the offending nail is clipped, and the patient is instructed to soak the foot in water containing Epsom salts and povidone-iodine thrice daily. Procedures used to separate the nail from the fold include inserting a piece of fabric (moistened with antiseptics), plastic, or metal between the nail and the fold until the nail grows out. Cryotherapy, in which the affected nail fold is frozen with liquid nitrogen, is also used. Cauterization (destruction of tissue using heat) may be performed to eliminate granulation tissue. A metal brace may be worn on the toe for several months to flatten overcurvature.

Surgical

In cases of severe ingrown nail or ineffective nonsurgical treatment, part or all of the nail is surgically removed. Most commonly, only a portion of the nail is removed. Ingrown nail recurs in 60%–80% of the patients. If nail regrowth is expected to cause a recurrence of ingrown nail, then the nail matrix (where nail growth occurs) is destroyed, which prevents nail regrowth. In most cases, only local anesthesia is needed for surgical treatment.

Expected results

Although natural remedies can be effective in healing minor ingrown nails, prevention is the best solution. Many cases of ingrown nail require surgical treatment.

Complications of ingrown toenail include infection, osteomyelitis (infection of the bone), and **gangrene** (tissue death). The elderly are at increased risk of complications because of decreased sensation resulting from such

---

KEY TERMS

Granulation tissue—Small red bumpy velvety-looking tissue produced during the healing of wounds.

Lateral nail fold—The fold of skin along the side of the nail.

Nail plate—The horny plate covering the tips of the fingers and toes. Commonly called the nail.

Onychocryptosis—The medical term for ingrown nail.

---

conditions as diabetes, **heart disease**, or arteriosclerosis (hardening of the arteries).

Prevention

Ingrown nails may be prevented by:

- clipping nails straight across
- leaving the nail edge slightly longer than the end of the toe
- not trimming the sides of nails
- wearing shoes with ample toe space
- not pulling or tearing at the toenails

Resources

BOOKS

Nails: Therapy, Diagnosis, Surgery, edited by Richard K. Scher et al. Philadelphia: W. B. Saunders Company, 1997.

PERIODICALS

Ikard, Robert W. "Onychocryptosis." *Journal of the American College of Surgeons,* 187 (July 1998): 96-102.

Belinda Rowland

Insect bites *see* **Bites and stings**

Insomnia

Definition

Insomnia is the inability to obtain an adequate amount or quality of sleep. The difficulty can be in falling asleep, remaining asleep, or both. People with insomnia do not feel refreshed when they wake up. Insomnia is a common symptom affecting millions of people

---

that may be caused by many conditions, diseases, or circumstances.

According to a 1999 American Medical Association (AMA) report, approximately 30% of adults in the United States suffer occasionally from insomnia and 10% experience chronic insomnia.

Description

Sleep is essential for mental and physical restoration. It is a cycle with two separate states: rapid eye movement (REM), the stage in which most dreaming occurs; and non-REM (NREM). Four stages of sleep take place during NREM: stage I, when the person passes from relaxed wakefulness; stage II, an early stage of light sleep; stages III and IV, which are increasing degrees of deep sleep. Most stage IV sleep (also called delta sleep), occurs in the first several hours of sleep. A period of REM sleep normally follows a period of NREM sleep.

Sleeplessness or insomnia is a symptom and may be caused by "stress, **anxiety**, **depression**, disease, **pain**, medications, sleep disorders, poor sleep habits .. [and] sleep environment and health habits," according to the National Sleep Foundation (NSF).

Women are 1.3 times more likely to report insomnia than men, according to the NSF. Women may experience sleeplessness before and at the onset of the menstrual cycle, during **pregnancy**, and **menopause**. The foundation reported that people over the age of 65 are "more likely to complain of insomnia than younger people." Furthermore, people who are divorced, widowed, or separated are more likely to have the problem than those who are married. In addition, insomnia is more frequently reported by those with lower socioeconomic status.

Insomnia is classified both by its nightly symptoms and its duration. Sleep-onset insomnia refers to difficulty falling asleep. Maintenance insomnia refers to waking frequently during the night or waking early. Insomnia is also classified in relation to the number of sleepless nights. Short-term or transient insomnia is a common occurrence and usually lasts only a few days. Long-term or chronic insomnia lasts more than three weeks and increases the risk for injuries in the home, at the workplace, and while driving because of daytime sleepiness and decreased concentration. Chronic insomnia can also lead to mood disorders like depression.

Insomnia comes with a high price tag for the nation. NSF in 1999 reported that an estimated $14 billion was spent in one year on such direct costs as insomnia treatment, healthcare services, and hospital and nursing home care. Annual indirect costs like work loss, property damage from accidents, and transportation to and from health care providers were estimated at close to $28 billion. Furthermore, insomnia accounted for $18 billion in lost productivity, according to a 1997 National Sleep Foundation survey.

Causes & symptoms

Transient insomnia is often caused by a temporary situation in a person's life, such as an argument with a loved one, a brief medical illness, or **jet lag**. When the situation is resolved or the precipitating factor disappears, the condition goes away, usually without medical treatment.

Such prescription drugs as **asthma** medicine, steroids, and anti-depressants can cause insomnia. Sleeplessness may also be a side effect of over-the-counter products like nasal decongestants and appetite suppressants.

Chronic insomnia usually has different causes, and there may be more than one. These include:

• A medical condition or its treatment, including sleep apnea, arthritis, a heart condition, and asthma.

• Use of such substances as **caffeine**, alcohol, and nicotine.

• Psychiatric conditions like mood or anxiety disorders.

• **Stress** or depression, such as sadness caused by the loss of a loved one or a job.

• Disturbed sleep cycles caused by a change in work shift.

• Sleep-disordered breathing, such as snoring.

• Periodic jerky leg movements, *nocturnal myoclonus,*which happen just as the individual is falling asleep.

• Repeated nightmares or panic attacks during sleep.

Another cause is excessive worrying about whether or not a person will be able to fall asleep, which creates so much anxiety that the individual's bedtime rituals and behavior actually trigger insomnia. This is called psychophysiological insomnia.

Symptoms of insomnia

People who have insomnia do not start the day refreshed from a good night's sleep. They are tired. They may have difficulty falling asleep, and commonly lie in bed tossing and turning for hours. Or the individual may go to sleep without a problem but wakes in the early hours of the morning and is either unable to go back to sleep, or drifts into a restless, unsatisfying sleep. This is a common symptom in the elderly and those suffering from depression. Sometimes sleep patterns are reversed and the individual has difficulty staying awake during the day and takes frequent naps. The sleep at night is fitful and frequently interrupted.

Diagnosis

Insomnia, unlike some medical conditions, is easily recognizable. People know when they aren't getting enough sleep. The key to treating insomnia is determining its causes. Some people can identify sleep-inhibiting factors such as a death in the family or a hectic work schedule with too much caffeine consumption and not enough **exercise**. A doctor will take factors such as these into account when making a diagnosis.

The physician's diagnosis is based on the patient's reported signs and symptoms. The doctor may review a patient's health history or order tests to determine if a medical condition is causing the insomnia. The physician may ask if the patient is depressed, in pain, under stress, or taking medications, according to the National Sleep Foundation. The doctor may ask about disruptions in a patient's life such as working nontraditional shifts or traveling across different time zones.

It can be useful for the patient to keep a daily record for two weeks of sleep patterns, food intake, use of alcohol, caffeine, nicotine, medications, exercise, and any other information recommended by the physician. If the patient has a bed partner, information can be obtained about whether the patient snores or is restless during sleep. This record, together with a medical history and physical examination, can help confirm the doctor's assessment.

A wide variety of healthcare professionals can recognize and treat insomnia, but when a patient with chronic insomnia does not respond to treatment, or the condition is not adequately explained by the patient's physical, emotional, or mental circumstances, then more extensive testing by a specialist in sleep disorders may be warranted.

Treatment

In both alternative and conventional medicine, treatment of insomnia includes alleviating or coping with any physical and emotional problems that contribute to the condition. Also effective is exploration of changes in lifestyle that will improve the situation.

Changes in behavior

Patients can make changes in their daily routine that are simple and effective in treating insomnia. Eating a healthy diet rich in calcium, **magnesium**, and the B vitamins is also beneficial. A high protein snack like yogurt before going to bed is recommended.

Patients should go to bed only when sleepy and use the bedroom only for sleep. Activities like reading, watching television, or snacking should take place elsewhere. If people are unable to go to sleep, they should go into another room and do something like reading. People should return to bed only when sleepy. Patients should set the alarm and get up every morning at the same time, no matter how much they have slept, to establish a regular sleepwake pattern. Naps during the day should be avoided, but if absolutely necessary, than a 30-minute nap early in the afternoon may not interfere with sleep at night.

Another successful technique is called sleep-restriction therapy, restricting the time in bed to the actual time spent sleeping. This approach allows a slight sleep debt to build up, which increases the individual's ability to fall asleep and stay asleep. If a patient sleeps five hours a night, the time in bed is limited to 5–5.5 hours. The time in bed is gradually increased in small segments, with the individual rising at the same time each morning; at least 85% of the time in bed must be spent sleeping.

Mind and body relaxation

Incorporating **relaxation** techniques into bedtime rituals helps a person go to sleep faster and improves the quality of sleep. These, alone or in combination with other relaxation techniques, can safely promote sleepiness. Also effective are massage techniques such as the "cat stroke." The masseuse's hands move gently across the back. Four other types of stress-reducing bodywork were recommended in *Spontaneous Healing*, the book by **Andrew Weil**, M.D., who practices natural and preventative medicine. Weil recommended Feldenkrais, which includes movements, floor exercises, and body work; **Rolfing**, which involves firm pressure; shiatsu, the traditional Japanese form of body work; and Trager work.

Learning to substitute pleasant thoughts for unpleasant ones (imagery training) helps reduce worrying. Another technique is using audiotapes that combine the sounds of nature with soft relaxing music. Meditation, prayer, and breathing exercises can also be effective.

Many alternative treatments are effective in treating both the symptom of insomnia and its underlying causes. Much treatment is centered around herbal remedies. The herbs most often recommended for treating insomnia include **reishi mushroom**, **hops**, **valerian**, **skullcap**, passion flower, **lemon balm**, ginseng, St. John's wort, and kava, which is also known as **kava kava**. Herbs are "generally safe," but they have not been tested or classified in the United States by the U.S. Food and Drug Administration (FDA).

Herbal teas

Some people treat insomnia by sipping a warm cup of tea made with an herb such as **chamomile**, hops, passionflower, or St. John's wort.

Aromatherapy and hydrotherapy

Aromatherapy involves healing through **essential oils**, the aromatic extracts of plants. Essential oils may be used for a soothing bath; applied to the face, neck, shoulders, and pillow; or diffused in air.

Hydrotherapy consists of a warm bath, scented with an essence such as rose, **lavender**, marjoram, or chamomile. In the 1998 book *Healing Anxiety with Herbs* , Harold Bloomfield, M.D., recommended adding 2-15 drops of 10% essential oils into approximately 100°F (38° C) **water**. He also recommended using lavender and also suggested using ylang-ylang, neroli (orange blossom), geranium, and patchouli. The bath should be "approached in an unhurried and meditative state," Bloomfield wrote.

Dream pillows

Another form of aromatherapy involves sleeping on a dream pillow. Also known as a sleep pillow, it can be made by sewing together two 8-inch pieces of fabric. There should be an opening wide enough to insert a tablespoon. Herbs such as hops, chamomile, and lavender are spooned into the dream pillow, which is placed under the bed pillow.

Melatonin

Melatonin is a natural hormone that is secreted from the brain's pineal gland. The gland regulates a person's biological clock, particularly day and night cycles. When taken as a 3-mg dose one to two hours before bed for a maximum of four to five days per week, the dietary supplement melatonin is said to be effective in shortening the time before one falls asleep. The hormone can help to avoid jet lag and to establish sleep patterns for shift workers. However, melatonin is not regulated by the FDA, so there are no regulatory controls. Side effects may include mental impairment, drowsiness, severe headaches, and nightmares.

Traditional Chinese medicine

Traditional Chinese medicine (TCM) treatments for insomnia include **acupuncture** and herbal remedies. Acupuncture involves the insertion of needles to manipulate energy flows around the body. Acupuncture is also applied to the treatment of conditions including anxiety.

In TCM, herbs are used as remedies in teas and other preparations. Treatments for insomnia include reishi, a medicinal mushroom available in extract form.

Light therapy

In **light therapy**, natural or artificial light is used to boost serotonin, a neurotransmitter in the brain related to reducing anxiety. This therapy is used to treat seasonal affective disorder, a condition that some people experience when there is less sunlight or fewer daylight hours. Bright light therapy can be used for people whose insomnia is caused by jet lag or irregular work shifts. In the morning, the person is exposed to artificial lamps with a brightness of more than 2,000 lux. The treatment continues with avoidance of bright light during the evening.

Allopathic treatment

A physician may determine that drug therapy is necessary to treat insomnia. Drugs may be prescribed if the patient is undergoing a crisis or insomnia persists after a patient has made lifestyle changes. However, drug therapy is regarded as a short-term remedy, not a solution.

Conventional medications given for insomnia include sedatives, tranquilizers, and antianxiety drugs. All require a doctor's prescription and may become habit-forming. They can lose effectiveness over time and can reduce alertness during the day. The medications should be taken up to four times daily or as directed for approximately three to four weeks. This will vary with the physician, patient, and medication. If insomnia is related to depression, then an antidepressant medication may be helpful.

Drugs prescribed for improving sleep are called hypnotics. This category includes benzodiazepines, which are prescribed for anxiety and insomnia. Benzodiazepines most commonly prescribed for insomnia include Dalmane (fluazepam), Halcion (triazolam), Ativan (lorazepam), Xanax (alprazolam), Restoril (tempazepam), and Serax (oxazepam).

Insomnia is such a widespread problem that "people buy more over-the-counter and prescription sleeping medications than any other drug," according to CBS Health Watch. Many over-the-counter drugs have antihistamines as an active ingredient. While these products are not addictive, some experts believe they are not very effective in sustaining stage IV sleep and can affect the quality of sleep.

Over-the-counter sleep products include Nytol, Sleep-Eez, and Sominex. Antihistamines are used in combination with pain relievers in products including Anacin PM, Excedrin PM, Tylenol PM, Unison, and Quiet World.

Expected results

Insomnia has numerous causes and treatments, so the amount of time may vary before results are seen. A prescription drug may bring immediate results to someone coping with a spouse's death. An herbal remedy may not work immediately for a person who consumed excessive amounts of caffeine to stay awake at work after a sleepless night.

There has been research that provides information about when some treatments take effect:

- Melatonin: a dose of 3-5 mg taken within an hour of retiring will normalize sleep within 1-2 weeks.

- A combination of hops and valerian at bedtime can provide a good night's sleep.

- A combination of alternative therapies should bring a difference in disturbed sleep within two to four days.

- Valerian extract may take from two to three weeks before "significant benefits" are seen.

- St. John's wort can take two weeks to take effect.

- Combinations of treatments could more quickly bring about an uninterrupted night of sleep. The person who reduces caffeine intake, walks for 15 minutes and enjoys an herbal bath may discover that that combination brings restful sleep.

- Acupuncture: "A state of deep relaxation is often an immediate benefit of treatment for chronically anxious patients," William Collinge wrote in *The American Holistic Health Association Complete Guide to Alternative Medicine*. In addition, positive results were recorded in a study of people who had trouble falling asleep or remaining asleep, according to the an article in the October 1999 issue of the *Alternative Medicine Newsletter*. Patients received acupuncture for three to five sessions at weekly intervals. While acupuncture appeared effective, a "directive influence by the therapist cannot be excluded," according to the article.

- Light therapy usually results in earlier bedtimes.

Prevention

Prevention of insomnia centers around promotion of a healthy lifestyle. A balance of rest, recreation, and exercise in combination with stress management, regular physical examinations, and a healthy diet can do much to reduce the risk.

Walking is also recommended. However, exercise should be done no more than three hours before bedtime.

Drinks that contain caffeine such as coffee, tea and colas, chocolate (which contains a stimulant), and alcohol, which initially makes a person sleepy but a few hours later can have the opposite effect should all be avoided.

Maintaining a comfortable bedroom temperature, reducing noise, and eliminating light are also helpful.

Watching television should be avoided because it has an arousing effect. Weil wrote that the news with its "murder, mayhem, and misery" is a major source of tur-

---

KEY TERMS

Biofeedback—A training technique that enables an individual to gain some element of control over involuntary body functions.

Mood disorder—A group of mental disorders involving a disturbance of mood, along with either a full or partial excessively happy (manic) or extremely sad (depressive) syndrome not caused by any other physical or mental disorder. Mood refers to a prolonged emotion.

Sleep apnea—A condition in which a person stops breathing while asleep. These periods can last up to a minute or more, and can occur many times each hour. In order to start breathing again, the person must become semi-awake. The episodes are not remembered, but the following day the client feels tired and sleepy. If severe, sleep apnea can cause other medical problems.

Sleep disorder—Any condition that interferes with sleep. At least 84 have been identified, according to the American Sleep Disorders Association.

---

moil. He sometimes advises "news fasts" as part of a healing program.

Exercise, relaxation, and **nutrition** should be considered ongoing preventive measures. While life will bring unexpected stresses and pressures, the person who is familiar with relaxation techniques will be more prepared to cope with insomnia.

Resources

BOOKS

Albright, Peter. *The Complete Book of Complementary Therapies*. Allentown, PA: People's Medical Society, 1997.

Bloomfield, Harold. *Healing Anxiety with Herbs*. New York: HarperCollins, 1998.

Boyd, Mary Ann, and Mary Ann Nihart. *Psychiatric Nursing: Contemporary Practice*. Philadelphia, PA: Lippincott, 1998.

Bruce, Debra Fulghum and Harris H. McIlwain, *The Unofficial Guide to Alternative Medicine*. New York: Macmillan General Reference, 1998.

The Burton Goldberg Group. *Alternative Medicine: The Definitive Guide*. Fife, WA: Future Medicine Publishing, 1999.

Collinge, William. *The American Holistic Health Association Complete Guide to Alternative Medicine*. New York: Warner Books, 1996.

Frisch, Noreen Cavan, and Lawrence E. Frisch. *Psychiatric Mental Health Nursing*. Albany, NY: Delmar, 1988.

Keville, Kathi. *Herbs for Health and Healing*. Emmaus, PA: Rodale Press, Inc., 1996.

Nash, Barbara. *From Acupuncture to Zen: an encyclopedia of natural therapies.* Alameda, CA: Hunter House, 1996.

Ullman, Dana. *The Consumer's Guide to Homeopathy.* New York: G.P. Putnam Books,1995.

Weil, Andrew. *Spontaneous Healing.* New York: Random House, 1995.

ORGANIZATIONS

American Sleep Disorders Association. 6301 Bandel Road, Suite 101, Rochester, MN 55901. <http://www.asda.org>.

National Sleep Foundation. 1522 K St. NW, Suite 510, Washington, DC 20005. <http://www.sleepfoundation.org>.

OTHER

"Acupuncture and Insomnia." *Alternative Medicine Update* (October 1999). <http://www.healthmall.com>.

"Insomnia." CBS Health Watch. <http://www.cbshealthwatch.com>.

"Patient Information: Insomnia and What You Can Do to Sleep Better." *American Family Physician.* 49, no. 6 (May 1, 1994). <http://srvr.third-wave.com/tricounty/insomnia.html> (1998).

"Sleep Aids: Everything You Wanted to Know…But Were Too Tired to Ask." National Sleep Foundation, 1999. <http://www.sleepfoundation.org/publications/sleepaids.html>.

"What to Do When You Can't Sleep." Children's Hospital of Iowa. 1995. <http://www.vh.org/Patients/IHB/Family Practice/ AFP/January1995/Insomnia.html> (1998).

Willard, Terry. "Insomnia: Wake up to ten simple solutions." *Herbs for Health.* HealthWorld Online. <http://www. healthy.net/hfh/articlesHFH/sleep.htm>.

Liz Swain

Insulin resistance

Definition

Insulin resistance is a condition in which cells, particularly those of muscle, fat, and liver tissue, display "resistance" to insulin by failing to take up and utilize glucose for energy and metabolism (insulin normally promotes take up and utilization of blood glucose from the blood stream). In its early stages, the condition is asymptomatic, but may develop into Type II Diabetes. Although there are several established risk factors, the underlying cause is unknown.

It has been estimated that 30 to 33 million Americans are insulin resistant, and the number appears to be increasing.

Description

Insulin resistance is initially asymptomatic, and in its early stages can be detected only by laboratory tests. These tests will show an abnormally high blood sugar (glucose) level, but not high enough to be considered prediabetic or diabetic. While the condition does not always lead to further problems, the majority of people who reach the pre-diabetic level go on to develop Type II Diabetes (formerly called Maturity Onset Diabetes.

Causes & symptoms

The cause of insulin resistance is unknown, although the condition has been seen to run in families, indicating that there is a genetic association. Being overweight, and lack of **exercise** are also associated with insulin resistance, although the nature of the relationship is not clear. Risk factors for insulin resistance are:

• having a family history of diabetes

• having a low HDL (good) cholesterol level—and high serum lipids

• having high blood pressure

• having a history of diabetes during **pregnancy**, or having given birth to a baby weighing more than 9 pounds

• being a member of one of the racial groups that appear to have a high incidence of insulin resistance (African American, Native American, Hispanic American/Latino, or Asian American/Pacific Islander)

• having syndrome X

• being obese

In its mildest form, insulin resistance causes no symptoms, and is only recognizable on laboratory tests. In more severe cases, there may be dark patches on the back of the neck or even a dark ring around the neck. The dark patches are called *Acanthosis nigricans* and may also cause darkening of skin color in the elbows, knees, knuckles, and armpits.

There is a constellation of symptoms now called metabolic syndrome or insulin resistance syndrome that is linked to insulin resistance. This syndrome was formerly called syndrome X. Metabolic syndrome is defined by the National **Cholesterol** Education Program as the presence of any three of the following conditions:

• excess weight around the waistline (waist measurement of more than 40 inches for men and more than 35 inches for women)

• high levels of serum triglycerides (150 mg/dL or higher)

• low levels of HDL, or "good," cholesterol (below 40 mg/dL for men and below 50 mg/dL for women)

• high blood pressure (130/85 mm Hg or higher)

• high **fasting** blood glucose levels (110 mg/dL or higher)

Note that the numbers are those from an expert panel convened by the National Institutes of Health in

2001. Other panels of similarly qualified experts have given slightly different definitions.

Diagnosis

The only means of diagnosis for insulin resistance is laboratory tests. While there are several tests that may be performed, the two most common screening tests are the fasting blood sugar test and glucose tolerance test.

Fasting blood sugar measures the blood glucose level after a 12-hour fast (no food). A normal level, according to the United Sates National Institute of Diabetes and Digestive and Kidney Disease (NIDDK), should be below 100 mg/dL (milligrams of glucose in every deciliter of blood. A value in the n the 100 to 125 mg/dL range is considered evidence of insulin resistance, and is considered prediabetic. A value of 126 mg/dL is considered diabetic. (Blood sugar levels after a 12 hr fast are typically lower than this, and are controlled by pancreatic insulin secretion that transports blood glucose out of the blood and into the muscles, brain, organs, and other tissues.)

The glucose tolerance test is performed after the patient has had nothing but water for 10 to 16 hours. The patient has his blood drawn for a a baseline blood glucose level. Next, the patient drinks a special sweetened test drink that contains exactly 75 grams of glucose (pregnant women are normally given 100 grams of glucose.) Blood is drawn again at one-half hour and each of the next six hours to compare blood glucose levels and watch their pattern in response to the sweet drink. Normally the blood sugar levels is lower before the drink, rises quickly during the first few hours, and slowly drops again. In insulin resistance, the blood sugar level rises but stays abnormally high because it is resistant to being removed from blood into tissues by insulin. High blood sugar from food or the test glucose drink stimulates the pancreas to secrete insulin into the blood. However, in insulin resistance, the insulin is secreted but is only partially absorbed by the tissues. According to the National Diabetes Information Clearinghouse (NDIC) a normal level would be below 140 mg/dL 2 hours after the drink. If it is in the 140 to 199 mg/dL range 2 hours after drinking the solution, the diagnosis is impaired glucose tolerance (IGT) or prediabetes. A level of 200 or higher, if confirmed, represents a diagnosis of diabetes.

Treatment

Among the most important treatment modalities are diet and exercise, weight loss if obese, endocrine hormone correction if unbalanced. In 2001, the National Institutes of Health completed the Diabetes Prevention Program (DPP), a clinical trial designed to find the most effective ways of preventing type 2 diabetes in overweight people with prediabetes. The researchers found that lifestyle changes reduced the risk of diabetes by 58 percent. Also, many people with prediabetes showed a return to normal blood glucose levels.

According to the DDP results, a mere half hour of brisk walking or bicycling five days a week can significantly reduce the risk of developing type 2 diabetes. Patients should use diet and exercise to reduce their body mass index (BMI) to 25 or below.

Smoking has been associated with insulin resistance, as well as with some of the more severe problems associated with diabetes. Discontinuing smoking should be a top priority.

A healthful diet, in addition to assisting in weight loss, may reduce serum lipids and reduce some of the risk factors for diabetes. One study recommended the **Mediterranean diet** as being the most beneficial for people with insulin resistance. Diet improvements include reducing sweets, desserts and high glycemic meals; eating balanced meals that contain protein, complex carbohydrates, fiber, greens and healthy oils, eating at regular times, and avoiding excess junk food and sugar.

No complimentary or alternative therapies have been proven to cure insulin resistance. Although several herbal remedies have been traditionally used for treatment of diabetes, none have been adequately documented as effective. Among medicinal plants shown to help lower elevated blood sugar are the Asian **bitter melon** and the Navaho Optunia cactus. Such herbal **bitters** as **dandelion** root and **yellow dock** can improve digestive strength and sometimes help, though no herbal remedy alone "cures" insulin resistance or diabetes. Guar gum, glucomannan, and **psyllium** seed all have demonstrated some ability to lower blood sugar in insulin resistance or diabetes, but none have been shown to be reliably effective for use in treatment of humans.

Allopathic treatment

Insulin resistance does not normally require drug therapy; however, some studies have shown that the drugs used to treat type 2 diabetes may delay development of diabetes. Two classes of drugs now used to treat diabetes act by increasing insulin sensitivity, the biguanides and the thiazolidinediones; the other drugs used to treat diabetes act in different ways.

Although drugs from both classes have been effective in treatment of insulin resistance, neither drug has been as effective as a regimen of diet and exercise. Both classes of drugs have the potential for very severe adverse effects.They are also not approved by the FDA for control of insulin resistance, although physicians may prescribe them for this use if the condition appears to be getting worse without drug therapy. In one study, oral hypoglycemic drugs of various mechanisms that help reduce elevated blood blood glucose reduced the rate of disease progression from insulin resistance to diabetes by about one-third over a three-year period.

Expected results

In mild asymptomatic insulin resistance, proper treatment may lead to a complete reversal, with normalization of blood sugar.

Even if complete normalization is impossible, treatment will lead to control of the condition, and a significant reduction in its rate of progression to diabetes.

Prevention

In insulin resistance, prevention is even better than treatment. Maintaining a normal weight, eating a balanced diet, and keeping up a regular program of aerobic exercise are the best preventive measures.

Resources

BOOKS

Beers, M. H., and R. Berkow, eds. *The Merck Manual of Diagnosis and Therapy, 17th ed.* Whitehouse Station, New Jersey: Merck and Co., 2004.

Blumenthal, M., ed. *The Complete German Commission E Monographs.* Austin, TX: American Botanical Council, 1999.

Blumenthal, M., ed. *Herbal Medicine.* Austin, TX: American Botanical Council, 2000.

Hart, C. R., and M. K. Grossman. *The Insulin Resistance Diet.* Chicago: Contemporary Books, 2001

PERIODICALS

Brame, L., S. Verma, T. Anderson, A. Lteif, and K. Mather. "Insulin resistance as a therapeutic target for improved endothelial function: metformin." *Curr Drug Targets Cardiovasc Haematol Disord* (March 2004): 53–63.

Camp, H. S. "Thiazolidinediones in diabetes: current status and future outlook." *Curr Opin Investig Drugs* (April 2003): 406–11.

Cargo, D. M. "Association between smoking, insulin resistance and beta-cell function in a North-Western First Nation." *Diabet Med* (February 2004): 188–93.

Dzien, A., C. Dzien-Bischinger, F. Hoppichler, and M. Lechleitner. "The metabolic syndrome as a link between smoking and cardiovascular disease." *Diabetes Obes Metab* (March 2004): 127–32.

Nelson, M. R. "Managing 'metabolic syndrome' and multiple risk factors." *Aust Fam Physician* (April 2004): 201–5.

Osei, K, S. Rhinesmith, T. Gaillard, and D. Schuster. "Beneficial metabolic effects of chronic glipizide in obese African Americans with impaired glucose tolerance: implications for primary prevention of type 2 diabetes." *Metabolism* (April 2004): 414–22.

KEY TERMS

Acanthosis nigricans—A localized darkening of the skin that is associated with insulin resistance. This is not seen in all cases, and is considered a Rare Disorder.

Diabetes—Any of several metabolic diseases affecting the body's use of blood sugars or the intake and excretion of fluids. In Type 2 diabetes, formerly called maturity onset diabetes, there is sufficient insulin, but the insulin is unable to penetrate the cell membrane.

Insulin—A hormone, secreted by the pancreas, which is essential for the body's ability to use glucose to provide energy. Inadequate insulin supplies result in Type 1 diabetes.

Metformin—An anti-diabetic drug of the biguanide class. This drug increases the sensitivity of cells to insulin, but is capable of causing very severe adverse reactions, including lactic acidosis and anemia.

Pioglitazone—An anti-diabetic drug of the thiazolidinedione class. This drug increases the sensitivity of the cells to insulin, but is capable of causing severe adverse reactions, including congestive heart failure.

Scheen, J. "Current management strategies for coexisting diabetes mellitus and obesity." *Drugs* (2003): 1165–84.

Yamamoto, Y., I. Sogawa, A. Nishina, S. Saeki, N. Ichikawa, and S. Iibata. "Improved hypolipidemic effects of xanthan gum-galactomannan mixtures in rats." *Biosci Biotechnol Biochem* (October 2000): 2165–71.

ORGANIZATIONS

American Association of Clinical Endocrinologists (AACE). 1000 Riverside Avenue, Suite 205, Jacksonville, FL 32204.

National Organization for Rare Disorders. 55 Kenosia Avenue, PO Box 1968, Danbury, CT 06813-1968.

Samuel Uretsky, Pharm.D.

Iodine

Description

Iodine is a trace mineral required for human life. Humans require iodine for proper physical and mental development. It impacts cell respiration, metabolism of energy and nutrients, functioning of nerves and muscles, differentiation of the fetus, growth and repair of tissues, and the condition of skin, hair, teeth, and nails. Iodine is also needed for the production of thyroid hormones. The thyroid (a small gland in the front of the neck), which contains 80% of the body's iodine pool, converts iodine into the thyroid hormones thyroxine (T_4) and triiodothyronine (T_3). These hormones are released into the bloodstream, controlling the body's metabolism.

General use

As established by the National Research Council's Food and **Nutrition** Board, the revised 1989 Recommended Dietary Allowance (RDA) for iodine is 40 mcg for infants, increasing to 150 mcg for adults and children age 11 and older. The RDA for pregnant and lactating women increases to 175 and 200 mcg respectively. *Harrison's Principles of Internal Medicine* reports that average U.S. iodine daily intake ranges from approximately 0.5–1.0 mg. According to the *Merck Manual of Diagnosis and Therapy*, less than 20 mcg per day of iodide results in iodine deficiency; iodide intake 20 times greater than the daily requirement (2 mg) results in chronic iodine toxicity.

Iodine is available from a variety of food sources, drugs, and most commercial vitamin preparations. Some seafood and sea vegetables provide good sources of dietary iodine, including: canned sardines, canned tuna, clams, cod, haddock, halibut, herring, lobster, oyster, perch, salmon, sea bass, and shrimp. Dulse, **kelp**, and seaweed are also sources of dietary iodine. If grown in iodine-rich soil, foods including asparagus, green peppers, lettuce, lima beans, mushrooms, pineapple, raisins, spinach, summer squash, Swiss chard, turnip greens, and whole wheat bread may provide good sources of dietary iodine. Animal products can also provide a source of iodine, especially if the animals are fed iodine-enriched foods or salt: beef, beef liver, butter, cheddar cheese, cottage cheese, cream, eggs, lamb, milk, and pork. Some foods such as breads may contain iodine additives.

Another source of dietary iodine is iodized salt. Iodized table salt was introduced in the United States in 1924 and significantly reduced the incidence of iodine deficiency. Providing iodized salt licks for livestock adds iodine to animal products. In some parts of the world, iodized oil supplements and water iodination provide other means of iodine supplementation. Many countries, however, still have insufficient iodine supplementation programs.

Iodine has several medical applications. Typically, in conjunction with drug therapy, iodine may be used to treat goiter (an enlargement of the thyroid gland), symptoms of **hypothyroidism** (diminished production of thyroid hormone), and hyperthyroidism (increased production of the thyroid gland). It may also be used as an expectorant in **cough** medications. Applications of iodine to conditions including arteriosclerosis, arthritis, and **angina** pectoris have also been noted. Iodine tinctures (dilute mixtures of alcohol and iodine) or Betadine are used as antiseptics to kill bacteria in skin cuts. Atomidine (a product containing iodine trichloride and other unlisted ingredients) is also sold as an antiseptic. Atomidine taken orally in minute cyclic doses is also recommended as a glandular stimulant and purifier.

Some research has shown that oral iodine supplements have antifibrotic and anti-inflammatory effects. Commonly reported studies have also suggested that iodine deficiency may be a factor in fibrocystic breast disease (FBD), a catch-all term that describes general, often normal, lumpiness of the breast. Clinical trials on women diagnosed with FBD found that, even in women showing normal thyroid function, thyroid hormone supplementation produced results including decreased breast **pain** and decreased breast nodules. Some early research also correlated higher incidence of breast, endometrial, and ovarian cancers with hypothyroidism and/or iodine deficiency. However, others have noted that low levels of **selenium**, which is more classically associated with **cancer**, were also present in the women in these studies.

Iodine is used in several compounds for a variety of medical testing. For example, it may be used in x-rays of the gallbladder or kidneys or in cardiac imaging. It is used as a diagnostic tool to examine the thyroid gland's output. A common test measures thyroid radioactive iodine uptake (RAIU). Trace amounts of radioactive iodine (I^{123} or I^{131}) are used to test thyroid function. Together with blood tests, examining how much iodine is taken up by the thyroid gland helps physicians diagnose hypothyroid conditions (when the thyroid takes up too little iodine) and hyperthyroid conditions (when it takes up too much). Radioactive iodine therapy is also used for treating thyroid disease and cancer. Radioactive iodine can cross the placenta, causing severe dysfunction and damage to the fetus's thyroid gland. *Current Medical Diagnosis and Treatment 2000* notes that nursing mothers should discontinue nursing for a period of time after receiving test or treatment doses of radioactive iodine. One study published in the *Journal of the American Medical Association (JAMA)* in May 2000 reported radiation exposure to family members of non-pregnant, non-nursing outpatients from I^{131} treatment to be well below limits mandated by U.S. Nuclear Regulatory Commission (NRC) guidelines. Medical professionals may also prescribe low iodine **diets** in combination with radioactive iodine tests or treatments.

Precautions

Too much or too little iodine intake results in a wide spectrum of disorders that are addressed by adjusting iodine intake. Too much iodine can result in toxicity.

Iodine deficiency disorders (IDDs) are preventable, but not curable, by ensuring adequate iodine intake. Only a small amount of iodine is required over the human life span. The body, however, does not store iodine for long periods, so the intake must be regular. Too little iodine intake can result in cold feet, **fatigue**, insomnia, problems with skin, nails, and hair, and weight gain. Goiter can result from iodine deficiency. Certain substances called goitrogens can also induce goiter by interfering with thyroid functioning. Some foods have goitrogenic tendencies, as do certain drugs, for example, thiourea, sulfonamides, and antipyrine. As listed by *Prescriptions for Nutritional Healing* and other sources, foods containing substances that can prevent the utilization of iodine when eaten in large quantities include Brussels sprouts, cabbage, cauliflower, kale, millet, mustard, peaches, peanuts, pears, pine nuts, soybeans, and turnips. Limiting consumption of these foods may be recommended for persons with an underactive thyroid.

Iodine deficiency can also result in serious irreversible disorders and, as of May 2000, is considered a major global health problem by organizations such as the World Health Organization (WHO) and the United Nations Children's Fund (UNICEF). According to the International Council on Control of Iodine Deficiency Disorders (ICCIDD), IDDs are the most common cause of preventable brain damage and mental retardation worldwide. IDD results in cretinism (a form of stunted growth) and problems in movement, speech, and hearing. A pregnant woman with an iodine deficiency risks miscarriage, stillbirth, and mental retardation of her baby. As of 1999, the WHO called IDD a significant public health problem in 130 countries. The ICCIDD reported 1.6 billion people worldwide at risk for IDDs, and 50 million children suffering from some degree of IDD. Although not common, iodine deficiency is on the rise in the United States.

In 2002, the United Nation's Children's Fund announced a pledge to eliminate iodine deficiency in the world by 2005, citing the problem as a major cause of psychiatric and learning disabilities.

Side effects

Excess iodine is typically excreted, and output can be measured in the urine. Regular excessive iodine intake is needed for toxicity. Excess iodine, when used as a supplement or in drug therapy, may reduce thyroid function. Although more commonly associated with iodine deficiency, goiter can also result from too much iodine due to thyroid hyperactivity. Additionally, high amounts of iodine from sources such as overuse of iodized salt, vitamins, cough medications, kelp tablets, or from medical testing can cause effects including rapid pulse, nervous-

ness, headaches, fatigue, a brassy taste in the mouth, excessive salivation, gastric irritation, and hypothyroidism. **Acne** can appear or become worse. Some iodine-sensitive individuals may have an allergic reaction to iodine, often a skin rash. A physician may recommend that high iodine foods be removed from the diet of those who are iodine-sensitive. Similar side effects have also been observed in some women participating in studies on iodine and diagnosed FBD. Radioactive iodine has been implicated in producing thyroid dysfunction and thyroid cancer.

Resources

BOOKS

The Merck Manual of Diagnosis and Therapy. 17th ed. Edited by Mark H. Beers and Robert Berkow. Whitehouse Station, N.J.: Merck Research Laboratories, 1999.

National Research Council. *Recommended Dietary Allowances.* 10th ed. Washington, D.C.: National Academy Press, 1989.

PERIODICALS

"In Case you Haven't Heard." *Mental Health Weekly* (July 1, 2002): 8.

ORGANIZATIONS

International Council for Control of Iodine deficiency Disorders (ICCIDD). Prof. Jack Ling. Director, ICEC. 1501 Canal Street, Suite 1304, New Orleans, LA 70112. (504)584–3542 Fax: (504)585–4090. ICEC@mailhost.tcs. tulane.edu. <http://www.people.virginia.edu/~jtd/iccidd/>.

U.S. Fund for UNICEF. 333 East 38th Street NY, NY 10016. webmaster@unicefusa.org. <http://www.unicefusa.org/issues99/sep99/learn.html>.

World Health Organization (WHO). Avenue Appia 20 1211 Geneva 27, Switzerland. (+00–41–22)791–21–11. Fax: (+00–41–22)791–311. info@who.int. <http://www.who.int/inf-fs/en/fact121.html>.

OTHER

HealthWorld Online. <http://www.healthy.net>.

Kathy Stolley
Teresa G. Odle

Ipecac

Description

There are two categories of ipecac preparations— a syrup used in standard medical practice and a homeopathic remedy. They are given for different purposes. The medicinal effects of ipecac were recognized centuries ago by the Portuguese who settled in South America. They found a plant that can make people vomit and appropriately named it *Cephalis ipecacuanha*, meaning sick-making plant. Nowadays, ipecac is used to treat a variety of conditions. Its most widely accepted use is to induce **vomiting** in cases of accidental poisoning. When ipecac is swallowed, a substance in it called cephaeline irritates the stomach and causes vomiting. Syrup of ipecac is now considered the safest drug to treat poisoning and is often the most effective. There are different types of ipecac preparations that vary greatly in strength. Syrup of ipecac is best for use at home to treat accidental poisoning. Ipecac fluid extract and ipecac tincture should be avoided, as they are much stronger compounds and can be toxic.

Ipecacuanha is a homeopathic remedy made from ipecac by a process of dilution and succussion (shaking). In contrast to syrup of ipecac, it is given to relieve vomiting.

General use

Treatment of poisoning

Standard medical practice uses ipecac to cause vomiting in cases of poisoning in order to remove the toxic substance from the stomach before absorption occurs. It can be used on animals as well as humans. Ipecac is safer and more effective than many other methods for inducing vomiting, such as sticking a finger down a child's throat or using saltwater. There are times, however, when ipecac should not be used because it can make certain kinds of poisoning worse. Syrup of ipecac should *not* be used if the poison is one of the following.

- strychnine
- alkalis (lye)
- strong acids
- kerosene
- fuel oil
- gasoline
- coal oil
- paint thinner
- cleaning fluid

Poisoning is a potentially serious condition. It is best to contact a local poison control center, local hospital emergency room, or the family doctor for instructions before using syrup of ipecac.

Ipecac's reputation for inducing vomiting has encouraged some bulimics to take it on a regular basis in order to purge the contents of the stomach after an eating binge. This misuse of ipecac is extremely dangerous; it can cause heart problems, tears in the esophagus or stomach lining, vomiting blood, seizures, or even death.

Homeopathy

The homeopathic remedy made from ipecac is called *Ipecacuanha*. Homeopathic preparations are given for a reason completely opposite from that of standard allopathic treatment. In **homeopathy**, ipecac is given to stop vomiting rather than to induce it. According to Hahnemann's law of similars, a substance that would cause vomiting in large doses when given to a healthy person will stimulate a sick person's natural defenses when given in extremely diluted and carefully prepared doses. *Ipecacuanha* is a favorite homeopathic remedy for **morning sickness** associated with **pregnancy**. It is also given to stop **nausea** that is not relieved by vomiting; when the vomitus is slimy and white; when there is gagging and heavy salivation; when the tongue is clean despite the patient's feelings of nausea; and when the patient is not thirsty. The nausea may be accompanied by a **headache**, **cough**, or heavy menstrual bleeding. The modalities (circumstances) that suggest *Ipecacuanha* as the appropriate homeopathic remedy is that the patient feels worse lying down; in dry weather; in winter; and when exercising or moving about.

A homeopathic practitioner would not necessarily prescribe ipecac for all cases of nausea. *Arsenicum* would be given when the nausea is caused by **food poisoning** and accompanied by strong thirst, *Nux vomica* when the nausea is the result of overindulgence in food or alcohol and accompanied by **gas** or **heartburn**. A sick child might be given *Pulsatilla*, particularly if rich foods have been eaten.

On the other hand, a homeopathic practitioner may prescribe ipecac for any of the following conditions that are not related to nausea and vomiting.

- nosebleeds producing bright red blood
- dental bleeding
- diarrhea with cramping abdominal **pain**. The stools are green with froth or foam.
- Asthma of sudden onset. The patient has to sit up in order to breathe, but cannot bring up any mucus in spite of violent coughing.
- hoarseness or loss of voice following a cold
- physical or mental exhaustion

Preparations

Syrup of ipecac

Syrup of ipecac is made from the dried roots and rhizomes (underground stems) of *Cephaelis ipecacuanha*. It is available over the counter in 0.5–1 oz bottles. Larger bottles require a doctor's prescription. The dosage for infants under 6 months old should be prescribed by the family doctor or poison control center. For children six months to one year, the usual dose is 5–10 ml or 1–2 tsp. One-half or one full glass (4–8 oz) of water should be taken immediately before or after the dose. The dose may be repeated once after 20–30 minutes if vomiting does not occur. For children one to 12 years of age, the usual dose is 15 ml (1 tbsp) to be taken with one full glass (8 oz) of water. Adults and teenagers should take 15–30 ml of ipecac with at least 1 full glass of water. Syrup of ipecac should not be taken with milk or soda drinks as these foods may prevent it from working properly. If vomiting does not occur within 20–30 minutes after the first dose, a second dose may be needed. If the second dose fails to induce vomiting, the patient should be taken to a hospital emergency room.

If both **activated charcoal** and syrup of ipecac are recommended to treat poison, ipecac must be used first. Activated charcoal should not be taken until 30 minutes after taking syrup of ipecac, or until the vomiting caused by ipecac stops.

Homeopathic preparations

Ipecacuanha is available as an over-the-counter remedy in 30x potency. This is a decimal potency, which means that one part of ipecac has been mixed with nine parts of alcohol or water; 30x means that this decimal dilution has been repeated 30 times. The dilute solution of ipecac is then added to sugar tablets so that the remedy can be taken in tablet form.

Precautions

Syrup of ipecac

For inducing vomiting in cases of accidental poisoning, only the syrup form of ipecac should be used. Syrup of ipecac should not be mixed with milk or carbonated drinks as they may prevent vomiting. If syrup of ipecac is not immediately available in the home, it generally cannot be used. A 2002 report studied parents' attempts to administer the syrup upon calling a poison center when they felt they could obtain it within 15 minutes. However, actual time to administration was generally closer to 30 minutes. The report recommended that parents not be referred to purchase ipecac when their children have ingested a significant amount of a poisonous substance and the syrup is not already available in the home.

Syrup of ipecac should *not* be used in the following situations (contact poison control center or family doctor for alternative treatments).

- Poisoning caused by strychnine; sustained-release theophylline; such corrosive substances as strong alka-

lis (lye); strong acids (such as toilet bowl cleaner); and such petroleum products as kerosene, gasoline, coal oil, fuel oil, paint thinner, or cleaning fluids.

- Overdoses of medications given for depression.
- Excessive vomiting.
- A serious heart condition.
- Timing. Do not give ipecac more than 4–6 hours after the poison was ingested.
- Pregnancy.
- Very young children (less than six months old). Infants and very young children may choke on their own vomit or get vomit into their lungs.
- Drowsy or unconscious patients.
- Seizures.

Homeopathic preparations

Ipecacuanha should not be given after *Arsenicum* or *Tabac* because these remedies will counteract it.

Side effects

The following side effects have been associated with the use of syrup of ipecac.

- Loose bowel movements.
- Diarrhea.
- Fast irregular heartbeat.
- Inhaling or choking on vomit.
- Stomach cramps or pains.
- Coughing.
- Weakness.
- Aching.
- Muscle stiffness.
- Severe heart problems often occur in cases of ipecac abuse. Because ipecac stays in the body for a long time, damage to the heart frequently occurs in persons who repeatedly take ipecac to induce vomiting.
- Seizures. These are most likely to occur in patients who accidentally swallow ipecac or in ipecac abusers.
- Death. Deaths have been reported due to ipecac abuse in bulimic persons.

Homeopathic *Ipecacuanha* has been highly diluted and is relatively nontoxic.

Interactions

Ipecac should not be given together with other drugs because it can decrease their effectiveness and increase their toxicity. If both syrup of ipecac and activated charcoal are needed to treat suspected poisons, ipecac should be given first. Activated charcoal should not be given until vomiting induced by ipecac has stopped. Soda should also be avoided because it can cause the stomach to swell. The person should lie on the stomach or side in case vomiting occurs.

Homeopathic *Ipecacuanha* is considered complementary to *Arnica* and *Cuprum*. It is counteracted by *Arsenicum* and *Tabac*.

Resources

BOOKS

Cummings, Stephen, MD, and Dana Ullman, MPH. *Everybody's Guide to Homeopathic Medicines.* New York: G. P. Putnam's Sons, 1991.

Ellenhorn's Medical Toxicology, 2nd ed. Baltimore: Williams & Wilkins, 1997.

Hammond, Christopher. *The Complete Family Guide to Homeopathy: An Illustrated Encyclopedia of Safe and Effective Remedies.* New York: Penguin Studio, 1995.

PDR Nurse's Drug Handbook. Montvale, NJ: Delmar Publishers, 2000.

PERIODICALS

J. Garrison, et al. "Effectiveness of Home Ipecac Syrup Administration When It Is Not Initially Available." *Journal of Toxicology:Clinical Toxicology* (August 2002): 618.

ORGANIZATIONS

American Foundation for Homeopathy. 1508 S. Garfield, Alhambra, CA 91801.

Homeopathic Educational Services. 2124B Kittredge St., Berkeley, CA 94704. (510) 649-0294. Fax: (510) 649-1955.

Mai Tran
Teresa G. Odle

Ipraflavone *see* **Ipriflavone**

Ipriflavone

Description

Ipriflavone (IP), also called ipraflavone, is a mass-produced synthetic derivative of genistein (genistin) or daidzein. Genistein and daidzein are unique plant compounds called isoflavones, which are primarily found in soy products. Isoflavones belong to a larger category known as flavonoids, which are natural plant components that have antioxidant, anti-inflammatory, anti-allergy, and anticancer properties. Although most soy isoflavones are classified as plant estrogens (phytoestrogens), ipriflavone does not have estrogenic activity, and does not activate any estrogen receptors in the body. However, it may prevent or treat bone loss—osteoporosis—associated with **menopause** (the cessation of **menstruation**) and **aging**.

Ipriflavone contains three carbon rings. Its chemical names are:

- 7-isopropoxyisoflavone
- 7-isopropoxy-3-phenyl-4H-1-benzopyran-4-one
- 7-(1-methylethoxy)-3-phenyl-4H-1-benzopyran-4-one
- 7-isopropoxy-3-phenylchromone

One source notes that ipriflavone is found in foods, but only in trace amounts. In addition to soy products (including some soy sauces), trace amounts are found in **alfalfa** and other foods. It is also found in propolis, a resin that bees collect from tree buds for use as a hive cement. Ipriflavone is a solid that dissolves only slightly in **water**.

The liver metabolizes ipriflavone into 7-hydroxy-ipriflavone and 7-(1-carboxy-ethoxy)-isoflavone. IP and its derivatives are bound to albumin, a blood protein, and distributed to tissues throughout the body.

Ipriflavone may be one of the best-studied compounds in the natural health industry. However, the results of these studies are not clear with regard to efficacy in increasing bone density, its primary claim. Ipriflavone was first isolated at a Hungarian pharmaceutical company in 1969. Since the 1980s, it has been a registered prescription drug for the prevention and treatment of **osteoporosis** in Japan, Argentina, and Europe.

General use

Like other cells in the human body, bone cells are constantly being replaced. Furthermore, bones serve as a **calcium** bank because they are a source of calcium used for other functions, such as buffering the blood. Osteoporosis is a net loss of bone mass, caused either by excessive bone-resorping (dissolving) or low bone-forming activities. These activities are often related to the increased bone turnover rate that accompanies menopause.

Women have a lifetime risk of 40% for developing osteoporosis. One-half of all women over the age of 50 will develop the disease. One in eight men experience bone **fractures** as a result of osteoporosis. Hip fractures caused by osteoporosis are a direct or indirect cause of death in one-quarter of elderly Americans. Bone building and breakdown are influenced by the following:

- hormones, including estrogen and calcitonin (from the parathyroid gland)
- such minerals as **magnesium**, **phosphorus**, **boron**, **zinc**, **silica**, and vanadium
- vitamins, including vitamin D.
- such other factors as corticosteroid use, sunlight, dietary acidity, physiologic pH, and overall bodily health

Numerous studies have indicated that ipriflavone maintains or increases bone mineral density in osteoporosis, particularly in conjunction with calcium supplementation. Clinical studies have demonstrated that ipriflavone supplementation may:

- prevent rapid bone loss immediately following menopause
- increase bone density in postmenopausal women by as much as 3%
- increase bone mineral density in women with osteoporosis by up to 6%
- decrease the incidence of bone fractures among postmenopausal women
- reduce bone **pain** caused by osteoporosis
- increase mobility in women with osteoporosis
- stimulate the synthesis and secretion of calcitonin, a hormone that controls calcium metabolism
- lower the high **cholesterol** levels associated with menopausal estrogen deficiency
- have some activity against **cancer**

Ipriflavone also slows bone loss in women whose ovaries have been removed, although it does not appear to prevent acute bone loss immediately following ovariectomy. Further studies in this area have not obtained the same conclusions, except under very specific conditions including younger age and active bone loss. Therefore, the presence of osteoporosis alone does not appear to be sufficient for obtaining good results, even with calcium supplementation.

The mechanisms of ipriflavone activity are not understood. *In vitro* and animal studies have indicated that:

- Genistein inhibits the breakdown of bone.
- Ipriflavone inhibits bone resorption (the breakdown and recycling of bone tissue).
- Ipriflavone may stimulate bone formation.

In contrast, one large study of postmenopausal women with slight osteoporosis found no significant bone density changes between the group taking calcium supplements alone and those taking calcium plus ipriflavone.

Since ipriflavone does not have estrogenic activity, it may be appropriate for treating bone loss in men, particularly in those with **prostate cancer** who are receiving therapies that reduce androgen (masculinizing hormone) levels.

Preparations

Ipriflavone is available over-the-counter (OTC) in many generic and brand name forms (e.g. Ostivone, Natrol, and Bone Support Ipriflavone Blend). It is supplied in capsules, each containing 100, 200, or 300 mg. A typical IP dose for the management of osteoporosis is 200 mg, two to three times daily. Almost all studies consistently used 600 mg daily. A two-month supply costs about $20.

Food items, particularly those containing lipids, increase the small intestine's absorption of ipriflavone. IP supplements are more effective if combined with calcium and other supplements that help to diminish bone loss during menopause and aging. Ipriflavone sometimes is combined with low-dose estrogen preparations.

Natural isoflavone supplements isolated from soy do not appear to have the same benefits or phytoestrogen neutral qualities as ipriflavone.

Precautions

Ipriflavone has not been subjected to long-term safety studies. In one study, a consistent precaution resulting from research that spanned as much as three years is that ipriflavone appears to decrease lymphocyte (disease-fighting white-blood-cell) levels in a significant number of postmenopausal women with minor osteoporosis. Additionally, since ipriflavone is metabolized by the liver, those with liver disease are advised to avoid it unless directed otherwise by a healthcare professional. Other contraindications include **pregnancy** and breastfeeding, gastric or duodenal ulcers, and kidney disease. Ipriflavone is not recommended for small children.

Side effects

No significant side effects have been observed with ipriflavone, although there are reports of **heartburn**, **nausea**, **diarrhea**, or other mild gastrointestinal disturbances. These side effects may be avoided by taking the supplement with food. One source noted that the percentage of perceived side effects was actually less among the IP users than in the placebo group. Generally, ipriflavone is considered to be well tolerated, to have no effect on fertility, and to not promote precancerous cellular changes (mutagenicity). Approximately 13% of women studied had a decrease in white blood cell count, usually within the first six months. However, this group did not become more susceptible to disease or illness. Their normal white blood cell counts returned within one to two years of discontinuing the IP. There were occasional reports of hypersensitivity reactions and increases in liver function test scores.

Interactions

Similar to grapefruit juice, IP has an inhibiting effect on a liver **detoxification** pathway involving an enzyme known as cytochrome P450. This effect increases both the blood levels and the effects of these drugs:

- theophylline: IP and 7-hydroxy-ipriflavone may inhibit the metabolism and elimination of this **asthma** drug, leading to elevated—and potentially toxic—blood levels
- zafirlukast (Accolate), an asthma medication
- antipsychotic medications
- caffeine
- celecoxib (Celebrex), a pain reliever for arthritis
- cyclobenzaprine (Flexeril), a muscle relaxant
- nifedipine
- nonsteroidal anti-inflammatory medications and pain relievers
- tacrine (Cognex), a medication for Alzheimer's disease
- tamoxifen (Nolvadex), for cancer prevention and treatment
- tolbutamide levels are increased by both ipriflavone and 7-hydroxy isoflavone

- warfarin (Coumadin), a blood-thinner

The effects of ipriflavone may be additive with the effects of these drugs:

- bisphosphonates for the treatment of osteoporosis
- calcitonin
- estrogen
- selective estrogen receptor modulators (SERMs)

During the management of osteoporosis, ipriflavone effects may be additive with the effects of the following nutritional supplements:

- boron
- calcium
- fluoride
- vitamin D
- vitamin K

Resources

BOOKS

Girman, A., and C. Poole. *Preventing Osteoporosis with Ipriflavone: Discover the Proven, Safe Alternative to Estrogen Replacement Therapy.* Roseville, CA: Prima Publishing, 2000.

PDR for Nutritional Supplements. Montvale, NJ: Thomson PDR, 2001.

PERIODICALS

Alexandersen, Peter, et al. "Ipriflavone in the Treatment of Postmenopausal Osteosporosis: A Randomized Controlled Study." *Journal of the American Medical Association* 285, no. 11 (March 21, 2001): 1482–8.

"Can Ipriflavone Help Save Your Bones From Osteoporosis?" *Environmental Nutrition* 2415 (May 2001): 7.

Fuchs, Nan K. "Ipriflavone Limitations." *Women's Health Letter* 813 (March 2002): 7.

Glazier, M. Gina, and Marjorie A. Bowman. "A Review of the Evidence for the Use of Phytoestrogens as a Replacement for Traditional Estrogen Replacement Therapy." *Archives of Internal Medicine* 161 no. 9 (May 14, 2001): 1161–72.

Schelonka, E. P., et al. "Ipriflavone and Osteoporosis." *Journal of the American Medical Association* 286 no. 15 (October 17, 2001): 1836.

"Total Health Resource Guide: Ipriflavone—A Foundation for Healthy Bones." *Total Health* 24, no. 5 (November/December 2002): S24–5.

Walsh, Nancy. "Dietary Supplement Ipriflavone Stems Bone Loss." *Family Practice News* 31, no. 8 (April 15, 2001): 32.

ORGANIZATIONS

National Osteoporosis Foundation. 1232 22nd Street N.W., Washington, DC 20037-1292. (202) 223-2226. <http://www.nof.org>.

KEY TERMS

. . . .

Calcitonin—A hormone that inhibits bone resorption in response to high blood levels of calcium.

Daidzein—A soy isoflavone used to produce ipriflavone.

Genistein—A plant isoflavone found as genistin in soy that is used to produce ipriflavone.

Isoflavones—Compounds, including plant estrogens, with two phenolic rings, that are found in significant quantities in soybeans and soy foods. Isoflavones belong to the larger category of flavonoids, plant compounds that are often a source of the plant fruit or flower color, and possess anticancer, anti-inflammatory, anti-allergy, and antioxidant qualities.

Menopause—The cessation of menstruation.

Osteoporosis—A progressive disease characterized by loss of bone density and increased bone fragility.

Resorption—The dissolution of bone tissue.

OTHER

Brown, Susan E. Ph.D., CCN, *Ipriflavone, Osteoporosis Education Project Analysis.* The Osteoporosis Education Project (OEP), 2000. [cited May 28, 2004]. <http://www.betterbones.com>.

Ipriflavone. Healthnotes, Inc. 2004. [cited May 28, 2004]. <http://www.healthwell.com/healthnotes>.

Ipriflavone. National Nutritional Foods Association, 2001. [cited May 28, 2004]. <http://www.nnfa.org/services/science/bg_ipriflavone.htm>.

Mercola, Joseph. *Ipriflavone Has No Effect on Bone Density.* 2004. [cited May 28, 2004]. <http://www.mercola.com/2000/oct/8/ipriflavone.htm>.>

Margaret Alic

Iridology

Definition

Iridology, also called iris analysis or iris diagnosis, is the study of the iris (the colored part of the eye). Iris "readings" are made by iridologists to assess a person's health picture (physical, emotional, mental, and spiritual) and guide them to take measures to improve their health.

Origins

The basic concept of iridology has existed for centuries. The medical school of the University of Salerno in Italy offered training in iris diagnosis. A book published by Philippus Meyers in 1670, called *Chiromatica medica*, noted that signs in the iris indicate diseases. Dr. Ignatz von Peczely, however, is generally considered the father of iridology, with the date of his discovery given as 1861. Von Peczely was a Hungarian physician. As a child, he accidentally broke an owl's leg. He observed that a black line formed in the owl's lower iris at the time of the injury. After the owl's leg healed, the young von Peczely noted that the black streak had changed appearance. As a physician, he treated a patient with a broken leg in whose eye he observed a black streak in the same location as on the injured owl's iris. Von Peczely became intrigued by the possibility of a connection between diseases and eye markings. Through observing his patients' eyes, he became convinced of this connection and developed a chart that mapped iris-body correlations. After several decades of comparative study, von Peczely mapped organs across zones identified by hours and minutes on a clock face superimposed over drawings of the eyes. In 1881, he published his theories in a book called *Discoveries in the Field of Natural Science and Medicine: Instruction in the Study of Diagnosis from the Eye.*

A Swedish pastor and homeopath named Nils Liljequist also developed the concept of iris-body correlations at roughly the same time but independently of von Peczely's work. He was the first iridologist to identify the effects of such drugs as **iodine** and quinine on the iris. Liljequist based his initial observations on changes in his own irises after illnesses and injuries, publishing writings and eye drawings during the late nineteenth century. One of his students, Dr. Henry Lahn, brought the practice of iridology to the United States. A variety of practitioners, primarily European, have sought to popularize iridology since these early works. Dr. Bernard Jensen, a chiropractor, is the best-known contemporary American advocate of iridology.

Benefits

Iridologists claim that by studying the patterns of a person's iris, they can provide helpful and accurate health and wellness information. Iridology is a holistic endeavor in that it addresses the person's whole being in the reading. The range of information gleaned encompasses physical, emotional, mental, and spiritual aspects of the person's health picture. In addition to assessing the person's general level of health, readings can reveal other data, including energy quotients; internal areas of irritation, degeneration, injury, or inflammation; nutri-

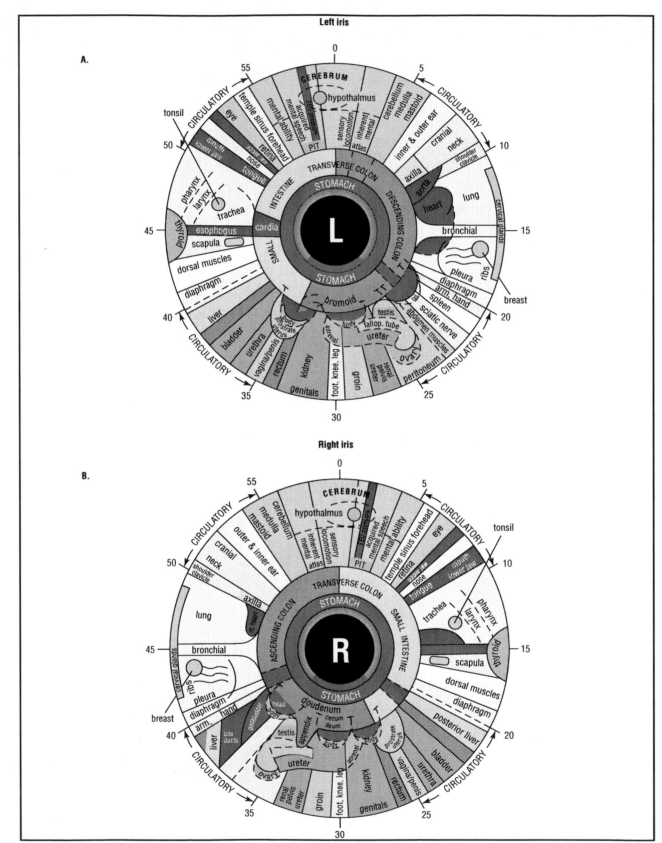

Iridology charts for left and right irises. (Illustration by GGS Information Services, Inc. The Gale Group.)

tional and chemical imbalances; accumulation of toxins; life transitions; and subconscious tensions. Iridologists maintain that the eyes reveal information about the person's physical and emotional constitution, such as inherited weaknesses and risks to which the person may be prone. Strengths may also be revealed, including inherited emotional tendencies from which the person derives particular talents. Cleansing and healing can be verified by changes in the iris. By looking for certain signs such as healing lines, iridologists obtain information about previous health problems and injuries and discover what may have gone wrong in the person's past.

An iridology reading reflects the causes of problems, not symptoms. It may, iridologists claim, reveal that organs or systems are overstressed or predisposed to disease before clinical symptoms even develop. By predicting future problems, iridology can be used as a preventive tool. People can use the information from iridology readings to improve their health and make better behavioral choices in the future, thereby heading off problems before they occur.

In North America, iridology is generally considered to be an assessment tool to be used in cooperation with other health specialties. Iridology is not a diagnostic tool (although it is more likely to be considered so by European iridologists) and should not be used to diagnose or name specific diseases. Not only would diagnosis represent an improper application of iridology according to many iridologists, as noted by the International Iridology Research Association (IIRA), it could also be construed in many countries as practicing medicine without a license.

Description

Iridology is generally based on the concept of neural pathways between the body and the iris. Although iridologists may differ on the exact mechanism, most maintain that the iris reflects what is happening throughout the body via nerve conduction from all parts of the body to the eye. The client's health is assessed by the iridologist, who interprets patterns, shapes, rings, colors and pigmentation markings, fibers, structures, and changes in the pupil and iris. Many iridologists also use sclerology (reading the lines in the white part of the eyes) in their health evaluation.

Iridology readings are typically performed by such holistically oriented practitioners as naturopaths, chiropractors, or nutritionists. The reading may be done using a bright light, a magnifying glass, and a notepad. The iridologist may also use various tools to better view the eye, a special camera to take pictures of the iris, and/or a computer.

Iridologists conduct their readings using charts on which each area of the iris is mapped to a specific body system or organ. Iridology charts vary, with at least 20 different ones in existence. Some charts are more widely used than others; however, many iridologists believe that there is more than one correct map and that each practitioner should become familiar with several charts. Some iridologists even develop their own charts. Differences also exist among practitioner techniques; among American, European, and other approaches; and in the interpretation of specific iris signs.

Iridology charts divide the iris into numerous zones corresponding to different parts of the body. Although the specifics may differ on each chart, all share a general pattern. The left eye is mapped to the left side of the body and the right eye to the right side. The top of the eye is mapped to the upper body (e.g., brain, face, neck, chest and heart). The center of the eye is mapped to the stomach and digestive organs, with other organs being represented by concentric circular zones moving outward toward the edge of the iris. The bottom of the eye is mapped to the legs and lower half of body. Paired organs (e.g., the kidneys) are mapped to both irises.

Using a holistic approach that considers each client as an individual with unique health patterns and concerns, behaviors, and experiences, the iridologist will examine the eyes and make a health assessment. Based on the results of that reading, the iridologist generally recommends a wellness program tailored to the individual's physical, emotional, and life situation. This program may incorporate various health improvement, maintenance, and prevention regimes. Recommendations may include vitamins, minerals, herbs, supplements, and/or diet and **nutrition**, among other suggestions.

Preparation

No special preparations are necessary before an iridology reading.

Precautions

An iridology reading is unlikely to cause any physical harm by itself, as it does not involve direct contact with the eye or applying eye drops of any kind. Critics of iridology, however, argue that iridology can be detrimental to health if a sick person delays treatment for a condition not suggested by the iridology reading; or that it can can cause anguish and unnecessary expense if a reading suggests a problem when there actually is none.

Research & general acceptance

Rita M. Holl, RN, PhD, states that "Within Western medicine, iridology is considered a controversial science at best and medical fraud at worst." Proponents of iridology argue that the practice is time-tested with proven results. Although critics acknowledge that certain symptoms of non-ocular disease do appear in the eyes (e.g., brain injury), there is, they argue, a lack of rigorous scientific testing and no evidence that iridology has any merit. Studies published in the *Australian Journal of Optometry*, the *British Medical Journal*, and the *Journal of the American Medical Association (JAMA)* have found iridologists' assessment of patients with diagnosed serious diseases including kidney and gall bladder disease to be inaccurate. Iridologists counter that the research itself was faulty, citing problems including poor-quality photos; the absence of important additional information including the ability to see/interview the client; and inappropriate expectations of diagnosing specific diseases, a task outside the parameters of iridology. A more recent study conducted to reevaluate *JAMA's* findings in regard to renal failure was published in the *Alternative Health Practitioner*. Acknowledging that the "study leaves several questions unanswered," the author reported both similarities and variations in the iridologists' readings and concluded that the iridologist's level of expertise is extremely important as well.

Training & certification

Iridologists receive training from various sources. They may learn their trade through books, tapes, correspondence courses, online classes, or live classes. According to the IIRA, "Iridology operates in a gray area in North America. In general, there are no laws defining or regulating the practice. In Europe, especially in Germany, Iridology is well recognized and routinely used by natural medicine practitioners." Also according to the IIRA, "Because Iridology has no official standards of practice, anyone can call themselves an Iridologist, often with little training or experience. There are also great differences in the Iridology information being taught, especially in North America."

Resources

BOOKS

Jackson, Adam J. *Iridology: A Guide to Iris Analysis and Preventive Health Care.* Boston: Charles B. Tuttle, 1993.

Jensen, Bernard. *Iridology: Science and Practice in Healing Arts,* Vol. II. Escondido, CA: B. Jensen, 1982.

Jensen, Bernard. *What is Iridology?* Escondido, CA: B. Jensen, 1984.

Jensen, Bernard and Donald Bodeen. *Visions of Health: Understanding Iridology.* Garden City Park, NY: Avery Publishing, 1992.

Worrall, Russell S. "Iridology: Diagnosis or Delusion?" in *Science Confronts the Paranormal,* ed. Kendrick Frazier. Buffalo, NY: Prometheus Books, 1986.

> ### KEY TERMS
> . . . .
> **Iris**—The colored portion of the eye.
>
> **Sclera**—A dense white fibrous membrane that, together with the cornea, forms the outer covering of the eyeball.

ORGANIZATIONS

Canadian Neuro-Optic Research Institute. P.O. Box 29053. 4324 Dewdney Ave. Regina, Saskatchewan S4T 7X3. Canada. (306) 359-7694. Fax: (306) 525-2659. cnricontacts@cnri.edu. http://www.cnri.edu/.

International Iridology Research Association. PO Box 1442. Solano Beach, CA 92075-2208. (888) 682-2208. IIRAOffice@aol.com. http://www.iridologyassn.org/.

OTHER

Quackwatch: Your Guide to Health Fraud, Quackery, and Intelligent Decisions. http://www.quackwatch.com/01QuackeryRelatedTopics/iridology.html.

Kathy Stolley

Iron

Description

Iron is a mineral that the human body uses to produce the red blood cells (hemoglobin) that carry oxygen throughout the body. It is also stored in myoglobin, an oxygen-carrying protein in the muscles that fuels cell growth.

General use

Iron is abundant in red meats, vegetables, and other foods, and a well-balanced diet can usually provide an adequate supply of the mineral. But when there is insufficient iron from dietary sources, or as a result of blood loss in the body, the amount of hemoglobin in the bloodstream is reduced and oxygen cannot be efficiently transported to tissues and organs throughout the body. The resulting condition is known as iron-deficiency **anemia**, and is characterized by **fatigue**, shortness of breath, pale skin, concentration problems, **dizziness**, a weakened immune system, and energy loss.

Iron-deficiency anemia can be caused by a number of factors, including poor diet, heavy menstrual cycles, **pregnancy**, kidney disease, **burns**, and gastrointestinal disorders. Individuals with iron-deficiency anemia should always undergo a thorough evaluation by a physician to determine the cause.

Children two years old and under also need adequate iron in their **diets** to promote proper mental and physical development. Children under two who are not breastfed should eat iron-fortified formulas and cereals. Women who breastfeed need at least 15 mg of dietary or supplementary iron a day in order to pass along adequate amounts of the mineral to their child in breast milk. Parents should consult a pediatrician or other healthcare professional for guidance on iron supplementation in children.

It has been theorized that excess stored iron can lead to **atherosclerosis** and ischemic **heart disease**. Phlebotomy, or blood removal, has been used to reduce stored iron in patients with iron overload with some success. Iron chelation with drugs such as desferrioxamine (Desferal) that help patients excrete excess stores of iron can be helpful in treating iron overload caused by multiple blood transfusions.

Iron levels in the body are measured by both hemoglobin and serum ferritin blood tests.

Normal total hemoglobin levels are:

- neonates: 17-22 g/dl
- one week: 15-20 g/dl
- one month: 11-15 g/dl
- children: 11-13 g/dl
- adult males: 14-18 g/dl (12.4-14.9 g/dl after age 50)
- adult females: 12-16 g/dl (11.7-13.8 g/dl after menopause)

Normal serum ferritin levels are:

- neonates: 25-200 ng/ml
- one month: 200-600 ng/ml
- two to five months: 50-200 ng/ml
- six months to 15 years: 7-140 ng/ml
- adult males: 20-300 ng/ml
- adult females: 20-120 ng/ml

Preparations

Iron can be found in a number of dietary sources, including:

- pumpkin seeds
- dried fruits (apricots)
- lean meats (beef and liver)
- fortified cereals
- turkey (dark meat)
- green vegetables (spinach, kale, and broccoli)
- beans, peas, and lentils
- enriched and whole grain breads
- molasses
- sea vegetables (blue-green algae and kelp)

Eating iron-rich foods in conjunction with foods rich in **vitamin C** (such as citrus fruits) and lactic acid (sauerkraut and yogurt) can increase absorption of dietary iron. Cooking food in cast-iron pots can also add to their iron content.

The recommended dietary allowances (RDA) of iron as outlined by the United States Department of Agriculture (USDA) are as follows:

- Children 0–3: 6-10 mg/day
- children 4–10: 10 mg/day
- adolescent–adult males: 10 mg/day
- adolescent–adult females: 10-15 mg/day
- pregnant females: 30 mg/day
- breastfeeding females: 15 mg/day

A number of herbal remedies contain iron, and can be useful as a natural supplement. The juice of the herb stinging **nettle** (*Urtica dioica*) is rich in both iron and vitamin C (which is thought to promote the absorption of iron). It can be taken daily as a dietary supplement. **Dandelion** (*Taraxacum officinale*), curled dock (*Rumex crispus*), and **parsley** (*Petroselinum crispum*) also have high iron content, and can be prepared in tea or syrup form.

In Chinese medicine, dang gui (**dong quai**), or *Angelica sinensis*, the root of the **angelica** plant, is said to both stimulate the circulatory system and aid the digestive system. It can be administered as a decoction or tincture, and should be taken in conjunction with an iron-rich diet. Other Chinese remedies include **foxglove** root (*Rehmannia glutinosa*), **Korean ginseng** (*Panax ginseng*), and **astragalus** (*Astragalus membranaceus*).

Ferrum phosphoricum (iron phosphate), is used in homeopathic medicine to treat anemia. The remedy is produced by mixing iron sulfate, phosphate, and **sodium** acetate, which is administered in a highly diluted form to the patient. Other homeopathic remedies for anemia include *Natrum muriaticum, Chinchona officinalis, Cyclamen europaeum, Ferrum metallicum,* and *Manganum aceticum.* As with all homeopathic remedies, the type of remedy prescribed for iron deficiency depends on the individual's overall symptom picture, mood, and temperament. Patients should speak with their homeopathic professional or physician, or healthcare professional before taking any of these remedies.

Iron is also available in a number of over-the-counter supplements (i.e., ferrous fumerate, ferrous sulfate, ferrous gluconate, iron dextran). Both heme iron and non-heme iron supplements are available. Heme iron is more efficiently absorbed by the body, but non-heme iron can also be effective if used in conjunction with vitamin C and other dietary sources of heme iron. Some multivitamins also contain supplementary iron. Ingesting excessive iron can be toxic, and may have long-term negative effects. For this reason, iron supplements should be taken only under the recommendation and supervision of a doctor.

Precautions

Iron deficiency can be a sign of a more serious problem, such as internal bleeding. Anyone suffering from iron-deficiency anemia should always undergo a thorough evaluation by a healthcare professional to determine the cause.

Iron overdose in children can be fatal, and is a leading cause of poisoning in children. Children should never take supplements intended for adults, and should receive iron supplementation only under the guidance of a physician.

Individuals with chronic or acute health conditions, including kidney infection, **alcoholism**, liver disease, **rheumatoid arthritis**, **asthma**, heart disease, colitis, and stomach ulcer should consult a physician before taking herbal or pharmaceutical iron supplements.

If individuals taking homeopathic dilutions of *ferrum phosphoricum* experience worsening of their symptoms (known as a homeopathic aggravation), they should stop taking the remedy and contact their healthcare professional. A homeopathic aggravation can be an early indication that a remedy is working properly, but it can also be a sign that a different remedy is needed.

Patients diagnosed with hemochromatosis, a genetic condition in which the body absorbs too much iron and stores the excess in organs and tissues, should never take iron supplements.

Side effects

Taking herbal or pharmaceutical iron supplements on an empty stomach may cause **nausea**. Iron supplementation may cause hard, dark stools, and individuals who take iron frequently experience **constipation**. Patients who experience dark bowel movements accompanied by stomach pains should check with their doctor, as this can also indicate bleeding in the digestive tract.

Other reported side effects include stomach cramps and chest **pain**. These symptoms should be evaluated by a physician if they occur.

Some iron supplements, particularly those taken in liquid form, may stain the teeth. Taking these through a

---

KEY TERMS

Chelation—The use of a medication or herbal substances to inactivate toxic substances in the body. Chelation is used to treat iron overload in some patients.

Decoction—An herbal extract produced by mixing an herb in cold water, bringing the mixture to a boil, and letting it simmer to evaporate the excess water. The decoction is then strained and consumed hot or cold. Decoctions are usually chosen over infusion when the botanical in question is a root or berry.

Ferritin—An iron storage protein found in the blood. High levels of serum ferritin may indicate iron overload.

Hemochromatosis—Also known as iron overload; a genetic condition in which excess iron is stored in the tissues and organs by the body where it can build up to toxic amounts.

Homeopathic remedy—Used to treat illnesses that manifest symptoms similar to those that the remedy itself causes, but administered in extremely diluted doses to prevent any toxic effects.

Infusion—An herbal preparation made by mixing boiling water with an herb, letting the brew steep for 10 minutes, and then straining the herb out of the mixture. Tea is made through infusion.

Thalassemia—A group of several genetic blood diseases characterized by absent or decreased production of normal hemoglobin. Individuals who have thalassemia have to undergo frequent blood transfusions, and are at risk for iron overload.

Tincture—A liquid extract of an herb prepared by steeping the herb in an alcohol and water mixture.

---

straw, or with a dropper placed towards the back of the throat, may be helpful in preventing staining. Toothpaste containing baking soda and/or hydrogen peroxide can be useful in removing iron stains from teeth.

Signs of iron overdose include severe **vomiting**, racing heart, bloody **diarrhea**, stomach cramps, bluish lips and fingernails, pale skin, and weakness. If overdose is suspected, the patient should contact poison control and/or seek emergency medical attention immediately.

Interactions

Iron supplements may react with certain medications, including antacids, acetohydroxamic acid (Lithostat), dimercaprol, etidronate, fluoroquinolones. In addition, they can decrease the effectiveness of certain tetracyclines (antibiotics). Individuals taking these or any other medications should consult their healthcare professional before starting iron supplements.

Certain foods decrease the absorption of iron, including some soy-based foods, foods with large concentrations of **calcium**, and beverages containing **caffeine** and tannin (a substance found in black tea). These should not be taken within two hours of using an iron supplement. Some herbs also contain tannic acid, and should be avoided during treatment with iron supplements. These include allspice (*Pimenta dioica*) and **bayberry** (*Myrica cerifera*, also called wax myrtle).

Individuals considering treatment with homeopathic remedies should also consult their healthcare professional about possible interactions with certain foods, beverages, prescription medications, aromatic compounds, and other environmental elements—factors known in **homeopathy** as *remedy antidotes*—that could counteract the efficacy of treatment for iron deficiency.

Resources

BOOKS

Medical Economics Company. *PDR 2000 Physicians' Desk Reference.* Montvale, NJ: Medical Economics Company, 1998.

Medical Economics Company. *PDR for Herbal Medicines.* Montvale, NJ: Medical Economics Company, 1998.

Ody, Penelope. *The Complete Medicinal Herbal.* New York: DK Publishing, 1993.

PERIODICALS

de Valk, B., and J.J.M. Marx. "Iron, Atherosclerosis, and Ischemic Heart Disease." *Archives of Internal Medicine* 159(i14): 1542.

Paula Ford-Martin

Irritable bowel syndrome

Definition

Irritable bowel syndrome (IBS) is a common intestinal condition characterized by abdominal **pain** and cramps; changes in bowel movements (diarrhea, constipation, or both); gassiness; bloating; **nausea**; and other symptoms. There is no recognized cure for IBS. Much about the condition remains unknown or poorly understood; however, dietary changes, drugs, and psychological treatment are often able to eliminate or substantially reduce its symptoms.

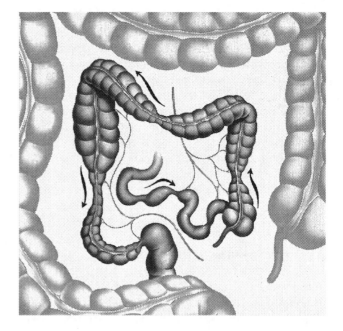

Normal and diseased (center) colons. Areas of constriction in the colon cause constipation, while areas of distention cause diarrhea. *(John Bavosi/Science Photo Library. Custom Medical Stock Photo. Reproduced by permission.)*

Description

IBS is the name people use today for a condition that was once called colitis, spastic colon, nervous colon, spastic bowel, and functional bowel disorder. Some of these names reflected the now-outdated belief that IBS is a purely psychological disorder and a product of the patient's imagination. Although modern medicine recognizes that **stress** can trigger IBS attacks, medical specialists agree that IBS is a genuine physical disorder or group of disorders with specific identifiable characteristics.

No one knows for sure how many Americans suffer from IBS. Surveys indicate a range of 10-20%, with perhaps as many as 30% of Americans experiencing IBS at some point in their lives. IBS normally makes its first appearance during young adulthood, and in half of all cases, symptoms begin before age 35. Women with IBS outnumber men by two to one, for reasons not yet understood. IBS is responsible for more time lost from work and school than any medical problem other than the **common cold**. It accounts for a substantial proportion of the patients seen by gastroenterologists, who are specialists in diseases of the digestive system. Yet only half—possibly as few as 15%—of IBS sufferers ever consult a doctor.

Causes & symptoms

The symptoms of IBS tend to rise and fall in intensity rather than grow steadily worse over time. They always include intestinal (abdominal) pain that may be relieved by defecation; diarrhea or constipation; or diarrhea alternating with constipation. Other symptoms, which vary from person to person, include cramps, gassiness, bloating, nausea, a powerful and uncontrollable urge to defecate (urgency), passage of a sticky fluid (mucus) during bowel movements, or the feeling after finishing a bowel movement that the bowels are still not completely empty. The accepted diagnostic criteria, known as the Rome criteria, require at least three months of continuous or recurrent symptoms before IBS is diagnosed. According to Christine B. Dalton and Douglas A. Drossman in the *American Family Physician,* an estimated 70% of IBS cases can be described as "mild"; 25% as "moderate"; and 5% as "severe." In mild cases the symptoms are slight. As a general rule, they are not present all the time and do not interfere with work and other normal activities. Moderate IBS disrupts normal activities and may cause some psychological problems. People with severe IBS may constantly fear the unpredictable need for a bathroom. They often find living a normal life impossible and experience crippling psychological problems as a result. For some, the physical pain is constant and intense.

Causes

Researchers remain unsure about the cause or causes of IBS. It is called a functional disorder because it is thought to result from changes in the activity of the major part of the large intestine (the colon). After food is digested by the stomach and small intestine, the undigested material passes in liquid form into the colon, which absorbs water and salts. This process may take several days. In a healthy person the colon is quiet during most of that period except after meals, when its muscles contract in a series of wavelike movements called peristalsis. Peristalsis helps absorption by bringing the undigested material into contact with the colon wall. It also pushes undigested material that has been converted into solid or semisolid feces toward the rectum, where it remains until defecation. In IBS, however, the normal rhythm and intensity of peristalsis is disrupted. Sometimes there is too little peristalsis, which can slow the passage of undigested material through the colon and cause constipation. Sometimes there is too much, which has the opposite effect and causes diarrhea. A Johns Hopkins University study found that healthy volunteers experienced six to eight contractions of the colon each day, compared with up to 25 contractions a day for volunteers suffering from IBS with diarrhea, and an almost complete absence of contractions among constipated IBS volunteers. In addition to differences in the number of contractions, many of the IBS volunteers experienced powerful spasmodic contractions affecting a larger-than-normal area of the colon—"like having a Charlie horse in the gut," according to one of the investigators.

DIET. Some kinds of food and drink appear to play a key role in triggering IBS attacks. Food and drink that healthy people can ingest without any trouble may disrupt peristalsis in IBS patients, which probably explains why IBS attacks often occur shortly after meals. Chocolate, milk products, **caffeine** (in coffee, tea, colas, and other drinks), and large quantities of alcohol are some of the chief culprits. Other kinds of food have also been identified as problems, however, and the pattern of what can and cannot be tolerated is different for each person. Characteristically, IBS symptoms rarely occur at night and disrupt the patient's sleep.

In 2002 a research study reported that some children had trouble absorbing certain sugars from some fruit juices, particularly apple and pear juices. When children with IBS went off these juices for one month, 46% saw improvement in their IBS symptoms. Apple and pear juice contain more fructose than glucose sugar, which may be the cause of the poor absorption in IBS sufferers' intestines. Yet white grape juice, which contains almost equal portions of fructose and glucose, is more easily absorbed.

STRESS. Stress is an important factor in IBS because of the close nervous system connections between the brain and the intestines. Although researchers do not yet understand all of the links between changes in the nervous system and IBS, they point out the similarities between mild digestive upsets and IBS. Just as healthy people can feel nauseated or have an upset stomach when under stress, people with IBS react the same way, but to a greater degree. Finally, IBS symptoms sometimes intensify during **menstruation**, which suggests that female reproductive hormones are another trigger. In fact, a study published in 2002 confirmed that IBS symptoms worsened in women and that rectal sensitivity changed with the menstrual cycle in women with IBS. It also was the first study to contrast these changes with those in healthy women.

Diagnosis

Diagnosing IBS is a fairly complex task because the disorder does not produce changes that can be identified during a physical examination or by laboratory tests. When IBS is suspected, the doctor (a family doctor or a specialist) needs to determine whether the patient's symptoms satisfy the Rome criteria. The doctor rules out other conditions that resemble IBS, such as **Crohn's disease** and ulcerative colitis. These disorders are ruled out by taking a standard medical history, performing a physical examination, and ordering laboratory tests. The patient may be asked to provide a stool sample that can be tested for blood and intestinal parasites. In some cases x rays, bowel studies, or an internal examination of the colon using a flexible instrument inserted through the anus (a sigmoidoscope or colonoscope) is necessary.

Patients may also be asked to keep a diary of symptoms for two or three weeks, covering daily activities including meals and emotional responses to events. The doctor can then review the diary with the patient to identify possible problem areas.

Treatment

Dietary adjustments are critical to controlling IBS. For some patients, a **high-fiber diet** including whole grain breads and cereals, dried and fresh fruits, spinach, and oat bran can reduce digestive system irritation. For others, a high-fiber diet aggravates the symptoms. Many patients with IBS also find that avoiding alcohol, caffeine, sugar, and fatty, **gas**-producing, or spicy foods can prevent symptoms.

To control IBS symptoms that are triggered or made worse by stress, several stress management therapies may be helpful. These include **yoga**, **meditation**, hypnosis, **biofeedback**, **exercise**, muscle **relaxation** training, **aromatherapy**, **hydrotherapy**, and **reflexology**. Reflexology is a foot massage technique that focuses on manipulating different regions of the foot in order to bring harmony to specific organs and body systems. Hydrotherapy is the therapeutic use of water, as in a whirlpool bath.

Biofeedback, which teaches an individual to control muscle tension and any associated pain through thought and visualization techniques, is also a treatment option for IBS. In biofeedback treatments, sensors placed on the forehead of the patient are connected to a special machine that allows the patient and healthcare professional to monitor a visual and/or audible readout of the level of muscle tension and stress in the patient. Through relaxation and visualization exercises, the patient learns to relieve tension and can actually see or hear the results of his or her efforts instantly through a sensor readout on the biofeedback equipment. Once the technique is learned and the patient is able to recognize and differentiate between the feelings of muscle tension and muscle relaxation, the biofeedback equipment itself is no longer needed and the patient has a powerful, portable, and self-administered treatment tool to deal with pain and tension.

To soothe an irritated or inflamed digestive tract, an herbalist or holistic healthcare practitioner may recommend one or more herbs, including **comfrey** root (*Symphytum officinale*), **hops** (*Humulus lupulus*), **Iceland moss** (*Cetraria islandica*), Irish moss (*Chondrus crispus*), **marsh mallow** root (*Althaea officinalis*), oats (*Avena sativa*), quince seed (*Cydonia oblonga*), and **slippery elm** (*Ulmus rubra*).

Herbs that relieve gas associated with IBS (known as carminatives) include **angelica** (*Angelica archangelica*), aniseed (*Pimpinella anisum*), caraway (*Carum carvi*), **cayenne** (*Capsicum annuum*), German **chamomile** (*Matricaria recutita*), **ginger** (*Zingiber officinale*), **thyme** (*Thymus vulgaris*), and **peppermint** (*Menthapiperata*).

An infusion of meadowsweet (*Filipendula ulmaria*) may be helpful in treating diarrhea related to IBS, and herbs such as **barberry** (*Berberis vulgaris*), **psyllium** ovata seed, **dandelion** root (*Taraxacum officinale*), **licorice** (*Glycyrrhiza glabra*), and **yellow dock** (*Rumex crispus*) have laxative properties that can help to relieve constipation. More powerful laxative herbs, such as **rhubarb root** (*Rheum palmatum*), **buckthorn** (*Rhamnus catharticus*), and cascara (*Rhamnus purshiana*) should only be taken under the direction of a healthcare professional.

Individuals with cramp-like pains, or **colic**, can benefit from antispasmodic herbs such as German chamomile (*Matricaria recutita*), **Valerian** (*Valeriana officinalis*), **lemon balm** (*Melissa officinalis*), ginger (*Zingiber officinale*), and wild yam (*Dioscorea villosa*).

Homeopathy uses highly-diluted remedies that cause similar effects to the symptoms they are intended to treat in an effort to stimulate the body's natural immune response. A homeopathic physician might recommend a remedy of **belladonna**, *colocynthis* (bitter cucumber), phosphate of magnesia *(Magnesia phosphorica)*, or wild hops (*Bryonia alba*) to relieve abdominal pain and cramping associated with IBS. As with all homeopathic remedies, the prescription depends on the individual's overall symptoms, mood, and temperament.

Acupuncture and **guided imagery** may be useful tools in treating IBS symptoms. Acupuncture involves the placement of thin needles into the skin at targeted locations on the body known as acupoints in order to harmonize the energy flow within the human body. An acupuncturist may also use **moxibustion**, which involves applying a heat source such as warm herbs to the acupoint, to treat IBS symptoms. Guided imagery techniques teach the patient to visualize a peaceful, soothing scene or situation to relax the body and better cope with the discomfort caused by IBS.

Allopathic treatment

Dietary changes, sometimes supplemented by drugs or **psychotherapy**, are considered the key to successful treatment. A drug called alosetron (Lotronex) was approved by the Food and Drug Administration (FDA) in 2002 for limited marketing for treating women with diarrhea-prominent IBS after some controversy in 2000 because of serious side effects from the drug. Its use should be limited to only those patients suffering from severe, chronic diarrhea-predominant IBS who have failed to respond to conventional therapy.

An individualized diet, low in saturated fats and foods that trigger the patient's reaction, can reduce symptoms for many IBS sufferers. Caffeine sources, sugar, and alcohol usually worsen symptoms. Bran or 15-25 grams a day of an over-the-counter psyllium laxative may also help both constipation and diarrhea. The patient can have milk or milk products if lactose intolerance is not a problem. Establishing set times for meals and bathroom visits may help people with irregular bowel habits, especially for constipated patients.

Although a high-fiber diet remains the standard treatment for constipated patients, such laxatives as lactulose or sorbitol may be prescribed. Loperamide and cholestyramine are suggested for diarrhea. Abdominal pain after meals can be reduced by taking antispasmodic drugs such as hyoscyamine or dicyclomine before eating.

Psychological counseling or **behavioral therapy** may be useful for some patients to reduce **anxiety** and to learn to cope with the pain and other symptoms of IBS. Relaxation therapy, hypnosis, biofeedback, and cognitive-behavioral therapy are examples of behavioral therapy.

When IBS produces constant pain that interferes with everyday life, antidepressant drugs can help by blocking pain transmission from the nervous system.

Expected results

IBS is not a life-threatening condition. It does not cause intestinal bleeding or inflammation, nor does it cause other bowel diseases or **cancer**. Although IBS can last a lifetime, in up to 30% of cases the symptoms eventually disappear. Even if the symptoms cannot be eliminated, with appropriate treatment they can usually be decreased so that IBS becomes merely an occasional inconvenience. Treatment requires a long-term commitment, however; six months or more may be needed before the patient notices substantial improvement.

Resources

BOOKS

Lynn, Richard B., and Lawrence S. Friedman. "Irritable Bowel Syndrome." In *Harrison's Principles of Internal Medicine,* edited by Anthony S. Fauci, et al. New York: McGraw-Hill, 1998.

PERIODICALS

"Can Fruit Juices Cause Irritable Bowel Syndrome?" *Child Health Alert* (June 2002):1.

Dalton, Christine B., and Douglas A. Drossman. "Diagnosis and Treatment of Irritable Bowel Syndrome." *American Family Physician* (February 1997): 875+.

Elliott, William T., and James Chan. "Alosetron Hydrochloride Tablets (Lotronex ™ GlaxoSmithKline) Reintroduction." *Internal Medicine Alert* (June 29, 2002): 94.

Houghton L.A. et al. "The Menstrual Cycle Affects Rectal Sensitivity in Patients with Irritable Bowel Syndrome but not Healthy Volunteers." *Gut* (April 2002): 471-474.

"Irritable Bowel Syndrome: Treating the Mind to Treat the Body." *Tufts University Health & Nutrition Letter* (September 1997): 4+.

Maxwell, P. R., M. A. Mendall, and D. Kumar. "Irritable Bowel Syndrome." *The Lancet* 350(1997): 1691+.

ORGANIZATIONS

International Foundation for Functional Gastrointestinal Disorders. PO Box 17864, Milwaukee, WI 53217. (888) 964-2001. http://www.execpc.com/iffgd.

National Digestive Diseases Information Clearinghouse. 2 Information Way, Bethesda, MD 20892-3570. http://www.niddk.nih.gov/health/digest/nddic.htm.

Paula Ford-Martin
Teresa G. Odle

> ## KEY TERMS
>
> **Anus**—The opening at the lower end of the rectum.
>
> **Crohn's disease**—A disease characterized by inflammation of the intestines. Its early symptoms may resemble those of IBS.
>
> **Defecation**—Passage of feces through the anus.
>
> **Feces**—Undigested food and other waste that is eliminated through the anus. Feces are also called fecal matter or stools.
>
> **Homeopathy**—A system of medical practice that treats a disease by administering diluted doses of a remedy that would, in a healthy person, cause symptoms like the illness being treated. Homeopaths believe that this treatment stimulates the body's natural healing processes.
>
> **Lactose**—A sugar found in milk and milk products. Some people are lactose-intolerant, meaning they have trouble digesting lactose. Lactose intolerance can produce symptoms resembling those of IBS.
>
> **Peristalsis**—The periodic waves of muscular contractions that move food through the intestines during the process of digestion.
>
> **Ulcerative colitis**—A disease that inflames and causes breaks (ulcers) in the colon and rectum, which are parts of the large intestine.

Ischemia

Definition

Ischemia is an insufficient supply of oxygenated blood to an organ, usually due to a blocked artery.

Description

Myocardial ischemia is an intermediate condition in coronary artery disease during which the heart tissue is slowly or suddenly starved of oxygen and other nutrients. Eventually, the affected heart tissue will die. When blood flow is completely blocked to the heart, ischemia can lead to a **heart attack**. Ischemia can be silent or symptomatic. According to the American Heart Association, up to four million Americans may have silent ischemia and be at high risk of having a heart attack with no warning.

Symptomatic ischemia is characterized by chest **pain** called **angina** pectoris. The American Heart Association estimates that nearly seven million Americans have angina pectoris, usually called angina. Angina occurs more frequently in women than in men, and more often in African-Americans and Hispanics than in Caucasians. It also occurs more frequently as people age—25% of women over the age of 85 and 27% of men between 80 and 84 years of age have angina.

People with angina are at risk of having a heart attack. Stable angina occurs during exertion, can be quickly relieved by resting or taking nitroglycerine, and lasts from three to 20 minutes. Unstable angina, which increases the risk of a heart attack, occurs more frequently, lasts longer, is more severe, and may cause discomfort during rest or light exertion.

Ischemia also can occur in the arteries of the brain, where blockages can lead to a **stroke**. About 80–85% of all strokes are ischemic. Most blockages in the cerebral arteries are due to a blood clot, often in an artery narrowed by plaque. Sometimes, a blood clot in the heart or aorta travels to a cerebral artery. A transient ischemic attack (TIA) is a "mini-stroke" caused by a temporary deficiency of blood supply to the brain, or by a blood clot briefly blocking a cerebral artery. It occurs suddenly, lasts a few minutes to a few hours, and is a strong warning sign of an impending stroke. Ischemia can also affect intestines, legs, feet, and kidneys. Pain, malfunctions, and damage in those areas may result.

Causes & symptoms

Ischemia almost always is caused by blockage of an artery, usually due to atherosclerotic plaque. Myocardial

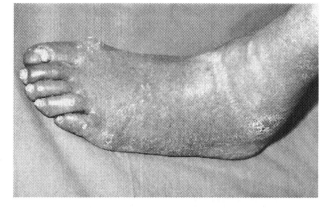

This patient's foot is affected with ischemia. Ischemia occurs when there is an insufficient supply of blood to a specific organ or tissue. (Photograph by Dr. P. Marazzi, Photo Researchers, Inc. Reproduced by permission.)

ischemia also is caused by **blood clots** (which tend to form on plaque), artery spasms or contractions, or any of these factors combined. Silent ischemia usually is caused by emotional or mental **stress** or by exertion, but there are no symptoms. Angina usually is caused by increased oxygen demand when the heart is working harder than usual, for example, during **exercise**, or during mental or physical stress. According to researchers at Harvard University, physical stress is harder on the heart than mental stress.

Risk factors

The risk factors for myocardial ischemia are the same as those for coronary artery disease, TIA, and stroke:

- Heredity. People whose parents have coronary artery disease are more likely to develop it. African-Americans also are at higher risk.

- Sex. Men are more likely to have heart attacks than women, and to have them at a younger age. Angina is more likely to occur in women.

- Age. Men who are 45 years of age and older and women who are 55 years of age and older are considered to be at risk. Risk also increases with age.

- **Smoking**. Smoking increases both the chance of developing coronary artery disease and the chance of dying from it. Secondhand smoke also may increase risk.

- High **cholesterol levels**. Risk of developing coronary artery disease increases as blood cholesterol levels increase. When combined with other factors, the risk is even greater.

- High blood pressure. High blood pressure makes the heart work harder, and with time, weakens it. When combined with **obesity**, smoking, high cholesterol levels, or diabetes, the risk of heart attack or stroke increases several times.

- High fibrinogen levels. Fibrinogens are the proteins involved in blood clotting and plaque formation.

- High homeocysteine levels. Homeocysteine also is involved in plaque formation.

- Oxidant damage, as indicated by high lipid peroxide levels. High lipid peroxide levels represent a high level of free radical damage and antioxidant deficiency.

- Lack of physical activity. Lack of **exercise** increases the risk of coronary artery disease.

- Diabetes mellitus. The risk of developing coronary artery disease is seriously increased for diabetics.

- Obesity. Excess weight increases the strain on the heart and increases the risk of developing coronary artery disease, even if no other risk factors are present. Obesity increases blood pressure and blood cholesterol, and can lead to diabetes.

- Stress and anger. Some scientists believe that stress and anger can contribute to the development of coronary artery disease. Stress increases the heart rate and blood pressure and can injure the lining of the arteries. Angina attacks often occur after outbursts of anger, as do many heart attacks and strokes.

Angina symptoms include:

- a tight, squeezing, heavy, burning, or choking pain that is usually beneath the breastbone—the pain may spread to the throat, jaw, or one arm

- a feeling of heaviness or tightness that is not painful

- a feeling similar to **gas** or indigestion

- attacks brought on by exertion and relieved by rest

If the pain or discomfort continues or intensifies, immediate medical help should be sought, ideally within 30 minutes.

TIA symptoms include:

- sudden weakness, tingling, or numbness, usually in one arm or leg or both the arm and leg on the same side of the body, as well as sometimes in the face

- sudden loss of coordination

- loss of vision or double vision

- difficulty speaking

- vertigo and loss of balance

Diagnosis

Diagnostic tests for myocardial ischemia include: resting, exercise, or ambulatory electrocardiograms; scintigraphic studies (radioactive heart scans); echocar-

diography; coronary angiography; and, rarely, positron emission tomography. Diagnostic tests for TIA include physician review of symptoms, computed tomography (CT) scans, carotid artery ultrasound (Doppler ultrasonography), and magnetic resonance imaging (MRI). Angiography is the best test for ischemia of any organ.

An electrocardiogram (ECG) shows the heart's activity and may reveal a lack of oxygen. Electrodes covered with conducting jelly are placed on the patient's chest, arms, and legs. Impulses of the heart's activity are recorded on paper. The test takes about 10 minutes and is performed in a physician's office. About 25% of patients with angina have normal electrocardiograms. Another type of electrocardiogram, the exercise stress test, measures response to exertion when the patient is exercising on a treadmill or a stationary bike. It is performed in a physician's office or an exercise laboratory and takes 15–30 minutes. This test is more accurate than a resting ECG in diagnosing ischemia. Sometimes an ambulatory ECG is ordered. For this test, the patient wears a portable ECG machine called a Holter monitor for 12, 24, or 48 hours.

Myocardial perfusion scintigraphy and radionuclide angiography are nuclear studies involving the injection of a radioactive material (e.g., thallium), that is absorbed by healthy tissue. A gamma scintillation camera displays and records a series of images of the radioactive material's movement through the heart. Both tests usually are performed in a hospital's nuclear medicine department and take about 30 minutes to an hour. A perfusion scan sometimes is performed at the end of a stress test.

An echocardiogram uses sound waves to create an image of the heart's chambers and valves. The technologist applies gel to a handheld transducer, then presses it against the patient's chest. The heart's sound waves are converted into an image on a monitor. Performed in a cardiology outpatient diagnostic laboratory, the test takes 30 minutes to an hour. It can reveal abnormalities in the heart wall that indicate ischemia, but it does not evaluate the coronary arteries directly.

Coronary angiography is the most accurate diagnostic technique, but it also is the most invasive. It shows the heart's chambers, great vessels, and coronary arteries by using a contrast solution and x-ray technology. A moving picture is recorded of the blood flow through the coronary arteries. The patient is awake, but sedated, and connected to ECG electrodes and an intravenous line. A local anesthetic is injected. The cardiologist then inserts a catheter into a blood vessel and guides it into the heart. Coronary angiography is performed in a cardiac catheterization laboratory and takes from 30 minutes to two hours.

Positron emission tomography (PET) is a noninvasive nuclear test used to evaluate the heart tissue. A PET scanner traces high-energy gamma rays released from radioactive particles to provide three-dimensional images of the heart tissue. Performed at a hospital, it usually takes from one hour to one hour and 45 minutes.

CT and MRI are computerized scanning methods. CT scanning uses a thin x-ray beam to show three-dimensional views of soft tissues. It is performed at a hospital or clinic and takes only minutes. MRI uses a magnetic field to produce clear, cross-sectional images of soft tissues. The patient lies on a table that slides into a tunnel-like scanner for about 30 minutes.

Treatment

Ischemia can be life-threatening. Although there are alternative treatments for angina, traditional medical care may be necessary. Prevention of the cause of ischemia, primarily **atherosclerosis**, is primary. This becomes even more important for people with a family history of **heart disease**.

Nutritional therapy

Dietary modifications are essential in the treatment and prevention of ischemic heart disease. The following dietary changes are recommended:

- Limiting intake of red meat and animal fats that contain high amounts of cholesterol and saturated fats.

- Eating a heart-wise diet with emphasis on fresh fruits and vegetables, grains, beans, and nuts. Increased fiber (found in fresh fruits and vegetables, grains, and beans) can help the body eliminate excessive cholesterol through the stools.

- Avoiding coffee (caffienated and decaffeinated) and smoking. Not smoking will prevent damage from smoke and the harmful substances (oxidants) it contains.

- Taking high-potency multivitamin/mineral supplement (one tablet daily). Heart patients may require higher amounts of **antioxidants**, such as vitamins C and E. They should aim for total daily intake of 500–1,000 mg of **vitamin C** and 400–800 IU of (natural) **vitamin E**. They also should take 1 tbsp of **flaxseed** oil or **fish oil** per day. Flaxseed oil is a good source of omega-3 oils. Numerous studies have demonstrated the cardio-protective effects of omega-3 fatty acids.

- Considering supplements for specific health problems. Individuals with diabetes might benefit from **chromium**, **garlic**, and pantethine supplements. **Niacin**, flaxseed oil, and garlic help treat elevated fibrinogen levels. For those with high homocysteine levels, vitamin B_6, B_{12}, and **folic acid** may be needed. Patients with high lipid peroxide

levels require more antioxidants to prevent free radical damage. Antioxidants, such as vitamins C and E, **selenium**, *Ginkgo biloba*, **bilberry** (*Vaccinium myrtillus*), and **hawthorn**, can help prevent initial arterial injury that can lead to the formation of plaque deposits. In fact, a 2001 report indicated that patients saw clinical improvements in exercise tolerance, **fatigue**, and shortness of breath when using hawthorn extract.

Herbal therapy

Western herbal medicine recommends hawthorn (*Crataegus laevigata* or *C. oxyacantha*) to help prevent long-term angina, since this herb strengthens heart muscles' ability to contract.

Homeopathy

Cactus grandiflorus is a homeopathic remedy made from night-blooming cactus and used for pain relief during an attack.

Ayurvedic medicine

Abana, a mixture of herbs and minerals used in Ayurvedic medicine, may reduce the frequency and severity of angina attacks.

Exercises

Exercise, particularly aerobic exercise, is essential for circulation health. It is recommended that the patient exercise for 20 minutes, three times a week.

Mind/body medicine

Mind/body **relaxation** techniques such as **yoga**, **meditation**, stress reduction, and **biofeedback** can help control strong emotions and stress.

Chelation therapy

The use of **chelation therapy**, a long-term injection by a physician of a cocktail of synthetic amino acid, ethylenediaminetetracetic acid, and anticoagulant drugs and nutrients, is controversial.

Allopathic treatment

Angina is treated with drug therapy and surgery. Drugs such as nitrates, beta-blockers, and **calcium** channel blockers relieve chest pain, but they cannot clear blocked arteries. In 2003, it was reported that administering testosterone to men with myocardial ischemia helped reduce the ischemia. Another study in patients with Type II diabetes used intensive therapy combining lifestyle interventions, aspirin and such dietary supplements as vitamins E and C, as well as certain prescribed drugs. These patients showed fewer cardiovascular events such as heart attack and stroke, than those treated more conservatively. Aspirin helps prevent blood clots. Surgical procedures include percutaneous transluminal coronary angioplasty and coronary artery bypass graft surgery.

Nitroglycerin is the classic treatment for angina. It quickly relieves pain and discomfort by opening the coronary arteries and allowing more blood to flow to the heart. Beta-blockers reduce the amount of oxygen required by the heart during stress. Calcium channel blockers help keep the arteries open and reduce blood pressure. Aspirin helps prevent blood clots from forming on plaques. Statins help reduce cholesterol levels, which can lessen ischemic events.

Percutaneous transluminal coronary angioplasty and coronary artery bypass graft surgery are invasive procedures that improve blood flow in the coronary arteries. Percutaneous transluminal coronary angioplasty is a nonsurgical procedure in which a catheter tipped with a balloon is threaded from a blood vessel in the thigh into the blocked artery. The balloon is inflated, compressing the plaque to enlarge the blood vessel and open the blocked artery. The balloon is deflated and the catheter is removed. Sometimes a metal stent is placed in the artery to prevent closing.

In coronary artery bypass graft, called bypass surgery, a detour is built around the coronary artery blockage with a healthy leg vein or chest wall artery. The healthy vein or artery then supplies oxygen-rich blood to the heart. Bypass surgery is major surgery appropriate for patients with blockages in two or three major coronary arteries or severely narrowed left main coronary arteries, as well as those who have not responded to other treatments.

There are several experimental surgical procedures: atherectomy, in which the surgeon shaves off and removes strips of plaque from the blocked artery; laser angioplasty, in which a catheter with a laser tip is inserted to burn or break down the plaque; and insertion of a metal coil, called a stent, that can be implanted permanently to keep a blocked artery open. This stenting procedure is becoming more common. An experimental procedure uses a laser to drill channels in the heart muscle to increase blood supply.

TIAs are treated by drugs that control high blood pressure and reduce the likelihood of blood clots and surgery. Aspirin is commonly used and anticoagulants are sometimes used to prevent blood clots. In some cases, carotid endarterectomy surgery is performed to help prevent further TIAs. The procedure involves removing arterial plaque from inside blood vessels.

Expected results

In many cases, ischemia can be successfully treated, but the underlying disease process of atherosclerosis is usually not "cured." New diagnostic techniques enable doctors to identify ischemia earlier. New technologies and surgical procedures can prevent angina from leading to a heart attack or TIA from resulting in a stroke. The outcome for patients with silent ischemia has not been well established.

Prevention

A healthy lifestyle, including eating a well-balanced diet, getting regular exercise, maintaining a healthy weight, not smoking, drinking in moderation, not using illegal drugs, controlling **hypertension**, and managing stress are practices that can reduce the risk of ischemia progressing to a heart attack or stroke.

A healthy diet includes a variety of foods that are low in fat (especially saturated fat), low in cholesterol, and high in fiber. Plenty of fruits and vegetables should be eaten and **sodium** intake should be limited. Fat should comprise no more than 30% of total daily calories. Cholesterol should be limited to about 300 mg and sodium to about 2,400 mg per day.

Moderate aerobic exercise lasting about 30 minutes four or more times per week is recommended for maximum heart health, according to the Centers for Disease Control and Prevention and the American College of Sports Medicine. Three 10-minute exercise periods also are beneficial. If any risk factors are present, a physician's clearance should be obtained before starting exercise.

Maintaining a desirable body weight also is important. People who are 20% or more over their ideal body weight have an increased risk of developing coronary artery disease or stroke.

Smoking has many adverse effects on the heart and arteries, and should be avoided. Heart damage caused by smoking can be improved by quitting. Several studies have shown that ex-smokers face the same risk of heart disease as nonsmokers within five to ten years after quitting.

Excessive drinking can increase risk factors for heart disease. Modest consumption of alcohol, however, can actually protect against coronary artery disease. The American Heart Association defines moderate consumption as one ounce of alcohol per day—roughly one cocktail, one 8-oz glass of wine, or two 12-oz glasses of beer.

Commonly used illegal drugs can seriously harm the heart and should never be used. Even stimulants like **ephedra** and decongestants like pseudoephedrine can be harmful to patients with hypertension or heart disease.

Treatment should be sought for hypertension. High blood pressure can be completely controlled through lifestyle changes and medication. Stress, which can increase the risk of a heart attack or stroke, should also be managed. While it cannot always be avoided, it can be controlled.

Resources

BOOKS

American Heart Association. *Heart Attack Treatment, Prevention, Recovery.* New York: Time Books, 1996.

"Angina." In *The Alternative Advisor: The Complete Guide to Natural Therapies & Alternative Treatments.* Alexandria, VA: Time-Life Books, 1997.

DeBakey, Michael E., and Antonio M. Gotto Jr. "Coronary Artery Disease Stroke." In *The New Living Heart.* Holbrook, MA: Adams Media Corporation, 1997.

Iskandrian, A.S., and Mario S. Verani. "Scintigraphic Techniques in Acute Ischemic Syndromes." In *Nuclear Cardiac Imaging: Principles and Applications.* 2nd ed. Philadelphia: F.A. Davis, 1996.

Murray, Michael T., and Joseph E. Pizzorno. "Heart and Cardiovascular Health." In *Encyclopedia of Natural Medicine.* 2nd ed. Rocklin, CA: Prima Publishing, 1998.

Tierney Lawrence M., Jr., Stephen J. McPhee, and Maxine A. Papadakis. "Coronary Heart Disease (Arteriosclerotic Coronary Artery Disease; Ischemic Heart Disease)." In *Current Medical Diagnosis & Treatment,* 36th ed. Stamford, CT: Appleton & Lange, 1997.

PERIODICALS

"Administration of Testosterone Reduces Myocardial Ischemia." *Cardiovascular Week* (March 31, 2003): 4.

Geraci, Ron, and Duane Swierczynski. "Short Strokes." *Men's Health* (September 1997): 56.

"How Mental Stress Taxes the Heart." *Harvard Health Letter* (March 1997): 2.

Huffman, Grace B. "Reducing Ischemic Events in Acute Coronary Syndrome." *American Family Physician* 64, no. 19 (November 1, 2001): 1613.

"Ischemic Heart Disease." *Heart* (April 2003): 471.

Walsh, Nancy. "Hawthorn Extract Limits CHF, Mild Heart Ailments." *Internal Medicine News* 34, no. 19 (October 1, 2001): 9.

ORGANIZATIONS

American Heart Association. National Center. 7272 Greenville Avenue, Dallas, TX 75231-4596. (214) 373-6300. <http://www.medsearch.com/pf/profiles/amerh>.

National Heart, Lung, and Blood Institute Information Center. P.O. Box 30105, Bethesda, MD 20824-0105. <http://www.nhlbi.gov/nhlbi/nhbli.htm>.

Texas Heart Institute Heart Information Service. P.O. Box 20345, Houston, TX 77225-0345. (800)292-2221. <http://www.tmc.edu/thi/his.html>.

Mai Tran
Teresa G. Odle

Italian diet *see* **Mediterranean diet**

Itching

Definition

Itching is an intense, distracting irritation or tickling sensation that may be felt all over the skin's surface or confined to just one area. The medical term for itching is pruritus.

Description

Itching leads most people instinctively to scratch the affected area. Different people can tolerate different amounts of itching, and anyone's threshold of tolerance can be changed due to **stress**, emotions, and other factors. In general, itching is more severe if the skin is warm, and if there are few distractions. This is why people tend to notice itching more at night.

Causes & symptoms

As of 2002, the recent discovery of itch-specific neurons (nerve cells) has given doctors a better understanding of the causes of the sensation of itching. Another factor that contributes to itching is the release of endogenous opioids in the body. While these chemicals function primarily to relieve **pain**, they also appear to enhance the sensation of itching. Although itching is the most noticeable symptom of many skin diseases, however, it doesn't necessarily mean that a person who feels itchy has a disease.

Stress and emotional upset can make itching worse, no matter what the underlying cause. If emotional problems are the primary reason for feeling itchy, the condition is known as psychogenic itching. Some people become convinced that their itch is caused by a parasite or some medical disorder. This conviction is often linked to burning sensations in the tongue, and may be caused by a major psychiatric disorder.

Generalized itching

Itching that occurs all over the body may indicate a medical condition such as **diabetes mellitus**, liver disease, kidney failure, **jaundice**, thyroid disorders, and rarely, **cancer**. Blood disorders such as **leukemia**, and lymphatic conditions such as **Hodgkin's disease** may sometimes cause itching as well.

Some people may develop an itch without a rash when they take certain drugs (such as aspirin, codeine, cocaine). Others may develop an itchy, red "drug rash" or **hives** because of an allergy to a specific drug.

A team of researchers in Texas has discovered that some people infected by *Helicobacter pylori*, a bacterium that causes **gastritis**, also develop itching that does not respond to usual treatments. When the bacterium is eradicated from the patient's digestive tract, the itching is relieved.

Itching also may be caused when hookworm larvae penetrate the skin. This type of itching includes swimmer's itch, creeping eruptions caused by cat or dog hookworm, and ground itch caused by the "true" hookworm.

Skin conditions that cause an itchy rash include:

- atopic **dermatitis**
- chickenpox
- **contact dermatitis**
- dermatitis herpetiformis (occasionally)
- **eczema**
- fungal **infections** (such as **athlete's foot**)
- hives (urticaria)
- insect bites
- lice
- lichen planus
- neurodermatitis (lichen simplex chronicus)
- **psoriasis** (occasionally)
- scabies

Itching all over the body can be caused by something as simple as bathing too often, which removes the skin's natural oils and may make the skin too dry and scaly.

Localized itching

Specific itchy areas may occur if a person comes in contact with soaps, detergents, and wool or other rough-textured, scratchy material. Adults who have **hemorrhoids**, anal fissures, or persistent **diarrhea** may notice pruritus ani (itching around the anus). In children, itching in this area is most likely due to **worms**.

Intense itching called pruritus vulvae (itching of the external genitalia in women) may be due to a **yeast infection**, hormonal changes, contact dermatitis, or the use of certain spermicides, vaginal suppositories, ointments, or deodorants.

It's also common for older people to suffer from dry, itchy skin (especially on the back) for no obvious reason. Moreover, older people are more likely to develop itching as a side effect of prescription medications. Younger people may notice dry, itchy skin in cold weather. Itching is also a common complaint during **pregnancy**.

Diagnosis

Itching is a symptom that is quite obvious to its victim. Someone who itches all over should seek medical care. Because itching can be caused by such a wide variety of triggers, a complete physical exam and medical history will help diagnose the underlying problem. A variety of blood and stool tests may help determine the underlying cause.

Treatment

In general, itchy skin should be treated very gently. While scratching may temporarily ease the itch, in the long run scratching just makes it worse. In addition, scratching can lead to an endless cycle of more itching and scratching.

To control the urge to scratch, a person can apply a cooling or soothing lotion or cold compress to the area. Itching may be relieved by applying a warm compress of diluted vinegar, preferably such herbal vinegars as **plantain**, violet, **lavender**, or rose.

The itching associated with mosquito bites can be reduced by applying meat tenderizer paste, table salt (to wet skin), or toothpaste. Any alkaline preparation (like a paste of baking soda and **water**) will help ease the itch.

Probably the most common cause of itching is dry skin. **Flaxseed** oil and **vitamin E** taken orally can help to rehydrate dry skin and can reduce itching. There are a number of simple things a person can do to relieve itching.

• Don't wear tight clothes.

• Avoid synthetic fabrics.

• Don't take long baths.

• Wash the area in lukewarm water with a little baking soda.

• Take a lukewarm shower for generalized itching.

• Try a lukewarm oatmeal (or Aveeno) bath for generalized itching.

• Apply bath oil or lotion (without added colors or scents) right after bathing.

Practitioners of Chinese medicine utilize a wide variety of herbs as well as **acupuncture** and ear acupuncture to treat itching based upon the cause. The medicine Xiao Feng Zhi Yang Chong Ji (Eliminate Wind and Relieve Itching Infusion) can be taken three times daily to relieve itching. For external treatment of itching, the patient may bathe in Zhi Yang Xi Ji (Relieve Itching Washing Preparation) and apply She Chuang Zi Ding (Cnidium Tincture) and Zhi Yang Po Fen (Relieve Itching Powder).

Emotional stress can trigger many different dermatoses, including certain itching **rashes**. Hypnosis has been helpful in treating atopic dermatitis, itching, psoriasis, hives, and other dermatoses.

In several small studies, transcutaneous electrical nerve stimulation (TENS) has been effective in temporarily relieving chronic itch associated with varying dermatoses. TENS is a treatment in which mild electrical current is passed through electrodes on the skin to stimulate nerves and block pain signals. Portable TENS units are available for home use.

Cutaneous field stimulation (CFS) was found to safely relieve experimentally induced itching for a longer time period than TENS. CFS electrically stimulates nerves in the skin to harmlessly mimic scratching and inhibit the itch sensation.

Herbal itch remedies

The following herbal remedies for itching are used externally:

• aloe vera

• bracken juice

• bird-of-paradise (*Strelitzia reginae*) flowers

• cabbage leaf poultice

• cattail (*Typha latifolia*) juice

• chickweed (*Stellaria media*) salve

• comfrey (*Symphytum officinale*) juice

• evening primrose (*Oenothera biennis*) oil

• heal-all (*Prunella vulgaris*) juice

• honeysuckle vine flowers and leaves

• marigold (*Calendula officinalis*)

• marsh mallow (*Althaea officinalis*) leaf poultice

• myrrh (*Commiphora* species) oil

• oats (*Avena sativa*) bath or poultice

• onion juice

• papaya fruit

• plantain (*Plantago major*) juice or poultice

• red pepper juice

• Sage (*Salvia officinalis*) leaves

• St. John's wort (*Hypericum perforatum*)

• tea tree (*Melaleuca alternifolia*) oil

• yellow dock (*Rumex crispus*) tea bath

Allopathic treatment

Specific treatment of itching depends on the underlying cause. Such antihistamines as diphenhydramine (Benadryl) can help relieve itching caused by hives but won't affect itching from other causes. Most antihistamines also make people sleepy, which can help patients sleep who would otherwise be awake from the itch. Newer antihistamines that do not make people drowsy as a side effect are also available to treat itching.

Creams or ointments containing cortisone may help control itching from insect bites, contact dermatitis, or eczema. Cortisone cream should not be applied to the face unless a doctor prescribes it, and should not be used over the body for prolonged periods without a doctor's approval.

A newer medication that relieves the itching associated with **burns** as well as speeding the healing process is called dexpanthenol. Dexpanthenol helps to relieve the itching by preventing the affected skin from drying out.

Expected results

Most cases of itching go away when the underlying cause is treated successfully.

Prevention

Soaps are often irritating and drying to the skin and can make an itch worse. They should be avoided or used only when necessary. People who tend to have itchy skin should:

- Avoid bathing daily.
- Use lukewarm water when bathing.
- Use mild soap.
- Pat (not rub) the skin dry after bathing, leaving some water on the skin.
- Apply a moisturizer immediately after the bath but avoid lanolin products.
- Use a humidifier, particularly during heating season in colder climates.

Eating **garlic** and onion and taking vitamin B supplements may help to repel mosquitoes. Application of cedar, sage, **pennyroyal**, **rosemary**, artemisia, or marigold to the skin may also repel mosquitoes

Resources

BOOKS

Turkington, Carol A., and Jeffrey S. Dover. *Skin Deep: An A to Z of Skin Disorders, Treatments and Health.* New York: Facts on File, 1998.

Ying, Zhou Zhong, and Jin Hui De. "Cutaneous Pruritus." *Clinical Manual of Chinese Herbal Medicine and Acupuncture.* New York: Churchill Livingston, 1997.

PERIODICALS

Black, A. K., and M. W. Greaves. "Antihistamines in Urticaria and Angioedema." *Clinical Allergy and Immunology* 17 (2002): 249-286.

Ebner, F., A. Heller, F. Rippke, and I. Tausch. "Topical Use of Dexpanthenol in Skin Disorders." *American Journal of Clinical Dermatology* 3 (2002): 427-433.

Kandyil, R., N. S. Satya, and R. A. Swerlick. "Chronic pruritus associated with *Helicobacter pylori.*" *Journal of Cutaneous Medicine and Surgery* 6 (March-April 2002): 103-108.

Nilsson, Hans-Jörgen, Anders Levinsson, and Jens Schouenborg. "Cutaneous Field Stimulation (CFS): A New Powerful Method to Combat Itch." *Pain* 71 (1997): 49-55.

Schmelz, M. "Itch—Mediators and Mechanisms." *Journal of Dermatologic Science* 28 (February 2002): 91-96.

Shenefelt, Philip D. "Hypnosis in Dermatology." *Archives of Dermatology* 136 (March 2000): 393-399.

Stander, S., and M. Steinhoff. "Pathophysiology of Pruritus in Atopic Dermatitis: An Overview." *Experimental Dermatology* 11 (February 2002): 12-24.

Tang, William Yuk Ming, Loi Yuen Chan, Kuen Kong Lo, and Tze Wai Wong. "Evaluation of the Antipruritic Role of Transcutaneous Electrical Nerve Stimulation in the Treatment of Pruritic Dermatoses." *Dermatology* 199 (1999): 237-241.

Yoon, S., J. Lee, and S. Lee. "The Therapeutic Effect of Evening Primrose Oil in Atopic Dermatitis Patients with Dry Scaly Skin Lesions Is Associated with the Normalization of Serum Gamma-Interferon Levels." *Skin Pharmacology and Applied Skin Physiology* 15 (January-February 2002): 20-25.

KEY TERMS

Atopic dermatitis—An intensely itchy inflammation often found on the face of people prone to allergies. In infants and early childhood, it's called infantile eczema.

Creeping eruption—Itchy irregular, wandering red lines on the skin made by burrowing larvae of the hookworm family and some roundworms. Also called cutaneous larva migrans.

Dermatitis herpetiformis—A chronic, very itchy skin disease with groups of red lesions that leave spots behind when they heal. It is sometimes associated with cancer of an internal organ.

Eczema—A superficial type of inflammation of the skin that may be very itchy and weeping in the early stages; later, the affected skin becomes crusted, scaly, and thick. There is no known cause.

Endogenous opioids—Natural pain relievers produced by the body that are also associated with the sensation of itching.

Hodgkin's disease—A type of cancer characterized by slowly enlarging lymph tissue; symptoms include generalized itching.

Lichen planus—A noncancerous, chronic, itchy skin disease that causes small flat purple plaques on wrists, forearm, and ankles.

Neurodermatitis—An itchy skin disease (also called lichen simplex chronicus) found in nervous, anxious people.

Psoriasis—A common, chronic skin disorder that causes red patches anywhere on the body.

Scabies—A contagious parasitic skin disease characterized by intense itching.

Swimmer's itch—An allergic skin inflammation caused by a sensitivity to flatworms that die under the skin, causing an itchy rash.

ORGANIZATIONS

American Academy of Dermatology. 930 N. Meacham Rd., PO Box 4014, Schaumburg, IL 60168. (708) 330-0230.

Belinda Rowland
Rebecca J. Frey, PhD

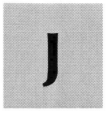

J

Japanese traditional medicine *see* **Kampo medicine**

Jaundice

Definition

Jaundice is a condition in which a person's skin and the whites of the eyes are discolored yellow due to an increased level of bile pigments in the blood resulting from liver disease. Jaundice is sometimes called *icterus*, from a Greek word for "the condition."

Description

In order to understand jaundice, it is useful to know about the role of the liver in producing bile. The most important function of the liver is the metabolic processing of chemical waste products like **cholesterol**, and excreting them into the intestines as bile. The liver is the premier chemical factory in the body—most incoming and outgoing chemicals pass through it. It is the first stop for all nutrients, toxins, and drugs absorbed by the digestive tract. The liver also collects chemicals from the blood for processing. Many of these outward bound chemicals are excreted into the bile. One particular substance, bilirubin, is yellow. Bilirubin is a product of the breakdown of hemoglobin, which is the protein inside red blood cells. If bilirubin cannot leave the body, it accumulates and discolors other tissues. The normal total level of bilirubin in blood serum is between 0.2 mg/dL and 1.2 mg/dL. When it rises to 3 mg/dL or higher, the person's skin and the whites of the eyes become noticeably yellow.

Bile is formed in the liver. It then passes into the network of hepatic bile ducts, which join to form a single tube. A branch of this tube carries bile to the gallbladder, where it is stored, concentrated, and released on a signal from the stomach. Food entering the stomach is the signal that stimulates the gallbladder to release the bile. The

tube, which is called the common bile duct, continues to the intestines. Before the common bile duct reaches the intestines, it is joined by another duct from the pancreas. The bile and the pancreatic juice enter the intestine through a valve called the ampulla of Vater. After entering the intestine, the bile and pancreatic secretions together help in the process of digestion.

Causes & symptoms

There are many different causes for jaundice, but they can be divided into three categories based on where they start—before (pre-hepatic), in (hepatic), or after (post-hepatic) the liver. When bilirubin begins its life cycle, it cannot be dissolved in water. Thus, the liver changes it so that it is soluble in water. These two types of bilirubin are called unconjugated (insoluble) and conjugated (soluble). Blood tests can easily distinguish between these two types of bilirubin.

Hemoglobin and bilirubin formation

Bilirubin begins as hemoglobin in the blood-forming organs, primarily the bone marrow. If the production of red blood cells (RBCs) falls below normal, the extra hemoglobin finds its way into the bilirubin cycle and adds to the pool.

Once hemoglobin is in the red cells of the blood, it circulates for the life span of those cells. The hemoglobin that is released when the cells die is turned into bilirubin. If for any reason the RBCs die at a faster rate than usual, then bilirubin can accumulate in the blood and cause jaundice.

Hemolytic disorders

Many disorders speed up the death of red blood cells. The process of red blood cell destruction is called hemolysis, and the diseases that cause it are called hemolytic disorders. If red blood cells are destroyed faster than they can be produced, the patient develops **anemia**.

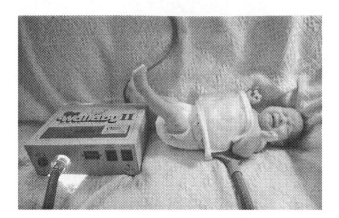

A newborn receives home health care to treat jaundice with Bilirubin Lights. *(Photograph by Cindy Roesinger, Photo Researchers, Inc. Reproduced by permission.)*

Hemolysis can occur in a number of diseases, disorders, conditions, and medical procedures:

- **Malaria**. The malaria parasite develops inside red blood cells. When it is mature it breaks the cell apart and swims off in the blood. This process happens to most of the parasites simultaneously, causing the intermittent symptoms of the disease. When enough cells burst at once, jaundice may result from the large amount of bilirubin formed from the hemoglobin in the dead cells. The pigment may reach the urine in sufficient quantities to cause "blackwater fever," an often lethal form of malaria.

- Side effects of certain drugs. Some common drugs can cause hemolysis as a rare but sudden side effect. These medications include some antibiotic and antituberculosis medicines; drugs that regulate the heartbeat; and levodopa, a drug used to treat Parkinson's disease.

- Certain drugs in combination with a hereditary enzyme deficiency known as glucose–6–phosphate dehydrogenase (G6PD). G6PD is a deficiency that affects more than 200 million people in the world. Some of the drugs listed above are more likely to cause hemolysis in people with G6PD. Other drugs cause hemolysis only in people with this disorder. Most important among these drugs are such antimalarial medications, as quinine, and vitamins C and K.

- Poisons. Snake and spider venom, certain bacterial toxins, **copper**, and some organic industrial chemicals directly attack the membranes of red blood cells.

- Artificial heart valves. The inflexible moving parts of heart valves damage RBCs as they flutter back and forth. This damage is one reason to recommend pig valves and valves made of other organic materials.

- Hereditary RBC disorders. There are a number of hereditary defects that affect the blood cells. There are many genetic mutations that affect the hemoglobin itself, the best known of which is sickle cell disease. Such hereditary disorders as spherocytosis weaken the outer membrane of the red cell. There are also inherited defects that involve the internal chemistry of RBCs.

- Enlargement of the spleen. The spleen is an organ that is located near the upper end of the stomach and filters the blood. It is supposed to filter out and destroy only worn-out RBCs. If it has become enlarged, it filters out normal cells as well. Malaria, other **infections**, cancers and leukemias, some of the hereditary anemias mentioned above, obstruction of blood flow from the spleen—all these and many more diseases can enlarge the spleen to the point where it removes too many red blood cells.

- Diseases of the small blood vessels. Hemolysis that occurs in diseased small blood vessels is called microangiopathic hemolysis. It results from damage caused by rough surfaces on the inside of the capillaries. The RBCs squeeze through capillaries one at a time and can easily be damaged by scraping against the vessel walls.

- Immune reactions to RBCs. Several types of **cancer** and immune system diseases produce antibodies that react with RBCs and destroy them. In 75% of cases, this reaction occurs all by itself, with no underlying disease to account for it.

- Transfusions. If a patient is given an incompatible blood type, hemolysis results.

- Kidney failure and other serious diseases. Several diseases are characterized by defective blood coagulation that can destroy red blood cells.

- Erythroblastosis fetalis. Erythroblastosis fetalis is a disease of newborns marked by the presence of too many immature red blood cells (erythroblasts) in the baby's blood. When a baby's mother has a different blood type, antibodies from the mother may leak into the baby's circulation and destroy blood cells. This reaction can produce severe hemolysis and jaundice in the newborn. Rh factor incompatibility is the most common cause.

- High bilirubin levels in newborns. Even in the absence of blood type incompatibility, the newborn's bilirubin level may reach threatening levels.

Normal jaundice in newborns

Normal newborn jaundice is the result of two conditions occurring at the same time—a prehepatic and a hepatic source of excess bilirubin. First of all, the baby at birth immediately begins converting hemoglobin from a fetal type to an adult type. The fetal type of hemoglobin was able to extract oxygen from the lower levels of oxygen in the mother's blood. At birth the infant can extract oxygen directly from his or her own lungs and does not need the fetal hemoglobin any more. So fetal hemoglobin is removed from the system and replaced with adult hemoglobin. The resulting bilirubin loads the system and places demands on the liver to clear it. But the liver is not quite ready for the task, so there is a period of a week or so when the liver has to catch up. During that time the baby is jaundiced.

In 2002 new studies found that infants younger than eight weeks old with jaundice often had hidden (asymptomatic) urinary tract infections. Previous studies have shown that newborn jaundice may be an early sign of bacterial infections in infants. The study recommended that pediatricians routinely test young infants with jaundice for urinary tract infections.

Hepatic jaundice

Liver diseases of all kinds threaten the organ's ability to keep up with bilirubin processing. Starvation, circulating infections, certain medications, **hepatitis**, and **cirrhosis** can all cause hepatic jaundice, as can certain hereditary defects of liver chemistry, including Gilbert's syndrome and Crigler-Najjar syndrome.

Post-hepatic jaundice

Post-hepatic forms of jaundice include the jaundices caused by failure of soluble bilirubin to reach the intestines after it has left the liver. These disorders are called obstructive jaundices. The most common cause of obstructive jaundice is the presence of **gallstones** in the ducts of the biliary system. Other causes have to do with birth defects and infections that damage the bile ducts; drugs; infections; cancers; and physical injury. Some drugs—and **pregnancy** on rare occasions—simply cause the bile in the ducts to stop flowing.

Symptoms and complications associated with jaundice

Certain chemicals in bile may cause **itching** when too much of them end up in the skin. In newborns, insoluble bilirubin may get into the brain and do permanent damage. Long-standing jaundice may upset the balance of chemicals in the bile and cause stones to form. Apart from these potential complications and the discoloration of skin and eyes, jaundice by itself is inoffensive. Other symptoms are determined by the disease producing the jaundice.

Diagnosis

Physical examination

In many cases, the diagnosis of jaundice is suggested by the appearance of the patient's eyes and complex-

ion. The doctor will ask the patient to lie flat on the examining table in order to feel (palpate) the liver and spleen for enlargement and to evaluate any abdominal **pain**. The location and severity of abdominal pain and the presence or absence of **fever** help the doctor to distinguish between hepatic and obstructive jaundice.

Laboratory tests

Disorders of blood formation can be diagnosed by more thorough examination of the blood or the bone marrow, where blood is made. Occasionally a bone marrow biopsy is required, but usually the blood itself will reveal the diagnosis. The spleen can be evaluated by an ultrasound examination or a nuclear scan if the physical examination has not yielded enough information.

Imaging studies

Disease in the biliary system can be identified by imaging techniques, of which there are many. X rays are taken a day after swallowing a contrast agent that is secreted into the bile. This study gives functional as well as anatomical information. There are several ways of injecting x-ray dye directly into the bile ducts. It can be done through a thin needle pushed straight into the liver, or through a scope passed through the stomach that can inject dye into the ampulla of Vater. CT and MRI scans are very useful for imaging certain conditions, such as cancers in and around the liver, or gallstones in the common bile duct.

Liver disease is usually assessed from blood studies alone, but again a biopsy may be necessary to clarify less obvious conditions. A liver biopsy is performed at the bedside. The doctor uses a thin needle to take a tiny core of tissue from the liver. The tissue sample is sent to the laboratory for examination under a microscope.

Assessment of jaundice in newborns

Newborns are more likely to have problems with jaundice if:

• They are premature.

• They are of Asian or Native American descent.

• They have been bruised during the birth process.

• They have lost too much weight during the first few days.

• They are born at a high altitude.

• The mother has diabetes.

• Labor had to be induced.

In 2003, research was continuing to find noninvasive methods to determine bilirubin levels in newborns so that physicians did not have to rely on visual examination alone to determine which infants should receive blood tests. Once these measurements of skin pigment can be shown effective and cost-effective in clinical practice, they may become more widely available. Another study used this measurement method incorporated into home health visits to monitor babies within 24 hours of discharge from the hospital following birth.

Treatment

Jaundice is often an early warning sign of serious liver damage. Alternative medicine treatments should not be used as a substitute for conventional medical treatment. Patients should contact their doctors for diagnosis and treatment immediately if experiencing signs and symptoms of jaundice. Alternative therapies may be helpful as complementary measures for patients who have an underlying disease that already has been diagnosed.

Nutritional therapy

Naturopaths or nutritionists may recommend the following dietary changes:

- Drinking fresh vegetable or fruit juices during the first several weeks after diagnosis and eating a diet consisting mostly of raw fruits and vegetables, seeds, and nuts during the next month. These fruits and vegetables are easy to digest and contain lots of **antioxidants**, vitamins and minerals. They help the body remove toxins from the blood, and decrease stress/strain on the liver for digestion/metabolism.

- **Fasting** intermittently.

- Eliminating alcohol from the diet for good, and avoiding foods that are processed and high in fat. These foods are bad for the liver.

- Drinking a cup of lemonade (without sugar) early in the morning to improve liver and bile function.

- Incorporating olive oil or lemon oil into the diet as a liver flushing regimen.

- Taking nutritional supplements, such as multivitamins or minerals, **vitamin C**, **vitamin B complex**, other antioxidant-containing supplements, supplements containing alpha lipoic acid, protein supplements, **essential fatty acids** (EFAs), and **digestive enzymes** with bile (for patients having pale stools).

Traditional Chinese medicine

Depending on a patient's specific condition, an expert Chinese herbalist may prescribe herbal remedies that can help improve liver function. Animal studies have shown the following Chinese herbs may have liver protective effects:

- *Bupleurum chinense*
- *Phellodendron wilsonii*
- *Clementis chinensis*

Herbal therapy

Patients should consult an experienced herbalist for specific herbal treatments that may include **milk thistle** or artichoke.

Homeopathy

For homeopathic therapy, patients should consult a homeopathic physician who will prescribe specific remedies based on knowledge of the underlying cause.

Juice therapy

Juice therapy helps the liver detoxify toxins to be eliminated from the body. Patients should mix one part of pure juice with one part of water before drinking. Daily consumption of the following juices may be helpful:

- carrot and beet juice with a touch of radish or **dandelion** root juice
- grapes, pear, and lemon
- carrot, celery, and parsley
- carrot, beet, and cucumber

Aromatherapy

Essential oils of **rosemary**, lemon, and geranium may help improve liver function and relax the body. They can be given as inhalants, a soothing bath, or soak.

Other therapies

Other alternative treatments that may be help improve liver function include fasting, Ayurveda, **hydrotherapy**, and **acupuncture**.

Allopathic treatment

Jaundice in newborns

Newborns are the only major category of patients in whom the jaundice itself requires attention. If there is reason to suspect increased hemolysis in the newborn, the bilirubin level must be measured repeatedly during the first few days of life. If the level of bilirubin shortly after birth threatens to go too high, treatment must begin immediately. Exchanging most of the baby's blood was the only way to reduce the amount of bilirubin until a few decades ago. Jaundiced babies are now fitted with eye protection and placed under bright fluorescent blue lights. The light chemically alters the bilirubin in the blood as it passes through the baby's skin so that it may be more easily eliminated in the urine. In 2003 researchers were testing a new drug called Stanate that showed promise in blocking bilirubin production. However, debate concerning the use of the drug for treatment of only those infants with jaundice or as a preventive measure was delaying its FDA approval and widespread use.

Hemolytic disorders

Hemolytic diseases are treated, if at all, with medications and blood transfusions, except in the case of an enlarged spleen. Surgical removal of the spleen (splenectomy) can sometimes cure hemolytic anemia. Drugs that cause hemolysis or arrest the flow of bile must be stopped immediately.

Hepatic jaundice

Most liver diseases have no specific cure, but the liver is so robust that it can heal from severe damage and regenerate itself from a small remnant of its original tissue.

Posthepatic jaundice

Obstructive jaundice frequently requires a surgical cure. If the original passageways cannot be restored, surgeons have several ways to create alternate routes. To create alternate passageways, a surgeon will sew an open piece of intestine over a bare patch of liver. Tiny bile ducts in that part of the liver will begin to discharge their bile into the intestine, and pressure from the obstructed ducts elsewhere will find release in that direction. As the flow increases, the ducts grow to accommodate it. Soon, all the bile is redirected through the open pathways.

Prevention

Erythroblastosis fetalis can be prevented by giving an Rh-negative mother a gamma globulin solution called RhoGAM whenever there is a possibility that she is developing antibodies to her baby's blood. G6PD hemolysis can be prevented by testing patients before giving them drugs that can cause it. Medication side effects can be minimized by early detection and immediate cessation of the drug. Malaria can often be prevented by taking certain precautions when traveling in tropical or subtropical countries. These precautions include staying in after dark; using such prophylactic drugs as mefloquine; and protecting sleeping quarters with mosquito nets treated with insecticides and mosquito repellents. In 2003, new studies showed promise for a possible vaccine against malaria. Early trials showed that vaccination combination

---

KEY TERMS

Ampulla of Vater—The widened portion of the duct through which the bile and pancreatic juices enter the intestine. *Ampulla* is a Latin word describing a bottle with a narrow neck that opens into a wide body.

Anemia—A condition in which the blood does not contain enough hemoglobin.

Biliary system/bile ducts—The gall bladder and the system of tubes that carry bile from the liver into the intestines.

Bilirubin—A reddish pigment excreted by the liver into the bile as a breakdown product of hemoglobin.

Crigler-Najjar syndrome—A moderate to severe form of hereditary jaundice.

Erythroblastosis fetalis—A disorder of newborn infants marked by a high level of immature red blood cells (erythroblasts) in the infant's blood.

Gilbert's syndrome—A mild hereditary form of jaundice.

Glucose–6–phosphate dehydrogenase (G6PD) deficiency—A hereditary disorder that can lead to episodes of hemolytic anemia in combination with certain medications.

Hemoglobin—The red chemical in blood cells that carries oxygen.

Hemolysis—The destruction or breakdown of red blood cells.

Hepatic—Refers to the liver.

Icterus—Another name for jaundice.

Microangiopathic—Pertaining to disorders of the small blood vessels.

Pancreas—The organ beneath the stomach that produces digestive juices, insulin, and other hormones.

Sickle cell disease—A hereditary defect in hemoglobin synthesis that changes the shape of red cells and makes them more fragile.

Splenectomy—Surgical removal of the spleen.

---

might stimulate T-cell activity against malaria, the best type of protection that researchers can hope to find. However, further studies will have to be done.

New research in 2002 linked a popular antidepressant drug called paroxetine (Paxil) to several newborn complications, including jaundice. Although research is preliminary, pregnant women might want to discuss use of the drug with their physicians to prevent complications like jaundice in their newborn babies.

Resources

BOOKS

Balistreri, William F. "Manifestations of Liver Disease." In *Nelson Textbook of Pediatrics,* edited by Waldo E. Nelson, et al. Philadelphia: W. B. Saunders, 1996.

"Jaundice." *Alternative Medicine: The Definitive Guide.* Tiburon, CA: Future Medicine Publishing, Inc., 1999.

"Jaundice." In *Sleisenger & Fordtran's Gastrointestinal and Liver Disease,* edited by Mark Feldman, et al. Philadelphia: W. B. Saunders, 1998.

Kaplan, Lee M., and Kurt J. Isselbacher. "Jaundice." In *Harrison's Principles of Internal Medicine,* edited by Kurt Isselbacher et al. New York: McGraw–Hill, 1998.

"Liver Problems." *The Hamlyn Encyclopedia of Complementary Health.* London, Reed International Books Limited.

McQuaid, Kenneth R. "Alimentary Tract." In *Current Medical Diagnosis and Treatment,* edited by Lawrence M. Tierney, Jr., et al. Stamford, CT: Appleton & Lange, 1996.

Scharschmidt, Bruce F. "Bilirubin Metabolism, Hyperbilirubinemia, and Approach to the Jaundiced Patient." In *Cecil Textbook of Medicine,* edited by J. Claude Bennett and Fred Plum. Philadelphia: W. B. Saunders, 1996.

PERIODICALS

Chin, Hui–Fen, Chun–Ching Lin, Chui–Ching Yang, and Fay Yang. "The Pharmacological and Pathological Studies on Several Hepatic Protective Crude Drugs from Taiwan." *American Journal of Chinese Medicine* XVI no. 3–4 (1988): 127–137.

Garcia, Francisco J., and Alan L. Nager. "Jaundice as an Early Diagnostic Sign of Urinary Tract Infection in Infancy." *Pediatrics* (May 2002): 846.

Grimm, David. "Baby Pigment Peril." *U.S. News & World Report* (July 28, 2003): 39.

Lawrence, David. "Combination Malaria Vaccine Shows Early Promise in Human Trials." *The Lancet* (May 31, 2003): 1875.

Morantz, Carrie, and Brian Torrey. "AHRQ Report on Neonatal Jaundice." *American Family Physician* (June 1, 2003): 2417.

"Paxil Linked to Complications in Newborns." *Psychopharmacology Update* (June 2002): 6.

Richmond, Glenn, Melissa Brown, and Patricia Wagstaff. "Using a Home Care Model to Monitor Bilirubin Levels in Early Discharged Infants." *Topics in Health Information Management* (January&-March 2003): 39–43.

ORGANIZATION

American Liver Foundation. 1425 Pompton Avenue, Cedar Grove, New Jersey 07009. (800) 223–0179.

Teresa G. Odle

Jet lag

Definition

Jet lag is a condition marked by **fatigue**, **insomnia**, and irritability that is caused by air travel through changing time zones. It is commonplace: a 2002 study of international business travelers (IBTs) found that jet lag was one of the most common health problems reported, affecting as many as 74% of IBTs.

Description

Living organisms are accustomed to periods of night and day alternating at set intervals. Most of the human body's regulating hormones follow this cycle, known as circadian rhythm. The word circadian comes from the Latin, *circa*, meaning about, and *dies*, meaning day. These cycles are not exactly 24 hours long, hence the "circa." Each chemical has its own cycle of highs and lows, interacting with and influencing the other cycles. Body temperature, sleepiness, thyroid function, growth hormone, metabolic processes, adrenal hormones, and the sleep hormone **melatonin** all cycle with daylight. There is a direct connection between the retina (the light-sensitive structure at the back of the eye) and the part of the brain that controls all these hormones. Artificial light has some effect but sunlight has much more. Disruption of circadian rhythms affects the sleep-wake cycles of night-shift workers as well as travelers.

When people are without clocks in a compartment that is completely closed to sunlight, most of them fall into a circadian cycle of about 25 hours. Normally, all the regulating chemicals follow one another in order like threads in a weaving pattern. Every morning the sunlight resets the cycle, stimulating the leading chemicals and thus compensating for the difference between the 24-hour day and the 25-hour innate rhythm.

When traveling through a number of time zones, most people reset their rhythms within a few days, demonstrating the adaptability of the human species. Some people, however, have upset circadian rhythms that last indefinitely.

Causes & symptoms

Traveling through a few time zones at a time is not as disruptive to circadian rhythms as traveling around the world can be. The foremost symptom of jet lag is altered sleep pattern—sleepiness during the day, and insomnia during the night. Jet lag may also include **indigestion** and trouble concentrating. Individuals afflicted by jet lag will alternate in and out of a normal day-night cycle.

Treatment

Exposure to bright morning sunlight cures jet lag after a few days in most people. A few will have prolonged sleep phase difficulties. For these, there is a curious treatment that has achieved success. By forcing one's self into a 27 hour day, complete with the appropriate stimulation from bright light, all the errant chemical cycles will be able to catch up during one week.

When selecting an international flight, individuals should try to arrange an early evening arrival in their destination city. When an individual is traveling to a destination in the east, he or she can try going to bed and waking up a few hours earlier several days before their flight. If travel is to the west, going to bed and waking up later than usual can help the body start to adjust to the upcoming time change. More specific recommendations are available as of 2002, tailored to whether the person is traveling through six time zones, 7–9 zones, or 10 or more.

The following precautions taken during an international flight can help to limit or prevent jet lag:

• Stay hydrated. Drink plenty of **water** and juices to prevent dehydration. Beverages and foods with **caffeine** should be avoided because of their stimulant properties. Alcohol should also be avoided.

• Stretch and walk. As much movement as possible during a flight helps circulation, which moves nutrients and waste through the body and aids in elimination.

• Stay on time. Set watches and clocks ahead to the time in the destination city to start adjusting to the change.

• Sleep smart. Draw the shade and sleep during the evening hours in the destination city, even if it is still daylight outside of the airplane. Earplugs and sleep masks may be helpful in blocking noise and light. Many airlines provide these items on international flights.

• Dress comfortably. Wear or bring comfortable clothes and slippers that will make sleeping during the flight easier.

Once arriving in their destination city, individuals should spend as much time outdoors in the sunlight as possible during the day to reset their internal clock and lessen the symptoms of jet lag. Bedtime should be postponed until at least 10 P.M., with no daytime naps. If a daytime nap is absolutely necessary, it should be limited to no more than two hours.

To promote a restful sleeping environment in a hotel setting, travelers should request that the hotel desk hold all phone calls. Because sleeping in too late can also prolong jet lag, an early wake up call should be requested if an alarm clock is not available. If the hotel room is noisy, a portable white noise machine can help to block outside traffic and hallway noises. A room air conditioner or fan can serve the same purpose. The temperature in the room should also be adjusted for sleeping comfort.

New information shows that **exercise** when at the destination can also help. When headed westbound, travelers should exercise for one hour in the evening. If going eastbound, they do best by exercising in the morning.

All **antioxidants** help to decrease the effects of jet lag. Extra doses of vitamins A, C, and E, as well as **zinc** and **selenium**, two days before and two days after a flight help to alleviate jet lag. Melatonin, a hormone that helps to regulate circadian rhythms, can also help to combat jet lag. Melatonin is available as an over-the-counter supplement in most health food stores and pharmacies. Reports in 2002 show that the drug is safe for short-term use and recommend 5 mg between 10 pm and midnight at the destination to help fall asleep and to sleep better.

If weather prevents an individual from spending time in the sunlight, **light therapy** may be beneficial in decreasing jet lag symptoms. Light therapy, or phototherapy, uses a device called a light box, which contains a set of fluorescent or incandescent lights in front of a reflector. Typically, the patient sits for 30 minutes next to a 10,000-lux box (which is about 50 times as bright as an ordinary indoor light). Light therapy is safe for most people, but those with eye diseases should consult a healthcare professional before undergoing the treatment.

In 2002, a team from Flanders University invented new jet lag sunglasses equipped with a vision device that used light to stimulate travelers' brains. They believed that wearing the glasses before and during flights could help the internal human clock adjust more easily to changing time zones. The researchers were looking for a commercial partner to help them further study the glasses and make them widely available. The effectiveness of glasses or other head-mounted light devices is still uncertain, however. A team of researchers at Columbia University reported in the fall of 2002 that the use of a head-mounted light visor yielded only modest improvement in the test subjects' symptoms of jet lag.

Allopathic treatment

In cases of short-term insomnia triggered by jet lag, a physician may recommend sleeping pills or prescription medication. Such medication should be taken only under the guidance of a health care professional.

A newer medication that is considered investigational is a melatonin agonist presently known as LY 156735. An agonist is a drug that stimulates activity at cell receptors that are normally stimulated by such naturally occurring substances as melatonin. LY 156735 was found to speed up the readaptation time of volunteer subjects following a simulated 9-hour time shift.

Another new area of research involves the genes that encode the proteins governing circadian rhythms. It is known as of late 2002 that differences among individuals in adaptability to time zone changes are to some extent genetically determined. Targeting the genes that affect this adaptability may yield new treatments for jet lag and other disorders of circadian rhythm.

Expected results

Jet lag usually lasts 24–48 hours after travel has taken place. In that short time period, the body adjusts to the time change, and with enough rest and daytime exposure to sunlight, it returns to normal circadian rhythm.

Prevention

Eating a high-protein diet that is low in calories before intended travel may help reduce the effects of jet lag.

Resources

BOOKS

Czeisler, Charles A., and Gary S. Richardson. "Disorders of Sleep and Circadian Rhythms." In *Harrison's Principles of Internal Medicine,* edited by Anthony S. Fauci, et al. New York: McGraw-Hill, 1998.

PERIODICALS

Boulos, Z., M. M. Macchi, M. P. Sturchler, et al. " Light Visor Treatment for Jet Lag After Westward Travel Across Six Time Zones." *Aviation, Space, and Environmental Medicine* 73 (October 2002): 953–963.

Garfinkel D. and N. Zisapel. "The Use of Melatonin for Sleep." *Nutrition* 14 (January 1998): 53–55.

"Jet Lag Sunglasses Help Body Clock Tick." *Optician* (August 2, 2002): 1.

Monson, Nancy. "What Really Works for Jet Lag." *Shape* (August 2002): 78.

Nickelsen, T., A. Samel, M. Vejvoda, et al. "Chronobiotic Effects of the Melatonin Agonist LY 156735 Following a Simulated 9h Time Shift: Results of a Placebo-Controlled Trial. " *Chronobiology International* 19 (September 2002): 915–936.

Parry, B. L. " Jet Lag: Minimizing Its Effects with Critically Timed Bright Light and Melatonin Administration." *Journal of Molecular Microbiology and Biotechnology* 4 (September 2002): 463–466.

Rogers, H. L., and S. M. Reilly. " A Survey of the Health Experiences of International Business Travelers. Part One—Physiological Aspects." *Journal of the American Association of Occupational Health Nurses* 50 (October 2002): 449–459.

Wisor, J. P. "Disorders of the Circadian Clock: Etiology and Possible Therapeutic Targets." *Current Drug Targets: Cns and Neurological Disorders* 1 (December 2002): 555–566.

ORGANIZATIONS

American Sleep Disorders Association. 1610 14th Street NW, Suite 300. Rochester, MN 55901. (507) 287-6006.

National Sleep Foundation. 1367 Connecticut Avenue NW, Suite 200. Washington, DC 20036. (202) 785-2300.

Paula Ford-Martin
Rebecca J. Frey, PhD

Jew's myrtle *see* **Butcher's broom**

Jock itch

Definition

Also known as *tinea cruris*, jock itch is a growth of fungus in the warm, moist area of the groin.

Description

Fungal infections are named for the affected part of the body. *Cruris* is derived from the Latin word for leg, hence *Tinea cruris*, for the fungal rash affecting the area where the leg joins the pelvis. Fungi seem to thrive in dark moist places. Jock itch has been found most often in males, especially those who wear athletic equipment and frequently use public showers and locker rooms. It is also thought that some fungal **infections** may be spread by towels that may be inadequately cleansed between gym/spa users, but this has not been clearly documented.

Fungal infections can invade or spread to various other areas of the body, and are named for the affected body part. For example, *Tinea capitis* is a fungal infection of the head, usually resulting in red, itchy areas that destroy the hair in the affected area. A fungal infection of the skin on the arms, legs or chest is called *Tinea corporis*. **Athlete's foot** or *Tinea pedis* is a fungal infection in the moist skin fold between the toes. Fungal infection affecting the toenails is called *Tinea unguium*, and causes thickened, crumbly toenails.

Causes & symptoms

The mode of transmission of fungal infections is not clear, but it seems that some individuals are more prone to development of the infection than others. An average of one in five people develops fungal infection at some point during their lifetime. Fungal infection can also be carried by household pets, such as cats and dogs, or by farm animals. In animals, fungal infection manifests itself as a missing area of fur. In humans, as the fungus grows, it spreads to surrounding tissues in a circular fashion, with the skin in the middle returning to a normal appearance. The borders of the affected area may look red and scaly, and the individual may complain of intense **itching** and/or burning. Because the borders develop a raised appearance, there may appear to be a worm beneath the skin and be referred to as ringworm. There is, however, no worm affecting the skin or underlying tissue in cases of fungal infections, including jock itch.

Diagnosis

Often a case of jock itch can be identified based on the characteristic description previously described. If assessed by a conventional doctor, the area of affected skin may be scraped onto a glass slide for definitive diagnosis under the microscope. In order to determine the exact type of fungus present, a small piece of affected skin may be sent to a laboratory for further study or cultured via scrapings from the affected area.

Treatment

Topical treatments include poultices of **peppermint**, oregano, or **lavender**. **Tea tree oil** diluted with a carrier oil of almond oil can be applied to the rash several times per day. Cedarwood and jasmine oils can relieve itching when applied in the same manner. **Grapefruit seed extract** can be taken as a strong solution of 15 drops in 1 oz of **water**.

Bupleurum, or **Chinese thoroughwax**, is an Asian plant that has been used in **traditional Chinese medicine** and Japanese Kampo formulations to treat jock itch and other fungal skin infections. Bupleurum contains compounds known as saikosaponins, which have anti-allergic and anti-inflammatory effects.

A good remedy for jock itch is to wash the groin area with the diluted juice of a freshly squeezed lemon, which can help dry up the rash. A hair dryer on the cool setting can also be used on the area after showering to dry it thoroughly. A warm bath relieves itching in many patients. The affected area should kept clean and dry, and patients are advised to wear loose-fitting pure cotton underwear. Fabrics that contain polyester or nylon hold moisture against the body.

Allopathic treatment

Typical conventional treatment for jock itch involves the use of an antifungal cream, spray, or powder twice a day for about two weeks. Two commonly used over-the-counter antifungal preparations are clotrimazole (Lotrimin) and tolnaftate (Tinactin). While the tendency to discontinue treatment once itching disappears is common, patients should use the antifungal preparation for a full two-week course in order to prevent recurrence of the infection. As of 2002, doctors recommend continuing the treatment for a full week following clinical clearance of the infection.

Expected results

Most tinea infections resolve without scarring or spread of infection below the skin's surface. Inflammation, however, may require the use of a combination antifungal/steroid medication.

Prevention

Careful attention to skin hygiene, including the maintenance of clean, dry, and intact skin, is the most important step in preventing the development of fungal infection. Light clothing should be worn during warm weather to decrease perspiration and allow dissipation of body heat. Clean and dry cotton underwear will wick perspiration away from the skin, and prevent jock itch from developing. Use baby powder to keep the area dry during **exercise**. Do not share towels at the gym. Dietary measures discussed under treatment will also prevent initial fungal infection and/or recurrence.

Resources

BOOKS

Gottlieb, Bill. *New Choices in Natural Healing*. Emmaus, PA: Rodale Press, Inc., 1995.

PERIODICALS

Park, K. H., J. Park, D. Koh, and Y. Lim. "Effect of Saikosaponin-A, a Triterpenoid Glycoside, Isolated from *Bupleurum falcatum* on Experimental Allergic Asthma." *Phytotherapy Research* 16 (June 2002): 359-363.

Weinstein, A., and B. Berman. "Topical Treatment of Common Superficial Tinea Infections." *American Family Physician* 65 (May 15, 2002): 2095-2102.

ORGANIZATIONS

American Academy of Dermatology. 930 East Woodfield Rd., PO Box 4014, Schaumburg, IL 60168. (847) 330-0230. <www.aad.org>.

American Association of Oriental Medicine. 5530 Wisconsin Avenue, Suite 1210, Chevy Chase, MD 20815. (301) 941-1064. <www.aaom.org>.

Kathleen Wright
Rebecca J. Frey, PhD

Jojoba oil

Description

Jojoba (pronounced ho-ho-ba) oil is a vegetable oil obtained from the crushed bean of the jojoba shrub (*Simmondsia chinenis*). The jojoba shrub is native to the Sonoran Desert of northwestern Mexico and neighboring regions in Arizona and southern California. It grows in dense stands throughout that region. The woody evergreen shrub may reach 15 ft (4.5 m) in height. Jojoba has flat gray-green leathery leaves and a deep root system that make it well adapted to desert heat and drought. It has a life span of 100–200 years, depending on environmental conditions. Jojoba grows best in areas with 10–18 in (25–45 cm) of annual rainfall where temperatures seldom fall below 25°F (-4°C) for more than a few hours at night. It can grow on many types of soils, including porous rocks, in slightly acid to alkaline soils, and on mountain slopes or in valleys.

Jojoba shrubs are dioecious, meaning plants are either male (staminate), producing pollen, or female (pistillate), producing flowers. The small flowers have no odor or petals and do not attract pollinating insects. The flowers are pollinated by wind in late March; the flowers

develop into fruit by August, with full maturation occurring by October. The green fruit dries in the desert heat, its outer skin shriveling and pulling back to expose a wrinkled brown soft-skinned seed (referred to as a nut or bean) the size of a small olive. These nuts, which resemble coffee beans, contain a vegetable oil that is clear and odorless but less oily to the touch than traditional edible oils. The oil comprises half of the weight of the nut. There are about 1,700 seeds in a pound; 17 lb (6.3 kg) of jojoba seeds are required to produce one gallon of oil.

Native Americans have used jojoba for hundreds of years. In the 1700s, Father Junipero Serra, the founder of 21 California missions, noted in his diary that the Native Americans were using the oil and the seeds for many different purposes: for treating sores, cuts, **bruises**, and **burns**; as a diet supplement and as an appetite suppressant when food was not available; as a skin conditioner, for soothing windburn and **sunburn**; as a cooking oil; as a hair or scalp treatment and hair restorative; and as a coffee-like beverage by roasting the seeds.

The chemical structure of jojoba oil is different from that of other vegetable oils. Rather than being an oil, it is actually is a polyunsaturated liquid wax that is similar to sperm whale oil, though without the fishy odor. It is made of fatty acids as well as esters composed entirely of straight chain alcohols. Both the acid and alcohol portions of jojoba oil have 20 or 22 carbon atoms, and each has one unsaturated bond. Waxes of this type are difficult to synthesize. As a wax, jojoba oil is especially useful for applications that require moisture control, protection, and emolliency. Jojoba oil is liquid at room temperature because of its unsaturated fatty acids. It does not oxidize or become rancid and does not break down under high temperatures and pressures. Jojoba oil can be heated to 370°F (188°C) for 96 hours without exhibiting degradation in general composition and carbon chain length. The stability shown by jojoba oil makes it especially useful for cosmetic applications.

When the United States banned the use of sperm whale oil (spermaceti wax) in 1974, the government began to fund efforts to investigate and cultivate jojoba as a replacement. Jojoba oil was found to be an adequate substitute for applications that had previously used sperm whale oil. The first commercial cultivation of jojoba was in the Negev Desert and Dead Sea areas of Israel, but by 1977, domestic cultivation had begun in the United States. In 2000, the International Jojoba Export Council expected the global jojoba production to increase 15% over a five-year period.

General use

Jojoba oil has many uses in a wide variety of industries. As a cosmetic, it is an effective cleanser, conditioner, moisturizer, and softener for the skin and hair. It is applied directly to the skin to soften the skin, to reduce

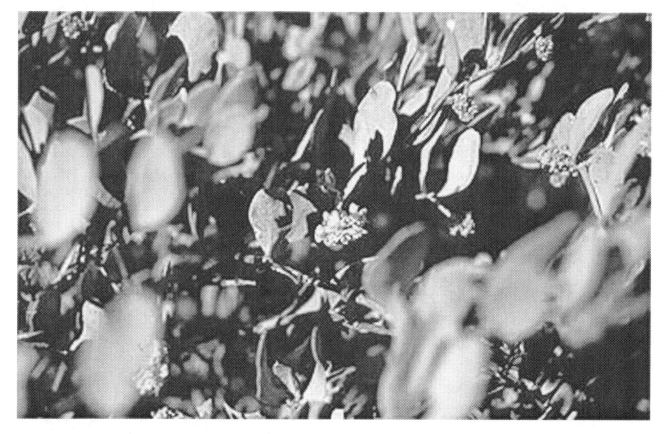

Jojoba plant (*Simmondsia chinensis*). *(Photo by Henriette Kress. Reproduced by permission.)*

wrinkles and stretch marks, to lighten and help heal scars, and to promote healthy scalp and hair. Jojoba oil is similar to, and miscible with, sebum, which is secreted by human sebaceous glands to lubricate and protect skin and hair. When sebum production decreases due to age, pollutants, or environmental stresses, jojoba oil can be used to replicate sebum oil. Jojoba oil can accumulate around hair roots, thereby conditioning hair and preventing it from becoming brittle and dull. If there is too much sebum buildup on the scalp, it dissolves and removes the sebum, leaving the hair clean. Jojoba oil as a solubilizing agent can also remove sticky buildup on hair from hair preparations as well as airborne particulates deposited on the hair. It forms a lipid layer on the skin, acting as a moisturizer, as well as penetrating and being absorbed by the outer layer of skin. It is widely used as an ingredient in shampoos, conditioners, facial, hand and body lotions, cuticle and nail care products, baby care lotions, creams and oils, cleansers, moisturizers, bath oils and soaps, sunscreen lotions, and makeup products. Jojoba oil is also used as a base in the manufacture of perfume.

The potential therapeutic uses of jojoba oil include the treatment of **acne**, cold sores, and such skin diseases as **psoriasis**.

Jojoba oil is also a registered (licensed for sale) pesticide for use on crops. It is used to control white flies on all crops and powdery mildew on grapes and ornamentals. It is applied as a spray containing 1% or less final concentration of jojoba oil. It acts as a pesticide by forming a physical barrier between an insect pest and the leaf surface. Because of its low toxicity and its rapid degradation in the environment, jojoba oil does not pose a risk to non-target organisms or the environment; though as an oil, it should not be disposed of in lakes or other bodies of water.

Preparations

Jojoba oil is prepared by pressing the jojoba seeds to extract the oil, followed by filtration. It is then pasteurized to ensure product safety. Four grades of jojoba oil are produced: (1) a pure, natural golden grade, a golden-yellow color oil that is produced by the basic production process; (2) refined and bleached jojoba oil, with color removed by bleaching and filtration; (3) a decolorized/deodorized grade, which is used in cosmetics requiring colorless and odorless oils; and (4) a molecular distilled grade, an expensive formulation produced in minimal quantities, with its use having mostly been replaced with decolorized/deodorized jojoba oil.

KEY TERMS

. . . .

Noncomedogenic—A substance that contains nothing that would cause blackheads or pimples to form on the skin. Jojoba oil is noncomedogenic.

Precautions

Jojoba oil is a nontoxic, noncomedogenic (does not clog pores), and hypoallergenic substance. It has been widely used for decades in cosmetics, with no reported adverse effects. If jojoba oil is ingested, most of it is eliminated in the feces, with little getting distributed in the body.

Side effects

No side effects are expected with the use of jojoba oil in recommended amounts, although allergic reactions are a rare possibility.

Interactions

Since jojoba oil does not oxidize or become rancid, it is added to other oils to extend their shelf life.

Resources

BOOKS

Baldwin, A.R. *Seventh International Conference on Jojoba and Its Uses.* American Oil Chemists Society, 1989.

Wisniak, Jaime. *The Chemistry and Technology of Jojoba Oil.* American Oil Chemists Society, 1987.

Judith Sims

Journal therapy

Definition

Journal therapy is the purposeful and intentional use of a written record of one's own thoughts or feelings to further psychological healing and personal growth. It is often used as an adjunct to many **psychotherapy** and recovery programs. Healthcare practitioners maintain that written expression fills a very important role in the therapeutic process by providing a mechanism of emotional expression in circumstances in which interpersonal expression is not possible or viable.

Origins

People have kept journals and diaries to record dreams, memories, and thoughts since ancient times.

Emotional expression has also long held a central role in the study and practice of psychology. Throughout history, psychologists have advocated the expression of emotions as essential for good mental and physical health. Since the early 1980s, interest in this topic has resulted in numerous research studies investigating the health benefits of expressive writing.

Benefits

Journal writing produces a number of benefits in healthy people—among other things, it enhances creativity, helps cope with **stress**, and provides a written record of memorable life experiences. Likewise, some researchers have found that journal writing has a number of psychological and physical health benefits for people who are ill.

Aside from a reduction in physical symptoms of disease, the psychological benefits include reconciling emotional conflicts, fostering self-awareness, managing behavior, solving problems, reducing **anxiety**, aiding reality orientation, and increasing self-esteem. Writing therapy has been used as an effective treatment for the developmentally, medically, educationally, socially, or psychologically impaired and is practiced in mental health, rehabilitation, medical, educational, and forensic institutions. Populations of all ages, races, and ethnic backgrounds are served by writing therapy in individual, couple, family, and group therapy formats.

The therapeutic use of expressive writing allows individuals to confront upsetting topics, thus alleviating the constraints or inhibitions associated with not talking about the event. The psychological drain of the inhibition is believed to cause and/or exacerbate stress-related disease processes. Researchers have found that emotional expression facilitates cognitive processing of the traumatic memory, which leads to emotional and physiological change. Specifically, written emotional expression promotes integration and understanding of the event while reducing negative emotions associated with it.

Description

Journal writing and other forms of writing therapy are based on the premise that the mind and the body are inseparably joined in the healing process. Although there are many methods of conducting journal writing therapy depending on the therapeutic technique of the psychologist or psychiatrist, the therapist often instructs the participant to write about a distressing or traumatic event or thought in one or more sessions.

Although researchers are uncertain about exactly how writing about traumas produces improvements in psychological well-being, traumatic stress researchers have pointed out that ordinary memories are qualitatively different from traumatic memories. Traumatic memories are more emotional and perceptual in nature. The memory is stored as a sensory perception, obsessional thought, or behavioral reenactment. It is associated with persistent, intrusive, and distressing symptoms, avoidance, and intense anxiety that results in observed psychological and biological dysfunction. Thus, one goal in treating traumatic memories is to find a means of processing them.

A narrative that becomes more focused and coherent over a number of writing sessions is often associated with increased improvement, according to several research studies. The memories become deconditioned and restructured into a personal, integrated narrative. Changes in psychological well-being after writing therapy may result from cognitive shifts about the trauma either during or after the writing process.

Preparations

In a health care setting, the participant often prepares for journal writing by receiving (from the therapist) a set of instructions regarding the length and focus of the writing session or sessions. Other instructions may include writing in a stream-of-consciousness fashion, without censorship or concern about grammar or style.

Precautions

It is advisable that journal therapy be conducted only by a licensed health professional, such as a certified **art therapy** practitioner or trained psychologist or psychiatrist. While journal writing classes available to the general public may perform a variety of useful functions, these classes are not intended to provide medical therapy. In journal therapy, the participant may, for example, uncover potentially traumatic, repressed, or painful memories. Therefore, a trained health professional may be necessary to supervise the process and treat these symptoms as they arise.

Side effects

There are no known side effects of journal or writing therapy.

Research & general acceptance

Therapeutic writing became an increasingly popular topic in the final decades of the twentieth century, not only among trained health care professionals, but also among self-improvement speakers without medical training. Seminars, workshops, and Internet sites purportedly offering therapy though expressive writing sprang up around the nation and gained popular acceptance. Despite the large body of research indicating that writing confers benefits on healthy people, the topic of writing therapy's affects on diseased individuals has not received a great deal of research attention. Although increasingly used by health care professionals as an adjunct to various therapeutic approaches, the practice has been criticized by some members of the health care community. Some researchers are distrustful of the findings that so much measurable improvement in health status can occur in just a few brief writing sessions.

In the United Kingdom, the focus of journal therapy has been on descriptive accounts and psychodynamic explanations for subjective improvements in the health status of participants. In the United States, on the other hand, the focus is on formal scientific research aimed at validating the impact of brief, highly standardized writing exercises on physical measures of illness. The research demonstrates that although physical measures of illness may change, the reasons for the change are not always clear.

In the United States, one study on the effects of writing about stressful experiences on symptom reduction in patients with **asthma** or **rheumatoid arthritis** found that after four months of writing therapy—in conjunction with standard pharmacotherapy—nearly half the patients enrolled in the study experienced clinically relevant improvement. A growing number of studies have documented symptom improvement in patients with psychiatric disorders as well, suggesting that addressing patients' psychological needs produces both psychological and physical health benefits.

Training & certification

Although journal therapy is often provided by certified instructors who receive variable amounts of training in a number of programs around the country, journal therapy is best administered by a licensed psychologist (who may also be an art therapist) or psychiatrist.

Educational, professional, and ethical standards for art therapists who conduct writing therapy are regulated by the American Art Therapy Association, Inc. The American Art Therapy Credentials Board, Inc., an independent organization, grants postgraduate supervised experience. A registered art therapist who successfully completes the written examination administered by the Art Therapy Credentials Board qualifies as Board Certified (ATR-BC), a credential requiring maintenance through continuing education credits.

Resources

BOOKS

Adams, Kathleen. *Journal to the Self.* New York: Warner Books, 1990.

PERIODICALS

Greenhalgh, Tricia. "Writing as Therapy." *British Medical Journal* (July 1999): 270-271.

Nye, Emily F. "Writing as Healing." *Qualitative Inquiry* (December 1997): 439-450.

Smyth, Joshua M. et al. "Effects of Writing About Stressful Experiences on Symptom Reduction in Patients With Asthma or Rheumatoid Arthritis." *Journal of the American Medical Association* (April 1999): 1304-1309.

Smyth, Joshua M. "Written Emotional Expression: Effect Sizes, Outcome Types, and Moderating Variables." *Journal of Consulting and Clinical Psychology* (1998): 174-184.

Spiegel, David. "Healing Words: Emotional Expression and Disease Outcome." *Journal of the American Medical Association* (April 1999): 1328-1329.

Walker, B. Lee, Lillian M. Nail, and Robert T. Croyle. "Does Emotional Expression Make a Difference in Reactions to Breast Cancer?" *Oncology Nursing Journal* (July 1999): 1025-1032.

ORGANIZATIONS

The American Art Therapy Association. 1202 Allanson Road. Mundelein, IL 60060-3808. http://www.arttherapy.org.

The Center for Journal Therapy. 12477 W. Cedar Drive, #102. Lakewood, CO 80228. http://www.journaltherapy.com.

Genevieve Slomski

Juice therapies

Definition

Juice therapy involves the consumption of the juice of raw fruit or vegetables. A person may drink juice preventively to stay healthy, to treat a medical condition like **cancer**, or to produce a certain outcome, such as strengthening the immune system. Three widely practiced juice therapies differ primarily in the amount of time that a person is involved in the therapy and whether other items are included in the person's diet.

For some people, adding fresh juice to their daily meal plan is sufficient. Others will embark on a juice fast for several days to cleanse their systems. Juice is also a major component of the so-called **Gerson therapy** diet that is used to treat cancer. This therapy usually starts with a stay of three to eight weeks in a clinic. Then therapy continues at home and may continue for years.

Origins

Fasting and juice consumption

The two components of most juice therapies, **fasting** and juice consumption, date back thousands of years. Fasting is a long-standing religious tradition described in the Bible and other sources. The medicinal use of juice can be traced back thousands of years to India. Proponents of Ayurveda, a healing system, believed that drinking juice strengthens body tissues.

In the centuries that followed, people recognized that eating fruit and vegetables produce many health benefits. Carrots were said to improve eyesight; and according to the adage, "An apple a day keeps the doctor away." During the twentieth century, fruit and vegetables became important components of healing therapy.

Gerson juice diet

During the 1940s, a German doctor named Max B. Gerson developed a therapy using juice to treat his migraine. His diet was based on the theory that excessive **sodium** in a person's system disrupts the immune system and the functions of the liver, pancreas, and thyroid gland. Gerson developed a low-salt organic diet that focuses on raw vegetable and fruit juices. The diet included nutritional supplements and coffee enemas to detoxify the liver and relieve **pain**. The therapy worked for Gerson, so he recommended it to patients. People diagnosed with cancer and **tuberculosis** said that the Gerson diet therapy produced positive results.

Advocates of juice therapies maintain that refraining from food boosts the body's ability to heal itself. Since the body is not spending time and energy on digesting high-fat food, it can concentrate on healing instead. That reasoning is the basis of juice fasts.

Juicing

Another form of juice therapy known as juicing involves extracting the juice from raw fruit and vegetables. From the 1970s on, people like "Juiceman" Jay Kordich popularized the concept of drinking fresh juice to boost energy, lose weight, and achieve other health benefits. Kordich provided recipes and sold juice extractors that are also known as "juicers."

VITAMINS AND MINERALS FOUND IN JUICES	
Type of Juice	**Vitamins and minerals**
Apple	Chromium, selenium
Asparagus	Vitamin E
Bok choy	Calcium
Broccoli	Folic acid, vitamin K
Brussel sprouts	Manganese
Cabbage	Chromium, manganese, vitamin C
Cantaloupe	Beta-carotene, potassium
Carrots	Beta-carotene, zinc
Celery	Potassium
Citrus fruits	Vitamin C
Collard greens	Calcium, vitamin K
Garlic	Selenium
Ginger	Zinc
Green peas	Zinc
Kale	Calcium, folic acid, vitamin B_6, vitamin K
Orange	Folic acid
Papaya	Beta-carotene
Peppers	Vitamin C
Spinach	Vitamin B_6, vitamin E
Sweet peppers	Chromium
Tomatoes	Potassium
Turnips	Selenium
Turnip greens	Manganese, vitamin B_6

Kordich toured the country and talked about juice ingredients that seemed exotic to a public used to tomato juice and orange juice. One beverage consisted of juiced potato, apple, carrot, and **parsley**.

Benefits

Research has shown that a diet rich in fruit and vegetables reduces the risk of such diseases such as **heart disease**, cancer, and diabetes. Furthermore, raw vegetables and fruit contain vitamins, food enzymes, minerals, **amino acids**, and natural sugars. Some of those benefits may be lost when commercial juice is purchased because juice sold in stores is pasteurized, which results in the loss of some nutrients. Fresh juice's benefits extend beyond its nutritional content, according to juice therapy advocates.

Proponents of juice therapies continue to study its benefits. In 2002, a physician reported to the American College of Cardiology that two cups of orange juice daily significantly lowered the blood pressure of hypertensive patients. A British study in the same year verified the positive effects of **cranberry** juice on urinary tract **infections**.

Juice is used in Ayurvedic treatment for such conditions as arthritis, **anemia**, and **constipation**. Juice is also a component of naturopathy, which is also known as the "whole body cure." A naturopathic doctor may prescribe a juice fast.

Supporters of fasting believe that the process releases a hormone that helps the body fight disease. A juice fast will strengthen the immune system, according to adherents. It may be part of naturopathic treatment for conditions including arthritis, cancer, and **AIDS**. The fast also allows the naturopathic physician to identify food sensitivities (allergens) as the patient begins eating food.

Juice therapy is part of the Gerson diet, a cancer therapy said to eliminate the buildup of toxins in the body by stimulating enzymes, improving the digestive system, and providing the correct balance of vitamins and minerals.

Description

Juice therapy can be as simple as extracting the juice from raw produce or as complicated as the Gerson diet. The therapies vary in the amount of commitment involved and the cost. Whether a therapy is covered by medical insurance will depend on the patient's health plan. The person who juices or fasts at home generally isn't covered. A juice fast administered as part of another treatment by a doctor or health practitioner might be covered. For Gerson therapy, some companies pay for part or all of costs, according to the Gerson Institute website.

Gerson therapy

The Gerson therapy treatment is based on drinking freshly pressed vegetable and fruit juice every hour. During a typical day at a Gerson clinic, a person would drink 13 glasses of raw carrot/apple and green-leaf vegetable juices. Vegetarian meals of organically grown food are served. During treatment, the patient receives **caffeine** enemas during the evening to detoxify the blood and tissues, according to the Gerson Institute website.

The institute does not operate facilities; instead it licenses such facilities as the Oasis of Hope Hospital in Tijuana, Mexico. The hospital opened a Gerson Therapy Center in September of 1999 that cost each patient $4,900 for a week of care. That figure included the cost of a companion's housing as well as follow-up consultations.

Fasting

A juice fast can be done at home with no help or under the direction of a practitioner such as a naturopathic doctor. The fast could also be part of the program at a retreat center.

Another option is a short-term cleansing diet lasting two to three days. One popular fast involves consumption of fruit and vegetable juice for several days. In some plans, herbal tea and broth are allowed. Another variation is the raw food diet, which involves eating uncooked fruit and vegetables. The diet is said to be useful in treating such conditions as heart disease and arthritis.

Juicing

Juicing involves the extraction of juice from raw fruit or vegetables. An extractor, fresh produce, and a commitment of time to juice the items are required. A blender isn't strong enough to juice raw produce, and extractors are priced from about $120–2,000. Juice should be consumed as soon as possible after extraction because when it's stored, juice loses its nutritional value.

BENEFICIAL JUICES. While most people know that orange juice is rich in vitamin C, the juice of other produce is believed to provide additional health benefits. The wide selection of juices offers benefits that include the following:

- An 8-oz (240 ml) glass of carrot juice contains more than 10 times the recommended daily allowance of vitamin C.

- Fresh fruit and vegetable juices, including wheatgrass juice, are consumed for ulcers. Ulcer remedies include raw potato juice for peptic ulcers. For a duodenal ulcer, raw cabbage juice can be mixed with carrot and celery juice.

- Cranberries help prevent and treat urinary infections.

- Beet juice can be diluted to stimulate the liver.

- Garlic lowers the blood pressure and cholesterol.

- Cantaloupe juice can be consumed for stress.

Preparations

People should consult a doctor, practitioner, or nutritionist before beginning a fast or treatment like Gerson therapy. The medical professional can determine whether it's safe to fast and how long the fast should last. The doctor may discover during the test that the person has a condition like diabetes. If that is the case, only a supervised fast would be recommended.

Precautions

Some caution should be taken with each form of juice therapy. Juicing removes much of the necessary dietary fiber found in fruits and vegetables. Since an adult diet should contain 20–25 g of fiber per day, a person should find other sources of fiber. Another caution is that carrot greens, rhubarb greens, and apple seeds can be toxic and should not be juiced.

Some health professionals advise against fasting, a process they say can produce weakness, **fatigue**, anemia, and other disorders. Other health professionals believe that fasts are safe but should not be undertaken by pregnant women, people who are diabetic, and those who have ulcers or a heart condition. In some cases, the doctor or practitioner may advise a supervised fast.

Critics of the Gerson diet maintain that its dangerous side effects include too much weight loss and poor resistance to disease. A person diagnosed with cancer should not abandon such other conventional treatments as chemotherapy in favor of alternative treatment, according to organizations such as the National Cancer Institute. Furthermore, the Gerson Institute advised that therapy should be conducted under the supervision of a Gerson practitioner when a patient is undergoing chemotherapy, is a diabetic, has severe kidney damage, or has breast implants.

Lastly, the juicing of fresh fruit and some vegetables can lead to the intake of considerable amounts of sugar. In some people, the sugar produces a quick rush of energy followed by a "crash."

Side effects

The side effects of fasting can include weight loss and fatigue.

In Gerson therapy, **diarrhea** and **nausea** are considered part of the healing process. During the treatment, a person may experience flu-like symptoms, loss of appetite, weakness, and **dizziness**. Other side effects may include **fever blisters**, perspiration and **body odor**, intestinal cramping, and a painful feeling in tumors.

Research & general acceptance

Studies of Gerson therapy indicated a higher rate of survival for cancer patients who received the treatment in comparison to those who didn't. That research included a 1995 study performed in Mexico. The therapy has not been researched extensively, however, and the Gerson diet is classified by the National Cancer Institute as not medically proven and potentially unsafe.

Some elements of the diet are beneficial—fruit, vegetables, and low-fat food. Most medical professionals believe, however, that less strenuous forms of therapy can be used to treat cancer.

Training & certification

Although there is no official training in juice therapy as such, those who administer it may have training and certification in other disciplines. A naturopathic doctor or medical doctors will have medical training; staffers at Gerson Clinics have been trained in that therapy.

Resources

BOOKS

Albright, Peter. *The Complete Book of Complementary Therapies*. Allentown, PA: People's Medical Society, 1997.

Bruce, Debra Fulghum, and Harris H. McIlwain. *The Unofficial Guide to Alternative Medicine*. New York: Macmillan General Reference, 1998.

Gottlieb, Bill. *New Choices in Natural Healing*. Emmaus, PA: Rodale Press, Inc., 1995.

Kordich, Jay. *The Juiceman's Power of Juicing*. New York: William Morrow & Co., 1992.

Nash, Barbara. *From Acupuncture to Zen: An Encyclopedia of Natural Therapies*. Alameda, CA: Hunter House, 1996.

PERIODICALS

Jancin, Bruce. "Juice Puts Squeeze on Blood Pressure in Pilot Study." *Family Practice News* (May 1, 2002): 13.

Kontiokari, T., K. Sundqvist., Nuutinen, M. "Regular Drinking of Cranberry–Lingonberry Juice Concentrate Reduced Recurrent Urinary Tract Infections in Women." *Evidence–Based Nursing* (April 2002): 43.

ORGANIZATIONS

American Cancer Society. http://www.cancer.org.

Gerson Institute. P.O. Box 430. Bonita, CA 91908-0440. (888) 4GERSON. http://www.gerson.org.

Liz Swain
Teresa G. Odle

Juniper

Description

Juniper (*Juniperus communis*) is an evergreen shrub found on mountains and heaths throughout Europe, Southwest Asia, and North America. The tree grows to a height of 6-25 ft (2-8 m) and has stiff, pointed needles that grow to 0.4 in (1 cm) long. The female bears cones that produce small round bluish-black berries, which take three years to fully mature.

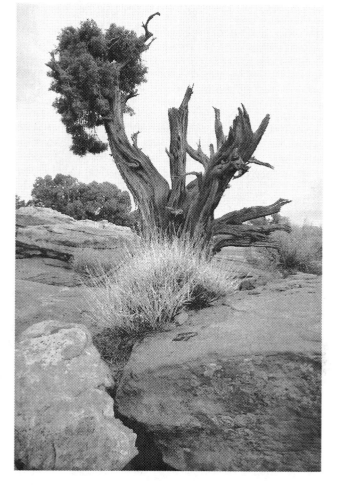

Juniper in Utah. *(Photograph by Robert J. Huffman. Field Mark Publications. Reproduced by permission.)*

Juniper belongs to the pine family (Cupressaceae). Juniper has diuretic, antiseptic, stomachic, antimicrobial, anti-inflammatory, and antirheumatic properties. The tree's therapeutic properties stem from a volatile oil found in the berries. This oil contains terpenes, flavonoid glycosides, tannins, sugar, tar, and resin. Terpinen-4-ol (a diuretic compound of the oil) stimulates the kidneys, increasing their filtration rate. The flavonoid amentoflavone exhibits antiviral properties. Test tube studies show that another constituent of juniper, desoxy-podophyllotoxins, may act to inhibit the herpes simplex virus. The resins and tars contained in the oil benefit such skin conditions as **psoriasis**.

For more than 300 years, juniper berries have been a popular flavoring agent for gin. The word gin comes from the Dutch word for juniper, "geniver." In addition to being an ingredient in alcohol, juniper also has medicinal properties. Ancient Egyptian doctors used the oil as a laxative as far back as 1550 B.C. The Zuni Native American people used the berries to assist them in **child-**

birth. Other Native Americans gathered juniper berries and leaves to treat **infections**, arthritis, and **wounds**. British herbalists used juniper to promote **menstruation**. Nineteenth-century American herbalists used juniper as a remedy for congestive heart failure, **gonorrhea**, and urinary tract infections.

Juniper has also been used as a traditional remedy for **cancer**, arthritis, **gas**, **indigestion**, **warts**, **bronchitis**, **tuberculosis**, **gallstones**, **colic**, heart failure, intestinal disease, **gout**, and back **pain**. The berries were often eaten to relieve rheumatism or to freshen **bad breath**. When treating patients, doctors often chewed juniper berries to prevent infection.

General use

Modern herbalists prescribe juniper to treat bladder infections, kidney disease, chronic arthritis, gout, rheumatic conditions, fluid retention, cystitis, skin conditions, inflammation, digestive problems, menstrual irregularities, and high blood pressure. The German Commission E has approved juniper berries for use in treating **heartburn** and dyspepsia (indigestion), belching, and other digestive disturbances.

Juniper is a powerful diuretic. The volatile oil contained in juniper is composed of compounds that stimulate the kidneys to remove fluid and bacterial waste products from the body. This diuretic action is useful in such conditions as congestive heart failure, urinary infections, and kidney disease.

The oil also has antiseptic properties, which makes it a useful disinfectant treatment for urinary and bladder infections. The German Commission E reported that juniper caused an increase in urine flow and smooth muscle contractions. Juniper may be combined with other herbs such as **uva ursi**, **parsley**, cleavers, or **buchu** to treat bladder infections. In fact, juniper may help treat bladder infections more effectively when combined with other herbs.

Juniper's anti-inflammatory properties help to relieve the inflammation, stiffness, and pain that are present in conditions like arthritis, rheumatism, and gout. The berries can be made into an ointment and rubbed on the affected joints and muscles. The tree needles may be crushed and added to a bath to ease aching muscles. Some people may find relief from the nerve, muscle, joint, and tendon pains of gout and **rheumatoid arthritis** by applying a compress made from an infusion of juniper berries.

Juniper is also warming to the digestive system and increases the production of stomach acid, stimulates the appetite, settles the stomach, and relieves gas.

A steam distillation process is used to extract the essential oil of juniper from the ripe dried berries. This aromatic oil has a light, fruity fragrance that is psychologically uplifting during periods of low energy, **anxiety**, and general weakness. Applied topically, essential oil of juniper has a warming effect on the skin and helps to promote the removal of fluid and waste products from tissues. External applications also help relieve sore muscles, joint and lower back pain, and can be used to clear up **acne**, **eczema**, and **varicose veins**. To stimulate menstruation, juniper oil can be added to a carrier oil and used in a sitz bath or massage. Steam inhalation of the essential oil may also help relieve coughs and lung conditions such as bronchitis.

Consumers should use juniper oil sparingly and should not use more than the recommended dose. Six or more drops of juniper oil can have a toxic effect. Any **aromatherapy** essential oil should be diluted in a carrier oil such as almond or grapeseed oil before external use.

Preparations

The ripe, berries and needles from the tree are used in herbal medicine. Juniper is available in bulk form as whole berries, or as a supplement in the form of capsules or tinctures.

The recommended tincture dosage is 10-20 drops four times daily.

Teas are often taken to relieve digestive problems. To make a tea, 1 cup of boiling **water** is poured over 1 tablespoon of juniper berries. The mixture is covered and steeped for 10-20 minutes. One cup can be drunk two times daily. The tea should not be used for longer than two weeks at a time. A clean cloth may be soaked in the cooled mixture to create a compress.

Precautions

Juniper should be used only for short periods of time. High doses or prolonged use of juniper may irritate the kidneys and urinary tract, causing damage. People with kidney problems should not use this herb.

Juniper stimulates contractions of the womb. Pregnant women should not use juniper. Breast-feeding women also should not use juniper.

Juniper may increase blood sugar levels in diabetics. Therefore, diabetics should consult with their doctor before using juniper.

When taking juniper for a **bladder infection**, consumers should see their doctor if the infection is still present after several days of use, or if lower back pain, **fever**, or **chills** develop.

Side effects

External application of juniper oil may cause a skin rash.

KEY TERMS

Diuretic—A substance that promotes urination.

Infusion—An herbal tea created by steeping herbs in hot water. Generally, leaves and flowers are used in infusions.

Sitz bath—A bath in which only the hips and buttocks are soaked.

Stomachic—A substance that increases the appetite.

People with **allergies** may experience allergy symptoms such as nasal congestion.

Symptoms of juniper overdose include **diarrhea**, purplish urine, blood in the urine, kidney pain, intestinal pain, elevated blood pressure, and a quickened heartbeat. If these effects occur, consumers should stop taking juniper and call their doctor immediately.

Interactions

Consumers should use juniper cautiously with other diuretic drugs or substances because excessive fluid loss may occur.

Resources

BOOKS

Time-Life Books. *The Alternative Advisor.* Alexandria, VA: Time Life Inc., 1997.

Lininger, Skye, D.C. *The Natural Pharmacy.* Virtual Health, LLC, 1998.

Jennifer Wurges

Juvenile rheumatoid arthritis

Definition

Juvenile **rheumatoid arthritis** (JRA) refers to a number of different conditions, all of which strike children, and all of which have immune-mediated joint inflammation as their major manifestation. JRA is also known as juvenile idiopathic arthritis or JIA. The European League Against Rheumatism, or EULAR, refers to the disorder as juvenile chronic arthritis, or JCA.

Description

The skeletal system of the body is made up of different types of strong, fibrous tissue known as connective tissue. Bone, cartilage, ligaments, and tendons are all forms of connective tissue that have different compositions, and thus different characteristics.

The joints are structures that hold two or more bones together. Some joints (synovial joints) allow for movement between the bones being joined (articulating bones). The simplest model of a synovial joint involves two bones, separated by a slight gap called the joint cavity. The ends of each articular bone are covered by a layer of cartilage. Both the articular bones and the joint cavity are surrounded by a tough tissue called the articular capsule. The articular capsule has two components: the fibrous membrane on the outside, and the synovial membrane (or synovium) on the inside. The fibrous membrane may include tough bands of fibrous tissue called ligaments, which are responsible for providing support to the joints. The synovial membrane has special cells and many capillaries (tiny blood vessels). This membrane produces a supply of synovial fluid that fills the joint cavity, lubricates it, and helps the articular bones move smoothly about the joint.

In JRA, the synovial membrane becomes intensely inflamed. Usually thin and delicate, the synovium becomes thick and stiff, with numerous infoldings on its surface. The membrane becomes invaded by white blood cells, which produce a variety of destructive chemicals. The cartilage along the articular surfaces of the bones may be attacked and destroyed, and the bone, articular capsule, and ligaments may begin to be worn away (eroded). These processes severely interfere with movement in the joint.

JRA specifically refers to chronic arthritic conditions that affect a child under the age of 16 years, and that last for a minimum of three to six months. JRA is often characterized by a waxing and waning course, with flares separated by periods of time during which no symptoms are noted (remission). Some literature refers to JRA as juvenile rheumatoid arthritis, although most types of JRA differ significantly from the adult disease called rheumatoid arthritis in terms of symptoms, progression, and prognosis.

Causes & symptoms

A number of different causes have been sought to explain the onset of JRA. There seems to be some genetic link, based on the fact that the tendency to develop JRA sometimes runs in particular families, and based on the fact that certain genetic markers are more frequently found in patients with JRA and other related diseases. Recent research has shown that several autoimmune diseases, including JRA, share a common genetic link. In other words, patients with JRA might share common

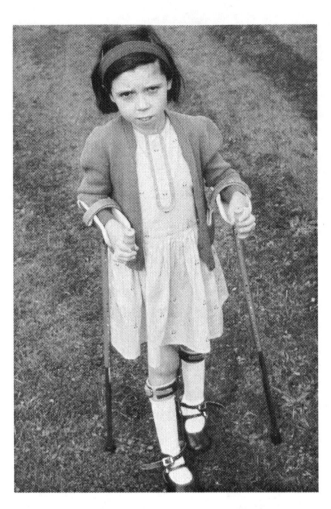

Girl with juvenile rheumatoid arthritis. The disease affects children under the age of 16 and lasts for at least three to six months. *(©John Moss/Photo Researchers Inc. Reproduced by permission.)*

genes with family members who have other autoimmune diseases like rheumatoid arthritis, systemic lupus, **multiple sclerosis**, and others.

Many researchers have looked for some infectious cause for JRA, but no clear connection to a particular organism has ever been made. JRA is considered by some to be an autoimmune disorder. Autoimmune disorders occur when the body's immune system mistakenly identifies the body's own tissue as foreign, and attacks those tissues, as if trying to rid the body of an invader (such as a bacteria, virus, or fungi). While an autoimmune mechanism is strongly suspected, certain markers of such a mechanism (such as rheumatoid factor, often present in adults with such disorders) are rarely present in children with JRA.

Joint symptoms of arthritis may include stiffness, **pain**, redness, warmth of the joint, and swelling. Bone in the area of an affected joint may grow too quickly or too slowly, resulting in limbs that are of different lengths. When the child tries to avoid moving a painful joint, the muscle may begin to shorten from disuse. This is called a contracture.

Symptoms of JRA depend on the particular subtype. According to criteria published by the American College of Rheumatology (ACR) in 1973 and modified in 1977, JRA is classified by the symptoms that appear within the first six months of the disorder:

- Pauciarticular JRA: This is the most common and the least severe type of JRA, affecting about 40–60% of all JRA patients. It affects fewer than four joints, usually the knee, ankle, wrist, and/or elbow. Other more general (systemic) symptoms are usually absent, and the child's growth usually remains normal. Very few children (less than 15%) with pauciarticular JRA end up with deformed joints. Some children with this form of JRA experience painless swelling of the joint. Others have a serious inflammation of structures within the eye, which if left undiagnosed and untreated could even lead to blindness. This condition is known as uveitis, and affects about 20% of children diagnosed with JRA. While many children have cycles of flares and remissions, in some children the disease completely and permanently resolves within a few years of diagnosis.

- Polyarticular JRA: About 40% of all cases of JRA are of this type. It is most common in children up to age three or after the age of 10, and affects girls more often than boys. Polyarticular JRA affects five or more joints simultaneously. This type of JRA usually affects the small joints of both hands and both feet, although other large joints may be affected as well. Some patients with arthritis in their knees will experience a different rate of growth in each leg. Ultimately, one leg will grow longer than the other. About half of all patients with polyarticular JRA have arthritis of the spine and/or hip. Others with polyarticular JRA will have other symptoms of a systemic illness, including **anemia** (low red blood cell count), decreased growth rate, low appetite, low-grade **fever**, and a slight rash. The disease is most severe in those children who are diagnosed in early adolescence. Some of these children will test positive for a marker present in other autoimmune disorders, called rheumatoid factor (RF). RF is found in adults who have rheumatoid arthritis. Children who are positive for RF tend to have a more severe course, with a disabling form of arthritis that destroys and deforms the joints. This type of arthritis is thought to be the adult form of rheumatoid arthritis occurring at a very early age.

- Systemic onset JRA: Sometimes called Still disease (after a physician who originally described it), this type of JRA occurs in about 10–20% of all patients with

JRA. Boys and girls are equally affected, and diagnosis is usually made between the ages of five and 10. The initial symptoms are not usually related to the joints. Instead, these children have high fevers; a rash; decreased appetite and weight loss; severe joint and muscle pain; swollen lymph nodes, spleen, and liver; and serious anemia. Some children experience other complications, including inflammation of the sac containing the heart (pericarditis), inflammation of the tissue lining the chest cavity and lungs (pleuritis), and inflammation of the heart muscle (myocarditis). The eye inflammation often seen in pauciarticular JRA is uncommon in systemic onset JRA. Symptoms of actual arthritis begin later in the course of systemic onset JRA, and they often involve the wrists and ankles. Many of these children continue to have periodic flares of fever and systemic symptoms throughout childhood. Some children will go on to develop a polyarticular type of JRA.

- Spondyloarthropathy: This type of JRA most commonly affects boys older than eight years of age. The arthritis occurs in the knees and ankles, moving over time to include the hips and lower spine. Inflammation of the eye may occur occasionally but usually resolves without permanent damage.

- Psoriatic JRA: This type of arthritis usually shows up in fewer than four joints, but goes on to include multiple joints (appearing similar to polyarticular JRA). Hips, back, fingers, and toes are frequently affected. A skin condition called **psoriasis** accompanies this type of arthritis. Children with this type of JRA often have pits or ridges in their fingernails. The arthritis usually progresses to become a serious, disabling problem.

As of 2003, there is some disagreement among specialists about the classification of JRA. Some prefer the EULAR classification, also introduced in 1977, to the ACR system. In 1997, the World Health Organization (WHO) met in Durban and issued a new classification system for JRA known as the Durban criteria, in an attempt to standardize definitions of the various subtypes of JRA. None of the various classification systems, however, are considered fully satisfactory as of early 2004.

Diagnosis

Diagnosis of JRA is often made on the basis of the child's collection of symptoms. Laboratory tests often show normal results. Some nonspecific indicators of inflammation may be elevated, including white blood cell count, erythrocyte sedimentation rate, and a marker called C-reactive protein. As with any chronic disease, anemia may be noted. Children with an extraordinarily early onset of the adult type of rheumatoid arthritis will have a positive test for rheumatoid factor.

Treatment

One of the best natural therapies for JRA is resistance exercises, according to a 1999 study at the University of Buffalo in New York. In the study, children did lower body exercises three times a week for an hour per session. After eight weeks, the children had a 40–60% increase in muscle strength, speed, and endurance. The less fit the child, the more improvement that was shown. Also, pain was reduced by 50% and medication use was cut by 25%. In a related study, researchers found **exercise** decreased inflammatory agents while increasing anti-inflammatory compounds in the body, thereby improving immune function. Diet is also believed to play a role in treating juvenile rheumatoid arthritis. A strict vegetarian diet low in fats and free of glutens can also be helpful, as well as an allergy **elimination diet**. A number of autoimmune disorders, including JRA, seem to have a relationship to food **allergies**. Identification and elimination of reactive foods may result in a decrease in JRA symptoms.

Alternative treatments that have been suggested for arthritis include **juice therapy,** which can work to detoxify the body, helping to reduce JRA symptoms. Some recommended fruits and vegetables to include in the juice are carrots, celery, cabbage, potatoes, cherries, lemons, beets, cucumbers, radishes, and **garlic**. Tomatoes and other vegetables in the nightshade family (potatoes, eggplant, and red and green peppers) are discouraged. As an adjunct therapy, **aromatherapy** preparations use cypress, **fennel**, and lemon. Massage oils include **rosemary**, benzoin, **chamomile**, camphor, **juniper**, **eucalyptus**, and **lavender**. Other types of therapy that have been used include **acupuncture**, **acupressure**, and body work.

Also shown to be effective in some cases are the essential fatty acids: **omega-3 fatty acids** in **fish oil**, and the omega-6 fatty acid gamma liolenic acid (GLA) found in **borage oil**, currant seed oil, and **evening primrose oil**. Several alternative medicine doctors suggest there may be some benefit in taking **cartilage supplements**, although no definitive studies have been done on this treatment. Anti-inflammatory spices such as tumeric, **ginger**, and **cayenne** may be helpful. Natural remedies such as **yucca, burdock root, horsetail, devil's claw**, sarsaparilla, and **white willow** bark also can be helpful since they have anti-inflammatory and analgesic properties.

Nutritional supplements that may be beneficial include large amounts of **antioxidants** (vitamins C, A, E, **zinc, selenium**, and flavenoids), as well as B vitamins and a full complement of minerals (including **boron, copper, manganese**). One study showed 1,800 International Units (IU) of **vitamin E** a day could be helpful in relieving symptoms. Other nutrients that assist in detoxifying the body, including **methionine**, cysteine, and other **amino acids**, may also be helpful. Constitutional **homeopathy** can also work to quiet the symptoms of JRA and bring about balance to the whole person.

Allopathic treatment

Treating JRA involves efforts to decrease the amount of inflammation, in order to preserve movement. Medications that can be used for this include nonsteroidal anti-inflammatory agents (such as ibuprofen and naproxen). Oral (by mouth) steroid medications are effective, but have many serious side effects with long-term use. Injections of steroids into an affected joint can be helpful. Steroid eye drops are used to treat eye inflammation. Other drugs that have been used to treat JRA include methotrexate, sulfasalazine, penicillamine, and hydroxychloroquine. Physical therapy and exercises are often recommended in order to improve joint mobility and strengthen supporting muscles. Occasionally, splints are used to rest painful joints and to prevent or improve deformities.

The FDA approved a new drug, etanercept, marketed under the brand name Enbrel, in 1999. It is the most dramatic advancement in treating JRA in recent years. A study by Children's Hospital Medical Center in Cincinnati, Ohio, released in 1999, showed the drug was effective in 75% of children with severe JRA. The drug eases joint pain, reduces swelling, and improves mobility.

In 2003, a group of Japanese researchers noted that the blood serum of patients with JRA contains elevated levels of interleukin-6, a cytokine (nonantibody protein) that is critical to regulation of the immune system and blood cell formation. Because interleukin-6 is also associated with inflammation, the researchers think that compounds inhibiting the formation of interleukin-6 might provide new treatment options for JRA.

Expected results

The prognosis for pauciarticular JRA is quite good, as is the prognosis for spondyloarthropathy. Polyarticular JRA carries a slightly worse prognosis. RF-positive polyarticular JRA carries a difficult prognosis, often with progressive, destructive arthritis and joint deformities. Systemic onset JRA has a variable prognosis, depending on the organ systems affected, and the progression to polyarticular JRA. About 1–5% of all JRA patients die of such complications as infection, inflammation of the heart, or kidney disease.

Prevention

Little is known about the causes of JRA, therefore there are no recommendations available for preventing it.

KEY TERMS

Articular bones—Two or more bones which are connected with each other via a joint.

Cytokine—A general term for nonantibody proteins released by a specific type of cell as part of the body's immune response.

Idiopathic—Of unknown cause or spontaneous origin. JRA is sometimes called juvenile idiopathic arthritis or JIA because its causes are still not fully known.

Joint—A structure that holds two or more bones together.

Rheumatology—The branch of medicine that specializes in the diagnosis and treatment of disorders affecting the muscles and joints.

Synovial joint—A particular type of joint that allows for movement in the articular bones.

Synovial membrane—The membrane that lines the inside of the articular capsule of a joint and produces a lubricating fluid called synovial fluid.

Uveitis—Inflammation of the pigmented vascular covering of the eye, which includes the choroid, iris, and ciliary body. Uveitis is a common complication of JRA.

Resources

BOOKS

Behrman, Richard, et al., eds. *Nelson Textbook of Pediatrics,* 16th ed. Philadelphia: W. B. Saunders Co., 2000.

"Juvenile Rheumatoid Arthritis." Section 19, Chapter 270 in *The Merck Manual of Diagnosis and Therapy*, edited by Mark H. Beers, MD, and Robert Berkow, MD. Whitehouse Station, NJ: Merck Research Laboratories, 2002.

Kredich, Deborah Welt. "Juvenile Rheumatoid Arthritis." In *Rudolph's Pediatrics,* edited by Abraham M. Rudolph. Stamford:McGraw-Hill, 2002.

Peacock, Judith. *Juvenile Arthritis.* Mankato, MN: LifeMatters Books, 2000.

PERIODICALS

de Boer, J., N. Wulffraat, and A. Rothova. "Visual Loss in Uveitis of Childhood." *British Journal of Ophthalmology* 87 (July 2003): 879–884.

Henderson, Charles W. "Etanercept a Dramatic Advancement in Treatment, Say Researchers." *Immunotherapy Weekly* (April 2, 2000).

Kotaniemi, K., A. Savolainen, A. Karma, and K. Aho. "Recent Advances in Uveitis of Juvenile Idiopathic Arthritis." *Survey of Ophthalmology* 48 (September-October 2003): 489–502.

Larkin, Marilynn. "Juvenile Arthritis Helped by Resistance Exercise." *Lancet* (November 20, 1999): 1797.

Manners, P., J. Lesslie, D. Speldewinde, and D. Tunbridge. "Classification of Juvenile Idiopathic Arthritis: Should Family History Be Included in the Criteria?" *Journal of Rheumatology* 30 (August 2003): 1857–1863.

Moran, M. "Autoimmune Diseases Could Share Common Genetic Etiology." *American Medical News* 44, no. 38 (October 8, 2001): 38.

Yokota, S. "Interleukin 6 as a Therapeutic Target in Systemic-Onset Juvenile Idiopathic Arthritis." *Current Opinion in Rheumatology* 15 (September 2003): 581–586.

ORGANIZATIONS

American College of Rheumatology. 1800 Century Place, Suite 250, Atlanta, GA, 30345. (404) 633-3777. acr@rheumatology.org. <http://www.rheumatology.org>.

Arthritis Foundation. P.O. Box 7669, Atlanta, GA 30357-0669. (800) 283-7800. <http://www.arthritis.org>.

National Arthritis and Musculoskeletal and Skin Diseases Information Clearinghouse. National Institutes of Health, 1 AMS Circle, Bethesda, MD 20892. (301) 495-4484. <http://www.nih.gov/niams>.

OTHER

MotherNature.com. "Rheumatoid Arthritis." [cited October 2002]. <http://www.mothernature.com/Library/Ency/Index.cfm?id=1257001>.

National Institute of Arthritis and Musculoskeletal and Skin Diseases (NIAMS). *Questions and Answers About Juvenile Rheumatoid Arthritis*. NIH Publication No. 01-4942. Bethesda, MD: NIAMS, 2001. <http://www.niams.nih.gov/hi/topics/juvenile_arthritis/juvarthr.htm>.

Ken R. Wells
Rebecca J. Frey, PhD

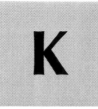

K

Kali bichromium

Description

Kali bichromium is a bright orange, caustic, corrosive compound used in the manufacture of dye, photography, and batteries. It is also used as a homeopathic remedy. In **homeopathy**, **potassium** bichromate is diluted to the point where it no longer retains any poisonous or caustic qualities. Homeopaths usually abbreviate kali bichromium as *Kali bich.* or as *Kali bi.*

General use

Homeopathic medicine operates on the principle that "like heals like." This principle means that a disease can be cured by treating it with products that produce the same symptoms as the disease. These products follow another homeopathic law, the Law of Infinitesimals. In opposition to traditional medicine, the Law of Infinitesimals states that the lower a dose of curative, the more effective it is. To achieve a low dose, the curative is diluted many, many times until only a tiny amount, if any, remains in a huge amount of the diluting liquid.

In homeopathic medicine, *Kali bichromium* is said to have an affinity for the mucous membranes and the skin. It is used primarily to treat stringy yellowish or greenish mucous discharges from any part of the body, including the nose, throat, larynx, vagina, urethra, and stomach. Its most common use is to treat colds that are accompanied by sinus congestion or evolve into sinusitis.

In these situations the patient feels pressure and fullness in the sinuses and experiences extreme **pain** at the root of the nose that improves when pressure is applied to the painful spot. *Kali bichromium* is also used to treat feelings of fullness and pressure in the middle ear and to treat sinus or migraine headaches that start at night.

In addition, *Kali bichromium* is used to treat a sore throat with swollen tonsils, swollen neck, and a discharge of pus. In the mouth, ulcers or a dry, burning feeling are treated by *Kali bichromium* when accompanied by intense pain at the root of the tongue or a dry, yellow-coated tongue.

Certain types of coughs are also treated with *Kali bichromium* when the voice is rough and hoarse, and the **cough** is dry. If the cough worsens when breathing damp, cold air, worsens in the early hours of the morning, and is better in warm air, these are also indications to the homeopath that kali bichromium is an appropriate remedy.

Kali bichromium is used to treat joint pains that appear and disappear suddenly or wander to different spots in the body causing severe pain. These pains, like the cough, are improved by warmth.

Kali bichromium is sometimes used for relief of distress in the digestive system such as **nausea** and vomiting of yellow mucus and bile. In homeopathic terminology, the effectiveness of remedies is proved by experimentation and reporting done by famous homeopathic practitioners. *Kali bichromium* was proved as a **vomiting** remedy by Dr. John H. Clark (1853–1931).

In homeopathic medicine the fact that certain symptoms get better or worse under different conditions is used as a diagnostic tool to indicate what remedy will be most effective. Symptoms that benefit from treatment with *Kali bichromium* get worse in the very early hours of the morning (2 a.m. to 5 a.m.), worsen in wet weather, are worse in the summer, are worse upon awaking, upon getting cold from undressing, and upon consuming alcohol (which often induces vomiting and **diarrhea** in patients that need this remedy). Symptoms improve with warmth, movement, pressure, and from eating. Patients needing *Kali bichromium* tend to get cold easily.

Homeopathy also ascribes certain personality types to certain remedies. The *Kali bichromium* personality is said to be listless with aversion to physical or mental **exercise.** People with *Kali bichromium* personalities also tend to be rigid and inflexible, doing most activities such as eating, sleeping, and working on a rigid timetable. They are very detail oriented. Morally, they tend to be very proper, rigid, and conservative, which results in a narrow-minded, self-centered personality.

Preparations

Kail bichromium is prepared by extensive dilutions of what is called a mother tincture of potassium dichromate dissolved in an alcohol/water mixture. There are two homeopathic dilution scales, the decimal (x) scale with a dilution of 1:10 and the centesimal (c) scale where the dilution factor is 1:100. Once the mixture is diluted, shaken, strained, then re-diluted many times to reach the desired degree of potency, the final mixture is added to lactose (a type of sugar) tablets or pellets. These are then stored away from light. *Kali bichromium* is available commercially in tablets or pellets in strengths of 6x, 12x, 30x, 200x, 6c, 12c, 30c, and 200c.

Homeopathic and orthodox medical practitioners agree that by the time the mother tincture is diluted to strengths used in homeopathic healing, it is likely that very few if any molecules of the original remedy remain. Homeopaths, however, believe that these remedies continue to work through an effect called potentization that has not yet been explained by mainstream scientists.

Precautions

No particular precautions have been reported when using *Kali bichromium*.

Side effects

When taken in the recommended dilute form, no side effects have been reported. However, concentrated quantities of this compound are corrosive.

Interactions

Studies on interactions between *Kali bichromium* given in homeopathic doses and conventional pharmaceuticals are nonexistent.

Resources

BOOKS

Cummings, Stephen and Dana Ullman. *Everybody's Guide to Homeopathic Medicines.* 3rd edition. New York: Putnam, 1997.

Hammond, Christopher. *The Complete Family Guide to Homeopathy.* London: Penguin Studio, 1995.

Lockie, Andrew, and Nicola Geddes. *The Complete Guide to Homeopathy.* London: Dorling Kindersley, 1995.

ORGANIZATIONS

Foundation for Homeopathic Education and Research. 21 Kittredge Street, Berkeley, CA 94704. (510) 649–8930.

International Foundation for Homeopathy. P. O. Box 7, Edmonds, WA 98020. (206) 776–4147.

National Center for Homeopathy. 801 N. Fairfax Street, Suite 306, Alexandria, VA 22314. (703) 548–7790.

ORGANIZATIONS

The British Institute of Homeopathy Canada. 1445 St. Joseph Blvd., Gloucester, ON K1C 7K9 Canada. (613) 830–4759. http://www.homeopathy.com.

OTHER

Holistic Medicine Online. http://www.holisticmed.com.

Tish Davidson

Kampo medicine

Definition

Kampo (sometimes spelled kanpo) is a Japanese variant of Chinese traditional medicine that involves the extensive use of herbs. The name is derived from the Japanese symbols *kan*, which means China and *po*, which means medicine. Kampo treatment has become very much integrated in the Japanese health care system. It is widely available from hospitals and physicians there, and is the most popular form of complementary health care in contemporary Japan. Kampo herbal preparations are sold by many Japanese pharmacies. The World Health Organization (WHO) reports that Japan has the highest per capita consumption of herbal medicine in the world. In addition to herbal treatments, Kampo practitioners may also administer **acupuncture**, **moxibustion**, and manipulative therapy.

Origins

Oriental traditional medicine has employed herbs for almost 4,000 years. Much of the earliest literature about the subject comes from ancient China, where wealthy families hired herbalists who were paid only when everyone in the family enjoyed good health. Kampo medicine is a form of traditional Chinese herbalism, which came to Japan about 16 centuries ago and was refined over the years by Japanese practitioners. At

Shoso-in, a famous historical site in western Japan, a 1,200-year-old cache of medicinal herbs was discovered, stored n air-tight wooden boxes. Researchers found that many of those samples still retained full medicinal potency. Western medicine started to enter Japan with Jesuit missionaries and Dutch traders during the sixteenth and seventeenth centuries, but never succeeded in fully displacing traditional practices. In recent years, there has been a considerable resurgence of Kampo's popularity.

Benefits

Kampo preparations are used to treat a wide variety of conditions, including **eczema**, atopic **dermatitis**, and gynecological problems. Other applications include allergies, **rheumatoid arthritis**, chronic **hepatitis**, diabetic retinopathy, bronchial **asthma**, endometrial cancer, collagen disease, bedwetting, colds, **nausea**, and high cholesterol levels.

Description

Like other forms of Oriental traditional medicine, Kampo is based on concepts quite foreign to Western medical thinking. These concepts include *In-You* (negative and positive); *Gogyou* (five lines); *Ki* (air); *Sui* (water); and *Ketu* (blood). Unlike Western medicine, which thinks largely in terms of diseases affecting specific organs, Kampo emphasizes identifying patterns of "whole body" symptoms.

Kampo herbal treatments are divided into three basic groups, related to urination, sweating, and defecation. Most prescriptions consist of a combination of crude drugs used to treat whatever disharmony is detected. Kampo remedies usually take longer to work than standard pharmaceuticals. A typical trial period for a new prescription is three months. Patients may continue taking some prescriptions for years. Examples of crude drugs used in Kampo preparations include glycyrrhiza (**licorice**), rhubarb, and ginseng.

Since the 1970s, Kampo has been recognized by Japan's medical regulators, and Kampo herbs are included in the list of reimbursable drugs under the country's national health insurance plan. During the 1990s and continuing into the new millennium, Japanese officials required recertification of a number of Kampo drugs, insisting that their safety and effectiveness be reevaluated. Japanese pharmacists are allowed to manufacture a limited number of drugs themselves. Of these licensed products, 50% are Kampo products, according to the Japan Pharmaceutical Association.

Precautions

As with all Oriental herbal remedies, persons should use only Kampo preparations obtained from a reliable source. Serious problems have arisen when Oriental herbal prescriptions were misidentified or contained adulterants. The Register of Chinese Herbal Medicine in the United Kingdom recommends that patent medicines mixing Western and Oriental herbs be avoided, together with any patent preparation containing heavy metals. Some patients have developed hepatitis after taking patent-medicine tablets based on traditional Oriental formulas. An investigation revealed that the tablets did not contain the complete herb, but rather a chemical isolated from a single herb. This practice contradicts the most basic principles of Oriental traditional medicine, which uses combinations of whole herbs. Because of Kampo's complexity, self-treatment is usually not advised; consulting a knowledgeable practitioner is essential. Some patients have experienced serious, even fatal, kidney or liver problems after treatment with Oriental herbs. Anyone with a history of disease in those organs should not be treated without accompanying blood tests to monitor their function. It has also been suggested that patients who consume considerable amounts of alcohol should receive liver function tests. It is important that patients be monitored after starting Oriental herb treatments to check for signs of liver or kidney problems.

Side effects

Because Kampo and other forms of Oriental traditional medicine are so old, practitioners say that most side effects were identified long ago and so are easily avoided by an experienced practitioner. Some Oriental herbal preparations, however, are known toxins that continue to be prescribed because of their beneficial effects. These must be used with extreme care, employing only low doses under the direction of a highly competent and certified practitioner. In most cases, these preparations should be used only in a hospital setting. In addition, some people may have an allergic hypersensitivity to certain herbs.

Research & general acceptance

In Japan, Kampo treatment is studied and frequently prescribed by medical doctors. As many as 70% of Japanese gynecologists are said to employ Kampo, particularly in menopausal patients.

Training & certification

In Japan, Kampo drugs are widely available from medical doctors and pharmacists. In the rest of the world, Kampo preparations and practitioners are largely unregulated.

Resources

PERIODICALS

Blackwell, Richard. "Adverse events following certain Chinese herbal medicines and the response of the profession." *Journal of Chinese Medicine.* 50:12.

ORGANIZATIONS

Japan Society for Oriental Medicine. Nihonbashi Nakadori Building 4F 2-2-20. Nihonbashi, Chuo-ku, Tokyo 103-0027. 81-3-3274-5060.

OTHER

Kampo Today. c/o Michael Solomon Associates, Inc. 516 Fifth Avenue, Suite 801. New York, NY 10036. (212) 764-4760. http://www.tsumura.co.jp/english/kthp/today.htm.

David Helwig

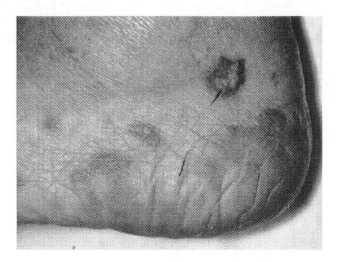

Kaposi's sarcoma. *Centers for Disease Control and Prevention.*

Kaposi's sarcoma

Definition

Kaposi's sarcoma (KS), also called multiple idiopathic hemorrhagic sarcoma, is a neoplastic disease associated especially with **AIDS**, usually affecting the skin and mucous membranes.

Description

Causes & symptoms

Kaposi's sarcoma (KS) is caused by herpesvirus 8. Malignant cells are found in the tissues under the skin or mucous membranes that line the mouth, nose, and anus. KS causes red or purple patches on the skin and/or mucous membranes and spread to other organs, such as the lungs, liver, or intestinal tract. KS is seen in three forms:

• indolent

• lymphadenopathic

• AIDS-related

The primary distinction between the three forms of KS is the rate of growth and the location of the lesions. In the past, the indolent form of Kaposi's sarcoma was the most common, and was most often seen in men over the age of 60 years of Jewish or Italian ancestry; in African men; and in patients who had organ transplants or had their immune systems impaired for other reasons. KS was frequently left untreated. Because of its slow growth, the **cancer** was not a threat to the patient. Since the 1980s, a far higher percentage of cases with rapid growth have been observed, usually accompanied by AIDS (HIV disease).

The aggressive form of KS is seen in about one-third of patients with AIDS, and has become endemic in equatorial African. In African nations, aggressive KS is seen most often among young men and children.

Lymphadenophic KS affects the lymph nodes as well as the skin structures.

Diagnosis

KS is traditionally diagnosed based on the red or purple patches on the skin or mucous membranes. A biopsy is usually performed in order to verify the diagnosis. Since other cancers may have a similar appearance to KS, it is often useful to test for the presence of human herpesvirus 8 in order to confirm the diagnosis.

Treatment

In indolent KS, localized treatment is often adequate. Superficial lesions may be removed surgically. Alternatives are radiation therapy, electrical curettage, in which the lesion is burned with an electrical current, or cryotherapy, in which a source of extreme cold, such as liquid nitrogen, is applied to the cancer in order to kill the cells.

Among patients who develop KS after an organ transplant, reduction in the dose of drugs used to control the immune response may be enough to control or eliminate the cancer, although this treatment increases the risk of transplant rejection. One report from the University of Barcelona in Spain states that a change of medication may resolve the problem of KS after transplantation.

In KS associated with AIDS, systemic chemotherapy is usually required.

The Gay Men's Health Crisis (GMHC) has reviewed a number of alternative therapies which have been tried in KS, but none have shown consistently favorable results. Among the treatments mentioned were shark cartilage, herbal and purifying massage therapies to enhance immune function, and transcendental **meditation**. **Homeopathy** has been tried, but here too the results have not been reliable.

Allopathic treatment

There are no current best-practice treatments for KS. For rapidly growing KS, a standard treatment is systemic chemotherapy with a combination of adriamycin, bleomycin, and vincristine (ABV); however, several studies have reported that single-agent treatments may be as effective as combinations. Single-agent treatments that have shown evidence of effectiveness are a liposomal form of adriamycin used alone; methotrexate, and trimetrexate. Interferon-alpha has also been reported to be effective in AIDS-related KS.

Expected results

The expected results depend primarily on the underlying condition of the patient. Those patients who have classic slow-growing KS may live many years, even in the absence of treatment. For patients with AIDS, a proposed staging system has divided patients into low-and high-risk groups, depending both on the extent of the sarcoma and their underlying immune function. Patients with well-functioning immune systems, no AIDS associated opportunistic **infections**, and KS confined to the skin have an estimated survival of about three years. Those with impaired immune systems, other infections, and more widespread KS have an estimated survival of about one year. Overall length of survival will depend on the patient's response to treatment.

Prevention

The United States Public Health Service (USPHS) guidelines for prevention of KS call for prophylactic administration of drugs that are effective against human herpesvirus-8. The primary drugs for this purpose are foscarnet and ganciclovir. In each case, the dose must be adjusted based on the patient's condition. While the USPHS recognizes that KS may affect children as well as adults, no formal recommendations for prevention have been published.

Resources

BOOKS

Abeloff M. D., J. O. Armitage, A. S. Lichter, and J. E. Niederhuber, editors. *Clinical Oncology, 2nd edition.* New York: Churchill Livingston, 2000.

PERIODICALS

Campistol, J. M., A. Gutierrez-Dalmau, and J. V. Torregrosa. "Conversion to sirolimus: a successful treatment for post-transplantation Kaposi's sarcoma." *Transplantation* (March 2004): 760–2.

Chao, S. C., J. Y. Lee, and C. J. Tsao. "Treatment of classical type Kaposi's sarcoma with paclitaxel." *Anticancer Res* (January-February 2001): 571–3.

Cheuk, W., K. O. Wong, C. S. Wong, J. E. Dinkel, D. Ben-Dor, and J. K. Chan. "Immunostaining for human herpesvirus 8 latent nuclear antigen-1 helps distinguish Kaposi sarcoma from its mimickers." *Am J Clin Pathol* (March 2004): 335–42.

"DaunoXome offers KS treatment alternative." *Aids Alert* (June 1996): 67–8.

OTHER

"Prevention of disease recurrence." *1999 USPHS/IDSA guidelines for the prevention of opportunistic infections in persons infected with HIV: Part III. United States Public Health Service/Infectious Diseases Society of America, 1999.*

"Prevention of the first episode of disease." *1999 USPHS/IDSA Guidelines for the Prevention of Opportunistic Infections in Persons Infected with HIV: Part II.* U.S. Department of Health and Human Services, Public Health Service, Centers for Disease Control and Prevention. U.S. Public Health Service/Infectious Diseases Society of America, 1999.

Samuel Uretsky, Pharm.D.

Kava kava

Description

Kava kava (*Piper methysticum*) is a tropical shrub that grows throughout the Pacific Islands. Kava kava belongs to the pepper family (Piperaceae) and is also known as kava, asava pepper, or intoxicating pepper. It grows to an average height of 6 ft (1.83 m) and has large heart-shaped leaves that can grow to 10 in (25.4 cm) wide. A related species is *Piper sanctum*, a native plant of Mexico that is used as a stimulant.

Kava kava has been used as a medicinal herb for hundreds of years and used by Pacific Islanders to treat rheumatism, **asthma**, **worms**, **obesity**, headaches, **fun-**

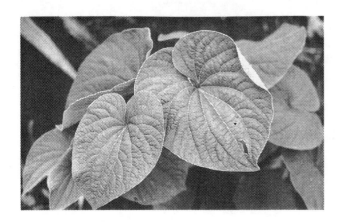

Kava kava leaves. *(Photo Researchers, Inc. Reproduced by permission.)*

gal **infections**, leprosy, gonorrhea, vaginal **infections**, urinary infections, menstrual problems, migraine headaches, and **insomnia**. It was also used as a diuretic, an aphrodisiac, to promote energy, and to bring about sweating during colds and fevers. Pacific Islanders consume a kava kava drink at social, ritual, and ceremonial functions. It is drunk at ceremonies to commemorate marriages, births, and deaths; in meetings of village elders; as an offering to the gods; to cure illness; and to welcome honored guests. Pope John Paul II, Queen Elizabeth II, and Hillary Rodham Clinton have all drunk kava kava during their island visits.

The drink is prepared by grinding, grating, or pounding the roots of the plant, then soaking the pulp in cold **water** or coconut milk. Traditionally the root was chewed, spit into a bowl, and mixed with coconut milk or water. That practice is no longer the standard.

Captain James Cook has been credited with the Western discovery of kava kava during his journey to the South Pacific in the late 1700s. The first herbal products made from kava kava appeared in Europe in the 1860s. Pharmaceutical preparations became available in Germany in the 1920s. Currently, kava kava has received widespread attention because of its reputation to promote **relaxation** and reduce stress.

General use

Kava kava has been prescribed by healthcare providers to treat a wide range of ailments, including insomnia, nervousness, and stress-related **anxiety** and anxiety disorders. It is also reported to relieve urinary infections, **vaginitis**, fatigue, asthma, rheumatism, and **pain**.

The active ingredients in kava kava are called kavalactones and are found in the root of the plant. Kavalactones cause reactions in the brain similar to phar-

maceutical drugs prescribed for depression and anxiety. Research has shown that kavalactones have a calming, sedative effect that relaxes muscles, relieves spasms, and prevents convulsions. Kavalactones also have analgesic (pain-relieving) properties that may bring relief to sore throats, sore gums, canker sores, and toothaches.

Kava kava is a strong diuretic that is reportedly beneficial in the treatment of **gout**, rheumatism, and arthritis. The diuretic effect of the herb relieves pain and helps remove waste products from the afflicted joints. Antispasmodic properties have shown to help ease menstrual cramps by relaxing the muscles of the uterus. Kava kava's antiseptic and anti-inflammatory agents may help relieve an irritable bladder, urinary tract infections, and inflammation of the prostate gland.

Preparations

Kava kava is available in dry bulk (powdered or crushed), capsule, tablet, tea, and tincture forms. Many of the products are made from the dried powder of the root. Western consumers have generally been advised to look for standardized extracts of kava kava that have a 70% kavalactone content. On the other hand, a report submitted to the Committee of Safety of Medicines (CSM) of the United Kingdom in April 2002 indicates that many of the side effects reported in connection with kava kava are due to the high concentration of the herb in commercial standardized extracts. The report suggested that kava preparations made according to traditional methods are relatively safe. It is likely that controversy over kava kava will continue.

Precautions

Before 2002, the usual precautions regarding kava kava stated that it should not be used by pregnant or lactating women, or when driving or operating heavy machinery. The American Herbal Products Association (AHPA) advised consumers in 1997 not to take kava kava for more than three months at a time, and not to exceed the recommended dosages. In light of more recent findings, however, it would be prudent for many adults to completely avoid preparations of or products containing kava kava.

As of March 25, 2002, the United States Food and Drug Administration (FDA) has recommended that people who have a history of liver disease or are taking medications that affect the liver should consult a physician before taking any preparations containing kava kava.

Side effects

Prior to 2002, most reports of side effects from kava kava concerned relatively minor problems, such as numbness in the mouth, headaches, mild **dizziness**, or skin **rashes**. Nineteenth-century missionaries to the Pacific islands noted that people who drank large quantities of kava kava developed yellowish scaly skin. A more recent study found the same side effect in test subjects who took 100 times the recommended dose of the plant.

As of 2002, however, kava kava has been associated with serious side effects involving damage to the liver, including **hepatitis**, **cirrhosis**, and liver failure. Most of the research on kava kava has been done in Europe, where the herb is even more popular than it is in the United States. By the late fall of 2001, there had been at least 25 reports from different European countries concerning liver damage caused by the plant. French health agencies reported one death and four patients requiring liver transplants in connection with kava kava consumption. On December 19, 2001, the MedWatch advisory of the U. S. Food and Drug Administration posted health warnings about the side effects of kava kava; and on January 16, 2002, Health Canada advised Canadians to avoid all products containing the herb. France banned the sale of preparations containing kava kava in February 2002. The U. S. National Center for Complementary and Alternative Medicine (NCCAM) put two research studies of kava kava on hold while awaiting further action by the FDA. NCCAM advised consumers in the United States on January 7, 2002 to avoid products containing kava. On March 25, 2002, the FDA issued a consumer advisory and a letter to health care professionals concerning the risk of severe liver damage from the use of products containing kava kava. While the most recent actions on the part of the FDA stop short of banning kava products from the U. S. market, the agency asks consumers as well as medical practitioners to notify its MedWatch hotline of any liver damage or other injuries associated with using kava kava. The MedWatch toll-free number is (800) 332-1088.

In addition to causing liver damage, kava kava appears to produce psychological side effects in some patients. Beverages containing kava kava have been reported to cause anxiety, **depression**, and insomnia. In addition, kava kava has caused **tremors** severe enough to be mistaken for symptoms of **Parkinson's disease** in susceptible patients.

Interactions

Kava kava has been shown to interact with beverage alcohol and with several categories of prescription medications. It increases the effect of barbiturates and other psychoactive medications; in one case study, a patient who took kava kava together with alprazolam went into a coma. It may produce dizziness and other unpleasant side effects if taken together with phenothiazines (med-

ications used to treat **schizophrenia**). Kava kava has also been reported to reduce the effectiveness of levodopa, a drug used in the treatment of Parkinson's disease.

Some interactions between kava kava and prescription medications, as well as some of the herb's side effects, have been attributed to synergy (combined effects) among the various chemicals contained in kava kava rather than to any one component by itself.

Resources

BOOKS

Cass, M.D., Hyla, and Terrence McNally. *Kava: Nature's Answer to Stress, Anxiety, and Insomnia.* Schoolcraft, MI: Prima Communications, Inc.,1998.

Connor, Kathryn M. and Donald S. Vaughan. *Kava: Nature's Stress Relief.* New York: Avon Books, 1999.

Lebot, Vincent, Mark Merlin, and Lamont Lindstrom. *Kava: The Pacific Elixir: The Definitive Guide to Its Ethnobotany, History, and Chemistry.* Rochester, VT: Inner Traditions International, Limited, 1997.

Robinson, Ph.D, Maggie Greenwood. *Kava: The Ultimate Guide to Nature's Anti-Stress Herb.* New York: Dell Publishing Company, Inc., 1999.

PERIODICALS

Almeida, J. C., and E. W. Grimsley. "Coma from the Health Food Store: Interaction Between Kava and Alprazolam." *Annals of Internal Medicine* 125 (1996): 940-941.

Ballesteros, S., S. Adan, et al. " Severe Adverse Effect Associated with Kava-Kava." *Journal of Toxicology: Clinical Toxicology* 39 (April 2001): 312.

Beltman, W., A. J. H. P van Riel, et al. "An Overview of Contemporary Herbal Drugs Used in the Netherlands. " *Journal of Toxicology: Clinical Toxicology* 38 (March 2000): 174.

Bilia, A. R., S. Gallon, and F. F. Vincieri. "Kava-Kava and Anxiety: Growing Knowledge About the Efficacy and Safety." *Life Sciences* 70 (April 19, 2002): 2581-2597.

Denham, A., M. McIntyre, and J. Whitehouse. "Kava— The Unfolding Story: Report on a Work-in-Progress." *Journal of Alternative and Complementary Medicine* 8 (June 2002): 237-263.

Ernst, E. "The Risk-Benefit Profile of Commonly Used Herbal Therapies: Ginkgo, St. John's Wort, Ginseng, Echinacea, Saw Palmetto, and Kava." *Archives of Internal Medicine* 136 (January 1, 2002): 42-53.

" France is Latest to Pull Kava Kava Prods." *Nutraceuticals International* (February 2002): np.

Humbertson, C. L., J. Akhtar, and E. P. Krenzelok. "Acute Hepatitis Induced by Kava Kava, an Herbal Product Derived from *Piper methysticum.*" *Journal of Toxicology: Clinical Toxicology* 39 (August 2001): 549.

Meseguer, E., R. Taboada, V. Sanchez, et al. "Life-Threatening Parkinsonism Induced by Kava-Kava." *Movement Disorders* 17 (January 2002): 195-196.

KEY TERMS

Analgesic—A medication or preparation given for pain relief.

Barbiturate—A group of drugs that have sedative properties. Barbiturates depress the body's respiratory rate, blood pressure, temperature, and central nervous system.

Diuretic—A substance that increases the flow of urine. Diuretics are given to lower the volume of liquid in the body.

Kavalactones—Medically active compounds in kava root that act as local anesthetics in the mouth and as minor tranquilizers.

Sedative—A drug that has a calming and relaxing effect. Sedatives are used to aid sleep and ease pain, and are often given as mild tranquilizers.

Standardized extract—A product that contains a specific amount of the active ingredients of the herb.

Synergy—Combined action or effects. Some researchers think that the side effects and interactions reported for kava kava are related to synergy among the various compounds in the herb.

Spinella, M. "The Importance of Pharmacological Synergy in Psychoactive Herbal Medicines." *Alternative Medicine Review* 7 (April 2002): 130-137.

ORGANIZATIONS

American Botanical Council (ABC). P.O. Box 144345, Austin, TX 78714-4345. (512) 926-4900. Fax: (512) 926-2345. <www.herbalgram.org.>.

FDA Center for Food Safety and Applied Nutrition (FDA/CFSAN). <www.fda.gov/medwatch/safety/2002/kava.htm.>.

NIH National Center for Complementary and Alternative Medicine (NCCAM) Clearinghouse. P. O. Box 8218, Silver Spring, MD 20907-8218. TTY/TDY: (888) 644-6226. Fax: (301) 495-4957. <www.nccam.nih.gov.>.

NIH Office of Dietary Supplements. Building 31, Room 1B25. 31 Center Drive, MSC 2086. Bethesda, MD 20892-2086. (301) 435-2920. Fax: (301) 480-1845. <www.odp.od.nih.gov/ods.>.

OTHER

FDA/CFSAN. *Consumer Advisory*, March 25, 2002. "Kava-Containing Dietary Supplements May be Associated with Severe Liver Injury." <www.cfsan.fda.gov/~dms/addskava.html>.

FDA/CFSAN. *Letter to Health Care Professionals*, March 25, 2002. "FDA Issues Consumer Advisory That Kava Products May be Associated with Severe Liver Injury." <www.cfsan.fda.gov/~dms/ds-ltr29.html>.

Jennifer Wurges
Rebecca J. Frey, PhD

Kegel exercises

Definition

Kegel exercises (Kegels) are exercises designed to strengthen the muscles of the lower pelvic girdle, or pelvic floor—the pubococcygeal (PC) muscles. The PC muscles support the bladder, urethra, and urethral sphincter—the muscle group at the neck of the bladder that acts as a spigot for controlling urine flow into the urethra—and the vagina, uterus, and rectum. Anything that puts pressure on the abdomen can weaken or damage these pelvic muscles. Such conditions include **pregnancy**, **childbirth**, excess weight, hormonal changes, and **aging**. Kegel exercises enable the PC muscles to better withstand increases in intra-abdominal pressure (pressure inside the abdomen). They make the bladder, urethra, and vagina more resilient, and improve bladder control and sexual relations.

Thirteen to 20 million American women suffer from **urinary incontinence**, primarily **stress** urinary incontinence (SUI)—urine leakage while laughing, coughing, sneezing, standing up suddenly, or exercising. SUI occurs when intra-abdominal pressure increases and the urethral sphincter opens inappropriately. During pregnancy, the fetus puts pressure on the bladder and the sphincter may relax and leak. Postpartum incontinence may result from muscle and nerve damage during childbirth due to delivery of a large baby, prolonged labor, excessive pushing, a forceps delivery, or an episiotomy (an incision made during delivery to prevent tearing of maternal tissue). About 40% of American women suffer from incontinence after childbirth, and the incidence increases by about 12% following each birth. Childbirth also increases the risk for incontinence later in life. During **menopause**, as a result of lower levels of estrogen, women with SUI may have thinning of the lining of the outer urethra, a sensation of having to urinate often, and recurrent urinary tract **infections** (UTIs). Beginning Kegels in midlife can help prevent urinary incontinence later.

Origins

In the 1930s, Dr. Joshua W. Davies hypothesized that strengthening the PC muscles could improve bladder control by assisting the closure of the urethral sphincter. By 1948, Dr. Arnold M. Kegel, a Los Angeles-area obstetrician and gynecologist, was having his patients practice vaginal contractions in preparation for childbirth. That same year he invented the Kegel perineometer, or pelvic-muscle sensor, to help prevent urinary incontinence (leakage) following childbirth.

Kegel's perineometer was the first **biofeedback** machine designed for clinical use. Employing a vaginal sensor, an air-pressure balloon, and a tire gauge, it enabled patients to verify that they were performing Kegel's correctly and to monitor their progress. The patients continued their practice at home. Kegel published numerous papers on his work and claimed to have cured incontinence in 93% of 3,000 patients. He produced a documentary movie to teach the procedure to other physicians. However, his perineometer was never marketed effectively and there was a widespread misconception that Kegels could not be performed without it. In the 1970s, more sensitive electromyography (EMG) perineometers became available for those with severely debilitated pelvic muscles.

Benefits

Kegel exercises strengthen the PC muscles and increase blood flow and nerve supply to the pelvic region, promoting or resulting in:

- increased pelvic support
- restoration of vaginal muscle tone and improved vaginal health
- protection from the physical stresses of childbirth
- restoration of sexual function and improved sexual response and pleasure
- increased vaginal-wall thickness and lubrication after menopause (cessation of menstruation)
- prevention or reversal of urinary leakage and rectal incontinence
- relief from pelvic **pain** or pain of vulvar vestibulitis (inflammation of the vaginal opening)

Description

Locating the PC muscles

The PC muscles can be felt by:

- stopping and starting urine flow to identify the forward PCs
- squeezing the vagina to identify the back of the PCs
- squeezing around two fingers placed in the vagina
- imagining sucking a marble up the vagina

- preventing a bowel movement or the passing of **gas** by tightening the muscles around the anus

There is a pulling sensation when the correct muscles are contracted. Weaker and stronger contractions are practiced until the PC muscles can be squeezed at will.

Practicing Kegels

There are numerous suggestions for practicing Kegels, which include:

- Contracting the PC muscles for three to 10 seconds and relaxing them three to 10 seconds for five to 15 repetitions, three to 12 times per day.
- Contracting the PC muscles strongly for one second, then releasing for one second, 20 times, three times per day, speeding up the contractions until there is a fluttery sensation.
- While emptying the bladder, stopping the urine flow at least three seconds, 10 times during each urination, which provides 60–80 contractions per day.

The complete **exercise** requires muscle contraction from back to front. It may take three to eight weeks for noticeable improvement. Once good muscle tone is achieved, Kegels may be performed just once a day.

The PC muscles can be exercised at almost any time—while lying down, sitting (in the car at a stop light, at work, etc.), squatting, standing, or walking—and varying the exercise position is said to be most effective. Sitting or standing adds weight to the exercise. It may be helpful to perform a Kegel squeeze before coughing, standing up, or lifting a heavy object. It may also be helpful to incorporate Kegels into a daily routine and keep a log. It is recommended that pregnant women practice Kegels regularly before, as well as after, childbirth.

Squeezing with two fingers in the vagina will confirm that only the vaginal muscles are contracting. Placing a hand on the lower abdomen is a reminder to keep the belly soft and relaxed, to refrain from tightening other muscles such as the stomach, buttocks, or leg muscles, or to hold the breath, all of which increase intra-abdominal pressure, working against the Kegels.

Vaginal cones

Kegels can be performed by the ancient Chinese technique of placing a weighted cone in the vagina and holding it in place up to 15 minutes twice a day. The practice is initiated using the heaviest cone that can be held easily for one minute. The cones weigh from 15–100 gm (0.04–0.3 lb). Brands include FemTone Weights, Kegel Weights, Kegel Kones, and Perineal Exerciser. Sequentially heavier cones are used until a maintenance program is established. This method automatically uses the correct muscles. Some of these products require a doctor's prescription.

Biofeedback devices and electrical stimulation

Nerve damage may prevent some people from performing Kegels properly. Vaginal or anal sensors and EMG perineometers with computerized visual or auditory feedback displays can measure the PC contraction. A handheld over-the-counter product (called the Myself pelvic muscle trainer) costs about $90. Another device can send mild electrical impulses to help locate the PC muscles.

With a vaginal sensor and biofeedback monitor, two 20-minute sessions per day for seven to nine months—with a specific goal such as holding 45-microvolts for 60 seconds—can relieve vulvar vestibular pain in the majority of women.

Insurance may not pay for EMG biofeedback therapy; however, Medicare will reimburse the patient if conventional Kegel exercises have failed.

Preparations

Training may be provided before initiating a Kegels routine.

Precautions

A temporary loss of muscle and nerve function following childbirth may make Kegels more difficult.

Kegel exercises do not work if abdominal, thigh, or buttock muscles are contracted. Furthermore, such contractions can increase pressure on the bladder, aggravating incontinence. Vaginal cones are not recommended in the presence of infection, neurological damage, diuretic medicines, or **caffeine**.

Side effects

There are no side effects to Kegel exercises.

Research & general acceptance

When performed properly and consistently, Kegels are usually helpful. The United States Agency for Health Care Policy and Research recommends that behavioral methods, including Kegels and biofeedback, be utilized to treat urinary incontinence before initiating drugs or surgery. Randomized controlled studies have shown that as many as 50–90% of women can reduce or overcome SUI with Kegels alone. However, reports of effectiveness vary since many people do not receive proper Kegel instruction. Consistent use of vaginal cones can improve or cure incontinence within four to six weeks in 70% of women.

The use of Kegels to improve urinary incontinence in men has not been extensively studied, although many clinicians report improvement. One study found that after the removal of a cancerous prostate, men who performed Kegels twice a day regained bladder control faster than those who did not do the exercises.

Training & certification

Patient training in Kegel exercises can be given by a knowledgeable healthcare provider.

Resources

BOOKS

Bladder Research Progress Review Group. *Overcoming Bladder Disease: A Strategic Plan for Research.* Bethesda, MD: National Institute of Diabetes and Digestive and Kidney Diseases, August 2002.

Hulme, Janet A. *Beyond Kegels: Fabulous Four Exercises and More—To Prevent and Treat Incontinence.* Missoula, MT: Phoenix, 2002.

Icon Health Publications. *Kegel Exercises: A Medical Dictionary, Bibliography, and Annotated Research Guide to Internet References.* Icon Health Publications, 2004.

National Kidney and Urologic Diseases Information Clearinghouse. *Exercising Your Pelvic Muscles.* NIH Publication No. 02-4188. Bethesda, MD: National Institute of Diabetes and Digestive and Kidney Diseases, April 2002.

National Kidney and Urologic Diseases Information Clearinghouse. *Treatments for Urinary Incontinence in Woman.* NIH Publication No. 03-5104. Bethesda, MD: National Institute of Diabetes and Digestive and Kidney Diseases, June 2003.

Northrup, Christiane. *The Wisdom of Menopause.* New York: Bantam, 2001.

PERIODICALS

Chiarelli, Pauline, and Jill Cockburn. "Promoting Urinary Continence in Women After Delivery: Randomized Controlled Trial." *British Medical Journal* 324, no. 7348 (May 25, 2002): 1241–4.

Perry, John D., and Leslie B. Talcott. "The Kegel Perineometer: Biofeedback Twenty Years Before Its Time." *Proceedings of the 20th Annual Meeting of the Association for Applied Psychophysiology and Biofeedback* (March 17–22, 1989): 169–72.

Resnick, Neil M., and Derek J. Griffiths. "Expanding Treatment Options for Stress Urinary Incontinence in Women." *Journal of the American Medical Association (JAMA)* 290, no. 3 (July 16, 2003): 395–7.

Singla, A. "An Update on the Management of SUI." *Contemporary Ob/Gyn* 45, no. 1 (2000): 68–85.

ORGANIZATIONS

American Foundation for Urologic Disease, Inc. 1000 Corporate Boulevard, Suite 410, Linthicum, MD 21090. (800) 828-7866. (410) 689-3990. memberservices@nafc.org. <http://www.afud.org>.

KEY TERMS

Biofeedback—An electronic monitoring technique for learning to control a body movement or function.

Electromyography (EMG)—The recording of electrical currents generated by muscle activity.

Incontinence—Inability to control the passage of urine or feces.

Perineometer—A device for measuring PC-muscle contraction.

Pubococcygeal (PC) muscles—The muscles of the lower pelvic girdle, or pelvic floor, which support the bladder, urethra, and urethral sphincter; the muscle group at the neck of the bladder that acts as a spigot for controlling urine flow into the urethra, vagina, uterus, and rectum.

Stress urinary incontinence (SUI).—Urine leakage upon straining, coughing, laughing, or sneezing.

Urethra—The tube that delivers urine from the bladder to the exterior.

Urethral sphincter—Circular muscle that controls the movement of urine from the bladder to the urethra.

Vaginal cone—A weighted cone held in the vagina for Kegel excercising.

Vulvar vestibulitis—Inflammation of the vestibule of the vulva or vagina.

Continence Restored, Inc. 407 Strawberry Hill Avenue, Stamford, CT 06902. (914) 493-1470.

National Association for Continence. P.O. Box 1019, Charleston, SC 292402-1019. 800-BLADDER. (843) 377-0900.

OTHER

Nerve Disease and Bladder Control. National Kidney and Urologic Diseases Information Clearinghouse. NIH Publication No. 03-4560. May 2003 [cited May 2, 2004]. <http://kidney.niddk.nih.gov/kudiseases/pubs/nervedisease/index.htm>.

Urinary Incontinence and Pelvic Muscle Rehabilitation Index. InContiNet. February 15, 2000 [cited May 2, 2004] <http:incontinent.com/articles/art_urin/index.htm>.

Urinary Incontinence in Men. National Kidney and Urologic Diseases Information Clearinghouse. NIH Publication No. 04-5280. March 2004 [cited May 2, 2004]. <http://niddk.nih.gov/kudiseases/pubs/uimen/index.htm>.

Margaret Alic

▮ Kelley-Gonzalez diet

Definition

The Kelley-Gonzalez diet consists of large amounts of raw fruits, juices, raw and steamed vegetables, cereals, and nuts. When combined with massive quantities of dietary supplements and freeze-dried pancreatic enzymes, together with a "detoxification" process involving coffee enemas, it is said to slow the growth of **cancer** tumors.

Origins

The Kelley-Gonzalez regimen is based on a belief that enzymes from the pancreas are capable, like chemotherapy, of killing cancer cells. The use of pancreatic enzymes to treat cancer was first proposed in 1906 by John Beard, a Scottish embryologist. This idea received some attention at the time but was largely abandoned after Beard died in 1923. During the 1960s, the concept was resurrected by William Donald Kelley, a controversial dentist from Grapevine, Texas. Kelley wrote a book titled *One Answer to Cancer* that outlined his five-pronged approach:

- Nutritional therapy: Beef pancreatic enzymes combined with numerous other dietary supplements.

- Diet: A carefully individualized diet, ranging all the way from vegetarian to all-meat.

- **Detoxification**: As few as three or as many as 52 weeks of enemas and laxative purging.

- Neurological stimulation: Various manipulations including **chiropractic**, osteopathic, mandibular, and physiotherapeutic.

- Spiritual therapy: Prayer and Bible reading.

In 1981, Nicholas Gonzalez, then a second-year medical student at Cornell University, began a five-year investigation of Kelley's work. Reviewing 10,000 patient records and interviewing 500 cancer patients, Gonzalez became convinced that many of Kelley's patients had survived significantly longer than would otherwise have been expected. "Despite the careful documentation and the five-year investment of time, my attempts at publication were met with scorn and ridicule," Gonzalez recalls. "It seemed no one in academic medicine could, at the time, accept that a nutritional therapy might produce positive results with advanced cancer patients."

In 1987, Gonzalez started practicing medicine in New York City and developing his own cancer regimen similar to Kelley's, except that he rejected the neurological and spiritual aspects of Kelley's treatment. In 1999, the journal *Nutrition and Cancer* published results from a pilot study of the Gonzalez regimen in 11 patients with inoperable pancreatic cancer. These results were promising, prompting the U.S. National Institutes of Health's (NIH) National Center for Complementary and Alternative Medicine (NCCAM) to sponsor a $1.4 million large-scale clinical study of the regimen.

Benefits

In his New York medical practice, Gonzalez uses his enzyme-based treatment on patients with pancreatic cancer, as well as a wide variety of other cancers. In addition, he uses variations of the Gonzalez regimen to treat a range of other illnesses, including **chronic fatigue syndrome**, arthritis, and **multiple sclerosis**.

Description

As currently practiced by Gonzalez, the regimen includes pancreatic enzymes taken orally every four hours and at meals for 16 days. Patients also take as many as 150 dietary supplements a day, including vitamins, minerals, **magnesium** citrate, papaya, trace elements, and glandular products from animals. Patients also receive frequent coffee enemas. They are placed on a strict diet including large quantities of fresh fruits, vegetable juices, cereals, and as many as 20 almonds a day. Red meat, white sugar, chicken, refined grain products, and soy are all forbidden. Fish is allowed only in limited quantities.

Precautions

The Kelley-Gonzalez diet is considered a highly experimental treatment for cancer, with only limited evidence of its effectiveness. It should therefore be undertaken only with competent medical advice and monitoring. Prospective patients should be aware that the diet requires considerable commitment and can almost be considered a full-time job. Initially, it can involve as many as eight enemas a day, as well as preparing four servings of fresh carrot juice and taking dietary supplements 10 times a day.

Side effects

At least two deaths have been linked to coffee enemas, attributed to hyponatremia and dehydration. With unqualified practitioners, there may also be a risk of contamination from unsanitary equipment used to administer enemas. For example, one outbreak of *Campylobacter* sepsis occurred among clients of a border clinic in Mexico that offered coffee enemas. In Colorado, an amebiasis outbreak was linked to fecal contamination of an enema-delivery system. Other side effects of the Kelley-Gonzalez treatment may include low-grade **fever**, muscle aches and pains, or **rashes**.

KEY TERMS

. . . .

Amebiasis—An infection or disease caused by amoebas.

Campylobacter—A genus of bacteria that can invade the lining of the intestine.

Hyponatremia—Abnormally low levels of sodium in the blood, often related to dehydration.

Sepsis—The presence of pus-forming micro-organisms or their toxins in the blood.

Research & general acceptance

For many years, the Kelley-Gonzalez Diet was rejected by orthodox medical practitioners. However, as described earlier, a 1999 pilot study by Gonzales has led to a clinical trial sponsored by the NIH.

Training & certification

Gonzalez offers his regimen from his medical practice in New York City. In a 1995 interview with *The Moneychanger,* he said that there are other practitioners "who say they do the Kelley therapy or the Gonzalez therapy, and I've never even met them." As of August 2000, the oncology and surgical oncology departments at New York's Columbia-Presbyterian Medical Center were seeking volunteers with advanced pancreatic cancer for a clinical trial of the Gonzalez regimen.

Resources

PERIODICALS

Gonzalez, Nicholas James, and Linda Lee Isaacs. "Evaluation of Pancreatic Proteolytic Enzyme Treatment of Adenocarcinoma of the Pancreas, with Nutrition and Detoxification Support." *Nutrition and Cancer.* 33 (2): 117-124.

"Innovative Clinical Trial for Advanced Pancreatic Cancer Patients." *Oncology News International.* 8 no. 7 (1999): 24.

OTHER

Nicholas J. Gonzalez, M.D., P.C. 36A East 36th St., Suite 204. New York, NY 10016. (212) 213-3337. www.dr-gonzalez.com.

David Helwig

Kelp

Description

Kelp (*Fucus vesiculosus*) is a type of brown seaweed, moderate in size, that grows in regions with cold

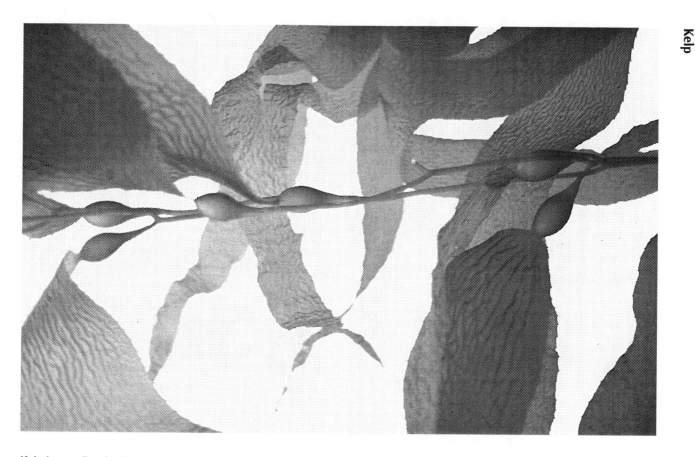

Kelp leaves floating in water. *(Photograph by Robert J. Huffman. FieldMark Publications. Reproduced by permission.)*

coastlines, including those of the northwestern United States and northern Europe. There are several varieties of kelp: true kelp, which thrives in cool seas; giant kelp, and bladder kelp, which grow in the North Pacific. Giant kelp is so named because it grows to 213 ft (65 m). Kelp anchors itself to rocky surfaces via tentacle-like roots. From these roots grows a slender stalk with long, leaf-like blades.

Kelp belongs to the Fucaceae family. Other names for *Fucus vesiculosus* are kelpware, black-tang, bladder-fucus, cutweed, and bladderwrack. The main constituents of kelp include phenolic compounds, mucopolysaccharides, algin, polar lipids, and glycosyl ester diglycerides. Kelp also contains protein, carbohydrates, and **essential fatty acids**.

Kelp contains approximately 30 minerals. It is a rich source of **iodine, calcium, sulfur**, and silicon. Other minerals include **phosphorus, iron, sodium, potassium, magnesium**, chloride, **copper, zinc, manganese**, barium, **boron, chromium**, lithium, nickel, silver, titanium, **vanadium**, aluminum, strontium, bismuth, chlorine, cobalt, gallium, tin, and zirconium. Kelp also contains vitamins C, E, D, K, and B complex. The highest concentrations of these vitamins and minerals are found in

the tissues of kelp. Since kelp is such a valuable source of nutrients, it is often recommended as a dietary supplement, particularly for people with mineral deficiencies.

Origins

Different kinds of kelp have been eaten for nutritional value for over a thousand years. The Chinese used kelp and other types of seaweed as medicine as far back as 3,000 B.C. The Greeks used kelp to feed their cattle around the first century B.C. Kelp has been a staple food of Icelanders for centuries, and ancient Hawaiian nobles grew gardens of edible seaweed. Kelp was also used in Europe and Great Britain as fertilizer to nourish soil and assist plant growth.

The largest consumer of kelp, however, has been Japan. The Japanese have incorporated kelp and seaweed into their **diets** for 1,500 years. During the seventh to ninth centuries, only the Japanese nobility consumed seaweed. In the seventeenth century, Japan began farming seaweed. The Japanese and other Asian cultures used kelp to treat uterine problems, genital tract disorders, and kidney, bladder, and prostate ailments.

Kelp is still an integral part of the Japanese diet. The Japanese include kelp in almost every meal, using it in salads or as a garnish, or cooking it in soups, sauces, and cakes. Noodles made from kelp are a staple of the Japanese diet. Until recently, kelp was eaten almost exclusively by the Japanese. Now the Western population is beginning to take note of this nutrient-rich seaweed. However, *Fucus vesiculosus* is not the kind of kelp that is eaten.

Eating dietary kelp may be responsible for the low rate of **breast cancer** among Japanese women, and also for the low rate of **heart disease**, respiratory disease, rheumatism, arthritis, high blood pressure, and gastrointestinal ailments. The occurrence of thyroid disease is also low in Japan.

General use

Many herbalist and naturopathic physicians recommend *Fucus vesiculosus* to treat thyroid disorders, arthritis, rheumatism, **constipation**, colds, high blood pressure, colitis, **eczema**, goiter, **obesity**, low vitality, poor digestion, nervous disorders, menstrual irregularities, glandular disorders, and water retention.

Fucus vesiculosus has a therapeutic effect on many systems of the body. It strengthens immune system function and increases resistance to infection and **fever**. Kelp is also beneficial to the nervous and endocrine systems. It enhances the function of the adrenal, thyroid, and pituitary glands, and supports brain health and function.

One of the main therapeutic uses of *Fucus vesiculosus* is for thyroid conditions such as **hypothyroidism** and goiter. Partly due to its high iodine content, this kind of kelp assists in the production of thyroid hormones, which help regulate the thyroid gland. People who don't eat dairy products, seafood, and salt may develop an iodine deficiency, which may result in low thyroid function. Kelp is a good source of iodine for those who may be deficient.

Thyroid hormones are also necessary to maintain a normal metabolism. *Fucus vesiculosus* helps boost metabolism, which helps to sustain normal weight (especially in people who are overweight because of a thyroid condition).

This type of kelp is also used to rid the body of and keep it from absorbing harmful chemicals, toxins, carcinogens, and such heavy metal pollutants as barium and cadmium. Algin, a fiber-like extract of kelp, helps prevent the body from assimilating these elements. Algin is used industrially in the production of tires and as an agent that prevents ice cream from crystallizing. Kelp also helps to prevent the body from absorbing radioactive elements such as strontium 90, a dangerous radioactive substance created by nuclear power plants. However, since *Fucus vesiculosus* absorbs toxic chemicals, it must be harvested from clean waters or it may contain toxins.

Kelp also reduces **cholesterol** levels by inhibiting bile acid absorption. The diuretic effect of kelp is beneficial to an irritated or infected bladder since it helps to flush out harmful bacteria. Kelp helps reduce inflammation in injured tissues and ease painful joints in rheumatism and **rheumatoid arthritis**. Kelp may also reduce an enlarged prostate in men, and is also used to strengthen fingernails, prevent **hair loss**, and regenerate hair if the follicle is still alive.

In addition to its medicinal uses, kelp contains natural **antioxidants** that make it useful to the food industry in retarding spoilage. The cosmetics industry is also studying the effects of a gel derived from kelp in improving the elasticity of human skin.

Preparations

The kelp used medicinally in modern times is generally harvested in kelp farms. These farms help preserve the natural balance of the sea, which is disrupted when large amounts of naturally growing seaweed are removed. Farming kelp also helps to ensure that the kelp retains its nutritional value. Kelp loses valuable nutrients when it is washed ashore. When kelp is harvested, it is cut, dried, then ground into powder. It is this powder that is encapsulated or pressed into tablets.

Kelp is available in bulk form either dried or as a ground powder. It is also sold as granules, capsules, tablets, or tinctures. Granulated or powdered kelp can be added to food as a salt substitute.

The recommended daily dose for adults is 10–15 mg. Kelp can also be made into a tea. To create an infusion, 1 cup of boiling water is poured over 2-3 tsp of dried or powdered kelp. The tea is steeped for 10 minutes, and can be drunk three times daily.

Precautions

People should not gather wild kelp because it may contain contaminants absorbed from the sea.

People with high blood pressure or a history of thyroid problems should consult their healthcare practitioner before using kelp. The high sodium content of *Fucus vesiculosus* may make high blood pressure worse. Kelp isn't recommended for people on a low-sodium diet.

Excessive consumption of kelp can provide the body with too much iodine and interfere with thyroid function. Consumers should use it only as directed.

Side effects

There are no known side effects, but some people may be sensitive or allergic to kelp. Common allergic symptoms include mild stomachache.

KEY TERMS

. . . .

Diuretic—A substance that promotes urination.

Goiter—An enlargement of the thyroid gland.

Hypothyroidism—A condition resulting from an underactive thyroid gland.

Infusion—An herbal tea created by steeping herbs in hot water. Generally, leaves and flowers are used in infusions.

Interactions

Fucus vesiculosus shouldn't be taken with thyroid medications.

Resources

BOOKS

Time-Life Books. *The Alternative Advisor.* Alexandria, VA: Time Life, Inc., 1997.

Lininger, D.C., Skye. *The Natural Pharmacy.* Virtual Health, LLC, 1998.

PERIODICALS

Fujimura, T., K. Tsukahara, S. Moriwaki, et al. "Treatment of Human Skin with an Extract of *Fucus vesiculosus* Changes Its Thickness and Mechanical Properties." *Journal of Cosmetic Science* 53 (January-February 2002): 1-9.

Ruperez, P., O. Ahrazem, and J. A. Leal. "Potential Antioxidant Capacity of Sulfated Polysaccharides from the Edible Marine Brown Seaweed *Fucus vesiculosus.*" *Journal of Agricultural and Food Chemistry* 50 (February 13, 2002): 840-845.

Jennifer Wurges
Rebecca J. Frey, PhD

Kidney infections

Definition

Kidney infection is a general term used to describe infection of the kidney by bacteria, fungi, or viruses. The infecting microbe may have invaded the kidney from the urinary bladder or from the bloodstream. The disease is characterized by **fever, chills,** back **pain,** and, often, the symptoms associated with **bladder infection.**

Description

As the principle part of the urinary system, the kidneys process the fluid component of blood (called plasma) to maintain appropriate water volume and concentrations of chemicals. The waste product formed from this process is called urine. Urine travels from the kidney, through tubes called ureters, to the urinary bladder, and is eliminated from the body through a tube called the urethra. The kidneys and ureters comprise the upper urinary tract, and the bladder and urethra comprise the lower urinary tract.

Kidney infection, also called pyelonephritis and upper urinary tract infection, occurs when microbes, usually bacteria, invade the tissues of the kidney and multiply. One or both kidneys may be infected. Infection originating directly from the bladder is called an ascending infection.

Inflammation occurs in response to the infection. As a result of the infection and inflammation, scarring and other tissue damage may occur. Most cases of acute kidney infection resolve without any permanent kidney damage. In severe cases, kidney damage is so extensive that the kidneys can no longer function, a state called renal failure.

Types of kidney **infections**:

- Acute pyelonephritis: uncomplicated kidney infection that has a short and relatively severe course.

- Chronic pyelonephritis: long-standing disease associated with either active or inactive (healed) kidney infection.

- Emphysematous pyelonephritis: acute infection associated with **gas** in and around the kidney. This type almost always occurs in persons with diabetes.

- Pyonephrosis: acute or chronic pyelonephritis associated with blockage of the ureter.

- Renal and perinephric abscesses: abscesses (pockets of pus) in and around the kidney.

Kidney infections occur most often in adult females who are otherwise healthy. Urinary tract infections are uncommon in males until old age, when bladder catheterization and other urinary procedures are more commonly performed.

Causes & symptoms

Kidney infection is usually caused by bacteria, although infection by fungi (yeasts and molds) or viruses does occur. The bacteria *Escherichia coli (E. coli)* is responsible for about 85% of the cases of acute pyelonephritis. Other common causes include *Klebsiella, Enterobacter, Proteus, Enterococcus,* and *Pseudomonas* species. Infection by *Proteus* species can lead to the formation of stones. *E. coli* causes only 60% of the acute pyelonephritis cases in the elderly. Kidney infection may also be caused by *Mycobacterium tuberculosis* or other *Mycobacterium* species or by the yeast *Candida*. Kidney infection can be caused by Group B streptococci in newborns.

Certain women are inherently more susceptible to urinary tract infections. Researchers have found that women who have recurrent infections possess certain markers on their blood cells. Also, the bacteria which commonly cause urinary tract infections stick more readily to the vaginal cells of women who have recurrent infections. Other risk factors for kidney disease include:

• bladder catheterization or instrumentation

• diabetes

• pregnancy

• urinary calculi (stones)

• urinary tract abnormalities

• urinary tract obstruction

The symptoms of kidney infection include fever, shaking chills, **nausea**, **vomiting**, and middle to lower back pain which may travel to the abdomen and groin. This pain may be severe. These symptoms may be preceded or accompanied by those associated with bladder infection—frequent, painful urination.

Infants and young children may show fever, irritability, straining on urination, and urine odor. Fewer than half of newborns have fever associated with kidney infection, which makes diagnosis difficult.

In more than 20% of elderly patients with kidney infection, the presenting symptoms are gastrointestinal or pulmonary (lung). Also, one-third of elderly patients do not develop fever.

Diagnosis

Kidney infections can be diagnosed by family doctors, OB/GYN doctors, and urologists (doctors who specialize in the urinary system). The diagnosis of kidney infection is based primarily on symptoms, urinalysis, and urine cultures. Blood tests may also be performed. Approximately 20% of patients have bacteria in the bloodstream, a condition called bacteremia. Urine dipsticks that detect signs of infection are often used right in the doctor's office. Urine would be examined with a microscope for the presence of bacteria and leukocytes (white blood cells). Urine culture would identify which microbe is causing the infection and may also be used to determine which antibiotic would be effective.

Other routine diagnostic procedures to look for signs of infection in the kidney may be used. An x ray of the abdomen may be taken. Ultrasound, which uses sound waves to visualize internal organs, may be used to examine the bladder and kidney. Less routinely performed are intravenous urograms, computerized tomography (CT scan), and scintillation scans.

Treatment

Delays in the diagnosis and treatment of kidney infection can lead to permanent kidney damage. Anyone who suspects kidney infection should seek professional care immediately. Alternative medicine may be used as an adjunct to the appropriate antibiotic treatment.

Dietary changes which may help to control and prevent kidney infection include:

• Drinking eight to 12 glasses of water daily helps to wash out bacteria (although this may also dilute antibacterial factors in the urine).

• Acidifying the urine by eating few alkaline foods (dairy and soda).

• Following a diet rich in grains, vegetables, and acidifying juices, like citrus.

• Eliminating high-sugar foods (sweet vegetables, fruits, sugar, and honey).

• Drinking unsweetened **cranberry** juice to acidify the urine and provide the antimicrobial agent hippuric acid. Cranberry capsules can substitute for the juice.

• Ingesting at least one clove of **garlic** (or up to 1,200 mg garlic as a tablet) daily for its anti-infective properties.

Magnesium may be helpful in treating renal disease. **Zinc** may boost the immune system. A study in rats with ascending pyelonephritis found that the addition of vitamins A and E to standard antibiotic therapy significantly reduced kidney inflammation as compared to antibiotic treatment alone.

Traditional Chinese medicine treats pyelonephritis with **acupuncture**, herbals, and patent medicines. The Chinese patent medicine Zhi Bai Di Huang Wan (**Anemarrhena**, Phellodendron, and Rehmannia Pill) is often used to treat kidney infections and disease and bladder infections. The patient can take eight pills three times daily. Treatment of urinary tract infection often uses one or more of the following herbs in doses of 30 g to 60 g taken once or twice daily (Patients should consult a traditional Chinese medical practioner for the treatment best suited for them.):

• *Herba commelinae*

• *H. plantaginis*

• *H. patriniae*

• *H. salviae plebeiae*

- *H. hedyotis seu oldenlandiae*
- *H. taraxaci*
- *H. andrographis*

Allopathic treatment

Initiating antibiotic therapy as soon as possible is critical to prevent or reduce damage to the kidneys. Historically, all pyelonephritis patients were treated in the hospital. This has been found to be unnecessary in many cases. Responsible patients who have mild kidney infection can be treated at home with antibiotics taken by mouth. Patients with high fever, vomiting, evidence of bacteria in the bloodstream, and/or dehydration would be hospitalized and treated with intravenous (IV) antibiotics and fluids. Severe illness, either with or without complications, would require hospitalization for treatment.

The recommended treatment for acute pyelonephritis is two weeks of therapy with the antibiotic combination trimethoprim/sulfamethoxazole. Fluoroquinolones (Cipro, Noroxin, NegGram), ceftriaxone (Rocephin), or gentamicin are other choices. Fluoroquinolones should not be used by pregnant women or children. With treatment, symptoms normally resolve within two to three days.

Abscesses may be resolved with percutaneous (by a needle through the skin) or surgical drainage. Emphysematous pyelonephritis may be treated with antibiotics; however, surgical removal of the kidney (nephrectomy) may be necessary. Because of the 75% death rate, nephrectomy is the treatment of choice in diabetics with emphysematous pyelonephritis. Urinary stones are eliminated by a percutaneous method which involves stone removal and shock wave treatment.

Expected results

Antibacterial therapy of kidney infection has a 90% cure rate. Severe or chronic infection can lead to kidney damage and renal failure. Renal failure requires hemodialysis, a process which uses a dialysis machine (an artificial kidney) to process the patient's blood. Patients with severe kidney damage requires kidney transplantation.

Prevention

Researchers are trying to develop a vaccine for UTIs, but as of early 2000, none are ready for human studies. The key to preventing kidney infection is to promptly treat bladder infection. Measures taken to prevent bladder infection may prevent subsequent kidney infection. These include:

- drinking large amounts of fluid

KEY TERMS

Ascending infection—Infection which begins in the urinary bladder and travels through the ureters up to the kidneys.

Hemodialysis—The blood processing procedure used when kidney function is lost. Blood is removed from a vein, processed through a dialysis machine (artificial kidney), and put back into a vein.

Nephrectomy—Surgical removal of a kidney.

Percutaneous—Medical procedure that is performed through the skin using a needle. Abscess drainage and urinary stones may be treated percutaneously.

Pyelonephritis—Infection and inflammation of the kidney.

Renal failure—A state when the kidneys are so extensively damaged that they can no longer function.

- reducing intake of sugar
- voiding frequently and as soon as the need arises
- proper cleansing of the area around the urethra (females), especially after sexual intercourse
- acupuncture (effective in preventing recurrent lower UTIs in women)
- avoiding use of vaginal diaphragms and spermicidal jelly (females) for contraception

The primary preventive measure specifically for males is prompt treatment of prostate infections. Chronic prostatitis may go unnoticed but can trigger recurrent UTIs. In addition, males who require temporary catheterization following surgery can be given antibiotics to lower the risk of UTIs.

Resources

BOOKS

Kunin, Calvin M. "Pyelonephritis and Other Infections of the Kidney." *Urinary Tract Infections: Detection, Prevention, and Management, 5th edition.* Baltimore: Willliams & Wilkins, 1997.

Kunin, Calvin M. "Pathogenesis of Infection — The Host Defenses." *Urinary Tract Infections: Detection, Prevention, and Management, 5th edition.* Baltimore: Willliams & Wilkins, 1997.

Ying, Zhou Zhong and Jin Hui De. "Genitourinary Diseases." In *Clinical Manual of Chinese Herbal Medicine and Acupuncture.* New York: Churchill Livingston, 1997.

PERIODICALS

Bennett, Robert T., Richard J. Mazzaccaro, Neeru Chopra, Arnold Melman, and Israel Franco. "Suppression of Renal Inflammation With Vitamins A and E in Ascending Pyelonephritis in Rats." *Journal of Urology* 161 (1999): 1681-1684.

Roberts, James A. "Management of Pyelonephritis and Upper Urinary Tract Infections." *Urologic Clinics of North America* 26 (1999): 753-763.

Belinda Rowland

Kidney stones

Definition

Kidney stones are solid accumulations of material that form in the tubal system of the kidney. Kidney stones cause problems when they block the flow of urine through or out of the kidney. When the stones move through the ureter, they cause severe **pain**.

Description

Urine is formed by the kidneys. Blood flows into the kidneys, and nephrons (specialized tubes) within the kidneys allow a certain amount of fluid from the blood, and certain substances dissolved in that fluid, to flow out of the body as urine. Sometimes, a problem causes the dissolved substances to become solid again. Tiny crystals may form in the urine, meet, and cling together to create a larger solid mass called a kidney stone.

Many people do not ever find out that they have stones in their kidneys. These stones are small enough to allow the kidney to continue functioning normally, never causing any pain. These are called "silent stones." Kidney stones cause problems when they interfere with the normal flow of urine. They can obstruct (block) the flow through the ureter (a tube) that carries urine from the kidney to the bladder. The kidney is not accustomed to experiencing any pressure. When pressure builds from backed-up urine, the kidney may swell (hydronephrosis). If the kidney is subjected to this pressure for some time, there may be damage to the delicate kidney structures. When the kidney stone is lodged further down the ureter, the backed-up urine may also cause the ureter to swell (hydroureter). Because the ureter is a muscular tube, the presence of a stone will cause the tube to go into a spasm,, causing severe pain.

About 10% of all people will have a kidney stone in their lifetime. Kidney stones are most common among male Caucasians over the age of 30, people who have previously had kidney stones, and relatives of kidney stone patients.

Causes & symptoms

Kidney stones can be composed of a variety of substances. The most common types of kidney stones are described here.

Calcium stones

About 80% of all kidney stones fall into this category. These stones are composed of either **calcium** and phosphate or calcium and oxalate. People with calcium stones may have other diseases that cause them to have increased blood levels of calcium. These diseases include primary parathyroidism, sarcoidosis, **hyperthyroidism**, renal tubular acidosis, multiple myeloma, hyperoxaluria, and some types of **cancer**.

Struvite stones

This type accounts for 10% of all kidney stones. Struvite stones are composed of **magnesium** ammonium phosphate. These stones occur most often in patients who have had repeated urinary tract **infections** with certain types of bacteria. These bacteria produce a substance called urease, which increases the urine pH and makes the urine more alkaline and less acidic. This chemical environment allows struvite to settle out of the urine, forming stones.

Uric acid stones

About 5% of all kidney stones are uric acid stones. These occur when increased amounts of uric acid circulate in the bloodstream. When the uric acid content becomes very high, it can no longer remain dissolved and solid particles of uric acid settle out of the urine. A kidney stone is formed when these particles cling to each other within the kidney, slowly forming a solid mass. About half of all patients with this type of stone also have deposits of uric acid elsewhere in their bodies, commonly in the joint of the big toe. This painful disorder is called **gout**. Other causes of uric acid stones include chemotherapy for cancer; certain bone marrow disorders in which blood cells are overproduced; and an inherited disorder called Lesch-Nyhan syndrome.

Cystine stones

These account for 2% of all kidney stones. Cystine is a type of amino acid, and people with this type of kidney stone have an abnormality in the way their bodies process **amino acids** in the diet.

Patients who have kidney stones usually do not have symptoms until the stones pass into the ureter. Prior to this development, some people may notice blood in their urine. Once the stone is in the ureter, however, most people will experience bouts of very severe pain. The pain is crampy and spasmodic, and is referred to as "colic." The pain usually begins in the flank region, the area between the lower ribs and the hip bone. As the stone moves closer to the bladder, a patient will often feel the pain radiating along the inner thigh. Women may feel the pain in the vulva, while men often feel pain in the testicles. **Nausea**, **vomiting**, extremely frequent and painful urination, and blood in the urine are common. **Fever** and **chills** usually mean that the ureter has become obstructed, allowing bacteria to become trapped in the kidney and cause a kidney infection (pyelonephritis).

Diagnosis

A diagnosis of kidney stones is based on the patient's history of the severe distinctive pain associated with the stones. Diagnosis includes laboratory examination of a urine sample and an x-ray examination. During the passage of a stone, examination of the urine almost always reveals blood. A number of x-ray tests are used to diagnose kidney stones. A plain x ray of the kidneys, ureters, and bladder may or may not reveal the stone. A series of x rays taken after injecting **iodine** dye into a vein is usually a more reliable way of seeing a stone. This procedure is called an intravenous pyelogram (IVP). The dye "lights up" the urinary system as it travels. In the case of an obstruction, the dye will be stopped by the stone or will only be able to get past the stone at a slow trickle. An ultrasound can also be used to detect renal blockage. Recently, the use of computed tomography (CT) scans has been added to the diagnosis of some kidney stones, more as a follow-up after treatment to detect how fragile or intact a stone might be.

When a patient is passing a kidney stone, it is important that all of his or her urine is strained through a special sieve to catch the stone. The stone can then be sent to a laboratory for analysis to determine the chemical composition of the stone. After the kidney stone has been passed, other tests are required to understand the underlying condition that may have caused the stone to form. Collecting urine for 24 hours, followed by careful analysis of its chemical makeup, can often determine the reason for stone formation.

Treatment

It is believed that stones may pass more quickly if the patient is encouraged to drink large amounts of water (2–3 quarts per day).

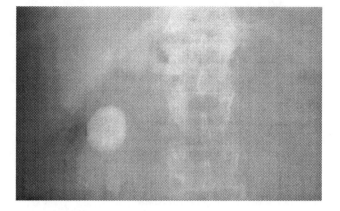

X ray showing a kidney stone. *(Custom Medical Stock Photo. Reproduced by permission.)*

Herbal remedies that have anti-lithic (stone-dissolving) action can assist in dissolving small kidney stones. These include gravel root (*Eupatorium purpureum*), hydrangea (*Hydrangea arborescens*), and wild carrot (*Daucus carota*). Starfruit (*Averrhoa carambola*) is recommended to increase the amount of urine a patient passes and to relieve pain. A Chinese herbal practitioner may use such herbs as *Semen Abutili seu Malvae, Semen Plantaginis,* and *Herba Lygodii Japonici* for urinary stones. Dietary changes can be made to reduce the risk of future stone formation and to facilitate the resorption of existing stones. Supplementation with magnesium, a smooth muscle relaxant, can help reduce pain and facilitate stone passing. **Guided imagery** may also be used to help relieve pain. Extremely large stones may require surgical intervention.

Allopathic treatment

A patient with a kidney stone will say that the most important aspect of treatment is adequate pain relief. Because the pain of passing a kidney stone is so severe, narcotic pain medications (such as morphine) are usually required. If the patient is vomiting or unable to drink fluids because of the pain, it may be necessary to provide intravenous fluids. If symptoms and urine tests indicate the presence of infection, antibiotics are required.

Although most kidney stones pass on their own, some do not. Surgical removal of a stone may become necessary when a stone appears too large to pass. Surgery may also be required if the stone is causing serious obstructions, pain that cannot be treated, heavy bleeding, or infection. Several alternatives exist for removing stones. One method involves inserting a tube into the bladder and up into the ureter. A tiny basket is then passed through the tube, and an attempt is made to snare the stone and pull it out. Open surgery to remove an obstructing kidney stone was relatively common in the past, but current methods allow the stone to be pulverized (crushed) with shock waves (called lithotripsy). These shock waves may be aimed at the stone from outside of the body by passing the necessary equipment through the bladder and into the ureter. The shock waves may be aimed at the stone from inside the body by placing the instrument through a tiny incision located near the stone. The stone fragments may then pass on their own or may be removed through the incision. These methods considerably reduce a patient's recovery time when compared to the traditional open operation. Some patients may have a follow-up CT scan to determine if the lithotripsy procedure successfully removed all stones.

Expected results

A patient's prognosis depends on the underlying disorder causing the development of kidney stones. In most cases, patients with uncomplicated calcium stones will recover very well. About 60% of these patients, however, will have other kidney stones. Struvite stones are particularly dangerous because they may grow extremely large, filling the tubes within the kidney. These are called staghorn stones and will not pass out in the urine. They will require surgical removal. Uric acid stones may also become staghorn stones.

Prevention

Prevention of kidney stones depends on the type of stone and the presence or absence of an underlying disease. In almost all cases, increasing fluid intake so that a person consistently drinks several quarts of water a day is an important preventative measure. Patients with calcium stones may benefit from taking a medication called a diuretic, which has the effect of decreasing the amount of calcium passed in the urine. While it was once believed that eating a low-calcium diet was helpful for patients with calcium oxalate stones, new research seems to prove otherwise. An Italian study published early in 2002 reported that a low-salt, low-meat diet

Other items in the diet that may encourage calcium oxalate stone formation include beer, black pepper, berries, broccoli, chocolate, spinach, and tea. Uric acid stones may require treatment with a medication called allopurinol. Struvite stones will require removal and the patient should receive an antibiotic. When a disease is identified as the cause of stone formation, treatment specific to that disease may decrease the likelihood of recurrent stones.

Resources

BOOKS

Asplin, John R., et al. "Nephrolithiasis." In *Harrison's Principles of Internal Medicine,* edited by Anthony S. Fauci, et al. New York: McGraw-Hill, 1998.

PERIODICALS

"CT Scans Reveal Structure of Stone." *Medical Update* (January 2002): 7.

DiLoreto, Stacy. "Which Diet Prevents Recurent Kidney Stones?." *Patient Care* (March 2002): 94.

Goshorn, Janet. "Kidney Stones: Strategies for Managing This Common, Excruciating Condition." *American Journal of Nursing* 96 no. 9 (September 1996): 40+.

Squires, Sally. "New Guidelines Issued for Kidney Stones." *The Washington Post* 120 no. 280 (October 7, 1997): WH7.

ORGANIZATIONS

American Foundation for Urologic Disease. 300 West Pratt St., Baltimore, MD 21201-2463. (800) 242-2383.

National Kidney Foundation. 30 East 33rd St., New York, NY 10016. (800) 622-9010.

Kinesiology *see* **Applied kinesiology**

Paula Ford-Martin
Teresa G. Odle

Kirlian photography

Definition

Kirlian photography creates a photographic image by placing the object or body part to be photographed on film or photographic paper and exposing it to an electromagnetic field.

Origins

Although experiments with photographing objects exposed to an electrical field are known to have been carried out as early as the 1890s, Kirlian photography is generally said to have originated with the work of a pair of Soviet scientists, Semyon and Valentina Kirlian, beginning around 1939. Over the next several decades at Kazakh State University, the Kirlians developed electrophotographic techniques that used neither a lens nor a camera. By the 1960s, their work had attracted public attention in the Soviet Union. Interest in Kirlian photography spread to the West during the 1970s, where attempts were made to replicate effects achieved in the photographs of Alexei Krivorotov, a well-known psychic healer in the U.S.S.R. In the United States, studies were carried out with psychic healers at the Jersey Society for Parapsychology and the UCLA Neuropsychiatric Institute.

Benefits

The most common therapeutic use of Kirlian photography is as a diagnostic tool. Variations in the shapes,

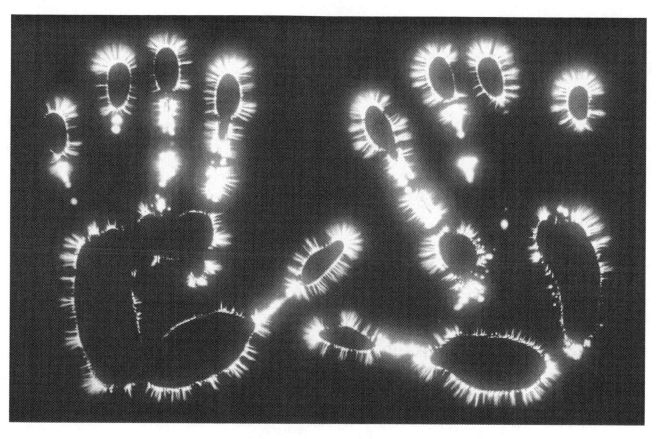

Kirlian photograph of the palms of a woman's hands. *(Photo Researchers, Inc. Reproduced by permission.)*

colors, and intensity of the images produced are said to provide clues to the patient's overall health and energy level and to indicate the presence or absence of disease, specific emotional states, and other physiological or psychological conditions.

Description

Practitioners most often photograph the patient's hand (or, less frequently, the foot), which rests on a photographic medium placed over an electrically charged metal plate. During the approximately one-minute exposure, the patient may feel tingling in the exposed surface. After developing the image, the practitioner interprets its significance and if necessary, refers the patient to a healthcare provider for treatment. Kirlian photography is also sometimes used to assess the effectiveness of treatments (such as **acupuncture**) by comparing before and after photographs of the patient.

Research & general acceptance

Although some have speculated that Kirlian photography actually records the aura long said by some mystics and psychic healers to exist around human beings, this is not a generally accepted viewpoint. A scientific explanation of these dramatic images is that they result from interactions between charged particles created by the electromagnetic field used to form the images. A 1976 *Science* article concluded that moisture is a principal determinant of the form and color of human Kirlian photographs.

It has also been noted that variations in a variety of factors, including the amount of pressure on the plate, the voltage and frequency, and the exposure time, moisture, and temperature, can all influence the images produced.

For these reasons, as well as claims of unreliability and a lack of research data supporting its use, Kirlian photography is not recognized as a legitimate diagnostic tool by the mainstream medical community.

Nevertheless, individual practitioners and researchers continue to experiment with Kirlian photography for diagnosis, especially in Russia and Eastern Europe. It has also been used for such nonmedical purposes as detecting flaws in metal and determining the viability of seeds.

Resources

BOOKS

Woodham, Anne, and Dr. David Peters. *DK Encyclopedia of Healing Therapies*. New York: DK Publishing, 1997.

PERIODICALS

Stanwick, M. "Aura Photography: Mundane Physics or Diagnostic Tool?" *Nursing Times* (June 1996): 19-25.

Peter Gregutt

Knee pain

Definition

Knee **pain** refers to any aching or burning pain in the knee joint. Knee pain can be a symptom of numerous conditions and diseases, including knee **stress**, **osteoarthritis**, injury, **gout**, infection, and **bursitis**.

Description

Knee pain is very common. Each year, millions of Americans visit the doctor for knee pain. It is the most frequent reason for visits to an orthopedist (bone and joint surgeon).

To understand the various causes of knee pain, it is important to know how the knee functions. The knee refers to the joint where the femur (thigh bone) meets the tibia (largest lower leg bone). In front of this joint lies the patella (knee cap). The joint is lined by a membrane called a synovial sac. The synovial sac produces synovial fluid which acts as a lubricant much in the way that oil lubricates the moving parts of machinery. Other tissues that make up the knee joint include cartilage, muscles, tendons, and ligaments. The upper end of the tibia has cartilaginous shock absorbers called menisci (singular meniscus). Other protective structures are the bursae, which cushion areas of friction in the joint. Most of the muscles involved with joint mobility originate in the thigh, cross the knee joint, and attach to the tibia.

The knee supports two to three times a person's body weight. It is a complex joint that allows for a considerable range in mobility. In addition to simple flexion (bending) and extension (straightening) movements, the knee joint is designed to allow for rotation, gliding, and rolling movements. To allow for complex mobility and joint stability, joint strength is sacrificed, making the knee vulnerable to injury.

Causes & symptoms

Knee pain is a symptom of many different diseases and conditions. Short-term knee pain may be the result of excess stress on the knee. Possible causes of knee pain include:

- Arthritis. Osteoarthritis (joint degeneration), **rheumatoid arthritis** (joint inflammation), and septic arthritis (joint infection) can cause knee pain.

- Bursitis. Inflammation of the bursae of the knee can cause knee pain. Bursitis, sometimes called housemaid's knee, can be caused by infection, gout, rheumatoid arthritis, injury, illness, or chronic irritation (crawling or kneeling).

- Cysts. A cyst is a fluid-filled sac. Cysts associated with the knee can cause swelling and knee pain or discomfort.

- Fracture. Breakage or crack in any of the bones associated with the knee joint can cause knee pain.

- Gout. A faulty chemical process leads to high levels of uric acid in the blood which causes inflammatory arthritis, crystal deposits in joints, joint destruction, and joint pain.

- Ligament injury or instability. The ligaments supporting the knee may be injured or strained by persons who participate in sports, particularly football, rugby, lacrosse, basketball, skiing, soccer, and volleyball. Other accidents can also cause ligament damage.

- Loose bodies. This condition refers to any loose objects that float around the knee and cause problems. They also are called "joint mice" because of their elusive nature.

- Meniscus conditions. Damage, usually in the form of a tear, to the menisci can result from degenerative changes associated with advancing age or sports-related injury. Sports that commonly cause menisci damage include football, basketball, soccer, tennis, lacrosse, and skiing.

- Osteonecrosis. Degeneration of the bones associated with the knee cause pain and deformity.

- Patellofemoral pain. Also known as anterior knee pain syndrome, this condition is characterized by pain around the knee cap. The exact cause of patellofemoral pain is unknown but is probably related to muscle inadequacy, lack of flexibility, rapid growth, or bone positioning.

Diagnosis

Knee pain can be diagnosed and treated by an orthopedic surgeon. Diagnosis is based primarily on medical history and physical exam. The diagnosis begins with a detailed medical history to fully characterize the knee pain. The knee will be bent to determine the range of motion and palpated (felt with the hands) to detect the presence of any abnormalities. The physical exam may include any of a number of different tests designed to detect injuries by manipulating the knee and leg. X rays may be taken. In some cases more advanced testing may be carried out using magnetic resonance imaging (MRI), computed tomography (CT), or contrast arthrography (x ray following injection of a contrast solution).

Treatment

Most alternative treatments for knee pain aim at reducing pain, inflammation, and stiffness. Persons experiencing long-term or severe knee pain should consult a physician to determine the underlying cause.

Herbals

Several herbal remedies are recommended to relieve knee pain. Some remedies are used externally, while others involve internal use of herbs.

The following herbs may relieve knee pain and/or associated symptoms when used externally:

- basil and **sage** oil rub: knee pain

- comfrey (*Symphytum officinale*) oil rub: joint stiffness and aching joints

- eucalyptus (*Eucalyptus globulus*) essential oil rub: swelling

- ginger (*Zingiber officinale*) root hot compress or bath: joint stiffness, arthritis, and degenerative joint disease

- lavender (*Lavandula officinalis*) essential oil rub: joint stiffness and aching joints

- mustard (*Sinapsis alba*) powder bath or paste (with alcohol): knee pain

- red pepper (*Capsicum*) lotion: arthritic pain and swelling

- St. John's wort (*Hypericum perforatum*) oil rub: joint stiffness and aching joints

- wintergreen (*Gaultheria procumbens*) oil rub: chronic pain

The following herbs may relieve knee pain and/or associated symptoms when used internally:

- celery (*Apium graveolens*) decoction or tincture: swollen joints and gout

- chamomile (*Matricaria recutita*): spasms and swelling

- deadly nightshade (*Atropa belladonna*) plaster: swollen joints

- devil's claw (*Harpagophytum procumbens*) tablets: swollen joints

- flaxseed (*Linus usitatissimum*) oil: lubricates joints

- geranium (*Pelargonium odoratissimum*): chronic pain

- Jamaican dogwood (*Piscidia erythrina*): pain and swelling

- lemon (*Citrus limon*) juice: swollen joints

- prickly ash (*Zanthoxylum americanum*) tea: joint pain

- white willow (*Salix alba*) tablets or decoction: swollen joints and joint pain

- wild lettuce (*Lactuca virosa*): pain and swelling

Other remedies

Various other alternative treatments that can be helpful in relieving knee pain include:

- Acupressure. Pressing the Stomach 36 point located below the knee caps tones muscles and relieves joint pain anywhere in the body. Pressing the Spleen 9 points located below the kneecap on the inside of each leg relieves knee pain.

- **Acupuncture**. Inflammation and pain may be relieved by acupuncture. The large intestine meridian is the most effective channel for pain relief. A National Institutes of Health consensus panel found that acupuncture may be an effective treatment for osteoarthritis pain.

- **Aromatherapy**. Aromatherapy with **essential oils** is sometimes recommended. The essential oil of **peppermint** relieves pain and decreases inflammation. The essential oil of **rosemary** relieves pain and relaxes muscles.

- Chinese medicine. Knee sprain and contusion (bruise) are treated by application of *Shang Ke Xiao Yan Gao* (Relieve Inflammation Paste of Traumatology) and ingestion of *Die Da Wan* (Contusion Pill). Once the initial pain and swelling have been reduced, the patient can apply *Shang Shi Zhi Tong Gao* (Relieve Damp-Inducing Pain Medicinal Plaster).

- **Exercise**. Regular moderate exercise can reduce pain by improving the strength, tone, and flexibility of muscles. The endorphins released while exercising may also be helpful.

- Food therapy. Following a **detoxification** diet may restore nutritional balance to the body and relieve joint pain. Animal proteins may induce joint pain caused by such inflammatory conditions as arthritis, so following a vegetarian diet may be helpful.

- Homeopathy. *Rhus toxicodendron* is recommended for joint and arthritis pain that is worse in the morning and relieved by warmth. *Kali bichromium* is indicated for persistent, severe pain. Other homeopathic remedies can be designed for specific cases by a homeopathic practitioner.

- Hydrotherapy. A warm compress can relieve joint stiffness and dull pain. A cold compress or ice pack can relieve sharp, intense pain.

- Magnetic therapy. Magnetic fields may increase blood flow and block pain signals.

- Massage. Joint pain may be relieved by massaging the area above and below the painful joint. Massaging with ice packs may interfere with pain signals and replace them with temperature signals.

- Reflexology. Knee pain may be relieved by working the knee reflex points.

- Rolfing. This deep, sometimes painful, **massage therapy** may speed healing and reduce pain.

- Supplements. Knee pain may be relieved by taking **vitamin C** to promote healing, the B vitamins to balance the nervous system, which reduces pain, and **calcium** to increase bone strength.

Allopathic treatment

Knee pain may be relieved by taking such nonsteroidal anti-inflammatory drugs as acetaminophen (Tylenol), ibuprofen (Advil, Motrin), or naproxen (Aleve). More severe pain may be treated with such prescription pain relievers as tramadol or a narcotic. Additional treatment for knee pain depends upon the underlying cause and may include injection of drugs into the knee, surgery, wearing a brace, and/or physical therapy. Surgical treatment depends on the cause; but in the case of osteoarthritis, some patients face actual replacement of the joint. However, in 2002, a new device was introduced that postponed the need to replace an arthritic knee. The device is made of chrome and fits between the natural structures of the knee.

Expected results

Most causes of knee pain respond well to conservative treatments and resolve within 4–6 weeks. Knee pain caused by injury or disease may require surgery and lengthy rehabilitation.

Prevention

Strengthening the leg muscles may help prevent knee pain caused by overworking the joint. In addition, a stronger knee may prevent injury to the joint. Squats are an easy exercise that will strengthen the quadriceps (front thigh muscles) and hamstrings (back thigh muscles). The **yoga** warrior posture strengthens the muscles around the knee and increases range of motion.

Resources

BOOKS

Dandy, David J., and Dennis J. Edwards. "Disorders of the Hip and Knee." In *Essential Orthopaedics and Trauma.*, 3rd edition. New York: Churchill Livingstone, 1998.

"Joint Pain." In *New Choices in Natural Healing: Over 1,800 of the Best Self-Help Remedies from the World of Alternative Medicine.* edited by Bill Gottlieb et al. Emmaus, PA: Rodale Press, Inc., 1995.

"Pain, Chronic." In *The Alternative Advisor: The Complete Guide to Natural Therapies and Alternative Treatments.* Alexandra, VA: Time-Life Books, 1997.

PERIODICALS

Brody, Lori Thein, and Jill M. Thein. "Nonoperative Treatment for Patellofemoral Pain." *Journal of Orthopaedics & Sports Physical Therapy* 28 (November 1998): 336-344.

Crowther, Christy L. "Approach to Knee Problems in Primary Care." *Lippincott's Primary Care Practice* 3 (1999): 355-375.

Jensen, Roar, Gothesen, Oystein, Liseth, Knut, and Anders Baerheim. "Acupuncture Treatment of Patellofemoral Pain Syndrome." *The Journal of Alternative and Complementary Medicine* 5 (1999): 521-527.

"Minimally Invasive Surgical Procedure for Arthritis May Delay Knee Replacement Surgery." *Medical Devices & Surgical Technology Week* (May 19, 2002):4.

Sullivan, Dana. "Sports Medicine's New Alternatives." *Women's Sports & Fitness* 2 (July/August 1999): 106+.

Belinda Rowland
Teresa G. Odle

Kneipp wellness

Definition

Kneipp wellness is a holistic system for overall health developed by Sebastian Kneipp, a nineteenth-century Bavarian priest. His approach included aspects of **hydrotherapy**, herbalism, and aerobic **exercise**.

FATHER SEBASTIAN KNEIPP 1821–1897

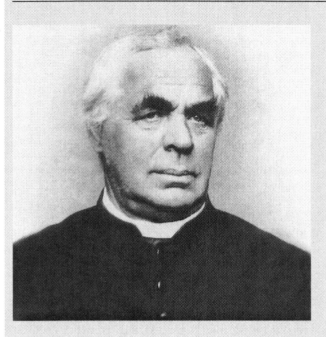

(Betmann/CORBIS. Reproduced by permission.)

Born in Stephansreid, Bavaria, Germany, of poor parents, Sebastian Kneipp's childhood was filled with labor, much of it learning weaving from his father. Even as a child, Kneipp wanted to become a priest. With the help of a priest who befriended him, Kneipp entered high school where he studied theology for five years. During this time, he contracted consumption (pulmonary tuber-culosis), usually a fatal disease at that time. While ill, he read an eighteenth-century book on hydrotherapy by Dr. Hahn. This book advised him to bathe two or three times a week in the icy Danube River to stimulate his immune system. His tuberculosis went into remission, his health improved, and in 1850, he entered a seminary in Munich. He continued his hydrotherapy and convinced other theological students to practice it. Kneipp was ordained a priest in 1852. During the next few years, he was called to the bedsides of many patients to perform the last rites. Instead he successfully treated a number of the patients with hydrotherapy.

He perfected his own system of hydrotherapy and his successful treatment of the poor attracted much attention. People came from throughout Germany to be healed by Kneipp's hydrotherapy. His success fostered resentment from physicians; at one point, he was charged in German courts with quackery, where he was subsequently acquitted. In 1886, he published *My Water Cure*, which was translated into several languages and became popular throughout Europe. He continued to refine his treatment from one of severity to milder versions. It consisted of bathing in and drinking cold water, going to bed and rising early, long barefoot walks in wet grass, and simple meals consisting of little meat and large quantities of whole-grain cereals. He continued his hydrotherapy practice at Wör-ishofen Monastery in the foothills of the Alps until his death. Kneipp's hydrotherapy is still practiced throughout the world, especially in Germany and the United States.

Ken R. Wells

Origins

Sebastian Kneipp was born to a poor family in Stephansreid, Bavaria, on May 17, 1821. He initially took up his father's trade of weaving, but longed to become a priest. With help from a sympathetic clergyman, he was admitted to high school as a mature student, but after five years of intensive studies, Kneipp became seriously ill with pulmonary **tuberculosis**. At that time, the disease was usually fatal, but Kneipp came across an eighteenth-century book about hydrotherapy that inspired him during the winter of 1849 to immerse himself several times a week in the icy Danube River. These brief exposures to cold **water** seemed to bolster his immune system, because Kneipp's tuberculosis went into remission and he was able to continue his theological studies in Munich. There, he convinced some of his fellow students to join his experiments with hydrotherapy.

Kneipp was ordained as a priest in 1852. In that capacity, he began using hydrotherapy to help some of his poorer parishioners. He broadened his approach to include herbalism, exercise, and other elements, and toned down his initial enthusiasm for shocking the body with cold water. "I warn all against too-frequent application of cold water," he later wrote. "Three times I concluded to remodel my system and relax the treatment from severity to mildness and thence to greater mildness still." Kneipp's reputation grew after a number of dying patients recovered when he was called to administer last rites and managed instead to restore them to health. In 1855 he was assigned to Worishofen, a village in the foothills of the Bavarian Alps that soon developed an international reputation as a place of healing. Kneipp summarized his teachings in two popular books, *My Water Cure* in 1886 and *So Sollt Ihr Leben (Thus Thou Shalt Live)* in 1889. Supporters of his techniques formed Kneipp Societies in Germany and the United States.

Father Kneipp was later named a monsignor by Pope Leo XIII. After his death in Worishofen on June 17,

1897, his wellness techniques became less popular, but interest in hydrotherapy increased again during the latter part of the twentieth century.

Benefits

Proponents of Kneipp therapy believe that it bolsters the immune system and results in improved overall wellness. In Germany, it is especially popular for treating **varicose veins**.

Description

Today, Kneipp physiotherapy is essentially a form of classical naturopathy. It is founded on five "pillars":

- Hydrotherapy. Hydrotherapy involves the use of hot and cold water to stimulate the nerves, blood vessels and internal organs. It uses baths, compresses, packs, and water jets.

- Phytotherapy. Plant therapy takes the form of medicinal herbs added to bath water and also administered as juices, lozenges, teas, or ointments, etc.

- Exercise therapy. This aspect of treatment involves long hikes, gymnastics, tennis, cycling, and other vigorous activities to amplify the effects of the water and herb therapies.

- Nutrition therapy, which employs a low-protein, **high-fiber diet**. Special Kneipp **diets** are also available for weight loss or such ailments as **gout**, diabetes, or metabolic problems.

- Health maintenance therapy. Patients in the Kneipp program are trained to adhere to their natural biorhythms.

Precautions

All forms of hydrotherapy may pose some risk of water-borne **infections**, and patients should make sure that baths and similar facilities are properly maintained and disinfected. In addition, persons with serious health problems should consult their physician before undertaking an exercise program.

Side effects

Side effects may vary, depending on the numerous herbs used in Kneipp therapy. When in doubt, it is best to consult a knowledgeable herbalist.

Research & general acceptance

Initially, Kneipp was rejected as a charlatan by the medical establishment. At one point, he was taken to court

---

KEY TERMS

Hydrotherapy—A family of therapies that treat illness by using water either externally or internally.

Phytotherapy—A form of treatment that uses plants or plant extracts either externally or internally.

---

for quackery, although the judge acquitted him after learning from Kneipp about the shortage of physicians in Alpine villages. Kneipp is now recognized by naturopaths as a founding father of their discipline. The benefits of immersion in water are wellknown to physiotherapists, but there is so far little conclusive evidence that Kneipp or other methods of hydrotherapy can increase the body's immunity. One German study published in 1977 found that immunological reactions to protein and bacterial antigens were significantly more intense in patients who had undergone Kneipp hydrotherapy, compared with a group of healthy volunteers. There is little doubt among medical doctors that patients should benefit from the vigorous exercise and high-fiber diet included in the Kneipp prescription for wellness.

Training & certification

The world center of Kneipp wellness is the village of Bad Worishofen in the foothills of the Bavarian Alps. There, the Kneipp *Kur* is offered by spas, physicians, and guest houses. Healer training is provided by the Sebastian Kneipp School of Physiotherapy. Elsewhere in the world, many adherents of Kneipp's writings treat themselves by using his techniques.

Resources

ORGANIZATIONS

Kneipp Corporation of America. 105-107 Stonehurst Court. Northvale, NJ 07647. (201) 750-0600 or (800) 937-4372. http://www.kniepp.com.

David Helwig

Kola nut

Description

The kola nut, or bitter cola, (*Cola vera, Cola acuminata, Cola nitida*) is a seed part from a tree from the Sterculiaceae family. The trees are native to Central and Western Africa, but are now found in the West Indies and

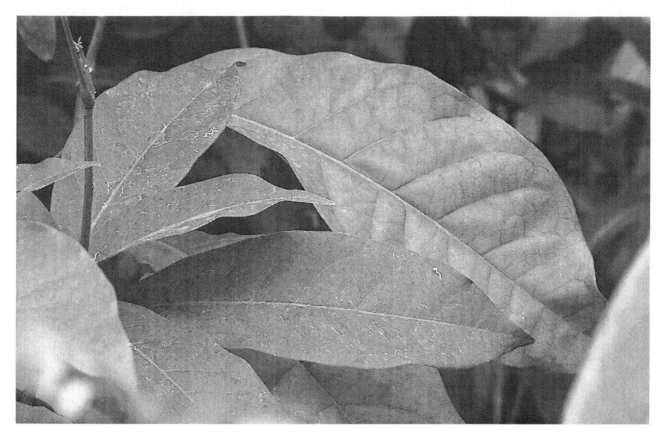

Kola nut plant. (© *PlantaPhile, Germany. Reproduced by permission.*)

Brazil, where they were introduced by African slaves. All three species are used as a stimulant and are prepared in the same manner. The kola tree grows to approximately 40 ft (12 m) in height, and has white to yellow flowers with spots that range from red to purple. The kola tree's leaves are 6–8 in long (15–20 cm) and the tree bears fruit that is shaped like a star. Inside the fruit, about a dozen round or square seeds can be found in a white seed shell.

General use

Kola nut, which contains high amounts of **caffeine**, helps combat **fatigue** and is most commonly used as a central nervous system stimulant that focuses on the cerebrospinal centers. It also contains theobromine, a stimulant found in chocolate as well as in **green tea**. Kola nut also contains tannins, phenolics, phlobaphens, kola red, betaine, protein, starch, fat, **thiamine, riboflavin**, and **niacin**. The *Journal of the American Medical Association* advocates the use of kola over other stimulants, because it is not addictive and does not lead to **depression**. Because kola nut is also a diuretic, its use has been suggested for those with renal diseases, cardiac or renal **edema** and rheumatic and rheumatoid conditions. Most people around the world are familiar with

kola; many have tasted it and do not even know it. In the 1800s, a pharmacist in Georgia took extracts of kola, sugar and coca and mixed them with carbonated water. His accountant tasted it and called it "Coca Cola." Today, Coca-Cola still uses kola in its original recipe.

Respiratory conditions

Kola is widely used as a treatment for **whooping cough** and **asthma**, as the caffeine acts as a bronchodilator, expanding the bronchial air passages. A *Journal of American Medicine* cites a study of kola nut's effects on asthma that showed "the attack being cut short and the child's condition rapidly improved."

Gastrointestinal disorders

In Africa, the fresh nuts are chewed as a ceremonial greeting, as a stimulant, and to help aid digestion, as kola nut stimulates gastric acid production. Kola nuts are also known to improve the taste of food and act as an appetite suppressant.

Other conditions

The kola nut is also used to treat migraine headaches, because the caffeine and theobromine act as cerebral vasodilators (increase blood flow in the head) and, when used in a poultice, can be applied to external cuts and scrapes.

More recently, an ephedra/caffeine preparation made from kola nut extract and a Chinese medication known as Ma Huang was tested for safety and efficacy as part of a weight reduction program. The study indicated that the preparation improved the subjects' rate of weight loss and reduction in body fat without undesirable side effects.

The flavor of kola nut in cola beverages appears to be more effective than other flavors in disguising the taste of **activated charcoal** when the charcoal must be given as an antidote for accidental poisoning.

Preparations

The part of the seed known as the kola nut is the cotyledon, which is also called the seed leaf. The cotyledons are white and bitter when they are fresh, but they turn reddish with almost no taste when they are dried. Fresh nuts are difficult to find outside of the tropical areas where they are grown. Sometimes, the nuts are sold at African markets in international cities, like Washington D.C. The dried cotyledons are 1–2 in (2.5–5 cm) long.

Dosage of kola nut should be 2–6 g per day, as 2.5–7.5 g of liquid extract or 10–30 g per day of tincture. Powdered cotyledons should be taken at 1-3 g per day, as a decoction, liquid extract, or tincture. For the decoction, boil 1-2 teaspoons in a cup of water and take three times a day. The liquid extract should be taken in a 1:1 solution of 60% alcohol at .6-1.2 ml three times a day. Tinctures in a 1:5 solution of 60% alcohol, with 1-4 ml of the cotyledons three times a day.

Precautions

Because of its use as a stimulant, kola nut should be used with caution. Patients should consult with their doctors, especially if they are taking other medications. Due to its caffeine content, kola nut should not be used by women who are pregnant or nursing a child. Also because of its caffeine content, it is not advisable for those suffering from **insomnia** or **anxiety** problems. In some cases, extreme restlessness and sleepnessness can occur. It should not be used by patients with a history of high blood pressure, heart trouble, palpitations, seizures, insomnia, **heart disease**, high **cholesterol**, or **stroke**. Research in Niger showed that the habitual chewing of kola nut can actually cause cardiac arrythmias, based on clinical trials using cats. Kola nut should not be used by those with stomach or duodenal ulcers because it increases gastric juice production and may add to gastrointestinal discomfort and disorders. Kola nut is also one of the top ten common food allergens, among cow's milk and chocolate. Kola nut is naturally very high in tannin, a white-to-yellow astringent powder that gets its name from its use as a textile and leather tanning agent. However, a University of Miami study shows that "tannins are increasingly recognized as dietary carcinogens and as antinutrients interfering with the system's full use of protein" and called for more studies correlating early death and regular kola nut use in third world countries. Kola nut should not be used for long periods of time.

Kola nut and cola beverages should be kept away from dogs, cats, and other domestic animals. The theobromine in kola nut (and in chocolate as well) can be fatal to these pets because they metabolize it much more slowly than humans.

Side effects

Kola nut may cause insomnia, anxiety, nervousness, gastrointestinal problems, and **tremors**. If there is any indication of an overdose, **diarrhea**, **nausea**, and/or cramps may follow. Oral **blisters** have also been known to form.

Heavy use of kola nut or drinking large quantities of cola beverages has been associated with bone loss in adults and inhibition of bone formation in adolescents. Some practitioners are recommending that teenagers should restrict intake of soft drinks containing cola in order to lower their risk of **osteoporosis** in later life.

Interactions

Kola nut should not be used with muscle relaxants, heart medications, high blood pressure medication, nitrates and calcium-channel blockers.

Clinical experiments indicate that beverages containing cola increase the rate and extent of absorption of carbamazepine (Tegretol), a drug used to treat **epilepsy** and some forms of **bipolar disorder**. Kola nut has been reported to interact with tricyclic antidepressant medications and with MAO inhibitors. In general, patients taking any medication for anxiety or depression should consult their physician before taking preparations containing kola nut.

Resources

BOOKS

Castleman, Michael. *The Healing Herbs*. New York: Bantam Books, 1995.

PERIODICALS

Boozer, C. N., P. A. Daly, P. Homel, et al. "Herbal Ephedra/Caffeine for Weight Loss: A 6-Month Randomized Safety and Efficacy Trial." *International Journal of Obesity and Related Metabolic Disorders* 26 (May 2002): 593-604.

Dagnone, D., D. Matsui, and M. J. Rieder. "Assessment of the Palatability of Vehicles for Activated Charcoal in Pediatric

KEY TERMS

Bronchodilator—A medicine that relaxes the bronchial muscles and opens up the air passages to the lungs.

Cardiac arrythmia—The irregular beating of the heart.

Cotyledon—A seed leaf, from the embryo of a seed plant.

Theobromine—A stimulant that occurs naturally in chocolate as well as in kola nut. Foods and drinks containing theobromine are poisonous to domestic pets.

Vasodilator—A drug or nerve that causes blood vessels to widen.

Volunteers." *Pediatric Emergency Care* 18 (February 2002): 19-21.

Malhotra, S., R. K. Dixit, and S. K. Garg. "Effect of an Acidic Beverage (Coca-Cola) on the Pharmacokinetics of Carbamazepine in Healthy Volunteers." *Methods and Findings in Experimental and Clinical Pharmacology* 24 (January-February 2002): 31-33.

Morton, J.F. "Widespread Tannin Intake Via Stimulants and Masticatories, Especially Guarana, Kola Nut, Betel Vine, and Accessories." *Basic Life Sciences* (1992): 739-65.

Reiling, Jennifer. "Therapeutics of Kola." *Journal of the American Medical Association,* (24 November 1999).

Root, A. W. "Bone Strength and the Adolescent." *Adolescent Medicine* 13 (February 2002): 53-72.

Speer, F. "Food Allergy: The 10 Common Offenders." *American Family Physician* (February 1976):106-12.

ORGANIZATIONS

Centre for International Ethnomedicinal Education and Research (CIEER). <www.cieer.org>.

OTHER

American Veterinary Medical Association (AVMA). "A Pet Owner's Guide to Common Small Animal Poisons." <www.avma.org/pubhlth/poisgde.asp>.

Katherine Kim
Rebecca J. Frey, PhD

Kombucha

Description

Kombucha is a fermented beverage prepared from a mushroom (*Fungus japonicus*). Known as kombucha tea, the drink is touted for its health-promoting properties. It is also called Manchurian mushroom tea, Manchurian fungus tea, Kwassan, combucha tea, and champagne of life. During fermentation and preparation, the kombucha membrane becomes a tough gelatinous cover composed of several different yeasts (one-celled fungi) and certain nontoxic bacteria derived from the air, similar to a sourdough bread starter. When the fungus is fermented in a mixture containing water, black or **green tea**, sugar, and vinegar (or other fermentation source), the microorganisms combine into a complex fermenting culture. This culture produces several compounds that have been considered health tonics over the centuries. Kombucha also contains several B vitamins and **vitamin C**. The tea is said to have a unique, but pleasant taste. The membrane surface of the kombucha is also edible.

In China, kombucha tea has been utilized as a health beverage for thousands of years, dating back to before 200 B.C. It has been consumed for centuries in Japan, Korea, and Russia. In the early 1900s, use of the tea spread from Russia into other European countries including Germany, where it was touted as a health elixir for many years. In the 1950s and 1960s, German and Italian researchers claimed that kombucha tea exhibited strong anticancer properties, and it was promoted as a miracle cure for **cancer**. Alexander Solzhenitzyn, the Nobel Prize winning Russian author, reported that kombucha tea, which he began to drink during a prison term, cured his stomach cancer. Proponents of kombucha tea continue to tout its possible anticancer and immunity-enhancing properties. However, controlled studies have failed to display conclusive evidence as to its efficacy in treating various medical conditions.

General use

Kombucha tea is taken as a general health tonic. Claims are made for its use as a remedy for specific health conditions and diseases. It is used to introduce and improve healthy intestinal flora and bacteria, as an energy-enhancing tonic, and as a detoxifier in helping to remove pollutants. It is taken to strengthen the immune system after an illness, stimulate hair growth, improve arthritis and skin conditions, and as a health tonic for cancer and autoimmune deficiency syndrom (**AIDS**) patients.

Kombucha tea contains significant amounts of the B complex vitamins, as well as vitamin C and minerals. It contains a small amount of alcohol (higher than 1%), which is produced during fermentation, and small amounts of methylxanthine stimulants. Teas do not contain **caffeine**, but they do contain methylxanthine alkaloids, a similar stimulant.

There is no large body of scientific evidence that supports the strong claims made by advocates of kombucha tea. Some European studies have pointed to positive results in cancer cases, but further research is needed to confirm these results. Its proposed anticancer and **detoxification** effects have been attributed to certain chemicals in the tea. However, more recent tests have failed to validate the presence of these chemicals in the beverage. One study did confirm improvements in liver function after a three-week treatment. Research in Russia demonstrated antibiotic effects caused by kombucha tea. There are many testimonial claims that the tea increases vitality and overall well-being. In general, properly fermented foods have been shown to aid in the growth of beneficial intestinal flora, reduce the growth of harmful yeasts and bacteria in the digestive tract, and improve digestion and absorption. Some testimonial claims have also been made by cancer and AIDS patients.

Preparations

Kombucha tea is available in several forms. Kits include the fungi and all ingredients, as well as directions to make the brew at home. The fungi may also be purchased separately. Dried kombucha is available in capsule form.

Making the tea from scratch is a process similar to preparing yogurt, sauerkraut, and other fermented foods. Instructions should be followed carefully. Particular care should be taken to maintain the cleanliness of the tea-making process, to avoid contamination by mold or unhealthy bacteria (a cause of health problems in those drinking poor-quality kombucha). **Smoking** in the same room as the mixture may contaminate it. Mold typically appears as green, pink, or black blotches in the culture, and should be thoroughly removed and discarded. The fermentation process is generally successful if the kombucha skin remains firm and rubbery. Care should be taken if the membrane becomes crumbly or discolored. On average, the fermentation of kombucha tea takes 12–14 days. After fermentation, new batches can be easily made from the existing culture.

When using the supplement in pill form, consumers can follow the manufacturer's recommended dosages. Users of the tea can drink up to three cups of the beverage per day with food or between meals.

Historically, kombucha was consumed as a tea. The health benefits of other forms of the supplement have not been compared with the original therapeutic beverage. There are reports of consumer illness from home-prepared kombucha. This may have been due to tea that was too old, infected with molds or other contaminants, or had other problems. Consumers must be alert to the risks of home-prepared fermentation methods.

Precautions

Several precautions concerning kombucha tea have been issued. Because the beverage is fermented at home, there is the risk that the liquid can become contaminated by such dangerous bacteria as anthrax. People with compromised immune systems must be extremely careful not

---

KEY TERMS

Anthrax—An infectious and potentially fatal bacterial disease. It takes its name from the Greek word for coal because it causes black boils on the patient's skin.

Intestinal flora—The beneficial bacteria that live in the digestive tract and aid digestion of food.

---

to consume contaminated fermentations. Due to the high acidity of the drink, the tea should not be placed in metal containers or in pottery that has a lead glaze finish. There have been reported cases of **lead poisoning** and anthrax due to drinking kombucha tea that has been improperly prepared. The United States Food and Drug Administration (FDA) issued a warning concerning the danger of lead poisoning from improperly made kombucha tea. Kombucha tea is not recommended for pregnant or nursing mothers.

Side Effects

Consumption of kombucha tea has been observed to cause stomach upset, yeast **infections**, allergic reactions, **nausea**, and **headache**. Persons with stomach ulcers may find that kombucha increases their symptoms. Due to harmful bacteria that can survive in the culture, ingesting contaminated tea can be dangerous or fatal.

Interactions

Kombucha tea is high in acidity and should not be consumed by those taking medications that make them susceptible to increased gastrointestinal acidity. The tea contains a small amount of alcohol and should not be consumed with any medications that interact unfavorably with alcohol. The tea should not be taken by people with stabilized **alcoholism**, to avoid aggravating the condition.

Some people report general and specific improved health from moderate use of kombucha tea. These reports await final validation by current research. There are risks associated with the use of poor quality or contaminated kombucha. Its use may be contraindicated in those who have medical conditions or require certain medications.

Resources

BOOKS

Chang, Shu-Ting. *Mushrooms: Cultivation, Nutritional Value, Medicinal Effect, and Environmental Impact.* Boca Raton, FL: CRC Press, 2004.

Hobbs, Christopher. *Medicinal Mushrooms: An Exploration of Tradition, Healing, and Culture.* Loveland, CO: Interweave Press, 1995.

Pascal, Alana and Lynne Van Der Kar. *Kombucha: How To and What It's All About*. Malibu, CA: Van Der Kar Press, 1995.
Pryor, Betsy and Sanford Holst. *Kombucha Phenomenon: The Miracle Health Tea*. Thriving Press, 1996.

OTHER
Kombucha Tea. <http://www.kombucha.org>.

Douglas Dupler

Kudzu

Description

Kudzu, whose botanical name is *Pueraria lobata*, is a member of the Fabaceae legume family. It is also known as Ge-gen, kudzu vine, mile-a-minute vine, foot-a-night vine, and the vine-that-ate-the-South. The latter names refer to this vine's property of rapid growth. This perennial trails, climbs, and winds its rough vines around tree poles and anything else it touches. It grows in shady areas, mountain areas, fields, roadsides and forests in China, Japan, and the southern United States, more so in the latter because when imported, its native insects did not tag along. Kudzu was first seen in the United States as an ornamental plant at the 1876 Philadelphia Centennial Exposition. During the **Depression**, the United States Department of Agriculture (USDA) imported kudzu for erosion control. In 1972, the USDA classified kudzu as a weed because the plant can reach 60 ft (18.29 m) in a single growing season. In June and July, the vines sport purple flowers and in autumn, the leaves shed.

The kudzu root, which can grow to the size of a human being, has a history of use in Chinese medicine. Kudzu contains daidzein, an isoflavone, and diadzin and puerarin, isoflavone glycosides. The isoflavone amount can range from 1.77–12.08%, based on kudzu's growing conditions. The highest isoflavone is puerarin with diadzin and daidzein, next in isoflavone amounts. A study at the University of Michigan compared legumes for their sources of the isoflavones of genistein and daidzein, The results showed the kudzu root as a good nutritional source of those two components.

The root also supports bacteria that grab nitrogen from the atmosphere and put it in the soil. This factor may explain kudzu's rapid growth and its success in feeding Angora goats raised by Tuskegee University researcher Dr. Errol G. Rhoden.

General use

Traditional uses

Traditional Chinese medicine has used kudzu, whose Chinese name is *ge gan*, for centuries. Kudzu's

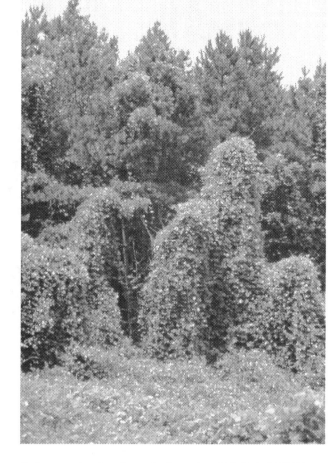

Kudzu growing in a forest in Georgia. *(U.S. Fish & Wildlife Service.)*

medicinal uses were first recorded in Shen Nong's herbal text, published around A.D. 100. Chinese medicine recommends kudzu for what it calls *wei*, or superficial syndrome, referring to a mild disease that appears just below the body's surface and is accompanied by a **fever**. Chinese medicine also indicates using kudzu for thirst, headaches (migraine and other types of headaches), **neck pain** from **hypertension**, **angina**, **allergies**, **diarrhea**, and speeding the progression of **measles** in children. In general, kudzu is used as a demulcent, or medication given to soothe irritated mucous membranes.

Cardiovascular disease

One alternative practitioner has stated that because kudzu improves the body's flow of blood and levels of oxygen and opens heart vessels, it might help the cardiovascular system. Another researcher, James Duke, refers to a Chinese clinical study that showed that kudzu can benefit angina sufferers. For a period of 1–6 months, 71 participants took 10–15 gm of kudzu root extract. The

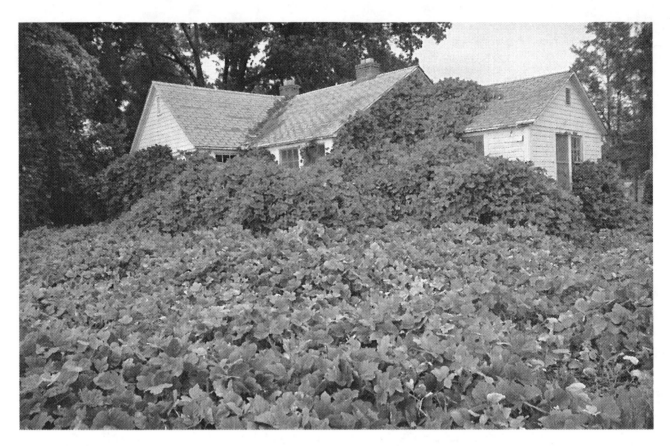

House and hill overgrown with kudzu. (*JLM Visuals. Reproduced by permission.*)

results indicated that 29 people had significant improvement, 20 had an intermediary amount of improvement, and the remaining 22 showed no improvement or only a slight improvement.

Duke cites another Chinese study showing that kudzu can lower blood pressure. For a period of 2–8 weeks, 52 people drank about 8 tsp of kudzu root in a tea. Seventeen people had their blood pressure decrease substantially, while the other 30 had some relief from hypertension.

Alcoholism

It is the Chinese medicinal use of kudzu in treating **alcoholism**, however, that is the focus of many studies on kudzu. In 1989, two associate research professors in the psychiatry department at the University of North Carolina tested rats for their alcohol cravings. In 1991 an organic chemist tested a tea containing seven herbs including kudzu on drunken rats. The rats had been injected with alcohol; when they ingested the herbal tea, their motor movements became more coordinated.

In further studies conducted in 1992, the rats were allowed to drink alcohol for an hour each day. The rats gulped down an enormous amount of alcohol; however,

after a week, when the herbal mixture containing kudzu was given to them 15 minutes before their happy hour, they drank much less alcohol. In another study, the rats were allowed to drink alcohol for the first 24 hours, then deprived for the next 24 hours. On day three, the rats' alcohol intake increased from 20% to 30%. Once injected with the herbal mixture, however, the rats either drank a normal or less than normal amount.

A 1995 study was also conducted at Harvard University using hamsters, because hamsters naturally choose alcohol over **water**. Thirty hamsters were given either daidzein, an active ingredient in kudzu; or disulfiram (Antabuse), a compound that stops ethanol craving in humans. Nine more hamsters were allowed to drink as much alcohol as they wanted without anything added. Hamsters receiving daidzein, dropped their alcohol intake by 70% and those receiving disulfiram had 80% less alcohol intake. The researchers concluded that daidzein, takes a less toxic metabolic route than disulfiram.

A double-blind random clinical study using human subjects was conducted at the Veterans' Affairs Medical Center in Prescott, Arizona. Thirty-eight middle-aged men suffering from chronic alcoholism were given either 1.2 g of kudzu root extract (21 men) or 1.2 g of a placebo

(17 men) twice daily for a month. The results of this test showed no significant difference in sobriety or alcohol cravings in either group.

Preparations

The problems of manufacturing kudzu root as a drug to treat alcoholism and other disorders were outlined in an article on traditional Chinese medicine by Dr. James Zhou. Zhou says that herbs lose their natural balance when manufacturers purify, refine, and treat them with chemicals. The daidzein, in kudzu could treat alcoholism, but the purification process destroys the isoflavone balance. Because it is the isoflavone puerarin in kudzu that stops cardiovascular damage impairment and may prevent an alcoholic side effect, liver damage, Zhou believes that the herb should be given in its natural state.

For angina pectoris, practitioners of traditional Chinese medicine recommend 30–120 mg of standardized tablets of kudzu root two to three times daily. Ten mg of a standardized tablet equals 1.5 g of the pure root. Tinctures of 1–2 ml three to five times daily are recommended in place of tablets. To help lower cravings for alcohol, the recommended dosage is 3–5 g of kudzu root three times daily or 3–4 ml of tincture three times daily. The *All-In-One-Guide to Natural Remedies and Supplements* recommends drinking kudzu tea to combat alcoholism. An alternative form of treatment involves taking 1500-mg supplements or cubes before or after the alcohol. The 1500 mg can be divided equally into three daily doses.

Kudzu also comes in supplements combined with **St. John's wort** to treat the symptoms of alcoholism. One capsule is taken with each meal on a daily basis.

Kudzu leaves can also be used in cooking, for example in quiches and as a deep-fried dish.

Precautions

Kudzu should not be taken by pregnant and lactating women. In traditional Chinese practice, people who sweat too much or have cold in their stomach should avoid kudzu because it is given for "wind-heat" illnesses.

KEY TERMS

Daidzein—An isoflavone contained in kudzu that appears to be useful in treating alcoholism.

Demulcent—A substance or medication given to soothe irritated or inflamed mucous membranes. Kudzu is used as a demulcent in traditional Chinese medicine.

Ethanol—Another name for the alcohol found in alcoholic drinks.

Extract—A concentrated form of the herb made by pressing the herb with a hydraulic press, soaking it in water or alcohol, then allowing the excess water or alcohol to evaporate.

Tincture—A liquid herbal preparation, made by soaking the herb in alcohol or a mixture of alcohol and water.

Side effects

As of 2000, no toxic side effects or damage to the liver have been reported from kudzu.

Interactions

Kudzu should not be taken in conjunction with prescription drugs. As with all medicinal supplements, it is best to check with a health care provider before taking kudzu.

Resources

BOOKS

Ali, Elvis, Dr., et al. *The All-In-One Guide to Natural Remedies and Supplements.* Niagara Falls, NY: AGES Publications, 2000.

Balch, James F., MD and Phyllis A. Balch, CNC. *Prescription for Nutritional Healing,* 2nd ed. New York: Avery Publishing Group, 1997.

Duke, James A., Ph.D. *The Green Pharmacy.* Emmaus, PA: Rodale Press, 1997.

Sharon Crawford